HYPERFINE INTERACTIONS

HYPERFINE INTERACTIONS

edited by

ARTHUR J. FREEMAN

and

RICHARD B. FRANKEL

NATIONAL MAGNET LABORATORY
MASSACHUSETTS INSTITUTE OF TECHNOLOGY
CAMBRIDGE, MASSACHUSETTS

ACADEMIC PRESS

New York · London   *1967*

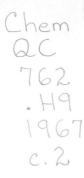
ACADEMIC PRESS INC.
111 Fifth Avenue, New York, New York 10003

United Kingdom Edition published by
ACADEMIC PRESS INC. (LONDON) LTD.
Berkeley Square House, London W.1

LIBRARY OF CONGRESS CATALOG CARD NUMBER: 67-21445

PRINTED IN THE UNITED STATES OF AMERICA

CONTRIBUTORS

A. ABRAGAM, Collège de France and Commissariat à L'Energie Atomique, France

B. BLEANEY, Clarendon Laboratory, Oxford, England

J. I. BUDNICK, Fordham University, Bronx, New York

M. J. CLAUSER, Physik Department, Technische Hochschule, Munich, Germany

S. G. COHEN, Department of Physics, The Hebrew University, Jerusalem, Israel

E. DANIEL, Institut de Physique, Strasbourg, France

A. J. DEKKER, Solid State Physics Laboratory, University of Groningen, The Netherlands

H. DE WAARD, Department of Experimental Physics, University of Groningen, The Netherlands

B. DODSWORTH, New York University, New York, New York

A. J. FREEMAN, National Magnet Laboratory, MIT, Cambridge, Massachusetts

S. GESCHWIND, Bell Telephone Laboratories, Murray Hill, New Jersey

U. GONSER, North American Aviation Science Center, Thousand Oaks, California

R. M. HOUSLEY, North American Aviation Science Center, Thousand Oaks, California

E. KARLSSON, Institute of Physics, Uppsala, Sweden

J. KIRSCH, Bell Telephone Laboratories, Murray Hill, New Jersey

O. V. LOUNASMAA, Technical University of Helsinki, Otaniemi, Finland

J. LUBBERS, University of Leiden, Kamerlingh Onnes Laboratory, The Netherlands

E. MATTHIAS, University of California, Lawrence Radiation Laboratory, Berkeley, California

C. M. MOSER, Centre de Mécanique Ondulatoire Appliquée, Paris, France

R. L. MÖSSBAUER, Physik Department, Technische Hochschule, Munich, Germany

D. MURNICK, Department of Physics and Laboratory for Nuclear Science, MIT, Cambridge, Massachusetts

A. NARATH, Sandia Laboratory, Alburquerque, New Mexico

J. F. REICHERT, Department of Physics and Condensed State Center, Western Reserve University, Cleveland, Ohio

P. G. H. SANDARS, Oxford University, Oxford, England

D. SHALTIEL, Microwave Division, Department of Physics, The Hebrew University, Jerusalem, Israel

S. SKALSKI, Fordham University, Bronx, New York

A. STEUDEL, Technische Hochschule, Hannover, Germany

N. J. STONE, Clarendon Laboratory, Oxford, England

J. C. WALKER, The Johns Hopkins University, Baltimore, Maryland

R. E. WATSON, Brookhaven National Laboratory, Upton, New York

PREFACE

Hyperfine interaction studies provide the single area of overlap between what have become two separate disciplines: the electronic structure of matter (atoms, molecules, and solids) and the structure of sub-atomic particles (nucleons and other elementary particles). As a result, there is an increasing need for scientists in each discipline to study and understand, at the very least, those techniques and experimental data of the other discipline which have become increasingly relevant to their own work. One example which may be cited stems from the need for polarized targets in both low and high energy nuclear physics experiments — a need now being fulfilled by the application of dynamic nuclear polarization methods. However, having polarized targets is not enough; the nuclear physicist must be able to measure the degree of polarization of his (crystalline solid or frozen liquid) target and he must understand the processes leading to the creation of the polarization and its destruction. Another example is the increasingly important role that the so-called nuclear techniques, i.e., those based on the observation of perturbed angular correlations of γ-rays and the Mössbauer effect, are playing in solid state investigations. A great advantage of these methods is their ability to work with small numbers of nuclei ($\sim 10^{12}$) as probes of electronic charge and spin densities. To make full and meaningful use of these tools the solid state physicist must master not only the experimental aspects, but must also understand the fundamental nuclear physics basic to the measurements.

This interdependence of information in the different disciplines may vary in degree but it is common to all hyperfine measurements. The reason is obvious: since hyperfine interaction experiments measure the product of a nuclear quantity (e.g. magnetic moment, electric quadrupole moment, nuclear radius) and an electronic quantity (the extranuclear electromagnetic fields and/or their gradients), knowledge of one factor in the product is essential if meaningful information about the other factor is to be determined. The chemist, or the solid state physicist, needs precise numerical values of nuclear moments in order to obtain precise values of the extranuclear electromagnetic fields originating in just the electronic structure of the system he is trying to understand. Until recently, the nuclear physicist considered these extranuclear fields a nuisance which prevented him from measuring with high accuracy the nuclear parameters he needs to know in order to understand nuclear structure. Today, many experimentalists recognize

vii

that far from being a nuisance these extranuclear (or hyperfine) fields can provide, in some cases, the means for carrying out nuclear physics experiments not previously thought possible or to an accuracy beyond that of previous work. Further, the combination of solid state resonance techniques with the conventional nuclear techniques promises to accelerate developments in the field of hyperfine interactions.

This book represents, in part, the proceedings of a NATO Advanced Study Institute held at Aix-en-Provence, France, August 8-26, 1966. The participants ranged from advanced predoctoral students to postdoctorals and more advanced researchers and had diverse backgrounds in physics and chemistry, not all in fields related to hyperfine interactions.

One aim of the Institute was to present the entire range of basic principles, current status and latest advances in the field of hyperfine interactions and associated relaxation phenomena. The different experimental techniques — nuclear magnetic resonance, atomic beams, Mössbauer effect, optical hyperfine, perturbed angular correlations, electron paramagnetic resonance, nuclear specific heats, etc. — were treated in great detail in order to clarify the relationships between them and to provide students, as well as specialists in any one technique, with an understanding of the types of information, their overlap and reliability, which are available from each of these diverse methods. The lecturers, eminent authorities in their fields, were asked to present a series of self-contained lectures which would provide, by means of a thorough explanation of fundamentals, the background necessary for an appreciation of the sophisticated and forward-looking treatment of their more advanced topics. Comprehensive critical discussions of the physical ideas and concepts inherent in all hyperfine interaction and relaxation studies served to unify these vast and rapidly expanding fields. Following two-and-one half weeks of these formal intensive lecture series, an Advanced Symposium was held during which lectures combining a tutorial and research nature were presented by leading specialists.

Our purpose as editors of this volume was to preserve and to transmit the aims and accomplishments of this Institute by means of written lectures presented with hoped-for textbook thoroughness. These chapters have been written solely for this book with this goal in mind and are not verbatim transcripts of the oral lectures. In this way the authors were able to incorporate into their presentation new ideas or illuminating material resulting from questions and discussion. Hence the chapters are, in a sense, the outgrowth of the Institute and for that reason are beyond it. The Institute lectures (Chaps. 1 to 13) and the Advanced Symposium lectures (Chaps. S.1 to S.12) also reflect, only in part, the format of the Institute. For clarity of presentation, the lecture format followed at the Institute was not retained here. In the process of editing this book, the overlap of subject matter was kept to a minimum, but was not entirely excluded in order to make each chapter as self-contained as possible. The editors accept responsibility for these actions and thank the authors for their full cooperation on these and other matters. A subject index allows for easy cross-referencing between the chapters. We hope that this book, just as the NATO Institute before it, will help to stimulate the interaction between researchers in the different disciplines and to promote future growth and a better understanding of theory and experiment in this exciting field of research.

One of us (A. J. F.) expresses his thanks to the NATO Science Council for their support of the Advanced Study Institute which he directed (C. M. Moser was Associate Director), Monsieur B. Guyon, Dean of the Faculté des Lettres et Sciences humaines d'Aix-en-Provence, for making the facilities of the University available, and Monsieur Deliau, Conseiller Administratif, for his gracious hospitality and full cooperation in making the Institute a success.

We are grateful to Mrs. Joan Latture who creatively and imaginatively carried out all aspects of the preparation, layout, and typing of this book, Mrs. Pam Dougherty, Mrs. Sue Luconi, and Miss Marcia Randlett for help with the technical typing, and Mr. Julian Brown for assistance with the graphical material. We thank Drs. N. Blum, S. Foner, G. Hoy, and D. Murnick for proofreading.

Arthur J. Freeman

Richard B. Frankel

Cambridge, Massachusetts
January 1967

CONTENTS

1. HYPERFINE STRUCTURE AND ELECTRON PARAMAGNETIC RESONANCE

B. Bleaney

Clarendon Laboratory
Oxford, England

Table of Contents

1

I. Magnetic Hyperfine Interaction

To illustrate the physical principles involved in the theory of hyperfine structure, we commence by giving a simple classical description of the interactions. The most important interaction in cases where the electrons of an ion or atom have a resultant electronic magnetic moment is the magnetic hyperfine structure resulting from the interaction of this moment with the nuclear magnetic moment. We may treat this as arising from the interaction of the nuclear magnetic moment with the magnetic field at the nucleus set up by the electron cloud, or as arising from the interaction of the electron magnetic moment with the magnetic field set up by the nuclear magnetic moment. A consistent treatment can be carried through either way, but there is no harm in using a mixture, as we shall do. The magnetic moment of the electrons is partly due to their orbital motion, and partly to their spin; we consider first the former.

A.   Interaction with the Electron Orbital Motion

The magnetic moment of the nucleus, regarded as a point dipole μ_I, sets up a magnetic vector potential

$$\mathbf{A} = \frac{\mu_0}{4\pi} \frac{(\mathbf{\mu}_I \times \mathbf{r})}{r^3} \tag{1}$$

at a point $\mathbf{r}$ in a co-ordinate system with the nucleus at the origin. We have here used the mks system of units; in cgs units (emu) the factor $(\mu_0/4\pi)$ should be set equal to unity. The energy of interaction with an electronic current density $\mathbf{J}_e$ is

$$W_\ell = -\int \mathbf{A} \cdot \mathbf{J}_e \, d\tau = \frac{\mu_0}{4\pi} \int \frac{(\mu_I \times \mathbf{r}) \cdot \mathbf{J}_e}{r^3} \, d\tau$$

$$= -\frac{\mu_0}{4\pi} \int \frac{\mu_I \cdot (\mathbf{r} \times \mathbf{J}_e)}{r^3} \, d\tau \tag{2}$$

where the integration is over the volume occupied by the electrons. The nuclear point dipole moment may be taken out of the integral, giving

$$W_\ell = -\frac{\mu_0}{4\pi} \, \mu_I \cdot \int \frac{(\mathbf{r} \times \mathbf{v})}{r^3} \, dq \tag{3}$$

since $\mathbf{J}_e \, d\tau = \mathbf{v} \, dq$, where $\mathbf{v}$ is the velocity of the charge element dq. For each electron the quantity $(\mathbf{r} \times \mathbf{v})$ can be related to its orbital momentum $m_0 (\mathbf{r} \times \mathbf{v}) = l\hbar$, which is a constant ($m_0$ = electronic mass); the integral can then be replaced by a summation over all electrons, with appropriate average values of $-e\langle r_\ell^{-3} \rangle = \int dq/r^3$. We have then

$$W_\ell = \frac{\mu_0}{4\pi} \sum_i 2\beta (\mu_I \cdot \ell_i) \langle r_\ell^{-3} \rangle_i \tag{4}$$

where $\beta = (e\hbar/2m_0)$ is the Bohr magneton. Both e and β are here taken as positive in sign. Electrons in orbits with the same quantum numbers n, ℓ are expected to have the same values of $\langle r_\ell^{-3} \rangle$, so that the sum will vanish for all closed shells, leaving only the contributions from electrons in unclosed shells. In LS-coupling we can then write

$$W_\ell = \frac{\mu_0}{4\pi} \, 2\beta \, (\mu_I \cdot \mathbf{L}) \langle r_\ell^{-3} \rangle$$

$$= \frac{\mu_0}{4\pi} 2\beta \, (\mu_I/I) \, (\mathbf{I} \cdot \mathbf{L}) \langle r_\ell^{-3} \rangle \tag{5}$$

on writing the nuclear moment μ_I as $(\mu_I/I)\mathbf{I}$, where $\mathbf{I}$ is the nuclear spin vector. Two small corrections are needed in more accurate work; the closed shells of electrons precess in the field of the nucleus, giving a diamagnetic shielding effect; the relativistic increase in mass reduces the magnetic moment of the electron (equivalent to a decrease in $\beta = (e\hbar/2m_0)$.

B.   Interaction with the Electron Spin

The interaction energy with the electronic magnetization associated with its intrinsic spin is conveniently expressed as

$$W = - \mu_I \cdot B_e \tag{6}$$

where B_e is the magnetic field at the nucleus due to the electron spin. It is simplest to consider separately the contributions to B_e which arise from the spin magnetization "outside" the nucleus and "inside" the nucleus. The former gives a simple dipolar contribution

$$B_e = - \frac{\mu_0}{4\pi} \int \frac{M_s - 3(M_s \cdot r_0)r_0}{r^3} \, d\tau \tag{7}$$

where M_s is the spin magnetization density at a point r, and r_0 is a unit vector parallel to r. We can write

$$M_s = - g_s \beta \sum_i s_i \, \rho_{si} \tag{8}$$

where s_i is the spin of the ith electron and ρ_{si} its spin density (i.e. the square of the amplitude of its wave function at the point r). Then

$$B_e = + \frac{\mu_0}{4\pi} g_s \beta \sum_i \frac{[s_i - 3(s_i \cdot r_0)r_0]}{r^3} \langle r_{sC}^{-3} \rangle_i \tag{9}$$

where

$$\langle r_{sC}^{-3} \rangle_i = \int \frac{\rho_{si}}{r_i^3} \, d\tau . \tag{10}$$

Here $g_s = 2.0023$ is the anomalous g-factor of the electron spin, and the negative sign in Eq. (8) arises from the negative charge on the electron. Once more there are small corrections due to diamagnetic effects and the relativistic increase of mass. It is generally convenient to absorb these and also the difference between g_s and 2 into an effective value of $\langle r^{-3} \rangle$, so that this part of the hyperfine interaction assumes the form

$$W_{sC} = - \frac{\mu_0}{4\pi} 2\beta (\mu_I/I) \sum_i \left\{ s_i \cdot I - 3(s_i \cdot r_0)(r_0 \cdot I) \right\} \langle r_{sC}^{-3} \rangle . \tag{11}$$

An important case where this interaction vanishes is that where the electron spin density has spherical symmetry; classically it is easily shown that the magnetic field at the center of a thin uniformly magnetized spherical shell is zero, since the integral involves the quantity

$$\int_0^\pi (1 - 3\cos^2\theta)\sin\theta\, d\theta = 0 \tag{12}$$

where θ is the angle between $\mathbf{M}_s$ and $\mathbf{r}_0$ in Eq. (7). It follows that the interaction (11) vanishes for a closed shell of electrons, and also (in LS-coupling) for a half-filled shell; in particular it vanishes for a single s-electron, but in this case we must consider also the electron magnetization "inside" the nucleus. Conceptually it is easiest at this point to regard the nuclear moment as due to an elementary current loop immersed in a magnetized medium arising from the spin magnetization density $\mathbf{M}_0$ at the nucleus. The latter gives rise to a magnetic field

$$B_e = \frac{2}{3}\mu_0\,\mathbf{M}_0 = \frac{\mu_0}{4\pi}\,\frac{8\pi}{3}\,\mathbf{M}_0 \tag{13}$$

and since for a single s-electron

$$\mathbf{M}_0 = -g_s\beta\mathbf{s}\,\rho_0 = -g_s\,\beta\mathbf{s}\,\left|\psi_s^{(0)}\right|^2 \tag{14}$$

where $\rho_0 = \left|\psi_s^{(0)}\right|^2$ is the electron spin density at the nucleus (square of the amplitude of the wave-function at the origin) and is here assumed to be uniform over the nuclear volume. Hence the energy associated with this "contact" interaction becomes

$$W_c = \frac{\mu_0}{4\pi}\,\frac{8\pi}{3}\,g_s\,\beta\,(\mathbf{\mu}_I\cdot\mathbf{s})\,\rho_0 \tag{15}$$

Since the dimensions of ρ_0 are r^{-3}, it is sometimes convenient to absorb the factors $(8\pi/3)$, $(g_s/2)$ and relativistic effects due to the change in mass with velocity (which are particularly important for s-electrons) into an effective value of $\langle r_c^{-3}\rangle$ for the "contact" interaction, writing

$$W_c = \frac{\mu_0}{4\pi}\,2\beta\,(\mathbf{\mu}_I/I)\,(\mathbf{I}\cdot\mathbf{s})\,\langle r_c^{-3}\rangle \tag{16}$$

Since an s-electron has no orbital momentum, and we have seen above that its spherically symmetric magnetization outside the nucleus produces zero magnetic field at the nucleus, Eq. (16) is the only interaction present for an s-electron.

C. Some Corrections

So far we have regarded the nuclear magnet as a point dipole or current loop of infinitesimal dimensions. We now consider the corrections arising from the fact that the nuclear magnetism is distributed over a small but finite volume. If the distribution of nuclear magnetization is spherically symmetric, its magnetic field outside the nucleus will be the same as that of a point dipole, and no correction is needed to W_ℓ or W_{sC}. If the distribution is not spherically symmetric, its interaction with the electronic magnetization can be expressed in a multipole expansion where the next term (the magnetic "octupole" term) is smaller by a factor of order (nuclear radius/electronic radius)^2 and has been detected in a few cases only by high precision atomic beam measurements. (The magnetic quadrupole operator does not conserve parity and therefore gives zero value for a pure parity state.)

A more important result of the finite distribution of nuclear magnetization arises from its interaction with the finite electronic magnetization within the nucleus. If the latter is uniform over the volume of the nucleus, then all the nuclear magnetization experiences the same value of the electronic field B_e (see Eq. (13)), and no correction is needed. The value of $|\Psi|^2$ is a maximum at the origin for an s-electron, but it may fall by a small but significant amount over the nuclear volume for heavier nuclei whose nuclear radii are larger and for which the electronic wave-functions are contracted because of the larger nuclear charge. Essentially we can allow for this by replacing Eq. (6) by

$$W = - \int B_e \cdot d\mu_I \tag{17}$$

and the change in the interaction due to the variation of B_e over the distribution of nuclear magnetization can be regarded as producing a change in the value of $\langle r_c^{-3} \rangle$. Experimentally a more important result arises from the fact that the distribution of nuclear magnetization may be quite different for different isotopes of the same element; if B_e is constant over the nuclear volume (as in a nuclear magnetic resonance experiment in an external field) it may be taken out of the integral (17) and the ratio of the hyperfine interactions for the two isotopes is the same as the ratio of the nuclear magnetic moments, since

$$\int d\mu_I = \mu_I .$$

When B_e varies over the nuclear volume this is not necessarily the case, and a "hyperfine anomaly" may be observed defined by a small quantity Δ such that

{ratio of hyperfine interactions}

$\quad$ = {ratio of nuclear magnetogyric factors (μ_I/I)} $(1+\Delta)$.

$$\tag{18}$$

The value of Δ is different from zero by an observable amount only for s-electrons, since other electrons have zero density at the origin. Experimentally Δ tends to be larger for the heavier elements, which have larger nuclear volumes and more contracted electronic wave functions.

D. Quantum Mechanical Formulation

$\quad$ Although we have treated the magnetic hyperfine interaction classically, it can be shown that the results obtained are valid on a quantum mechanical approach where we treat the angular momentum and other vector components as operators. We have then a hyperfine Hamiltonian of which the orbital term, for example, is [cf. Eqs. (3-5)]

$$\mathcal{K} = \frac{\mu_0}{4\pi} \, 2\beta(\mu_I/I) \sum_i (\mathbf{I} \cdot \boldsymbol{\ell}_i) \langle r_\ell^{-3} \rangle_i \tag{19}$$

which in LS-coupling becomes

$$\mathcal{K} = \frac{\mu_0}{4\pi} 2\beta(\mu_I/I)(\mathbf{I} \cdot \mathbf{L}) \langle r_\ell^{-3} \rangle \quad . \tag{20}$$

$\quad$ The "spin-dipolar" term equivalent to Eq. (11) is more tedious to evaluate, since it involves components of the unit vector $\mathbf{r}_0$. In electron spin resonance work it is customary to follow Abragam and Pryce (1951) in using an equivalent operator method where the components of $\mathbf{r}_0$ are replaced by those of the orbital angular momentum after allowing for the fact that the components of the latter do not commute while those of $\mathbf{r}_0$ do. Essentially this means that a product such as $xy = \frac{1}{2}(xy+yx)$ is replaced by $\frac{1}{2}(\ell_x \ell_y + \ell_y \ell_x)$, etc. The advantage of this is that the matrix elements of x, y, z can be replaced by those of ℓ_x, ℓ_y, ℓ_z (or, in LS-coupling, by those of L_x, L_y, L_z) with a constant of proportionality which is the same for all matrix elements of the same operator and which can be evaluated by direct calculation for one particular case. Thus for a single electron whose orbital quantum number is ℓ the operator

$$\{ -\mathbf{s} \cdot \mathbf{I} + 3(\mathbf{s} \cdot \mathbf{r}_0)(\mathbf{r}_0 \cdot \mathbf{I}) \} \tag{21}$$

can be replaced by

$$\frac{2}{(2\ell-1)(2\ell+3)} \left\{ \ell(\ell+1)(\mathbf{I}\cdot\mathbf{s}) - \frac{3}{2}(\boldsymbol{\ell}\cdot\mathbf{I})(\boldsymbol{\ell}\cdot\mathbf{s}) - \frac{3}{2}(\boldsymbol{\ell}\cdot\mathbf{s})(\boldsymbol{\ell}\cdot\mathbf{I}) \right\}$$

(22)

and in LS-coupling the sum of the terms (21) for the several electrons in the partly filled shell can be replaced by

$$\xi\left\{ L(L+1)(\mathbf{I}\cdot\mathbf{S}) - \frac{3}{2}(\mathbf{L}\cdot\mathbf{I})(\mathbf{L}\cdot\mathbf{S}) - \frac{3}{2}(\mathbf{L}\cdot\mathbf{S})(\mathbf{L}\cdot\mathbf{I}) \right\}$$ (23)

where

$$\xi = \frac{2\ell+1 - 4S}{S(2\ell-1)(2\ell+3)(2L-1)} \cdot$$ (24)

The Hamiltonian for the "spin dipolar" coupling with the nuclear magnetic moment is then

$$\mathcal{H} = \frac{\mu_0}{4\pi}\, 2\beta\,(\mu_I/I)\, \langle r^{-3} \rangle \times \text{Eq. (22) or (23)} .$$ (25)

In an atom or ion where $\mathbf{L}$ and $\mathbf{S}$ are coupled together to form a resultant $\mathbf{J}$ we must project the operators $\mathbf{L}, \mathbf{S}$ onto $\mathbf{J}$ to find the hyperfine operator for a manifold of states of given $\mathbf{J}$. For this purpose we replace $\mathbf{L}$ by a vector collinear with $\mathbf{J}$

$$\frac{(\mathbf{L}\cdot\mathbf{J})}{J(J+1)}\,\mathbf{J}$$ (26)

and similarly $\mathbf{S}$ by a vector collinear with $\mathbf{J}$

$$\frac{(\mathbf{S}\cdot\mathbf{J})}{J(J+1)}\,\mathbf{J}$$ (27)

where

$$(\mathbf{L}\cdot\mathbf{J}) = \tfrac{1}{2}\{J(J+1) + L(L+1) - S(S+1)\}$$

$$(\mathbf{S}\cdot\mathbf{J}) = \tfrac{1}{2}\{J(J+1) + S(S+1) - L(L+1)\}$$

and

$$(\mathbf{L}\cdot\mathbf{S}) = \tfrac{1}{2}\{J(J+1) - L(L+1) - S(S+1)\}$$

(28)

Thus (23) becomes

$$\frac{\xi}{J(J+1)}\{ L(L+1)(\mathbf{S}\cdot\mathbf{J}) - 3(\mathbf{L}\cdot\mathbf{J})(\mathbf{L}\cdot\mathbf{S})\}(\mathbf{J}\cdot\mathbf{I})$$ (29)

and the sum of the orbital and spin-dipolar contributions reduces to the simple form

$$\mathcal{K} = A_J (\mathbf{J} \cdot \mathbf{I}) \tag{30}$$

where

$$A_J = \frac{\mu_0}{4\pi} 2\beta(\mu_I/I)\frac{1}{J(J+1)}$$

$$\times [(\mathbf{L} \cdot \mathbf{J})\langle r_\ell^{-3}\rangle + \xi\{L(L+1) - 3(\mathbf{L} \cdot \mathbf{J})(\mathbf{L} \cdot \mathbf{S})\}\langle r_{sC}^{-3}\rangle]. \tag{31}$$

If the assumption is made that $\langle r_\ell^{-3}\rangle = \langle r_{sC}^{-3}\rangle$ and can be written simply as $\langle r^{-3}\rangle$, Eq. (31) can be written as

$$A_J = \frac{\mu_0}{4\pi} 2\beta(\mu_I/I) \langle r^{-3}\rangle \langle J\|N\|J\rangle \tag{32}$$

where $\langle J\|N\|J\rangle$ is a pure number which is tabulated by Elliott and Stevens (1953) for the ground states of the 4f ions.

To complete our enumeration of the magnetic hyperfine terms we need a term similar to (16), which in LS-coupling we write in the more general form

$$\mathcal{K} = \frac{\mu_0}{4\pi} 2\beta(\mu_I/I) (\mathbf{I} \cdot \mathbf{S}) \langle r_s^{-3}\rangle = A_S(\mathbf{I} \cdot \mathbf{S}) . \tag{33}$$

Here the value of $\langle r_c^{-3}\rangle$ embraces all contributions of the form $(\mathbf{I} \cdot \mathbf{S})$ (see below), whereas $\langle r_c^{-3}\rangle$ was restricted to those which arose from electrons which have a finite spin density at the nucleus (i.e. to the "contact" interaction).

When J is a good quantum number we can project S onto J as before, giving

$$\mathcal{K} = A_S'(\mathbf{I} \cdot \mathbf{J}) \tag{34}$$

where

$$A_S' = \frac{\mu_0}{4\pi} 2\beta(\mu_I/I) \langle r_s^{-3}\rangle \frac{(\mathbf{S} \cdot \mathbf{J})}{J(J+1)} . \tag{35}$$

Evaluation of two of the factors in Eq. (28) is simplified by expressing them in terms of the Landé factor g_J, whence

$$\frac{(\mathbf{L} \cdot \mathbf{J})}{J(J+1)} = 2 - g_J \left. \right\}$$

$$\frac{(\mathbf{S} \cdot \mathbf{J})}{J(J+1)} = g_J - 1 \left. \right\} \tag{36}$$

provided that g_S is taken as exactly two in the calculation of g_J. These last results follow readily from the operator equivalences

$$\mathbf{L} + 2\mathbf{S} \equiv g_J \mathbf{J} \left. \right\}$$

$$\mathbf{L} + \mathbf{S} \equiv \mathbf{J} \left. \right\} \tag{37}$$

E. The $\langle r^{-3} \rangle$ Parameters

In the formal development we have introduced three parameters dependent on the electron radial distribution, $\langle r_{\ell}^{-3} \rangle$, $\langle r_{sC}^{-3} \rangle$, and $\langle r_{s}^{-3} \rangle$. In origin they were connected with the interactions between the nuclear magnetic dipole moment and the electron orbit, the electron spin distribution outside the nucleus, and the electron spin density at the nucleus respectively. More generally they can be regarded as parameters which include all interactions which have the same operator form as the basic interactions from which we started. These arise from corrections which we now briefly outline. For additional detailed discussions of these $\langle r^{-3} \rangle$ parameters see Chapters 2 and 4 .

If the electron spin density is everywhere proportional to the electron charge density, as in a hydrogen-like atom with a single electron, we should have $\langle r_{\ell}^{-3} \rangle = \langle r_{sC}^{-3} \rangle$. In a many-electron atom, however, the resultant hyperfine structure is the sum of contributions from the individual electrons, and since we are summing vector quantities, the net effect depends on the balance between the positive and negative contributions. For example, in a closed electron shell we have

$$\sum_i s_i = 0 \tag{38}$$

but it does not necessarily follow that the sum

$$\sum_i s_i \langle r_s^{-3} \rangle_i = 0 \tag{39}$$

if different electrons in the same shell have different values of $\langle r_s^{-3} \rangle_i$. If all electron shells in the atom are closed, the sum in Eq. (39) and the corresponding sums involving $\langle r_{\ell}^{-3} \rangle$ and $\langle r_{sC}^{-3} \rangle$ are all zero, so that there is no hyperfine structure. If the atom has an open shell as well as closed shells, then the electrostatic repulsion between the electrons ("configuration interaction") gives rise to energy differences for electrons in the same shell which cause differences in their radial wave-functions and hence in their values of $\langle r^{-3} \rangle$. For example, the electrostatic repulsion gives rise (through the exclusion principle) to an exchange interaction between electrons in the open shell and electrons in the closed shell. If the net spin S of the electrons in the open shell is "up," then the electrons in the closed shells whose individual spins are "up" will have a slightly different energy from those whose spins are "down," and hence slightly different values of $\langle r^{-3} \rangle$.

The differences between $\langle r_\ell^{-3} \rangle$ and $\langle r_{SC}^{-3} \rangle$ which result from these causes are not large, though they cannot be neglected in the interpretation of accurate experimental results. A much more dramatic effect is the appearance of a contact term of the form (33) in cases where it would not be expected, such as open shells of p, d, f, ... electrons. This is mainly due to the effect of the exchange interaction on the s-electrons in the closed shells, giving different radial distributions from electrons with spin "up" and spin "down," and a non-zero value for the sum (39). The effect is especially important for s-electrons because a small degree of un-balance in (39) can give a rather large contribution to the hyperfine structure, and because the contribution [Eq. (33)] is different in form from the two terms [Eq. (31)] otherwise expected. The con-tribution is due to the magnetization of the closed shells or "core electrons," and is known as "core polarization."

Experimentally, differences of rather over 10 percent be-tween $\langle r_\ell^{-3} \rangle$ and $\langle r_{SC}^{-3} \rangle$ have been found by Harvey (1965) for the ground states of the oxygen atom ($2p^4$, ^3P) and the fluorine atom ($2p^5$, ^2P), as well as a finite value of $\langle r_s^{-3} \rangle$. These differences, however, may be exceptionally large. The most striking effect occurs in the case of half-filled shells, such as Mn^{2+}, $3d^5$, ^6S, where zero hyperfine interaction would be expected because L=0, the spin-dipolar interaction vanishes because of spherical sym-metry, and no unpaired s-electrons are present. In fact a con-siderable hyperfine interaction is observed of the form $(S \cdot I)$, whose explanation lies in the concept of "core-polarization."

Somewhat similar results may be produced by relativistic effects. In this case the energy difference is between electrons whose spins are parallel and anti-parallel to their orbits (i.e., electrons with $j = \ell + \frac{1}{2}$ and with $j = \ell - \frac{1}{2}$), giving rise to different values of $\langle r^{-3} \rangle$ for the different electrons in the same shell. Not only does this contribute to differences between $\langle r_\ell^{-3} \rangle$ and $\langle r_{SC}^{-3} \rangle$, but it may also contribute to a term of the form $(S \cdot I)$; for this reason Eq. (33) was written in the more general form which does not presuppose that it arises entirely from core-polarization.

The form of the relativistic effects in LS-coupling has been considered by Sandars and Beck (1965). They point out a signifi-cant difference between such effects and those due to core-polari-zation, in that the relativistic effects are single-electron effects. Thus in a half-filled shell such as $4f^7$ a term of the form $(S \cdot I)$ may arise from differences in $\langle r^{-3} \rangle$ for the electrons of the open

4f shell, which have zero density at the nucleus and hence cannot produce a hyperfine anomaly. On the other hand configuration interaction or core-polarization is a two-electron effect, in which the electrons of the open shell cause differences in $\langle r^{-3} \rangle$ amongst electrons in the closed shells, and in particular may unbalance the s-electrons with spin "up" and spin "down," giving a finite spin density at the nucleus and the possibility of a hyperfine anomaly. Measurements (Evans, Sandars, and Woodgate, 1965) on the europium atom (4f^7, ^{8}S) have shown that there is no hyperfine anomaly for the isotopes 151, 153, and the hyperfine interaction is attributed to relativistic effects, apart from a contribution from the breakdown of LS-coupling. On the other hand a considerably larger hyperfine interaction is observed for Eu^{2+} in CaF$_2$, which is also in a 4f^7, ^{8}S state and differs from Eu by lacking two 6s electrons; in this case Endor measurements reveal an appreciable hyperfine anomaly (Baker and Williams, 1962) and the larger hyperfine interaction is attributed mainly to core-polarization.

Finally we remark that it can be shown quite generally (Trees, 1953; Sandars and Beck, 1965) that the magnetic dipole hyperfine structure can be expressed as a sum of three terms of the form discussed above, and no term with a different angular dependence occurs. The subscripts we have used correspond to a notation in which the "spin-dipolar" term is written in the form $(sC^2)^1$, and the overall interaction may be expressed in the Hamiltonian

$$\mathcal{H} = \frac{\mu_0}{4\pi} \, 2\beta \, (\mu_I/I) \sum_i \left\{ \langle r_\ell^{-3} \rangle_i \, \ell_i - \langle r_{sC}^{-3} \rangle_i \sqrt{10} \, (sC^2)_i^1 + \langle r_s^{-3} \rangle_i \, s_i \right\} \cdot I \, .$$

$$(40)$$

Here (as before) the factor $(\mu_0/4\pi)$ appears in the mks system but not in the cgs (emu) system; β is the Bohr magneton, μ_I is the magnetic moment of the nucleus and I its spin; the summation is over electrons in the open shell. The parameters $\langle r_\ell^{-3} \rangle$, $\langle r_{sC}^{-3} \rangle$, $\langle r_s^{-3} \rangle$ can be determined separately by experiment if sufficient magnetic hyperfine constants are determined (e.g. for different states with the same values of L, S) and the nuclear magnetic moment is known independently from a measurement of its interaction with a known magnetic field (e.g. by nuclear magnetic resonance, ENDOR or the atomic beam triple resonance method). *

*From Sec. III onward we shall adopt the usual convention of cgs units and use **H** as the symbol for magnetic field rather than **B**.

II. Electrostatic Hyperfine Interaction

A. The Multipole Expansion for the Electrostatic Energy

The electrostatic interaction energy between the nucleus and an electron

$$W_E = \frac{1}{4\pi\epsilon_0} \int \int \frac{\rho_e \, \rho_N}{|r_N - r_e|} \, d\tau_e \, d\tau_N \tag{41}$$

may be expanded in spherical harmonics

$$W_E = \frac{1}{4\pi\epsilon_0} \sum_\ell \sum_m A_{\ell m} \, B_{\ell, -m} \tag{42}$$

where

$$A_{\ell, m} = \int \rho_N r_N^\ell \, C_{\ell, m} (\theta_N, \Phi_N) d\tau_N \tag{43}$$

$$B_{\ell, m} = (-1)^{|m|} \int \rho_e \, r_e^{-(\ell+1)} C_{\ell, m} (\theta_e, \Phi_e) d\tau_e \tag{44}$$

describe the multipole moments of order ℓ. (The factor $(1/4\pi\epsilon_0)$ occurs when the mks system of units is used, and is replaced by unity in the cgs (esu) system.) The quantities $C_{\ell, m}$ are related to spherical harmonics:

$$C_{\ell, m} = \left(\frac{4\pi}{2\ell+1}\right)^{\frac{1}{2}} Y_{\ell, m} . \tag{45}$$

Invariance under the parity operation excludes terms with odd values of ℓ, and the series is rapidly convergent because successive terms with even values of ℓ decrease as (nuclear radius/electronic radius)^2. Terms beyond the quadrupole term ($\ell = 2$) have been detected experimentally only in rare cases.

B. The Monopole Term

The first term ($\ell = 0$) is just the Coulomb interaction between the electron and a point charge Ze whose potential falls as r_e^{-1}. This requires modification for electrons with a finite charge density within the nuclear volume. Their energy is shifted by an amount

$$\int \delta V_N \, d\rho_e \tag{46}$$

where δV_N is the difference between the actual potential within the nucleus and the point charge value Ze/r_e (see Fig. 1); to this

Fig. 1: Variation of electrostatic
potential set up by nuclear charge
Ze, outside and inside the maximum nuclear radius $(r_N)_{max}$.
Outside the nucleus the potential
varies as Ze/r, apart from mutual repulsion of the electrons
in a many electron atom; inside
the nucleus the potential varies
less rapidly, in a manner dependent on the distribution of
nuclear charge density.

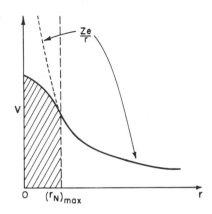

energy shift must be added a term from the region outside the
nucleus because of the overall change in the radial distribution of
electronic charge (equivalent to "normalization" of the electron
wave function). As far as hyperfine structure is concerned the
latter causes a change in the values of $\langle r^{-3} \rangle$ in the magnetic
hyperfine structure which we may regard as included in the
"parameterized" values of $\langle r^{-3} \rangle$ already employed. The energy
shift due to (46) is difficult to determine directly but is revealed
in two ways:

(a) Isotope Shift:* different isotopes of the same element
may have appreciably different distributions of nuclear charge, so
that δV_N depends on the isotope and electronic spectra of different isotopes are slightly shifted one from another.

(b) Isomer Shift:** different nuclear energy states of the same
isotope have different distributions of nuclear charge, so that δV_N
depends on the isomeric state and transitions between two nuclear
states (such as the Mössbauer effect) are shifted in energy in different substances where the electronic density at the nucleus is
different (an effect sometimes known as the "chemical shift").

C. The Quadrupole Term

We now consider the quadrupole interaction given by the
terms with $\ell = 2$. The quantities $A_{\ell, m}$, $B_{\ell, m}$ may be regarded

*For detailed discussion of this effect see Chap. 5 by A.
  Steudel.
**For detailed discussion of this effect see Chap. 11 by R.L.
  Mossbauer.

as tensor operators, one involving the nuclear co-ordinates, the other the electronic co-ordinates. The components of the nuclear electric quadrupole moment operator may be written in the form

$$
\left.
\begin{aligned}
A_{2,0} &= \int \rho_N \, r_N^2 \, C_{2,0} \, d\tau_N \\
A_{2,\pm 1} &= \int \rho_N \, r_N^2 \, C_{2,\pm 1} \, d\tau_N \\
A_{2,\pm 2} &= \int \rho_N \, r_N^2 \, C_{2,\pm 2} \, d\tau_N
\end{aligned}
\right\}
\tag{47a}
$$

where

$$
\left.
\begin{aligned}
r^2 \, C_{2,0} &= \tfrac{1}{2} r^2 \, (3\cos^2\theta - 1) = \tfrac{1}{2}(3z^2 - r^2) \\
r^2 \, C_{2,\pm 1} &= \mp (3/2)^{\frac{1}{2}} \cos\theta \sin\theta \exp(\pm i\Phi) = \\
&\qquad\qquad\qquad \mp (3/2)^{\frac{1}{2}} z(x \pm iy) \\
r^2 \, C_{2,\pm 2} &= (3/8)^{\frac{1}{2}} r^2 \sin^2\theta \exp(\pm i2\Phi) = \\
&\qquad\qquad\qquad (3/8)^{\frac{1}{2}} (x \pm iy)^2
\end{aligned}
\right\}
\tag{47b}
$$

.

The first integral

$$
\int \rho_N \, \tfrac{1}{2}(3 z_N^2 - r_N^2) \, d\tau_N
\tag{48}
$$

can be replaced by an equivalent expression in the nuclear spin co-ordinates

$$
A_{2,0} = \tfrac{1}{2}\alpha \left\{ 3 I_z^2 - I(I+1) \right\}
\tag{49}
$$

and the others by equivalent expressions

$$
A_{2,\pm 1} = \mp \tfrac{1}{2}(3/2)^{\frac{1}{2}} \alpha \, (I_z I_\pm + I_\pm I_z)
\tag{50}
$$

$$
A_{2,\pm 2} = (3/8)^{\frac{1}{2}} \alpha \, I_\pm^2 \, .
\tag{51}
$$

The value of the constant α is determined by our definition of the nuclear electric quadrupole moment. The usual definition is to represent by $\tfrac{1}{2}eQ$ the value of (48) in the nuclear state I, $I_z = I$, for which the equivalent expression (49) becomes

$$
\langle II | \tfrac{1}{2}\alpha \{ 3I_z^2 - I(I+1) \} | II \rangle = \tfrac{1}{2}\alpha \, I(2I-1)
\tag{52}
$$

so that the value of α is

$$\alpha = \frac{eQ}{I(2I-1)} \tag{53}$$

The components $B_{2,m}$ of the electronic tensor can be written out in a similar way, and replaced by operator equivalents involving the orbital angular momentum vector of each electron. This is then summed over all electrons, giving (since the electronic charge is $-e$)

$$\left.\begin{array}{l} B_{2,0} = -e \sum_i \langle \ell \| \alpha \| \ell \rangle \langle r_q^{-3} \rangle_i \tfrac{1}{2} \{3\ell_z^2 - \ell(\ell+1)\}_i \\[2ex] B_{2,\pm1} = \mp e \sum_i \langle \ell \| \alpha \| \ell \rangle \langle r_q^{-3} \rangle_i \tfrac{1}{2} (3/2)^{\frac{1}{2}} (\ell_z \ell_\pm + \ell_\pm \ell_z)_i \\[2ex] B_{2,\pm2} = -e \sum_i \langle \ell \| \alpha \| \ell \rangle \langle r_q^{-3} \rangle (3/8)^{\frac{1}{2}} (\ell_\pm^2) \end{array}\right\} \tag{54}$$

For a term in L,S coupling the sums can be replaced by operators involving the components of the total orbital angular momentum

$$\left.\begin{array}{l} B_{2,0} = -e \langle L \| \alpha \| L \rangle \langle r_q^{-3} \rangle \tfrac{1}{2} \{3L_z^2 - L(L+1)\} \\[2ex] B_{2,\pm1} = \mp e \langle L \| \alpha \| L \rangle \langle r_q^{-3} \rangle \tfrac{1}{2} (3/2)^{\frac{1}{2}} (L_z L_\pm + L_\pm L_z) \\[2ex] B_{2,\pm2} = -e \langle L \| \alpha \| L \rangle \langle r_q^{-3} \rangle (3/8)^{\frac{1}{2}} L_\pm^2 \end{array}\right\} \tag{55}$$

Thus in this case the electric quadrupole Hamiltonian takes the form

$$\mathcal{H}_Q = -\frac{e^2 Q}{I(2I-1)} \langle L \| \alpha \| L \rangle \langle r_q^{-3} \rangle$$

$$\times \left[\begin{array}{l} \tfrac{1}{4}\{3L_z^2 - L(L+1)\}\{3I_z^2 - I(I+1)\} \\[2ex] +\tfrac{3}{8}\{(L_z L_+ + L_+ L_z)(I_z I_- + I_- I_z) + (L_z L_- + L_- L_z) \\[2ex] (I_z I_+ + I_+ I_z)\} + \tfrac{3}{8}(L_+^2 I_-^2 + L_-^2 I_+^2) \end{array}\right] \tag{56}$$

The angular momentum operator expression in square brackets in Eq. (56) is in a form which is often most useful in calculations for paramagnetic ions; it is equivalent to the more usual form

$$\frac{1}{2} \{3(L \cdot I)^2 + \frac{3}{2}(L \cdot I) - L(L+1) \, I(I+1)\} \ . \tag{57}$$

In the notation of Abragam and Pryce (1951)

$$-\langle L \| \alpha \| L \rangle = \pm \eta \tag{58}$$

where the upper sign is used if the shell is less than half-full and the lower sign if it is more than half-full.

The constants $\langle \ell \| \alpha \| \ell \rangle$ and $\langle L \| \alpha \| L \rangle$ are found by a procedure such as the following. For a single electron with quantum numbers $\ell, \, \ell_z = \ell$ we have

$$\langle \ell\ell | \frac{3z^2 - r^2}{r^5} | \ell\ell \rangle = \langle r^{-3} \rangle \int |Y_\ell^\ell|^2 \, (3\cos^2\theta - 1)\mathrm{d}\tau$$

$$= -\langle r^{-3} \rangle \frac{2\ell}{2\ell+3} \tag{59}$$

and this is equivalent to

$$\langle \ell\|\alpha\|\ell \rangle \, \langle r^{-3} \rangle \, \langle \ell\ell | 3\ell_z^2 - \ell(\ell+1)|\ell\ell \rangle$$

$$= \langle \ell\|\alpha\|\ell \rangle \, \langle r^{-3} \rangle \, \ell(2\ell - 1) \ . \tag{60}$$

Hence

$$\langle \ell\|\alpha\|\ell \rangle = - \frac{2}{(2\ell - 1) \, (2\ell + 3)} \ . \tag{61}$$

For a ground state in LS-coupling obeying Hund's rules, so that S, L have their maximum values we proceed as follows. Suppose there are r electrons with orbital quantum number ℓ. Then for the state $L_z = L$, $S_z = S$,

$$L = \ell + (\ell - 1) + \dots \quad + (\ell - r + 1)$$

$$= \tfrac{1}{2} r \, (2\ell + 1 - r) \ . \tag{62}$$

Since we have single particle operators,

$$\sum \{3\ell_z^2 - \ell(\ell+1)\} = 3\{\ell^2 + (\ell - 1)^2 + \dots + (\ell - r + 1)^2\} - r\ell(\ell+1)$$

$$= \tfrac{1}{2} r(2\ell + 1 - r) (2\ell + 1 - 2r)$$

$$= L(2\ell + 1 - 2r) \ . \tag{63}$$

From the equivalence

$$\langle \ell \| \alpha \| \ell \rangle \sum \{3\ell_z^2 - \ell(\ell+1)\} = \langle L \| \alpha \| L \rangle \{3L_z^2 - L(L+1)\}$$

for this state we have then, since $L_z = L$,

$$\langle \ell \| \alpha \| \ell \rangle \, L(2\ell+1-2r) = \langle L \| \alpha \| L \rangle \, L(2L-1) \ .$$

If the shell is less than half filled ($2r \langle 2\ell+1 \rangle$), we have $r = 2S$ from Hund's rule, while if the shell is more than half full

$$2S = (2\ell-1) - r$$

and

$$2\ell+1-2r = 2\ell+1-2(2\ell+1-2S) = -(2\ell+1-4S) \ .$$

Hence

$$\langle L \| \alpha \| L \rangle = \pm \langle \ell \| \alpha \| \ell \rangle \frac{(2\ell+1-4S)}{2L-1}$$

$$= \mp \frac{2(\ell+1-4S)}{(2\ell-1)(2\ell+3)(2L-1)} \tag{64}$$

where the upper sign applies to a shell which is less than half-full of electrons, and the lower sign to a shell more than half-full.

When $\mathbf{L}$ and $\mathbf{S}$ couple to a resultant $\mathbf{J}$ formulae similar to (56) and (57) can be obtained for the quadrupole interaction in which $\mathbf{L}$ is replaced everywhere by $\mathbf{J}$ and $\langle L \| \alpha \| L \rangle$ by $\langle J \| \alpha \| J \rangle$. This representation is useful in electron paramagnetic resonance when considering ions of the rare earth group [for which the constants $\langle J \| \alpha \| J \rangle$ are tabulated by Elliott and Stevens (1953)], and is similar to that used in atomic beam measurements

$$\mathcal{H} = \frac{B}{2I(2I-1)J(2J-1)} \{3(I \cdot J)^2 + \frac{3}{2}(I \cdot J) - I(I+1)J(J+1)\} \tag{65}$$

where

$$B = -J(2J-1) \, e^2 Q \, \langle r_q^{-3} \rangle \, \langle J \| \alpha \| J \rangle \ . \tag{66}$$

In electron spin resonance work it is often convenient to have the quadrupole operator in a "Cartesian" form. The last term of Eq. (56) can be transformed as follows:

$$\frac{3}{8}(L_+^2 I_-^2 + L_-^2 I_+^2) = \frac{3}{4}(L_x^2 - L_y^2)(I_x^2 - I_y^2)$$

$$+ \frac{3}{4}(L_x L_y + L_y L_x)(I_x I_y + I_y I_x)$$

$$= -\frac{1}{12}\{3L_z^2 - L(L+1)\}\{3I_z^2 - I(I+1)\}$$

$$+ \frac{1}{6}\{3L_x^2 - L(L+1)\}\{3I_x^2 - I(I+1)\}$$

$$+ \frac{1}{6}\{3L_y^2 - L(L+1)\}\{3I_y^2 - I(I+1)\}$$

$$+ \frac{3}{4}(L_x L_y + L_y L_x)(I_x I_y + I_y I_x)\ .$$

Thus the electric quadrupole Hamiltonian can be written in the form

$$\mathcal{H}_Q = -\frac{e^2 Q}{I(2I-1)}\langle L\|\alpha\|L\rangle\langle r_q^{-3}\rangle$$

$$\times \begin{bmatrix} \frac{1}{6}\{3L_x^2 - L(L+1)\}\{3I_x^2 - I(I+1)\} \\[2mm] + \frac{1}{6}\{3L_y^2 - L(L+1)\}\{3I_y^2 - I(I+1)\} \\[2mm] + \frac{1}{6}\{3L_z^2 - L(L+1)\}\{3I_z^2 - I(I+1)\} \\[2mm] + \frac{3}{4}(L_x L_y + L_y L_x)(I_x I_y + I_y I_x) \\[2mm] + \frac{3}{4}(L_y L_z + L_z L_y)(I_y I_z + I_z I_y) \\[2mm] + \frac{3}{4}(L_z L_x + L_x L_z)(I_z I_x + I_x I_z) \end{bmatrix}\ . \tag{67}$$

D. The Sternheimer Effect

In these formulae we have written $\langle r_q^{-3} \rangle$ with a subscript q for the mean inverse third power of the electron radius to remind us that this quantity is only approximately but not exactly the same as the quantities $\langle r_\ell^{-3} \rangle$ and $\langle r_{SC}^{-3} \rangle$ involved in the magnetic hyperfine structure. In addition to computing $\langle r_q^{-3} \rangle$ for the open shell we have a rather considerable effect due to the fact that the closed shells of electrons are distorted ("quadrupolarized") by the field gradients to which they are subjected, and they may therefore also contribute to the field gradient at the nucleus. This "Sternheimer effect" is represented by multiplying $\langle r_q^{-3} \rangle$ for the open shell by a factor $(1 - R)$. The contributions to R are both positive (shielding) and negative (anti-shielding).

E. A Relativistic Correction

In a half-filled shell the electron charge distribution is expected to have spherical symmetry and the electric quadrupole interaction vanishes, corresponding to the fact that all orbits of different values of ℓ_z are singly occupied and the sum

$$\sum_{\ell_z=\ell}^{-\ell} \{3\ell_z^2 - \ell(\ell+1)\} = 0 \; . \tag{68}$$

This assumes however, that the values of $\langle r_q^{-3} \rangle$ are the same for every electron in the half-filled shell, but this is not exactly true owing to relativistic effects (see Sandars and Beck, 1965). The sum

$$\sum_{\ell_z=\ell}^{-\ell} \{3\ell_z^2 - \ell(\ell+1)\} \langle r_q^{-3} \rangle_{\ell_z}$$

does not then exactly equal zero, and a small quadrupole interaction of the form (65) with $J = S$ has been observed for Mn $(3d^5)$ and Eu $(4f^7)$ atoms (Evans, Sandars, and Woodgate, 1965), and also for the Eu^{2+} $(4f^7)$ ion in cubic symmetry in CaF_2 (Baker and Williams, 1962).

III. Paramagnetic Ions in Solids

A. The Ligand Interaction

   1. Interactions Internal to the Ion

      Paramagnetic ions in solids are subject to interactions with the neighbouring ions (the ligands), and this makes the theoretical treatment more complicated than that of a free many-electron atom. A perturbation approach is required in which terms must be considered in order of diminishing importance (i. e. diminishing interaction energy), and the ligand interaction must therefore be introduced at an appropriate point relative to the sequence of interactions internal to the paramagnetic ion. In order of interaction energy, the latter are, briefly —

     a. Interaction of an electron with the Coulomb field of the nucleus, which is reduced by the average field of the other electrons; this results in the grouping of the electronic levels into configurations, e. g. $3d^3$, with the ground configuration of order 10^5 cm^{-1} below the first excited configuration.

     b. The remaining mutual electrostatic repulsion of the electrons, not represented by the average field. This results in LS-coupling with energy splittings of order 10^4 cm^{-1} between terms of different L, S built from the same configuration. For example, Cr^{3+} ($3d^3$) has (by Hund's rules) a ground state ^4F, with S = 3/2, L = 3. This is $\sim 10^4$ cm^{-1} below the ^4P state belonging to the same ($3d^3$) configuration.

     c. The spin-orbit interaction then couples L, S to form a multiplet of levels with different values of the resultant J. The components of the multiplet are separated by $\sim 10^2$ cm^{-1} for 3d electrons and $\sim 10^3$ cm^{-1} for 4f electrons.

   2. Strength of the Ligand Interaction

      Paramagnetic ions normally belong to the "transition groups" with unpaired electrons in one of the 3d, 4d, 5d, 4f or 5f shells. In general they will have both unpaired spin and orbital angular momentum. The magnitudes of the ligand field interactions differ between the groups, which are therefore discussed separately.

     a. 4f (and to a somewhat lesser extent 5f) electrons are, crudely speaking, not valence electrons but "inner"

electrons. The interaction with the ligands is
$\sim 10^2$ cm^{-1} which is smaller than the spin-orbit
coupling, and to first approximation the effect of the
ligand interaction is to raise the $2J+1$ fold degeneracy of each member of a multiplet. Exceptions arise
for complex ions of the 5f group, e. g. $[UO_2]^{++}$, in
which the 5f electrons are involved in bond formation
with the oxygens of the O-U-O complex, and must be
treated as in c below.

b. 3d electrons: These are valence electrons and their
interaction with the ligands produces splittings of
order 10^4 cm^{-1}, comparable with the LS-coupling
energy. In the "weak field approximation" this is
considered as an interaction with the orbital motion
only, lifting the $2L+1$ degeneracy of the lowest L, S
state. Since the ligand interaction is comparable
with the LS-coupling energy, admixtures of excited
L, S states may be needed in the ground state.

c. 4d, 5d electrons, and some 3d compounds such as the
complex cyanides of type $K_3 Fe(CN)_6$. For these the
ligand interaction is much stronger than LS-coupling,
and the treatment necessitates a return to single
electron states, strongly split by the ligand field, and
to a lesser extent by the electrostatic and spin-orbit
couplings within the paramagnetic ion.

3. Representation of the Ligand Interaction by a Crystalline
Potential

The simplest method is to consider the ligand field as a
purely electrostatic interaction. The ligands are regarded simply
as charged ions, located on given lattice points, and giving rise to
a crystalline potential which reflects the symmetry of the ionic
environment. This results in splittings of the electronic levels
due to a "Stark effect" with a rather complex electric potential.
In this formalism three cases arise:

a. If the splittings are small compared with spin-orbit
coupling we can work in terms of J with, if necessary,
corrections for coupling to states of different J.
(Usually the first excited state, $J \pm 1$, will suffice.)
Then if, as in paramagnetic resonance, we have an
external applied field H, the diagonal Zeeman interaction is of the form

$$\mathcal{K} = g_J \beta (\mathbf{H} \cdot \mathbf{J}) \tag{69}$$

(for $\mathbf{H}$ of a few kilogauss the splittings produced are ≤ 1 cm^{-1}); we may also use the hyperfine interaction formulae given in terms of $\mathbf{J}$, e.g.,

$$\mathcal{K} = A(\mathbf{J} \cdot \mathbf{I}). \tag{70}$$

b.　If the spin-orbit coupling < crystal field splitting < electrostatic interactions within the ion, we may work in terms of L, S states with, if necessary, corrections for coupling to states of different L. The diagonal Zeeman interaction is

$$\mathcal{K} = \beta \{ \mathbf{H} \cdot (\mathbf{L} + g_S \mathbf{S}) \tag{71}$$

and the hyperfine interactions must be expressed in terms of $\mathbf{L}$ and $\mathbf{S}$ rather than $\mathbf{J}$.

c.　For the strongest ligand field splittings (> LS coupling) we must work in terms of single electron states 1, s. The effect of an applied field is then given by

$$\mathcal{K} = \beta \left\{ \mathbf{H} \cdot \sum_i (\ell_i + g_S s_i) \right\}. \tag{72}$$

In using the crystalline potential approach it is assumed that the values of the spin-orbit coupling constant, $\langle r^{-3} \rangle$, etc. are the same as for the free ion.

4.　Molecular Orbital Treatment

　　　The crystal field formulation outlined above is fairly successful in the interpretation of observed level splittings but attempts to calculate the crystal field from a simple electrostatic model give poor agreement with experiment. For a better representation a more complex model is necessary treating the transition group ion and ligand ions as a complex and including σ- and π-bonding between them using molecular orbitals. The calculation must start from single electron states, making it especially complex for ions with several electrons.

　　　In this case the Zeeman interaction is clearly given by Eq. (72) but now this and other interactions must be evaluated for molecular orbitals. We can summarize the results of this treatment as follows:

a.　The effect of transfer of electrons from the central ion to the ligand is to reduce the effective orbital

angular momentum of the central ion, i. e. the
Zeeman interaction becomes

$$\mathcal{H} = \beta \left\{ \mathbf{H} \cdot \sum_i (k\ell_i + g_s \, s_i) \right\} \tag{73}$$

where $k < 1$ and is normally anisotropic except for
cases of cubic symmetry.

b. The electron transfer reduces the effective spin-orbit
    coupling constant.

c. The electron transfer reduces the effective value of
    $\langle r^{-3} \rangle$ for hyperfine interactions with the nucleus of
    the central ion.

d. When nuclei of the ligand ions have spin, additional
    "ligand hyperfine structure" may be observed.

These effects reflect the fact that the magnetic electrons
spend only part of their time on the central paramagnetic ion, and
part on the ligand ions.

B. The Spin Hamiltonian

Whatever theoretical approach is adopted the result is a
splitting of levels leaving groups of rather small degeneracy. In
the case of local cubic symmetry, groups of 1, 2, 3, or 4 degenerate levels are found, but in cases of lower symmetry levels may
be only single or degenerate in pairs. An important overriding
theorem concerning the residual degeneracy is due to Kramers; in
a system containing an odd number of electrons, at least two-fold
degeneracy must remain in the absence of a magnetic field. The
pairs of states ("Kramers doublets") involved are time-conjugate,
one being obtained from the other by time-reversal and are thus
not split by an electrostatic perturbation, which is even under time
reversal.

In most electron paramagnetic resonance (EPR) studies of the
ionic energy levels we examine their properties through the excitation of magnetic dipole transitions at frequencies up to about 10^{11}
c/s between levels split by the Zeeman effect by at most a few
cm^{-1}. Hence we are immediately interested only in groups of
levels degenerate (or split by amounts of this order) in zero magnetic field. A full theoretical treatment of each system is lengthy,
and a convenient method is needed to represent the behaviour of
the group of levels immediately concerned. This method makes use
of an "effective spin" $\tilde{\mathbf{S}}$, a fictitious angular momentum such that

the degeneracy of the group of levels involved is set equal to $2\tilde{S}+1$. Thus for an isolated Kramers doublet with just two levels we take a value of $\tilde{S} = \frac{1}{2}$. The procedure followed is to set up an "effective spin Hamiltonian," which must give a correct description of the behaviour of this group of levels (determined, of course, by the strong interactions outlined above), in terms of the effective spin.

In some cases a theoretical justification of the effective spin Hamiltonian can be given; in others we assume it to consist of a plausible number of terms and try empirically to fit these to the observed EPR spectra. As an example we consider first the Zeeman interaction for the electronic levels; later we shall discuss the form of the magnetic and electric hyperfine interactions in the effective spin formulation. For a free ion or atom in a state J the Zeeman interaction is given by

$$\mathcal{H} = g_J \beta \, (\mathbf{H} \cdot \mathbf{J}) \tag{74}$$

and is independent of the direction of $\mathbf{H}$ because a free atom has rotational symmetry. In a solid, however, there may be anisotropy so that the size of the interaction depends upon the orientation of $\mathbf{H}$ with respect to the crystal axes. The most general form, in terms of $\tilde{S}$ is

$$\mathcal{H} = \beta(\mathbf{H} \cdot g \cdot \tilde{\mathbf{S}}) \tag{75}$$

which is a short-hand notation for

$$\mathcal{H} = \beta \left\{ \begin{aligned} & g_{xx}H_x\tilde{S}_x + g_{yy}H_y\tilde{S}_y + g_{zz}H_z\tilde{S}_z \\ & + g_{xy}H_x\tilde{S}_y + g_{yx}H_y\tilde{S}_x \\ & + g_{yz}H_y\tilde{S}_z + g_{zy}H_z\tilde{S}_y \\ & + g_{zx}H_z\tilde{S}_x + g_{xz}H_x\tilde{S}_z \end{aligned} \right\} . \tag{76}$$

Now, if, as is often true, $g_{xy} = g_{yx}$ etc., cross terms can be eliminated by a suitable choice of axes, known as the "principal axes," leaving

$$\mathcal{H} = \beta \{g_{xx}H_x\tilde{S}_x + g_{yy}H_y\tilde{S}_y + g_{zz}H_z\tilde{S}_z\} . \tag{77}$$

It is important to note that since $\tilde{S}$ is not the true angular momentum of the system, g is not the true magneto-gyric ratio as would be measured in a classical experiment of the Barnett or Einstein-de Haas type. For this reason g is sometimes known as the "spectroscopic splitting factor."

C. Hyperfine Interaction and the Spin Hamiltonian

The Zeeman interaction represented by Eq. (76) corresponds to the interaction of an anisotropic electronic magnetic moment with an external field H. The magnetic hyperfine interaction is the result of the interaction between this anisotropic electronic magnetic moment and the magnetic field due to the nuclear magnetic dipole moment. We may therefore expect to represent it by an effective spin Hamiltonian which is an extension of the operator for a free atom

$$\mathcal{K} = A(\mathbf{J} \cdot \mathbf{I}) \tag{78}$$

similar to the extension needed for the Zeeman interaction; i.e. we write

$$\mathcal{K} = (\widetilde{\mathbf{S}} \cdot A \cdot \mathbf{I}) \tag{79}$$

$$\left.\begin{aligned}
&= A_{xx}\widetilde{S}_x I_x + A_{yy}\widetilde{S}_y I_y + A_{zz}\widetilde{S}_z I_z \\
&\quad + A_{xy}\widetilde{S}_x I_y + A_{yx}\widetilde{S}_y I_x \\
&\quad + A_{yz}\widetilde{S}_y I_z + A_{zy}\widetilde{S}_z I_y \\
&\quad + A_{zx}\widetilde{S}_z I_x + A_{xz}\widetilde{S}_x I_z
\end{aligned}\right\} \tag{80}$$

Provided $A_{xy} = A_{yx}$, etc. (which is true in most cases) we can find a special set of axes (the "principal axes") where the cross terms vanish, leaving

$$\mathcal{K} = A_{xx}\widetilde{S}_x I_x + A_{yy}\widetilde{S}_y I_y + A_{zz}\widetilde{S}_z I_z . \tag{81}$$

In the case of the nuclear electric quadrupole operator discussed in Sec. II we note that the components of the electronic angular momentum [see Eq. (54 or 55)] occur always in the second degree.

For a paramagnetic ion in the solid state, energy levels appear as doublets only in cases where one of a pair of states is obtained from the other by reversing the angular momentum components. Thus the quantities $B_{2,m}$ in Eqs. (54 or 55) arc the same for each state of an electronic doublet, and become parameters multiplying the nuclear spin operators $A_{2,m}$. Hence for such a doublet the nuclear electric quadrupole interaction can be represented by a sum of terms $A_{2,m}$ with suitable parameters. In Cartesian co-ordinates this sum can be written in the form

$$
\begin{aligned}
I \cdot P \cdot I = P_{xx}I_x^2 &+ P_{yy}I_y^2 + P_{zz}I_z^2 \\
&+ P_{xy}I_xI_y + P_{yx}I_yI_x \\
&+ P_{yz}I_yI_z + P_{zy}I_zI_y \\
&+ P_{zx}I_zI_x + P_{xz}I_xI_z
\end{aligned}
\Bigg\} \qquad (82)
$$

From, for example, Eq. (67) we may expect this to be a symmetric tensor ($P_{xy} = P_{yx}$, etc.), and by a suitable choice of axes it can be reduced to the form

$$
P_{xx}I_x^2 + P_{yy}I_y^2 + P_{zz}I_z^2 \qquad (83)
$$

which can also be written as

$$
P_{\parallel}\left[\left\{I_z^2 - \tfrac{1}{3}I(I+1)\right\} + \tfrac{1}{3}\eta\,(I_x^2 - I_y^2)\right] \qquad (84)
$$

where

$$
P_{\parallel} = 3P_{zz}/2 \ , \quad \eta = (P_{xx} - P_{yy})/P_{zz} \ . \qquad (85)
$$

Since the nomenclature used here is somewhat different from that used in other branches of radio-spectroscopy, we note that

$$
P_{\parallel} = \frac{3eQq}{4I(2I-1)} = \frac{3eQ}{4I(2I-1)}\,(\partial^2 V/\partial z^2) \qquad (86)
$$

where $q = (\partial^2 V/\partial z^2)$ is the field gradient at the nucleus in axial symmetry.

In the solid state the electric field gradient at the nucleus will be modified by the quadrupolarization of the electron core (the "Sternheimer effect"), which can be represented by multiplying the value of $\langle r_q^{-3}\rangle$ for the open shell by a factor $(1-R)$. In addition, if the surroundings of the paramagnetic ion do not have cubic symmetry, they may set up a field gradient which interacts with the nuclear electric quadrupole moment of the central ion. This gradient is also modified by quadrupolarization of the electron cloud, but the factor is different because the polarizing source is different and because all the electrons take part and not just the closed shells of the electron core. If (in axial symmetry) the crystal field contains a term $A_2^0\,(3z^2 - r^2)$ in the nomenclature of

Elliott and Stevens, the additional contribution to the nuclear electric quadrupole interaction is

$$P_{\parallel}(\text{lattice}) = -\frac{3QA_2^0}{I(2I-1)}(1-\gamma_\infty) \tag{87}$$

where the values of $(1-\gamma_\infty)$ may be of order 100 for the 4f series
(see Edmonds, 1963; Barnes, Mössbauer, Kankeleit, and
Poindexter, 1964). This greatly enhances the importance of the
lattice contribution relative to that of the paramagnetic ion, for
which $(1-R)$ appears to be < 1 for the 4f group. For Nd^{3+} in
$LaCl_3$ the lattice contribution appears to be so large that it out-
weighs (and is of opposite sign to) the contribution from the 4f
electrons (see Bleaney, 1964).

Finally, we have a term $-\beta H \cdot g^{(I)} \cdot I$, which represents the
interaction between the nuclear magnetic moment and the external
field H. If this were a simple direct interaction, $g^{(I)}$ would be a
scalar quantity, equal to the ordinary nuclear g-factor. However,
when an external magnetic field is applied the electronic wave
function is changed by an amount which is in first approximation
proportional to H, and the electronic field at the nucleus is similarly modified, producing the equivalent of a paramagnetic shielding (or anti-shielding). This effect can be quite large, and when
low-lying excited electronic states are present so that the electronic wave-function is appreciably modified in a magnetic field,
the anti-shielding correction may far outweigh the direct interaction. For example, Lewis and Sabisky (1963) found that for the
Ho^{2+} ion in CaF_2, the apparent value of $g^{(I)}$ was 40 times larger
than the true value. When the electronic ground state is anisotropic, the anti-shielding will also be anisotropic, so that $g^{(I)}$
becomes a tensor with the same principal axes as the g-factor.

The term just considered may be called the "pseudo-nuclear
Zeeman effect," and its importance was pointed out by Baker and
Bleaney (1958). They also drew attention to other second-order
effects of the magnetic hyperfine structure, which produce a
"pseudo-nuclear electric quadrupole" interaction and also modify
the magnetic hyperfine interaction itself. We shall not give general expressions for these, but they are illustrated later in the
simple example discussed below. We say "illustrated" because
the formulae are derived for a special case and must not be taken
as general formulae, though the extension to the latter should not
be difficult.

D. A Simple Example: a $4f^1$ Ion in a Ligand Field of Axial Symmetry

In the foregoing discussion we have not attempted to justify the spin Hamiltonian in any way; this would require a lengthy procedure which would be inappropriate and not easy to follow. Instead we choose a specific example which shows how the effective spin Hamiltonian is related to the free ion Hamiltonian in a simple case. We shall consider first the electronic Zeeman effect, the magnetic dipole and electric quadrupole hyperfine interactions as first order perturbations, and then deduce some second order effects which give rise to "pseudo" contributions to the hyperfine interactions and to the nuclear Zeeman interaction.

1. The Electronic Zeeman Interaction

As an example we take a $4f^1$ ion such as Ce^{3+}, whose ground state is $^2F_{5/2}$. In a crystalline field of axial symmetry the six-fold $J = 5/2$ manifold splits into three doublets, characterized by $J_z = \pm 5/2$, $\pm 3/2$ and $\pm 1/2$ respectively. We call these three doublets $X^{\pm}$, $Y^{\pm}$, $Z^{\pm}$ and assume they are separated in energy by an amount small compared with that of the excited $J = 7/2$ state (at ca. 2250 cm^{-1} for Ce^{3+}) but large compared with the Zeeman energy in an external field. The latter is given by the matrix elements of the operator

$$\mathcal{K} = g_J \beta (\mathbf{H} \cdot \mathbf{J}) \tag{88}$$

which are

	$\langle \pm \lvert g_J \beta H J_z \rvert \pm \rangle$	$\langle \pm \lvert g_J \beta H J_\pm \rvert \mp \rangle$
X	$\pm \dfrac{5}{2} g_J \beta H$	0
Y	$\pm \dfrac{3}{2} g_J \beta H$	0
Z	$\pm \dfrac{1}{2} g_J \beta H$	$3 g_J \beta H$

$$\tag{89}$$

These can be compared with those of an effective spin Hamiltonian with $\widetilde{S} = 1/2$ for each doublet

$$\mathcal{K} = \beta \{ g_{\parallel} H_z \widetilde{S}_z + g_{\perp}(H_x \widetilde{S}_x + H_y \widetilde{S}_y) \} \tag{90}$$

for which we have in a corresponding table

$\langle\pm\lvert g_{\parallel}\beta H\widetilde{S}_z\rvert\pm\rangle$	$\langle\pm\lvert g_{\perp}\beta H\widetilde{S}_{\pm}\rvert\mp\rangle$
$\pm\dfrac{1}{2}\,g_{\parallel}\,\beta H$	$g_{\perp}\beta H$

(91)

from which we see that the values of $g_{\parallel}$, $g_{\perp}$ for each doublet are

	$g_{\parallel}$	$g_{\perp}$
X	$5g_J$	0
Y	$3g_J$	0
Z	g_J	$3g_J$

(92)

No resonance transitions are allowed within the first two doublets, but the last gives a resonance with a rather anisotropic g-factor.

2. The Magnetic Hyperfine Interaction

In the same approximation where we can neglect matrix elements between states belonging to $J = 5/2$ and $J = 7/2$ the magnetic hyperfine operator is

$$\mathcal{H} = A_J(\mathbf{J}\cdot\mathbf{I})$$ (93)

whose matrix elements within each doublet can be related to those of a term in the effective spin Hamiltonian with $\widetilde{S} = 1/2$

$$\mathcal{H} = A_{\parallel}\widetilde{S}_z I_z + A_{\perp}(\widetilde{S}_x I_x + \widetilde{S}_y I_y)\ .$$ (94)

It is clear that the matrix elements needed are exactly the same as those for the Zeeman interaction, so that we have the following tables:

	$A_{\parallel}$	$A_{\perp}$
X	$5A_J$	0
Y	$3A_J$	0
Z	A_J	$3A_J$

(95)

The fact that

$$A_{\parallel}/g_{\parallel} = A_{\perp}/g_{\perp} = A_J/g_J$$ (96)

or more generally

$$A_x/g_x = A_y/g_y = A_z/g_z = A_J/g_J$$ (97)

holds always for the 4f, 5f groups provided we can neglect matrix elements between manifolds of different J.

3. The Electric Quadrupole Hyperfine Interaction

We now consider the electric quadrupole interaction. As pointed out in Sec. II, we use for this a Hamiltonian equivalent to Eq. (56) in which $\mathbf{L}$ is everywhere replaced by $\mathbf{J}$ and $\langle L\|\alpha\|L\rangle$ by $\langle J\|\alpha\|J\rangle$. From the tables of Elliott and Stevens (1953) we have $\langle J\|\alpha\|J\rangle = -2/35$ for $4f^1$ in the $J = 5/2$ state. It is easily seen that all the matrix elements of this electric quadrupole operator within each doublet X, Y, Z vanish except those of $\{3J_Z^2 - J(J+1)\}$, which are

	$3J_Z^2 - J(J+1)$
X	$3(5/2)^2 - (35/4) = +10$
Y	$3(3/2)^2 - (35/4) = -2$
Z	$3(1/2)^2 - (35/4) = -8$

(98)

Hence for each doublet the electric quadrupole interaction has the form

$$\mathcal{H} = P_\| \left\{ I_z^2 - \frac{1}{3} I(I+1) \right\} \tag{99}$$

where

$$P_\| = -\frac{3e^2Q}{4I(2I-1)} \langle r_q^{-3} \rangle \langle J\|\alpha\|J\rangle \langle \pm\|3J_Z^2 - J(J+1)\|\pm\rangle \tag{100}$$

in which the value of $\langle J\|\alpha\|J\rangle$ is given above and those of $\langle \pm\|3J_Z^2 - J(J+1)\|\pm\rangle$ are listed in Eq. (98).

4. Pseudo Nuclear Electric Quadrupole Interaction

In some cases off-diagonal elements of the hyperfine operator may produce extra terms which cannot be neglected. From the magnetic hyperfine operator we have, for example, a term

$$\frac{\langle z|A_J(\mathbf{J}\cdot\mathbf{I})|y\rangle \langle y|A_J(\mathbf{J}\cdot\mathbf{I})|z\rangle}{W_z - W_y} \tag{101}$$

where y, z are states belonging to different electronic doublets. We evaluate this term for the doublet $Z^\pm (J_z = \pm 1/2)$, for which the only matrix elements are clearly those with the doublet $Y^\pm (J_z = \pm 3/2)$. We have then

$$\frac{\langle \pm\frac{1}{2} \mid \frac{1}{2} A_J J_\mp I_\pm \mid \pm\frac{3}{2}\rangle \langle \pm\frac{3}{2} \mid \frac{1}{2} A_J J_\pm J_\mp \mid \pm\frac{1}{2}\rangle}{W_Z - W_Y} \qquad (102)$$

which gives

$$\{2A_J^2/(W_Z - W_Y)\}\, I_+ I_- \qquad \text{for the } Z^+ \text{ state}$$

and

$$\{2A_J^2/(W_Z - W_Y)\}\, I_- I_+ \qquad \text{for the } Z^- \text{ state} \qquad (103)$$

Since

$$I_+ I_- = I_x^2 + I_y^2 - i(I_x I_y - I_y I_x) = I_x^2 + I_y^2 + \hbar I_z$$

while

$$I_- I_+ = I_x^2 + I_y^2 - \hbar I_z \qquad (104)$$

we have contributions of two types, one of which has the same sign for each component of the doublet and the other which has the opposite sign.

For the first of these we can write

$$I_x^2 + I_y^2 = I(I+1) - I_z^2 = \frac{2}{3}I(I+1) - \{I_z^2 - \frac{1}{3}I\,(I+1)\} \qquad (105)$$

which, apart from a term in $I(I+1)$ which moves all levels up or down together, represents an additional term of the same form as the nuclear electric quadrupole interaction of magnitude

$$\Delta P_{\parallel} = -2A_J^2/(W_Z - W_Y) \qquad (106)$$

The other contribution, linear in I_z and of opposite sign for the two components of the electronic doublet, represents an additional term of the same form as the magnetic hyperfine interaction of magnitude

$$\Delta A_{\parallel} = 4A_J^2/(W_Z - W_Y) \qquad (107)$$

where the extra factor 2 appears because we relate it to an operator $\Delta A_{\parallel} S_z I_z$ whose value is $\pm\frac{1}{2} \Delta A_{\parallel} I_z$ for the two components of the electronic doublet.

The magnitude of these additional terms needs to be evaluated in interpreting precise hyperfine measurements to find nuclear moments; note also in comparing values for two isotopes that their presence complicates the analysis, in that the ratio of the magnetic hyperfine interactions is not equal to the ratio of the nuclear magnetic moments (apart from any real hyperfine anomaly), and similarly the ratio of the nuclear electric quadrupole interactions will not equal the ratio of the nuclear electric quadrupole moments, because of the additional terms which vary as A_J^2.

5. Pseudo Nuclear Zeeman Effect

In addition to terms quadratic in the hyperfine structure, which are usually rather small compared with the first order hyperfine interactions, there are cross terms involving products of electronic and hyperfine terms. One such term involves the electronic Zeeman interaction and the magnetic hyperfine interaction, and has the general form

$$\frac{\langle z|A_J(\mathbf{J}\cdot\mathbf{I})|y\rangle\langle y|g_J\beta(\mathbf{H}\cdot\mathbf{J})|z\rangle}{W_z - W_y} + \frac{\langle z|g_J\beta(\mathbf{H}\cdot\mathbf{J})|y\rangle\langle y|A_J(\mathbf{J}\cdot\mathbf{I})|z\rangle}{W_z - W_y}.$$

$$(108)$$

For the doublet $Z^{\pm}$ ($J_z = \pm 1/2$) the matrix elements are again those with the doublet $Y^{\pm}$, and can be evaluated as before. We obtain

$$\{2g_J\beta A_J/(W_Z-W_Y)\}\,\{(H_x \pm iH_y)\,I_{\mp} + I_{\pm}\,(H_x \mp iH_y)\}$$

$$= \{4g_J\beta A_J/(W_Z - W_Y)\}\,(H_x I_x + H_y I_y). \quad (109)$$

This represents a term whose form is that of an anisotropic nuclear Zeeman effect

$$-\beta\left(\Delta g_{\perp}^{(I)} H_x I_x + \Delta g_{\perp}^{(I)} H_y I_y\right) \tag{110}$$

which is present in addition to the true nuclear Zeeman interaction $-g_I\beta(\mathbf{H}\cdot\mathbf{I})$. If we incorporate the latter into the more general expression $-\beta(\mathbf{H}\cdot g^{(I)}\cdot\mathbf{I})$ we have in the present case

$$\left.\begin{aligned}g_x^{(I)} &= g_y^{(I)} = g_I - 4g_J\beta A_J/(W_Z - W_Y)\,, \\[2mm] g_z^{(I)} &= g_I \end{aligned}\right\} \,. \tag{111}$$

Since g_I is about $1/1000$ of g_J, the "pseudo-nuclear Zeeman effect" may easily outweigh the true nuclear Zeeman effect if the separation of the electronic doublets Z and Y is not too large.

IV. The Paramagnetic Resonance Spectrum

In the last sections we have indicated the form which the electronic Zeeman interaction, the hyperfine interactions and the nuclear Zeeman interaction take for a paramagnetic ion whose electronic ground state is a Kramers doublet. (In other cases such terms do not always suffice — see, for example, Appendix II.) In the presence of so many terms, and the complications caused by anisotropy, it is nòt possible to give a general treatment relating the spin Hamiltonian to the spectrum. Instead the discussion will be confined to some simple cases which illustrate the main features of the electron paramagnetic resonance spectrum. Since we shall be dealing only with the effective spin Hamiltonian, we can drop the tildas on S which were used above to distinguish the effective spin from the true spin; for simplicity of notation we also write g_x for g_{xx}, and similarly for other terms.

A.   The Electronic Zeeman Interaction

Electron paramagnetic resonance spectra are normally observed by working at constant frequency (with consequent simplification of the spectrometer) and varying the magnetic field. In most cases the field strength is such that the electronic Zeeman interaction energy is large compared with any hyperfine terms, and we therefore follow a perturbation approach in which the electronic Zeeman term in the Hamiltonian is considered first; i.e. we start with the single interaction

$$\mathcal{K} = \beta(g_x H_x S_x + g_y H_y S_y + g_z H_z S_z) \tag{112}$$

which is the form of the anisotropic Zeeman interaction when referred to the special axes (x, y, z) which constitute the principal axes. In the special case where H is applied along one of these principal axes, which for convenience we take to be the z-axis, the Hamiltonian reduces to

$$\mathcal{K} = g_z \beta H S_z \tag{113}$$

whose energy matrix is diagonal, the energy for the state whose magnetic quantum number M is equal to a particular value of S_z being

$$W_M = g_z \beta H M . \tag{114}$$

An oscillatory magnetic field is applied which acts on the magnetic dipole moment of the system; under suitable conditions of frequency and orientation it may induce transitions to other states with different values of M according to the selection rule $\Delta M = \pm 1$. For the transition $M \leftrightarrow (M-1)$ this requires a quantum of radio-fre-quency energy

$$h\nu = W_M - W_{M-1} = g_z \beta H .\qquad(115)$$

If there are only two electronic levels $(S = 1/2)$, only one transi-tion $(+1/2 \leftrightarrow -1/2)$ is possible; if more than two levels exist, and Eq. (112) is the only term in the Hamiltonian, the levels are equally separated in energy (cf. Fig. 2) and the allowed transitions between successive levels all coincide, corresponding to the fact that Eq. (115) is independent of M. A measurement of the fre-quency ν and the magnetic field H required for resonance gives the value of g_z.

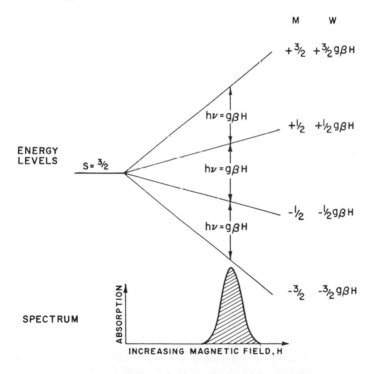

Fig. 2: Energy levels and spectrum of an ion for which S = 3/2 and the Hamiltonian contains only the electronic Zeeman interaction $\mathcal{H} = \beta(\mathbf{H} \cdot \mathbf{g} \cdot \mathbf{S})$. The energy levels are equal-ly spaced and the allowed transitions $M \leftrightarrow (M-1)$ coincide at $h\nu = g\beta H$, where g is given by Eq. (118).

In the general case where the steady field H is applied in an arbitrary direction whose direction cosines are (ℓ, m, n) with respect to the principal axes of the Zeeman interaction, the latter becomes

$$\mathcal{K} = \beta H(\ell g_x S_x + m g_y S_y + n g_z S_z) \; . \tag{116}$$

This can be diagonalized by a suitable transformation (see Appendix I) to give

$$\mathcal{K} = g\beta H S_z' \tag{117}$$

where

$$g^2 = \ell^2 g_x^2 + m^2 g_y^2 + n^2 g_z^2 \; . \tag{118}$$

Equation (117) is similar in form to Eq. (113); the energy levels are given by

$$W_M = g\beta H M \; , \tag{119}$$

and all transitions allowed are of the type $M \leftrightarrow (M-1)$ and require a quantum

$$h\nu = g\beta H \; . \tag{120}$$

The spectrum is similar to that in Fig. 2, but the value of H required for resonance at a given frequency depends on its orientation relative to the principal axes. The value of g is found from the resonance value of $(h\nu/\beta H)$, and its variation with the orientation of H can be plotted out. The positions of the principal axes (if not already known from details of the crystal structure of the paramagnetic solid) can be found, together with the principal values g_x, g_y, g_z, which are sufficient to specify the anisotropic behaviour. Clearly a single crystal is needed if anisotropy is present, otherwise the spectrum will be smeared out over a range of field.

B.   Electronic "Fine Structure" Terms

In the absence of an external magnetic field the Zeeman interaction (112) is zero and all levels would have the same energy. In practice higher order effects of the ligand interaction and the spin-orbit coupling may produce a ground state in which the levels are not exactly degenerate in zero magnetic field, except in the special case of a Kramers doublet. When such zero-field splittings are present the levels will no longer be equally spaced in an external magnetic field, so that the various magnetic resonance transitions no longer coincide and a series of lines is observed.

This may be called a "fine structure" (though it has nothing to do with the fine structure in ordinary atomic spectra), and it produces complications which will not be discussed here since our primary concern is with hyperfine structure. In the limit of an external magnetic field strength such that the Zeeman interaction $g\beta H$ is large compared with any zero-field splitting, the strongly allowed transitions are still of the type $M \leftrightarrow (M-1)$, giving a spectrum of $2S$ transitions between pairs of the $(2S+1)$ levels whose values of M differ by unity. The intensity of the various lines varies according to the rule that for the transition $M \leftrightarrow (M-1)$ the intensity is proportional to

$$\langle M-1|S_-|M\rangle^2 = (S+M)(S-M+1) . \qquad (121)$$

This is illustrated by the special case shown in Fig. 3. In the

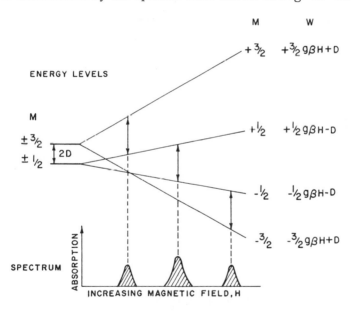

Fig. 3: Energy levels and spectrum of an ion for which $S = 3/2$ and the spin Hamiltonian is $\mathcal{H} = \beta(\mathbf{H} \cdot g \cdot \mathbf{S}) + D\{S_z^2 - \tfrac{1}{3}S(S+1)\}$. The diagram is drawn for the special case where H is along the z-axis. For other directions the levels do not vary linearly with H, but when g is isotropic and $g\beta H \gg D$, the energy levels vary approximately as $W = g\beta HM + \tfrac{1}{2} D(3\cos^2 \theta - 1)\{M^2 - \tfrac{1}{3}S(S+1)\}$ when H is at an angle θ to the z-axis.

limit of a strong magnetic field the spectrum is centered on the point $h\nu = g\beta H$ determined by Eqs. (118 and 120), but even when g is isotropic the separation between the various lines in the spectrum is a function of the orientation of the magnetic field characteristic of the interaction causing the zero-field splitting. This variation in the splitting gives information about the nature of the interaction, and the characteristic variation in intensity of the different lines makes it possible to differentiate easily between splittings due to such purely electronic effects and those due to hyperfine structure (see below).

C. The Hyperfine Spectrum

We now consider briefly the spectrum of an ion with an electronic doublet ground state (S = 1/2) and a hyperfine Hamiltonian

$$\mathcal{K} = (S \cdot A \cdot I) + (I \cdot P \cdot I) - \beta(H \cdot g^{(I)} \cdot I) . \tag{122}$$

We assume that where anisotropy is present the principal axes of all these terms coincide with those of the electronic Zeeman term (112); this is generally true when the hyperfine interaction is due to the nucleus of the paramagnetic ion itself, (but not usually when it is due to the nucleus of a ligand ion). In a typical case the strength of the interactions are roughly $A \sim 10^{-2}$ cm^{-1}; $P \sim 10^{-3}$ cm^{-1} or less; nuclear Zeeman term $\sim 10^{-4}$ cm^{-1}. All these terms are small compared with the electronic Zeeman interaction (~ 1 cm^{-1}), which is therefore diagonalized first. Normally, we cannot then diagonalize all the hyperfine terms, and we approximate using first order perturbation theory. For the first term in (122), the magnetic hyperfine interaction, this requires the retention of all terms involving S_z'; by a suitable transformation of the nuclear coordinates (see Appendix I) these terms assume the simple form

$$A S_z' I_z' \tag{123}$$

where A is given by the formula

$$g^2 A^2 = \ell^2 g_x^2 A_x^2 + m^2 g_y^2 A_y^2 + n^2 g_z^2 A_z^2 . \tag{124}$$

The energy of the state (M, m), where m is the nuclear magnetic quantum number, is (in first order)

$$W = g\beta HM + AMm . \tag{125}$$

The strongly allowed transitions are again those in which $\Delta M = \pm 1$, but since the oscillatory magnetic field has only a weak interaction with the comparatively small nuclear magnetic moment, we have the selection rule $\Delta m = 0$. Thus, for the strong transition (M, m) $\leftrightarrow$ (M-1, m) we require a quantum of energy

$$hv = g\beta H + Am \ .\tag{126}$$

At ordinary temperatures where $A \ll kT$, the population of all nuclear states is equal, so that we have one hyperfine line for each value of m, giving $(2I+1)$ lines in all, equally spaced in our approximation. When the experiment is carried out at constant frequency and variable magnetic field H, the energy levels and allowed transitions are as shown in Fig. 4.

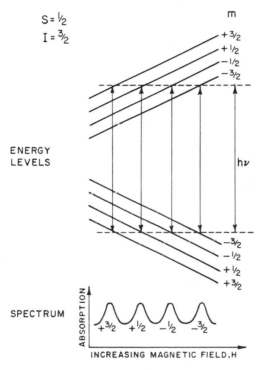

Fig. 4: Energy levels and spectrum of an ion for which $S = 1/2$, $I = 3/2$ and the spin Hamiltonian is $\mathcal{H} = \beta(\mathbf{H \cdot g \cdot S}) + (\mathbf{S \cdot A \cdot I})$. The hyperfine levels are equally spaced when $g\beta H \gg A$, giving four equally spaced hyperfine transitions of equal intensity, according to the selection rule $\Delta m = 0$.

The physical significance of this result is that the electron is subjected to a magnetic field, set up by the nuclear magnetic moment, which is small compared with the external field H but which has a steady component H_N parallel to H, so that the resonence condition becomes

$$h\nu = g\beta(H + H_N) \tag{127}$$

or

$$H = (h\nu/g\beta) - H_N . \tag{128}$$

There are $(2I+1)$ equally probable values of $H_N = (Am/g\beta)$, equally spaced from $+(AI/g\beta)$ to $-(AI/g\beta)$, so that the electron resonance line is centered on $H = (h\nu/g\beta)$ but split into $(2I+1)$ lines of equal intensity.

The formulae given above should be regarded as part of a series expansion where the next term is of order $(A^2/g\beta H)$ in energy. When this term is included, the hyperfine lines are not quite equally spaced, and other transitions are weakly allowed in which $\Delta m = \pm 1$, whose intensity is smaller than those of the main hyperfine lines by a factor of order $(A/g\beta H)^2$.

D. The Quadrupole and Nuclear Zeeman Terms

As pointed out above, these terms are generally small compared with the magnetic hyperfine energy A, and in a first approximation we retain only those parts of these interactions which contain I_z and are thus diagonal in the nuclear co-ordinate system used to give Eq. (123). The terms which remain in this approximation are of the form

$$P\{I_z'^2 - \tfrac{1}{3}I(I+1)\} - G_I I_z' \tag{129}$$

where it can be shown that

$$g^2 A^2 P = \frac{3}{2} (\ell^2 g_x^2 A_x^2 P_x + m^2 g_y^2 A_y^2 P_y + n^2 g_z^2 A_z^2 P_z) \tag{130}$$

and

$$gAG_I = \beta H(\ell^2 g_x A_x g_x^{(I)} + m^2 g_y A_y^{(I)} + n^2 g_z A_z g_z^{(I)}) , \tag{131}$$

where g is given by Eq. (118) and A by Eq. (124).

The two terms in Eq. (129) involve only I_z' and not S_z'. Hence in the strongly allowed transitions of the type $(M, m) \leftrightarrow (M-1, m)$ in which S_z' changes but I_z' does not, the quantum of energy required is independent of P and G_I because the transition is between two nuclear levels which are equally displaced in the same direction by the quadrupole and nuclear Zeeman interactions. Thus in the first approximation the spectrum is again a set of equally spaced lines whose separation is determined by A; it follows that values of P and G_I cannot be determined from such a spectrum.

Since the energy levels are displaced by the terms in Eq. (129) by amounts proportional to m^2 and m, transitions in which the nuclear quantum number m changes ($\Delta m \neq 0$) are displaced in first order. Such transitions are weakly allowed through second order effects; these arise both from the magnetic hyperfine interaction, giving weak transitions of relative intensity $(A/g\beta H)^2$ as mentioned above, or from the terms neglected above in the quadrupole interaction, which give different weak transitions of relative intensity $(P/A)^2$. Such transitions have been observed and measured in a few cases (see for example, experiments on Cu^{2+} by Bleaney and associates, 1955); the analysis is complicated and high accuracy is difficult to obtain. There are also second order displacements in the energy levels of order (P^2/A) which shift the transitions slightly.

E. Main Features of Electron Paramagnetic Resonance

(1) Spectrometer sensitivity is high — under favourable circumstances as few as 10^{11} ions will give a detectable signal, though in most cases the concentrations used are rather higher by a few orders of magnitude.

(2) Single crystals are almost invariably needed because of anisotropy in the spectrum.

(3) Spectrometers are commonly operated at low temperatures to avoid broadening of the resonance lines through interaction with the thermal lattice vibrations ("spin-lattice relaxation"). Higher sensitivity is also thereby obtained because the intensity is proportional to the difference of population between the lower and upper levels between which a transition is being observed.

(4) Magnetically dilute substances are used to minimize broadening through interactions with other magnetic ions ("spin-spin interaction").

(5) Though an appreciable amount of nuclear information has been obtained from electron paramagnetic resonance in the past (e. g. values of nuclear spin I from the number of hyperfine lines = 2I+1), nuclear moments can be estimated from hyperfine interactions with only limited accuracy because of complications in theoretical analysis and lack of precision in electronic wavefunctions. Electron paramagnetic resonance has developed primarily into a tool for investigation of effects in the solid state, in which additional information is provided by hyperfine structure; for example the latter can identify the nucleus (or nuclei) with which magnetic electrons interact, and give the strength of the interaction.

(6) Precision measurements of hyperfine interactions are made whenever possible by means of ENDOR, in which the excitation of the weak,(almost) purely nuclear transitions of the type $\Delta M = 0$, $\Delta m = \pm 1$ is detected through the consequent changes in the intensity of the much stronger electronic transitions discussed above ($\Delta M = \pm 1$, $\Delta m = 0$). Such changes are observable when the populations of the energy levels involved are disturbed from the normal thermal equilibrium values through the application of strong radio-frequency driving power.

Observation of ENDOR signals gives direct measurement of the separations of the nuclear levels, and hence of the hyperfine interactions (including the electric quadrupole and nuclear Zeeman interactions). In favourable cases ENDOR measurements can be made with a precision of the order of kc/sec rather than the Mc/sec typical of electron paramagnetic resonance. *

Appendix I

DERIVATION OF FORMULAE USED IN SECTION IV

In the previous section we have quoted formulae without deriving them, in order to give a simple discussion of the paramagnetic resonance spectrum under conditions most often encountered in practice. The formulae can be derived in various ways, one method being outlined in this Appendix.

The Hamiltonian from which we start is the same as in Sec. IV and can be written in the convenient notation

$$\mathcal{H} = \beta(\mathbf{H} \cdot g \cdot \mathbf{S}) + (\mathbf{S} \cdot A \cdot \mathbf{I}) + (\mathbf{I} \cdot P \cdot \mathbf{I}) - \beta(\mathbf{H} \cdot g^{(I)} \cdot \mathbf{I}) \, . \qquad (A.1)$$

We shall assume that all the anisotropic quantities have the same principal axes, and that the first term in (A.1), the electronic Zeeman term, is much larger than any of the following (hyperfine) terms. This is the strong field case, analogous to the Back-Goudsmit region in optical hyperfine spectroscopy. The electronic term is then considered first and diagonalized exactly. The hyperfine terms cannot then in general be diagonalized exactly, but are treated by a method equivalent to first order perturbation theory, the perturbations being introduced in descending order of magnitude.

*ENDOR is discussed in Chap. 6 by S. Geschwind.

In considering the electronic Zeeman term we shall also indicate how the transition probabilities may be calculated.

A.   The Electron Zeeman Interaction and Transition Probability

We consider first the Zeeman interaction of a paramagnetic ion with an external magnetic field, starting with the case of no anisotropy. If the direction cosines of the external field H are (l, m, n) with respect to an arbitrary set of axes (x, y, z), the Hamiltonian is

$$\mathcal{H} = g\beta H(l S_x + m S_y + n S_z) \ . \tag{A.2}$$

By changing to a new set of axes (x_e, y_e, z_e) where the z_e axis is parallel to H, the Hamiltonian reduces to

$$\mathcal{H} = g\beta H \, S_z' \tag{A.3}$$

which corresponds to a set of $(2S+1)$ levels equally spaced in energy by $g\beta H$.

If an oscillatory magnetic field is now applied, linearly polarized along a direction with direction cosines (l_1, m_1, n_1), its interaction with the magnetic dipole moment is

$$\mathcal{H}' = -(l_1 \mu_x + m_1 \mu_y + n_1 \mu_z) H_1 \cos \omega t$$

$$= -\tfrac{1}{2}(l_1 \mu_x + m_1 \mu_y + n_1 \mu_z) H_1 \{\exp(i\omega t) + \exp(-i\omega t)\} \ . \tag{A.4}$$

The transition probability between states i and j depends on the square of the matrix element of the dipole moment operator between these states:

$$\mu_{ij} = \langle \mu_j | l_1 \mu_x + m_1 \mu_y + n_1 \mu_z | \mu_i \rangle \tag{A.5}$$

and the dipole moment operator may be written as

$$\tfrac{1}{2}(l_1 - im_1)\mu_+ + \tfrac{1}{2}(l_1 + im_1)\mu_- + n_1 \mu_z \ . \tag{A.6}$$

If we assume at once that the steady magnetic field H is directed along the z-axis, the transition probabilities involve only the matrix elements of μ_+, μ_-. Here the quantities μ_+, μ_- are defined by

$$\mu_\pm = \mu_x \pm i\mu_y \ . \tag{A.7}$$

The square of the matrix element for the transition $S_z = M \leftrightarrow M-1$ is

$$|\mu_{M,M-1}|^2 = \tfrac{1}{4}(\ell_1^2 + m_1^2)\,\langle M-1|\mu_-|M\rangle^2$$

$$= \tfrac{1}{4}(\ell_1^2 + m_1^2)\,g^2\beta^2\,\langle M-1|S_-|M\rangle^2$$

$$= \tfrac{1}{4}g_1^2\,\beta^2\,\langle M-1|S_-|M\rangle^2 \tag{A.8}$$

where we have defined a quantity g_1 such that

$$g_1^2 = (\ell_1^2 + m_1^2)g^2\ . \tag{A.9}$$

The value of g_1 is clearly a maximum if H_1 is normal to H, when $(\ell_1^2 + m_1^2) = 1$ and $g_1 = g$.

When anisotropy is present, it is simplest to assume that the (x, y, z) axes are the principal axes of the g "tensor," so that Eq. (A.2) is replaced by

$$\mathcal{K} = \beta H(\ell g_x S_x + m g_y S_y + n g_z S_z)\ . \tag{A.10}$$

To find the energy levels, we can write out the energy matrix and diagonalize it. This is equivalent to changing to a new set of axes (x_e, y_e, z_e) in which only terms in S_z' occur, as in Eq. (A.3). Now we can write Eq. (A.9) in the form

$$\mathcal{K} = g\beta H\,(\ell' S_x + m' S_x + n' S_z) \tag{A.11}$$

where $g\ell' = g_x\ell$, etc. If we now make $(\ell'^2 + m'^2 + n'^2) = 1$, Eq. (A.11) is identical with Eq. (A.2) and is equivalent to that for an ion with spectroscopic splitting factor g in a field with direction cosines (ℓ', m', n'). The allowed transitions are those in which the component S_z changes by one unit, requiring a quantum of energy

$$h\nu = g\beta H \tag{A.12}$$

where the value of g^2 follows from the normalization condition on the apparent direction cosines (ℓ', m', n')

$$g^2 = g^2(1'^2 + m'^2 + n'^2) = g_x^2\ell^2 + g_y^2 m^2 + g_z^2 n^2\ . \tag{A.13}$$

Although we have spoken above of changing to a new set of axes (x_e, y_e, z_e), only the direction of z_e is defined. Its direction cosines are (ℓ', m', n'), or $(g_x\ell/g, g_y m/g, g_z n/g)$. If there is no anisotropy, the direction cosines of z_e are simply (ℓ, m, n), so that z_e is parallel to the external field H in Eq. (A.2). When anisotropy is present, the direction of z_e coincides with that of H only when H is along one of the principal axes (x, y, z).

Evaluation of the transition probability is more complicated when anisotropy is present. Since normally $H >> H_1$, we must transform the oscillatory Hamiltonian to the set of axes (x_e, y_e, z_e) in which the static Hamiltonian is diagonal. The transition probabilities are again obtained from the square of the matrix elements $|\mu_{M,M-1}|^2$, and the selection rules are the same as for an ion with no anisotropy. A quantity g_1 can be defined which is more complicated than Eq. (A.9) since it contains both sets of direction cosines (ℓ, m, n) and (ℓ_1, m_1, n_1); i. e. it depends on the orientation of both H and H_1 with respect to the principal axes of anisotropy defined in the crystal. It can be shown that for maximum transition probability H_1 should again lie in the plane normal to H; but, because of the anisotropy, a specific orientation in this plane gives the optimum value. A detailed discussion for the special case of axial symmetry is given by Bleaney (1960), where the question of determination of the signs of the principal g-values is also discussed.

B. The Magnetic Hyperfine Term

If the electronic Zeeman interaction $\beta(\mathbf{H} \cdot g \cdot \mathbf{S})$ is the largest interaction, it must be diagonalized first; e. g. by a transformation to axes (x_e, y_e, z_e) as in the previous section for the components of **S**. When this new system of axes is introduced into the magnetic hyperfine term

$$\mathcal{H} = \mathbf{S} \cdot \mathbf{A} \cdot \mathbf{I} \tag{A.14}$$

the resultant will be in general a sum of products containing all combinations of the components of I and S'. Those containing S_x', S_y' are off-diagonal and connect levels separated by the Zeeman energy; they can be treated by second order perturbation theory, giving energy displacements of order $(A^2/g\beta H)$. The term in S_z' is

$$S_z'(\ell' A_x I_x + m' A_y I_y + n' A_z I_z) =$$
$$S_z'(\ell g_x A_x I_x + m g_y A_y I_y + n g_z A_z I_z)/g \tag{A.15}$$

and must be treated differently, in a manner analogous to the electronic Zeeman energy. The coefficients of I_x, etc., can be regarded as a set of direction cosines, if suitably normalized; then by changing to a new set of axes (x_n, y_n, z_n) for the components of the vector I, the first order hyperfine energy term (A.15) can be reduced to the form

$$A S_z' I_z' \tag{A.16}$$

where the primes indicate that S_z' refers to the electronic co-ordinate system (x_e, y_e, z_e) and I_z' to the nuclear co-ordinate system (x_n, y_n, z_n). The normalization requirement gives

$$g^2 A^2 = \ell^2 g_x^2 A_x^2 + m^2 g_y^2 A_y^2 + n^2 g_z^2 A_z^2 \tag{A.17}$$

and the direction z_n then has the direction cosines $(\ell g_x A_x/gA, m g_y A_y/gA, n g_z A_z/gA)$. Hence z_n is not parallel to z_e unless A is isotropic (this rarely occurs unless g is also isotropic).

Note that, unlike the electronic Zeeman interaction, the magnetic hyperfine interaction has not been diagonalized completely since we still have terms containing S_x', S_y' which are equivalent physically to the interaction of the nuclear magnetic moment with precessing components of the electronic magnetic field at the nucleus. We have diagonalized only the first order term, equivalent to the interaction of the nuclear magnetic moment with the steady component of the electronic magnetic field.

C. The Quadrupole and Nuclear Zeeman Terms

When referred to the principal axes (x, y, z) the electric quadrupole interaction term (83) is (writing P_x for P_{xx}, etc.)

$$P_x I_x^2 + P_y I_y^2 + P_z I_z^2 \ . \tag{A.18}$$

It is convenient to take $P_x + P_y + P_z = 0$; if this is not already the case it can be made so by subtracting a constant quantity $\frac{1}{3}(P_x + P_y + P_z)(I_x^2 + I_y^2 + I_z^2) = \frac{1}{3}(P_x + P_y + P_z) I(I+1)$ which just moves all the energy levels up or down together and does not affect the transitions.

On the assumption that $P << A$, the quadrupole term must be transformed to the axes (x_n, y_n, z_n) defined in the previous section. This gives a term in $I_z'^2$ of magnitude

$$P_z' I_z'^2 = \{(\ell g_x A_x/gA)^2 P_x + (m g_y A_y/gA)^2 P_y +$$

$$(n g_z A_z/gA)^2 P_z\} I_z'^2 \tag{A.19}$$

together with terms in $I_x'^2$, $I_y'^2$ and cross terms. The diagonal terms are

$$P_z' I_z'^2 + \frac{1}{2}(P_x' + P_y')(I_x'^2 + I_y'^2) = \frac{1}{2} P_z'(2I_z'^2 - I_x'^2 - I_y'^2)$$

$$= \frac{3}{2} P_z' \{I_z'^2 - \frac{1}{3}I(I+1)\} \tag{A.20}$$

where we have used the fact that $P_x' + P_y' + P_z' = P_x + P_y + P_z = 0$

since the spur of the energy matrix is invariant. Combining Eqs. (A. 19) and (A. 20) we obtain for the diagonal part of the quadrupole interaction

$$P\{I_z'^2 - \tfrac{1}{3} I(I+1)\} \tag{A. 21}$$

where

$$g^2 A^2 P = \tfrac{3}{2} (\ell^2 g_x^2 A_x^2 P_x + m^2 g_y^2 A_y^2 P_y + n^2 g_z^2 A_z^2 P_z) . \tag{A. 22}$$

The generalized form of the nuclear Zeeman energy, including the pseudo-nuclear Zeeman effect mentioned in Sec. III. D. 5. is

$$-\beta(\mathbf{H} \cdot \mathbf{g}^{(I)} \cdot \mathbf{I}) = -\beta H \left(\ell g_x^{(I)} I_x + m g_y^{(I)} I_y + n g_z^{(I)} I_z \right) \tag{A. 23}$$

if the external magnetic field H is applied in the direction (ℓ, m, n). On transforming to the axes (x_n, y_n, z_n) this becomes

$$\beta H \left(\ell^2 g_x A_x g_x^{(I)} + m^2 g_y A_y g_y^{(I)} + n^2 g_z A_z g_z^{(I)} \right) I_z' (gA) \tag{A. 24}$$

together with terms in I_x', I_y' which are off-diagonal.

Appendix II

PARAMAGNETIC IONS IN CUBIC SYMMETRY

A. The Electronic Zeeman Interaction

For a paramagnetic ion subject to a ligand interaction of cubic symmetry the principal values of quantities such as g and A along the cubic axes (x, y, z) must obviously be equal; i. e.,

$$g_x = g_y = g_z \tag{A. 25}$$

and

$$A_x = A_y = A_z . \tag{A. 26}$$

Under these conditions the electronic Zeeman interaction and magnetic hyperfine interaction become simply

$$\mathcal{K} = g\beta(\mathbf{H} \cdot \mathbf{S}) + A(\mathbf{S} \cdot \mathbf{I}) \tag{A. 27}$$

which are identical with those for a free ion, so that the spectrum is independent of the direction of H relative to the cubic axes. However a free ion has full rotational symmetry; this is a higher symmetry than cubic and terms may appear in the latter case

which are ruled out in the former, as pointed out by Koster and
Statz (1959). An important example is the Γ_8 quartet of levels,
one of the degeneracies possible under cubic symmetry. If we
wish to represent the behaviour of this group of four levels by
means of a spin Hamiltonian with effective spin S = 3/2, it is
found that the electronic Zeeman interaction has the more complicated form

$$\mathcal{K} = g\beta(\mathbf{H}\cdot\mathbf{S}) + f\beta(H_x S_x^3 + H_y S_y^3 + H_z S_z^3) \qquad (A.28)$$

where f is an additional constant, The extra term clearly has
cubic symmetry in that the coefficients of the terms in x, y, z are
equal. Although the energy levels still diverge linearly with H,
the presence of the extra term in (A.28) means that they are no
longer equally spaced (as they are in Fig. 2), and the spacing
varies with the orientation of H with respect to the cubic axes
(x, y, z). The selection rules for magnetic resonance transitions
between the levels, and their intensities are also more complex
when the extra term is present (see, for example, Bleaney (1959),
where a specific example is given where f is of the same order
as g).

The terms in the effective spin Hamiltonian may be grouped
in different ways. For example, instead of a simple term in S_z^3
it may be more convenient to use the operator

$$S_z^3 - \tfrac{3}{5} S(S+1)S_z + \tfrac{1}{5} S_z \qquad (A.29)$$

which has the advantage that it vanishes for values of S < 3/2.
Then the Zeeman interaction takes the form

$$\mathcal{K} = g'\beta(\mathbf{H}\cdot\mathbf{S})$$
$$+ f\beta\left[H_x S_x^3 + H_y S_y^3 + H_z S_z^3 - \tfrac{1}{5}(\mathbf{H}\cdot\mathbf{S})\{3S(S+1) - 1\}\right].$$
$$(A.30)$$

B. Magnetic Hyperfine Interaction

The magnetic hyperfine interaction arises from the effect
on the electronic magnetic moment of the magnetic field of the
nucleus, and for a Γ_8 quartet we may expect additional terms
similar to those for the electronic Zeeman interaction. The
effective spin Hamiltonian in this case becomes

$$\mathcal{K} = A(\mathbf{S}\cdot\mathbf{I})$$
$$+ A'\left[S_x^3 I_x + S_y^3 I_y + S_z^3 I_z - \tfrac{1}{5}(\mathbf{S}\cdot\mathbf{I})\{3S(S+1) - 1\}\right].$$
$$(A.31)$$

C. Electric Quadrupole Interaction

For a doublet electronic state the quadrupole interaction has the form

$$\mathcal{H} = P_x I_x^2 + P_y I_y^2 + P_z I_z^2 \tag{A.32}$$

and since in cubic symmetry we must have $P_x = P_y = P_z$ this reduces to

$$\tfrac{1}{3}(P_x + P_y + P_z)(I_x^2 + I_y^2 + I_z^2) = \tfrac{1}{3}(P_x + P_y + P_z)I(I+1) \tag{A.33}$$

which is just a constant, or zero if $P_x + P_y + P_z = 0$. Obviously this is true also for manifolds of higher electronic multiplicity, and it is often assumed that the nuclear electric quadrupole interaction must vanish in the case of cubic symmetry. That this is not necessarily the case follows from the fact that a free ion, which has full rotational symmetry, can have a nuclear electric quadrupole interaction, provided that it has an electronic angular momentum of $J = 1$ or more. The interaction is then, of course, not of the type in Eq. (A.32) which does vanish in cubic symmetry, but of the type considered in Sec. II. Such an interaction has been shown to exist for ions in the $4f^7$ state (Eu^{2+}, Gd^{3+}, Tb^{4+}) in the solid (see, for example, Baker and Williams (1962)). These ions have a half-filled shell, where the ligand interaction has relatively little effect; in other cases where the ligand interaction is strong, electronic degeneracies of three or four, corresponding to effective spins of 1 or 3/2, may remain under conditions of cubic symmetry. A nuclear electric quadrupole interaction may then exist similar to that for a free ion, with the effective spin S taking the place of J, but with an important modification.

To discuss this modification, we take the quadrupole operator in the form given in Eq. (67). For a free ion the size of the interaction is determined by a single parameter, since the requirement of full rotational symmetry determines the relationship between the numerical coefficients of all the terms. For the more restricted case of cubic symmetry, invariance under the transformation $x \to y \to z$ requires that the first three terms in Eq. (67) must each have the same numerical coefficient, and similarly for the last three terms, since (for example)

$$\{3L_x^2 - L(L+1)\} \to \{3L_y^2 - L(L+1)\} \to \{3L_z^2 - L(L+1)\}$$

and

$$(L_x L_y + L_y L_x) \to (L_y L_z + L_z L_y) \to (L_z L_x + L_x L_z).$$

However the cubic transformation does not turn terms of the first set into terms of the second set, so that the coefficients of the two sets of terms are not necessarily related. For cubic symmetry the quadrupole interaction, in terms of the effective spin S, may therefore have the more general form

$$\mathcal{K} = -\frac{e^2 Q}{I(2I-1)} \langle r_q^{-3} \rangle \times$$

$$\times \begin{bmatrix} \frac{m}{6}\{3S_x^2 - S(S+1)\}\{3I_x^2 - I(I+1)\} \\[2mm] +\frac{m}{6}\{3S_y^2 - S(S+1)\}\{3I_y^2 - I(I+1)\} \\[2mm] +\frac{m}{6}\{3S_z^2 - S(S+1)\}\{3I_z^2 - I(I+1)\} \\[2mm] +\frac{3n}{4}(S_x S_y + S_y S_x)(I_x I_y + I_y I_x) \\[2mm] +\frac{3n}{4}(S_y S_z + S_z S_y)(I_y I_z + I_z I_y) \\[2mm] +\frac{3n}{4}(S_z S_x + S_x S_z)(I_z I_x + I_x I_z) \end{bmatrix}. \qquad (A.34)$$

where m is not necessarily equal to n.

Acknowledgement

The author wishes to thank Dr. N. J. Stone for his very considerable assistance and constructive suggestions for improving the content and presentation of this article.

References

Abragam, A. and Pryce, M. H. L. (1951). Proc. Roy. Soc. A205, 135; ibid, A206, 164 and 173.

Baker, J. M. and Bleaney, B. (1958). Proc. Roy. Soc. A245, 156.

Baker, J. M. and Williams, F. I. B. (1962). Proc. Roy. Soc. A267, 283.

Barnes, R. G., Mössbauer, R. L., Kankaleit, E., and Poindexter, J. M. (1964). Phys. Rev. 136, A175.

Bleaney, B. (1959). Proc. Phys. Soc. 73, 937 and 939.

Bleaney, B. (1960). Proc. Phys. Soc. 74, 621.

Bleaney, B. (1964). Proc. Third International Symp. on Quantum Electronics (Columbia University Press, New York).

Bleaney, B., Bowers, K. D., Ingram, D. J. E., Trenam, R. S., and Pryce, M. H. L. (1955). Proc. Roy. Soc. A228, 147, 157, and 166.

Edmonds, D. T. (1963). Phys. Rev. Letters 10, 129.

Elliott, R. J. and Stevens, K. W. H. (1953). Proc. Roy. Soc. A218, 553; ibid., A219, 387.

Evans, L., Sandars, P. G. H., and Woodgate, G. K. (1965). Proc. Roy. Soc. A289, 108 and 114.

Harvey, J. S. M. (1965). Proc. Roy. Soc. A285, 581.

Koster, G. F. and Statz, H. (1959). Phys. Rev. 113, 445; ibid., 115, 1568.

Lewis, H. R. and Sabisky, E. S., (1963). Phys. Rev. 130, 1370.

Sandars, P. G. H. and Beck, J. (1965). Proc. Roy. Soc. A289, 97.

Trees, R. E. (1953). Phys. Rev. 92, 308.

2. HARTREE-FOCK THEORY OF ELECTRIC AND MAGNETIC HYPERFINE INTERACTIONS IN ATOMS AND MAGNETIC COMPOUNDS

R.E. Watson
Brookhaven National Laboratory *
Upton, New York

A.J. Freeman
National Magnet Laboratory **
Massachusetts Institute of Technology
Cambridge, Massachusetts

Table of Contents

Supported by the U.S. Atomic Energy Commission.
**Supported by the U.S.A.F. Office of Scientific Research.*

I. Introduction

The rapid growth in recent years of interest in Hartree-
Fock theory may be attributed, in part to its well known successes
in predicting a wide array of experimental observables, in part
to the physically transparent nature of the one-electron approximation it employs and in part to the fact that it provides the most
rigorous solutions of the many-electron Schrödinger equation
available to date for systems with more than ten or twenty electrons.   Interest in transition metal and rare-earth hyperfine effects has necessarily centered on Hartree-Fock theory in order
to interpret experiments (and in order to understand the shortcomings of the theory in its various forms).   To date, accurate
Hartree-Fock solutions are available only for free atoms (and
small molecules) — a situation which has encouraged the practice
of using these free atom results to interpret experiments in
solids.   This practice as well as the predictions and properties
of Hartree-Fock theory were studied in an earlier review (Freeman
and Watson, 1965) and the inspection is extended and brought up
to date here.

In this chapter, we review some basic aspects of Hartree-
Fock theory, and the so-called unrestricted Hartree-Fock approximations, as related to magnetic and electric quadrupole
hyperfine interactions.   Emphasis will be on new developments
(i. e. those which have taken place since our earlier review) involving the various "unrestricted" Hartree-Fock approximations
and the experimental consequences of core polarization effects
(closed shell distortions) for both magnetic and electric hyperfine
fields.   We also discuss recent aspects of the theory of magnetic
hyperfine interactions in magnetic ionic compounds (transferred
hfs and "super-transferred" hfs).   Finally, the relevance of some
of these matters to hyperfine effects in metals will be briefly
noted.

II. Hartree-Fock Theory

Simple *Hartree* theory approximates the wave function of the many electron system by a product of one-electron spin-orbitals

$$\Psi_H(\mathbf{x}_1, \mathbf{x}_2 \cdots \mathbf{x}_N) = \varphi_1(\mathbf{x}_1)\varphi_2(\mathbf{x}_2) \cdots \varphi_N(\mathbf{x}_N) \tag{1}$$

where $\mathbf{x}_1$ denotes space and spin coordinates of the ith electron. The expectation value of the energy then becomes

$$E = \sum_i \int \varphi_i^*(\mathbf{x}_1) K_{op} \varphi_i(\mathbf{x}_1) d\tau_1 + \sum_{i<j} \int \int |\varphi_i(\mathbf{x}_1)|^2 |\varphi_j(\mathbf{x}_2)|^2 \, d\tau_1 \, d\tau_2. \tag{2}$$

The first term represents the one-electron part of the energy (kinetic energy and potential energy due to nuclear attraction), and the second term is the mutual interelectronic Coulomb repulsion of the electrons. In this model, each electron sees an average potential due to the charge density of the other electrons as is shown in Fig. (1a).

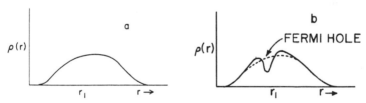

Fig. 1: Schematic of charge density as seen by an electron at $\mathbf{r}_1$. (For description and discussion see text).

The obvious shortcoming of the Hartree model is that the Pauli exclusion principle is not obeyed. Therefore one anti-symmetrises the Hartree product and arrives at the Hartree-Fock function, which can be written as a Slater determinant

$$A \, \Psi_H = \Psi_{HF} = \frac{1}{\sqrt{N}} \begin{vmatrix} \varphi_1(\mathbf{x}_1)\varphi_2(\mathbf{x}_1) \cdots \varphi_N(\mathbf{x}_1) \\ \varphi_1(\mathbf{x}_2)\varphi_2(\mathbf{x}_2) \cdots \varphi_N(\mathbf{x}_2) \\ \vdots \\ \varphi_1(\mathbf{x}_N)\varphi_2(\mathbf{x}_N) \cdots \varphi_N(\mathbf{x}_N) \end{vmatrix} \tag{3}$$

for which the Pauli exclusion principle is fulfilled.* If the φ_i, from which Ψ_{HF} is constructed, are not orthogonal, they can be orthogonalized, e. g. by the Schmidt process. This does not change the value of the determinant,** nor the matrix element of any physical operator calculated with this determinant. In general, any mixing of one occupied orbital, say φ_i, into any other occupied orbital, φ_i, similarly has no effect on the determinant nor on the expectation value of any operator evaluated with it. Only the mixing of an unoccupied orbital φ_i with an occupied φ_j (and vice versa) has any effect on physical predictions.†

With Ψ_{HF} constructed from orthogonal φ_i, the Hartree-Fock energy adds an additional term to the Hartree energy (Eq. (2)), namely the so-called exchange energy,

$$-\sum_{i<j}\sum \delta(m_{s_i},m_{s_j}) \int \int \varphi_i^*(1)\varphi_j^*(2)\frac{1}{r_{12}} \varphi_i(2)\varphi_j(1)d\tau_1 d\tau_2 \quad (4)$$

where the minus sign is associated with the antisymmetry of Ψ_{HF} and the delta function is included to remind us that the integrations are actually over spin as well as space leading to non-zero exchange interactions between spin orbitals having common spin. Since the self-energy (i = j) Coulomb and exchange terms are equal but have opposite sign, we may rewrite the combined Coulomb and exchange interaction as

$$\frac{1}{2}\sum_i\sum_j \int \int \varphi_i^*(1)\varphi_j^*(2)\frac{1-P_{12}}{r_{12}} \varphi_i(1)\varphi_j(2) \, d\tau_1 d\tau_2 \quad (5)$$

---

*This can be seen by setting either a pair of coordinates (rows) or a pair of φ (columns) equal, in which case Ψ_{HF} becomes zero valued.

**Adding a constant times one column (or row) to another column (or row) makes a zero contribution to the determinant's value.

†We mention this because one is frequently involved with theories of a perturbed many-electron system (as described in Chap. 9) in which an observable perturbation is occasionally attributed to mixing among only occupied (or only unoccupied) φ. This is a wrong result, usually due to incorrectly accounting for all terms of a given order in perturbation theory.

where the permutation operation P_{12} interchanges coordinates 1 and 2 on its right. The exchange terms, acting on φ_j, can be written as an effective potential

$$V_{exch}(1)\varphi_j(1) = -\sum_i \int \varphi_i^*(2) \frac{P_{12}}{r_{12}} \varphi_i(2)\varphi_j(1)d\tau_2 \quad, \tag{6}$$

$$V_{exch}(1) \equiv -\left\{ \sum_i \frac{\int \varphi_i^*(2)(1/r_{12})\varphi_i(1)\varphi_j(2)d\tau_2}{|\varphi_j(1)|^2} \right\}\varphi_j^*(1) \tag{7}$$

which can be associated with an effective charge density

$$\rho_{exch} = \frac{-\sum_i \delta(m_{s_i}, m_{s_j})\,\varphi_j^*(1)\varphi_i^*(2)\varphi_i(1)\varphi_j(2)}{|\varphi_j(1)|^2} \tag{8}$$

This density has three properties of interest: (i) Integration over coordinates 1 yields unity, i.e. a total of one electron charge is associated with it. (ii) This "charge" is associated with electrons having the same spin as φ_j. (iii) Setting $r_1 = r_2$

$$\rho_{exch} = -\sum_i \delta(m_{s_i}, m_{s_j})|\varphi_i(1)|^2 \tag{9}$$

or in other words, minus the total density of orbitals of spin common to φ_j.

The combined Coulomb* plus exchange density is plotted in Fig. 1b, the exchange term contributing an exchange or Fermi "hole" — the manifestation of electrons of like spin staying away from position r_1 where the jth electron is located. This correlation, in coordinates, of electrons of like spin is entirely due to the exclusion principle; its range is generally small compared with an overall atomic charge distribution. The non-zero density at the position of electron j reflects the fact that there is no such correlation between electrons of antiparallel spin. The repulsive interelectronic $1/r_{12}$ interaction induces further correlation effects, which are quite outside the Hartree-Fock description, and which contribute a further correlation hole to the density of Fig. 1b. The exchange hole, by its existence, provides some of the necessary interelectronic correlation between like spins, but, by providing nothing between antiparallel spins, it makes an *imbalance* in spins in its partial introduction of a correlation type hole. When considering spin or exchange polarization, as we will shortly, there then arises the question of the role played by such
Here this includes the self Coulomb term.

such an imbalance in the results.*

Traditional Hartree-Fock theory, as embodied in the bulk of existing calculations, imposes four restrictions on the spin orbitals (for a fuller discussion see Freeman and Watson, 1965): (i) The spin orbitals are constrained to be a product of a space function times a spin function,

$$\varphi_i(\mathbf{x}) = \psi_i(\mathbf{r})\chi_i(\sigma) \tag{10}$$

implying a fixed spin, independent of spatial coordinates.** (ii) For atoms, the $\psi(\mathbf{r})$ are restrained to be separable into a radial and angular part

$$\psi(\mathbf{r}) = R_{n\ell}(r)Y_{\ell m}(\theta, \varphi) \equiv 1/r\, P_{ne}(r)\, Y_{\ell m}(\theta, \varphi) \tag{11}$$

where the n and ℓ are the principle quantum numbers of the atomic shell in question (the extension to a molecule or solid is obvious here and below). (iii) The $R_{n\ell}$ are independent of m_ℓ quantum number within an $n\ell$ shell. (iv) The $R_{n\ell}$ are independent of m_s quantum number within an $n\ell$ shell.

Restraints (ii) and (iii) effectively assume a spherically symmetric potential, and (iv) assumes no significant net spin in the system. Relaxing one or several of these constraints leads to an "unrestricted" Hartree-Fock theory. For example, the exchange or spin polarized Hartree-Fock formalism for systems with a net spin, which is simply a relaxation of restriction (iv), allows orbitals of spin parallel (say up) and antiparallel (down) to the net spin to differ in their spatial behavior, thereby responding to the fact that all up spin electrons have an exchange interaction with the electrons contribution to the net spin, while those of down spin do not.

*Schrieffer and co-workers, for example, have been recently arguing that the criteria for the occurrence of local moments in metals developed by Anderson, Clogston, and Wolff are not complete since they are Hartree-Fock treatments of exchange effects which largely ignore correlation.

**The Overhauser (1961) spin density waves in metals are an example of abandoning this restraint. They are also an example of the possible dangers of employing Hartree-Fock theory since they can be formally shown to exist for a Hartree-Fock electron gas but seem to disappear when correlation effects are accounted for (Hammon and Overhauser, 1966).

One virtue of the free ion restricted HF functions is that they are eigenfunctions of the spin (S^2) and orbit (L^2) operators which commute with the Hamiltonian. By relaxing a restraint one produces a UHF function which, in general loses this symmetry. As discussed in an earlier review (Freeman and Watson, 1965), there is considerable controversy as to the implications of this loss of symmetry and what, if anything, should be done about it, within, and outside of, the Hartree-Fock picture. While considerable new thinking has gone on, no consensus has been reached and we will not review matters here.

It is wise to worry about symmetry *and* correlation problems simultaneously, both in themselves and when attempting to learn what can and should be asked of Hartree-Fock theory. Since many-electron treatments rapidly become formidable as the number of electrons increase, results have been largely limited to the special three-electron case of Li. Employment of modern perturbation theory, for example the application of Bethe-Goldstone theory by Nesbet (1966), promises to extend the size of the systems studied. * It is not obvious that it will be computationally practicable in the near future to work with systems the size of P (the outstanding case where s electron exchange polarization appears in trouble) much less with the transition and rare-earth ions. Therefore, not only is the one-electron picture of Hartree-Fock theory intuitively transparent, but we will very likely be constrained to employ some version or minor extension of it for these metal ions for some time to come.

III. Core Polarization and the Exchange Polarized Hartree-Fock Approximation

A. Description of Exchange Polarization Effects

Given the Hartree-Fock restrictions just discussed, spherical half-filled shell S state ions such as $N(2p^3)$, $P(3p^3)$, $Mn^{2+}(3d^5)$, and $Eu^{2+}(4f^7)$ would have zero valued magnetic hyperfine interactions whereas, in fact, they have quite large ones. The lighter ions remain effectively spherical, ** the hyperfine interaction

*See also the work of Szasz (1960-1962), Sinanoglu (1961), and Kelley (1963).

**Heavy ions such as Eu may suffer distortions from spin-orbit coupling which contribute to the hyperfine interaction — a matter discussed by Bleaney in Chap. 1 and by Sandars and Dodsworth in Chap. 4. These terms are relatively small for the rare earths.

arising from a contact interaction involving a net electronic spin density at the nucleus. The existence of this "core polarization" effect is well established experimentally.

In the first theoretical investigation of this effect Fermi and Segré (1933) employed configuration interaction techniques to estimate the effect of exchange in producing a contact term in the closed 6s shell of Tl. This was, in effect, a Hartree-Fock estimate of the difference in spin ↑ and spin ↓ spatial character induced by exchange in the 6s shell. Since then there has been a continuing and growing body of work, employing perturbation, configuration interaction and Hartree-Fock calculations. Two efforts in this body of work require mention.

First, Sternheimer (1952) pointed out that the induced contact terms are liable to be of the same order of magnitude for all the s shells of an ion; hence all shells must be accounted for. Secondly, in a series of important papers Abragam and Pryce (1951) systematically studied the role of core polarization in the hyperfine interactions of iron series ions in salts where near cubic environments largely wash out orbital and spin dipolar terms. With this work, the importance of core polarization to solid state as well as atomic hyperfine effects became apparent.

The lowest order description of core polarization has already been indicated, namely, Hartree-Fock theory with the fourth restriction dropped. The result of such an exchange polarized Hartree-Fock (EPHF) calculation is to produce a spin density

$$\sum_{n\ell} \left\{ |\psi_{n\ell\uparrow}(\mathbf{r})|^2 - |\psi_{n\ell\downarrow}(\mathbf{r})|^2 \right\}$$

in the closed electron shells of the atom. Such a spin density, induced in the closed 2s and 4s shells of neutral Fe, is seen in Fig. 2. The integrated spin densities are, of necessity, zero and the nodes are associated with the noded character of the shells. The electron with spin parallel to that of the open $3d^6$ shell (spin ↑) is attracted into the 3d region (the 2s outward, the 4s inward), the regions outside then having antiparallel spin. (The exchange polarized spin density at an atomic nucleus of an open p, d, or f shell atom is therefore almost inevitably antiparallel that of the open shell.) In producing this spin behavior, the exchange interaction is acting like an attractive interaction (note the minus sign of Eq. (4)). It is actually a reduction in the excess repulsion, due to lack of correlation, in the Hartree potential.

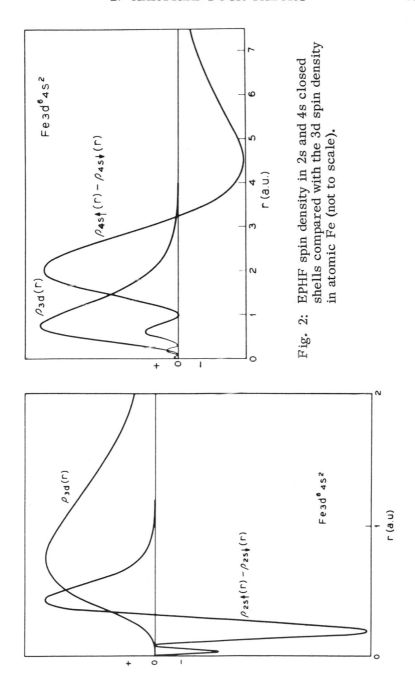

Fig. 2: EPHF spin density in 2s and 4s closed shells compared with the 3d spin density in atomic Fe (not to scale).

This becomes obvious if one notes that exchange and correlation holes have dimensions which are small with respect to atomic size.

Another important example of this attraction is seen in Fig. 3 where the spin density predicted for the closed shells of $Gd^{3+}(4f^7)$ is plotted. The open 4f shell is inside the closed 5s and 5p shells of the ion leading to a negative spin density in the outer reaches of the ion as well as at the nucleus (Watson and Freeman, 1961a). Very similar spin density behavior will be seen in Chap. 9.

As is well known, this core polarized spin density results in a net spin density at the nucleus for each closed s shell, with the resulting hyperfine field H_c just the superposition of contributions from all the s electron shells, i.e.,

$$H_c = (8\pi/3) g\mu_0 S \sum_{ns} \left\{ |\psi(o)|^2_{ns\uparrow} - |\psi(o)|^2_{ns\downarrow} \right\} \tag{12}$$

where S is the total spin of the ion in question. In what follows we shall use as a convenient measure of the hyperfine interaction the field per unit spin (Abragam and Pryce, 1951)

$$\chi = 4\pi/2S \sum_{ns} \left\{ |\psi(o)|^2_{ns\uparrow} - |\psi(o)|^2_{ns\downarrow} \right\}$$

with χ given in atomic units (a.u.), H_c is found in gauss by using the conversion factor 1 a.u. $= 4.21 \times 10^4$ gauss times twice the spin of the ion.

Phosphorous is the one case where the unrestricted Hartree-Fock approach has predicted the wrong sign for the core polarization, as have configuration interaction calculations* (cf discussion by Moser in Chap. 3). It should be noted also that the observed sign of the core polarization is as annoying to analyses of Knight shifts in metals as it has been embarrassing to the theoretical calculations. This is because it has been standard practice to assume an essentially constant value for χ, across a row in the periodic table — a practice suggested by the original iron series ion results of Abragam et al. (1955) which we discuss below. The experimental sign for P and the assumption of a constant χ makes a variety of Knight shift data hard to rationalize.

---

*One important point does stand out for this case, viz., the polarization is small and so the absolute error is not large.

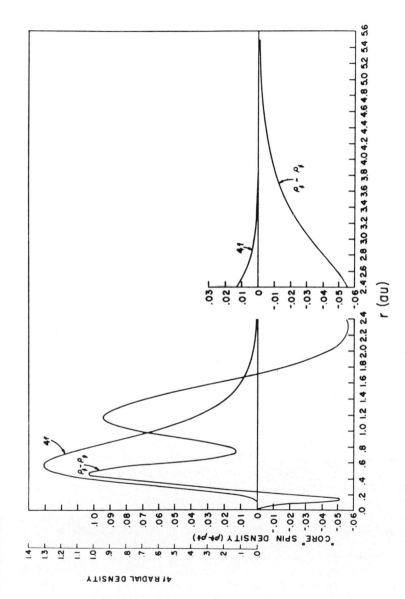

Fig. 3: Comparison of core closed shell EPHF spin density with 4f density in Gd^{3+}. Note change of scale to common scale in right side of figure.

B. Recent Developments: Comparison Between Theory and Experiment

At this point we would like to inspect some experimental and computational results which have become available since an earlier review (Freeman and Watson, 1965).

1. 3d Transition Metal Ions and Free Atoms

The exchange (or spin) polarized Hartree-Fock (EPHF) method has had perhaps its greatest success in accounting for the large negative hyperfine fields observed in the metals and ionic compounds of the 3d elements (Freeman and Watson, 1965). This has been remarkable in view of the fact that (1) the experimental data were taken on solids, while the calculations were done for free ions and (2) the EPHF method is known to be only approximate and the calculations rely on the numerical differencing of large numbers to yield a final result which is many times smaller.

Abragam et al. (1955) noted a crude experimental constancy for $\chi (\simeq -3$ au) for the divalent 3d ions. The minus sign indicates that the hyperfine field is found to be negative or antiparallel to the net (spin) magnetic moment on the ion. EPHF calculations (Watson and Freeman, 1961b) subsequently yielded consistent results but showed a distinct, though small, tendency for χ to increase in magnitude with increasing Z. On careful examination of more modern and more extensive experimental data, Locher and Geschwind (1963) observed that χ does increase with Z (by ~ 25 percent on going from the $3d^3$ to the $3d^8$ configuration). The EPHF indication of this trend before the fact represents one of the striking successes of the formalism to date.

Despite these successes for the divalent transition metal ions the EPHF calculations gave results for the neutral 3d atoms which appeared to be poor when compared with Abragam's and Pryce's values deduced from pre-World War II experiments. The more precise experimental data which have become available in recent years are shown in Fig. 4. These data, first collected and compared to experiment by Winkler (1966), provide us once again with a very remarkable success for the EPHF scheme rather than, as thought previously, a failure. As seen from the figure, not only the sign but also the magnitude and the trend along the iron series had been rather well predicted by the exchange polarized calculations. (Such good agreement in sign, magnitude and trend is very surprising because the calculated χ values are very small — the positive 4s contribution almost completely cancels the negative contribution from the inner 1s, 2s, and 3s shells — and so are very sensitive to any small errors.)

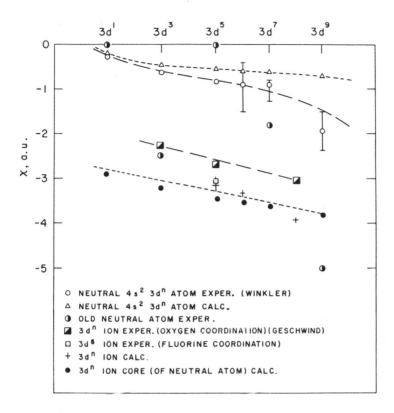

Fig. 4: Comparison of iron series EPHF results with experiment (see text).

Along with these neutral atom data, theoretical results for some divalent ions are also shown in Fig. 4 and compared with Geschwind's recently refined analyses of core polarization of these ions in salts. * These theoretical results consist of EPHF calculations for the divalent ions shown in Table A, augmented by the χ values for the core (1s, 2s, and 3s) electrons taken from the neutral atom calculations referred to above. As experimental data, we have plotted Geschwind's three points for ions in oxide environments and one for $3d^5$ ions in fluoride environments. Upon accounting for the tendency for covalency to reduce core polarization,**

*See discussion by S. Geschwind, Chap. 6.
**Crude subtraction of covalent effects lowers the experimental points to a level at, or slightly below, the computed values.

the calculations again appear in excellent agreement in both magnitude and trends with divalent ion experiment.

2. The 4d Ions

The agreement between experiment and EPHF theory for the 3d transition metals, which is beyond reasonable expectation, raises the obvious question as to how well the method does for heavier elements for which the more refined theories are not practicable. For this reason and in order to stimulate experiment, EPHF predictions for a series of 4d ion χ values have been obtained (Freeman et al., 1966; Bagus et al., 1967) and appear in Table I. The resulting χ's are again negative with a magnitude (equivalent to ~ 375 kG per unpaired electron) three times that seen for the 3d elements. The χ's are found to be more nearly constant with varying Z and degree of ionicity than are their 3d counterparts.

Table I: Core polarization hyperfine field per unit spin, χ, as predicted by EPHF calculations for various 4d ions.

Ion	χ (a. u.)	Ion	χ (a. u.)
Y^{2+} $(4d)^1$	-7. 96	Tc^{2+} $(4d)^5$	-8. 81
Zr^{2+} $(4d)^2$	-8. 42	Ru^{3+} $(4d)^5$	-8. 58
Nb^{2+} $(4a)^3$	-8. 60	Pd^{2+} $(4d)^8$	-8. 90
Nb^{3+} $(4d)^2$	-8. 36	Pd^{3+} $(4d)^7$	-8. 62
Mo^+ $(4d)^5$	-8. 75		

The net individual s-electron shell contributions to χ for a typical 4d ion, Mo^+, appear in Table II as do similar results for Mn which are shown for comparison. It is clear that the dominant Mo^+ contributions come from the 2s and 4s shells which are both negative. The negative 1s and positive 3s contributions are each very small; their algebraic sum is entirely negligible. For the divalent ion core of our 3d example, Mn, the 2s contribution is largest and negative, the 3s is positive and about 1/2 the 2s value and the 1s is negligibly small and negative Such results were previously understood in terms of the attractive nature of the exchange force and the position of the positive 3d spin density relative to the wave functions of the 1s, 2s, and 3s shells. The fact that the two dominant contributions to χ in the 4d ions are both of the same sign, unlike the 3d case, arises because of the different spatial relationship between the s electron wave functions and the different *parts* of the 4d wave function, which unlike the 3d orbital, is

Table II: Comparison of s-shell contributions to χ with d exchange and "overlap integrals" for Mn and Mo^+.

		χ (a. u.)	G^2 (d, ns)	$\int P_d P_{ns} dr$	r_{max}(a. u.)
Mn	1s shell	-0.03	0.003	0.024	0.04
	2s shell	-6.63	0.265	0.35	0.23
	3s shell	+3.23	0.802	0.87	0.75
	4s shell	+2.89	0.063	0.27	2.7
Mo^+	1s shell	-0.10	0.0008	-0.013	0.025
	2s shell	-2.10	0.035	-0.12	0.13
	3s shell	+0.67	0.020	+0.024	0.4
	4s shell	-7.21	0.249	+0.83	1.0

Mn: r_{max}(3d) = 0.80 $\qquad$ Mo^+ $\begin{cases} r_{max} \text{ (4d)} = 1.4 \\ r_{node} \text{ (4d)} = 0.5 \\ r_{max} \text{ (4d)} = 0.27 \end{cases}$

noded. As in the 3d case, the 1s and 2s contributions are negative (due to the inner loop of the 4d function), but the 3s contribution which remains positive (as expected) has been greatly reduced. For the 4d ions, the 4s contribution is *negative* and large, unlike what might be expected by comparison with the 3s shell of Mn. * Despite this difference the 4d, as well as the 3d, results appear consistent with the simple idea of exchange acting as an attractive force.

Our reasons for this assertion become clear upon inspection of Table II which gives the s-d exchange and overlap integrals and the radii at which the different s and d electrons have their (main) maxima. The Mn radii illustrate exchange acting as an attractive force, the radii inside (outside) r(3d) being associated with outward (inward) shifts of spin ↑ electrons into the region where the 3d shell is concentrated. The large 3d-3s overlap and exchange integral results in a reduced χ because of competing tendencies for expansion and contraction. The data for $Mo^+(4d^5, {}^6S)$ includes the position of the node of the 4d electron (r_{node}) and the value of the maximum of the inner loop of the 4d function. For the 1s and 2s electrons, the inner loop of the 4d function provides the attractive force for spin

*For the 3d neutral atoms, the 4s contribution is seen to be positive and large. While no neutral 4d atom calculations were performed, one expects, by extrapolation from the 4s behavior in the 3d case, that the 5s contribution will be large and positive.

up electrons thus leaving a net negative spin density at the origin. The 3s electron (with its $r_{max} = 0.4$) is "outside" the inner loop of the 4d function (with its $r_{max} = 0.27$) and so its spin up electron is attracted to a region closer to the nucleus thereby producing a net positive spin density at the nucleus; the outer loop of the 4d function ($r_{max} = 1.4$) has the opposite but weaker effect on the 3s electron thus accounting for the reduction in its contribution to χ relative to that seen for the case of Mn. Similarly, the 4s electron with spin up ($r_{max} = 1.0$) is attracted out toward the major part of the 4d function ($r_{max} = 1.4$) thus giving rise to its negative contribution to χ. The exchange and overlap integrals correlate well with this picture and the magnitude of the individual contributions to χ.

The divalent ion results of Table I show the same definite increase with Z, but only about half the percentage increase, shown by the 3d ions. This greater constancy is most certainly due to the fact that the dominant 2s and 4s contributions have the same sign. In this way the sensitive differencing problem, and hence the greater computational uncertainty obtained in the 3d ion results, is avoided here. Unlike the case of the 3d ions, we also see a strong tendency for χ to be independent of the degree of ionicity — at least for the +1, +2, and +3 ions.

One experimental 3d constancy (Locher and Geschwind, 1963) requires mention: in a given crystalline environment χ is independent of ionicity for a given $3d^n$ configuration (e. g. for V^{2+}, Cr^{3+}, and Mn^{4+} in six-fold oxygen coordination) and it is such *sets* of results which are plotted in Fig. 4. Now since χ is known to be sensitive to covalent effects and since there is considerable evidence of varying covalency for such sequences of ions (e. g., from g factors), the observation of this constancy implies that χ varies systematically for the free ion sequences. The 3d EPHF calculations have not yielded the appropriate variation.

Finally, it is interesting to compare the 4d results with experiment. Unfortunately, relatively little is known experimentally about χ in these ions. The electron spin resonance results compiled by Al'tshuler and Kozyrev (1964) for a variety of di- and trivalent 4d ions in salts can be crudely analyzed (Jones, 1966) to yield χ values which are 50 to 95 percent of the computed values. Covalent effects would, of course, cause a lowering of these experimental results. Since little is known of such effects one can at best, and pessimistically, say that the EPHF χ are within $\pm 30\%$ of experiment. Recently Low (1966) has reported a

χ for Mo^{5+} (4d) in $K_2 SnCl_6$ which is 30 percent *greater* than the results tabulated in Table I. The reasons for this result, and whether it is associated with the extreme degree of ionization are not known. The accuracy and trends of the results of Table I await further experimental investigation of the 4d salts. Such results will be invaluable, not only for the light they cast on theory, but because of the increasing interest in hyperfine effects in 4d metals and alloys.

One metal which has been investigated is pure Pd. Seitchik et al. (1964) determined that the field per unpaired spin equal -345 ± 10 kG/unpaired spin (a χ of -8.2 a.u.). This result is in very good (10 percent) agreement with the calculated results of Table I. This agreement is quite surprising in view of the complex experimental analysis involved (see Chap. 7), the uncertainties inherent in the EPHF method and arguments concerning hyperfine field contributions in the metal. One body of theory argues for substantial ($\sim$50 percent) hyperfine field contributions to arise from the s-like components of the conduction bands. Such arguments are difficult to verify or deny (see Chap. 9) and await further experimental and theoretical developments.

3. The 4f (Rare-Earth) Ions

Unlike the 3d or 4d ions, for which the orbital angular momentum is quenched, the dominant contributions to the hyperfine field at the nuclei of rare-earth ions in crystals arise from the angular momentum (spin and orbital) of the 4f electrons which are of the order of 10^6 to 10^7 gauss. Only in the ^{8}S state ions (Gd^{3+} and Eu^{2+}) is the core polarization field, H_c, dominant (and of the order of -350 to -300 kG). However, for the non-^{8}S state ions, the core polarization term is important when one is interested in studying the small changes induced in the measured hyperfine field by the environment. Since the core polarization field is relatively insensitive to environment, it can be treated as a constant (for a particular ion) and, provided some estimate can be made for its value, the environmental effects can be ascertained. A common practice, introduced by Bleaney and by Freeman and Watson, is to make the Abragam et al. (1955) assumption discussed earlier, i.e., to assume that χ is constant and hence that H_c is proportional to the spin on the ion. From the observed value of H_c for Eu^{2+} in CaF_2 one would estimate that $\chi \approx -1.1$ a.u., or that for any rare-earth ion

$$H_c \approx (-90 \text{ kG}) \times (g-1) J \tag{14}$$

where $(g-1)J$ is the projection of S along J. Because of the small relative magnitude of this term, it has not proved possible to confirm Eq. (14) experimentally and EPHF estimates become of interest. EPHF calculations for rare earth ions are limited to that of Watson and Freeman (1961) for Gd^{3+} (whose resulting spin density is plotted in Fig. 3), and more recent and more accurate results of Bagus et al. (1966) for Sm^{3+}, Gd^{3+}, Dy^{3+}, and Tm^{3+}. The calculations have yielded a fairly constant χ, suggesting that Eq. (14) is valid, with a value of ~ -1.2 a.u., which is in striking agreement* with the observed Eu^{2+} value of -1.1 a.u.

The observation of rare earth hyperfine effects in metals has been the object of increasing investigation** and a few comments are in order here. We have seen that rare earth core polarization effects are roughly one-third of their 3d counterparts, whereas orbital and spin dipolar hyperfine effects are roughly 50 percent larger.† Much discussion of the metals, as well as non-metals, has centered on these terms, but there are of course other contributions. Since the conduction bands at rare earth sites are of predominantly 5d and 6s character, both components will have associated core polarization effects (which we expect are smaller in magnitude than those induced by the 4f shell); the 6s will, of course, also interact directly with the nucleus via the contact interaction. Neutral atom calculations indicate that an unpaired 6s electron produces a hyperfine field of ~ 5 megagauss,†† a field of the order of the 4f orbital interaction, and roughly a factor five greater than that of its 4s (conduction) electron counterpart in iron series metals. The 6s field can be larger because it is sensitive to the outer atomic configuration; for example, the 6s field for the Gd^{2+} $4f^7$ 6s configuration approaches 20 megagauss. These observations suggest that s conduction electron fields in the rare earth metals are an order of magnitude more important, relative to core polarization, than those of the iron series metals. Experimentally something of this sort appears to be going on. As

---

Since these calculations are nonrelativistic one must question the role of relativistic effects in addition to the potential shortcomings of EPHF theory discussed earlier.
**See Budnick and Skalski, Chap. S.10.
† This is seen on inspection of the (r^{-3}) integrals tabulated in the Appendix of Freeman and Watson (1965).
†† This value is based on nonrelativistic functions; relativistic effects will increase the contribution.

discussed by Budnick and Skalski (Chap. S. 10) some Gd intermetallic compounds display Gd hyperfine fields close to the ion core polarization value while others do not. $GdFe_2$ (and other RFe_2 compounds) appears to have a +800 kG field associated with conduction bands. This result is readily rationalized if the 6s band character has an associated hyperfine field of the order of 5 or 10 megagauss per unpaired spin. Another possibly significant contribution to rare earth hyperfine fields in such compounds will be discussed toward the end of this chapter.

IV. Contributions of Closed Shells to Magnetic and Electric Hyperfine Interactions

Just as the closed shells make an important contribution to a hyperfine field via the Fermi contact part of the hyperfine interaction Hamiltonian, aspherical distortions of these shells leads to additional magnetic and electric quadrupole hyperfine contributions via the remaining terms in the Hamiltonian. We here describe the different physical origin of these contributions which has led to the use of different parameters, $\langle r^{-3} \rangle_{eff}$, to fit experimental data. * Most of the basic ideas are due to the well-known work of Sternheimer (1950-1966).

A. Electric Field Gradients and Quadrupole Interactions

For ions in solids, there are two sources of electric field gradients (EFG): (1) the EFG due to any external crystalline field, q_c, and (2) the EFG arising from any aspherical outer (or valence) shell electrons, q_v. The EFG actually seen by a nucleus is the sum of q_c and q_v and the EFG's associated with the distortions induced in the closed electron shells by the perturbing electrostatic fields. The total EFG may be written, in low order, as

$$q = q_c (1 - \gamma_\infty) + q_v (1 - R_q) \tag{15}$$

where γ_∞ and R_q are certain proportionality factors, called Sternheimer antishielding factors, which account for the contributions from the induced distortions. Calculations show $|R_q| < 0.2$, whereas $-7 > \gamma_\infty > -100$ (except for small ions which have only s electrons). **

See related descriptions in Chaps. 1, 3, 4.
**Strong overshielding effects can arise from the response of a metal's conduction electrons to a lattice field (Watson et al., 1965).*

1. External EFG's

Consider the case of a spherical ion, e. g. , Cl^- or Cu^+, in a lattice which gives rise to an EFG. The Hamiltonian one uses to describe the ion in this environment may be taken as $H = H_0 + H_1$ where H_0 is the free ion Hamiltonian whose solutions are assumed known and H_1 is some perturbing potential due to the rest of the lattice. In general, if the ions are far enough apart from each other, one uses the point charge multipole expansion between any two charges separated by a distance r_{12},

$$\frac{1}{r_{12}} = \sum_{\ell, m} \frac{4\pi}{2\ell + 1} \frac{r_<^\ell}{r_>^{\ell+1}} Y_\ell^m (\theta_1, \varphi_1) Y_\ell^{-m}(\theta_2, \varphi_2)$$

$$\equiv \sum_{\ell, m} \frac{r_<^\ell}{r_>^{\ell+1}} C_{\ell m} C_{\ell - m} \qquad (16)$$

(where $>$ and $<$ denote the greater or lesser of coordinate r_1 and r_2 respectively), to obtain H_1 from the sum of all such interactions. * For the EFG problem at hand, one retains only the quadrupole $(\ell = 2)$ term of H_1 and, if one assumes the external charges to be completely outside the ion considered, the form of the perturbing potential is then simply

$$V_2 = \text{Const. } r^2 P_2 (\cos \theta) = \frac{q}{2} r^2 P_2 (\cos \theta) \qquad (17)$$

Here the axis of quantization is defined as the principle axis of the external potential and the usual Legendre function notation has been followed.

The potential V_2 distorts the electron shells which then produce an EFG at the nucleus. In perturbation theory this is expressed as sums of terms

$$\langle gr | V_2 | ex \rangle \langle ex | \frac{2P_2 (\cos \theta)}{r^3} | gr \rangle \qquad (18)$$

where $| gr >$ and $| ex >$ denote ground and excited states which differ by a single orbital. A perturbation of $P_2 (\cos \theta)$ symmetry mixes orbitals which either have ℓ quantum numbers equal or which differ by ± 2. Thus, $s \rightarrow d$; $p \rightarrow p$ and f; $d \rightarrow s$, d and g, are allowed mixings. The contributions of terms with ℓ

*The second form of Eq. (16) is written in Bleaney's notation (see Chap. 1).

unchanged are called radial shielding because the distortion is of radial character of the orbitals, the angular character remaining unchanged; contributions from terms with differing ℓ are called angular shielding because the angular character is perturbed. This single orbital mixing is exactly equivalent to relaxing conventional Hartree-Fock restrictions and, in fact, can be estimated by unrestricted Hartree-Fock calculations where radical shielding is associated with relaxing the third restriction, (iii), and angular shielding the second, (ii). The two types of shielding tend to make contributions of opposite sign, with the radial terms enhancing (anti-shielding) and the angular terms generally shielding the interaction. Typical values of the computed results for γ_∞ are shown in Table III along with their experimental counterparts.

Table III: Theoretical and Experimental Values of γ_∞

Ion	Computed	Experimental
Cu^+	-17	-12 to -15
Cl^-	-55 to -90	-12 to -15
Rare-earths	~ -75	~ -75

We see that this antishielding may enhance an electric quadrupole interaction by better than an order of magnitude and thus is experimentally very significant. Some comments on these results are in order: (i) Agreement between computed and experimental values of γ_∞ for Cl^- (and other negative ions) is poor. Now, the largest contribution to γ_∞ comes almost entirely from the outermost shell (3p in Cl^-). In view of the large overlap between the negative ion and its neighbors, the disagreement with experiment is not a surprising result because the multipole expansion [Eq. (16)] and the associated assumption of the source being external to the ion are seen to break down. The outer part of the 3p shell should not be weighted by $r^2_<$ and taking this into account drastically reduces the estimated contribution from this shell. (ii) Since the outermost shell contributes so strongly (~ 90 percent of the total or 50 times the source EFG in Cl^-), one would expect the inner shells to feel, from self-consistency, a larger field from this, than from V_2 directly. For example, should one not expect the 2p radial contribution to be enhanced by this factor of 50? This is not the case, again because of overlap and the effect of the multipole $r^2_</r^3_>$ operator. The distorted 3p shell is weighted by r^{-3} when interacting with the nucleus; its *innermost* part is almost entirely responsible for the large gradient. When interacting with other electrons, this innermost part being *inside* the bulk of the ion's charge, is largely weighted by r^2, thus greatly reducing its ability to perturb the charge of the other electrons. In fact, self-consistent H-F calculations (Watson and Freeman, 1963) show an eight-fold increase in the 2p contribution for Cl⁻ (vs. the 50 "expected") and a two-fold increase in the 2p contribution for Cu⁺ (vs. the eight "expected" from the 3p or 3d shell's contribution to γ_∞). (iii) Large magnitudes of γ_∞ for the rare-earths so enhance the crystalline EFG that it becomes significant, relative to the strong EFG due to the open 4f shells. The analysis of the temperature dependence of electric quadrupole splittings by means of Mössbauer experiments has yielded values of the two shielding terms which agree well with theoretical results. *

2. Internal EFG's

Consider an ion with an open valence shell of electrons which produces an EFG at the nucleus. The valence shell interacts with the closed shells via a Coulomb field and the distorted closed shells then produce an additional EFG. This added EFG (expressed by the Steinheimer factor, R_q) is small for the same reason (ii) given above, namely, that the perturbing charge density overlaps the perturbed shells and is weighted by an $(r_<^2/r_>^3)$ factor. Calculations typically show $|R_q| \leq 0.2$ and to have either sign. The importance of R_q lies in the fact that while small it multiplies a large EFG (given by q_V). It is of particular interest when $q_C(1 - \gamma_\infty) \approx q_V(1 - R_q)$ as for certain rare-earth ions measured in salts at higher temperatures. Since q_V is proportional to the $\langle r^{-3} \rangle$ integral we may define an effective parameter

$$\langle r^{-3} \rangle_{eff, q} \equiv \langle r^{-3} \rangle (1 - R_q) \tag{19}$$

B. Closed Snell Distortions and Induced Magnetic Hyperfine Interactions

Closed shell distortions also contribute to the magnetic hyperfine interaction via both the orbital and the spin dipolar parts of the hyperfine Hamiltonian. ** These effects may be as much as 10 percent of the direct open shell contribution and lead to $\langle r^{-3} \rangle_{eff}$ values which are different for the orbital and spin dipolar terms and of course for the electric quadrupole $\langle r^{-3} \rangle_{eff, q}$ value considered above.

---

*See Mössbauer and Clauser, Chap. 11.
**See Bleaney, Chap. 1.

Unlike the case of electric quadrupole effects, Coulomb interactions alone (between the open and closed shells) will not lead to closed shell contributions to the magnetic $\langle r^{-3} \rangle_{eff}$ values. In the case of the spin dipolar term, not only must the closed shell be aspherically distorted (whether by Coulomb and/or exchange interactions), but pairs of orbitals differing in their m_s quantum number must have different spatial behavior. What is required is an imbalance in open shell exchange terms responsible for the distortion. Just as in the quadrupole case, all electrons contribute to the spin dipolar $\langle r^{-3} \rangle_{eff}$ values.

For the orbital $\mathbf{L} \cdot \mathbf{I}$ terms, however, Coulomb interactions treat a pair of orbitals with $+m_\ell$ and $-m_\ell$ identically because their charge density is independent of m_ℓ. Hence, the resulting contributions to this interaction term cancel identically. Exchange interactions, on the other hand, can be non-symmetric in treating $+m_\ell$ and $-m_\ell$ electrons, thus inducing non-zero closed shell $\mathbf{L} \cdot \mathbf{I}$ terms.

A requirement for an open valence shell to induce a closed shell contribution to a particular $\langle r^{-3} \rangle_{eff}$, is that the valence shell electrons already contribute a hyperfine interaction of that type. This is trivially obvious for the quadrupole case and only slightly less so, for the magnetic orbital and spin dipolar terms. The situation differs markedly with core s-shell exchange polarization, which is induced by any valence shell with net spin, whether or not it has an associated contact term. Another important property of $\langle r^{-3} \rangle_{eff}$ shielding is the tendency for distortions *within* the open valence shell to be as or more important, than those of closed shells, in causing $\langle r^{-3} \rangle_{eff}$ values to differ from restricted Hartree-Fock integrals.

Calculations of these terms are relatively limited. An m_ℓ plus m_s UHF calculation for Fe^{2+} (Freeman and Watson, 1963), for example, yielded

$$\langle r^{-3} \rangle_{eff, q} = 4.93 \text{ a.u.}$$
$$\langle r^{-3} \rangle_{eff, SD} = 4.55$$
$$\langle r^{-3} \rangle_{eff, LI} = 4.59$$

which are to be compared with the restricted HF $\langle r^{-3} \rangle$ of 5.08 a.u. Having relaxed only restrictions (iii) and (iv) implies that radial but *not* angular shielding was accounted for here. The missing angular terms will further (and significantly) perturb the result. Experimentally, Harvey (1965) has obtained a ten percent difference in the spin dipolar and orbital $\langle r^{-3} \rangle_{eff}$ of atomic O and F and recently Woodgate (1966) has seen a one percent difference in the same parameters for Sm. Since the two magnetic hyperfine interactions were acting simultaneously, the above experimental $\langle r^{-3} \rangle_{eff}$ values are obtained from fits assuming common $\langle r^{-3} \rangle_{eff}$ behavior in several levels. While we believe that the assumption is well justified, one must be alert to the fact that it has been made.

C.   Rare-Earth and Transition Series $\langle r^{-3} \rangle_{eff}$ Behavior as Inferred from LS Coupling

Uncertainties in our knowledge of nuclear magnetic moments (nmm's) are responsible for the current uncertainties in experimental determinations of the effective magnetic fields at the nuclei of rare-earth ions. Direct measurements of the nmm would obviously eliminate these difficulties, but to date this has been done for relatively few nuclei. In general, most of the rare-earth nmm data are still based on estimates of 4f shell hyperfine field behavior, and, in particular, on the $4f\langle r^{-3} \rangle$ (or $\langle r^{-3} \rangle_{eff}$) value associated with the (dominant) orbital contribution to the hyperfine field. Obviously, theoretical computations of this quantity represent potential sources of error in the estimated moments.

Traditionally, spin-orbit coupling parameters, ζ_{4f}'s, have been utilized to estimate values of $\langle r^{-3} \rangle$ — a procedure which assumes, however, a relationship between the two quantities, an assumption which is justified when the ion potential, $V(r)$, is taken to be Coulombic. Analytic expressions for $\langle r^{-3} \rangle$, based on optical spin-orbit measurements and a modified hydrogenic relationship for the quantities $\langle r^{-3} \rangle$ and ζ, have been worked out by Elliott and Stevens (1953a and 1953b), Bleaney (1955) and others, and a good deal of useful work and valuable information has resulted from these early efforts. More recently, Judd and Lindgren (1961) and Lindgren (1962) have used a modified hydrogenic function to match experimental spin-orbit coupling measurements. From this they determined $\langle r^{-3} \rangle$ values and, hence, nuclear magnetic moments (nmm's). Lindgren has refined and extended this procedure to yield a set of predicted nmm's for the entire rare-earth series.

These efforts have been criticized on a number of grounds (Freeman and Watson, 1965; Blume et al., 1964), several of which will become apparent from the discussion which follows.

We are concerned with this problem here because even with non-relativistic Hartree-Fock estimates (Freeman and Watson, 1962) of the $\langle r^{-3} \rangle$ integrals there remains the question of how these differ from the exact $\langle r^{-3} \rangle_{eff}$ values. Bleaney (cf Chap. 1) has discussed some aspects of the current state of theoretical vs. experimental $\langle r^{-3} \rangle_{eff}$ values and we shall return to this problem shortly. Our major interest concerns the suggestion by Judd (1963) that one can infer detailed information about $\langle r^{-3} \rangle_{eff, LI}$ behavior from studies of the contribution of closed shell distortions to observed spin-orbit parameters. *

Judd was struck by the fact that just as the restricted Hartree-Fock $\langle r^{-3} \rangle$ values overestimate the observed $\langle r^{-3} \rangle_{eff, LI}$ values, the spin-orbit coupling parameters determined from H-F wave functions as the expectation value of the familiar and commonly used one-electron operator

$$V'_{so} = \frac{\alpha^2}{2} \frac{1}{r} \frac{\partial V}{\partial r} \, \boldsymbol{\mathit{l}} \cdot \mathbf{s} \tag{20}$$

are also overestimated. Here V is the ion's direct Coulomb (i.e., Hartree) potential. Now, Eq. (20) may be approximately written as

$$V'_{so} \sim \frac{\alpha^2}{2} \frac{Z_{eff}}{r^3} \, \boldsymbol{\mathit{l}} \cdot \mathbf{s} \tag{21}$$

with Z_{eff} some appropriately chosen constant and α the fine structure constant. Judd emphasized the similarity of (21) to the orbital hyperfine operator, $\boldsymbol{\mathit{l}} \cdot \mathbf{I}/r^3$, and by comparing computed spin-orbit parameters with experiment he estimated the shielding appropriate to $\langle r^{-3} \rangle_{eff, LI}$ for the rare-earths.

Unfortunately, as emphasized by Blume and Watson (1962; 1963) the spin-orbit operator is not of the simple form given by Eq. (20) but is more exactly given by

$$V_{so} = \frac{\alpha^2}{2} Z \sum_i \frac{1}{r_i^3} \, \boldsymbol{\mathit{l}}_i \cdot \mathbf{s}_i - \frac{\alpha^2}{2} \sum_{i \pm j} \frac{(\mathbf{r}_{ij} \times \mathbf{p}_i)}{r^3_{ij}} \cdot (\mathbf{s}_i + 2\mathbf{s}_j) \tag{22}$$

The distortion of the outer closed 5s and 5p shells of the rare-earth ions appears to introduce a significant modification of the electrostatic interaction of an open 4f shell with the ion's external environment. While interesting, this is outside the province of this volume. See Watson and Freeman (1967) for a recent discussion and references.

Since V_{so} is a *two-electron operator*, its expectation value computed with a H-F determinantal function will contain direct Coulomb terms, as in Eq. (20), but also inter-electronic exchange, and certain valence electron-valence electron, terms.

Experimental and computed values of the many-electron spin-orbit parameter λ, appropriate to $\lambda \mathbf{L} \cdot \mathbf{S}$, are compared for 3d ions in Table IV. The experimental values are compared with the full result, λ_{HF} (including exchange and two-electron effects), obtained with Eq. (22) and with the traditionally employed expression, Eq. (20) (both equations being evaluated with the same Hartree-Fock wave functions).

Table IV: Calculated and experimental values of the spin-orbit parameter λ (in cm^{-1}) for some 3d ions.

Ion	Sc^{2+}	V^{2+}	Cr^{2+}	Cr^{3+}	Fe^{2+}	Co^{2+}	Ni^{2+}	Cu^{2+}
Configuration	$3d^1$	$3d^3$	$3d^4$	$3d^3$	$3d^6$	$3d^7$	$3d^8$	$3d^9$
$\lambda[(1/r)(\partial V/\partial r)]$	107	73	73	114	-123	-206	-382	-933
λ_{HF}	85.7	57	59	91	-114	-189	-343	-830
λ_{exp}	79	56	54 to 61	88 to 97	-94 to -109	-166 to -186	-303 to -340	-829

The λ_{HF} values, which are in good agreement with the experimental ranges, suggest that theory may be one or a few percent high. More accurate experimental fits are needed here.* The spin orbit comparisons in turn imply that the 3d ion restricted HF integrals, $\langle r^{-3} \rangle_{RHF}$, are but one, or a few, percent larger than the $\langle r^{-3} \rangle_{eff, LI}$ values appropriate to orbital hyperfine experiments. The extent of the agreement between restricted Hartree-Fock theory and experiment for spin-orbit and, by implication, orbital hyperfine effects, is surprising. It is important to note that $\lambda[(1/r)(\partial V/\partial r)]$ results for the 3d ions are significantly larger in magnitude than their more exact Hartree-Fock counterparts (λ_{HF}).

These would require careful accounting of two-electron effects which are important in the 3d series (Blume and Watson, 1963) and which, to our knowledge, have yet to be included in the fits for these ions.

Table V: Comparison of calculated and experimental values of the
spin-orbit coupling parameter (in cm^{-1}) for some 4f ions.

	Pr^{3+}	Nd^{3+}	Sm^{3+}	Tb^{3+}	Dy^{3+}	Ho^{3+}	Er^{3+}	Tm^{3+}	Yb^{3+}
$\zeta[(1/r)(\partial V/\partial r)]$	981	1138	1432	2097	2323	2572	2837	3109	3423
ζ_{HF}		878	1024	1342	1915	2182	2360	2610	2866	3161
Experimental ζ	$\begin{cases}750\\780\end{cases}$	900	$\begin{cases}1180\\1200\end{cases}$	$\begin{cases}1620\\1700\end{cases}$	$\begin{cases}1800\\1900\end{cases}$	$\begin{cases}2080\\2160\end{cases}$	$\begin{cases}2450\\2470\end{cases}$	$\begin{cases}2570\\2750\end{cases}$	$\begin{cases}2950\\3400\end{cases}$

The same behavior is seen for the rare earths in Table V
where, following custom, we inspect the one-electron parameters*
ζ appropriate to $\zeta \boldsymbol{l} \cdot \mathbf{s}$. (The ranges of experimental values reflect
various worker's opinions rather than any assessment of experi-
mental uncertainities.) Here the true Hartree-Fock parameters,
ζ_{HF}, are 10 ± 5 percent larger than experiment, lying approximately half-way between the $(1/r) \partial V/\partial r$ results and experiment.
While the effect of exchange, causing ζ_{HF} to be less than
$\zeta[(1/r)(\partial V/\partial r)]$, was known, the rare-earth ζ_{HF} were not available
when Judd (1963) estimated shielding and so he   employed the
$\zeta[(1/r)(\partial V/\partial r)]$ values. As a result, half of his estimated shielding was, in reality, spin-orbit exchange and it becomes useful to
revise his estimate.

Now the ζ_{HF} values were computed with non-relativistic
Hartree-Fock functions and it is our opinion that a large fraction
of the remaining disagreement with experiment is due indirectly
to relativistic mass effects. A comparison of relativistic and non-
relativistic Hartree-Fock-Slater atomic calculations, indicates
that inner shells undergo a relativistic contraction. This increases
the shielding of the nuclear charge as seen by d and f shells, and
causes them to expand resulting in f shell $\langle r^{-3} \rangle$ values which decrease by five or ten percent in the process. For either indirect
relativistic effects or Sternheimer shielding *within* the 4f shell,
one would expect

$$R_{LI} = R_{SO} \tag{23}$$

where

$$\langle r^{-3} \rangle_{eff, LI} \equiv \langle r^{-3} \rangle_{RHF} (1 - R_{LI}) \tag{24}$$

and

*This is a cruder measure of spin-orbit coupling than λ since
certain two-electron effects are omitted of necessity
(Blume et al., 1964).*

$$\zeta_{exper.} \equiv \zeta_{HF}(1 - R_{SO}) . \tag{25}$$

Alternatively if one ascribes the effects to p shell distortions, as was done by Judd, one would employ

$$R_{LI} = R_{SO} Z_{4f} / Z_p \tag{26}$$

where the Z's are the 4f and p shell values appropriate to Eq. (21). The Z_{4f} values can be obtained by comparing computed ζ_{HF} and $\langle r^{-3} \rangle_{HF}$ while the Z_p is crudely but adequately given by the nuclear charge minus two (Blume and Watson, 1963). Estimates of $\langle r^{-3} \rangle_{eff, LI}$ obtained with the results of Table V and Eqs. (23) and (26) are given in Table VI. With the exception of Woodgate's (1966) Sm result, the experimental values quoted here are crude, the worst values (which are extrapolations and interpolations) are given in parenthesis. No clear picture emerges from the table and what agreement there is, is at best crude. There is a suggestion that p shell effects are more important for the lighter elements and 4f shell effects for the heavier. The data for Sm, a light ion and the case of relatively high experimental accuracy, suggest that 4f effects dominate. We believe that comparisons such as this will eventually supply valuable insight into the $\langle r^{-3} \rangle_{eff, LI}$ shielding (and hopefully in turn for the other $\langle r^{-3} \rangle_{eff}$ for various sequences of ions). Unfortunately, these require far better experimental spin-orbit and hyperfine data than is available to date.

Table VI: Comparison of $\langle r^{-3} \rangle_{eff, LI}$ values (in a. u.).

	Pr^{3+}	Nd^{3+}	Sm^{3+}	Tb^{3+}	Dy^{3+}	Ho^{3+}	Er^{3+}	Tm^{3+}	Yb^{3+}
$\langle r^{-3} \rangle_{eff, LI}$ invoking 4f effects (Eq. 23)	4. 7 ±. 1	5. 3	6. 5	8. 3 ±. 2	8. 75 ±. 15	9. 9	11. 3 ±. 1	12. 0 ±. 4	12. 75 ±. 15
$\langle r^{-3} \rangle_{eff, LI}$ assuming p shell shielding (Eq. 26)	5. 0 ±. 1	5. 6	6. 9	8. 9 ±. 2	9. 45 ±. 15	10. 4	11. 5 ±. 1	12. 25 ±. 25	13. 15 ±. 1
experimental $\langle r^{-3} \rangle_{eff, LI}$	(5. 0)	5. 6	6. 38	8. 4 ±. 2	10. 4 ±. 2	10. 6	10. 9	11. 7 ±. 1	12. 8 ±. 3
$\langle r^{-3} \rangle_{HF}$	5. 4	6. 0	7. 4	9. 6	10. 3	11. 2	12. 0	12. 9	13. 8

V. Hyperfine Interactions in Magnetic Compounds

The measurement of magnetic hyperfine interactions has become a most useful source of information concerning the electronic properties of magnetic compounds involving transition and rare earth ions. Of particular interest in recent years has been the investigation of the role of covalency (or "chemical bonding") in determining observed optical and magnetic properties. One reason for this is the hope that such studies may lead to a deeper understanding of the superexchange coupling essential to the anti-ferromagnetism in these systems. Since, as we shall see, the measurement of both the metal ion hyperfine interaction and the transferred hyperfine interactions (i.e., the induced hyperfine field at the nucleus of a normally nonmagnetic ion like F^-), involve covalency in a direct and important way, we shall describe briefly the way in which the theory of metal complexes describes these experiments and how useful information has been gained for transition metal ions but not for the rare earth ions.

In much of the experimental work considered, the metal ion is an iron series element with an open shell of 3d electrons and sits in site of high symmetry, often octahedral. In most of the theoretical work done to data one considers a cluster, consisting of the metal ion surrounded by the first nearest neighbor shells of ions, or ligands. In this so-called ligand field theory approach, originated by Van Vleck (1932; 1939) the mixing between the 3d orbitals and the electrons of (say) the F^- ion (2p, 2s, and 1s) is taken into account. This mixing was shown by Van Vleck to contribute to the optical crystal field splitting parameter, 10 Dq, and by subsequent authors to other parameters such as spin-orbit coupling. In the following, we first describe the effect arising from the overlap of neighboring ions and then inspect the way covalency, or bonding, effects are introduced in order to properly account for electron transfer. These mechanisms perturb the system's charge and spin densities and in turn affect the hyperfine fields at the metal and neighboring non-metal sites. After considering these we will inspect the effect of overlap and covalency on the hyperfine fields induced at one metal ion site by the other metal ions, a case of considerable current interest since it is important to the analysis of NMR spinwave studies in these compounds.

A. Overlap, Covalency, and their Role in Metal Ion and Transferred Hyperfine Interactions

The concepts of overlap and covalency follow directly from the model one uses to describe a transition metal or rare-earth salt — namely, a Hartree-Fock description of the solid constructed from free ion (or from essentially free ion) wave functions. Given "free ion" one-electron orbitals, $\psi_{n,\,i_n}$ [where n denotes the ion site, and i_n an orbital at that site], one constructs a familiar many-electron Slater determinant Ψ which gives the proper antisymmetry of the many-electron function.

1. Overlap Effects

Consider the implications of such a construct for a simple cluster in which the metal ion has a single open shell orbital, φ, occupied with, say, spin $\uparrow$ and the neighboring closed shell ions, fixed in an octahedral array, have an occupied pair of "molecular orbitals," $\chi_\uparrow$ and $\chi_\downarrow$ of the same spatial symmetry* as $\varphi_\uparrow$, i. e. , we have

$$\varphi_\uparrow \; ; \; \chi_\uparrow \; ; \; \chi_\downarrow \; .$$

Having been inserted into the determinant Ψ, any mixing of the two occupied orbitals, say $\varphi_\uparrow$ and $\chi_\uparrow$ between themselves has no effect on the value of Ψ, and hence on any observable obtained with it (see Sec. II). This follows mathematically for any pair of occupied orbitals from the properties of a determinant and physically from the antisymmetry. Since the $\varphi_\uparrow$ and $\chi_\uparrow$ are orbitals appropriate to the free ions, they will in general not be orthogonal, but will have an overlap integral $S \neq 0$ between them. One can Schmidt orthogonalize these orbitals obtaining the set:

$$(1 - S^2)^{-\frac{1}{2}} \, [\varphi_\downarrow - S \chi_\uparrow] \; ; \; \chi_\uparrow \; ; \; \chi_\uparrow \tag{27}$$

without affecting the value of Ψ. [The $(1 - S^2)^{-\frac{1}{2}}$ is a normalization constant.] Whether one orthogonalizes them ($\varphi_\uparrow$ to $\chi_\uparrow$ as done here, or vice versa) or simply constructs Ψ from $\varphi_\uparrow$, $\chi_\uparrow$, and $\chi_\downarrow$ and then accounts for nonorthogonality when evaluating Ψ, one obtains for the system's charge density $|\Psi|^2$, an "overlap" term, $\Delta\rho_{ov\uparrow}(\mathbf{r})$, in addition to a simple superposition of the original free ion densities. To second order in S,

$$\Delta\rho_{ov\uparrow}(\mathbf{r}) = S^2 \left[|\varphi_\uparrow(\mathbf{r})|^2 + |\chi_\uparrow(\mathbf{r})|^2 \right]$$

$$- S \left[\varphi_\uparrow^*(\mathbf{r}) \, \chi_\uparrow(\mathbf{r}) + \varphi_\uparrow(\mathbf{r}) \chi_\uparrow^*(\mathbf{r}) \right] \; . \tag{28}$$

Note that this density is associated with spin $\uparrow$ electrons; spin orthogonality keeps $\chi_\downarrow$ from being involved.

*Here χ may be viewed as some appropriate linear combination of the ligand wave functions (LCAO's).

2. Covalent Effects

While the mixing of occupied orbitals with one another has no effect on Ψ, and in turn on any predicted observable, any mixing of *unoccupied* orbital character into an occupied orbital does. The obvious mixing is between the empty $\varphi_\downarrow$ and the occupied $\chi_\downarrow$ giving us instead of Eq. (27) the set of orbitals:

$$(1-S^2)^{-\frac{1}{2}} [\varphi_\uparrow - S\chi_\uparrow] \; ; \; \chi_\uparrow \; ;$$

$$(1+2S\gamma + \gamma^2)^{-\frac{1}{2}} [\chi_\downarrow + \gamma\varphi_\downarrow] \; . \tag{29}$$

This mixing corresponds to letting the neighboring, or ligand, ion spin $\downarrow$ electron spend time in the spin $\downarrow$ hole on the metal ion site; γ is the weighting or "covalent" mixing factor.

This "covalent" mixing will occur to the extent that it stabilizes the energy of the many-electron system. One can estimate the mixing and associated "bonding" energy in terms of the above occupied "bonding" orbital or equivalently in terms of the energy increase and mixing in the unitarily related hole state. (For example, in the cases of $Cu^{2+}3d^9$ and $Tm^{2+}4f^{13}$ with their single valence shell holes, the latter procedure is more convenient.) The covalent mixing contributes additional terms to the charge density of the system and gives, to second order in γ and S, the contribution

$$\Delta\rho_{c\downarrow}(\mathbf{r}) = \gamma^2 \left[|\varphi_\downarrow(\mathbf{r})|^2 - |\chi_\downarrow(\mathbf{r})|^2 \right]$$

$$- \gamma \left[\varphi_\downarrow^*(\mathbf{r})\chi_\downarrow(\mathbf{r}) + \varphi_\downarrow(\mathbf{r})\chi_\downarrow^*(\mathbf{r}) - 2S|\chi_\downarrow(\mathbf{r})|^2 \right] . \tag{30}$$

The first line shows explicitly the shift of charge off the ligands, onto the metal.

One adds $\Delta\rho_{c\downarrow}(\mathbf{r})$ to $\Delta\rho_{ov\uparrow}(\mathbf{r})$ when one wants to obtain the charge density, but *subtracts* it (because of its spin $\downarrow$ character) when estimating the system's spin density. The interplay of covalent and overlap effects is indicated in Fig. 5. Here the spin and charge densities are plotted along a metal-ligand internuclear line for a Ni^{2+} 3d orbital and a neighboring F^- 2p appropriate to $KNiF_3$ as a function of γ/S for a fixed spin density distribution at the ligand site. Two facts are to be seen by inspecting either the figure or Eqs. (28) and (30). First, overlap and covalent mixing act *cooperatively* in producing a spin density change at the ligand sites and a charge shift at the metal site, but act *destructively*

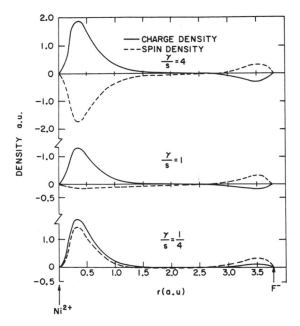

Fig. 5: Overlap plus covalent charge (solid curve) and spin
(dashed) densities plotted along a metal-ligand nuclear
line as a function of γ/S (see text).

for the charge change at the ligand site and spin shift at the metal.
Secondly, *overlap and covalent effects convey a spin density
onto ligand sites whose spin direction is parallel to that
of the local metal moment.* (Weaker covalent effects such as
the promotion of local moment electrons out onto empty neighboring ion shells (e.g., into the 3s of F^-) also preserve this sign
sense.) This sign prediction is one of the keys in interpreting
experimental data, as we shall see shortly.

So far, for illustration purposes, we have considered simple
mixing between a single 3d function and a single shell on the ligand
ion (using as example F^-) to obtain the results given as Eqs. (28)
and (30).

In the actual case of Ni^{2+} surrounded by F^- ions, there will
be overlap and covalent spin density effects involving the 1s, 2s,
and 2p shells of the ligand ions each of which contributes to the
hyperfine effects at ligand and metal sites. The s shells, of
course, interact with the F nuclei via the contact interaction and the
2p spin dipolar terms (the local symmetry in $KNiF_3$ leads to zero

valued orbital terms). With several such shells, one must be alert to cross terms, here in particular between χ_{2s} and χ_{1s}, terms such as $S_{2s}S_{1s}\chi_{2s}\chi_{1s}$ in the overlap density ρ_{ov}. Too often these are left out of the analyses of the experimental data because, as is well known, $S_{1s} < S_{2s}$; Freeman and Watson (1961) and Marshall and Stuart (1961) pointed out that while this is certainly true, $\chi_{1s}(o)$ is an order of magnitude greater than $\chi_{2s}(o)$ thus making the cross product term appreciable (some 30 percent of the direct $S^2_{2s}|\chi_{2s}(o)|^2$ contact term hyperfine contribution), and *negative* (because of the different phases of the s functions). This simple example points out the need for considering, and including, *all* terms arising from the determinantal nature of the many electron wave function.

3. Contributions to the Metal Ion Hyperfine Interaction

The results plotted in Fig. 5 allow us to discuss the difficulties involved in trying to predict, or to analyse, experimental data relevant to the hyperfine interaction on the metal ion site. From Eqs. (28) and (30) it is clear that the change in spin density, of purely φ_{3d} character has the form

$$\sum_i \sum_j (S_i^2 - \gamma_i^2)\varphi_j^2 \tag{31}$$

where the i sum is over ligand χ_i with symmetry common to a particular φ_j and the j sum is over unpaired occupied 3d orbitals (or holes), φ_j.

The competing signs of the overlap and covalent terms make it difficult to predict accurately the resulting net spin. There is a buildup of spin in the interior of the ion if $S > \gamma$, whereas there is a reduction if $\gamma > S$. As discussed at length in Sec. III, the hyperfine field at the metal ion's nucleus arises almost entirely from core polarization and seems to scale linearly with 3d spin. Experimentally, one finds that H_{eff} decreases with increasing "covalency." Unfortunately, not only do theoretical calculations*

*The discussion of these ab initio calculations lies outside the domain of this chapter. The traditional approaches employing free atom wave functions (for φ and χ) have been found to be inadequate (Sugano and Shulman, 1963; Watson and Freeman, 1964; Simanek and Sroubek, 1964; Ellis et al., 1965; Hubbard et al., 1966). Improvements have proceeded in two directions: (a) molecular orbital H-F calculations which aim at the best single determinant self-consistent-field solutions of the H-F equations (Ellis et al., 1967) and (b) limited configuration interaction Heitler-London calculations which introduce correlation effects (Hubbard et al., 1966).

have difficulty in accurately predicting the $(S^2 - \gamma^2)$ differences but it appears impossible to correlate the observed hyperfine field shifts with Eq. (31) (if the overlap integrals are evaluated with free ion orbitals and the γ's are inferred from other experiments). There are a variety of reasons why this is not altogether surprising. Environmental charge effects are stronger than spin effects and these will distort the 3d (and other orbital) *shapes*, thereby modifying the 3d spin distribution and the computed overlap integral (and, in turn, changing the experimental estimate of the γ's). Also, the $\varphi\chi$ cross terms in Eq. (30) contribute to the spin density at the metal site, further distorting the spin distribution and also causing the net change in spin "on" the metal site to differ from that indicated by Eq. (31). It therefore appears that one must inquire how H_{eff} varies with the shape of the spin distribution. This sort of detailed dependence is outside the capabilities of UHF calculations, but crude calculations (Freeman and Watson, 1960) suggest that H_{eff} should be sensitive to the shape of the "3d" spin density.

The situation seen for metal site hyperfine effects contrasts sharply with transferred hyperfine interactions which, following the work of Shulman et al., have given us some of our best information concerning transition metal covalency. These involve ligand orbital spin density terms of the form $(S+\gamma)^2 \chi^2$ where overlap and covalent mixing contribute *cooperatively* and yield a result which usually predominates over other ligand hyperfine field contributions. Dealing with transferred hyperfine effects has the added advantage that they are added to a zero valued first order (S state ion) field whereas the metal site terms are added to a large, essentially free ion term. The difficulties encountered when attempting a crude understanding of the metal fields makes it impossible to rationalize the observed constancies in 3d ion hyperfine field behavior discussed by Geschwind (Chap. 6) — constancies which appear to be associated with extraordinary concellations among terms which vary systematically.

B. Other Contributions to Transferred Hyperfine Effects in 3d and 4f Compounds

We have seen that overlap and covalent mixing involving an open d or f shell always convey a positive spin density off the metal ion site, a tendency reflected in the majority of transferred hyperfine data. There are, however, a number of experiments which have indicated negative contact term hyperfine fields at ligand nuclei; these include (i) F^{19} in K_2NaCrF_6 and other $Cr^{3+}-F^-$ complexes (Shulman and Knox, 1960); (ii) Rb in $RbMnF_3$ (Payne et al., 1965) (where Rb^+ is the second nearest neighbor to Mn^{2+} ions); and (iii) F^- or O^{2-} sites near rare-earth ions. Case (i) is special in that there are no occupied 3d orbitals which have the proper symmetry to produce ligand s-electron overlap and co-valent mixing and hence there are no associated contact terms. In the other two cases, there are metal ion orbitals of appropriate symmetry and we must conclude that there are other contributions which overpower the overlap and covalency terms and yield the observed net negative fields. Some additional possible contribu-tions are considered below; although discussed separately we should keep in mind that these may all occur at the same time.

(i) Consider the case of Cr^{3+} surrounded by an octahedron of ligand ions as discussed earlier. The three 3d spin ↑ electrons occupy the so-called t_{2g} symmetry states (i.e. xy, yz, and xz) which, by their symmetry cannot be involved in overlap or covalency with the ligand ion s shells. There is covalent mixing between χ_s and the 3d (↑ and ↓) holes of e_g symmetry ($x^2 - y^2$ and $3z^2 - r^2$) and if this mixing is exchange polarized, i.e., $\gamma_\uparrow (e_g) \neq \gamma_\downarrow (e_g)$, there will be a net contact term. Naively, one expects that the 3d exchange will encourage spin ↑ electrons on the F^- sites to be attracted relatively more into the Cr^{3+} e_g holes than those of spin ↓. This yields a net negative s-electron spin density at the F^- nucleus and hence a negative hyperfine field. While the argument given (Watson and Freeman, 1964) is danger-ously oversimplified, actual calculations (Danon et al., 1966) do show just this trend.

(ii) Similarly, one would expect the open 3d shell to ex-change polarize the closed electron shells on the ligands. Calcu-lations by the authors (Freeman and Watson, 1963) have indicated large negative spin densities suggesting that these effects are significant; the calculations themselves suffer from the usual difficulties associated with EPHF theory.

(iii) As discussed in an earlier section, the rare-earths have closed 5s and 5p shells which lie external to the open 4f shell. These are important for any understanding of crystal field split-tings, of covalent effects and of transferred hyperfine effects. For the latter, we must recall the results of exchange polarization of the ion's closed shells. The computed "core" electron spin density ($\rho_\uparrow - \rho_\downarrow$) for all electrons other than the 4f shell and, for comparison, the 4f density as well, was shown for Gd^{3+} in Fig. 3. (Note the change of scales at r = 3.0 atomic units (a.u.) to a common scale for both $\rho_\uparrow - \rho_\downarrow$ and the 4f density.) The two nega-tive regions indicate densities associated with a spin antiparallel to the net spin of the ion. The region near the nucleus produces the negative effective fields of the type already discussed. The outer region is important for interactions with neighboring atoms.

Let us consider the application of the overlap type of analysis, described above, to a rare-earth salt such as GdF_3 in order to explore the consequences of the negative spin density in the outer region of the Gd^{3+} ion. Since the "paired" orbitals (5s and 5p) have different radial distributions, they will overlap the fluoride orbitals differently, and it is this *difference* in their overlaps which gives rise to a hyperfine interaction with the fluorine nucleus. Denoting the Gd^{3+} 4f shell spin as up (↑), then the extent of the interaction is measured by $S_i^2(\uparrow) - S_i^2(\downarrow)$ where i denotes some pair of electrons. In Table VI we list the squares of the overlap integrals between the Gd^{3+} 4f(↑), 5s (↑ and ↓), and 5p (↑ and ↓) and the F^- Hartree-Fock 2s orbital at the observed nearest neighbor distance of 4.4 a.u. (Watson and Freeman, 1961).

Table VII: S^2 values between Gd^{3+} 4f(↑), 5s (↑ and ↓) and 5p (↑ and ↓) orbitals and the F^- 2s orbital.

	$S_\uparrow^2$		$S_\downarrow^2$
4f↑ - 2s	0.012×10^{-2}		
5p↑ - 2s	0.365×10^{-2}	5p↓ - 2s	0.483×10^{-2}
5s↑ - 2s	0.085×10^{-2}	5s↓ - 2s	0.107×10^{-2}
	$\Sigma S_\uparrow^2 = 0.462 \times 10^{-2}$		$\Sigma S_\downarrow^2 = 0.590 \times 10^{-2}$

Net effect = $\Sigma S_\uparrow^2 - \Sigma S_\downarrow^2 = 0.128 \times 10^{-2}$ *(equivalent to −7200 gauss at the F^- nucleus). Contribution from the 4f shell alone* = $+0.012 \times 10^{-2}$ *(equivalent to +700 gauss).*

We see that the sum of $S_\uparrow^2$ minus that of $S_\downarrow^2$ gives an effect which is ten times as large as, and *opposite in sign* to, that obtained by considering the 4f overlap alone. In other words, the spin-polarized functions predict that a Gd^{3+} ion, as seen by a nearest neighbor F^- ion, appears (in its transferred hyperfine interactions) to have a spin which is antiparallel to the actual Gd^{3+} spin. Including the $S_{1s}S_{2s}\chi_{1s}(o)\chi_{2s}(o)$ cross terms in the analysis brings the theoretical predictions into very good quantitative agreement with the experimental results of Baker and Hurrell (1963).

What is clear, and of importance to us here, is the fact that direct 4f covalent and overlap contributions to rare-earth transferred hyperfine interactions are very small and effects such as the polarized outer closed shells play the dominant role. In all

cases where the sign of a rare-earth transferred hyperfine interaction has been obtained (Shulman and Wyluda, 1959; Lewis et al.,
1962; Saraswati and Vijayaraghavan, 1966) it has been found to be
negative. The theoretical situation is more complicated for the
aspherical ($4f^1$ to $4f^6$ and $4f^8$ through $4f^{11}$) configurations where
mixing may occur in which 5p electrons spend time in 4f shell
holes. This leads to aspherical positive spin density contributions
in the outer reaches of the 5p shell. The general observation of
negative transferred hyperfine terms* suggests that the exchange
polarization effect predominates.

In our opinion, the factors discussed above satisfactorily
explain the negative terms observed for the rare earth and
$K_2 NaCrF_6$ compounds but it is not obvious that they account for
the negative Rb fields. An understanding of this awaits further
experimental and theoretical work.

The terms discussed in this section (there are others as
well, cf Marshall, 1962) have their analogs for other systems
where the hyperfine fields associated with ρ_{ov} and ρ_c predominate. In such cases (e.g., the F^{19} results in $KMnF_3$ and $KNiF_3$)
these additional terms are, of necessity, omitted from the analysis which yields estimates of the γ's. Their presence implies
larger uncertainties in the resultant "experimental" γ's than are
normally indicated in the literature.

C. Contribution of Metal Ion-Metal Ion Interactions to their
   Hyperfine Fields: "Supertransferred Hyperfine Interactions"

Recently, the change in hyperfine field at one metal site
produced by nearest neighboring metal ions in compounds such as
MnF_2 has aroused great interest by accounting for an apparent
contradiction between NMR experiments and the predictions of
spin-wave theory at low temperatures (Owen and Taylor, 1966;
Huang et al., 1966; 1967). Experimentally, the metal ion hyperfine field H_{eff} in a concentrated antiferromagnet was found to be
about equal to H_{eff} for the dilute (paramagnetic) salt. If one
assumes that in both cases the hyperfine coupling constant A is
the same (i.e., $A_c = A_d$) this then implies that the expectation
value of the spin $<S>$ equals the total spin, S, in disagreement
with spin wave theory which, because of zero point motion,
predicts a decrease in $<S>$ from S of 3 to 4 percent. Owen and
Taylor (1966) and Huang et al. (1966) showed that $A_c > A_d$, thus
allowing for a compensation for the decrease in $<S>$ predicted

*For an earlier and somewhat different theoretical discussion
see Lewis et al., 1962).

by spin wave theory.

These authors considered a linear three atom system, M_1 - L - M_2, where M_1 and M_2 are magnetic metal ions with opposite spins and L is a ligand ion which couples the two. Two mechanisms were considered. One arises from the unpairing of the core s-electrons on M_2 by overlap with the spin density at the ligand site associated with overlap and covalent mixing with M_1. The second takes account of a 3d electron transfer from M_1 to the empty 4s-like shells of M_2 by either a direct process or by an indirect process involving electron transfer from L to M_2 and another simultaneous transfer from M_1 to L. Since in the antiferromagnetic state the spin of M_1 will be antiparallel to that of M_2, the unpaired spin in the s orbitals of M_2 is *antiparallel* to the 3d spins of M_2. This process results in an enhanced H_{eff} because the 3d and s-electrons now contribute terms of the same sign (i.e., the 3d field is, of course, negative because of core polarization and the antiparallel s-electron contribution is also negative). The resulting increase is of the order of the decrease associated with zero point motion and therefore must be estimated with accuracy when employing NMR results as tests of spin wave theory. While a few puzzles remain (see Huang et al., 1967) these effects appear satisfactorily described by a straightforward extension of the model described in part A of this section.[*]

D. Relevance to Metals and Alloys

We have inspected a number of aspects of hyperfine effects in atoms and nonmetallic magnetic compounds, concentrating most heavily on developments which have emerged subsequent to our earlier review (Freeman and Watson, 1965). In closing, we would like to point out that almost everything that has been said, has relevance to hyperfine investigations in metals, either directly or upon subtle modification. For example, consider an alloy or intermetallic compound where one constituent is more magnetic than others, i.e., more spin resides on it than on its neighbors in a magnetically ordered system *or* on application of a magnetic field (as in a Knight shift experiment). The V_3 X compounds (where X = Si, Ga, Ge, Sn, etc.), for which there seems to be three times as much spin on a V site as on an X (Matthiess, 1965), are examples of such intermetallics and the Fe-Pd and Mn-Cu systems are examples of such alloys. The less magnetic sites can be significantly affected by transferred hyperfine contributions, the obvious leading, but by no means only, term being the Ruderman-Kittel-Kasuya-Yosida interaction discussed in Chap. 9.

[*]*See S. Geschwind, Chap. 6, Sec. IV.*

One can for example, expect at least some polarization of a less magnetic ion's core by the spin density situated on a neighboring, more magnetic, site and one might expect such an effect to become significant if either the spin difference is great (as for a Mn-Cu pair) or if a less magnetic site has a large number of the more magnetic ions as near neighbors (an X site has twelve near neighbor V atoms in the V_3 X compounds).

Another example would be the transferred hyperfine spin unpairing of the outer closed 5s shell of a rare-earth ion in a rare-earth intermetallic compound such as $GdFe_2$ (discussed by Budnick and Skalski, Chap. S-10). The spin unpairing can be very small and yet contribute a substantial hyperfine term since the 5s hyperfine field is of the order of 40 megagauss per unpaired 5s electron. Hence this unpairing, as well as the 6s "conduction" electron terms discussed earlier, can make significant contributions to the observed hyperfine fields which are of the order hundreds to thousands of kilogauss in various metals. (This suggests yet another effect associated with the traditionally inert outer 5s and 5p shells of the rare earths.)

The two types of terms described above are typical of many which can arise and which, of necessity, have been omitted from experimental analyses to date. Despite the complications they present, we believe that the state of the art has been refined to the point where workers must be alert to their presence and in some cases explicitly account for them.

References

Abragam, A. and Pryce, M. H. L. (1951). Proc. Roy. Soc. A205, 135; ibid. A206, 164, 173.

Abragam, A., Horowitz, J., and Pryce, M. H. L. (1955). Proc. Roy. Soc. A230, 169.

Al'tshuler, S. A. and Kozyrev, B. M. (1964). "Electron Paramagnetic Resonance," (Academic Press, N. Y.).

Bagus, P., Freeman, A. J., and Watson, R. E. (1967). to be published.

Bagus, P., Freeman, A. J., and Watson, R. E. (1966). unpublished.

Baker, J. M. and Hurrell, J. P. (1963). Proc. Phys. Soc. 82, 742.

Bleaney, B. (1955). Proc. Phys. Soc. A68, 937.

Blume, M., Freeman, A. J. and Watson, R. E. (1964). Phys. Rev. 134, A320.

Blume, M. and Watson, R. E. (1962). Proc. Roy. Soc. A270, 127.

Blume, M. and Watson, R. E. (1963). Proc. Roy. Soc. A271, 565.

Danon, J., Panepucci, H., Misetich, A. (1966). J. Chem. Phys. 44, 4154.

Elliott, R. J. and Stevens, K. W. H. (1953a). Proc. Roy. Soc. A218, 553.

Elliott, R. J. and Stevens, K. W. H. (1953b). Proc. Roy. Soc. A219, 387.

Ellis, D. E., Freeman, A. J. and Watson, R. E. (1965). International Conference on Magnetism, Nottingham, England (Inst. of Phys. and Phys. Soc. of London). p. 335.

Ellis, D. E., Freeman, A. J., and Ros, J. (1967). J. Appl. Phys. (to appear).

Fermi, E. and Segré, E. (1933). Rend. Accad. Nazl. Lincei 4, 18; Z. Physik 82, 729.

Freeman, A. J., Bagus, P., and Watson, R. E. (1966). Colloque CNRS Sur la Structure Hyperfine des Atoms et des Molecules, Paris.

Freeman, A. J. and Watson, R. E. (1965). "Hyperfine Interactions in Magnetic Materials," Treatise on Magnetism, Vol. IIA (Suhl-Rado, editors, Academic Press, N. Y.).

Freeman, A. J. and Watson, R. E. (1960). Phys. Rev. Letters 5, 498.

Freeman, A. J. and Watson, R. E. (1961). Phys. Rev. Letters 6, 343.

Freeman, A. J. and Watson, R. E. (1962). Phys. Rev. 127, 2058.

Freeman, A. J. and Watson, R. E. (1963). Phys. Rev. 131, 2566.

Hammon, D. R. and Overhauser, A. W. (1966). Phys. Rev. 143, 183.

Harvey, J. S. M. (1965). Proc. Roy. Soc. A285, 581.

Huang, N. L., Orbach, R. and Simanek, E. (1966). Phys. Rev. Letters 17, 134.

Huang, N. L., Orbach, R., and Simanek, E., Owen, J., and Taylor, D. R. (1967). Phys. Rev. (to be published).

Hubbard, J., Rimmer, D. E. and Hopgood, F. R. A. (1966). Proc. Phys. Soc. 88, 13.

Jones, E. D. (1966). unpublished.

Judd, B. R. (1963). Proc. Phys. Soc. 82, 874.

Judd, B. R. and Lindgren, I. (1961). Phys. Rev. 122, 1802.

Kelley, H. P. (1963). Phys. Rev. 131, 684.

Lewis, W. B., Jackson, J. A., Lemons, J. F., and Taube, H. (1962). J. Chem. Phys. 36, 694.

Lindgren, I. (1962). Nucl. Phys. 32, 151.

Locher, P. R. and Geschwind, S. (1963). Phys. Rev. 123, 2027.

Low, W. (1967). (to be published).

Marshall, W. and Stuart, R. (1961). Phys. Rev. 123, 2048.

Marshall, W. (1962). Paramagnetic Resonance, Vol. I (W. Low, editor, Academic Press, N. Y.).

Matthiess, L. F. (1965). Phys. Rev. 138, A112.

Nesbet, R. K. (1966). Colloque CNRS, "La Structure Hyperfine Magnétique des Atomes et des Molecules," Paris.

Overhauser, A. W. (1961). Phys. Rev. 128, 1437.

Owen, J., Taylor, D. R. (1966). Phys. Rev. Letters 16, 1164.

Payne, R. E., Forman, R. A. and Kahn, A. H. (1965). J. Chem. Phys. 42, 3806.

Saraswati, V. and Vijayaraghavan, R. (1966). Phys. Letters 21, 363.

Seitchik, J. A., Gossard, A. C., and Jaccarino, V. (1964). Phys. Rev. 136, A1119.

Shulman, R. G. and Knox, K. (1960). Phys. Rev. Letters 4, 603.

Shulman, R. G. and Wyluda, B. J. (1959). J. Chem. Phys. 30, 335.

Simanek, E. and Sroubek, Z. (1964). Phys. Acta. Solidi 4, 251.

Sinanoglu, O. (1961). Proc. Roy. Soc. A260, 376; Phys. Rev. 122, 491, 493; J. Chem. Phys. 34, 1078, 1237.

Sternheimer, R. M. (1950). Phys. Rev. 80, 102; (1951). Phys. Rev. 84, 244; (1952). Phys. Rev. 86, 316; (1954). Phys. Rev. 95, 736; (1957); Phys. Rev. 105, 158; (1959). Phys. Rev. 115, 1198; (1963). Phys. Rev. 132, 1637; (1966). Phys. Rev. 146, 140.

Sugano, S. and Shulman, R. G. (1963). Phys. Rev. 130, 517.

Szasz, L. (1960). Z. Naturforsch 15a, 909; (1961). J. Chem. Phys. Rev. 35, 1072; (1932). Phys. Rev. 41, 208.

Van Vleck, J. H. (1932). Phys. Rev. 41, 208.

Van Vleck, J. H. (1939). J. Chem. Phys. 7, 72.

Watson, R. E. and Freeman, A. J. (1961a). Phys. Rev. Letters 6, 277.

Watson, R. E. and Freeman, A. J. (1961b). Phys. Rev. 123, 2027.

Watson, R. E. and Freeman, A. J. (1963). Phys. Rev. 131, 250.

Watson, R. E. and Freeman, A. J. (1964). Phys. Rev. 134, A1526.

Watson, R. E., Gossard, A. C., and Yafet, Y. (1965). Phys. Rev. 140, 375.

Winkler, R. (1966). Phys. Letters 23, 301.

Woodgate, G. K. (1966). Proc. Roy. Soc. A293, 117.

3. CALCULATIONS OF MAGNETIC HYPERFINE CONSTANTS FOR THE GROUND STATES OF SOME LIGHT ATOMS

C.M. Moser

*Centre de Mécanique Ondulatoire Appliquée
Paris, France*

Table of Contents

I. Introduction

In this chapter we discuss some of the *ab initio* calculations that have been carried out on the magnetic hyperfine constants of the ^2S ground state of Li, the ^4S ground state of N and the ^3P ground state of O. A considerable amount of work has been done in recent years, thanks to the availability of large and rapid computers, and so the discussion will have to be extremely brief. * The discussion will be sufficiently critical to enable the reader, who may not be particularly interested in carrying out calculations himself, to have a feeling for the accuracy and the values of the calculations which are used to interpret experimental results.

It is known that the Schroedinger non-relativistic equation cannot be solved directly for even very small systems (although, e. g. , very good wave functions are known for the ^2S ground state of Li). As is the usual procedure in science, a very large effort has been put forth to develop approximate methods and models. If these prove to be sufficiently accurate for small systems, then we hope they may still be useful for larger systems. This is a pious hope, which, in the history of wave mechanics, has not always been justified.

The models serve two purposes — one uses them mathematically "to calculate," but even more often one uses them "to get physical insight," or to "understand the physics" of the problem. So we believe that even if a system is too complicated to carry out calculations we can at least "understand" what is going on. This is widely done and is an extremely dubious procedure, to our way of thinking. While one cannot solve the Schroedinger equation, he can in certain circumstances solve the Hartree-Fock equations, spin polarized equations, etc. for certain systems. But it does not at all follow that what is mathematically feasible has necessarily any real physical significance.

There will be no need to remind the reader that all discussion in terms of orbitals is inherently wrong because all electrons are indistinguishable. There are neither s electrons nor p electrons. There is certainly no physical validity in talking about a single configuration like s^2 or $p^3 d^5$. But even though we are all aware that neither orbitals nor configurations have physical significance, we will continue to discuss physical problems in terms of these concepts for a long time to come.

See Chap. 2 by R.E. Watson and A.J. Freeman for a description of work on heavier atoms and ions.

There are other enormous problems in using approximate methods which we can only touch on here. We would like, e. g. , these methods to at least obey the cardinal principles of the variational theorem and the symmetry properties of the wave function. Alas, in the method which has been the most used until now, we must sacrifice one or the other of these principles.

We will not derive the usual hyperfine Hamiltonian here, but as Z gets larger it is incomplete, to say the least. As Z gets larger, wave functions certainly become very much less accurate than those which are available. for Li. To add to our difficulties the hyperfine experiments are rather more often carried out on "atoms" in the solid state rather than "free" atoms but one used "free" (or nearly so) atom functions. In other words, we pile approximation on approximation and then the experimentalist is unpleasantly surprised when the agreement is not perfect.

But we haven't yet mentioned the most difficult aspect of all this. It isn't really all that important whether an approximate method is or isn't in agreement with experiment. It is, however, very important and necessary that the error be more or less constant. As we shall see in the detailed discussion this simply is not so — sometimes the agreement, using a given method, is very good and sometimes very poor indeed. We do not yet understand why this is so.

The usual one-electron Hamiltonian for the magnetic hyperfine constant has been derived classically by Prof. Bleaney. * The derivation from the Dirac equation has been given by Blinder (1965) who gives a critical and illuminating presentation.

If we assume that we can treat the problem of magnetic hfs by second order perturbation theory and that the atomic state is well represented by Russel-Saunders coupling, then the matrix element of the usual expression for the Hamiltonian has the form:

$$A(J,J') = 2\beta_n\beta_e\left\{\lambda_\ell(J,J')\alpha_\ell + \lambda_d(J,J')\alpha_d + \lambda_c(J,J')\alpha_c\right\} \qquad (1)$$

where β_n and β_e are the nuclear and electronic magnetic moments. The reduced matrix elements α_ℓ, α_d, and α_c are defined as follows:

$$\alpha_\ell = \langle LS \| \sum_i \frac{\ell_i}{r_i^3} \| LS \rangle \qquad (2)$$

$$\alpha_d = \langle \, LS \, \| \sum_i \frac{\mathbf{s}_i}{r_i^3} - \frac{3\mathbf{r}_i(\mathbf{s}_i - \mathbf{r}_i)}{r_i^5} \, \| \, LS \, \rangle \, , \qquad (3)$$

$$\alpha_c = \frac{8\pi}{3} \langle \, LS \, \| \sum_i \delta(r_i) \, \mathbf{s}_i \, \| \, LS \, \rangle \, . \qquad (4)$$

The λ's can be expressed in terms of 3j, 6j, and 9j Wigner coefficients. Their general form can be found in many places, e. g. in an article by Trees (1953).

The constants which are measured experimentally are

$$a_J = (IJ)^{-1} \, A(J,J) \, , \qquad (5)$$

$$a'_J = I^{-1} \, (2J-1)^{-\frac{1}{2}} \, A(J,J-1) \, , \qquad (6)$$

where I is the spin of the nucleus. The terms in the brackets in (1) are often called the orbital magnetic dipole and contact (or Fermi) contributions, respectively, to the magnetic constants; the non-zero terms for the first two terms in the brackets arise from non-s orbitals and the last term (contact term) is only non-zero for s orbitals.

Essentially then the work we shall talk about is concerned with calculating the *reduced matrix elements* (Eqs. (2-4)). We will make no mention of the methods used for deducing these experimentally.

II. Hyperfine Structure of ^{2}S Ground State of Li

A. Restricted Hartree-Fock Method

Lithium is the first atom in the periodic table, after the hydrogen atom, in which there is a magnetic hyperfine structure associated with the ground state. (He has a ^{1}S ground state so there is no hyperfine structure associated with the ground state. There is a large hyperfine structure associated with some of the excited states, but this is a somewhat more complicated problem than we will treat in this chapter.) The configuration of the ground state of Li is in conventional Hartree-Fock (HF) notation $(1s)^2$ 2s. That is, the 1s shell is doubly filled, the radial part of $(1s\alpha) =$ radial part of $(1s\beta)$ and then there is the half filled 2s shell. When we talk about the radial part of an orbital, we are referring, of course, to the numerical function one would find in solving the

Hartree-Fock equations. But for practical purposes it is often easier not to construct the numerical tables but to use an expression which is an expansion in terms of analytical functions,

$$\Phi = \sum_i r^{n_i} \exp(-\alpha_i r) \, Y(\theta, \varphi) \, . \tag{7}$$

Everything one does with analytical functions can be done with numerical functions and vice versa. The pros and cons of using these two types of functions have been discussed in a recent review by Freeman and Watson (1965).

For a very detailed and clear exposition of the Hartree-Fock method the reader is referred to a recent book by Slater (1960). One can divide the atomic states into those which are associated with a completely closed shell configuration and those which are associated with a partly open shell configuration. In the closed shells the radial part of spin α = radial part of spin β. For a closed shell configuration like the ^1S ground state of Be, which is $(1s)^2 (2s)^2$ in the usual notation, the Hartree-Fock equations take a very simple form

$$H^{SCF} \, \Phi_{1s} = \epsilon_{1s} \, \Phi_{1s}$$
$$H^{SCF} \, \Phi_{2s} = \epsilon_{2s} \, \Phi_{2s} \tag{8}$$

where

$$H^{SCF} = -\tfrac{1}{2} \nabla^2 - \frac{Z}{r} + 2J_{1s} - K_{1s} + 2J_{2s} - K_{2s} \tag{9}$$

$-\tfrac{1}{2} \nabla$ is the kinetic energy operation, Z/r is the nuclear attraction operator and J and K are called Coulomb and exchange operators respectively and are defined as follows:

$$J_b(1) \, \Phi_a(1) = \left\{ \int \Phi_b(2) \frac{1}{r_{12}} \, \Phi_b(2) \, d\tau_2 \right\} \Phi_a(1)$$
$$K_b(1) \, \Phi_a(1) = \left\{ \int \Phi_a(2) \frac{1}{r_{12}} \, \Phi_b(2) \, d\tau_2 \right\} \Phi_b(1) \, . \tag{10}$$

Since the ground state of Li has the s shells filled and half-filled the solution of the Hartree-Fock equations is rather more complicated than that for the ground state of Be. The 1s and 2s orbitals in Li are solutions of different Hamiltonians:

$$H'^{SCF} \Phi_{1s} = \epsilon_{1s} \Phi_{1s} + \epsilon_{2s,1s} \Phi_{2s}$$

$$H''^{SCF} \Phi_{2s} = \epsilon_{2s} \Phi_{2s} + 2\epsilon_{2s,1s} \Phi_{1s}$$

(11)

where

$$H'^{SCF} = -\tfrac{1}{2}\nabla^2 - \frac{Z}{r} + 2J_{1s} - K_{1s} + \tfrac{1}{2}(2J_{2s} - K_{2s})$$

and

$$H''^{SCF} = -\tfrac{1}{2}\nabla^2 - \frac{Z}{r} + 2J_{1s} - K_{1s} .$$

(12)

In Eq. (11) $\epsilon_{2s,1s}$ is an off-diagonal Lagrangian multiplier which ensures that $\langle \Phi_{1s} | \Phi_{2s} \rangle = 0$ even though Φ_{1s} and Φ_{2s} are solutions of different Hamiltonians.

What has been done for Li?

(i)   The problem can be solved exactly. Roothaan and Bagus (1963) have written a program which solves the problem for configurations of the type: (closed shells) $s^m p^n d^q$.

(ii) One can reduce this problem to an eigenvalue problem by using a Hamiltonian which is a compromise between those given in Eq. (11). This can be written

$$H_s'''^{SCF} = -\tfrac{1}{2}\nabla^2 \frac{Z}{r} + 2J_{1s} - K_{1s} + J_{2s} - AK_{2s} .$$

(13)

If $A = 1$ then this is called using the "equivalence restriction" in the Hartree-Fock Hamiltonian (Nesbet, 1955; Freeman and Watson, 1965). Some workers have suggested using $A = \tfrac{1}{2}$.

Nomenclature gets a bit difficult here. One usually says the restricted Hartree-Fock method is the one where the radial part of $nl\alpha$ is forced to be the same as $nl\beta$. But there is the added difficulty of how one treats the open shell problem — "exactly" or "traditionally."

In any event for our purposes we need to see how important these "restrictions" are in calculating the magnetic hfs constant from the one determinant HF function. The results of Sachs (1960) using method (i) and Nesbet (1960) using method (ii) with $A = 1$, are given in Table I and the results are not very different. Without a fairly large number of examples it is perhaps imprudent to conclude that the hyperfine constants calculated by (i) and (ii) are not very different. The constant is in better agreement with experiment using (ii) but the energy is higher. Unfortunately, as one

Table I: Hyperfine Intervals Calculated for Li

Wave Function	Energy (a. u.)	hfs Intervals (Mc/sec)	Ref.
Experiment	-7. 47807	803. 512	(a)
Restricted Hartree-Fock (i)	-7. 4327	579. 1	(b)
Restricted Hartree-Fock (ii)	-7. 4318	627. 0	(c)
Configuration Interaction: Nesbet	-7. 4318	794. 1	(c)
Weiss	-7. 4771	715. 1	
UHF	-7. 4328	781. 1[d]	(b)
PUHF		648. 3 [e]	(b)
James and Coolidge	-7. 4763	794. 0	(f)
Bethe-Goldstone	-7. 4769	801. 0	(g)

(a) *Kusch and Taub (1949).*
(b) *Sachs (1960).*
(c) *Nesbet (1960).*
(d) *H. Lefebvre (private communication) has repeated the UHF calculation using the basis of Clementi (1965) and finds a constant of 803 Mc/sec.*
(e) *There is an error in the table for this entry in the paper by Sachs (1960).*
(f) *Berggren and Wood (1963).*
(g) *Nesbet (1966).*

improves a wave function energetically there is no assurance in using approximate wave mechanical methods that one will improve the value of any other operator.

B. Configuration Interaction

The difference in energy between the experimental value and the energy found from the restricted Hartree-Fock function (i), about 0. 046 a. u. , is generally called the correlation energy. If we had a wave function which included all the correlation energy, we would have a very good wave function which would be able to describe all properties accurately (though this is not absolutely certain). The calculation of correlated functions is one of the central problems in wave mechanical calculations at the present time. If, in principle, we know several ways of solving the problem, it is quite another matter, in practice, even with the help of very large computers. In principle then we can expand the solution of the non-relativistic Schroedinger equation in terms of configurations where the dominant term is the Hartree-Fock configuration and the other terms are an infinite number of other configurations, all of which have ^{2}S symmetry.

The choice of these configurations is very troublesome because in practice, of course, one can only deal with a finite number of configurations. Naturally, the orbitals which are used to describe the configurations need not be restricted to those where $\ell = 0$. The important point is simply that the total symmetry be ^{2}S, so we should add orbitals where $\ell = 1, 2, 3 \ldots$ With only a little imagination you can see that the problem gets out of hand quickly. One can divide the configurations into two categories. Those which have a first order effect on the hfs and those which have a second or higher order effect. As the Hamiltonian [Eq. (1)] is a mono-electronic operator, then the first order terms will be those which differ from the Hartree-Fock configuration by only one orbital. The second and higher order terms will arise from all the other configurations.

In practice what one does is the following. One chooses a list of configurations, writes down the corresponding determinants, finds the proper symmetry combinations and from these combinations calculates the matrix elements of the electrostatic (or "total") Hamiltonian

$$ H = -\tfrac{1}{2} \nabla^2 - \frac{Z}{r} + \sum_{i \neq j} \frac{e^2}{r_{ij}} \tag{14} $$

and diagonalizes the corresponding matrix. By property symmetry combination we mean the linear combination of determinants which are simultaneously eigenfunctions of the operators S_z, S^2, L_z, and L^2. As there are methods available for diagonalizing very large matrices, one can simply write down the determinants which are an eigenfunction of S_z and L_z and diagonalize the complete set of these; one will automatically obtain eigenfunctions of S^2 and L^2.

Two configuration interaction (CI) calculations should be mentioned here. One by Nesbet (1960), which includes only singly substituted s configurations, and the other by Weiss and Martin (1964), which includes a very large number of configurations and which gives an important part of the correlation energy. Here again we note there is no correlation between a much better energy and the expectation value of the hyperfine operator (cf. Table I).

C. The Hartree-Fock Method and the Projected Unrestricted Hartree-Fock Method

In Sec. II-A, we restricted the freedom of the spin orbitals such that the radial part of $1s\alpha$ = radial part of $1s\beta$. One can relax this restriction and then we would have the one determinant "unrestricted Hartree-Fock" function for lithium,

$$\Psi_{UHF}(Li) = |1s\uparrow\ 1s\downarrow\ 2s\uparrow| \tag{15}$$

where $\uparrow$ indicates the orbitals which are a solution of one equation and $\downarrow$ indicates eigenfunctions of another Hamiltonian. These operators have the form

$$H\uparrow = -\tfrac{1}{2}\nabla^2 - \frac{Z}{r} + J_{1s}^{\alpha} - K_{1s}^{\alpha} + J_{2s}^{\alpha} - K_{2s}^{\alpha} + J_{1s}^{\beta}$$

$$H\downarrow = -\tfrac{1}{2}\nabla^2 - \frac{Z}{r} + J_{1s}^{\alpha} + J_{2s}^{\alpha} + J_{1s}^{\beta} - K_{1s}^{\beta} \tag{16}$$

The evident difficulty is that as the orbitals $\uparrow$ are not orthogonal to the orbitals $\downarrow$, the one determinant wave function is not an eigenfunction of S^2. What is one to do?

(i) One can ignore the fact that the UHF function for lithium is not exactly a doublet but in fact a mixture of a doublet and quartet; the function Eq. (15) is, in the basis set used by Sachs (1960), about 99.9979% doublet. One can then simply calculate the hfs constant for Li from the UHF function.

(ii) One can project out the doublet by the projection technique and calculate the constant from the projected function (PUHF).

Results of various calculations are given in Table I. The constant calculated from the UHF function is in much better agreement with experiment than the constant calculated from the projected function, and so it would be, evidently, very agreeable if one could propose a valid reason not to calculate the constant from the projected function. Marshall (1961) and Bessis et al. (1961) have given strong arguments why one should calculate the constant from the UHF and not from the PUHF method. Without going into the arguments in any detail it can be shown that the constant calculated from the UHF function should be equivalent, to *first order,* to the constant calculated from what Löwdin (1955) has called the extended-Hartree-Fock function (EHF) (and which should be a very good function). The constant calculated from UHF should be very close to the constant calculated from the configuration interaction function obtained from the Hartree-Fock configuration plus singly excited configurations. Even though PUHF is an eigenfunction of S^2 and EHF and CI are also eigenfunctions of S^2 one cannot show the first order equivalence for the hfs constant.

The extended Hartree-Fock (EHF) is the function obtained by a minimization process *after* one has carried out the projection. In the PUHF the minimization process is carried out *before* projection. As far as we know, no one has in fact calculated even a limited EHF function, i.e. limiting the spin orbitals to $\ell = 0$, for the ^2S ground state of Li. So there is good reason not to project out the eigenfunction of S^2 to calculate the hfs constant and it is agreeable that this is in better agreement with experiment, which is of considerable importance. (The problem is not as simple as all this in calculating the constant for nitrogen as we shall see later.)

If one wants to calculate the constant from the PUHF one does not have to carry out the projection completely, which is very tedious. To a high degree of approximation (Bessis et al., 1963)

$$a_s(\text{PUHF}) = \frac{S}{S+1} \, a_s(\text{UHF}) \cdot \qquad (17)$$

This holds only for the polarized part, i.e. that which is *in addition* to the constant calculated from the RHF function. Finally, even though the UHF function gives quite good agreement with experiment for the ground state of Li and in a number of other cases, * one must be on guard against assuming this to have some fundamental significance. There are a large number of examples where the method seems to work very poorly, and we shall see one in the next section.

If one calculates the constant for Li from a very good function of the type of James and Coolidge (1936) where the interelectronic coordinates are introduced in the wave function one finds (Berggren and Wood, 1963) a very good energy and extremely good agreement for the constant as is indicated in Table I. The good agreement is due to the fact that one has a highly correlated function, not to any open shell character of the wave function.

D. Bethe-Goldstone Equation

The catalogue, which we have presented here, of different types of wave functions which have been applied to Li is quite

*See Freeman and Watson (1965) for a long discussion.

incomplete. * But we do wish to discuss briefly a very recent calculation by Nesbet (1966) using an extension of the Bethe-Goldstone
(B-G) equation (Bethe and Goldstone, 1957). The B-G equation
allows one to solve the Schroedinger equation for two particles of
an N particle system. The interaction of the two particles with
the remaining N-2 particles is represented by a self-consistent
field and the function for the two particles is forced to be orthogonal to the surrounding "sea." By extending the Bethe-Goldstone
equation to an N particle equation one can obtain an exact solution
of the Schroedinger equation.

The two particle equation for $1s\alpha$ and $1s\beta$ in Li is in fact
obtained by diagonalizing the matrix where in the HF function
Φ_0 ($1s\alpha$ $1s\beta$ $2s\alpha$) one successivley replaces the particles ($1s\alpha$),
($1s\beta$), and ($1s\alpha$ $1s\beta$) by, in principle, an infinite set of holes, but,
in practice, the holes can be judiciously chosen so that there are
only a tractable number. One can use any operator F to construct
the matrix and not just the electrostatic energy operator. Nesbet
(1966) defines a net increment f_{ij} as the difference between the
gross increment

$$\Delta F_{ij} = \sum_{\mu, \nu} (F_{\mu\nu} - F_{oo} \delta_{\mu\nu}) c_\mu^* c_\nu \Big/ \sum_\mu c_\mu c_\mu$$

and the sum of net increments of all order less than ij that are
contained in the set ij. For example if we are interested in the
net energy increment of $1s\alpha$ $1s\beta$ in Li starting with HF as Φ_0 we
find

$$\epsilon_{12} = \Delta E_{12} - \epsilon_2 - \epsilon_1 .$$

If we restrict the calculation to s-like orbitals we find

$$\epsilon_{12} \approx -0.0135 \text{ a. u.}$$

which is an appreciable improvement.

The Fermi contact increments from the best available computations are given in Table II. It turns out that if ϵ_{123} is perfectly negligible, f_{123} (contact term) is by no means negligible.
Thus the variational theorem which deals only with energy is by
no means a sufficient criterion to determine a satisfactory function
for the contact operators. We need to work much harder to get a
"better" function. If the results are encouraging, i.e., if it is
possible to get very accurate results for the contact term, it
means a very considerable computational effort.

*Burke (1964) discusses no less than 16 different calcula-
tions of the ground state of Li.

Table II: Computed Fermi Contact Increments for Li
(best calculation)

f_o (a)	572. 452 Mc/sec
$\Sigma_i\, f_i$	174. 840
$\Sigma_{ij}\, f_{ij}$	77. 099
f_{ijk}	-22. 787
f total	800. 604

(a) *Parameters taken from E. Clementi (1964).*

III.   Hyperfine Structure of ^{4}S Ground State of N

Since we have described in some detail the methods used for Li, it will only be necessary to give results for N here. As N has a relatively large number of electrons, fewer calculations have been carried out than for Li. As in the case of Li only the contact term contributes to the magnetic hyperfine constant.

A.   Restricted Hartree-Fock Calculation

As seen from Eq. (4) the contact term contains the operator S_i; thus, only open s shells contribute. But as N has the configuration $1s^2\, 2s^2\, 2p^3$ there are no open s shells. The restricted Hartree-Fock function then predicts a zero magnetic hfs. While the constant is small (10. 45 Mc/sec)(Anderson et al., 1959), it is not zero. Thus, the RHF function for Li gave nearly 3/4 of the experimental value, the RHF function is completely useless for nitrogen. We must calculate a function which gives an unpaired spin density at the nucleus.

B.   Configuration Interaction

Configuration interaction calculations have been carried out using (i) only singly excited $s \rightarrow s'$ configurations and (ii) adding to (i) important doubly-excited configurations. The results, as one might expect, are somewhat dependent on the basis set chosen; the calculated constant varies rapidly with energy. Using only $s \rightarrow s'$ configurations (cf. Table III) gives 50 - 80 percent of the experimental value; adding doubly-excited configurations gives results which are in much better agreement with experiment.

Table III: Hyperfine Constant Calculated for N

	Energy (a. u.)	hfs Constant	Ref.
Experiment	-54. 627	10. 45	(a)
HF	-54. 401	0	
Configuration interaction (i) only s → s′ single excitations	-54. 401	5	(b)
(ii) (i) plus double excited functions	-54. 411	11	(b)
UHF (a)		33	(b)
(b)		20. 2	(c)
PUHF (a)		19. 8	(b)
(b)		12. 0	(c)
Bethe-Goldstone (incomplete)	-54. 456	10. 85	(d)

(a) *Anderson et al. (1959).*   (c) *Goodings (1961).*
(b) *Bessis et al. (1961).*   (d) *Nesbet (1966).*

C. Spin Polarized Calculations

The presence of the three 2p orbitals all with the same spin (say ↑) will mean that one can write a spin polarized function for N

$$\Psi_{UHF} = \left| 1s\uparrow\ 1s\downarrow\ 2s\uparrow\ 2s\downarrow\ 2p^3\uparrow \right| \qquad (18)$$

where

$$H_{s\uparrow} = -\tfrac{1}{2}\nabla^2 - \frac{Z}{r} + J^\alpha_{1s} - K^\alpha_{1s} + J^\beta_{1s} + J^\alpha_{2s} - K^\alpha_{2s} +$$

$$J^\beta_{2s} + 3J_{2p} - 3K_{2p}\ ,$$

$$\qquad\qquad\qquad\qquad\qquad\qquad (19)$$

$$H_{s\downarrow} = -\tfrac{1}{2}\nabla^2 - \frac{Z}{r} + J^\alpha_{1s} + J^\alpha_{2s} + J^\beta_{1s} - K^\beta_{1s} + 3J_{2p} +$$

$$J^\beta_{2s} - K^\beta_{2s}\ .$$

The formula for calculating the magnetic constant from the projection of the UHF function (PUHF) is

$$a_{(PUHF)} \simeq \frac{3}{5} \, a_{(UHF)}$$

The results here are also sensitive to the basis set. Two extreme values are given in Table III, one from analytic functions (Bessis et al., 1961), one from numerical functions (Goodings, 1961). The precise numbers are not extremely important in themselves because of this sensitivity. The point to be gained is that, contrary to what happened for Li, the constant calculated for N from the UHF function is 2-3 times larger than the experimental constant. The constant calculated from PUHF is evidently in much better agreement with experiment.

It is extremely difficult to say whether or not the projection *should* be made. As mentioned there are theorems which say that one should *not* since the constant calculated from UHF is a *first order* approximation to the constant calculated from EHF. But as there is only a first order relationship, it is certainly not a minor argument to say one gets better agreement with experiment by calculating the constant from the projected function. The problem as we see it is two fold: (i) should one or should one not use the projected function and (ii) why is it that in Li the polarization given by the UHF function is in extremely good agreement with experiment while in N it so poor. This is particularly disturbing since in a recent article Burke (1964) affirms that physically the concept of core-polarization by non-s electrons is much more valid than by s electrons. *

D.   Bethe-Goldstone Equations

By the time one gets to nitrogen, solving the Nth order Bethe-Goldstone equations becomes an enormous task — particularly if one must go to 7th order. Nesbet (1966) has investigated the problem of energy and hyperfine structure to second order (nearly completely in both s and p basis and has added d and f orbitals) and hyperfine structure in third order only in the Hartree-Fock basis. These results are given in Table III. The agreement with experiment is very good but the third order term contribution to the hfs is very large (and incomplete). We will have to await developments on this method. In principle it is obviously possible to

---

Here is an important example which points out the main purpose of these lectures which is not to present "solved" problems but rather to tempt the reader to use his own imagination and intelligence to "solve" problems which exist.

get very accurate results. But the amount of machine time necessary is also, at the present time, extremely large.

IV. Hyperfine Constants for the ^3P Ground State of Oxygen

Oxygen is an extremely interesting case for not only is the restricted Hartree-Fock configuration $1s^2 \, 2s^2 \, 2p^4$ but also because of very recent experimental* work by Harvey (1965) we know four constants for this state: a_2, a_2', a_1, and a_1'. Only two calculations have been published (Bessis et al. , 1962; 1963).

A. <u>Restricted Hartree-Fock Functions</u>

The results are given in Table IV. As almost all the hfs is due to the open p shells and as the contribution from the orbital and dipole terms in Eq. (1) are considerably larger than the contact term (which is zero in the HF function), the agreement with experiment is fair. The main additional difficulty using Hartree-Fock functions is that the parameters

$$\langle r^{-3} \rangle = \lambda_\ell \, (2,2) \, \alpha_\ell$$

$$\langle r^{-3} \rangle' = 5 \lambda_d \, (2,2) \, \alpha_d \qquad (20)$$

(where the λ's and α's were defined in Eq. (1)) are equal. The considerable importance of Harvey's work is to show this is not so.

Table IV: Hyperfine Constants for O^{17}

Mc/sec	HF	UHF	PUHF	CI	Exp.
a_2	-251. 7	-236. 5	-219. 8	-216. 1	-218. 6
a_2'	-145. 3	-117. 3	-127. 5	-131. 9	-126. 6
a_1	0	- 28. 3	- 8.6	- 3. 8	4. 74
a_1'	-146. 8	- 76. 8	-102.	-113. 1	- 91. 8
E(a. u.)	- 74. 8083	- 74. 8118		- 74. 8132	- 75. 105
a_S	0	- 34.	-17.	- 11. 5	- 18.
$\langle r^{-3} \rangle \, 10^{25}$ cm^{-3}	3. 36	3. 13	3. 13	3. 16	3. 06
$\langle r^{-3} \rangle' \, 10^{25}$ cm^{-3}	3. 36	3. 24	3. 29	3. 30	3. 46

*See discussion in Chaps. 1,2, and 4.

B. Unrestricted Hartree-Fock

The unrestricted Hartree-Fock equations are considerably more complicated here. In the ordinary restricted Hartree-Fock not only does one assume that the radial part of $ns\alpha$ = radial part $ns\beta$, but one also forces the radial part of $n\ell m\alpha$ = radial part of $n\ell m\beta$ and also the radial part of $n\ell m'\alpha$ = radial part of $n\ell m'\beta$ etc. That is, e. g. , in neon, all six 2p functions have the same radial parts.

There is considerable choice as to what can be done. One can simply spin polarize the p orbitals as one did the s (Bessis et al. , 1962) but this does not really make much sense. One can take all radial functions to be different for the four p functions in O, but this is doing in part useless calculation since it can be shown (Lefebvre-Brion et al. , 1966) that the best choice of the Hamiltonian has the radial part of $p+^{\alpha}$ = radial part of $p\cdot^{\alpha}$ with p_0^{α} and $p+^{\beta}$ each having different radial parts. One needs to calculate then three different radial p functions and two different radial s functions (s^{α} and s^{β}). The results are given in the second column of Table IV.

Another problem comes up here which did not occur when we were considering the core polarization of Li or N. What is one to do when calculating a_J if J is not maximum? There is no unanimity on this subject but it seems to us the only reasonable (sic.) thing to do is to calculate the reduced matrix elements for $J = J_{(max)}$ and then calculate all the other a_J's from the Wigner coefficients [Eq. (1)]. Needless to say not all workers have not always been so reasonable and this simply illustrates another difficulty in the UHF method.

The projection of the UHF for oxygen is more complicated and it is not possible to write a simple relation between the dipole and orbital constants obtained from UHF and PUHF functions as was true for the contact term. But the problem is tractable if one makes the following approximation for the overlap integrals

$$\langle \varphi_{i\uparrow} | \varphi_{i\downarrow} \rangle = \delta_{ij} \tag{21}$$

and assumes that the matrix element of a single electron operator takes the form

$$\langle \varphi_{i\uparrow} \| \varphi_{i\downarrow} \rangle = \tfrac{1}{2} \left[\langle \varphi_{i\uparrow} \| \varphi_{i\uparrow} \rangle + \langle \varphi_{i\downarrow} \| \varphi_{i\downarrow} \rangle \right]. \tag{22}$$

The results are in rather better agreement with experiment than projection.

The corresponding configuration interaction calculation is obtained from single $s \rightarrow s'$ and $p \rightarrow p'$ excitations conserving all three independent functions obtained from the latter excitations.

V. Conclusions

It is a bit foolhardy to try and draw any general conclusions from only three examples. But we feel that they are sufficiently representative so that this can be done with some justification. One can, as is pretty much always true with *ab initio* calculations adopt either a pessimistic or optimistic attitude. Pessimism is surely the proper attitude if one is looking for an error of less than 1 percent. Our own point of view is, on the contrary, one of optimism. It is perfectly obvious to us that as far as we can see in the future accurate numerical values of hyperfine constants will be obtained from experiments, not calculations. This being so where is the place for the calculation? Up to now, much of the experimental work has been on the constants of the ground state of atoms. In the future, there will certainly be much more done on the excited states of atoms and ions. Here the experiments will likely be more difficult to interpret and the calculations may provide an extremely useful qualitative guide to an interpretation.

An example may help to explain what we mean. A few years ago a group at the Ecole Normale in Paris (Decomps et al. , 1960) carried out EPR experiments on the n^1D states of He^3. They were very agreeably surprised to find, notwithstanding the well established concept in the literature that there is no hyperfine structure associated with singlet states, that there is a very large hyperfine structure in these n^1D states. For the 4^1D_2 state it was estimated to be "larger than 600 Mc/sec." This is sufficiently large that it ought to be observable in an optical experiment. But when the hyperfine structure of the 4^1D_2 of He^3 was studied at Bellevue by Professor Brochard, no hfs was observed at all. This did not necessarily mean that there was no hfs associated with these states but it did suggest it was rather smaller than the original estimate.

Lefebvre-Brion et al. (1964a) later became interested in the problem and calculated the hfs. Briefly, there is a hyperfine structure associated with these states because the singlet states are very close to the triplets which themselves have extremely large constants and there is enough mixing of the singlet and the triplet states to produce non-zero constants for the singlet. The calculations gave the magnetic hyperfine constant as 110 ± 3 Mc/sec. The problem was then reinvestigated at the Ecole Normale at several different frequencies and the constant for 4^1D_2 state was found to be 60 ± 20 Mc/sec (Decoubes et al., 1964). One sees that the calculated value is in quite good qualitative agreement with the correct experimental value. We certainly believe that the future lies in this kind of collaboration between calculations and experiment.

Honesty compels us to point out that, while we generally believe that when there is a difference between computed and calculated values that it is not always the computed value which is wrong, there is a glaring example of an ignominious error on the part of calculations. The hfs constant for ^4S state of P was determined by Lambert and Pipkin (1962) in an optical pumping experiment to be $+ 55$ Mc/sec. While the absolute value is undoubtedly correct the determination of sign from this experiment is rather involved. Calculations (Bessis et al., 1964b) have given -42 to -132 Mc/sec, i.e. with the opposite sign. Unfortunately for us a beam experiment (Pendlebury and Smith, 1964) has confirmed the sign determined from the optical pumping experiment. If the error in our calculations seems large it is really no larger than in N. So there are defeats to match against the victories, but we do not doubt that there will be many victories in the future.

References

Anderson, C. W., Pipkin, F. M., Baird, J. C. (1959). Phys. Rev. 116, 87.

Berggren, K. F. and Wood, R. F. (1963). Phys. Rev. 130, 198.

Bessis, N., Lefebvre-Brion, H., and Moser, C. M. (1961). Phys. Rev. 124, 1124; (1962). Phys. Rev. 128, 213; (1963). Phys. Rev. 130, 1441; (1964a). Phys. Rev. 135, A957.

Bessis, N., Lefebvre-Brion, H., Moser, C. M., Freeman, A. J., and Watson, R. E. (1964b). Phys. Rev. 135, A588.

Bethe, H. A. and Goldstone, J. (1957). Proc. Roy. Soc. (London) A238, 551.

Blinder, S. M. (1965). "Theory of Atomic Hyperfine Structure," in Advances in Quantum Chemistry, Vol. II, (Academic Press, New York), p. 47.

Burke, E. A. (1964). Phys. Rev. 135, A621.

Clementi, E. (1964). J. Chem. Phys. $\underline{40}$, 1944; (1965). IBM J. Res. Dev. $\underline{9}$, Supp. Table 4-1.

Decomps, B., Pebay-Peyroula, J. C., and Brossel, J. (1960). C. R. Acad. Sci. $\underline{251}$, 9141.

Decoubes, J. P., Decomps, B., and Brosell, J. (1964). C. R. Acad. Sci. $\underline{258}$, 4005.

Freeman, A. J. and Watson, R. E. (1965). in Magnetism, Vol. IIA, edited by Rado and Suhl, (Academic Press, New York).

Goodings, D. A. (1961). Phys. Rev. $\underline{123}$, 1706.

Harvey, J. S. M. (1965). Proc. Roy. Soc. $\underline{A285}$, 581.

James, H. M. and Coolidge, A. S. (1936). Phys. Rev. $\underline{49}$, 688.

Kusch, P. and Taub, H. (1949). Phys. Rev. $\underline{75}$, 1477.

Lambert, R. H. and Pipkin, F. M. (1962). Phys. Rev. $\underline{128}$, 198.

Lefebvre-Brion, H., Wajsbaum, J., and Bessis, N. (1966). Colloque CNRS, "La Structure Hyperfine Magnetique des Atomes et des Molécules," Paris.

Löwdin, P. O. (1955). Phys. Rev. $\underline{97}$, 1474.

Marshall, W. (1961). Proc. Phys. Soc. $\underline{78}$, 113.

Nesbet, R. K. (1955). Proc. Roy. Soc. $\underline{A230}$, 312; (1960). Phys. Rev. $\underline{118}$, 681; (1966). Colloque CNRS, "La Structure Hyperfine Magnetique des Atomes et des Molécules," Paris.

Pendlebury, J. M. and Smith, K. F. (1964). Proc. Phys. Soc. $\underline{84}$, 849.

Roothaan, C. C. J. and Bagus, P. S. (1963). Meth. Comp. Phys. $\underline{2}$, 47.

Sachs, L. M. (1960). Phys. Rev. $\underline{117}$, 1504.

Slater, J. C. (1960). in Quantum Theory of Atomic Structure, Vol. I, (McGraw-Hill, New York).

Trees, R. E. (1953). Phys. Rev. $\underline{92}$, 308.

Weiss, A. W. and Martin, J. B. (1964). cited in Freeman and Watson (1965).

4. HYPERFINE STRUCTURE IN ATOMIC BEAM RESONANCE

Lectures by P.G.H. Sandars

Oxford University
Oxford, England

Prepared by Barbara Dodsworth

New York University
New York, N.Y.

Table of Contents

I. Introduction

Resonance in atomic beams is one of the oldest techniques for the study of hyperfine interactions in atoms. The basic theory and experimental technique has been thoroughly discussed in the well known book by Kopferman (1958). In this chapter, we will consider some current experimental techniques and applications of atomic beam resonance and will discuss the theory of hyperfine structure (hfs) in free atoms.

An atomic beam machine may be used to detect either optical or radio frequency resonances. The method differs from other resonance techniques in that the radiation emitted or absorbed is not detected, but the atoms which have undergone a transition are detected.

Figure 1 shows the essential elements of an atomic beam apparatus in a schematic diagram. The apparatus consists of a

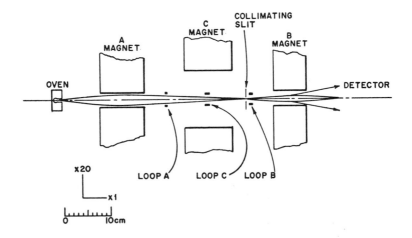

Fig. 1: Schematic diagram of a symmetric atomic beam machine.

source and detector, two inhomogeneous deflecting fields A and B which act as polarizer and analyzer respectively, and a homogeneous C field in which the resonances take place. The gradients of the A and B fields may be in opposite directions, in which case a transition in the C magnet that changes the sign of the atomic magnetic moment will cause an atom to be deflected away from the detector; the resonance is detected by a decrease in the number of atoms arriving at the detector. This is known as a "flop-out". If the gradients are in the same direction, then the same transition in the C magnet will cause the atoms undergoing the transition to be focussed onto the detector at resonance and is known as "flop-in".

The advantage of the atomic beam method is that one detects the atoms rather than the resonant frequency energy which typically may be of the order of 1 mc or $\approx 10^{-8}$ ev. If the atom is ionized, accelerated through a voltage of, for example, 10^4 volts and then passed through an electron multiplier, an energy of some 10^6 ev, or a gain of 10^{14} in energy, can be obtained. Hence the r.f. energy acts as a "trigger" to initiate the process. This means one can detect a resonance in which only a few atoms are involved. The second main advantage of the atomic beam method is that the atom is free and the precision of the measurement can be high. The linewidth is basically determined by the uncertainty principle

$$\Delta \nu \Delta t \geq 1$$

where $\Delta t = L/v$ is the time the atom spends in the resonance region, L being the length of the resonance and v the velocity of the atom. Therefore

$$\Delta \nu \frac{L}{v} \geq 1 \qquad \text{or} \qquad \Delta \nu \geq \frac{v}{L}$$

The linewidth can therefore be reduced by making L long.

II. Modern Atomic Beam Experiments

The present situation in atomic beams measurements can be broken up into two categories: The standard and the non-standard experiments.

A. Standard Experiments

The standard experiments are those performed on a conventional atomic beam machine for the purpose of measuring the magnetic dipole, electric quadrupole and magnetic octupole hyperfine constants as well as the electronic magnetic moment μ_J and to a lower precision the nuclear magnetic moment μ_I. These experiments can now be performed on all elements with paramagnetic ground states. Measurements in metastable atomic states are feasible if the half life is sufficient for the atom to get down the length of the atomic beam machine, i.e., $\tau_1 > 10^{-4}$ sec, and the energy ΔE of the metastable state relative to the ground state satisfies either of two conditions:

    i) ΔE is less than 1 e.v. in which case the metastable state may be achieved by thermal excitation in the oven;

    ii) ΔE is greater than 3 e.v., in which case the metastable state may be excited by electron bombardment. In this energy range the metastable atoms have sufficient energy to eject an electron from a surface upon which they are allowed to impinge and are thus detected.

B. Non-Standard Experiments

1. Triple Resonance

    The disadvantage of standard atomic beam experiments is that μ_I cannot be measured directly. This can easily be seen by looking at an energy level diagram in high field for $J = \frac{1}{2}$, $I = \frac{1}{2}$, shown in Fig. 2. The observable transitions are the ones for

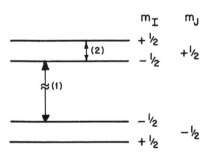

Fig. 2: Level diagram for $J = \frac{1}{2}$, $I = \frac{1}{2}$ and transitions illustrating atomic beam resonance.

which m_J changes. Precision measurement of the nuclear moment using such a transition is difficult because of the much larger interaction of the atomic moment with the field. One would like to observe a transition such as line (2) in Fig. 2, but since this does not lead to a change in the sign of the atomic magnetic moment, it cannot be observed. The triple resonance technique (Woodgate and Sandars, 1958)) is designed to allow direct detection of transitions between levels of different m_I, but the same m_J. In this method the atom passes successively through three separate r.f. loops, designated by A, C and B. If we designate the transition possibilities in each of the three loops by a, c, and b, then with loop A alone inducing transitions between the $(-\frac{1}{2}, -\frac{1}{2}) \leftrightarrow (-\frac{1}{2}, +\frac{1}{2})$ states, where the bracket gives the m_I and m_J numbers as (m_I, m_J) the relative height of the resonance at the detector would be proportional to 2a. If the same transition is observed, first in the A loop and then in the B loop, the relative resonance height at the detector will be proportional to 2a + 2b (1 - 2a). If all three loops are used, A and B for the $(-\frac{1}{2}, \frac{1}{2}) \leftrightarrow (-\frac{1}{2}, -\frac{1}{2})$ transition and C for the transition which changes the nuclear moment $(\frac{1}{2}, \frac{1}{2}) \leftrightarrow (-\frac{1}{2}, \frac{1}{2})$ then the resonance height will be proportional to 2a + 2b(1 - 2a) + 2abc. Table I shows the resonance heights at the detector for the case where a = b = c = 0.9.

Table I: Intensity at the detector for a = b = c = 0.9.

A alone	1.8
B alone	1.8
A and B together	0.36
A + B + C	1.8

Thus the previously unobservable $(-\frac{1}{2}, -\frac{1}{2}) \leftrightarrow (-\frac{1}{2}, +\frac{1}{2})$ transition and (transition (2) in Fig. 2) in the C loop produces a change of ~ 1.44 in the signal at the detector.

The precision of a normal nuclear moment measurement depends on the accuracy with which the magnetic field is known. However, it is not necessary to measure the magnetic field directly, since the frequency of the transition as a function of field is as follows:

$$\nu = \nu_0 + g_I H + \frac{\lambda}{H^2} \tag{1}$$

The last term is due to the breakdown of high field quantum numbers by the hyperfine interaction; λ and ν_0 are known. A plot of frequency vs field is shown in Fig. 3 with the maximum (or minimum depending on the sign of g_I) frequency occuring at

$$\nu_{min} = \nu_0 + \frac{3}{2}(2\lambda g_I^2)^{\frac{1}{3}} \tag{2}$$

or
max

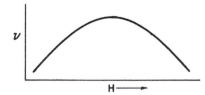

Fig. 3: Frequency versus magnetic field curve in the determination of a nuclear g-factor (see text).

This measurement of the maximum or minimum frequency yields a direct determination of g_I. An additional advantage is that at the turning point the frequency is field independent and the field inhomogeneities have minimum effect. One does not need to know the value of the magnetic field because one is really measuring the ratio of g_I/g_J.

For example, using this method, the moments of Eu isotopes* (Evans et al., 1965) were measured to be:

$$\mu\ (^{151}\text{Eu}) = 3.4391\ (6)\ \text{n.m.}$$

$$\mu\ (^{153}\text{Eu}) = 1.5186\ (8)\ \text{n.m.}$$

To obtain the ratio of moments, the value of the field is again not necessary, and measurements can be made at higher fields for greater accuracy. The ratio of the two moments was found to be

$$\mu\ (^{151}\text{Eu})/\mu\ (^{153}\text{Eu}) = 2.26505\ (42)$$

compared with the ENDOR measurement (Baker and Williams, 1962) of:

$$\mu\ (^{151}\text{Eu})/\mu\ (^{153}\text{Eu}) = 2.2632\ (26)$$

2. Isotope Shift in Atomic Beams

Because of the uncertainty in the electronic part of the interpretation of isotope shifts,* the most informative experiments are those in which one can measure the relative shifts for a range of isotopes of the same element. Up to the present time the range of isotopes has been restricted to those that are stable or very long-lived. Recently Marrus and McColm (1965) at the University of California have introduced a technique which will allow measurements of a wider range of radioactive elements.

The method involves the use of light in the C field instead of the conventional radio-frequency field. If the light comes from a lamp containing the same element and isotope as the beam, a light flop will result. What occurs is illustrated in Fig. 4 for an atom with ground state $J = \frac{1}{2}$ and no hyperfine structure (for simplicity). An atom initially in the $m_I = +\frac{1}{2}$ state will be excited to an excited level by the filtered light so that only one excited level is allowed. However, when the atom decays, for example from the $m_J = \frac{1}{2}$ level, there is a probability of both $\Delta m = 0$ and $\Delta m_J = +1$ transitions

*For detailed discussion see A. Steudel, Chap. 5.

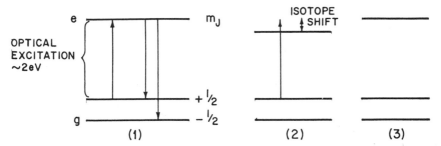

Fig. 4: Level scheme illustrating isotope shift measurement in an atomic beam (see text).

occurring. Hence an atom initially in the $m_J = +\frac{1}{2}$ ground state has a probability of ending up in the $m_J = -\frac{1}{2}$ ground state. If the apparatus is set to detect atoms which have undergone this transition, the result of turning the light on will be a signal at the detector.

However, if the isotope in the beam differs from that in the lamp, the light will not correspond to the resonance frequency as shown in diagram (2) of Fig. 4 and the light flop will not take place. In order to measure the isotope shift, Marrus and McColm applied an electric field to the beam atom which shifts its levels through the quadratic Stark effect. When the field is adjusted to bring the level separation back into coincidence with the radiation from the lamp, then the light flop will again occur and a signal at the detector will result (cf. Fig. 5). This assumes, of course, that the

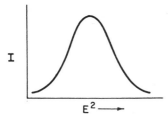

Fig. 5: Intensity versus the square of the applied electric field in the determination of isotope shifts.

relative isotope shift is large with respect to the width of the exciting radiation. The energy separation between levels, ΔW is

$$\Delta W = -\tfrac{1}{2} \alpha E^2 = \delta W \qquad (3)$$

where α is the difference in polarizability between levels and E is the value of the electric field obtained from the resonance curve. Then, if the polarizability is known, the isotope shift δW can be obtained. The usefulness of the method is that the beam can consist of any radioactive isotope conveniently handled by atomic beam techniques.

3. Ramsey Double Loop Methods

One of the biggest single improvements in beam techniques has been the introduction by Ramsey (1955) of the double loop method. Instead of passing through only one loop, the atom passes through two loops fed coherently from the same RF oscillator. Each loop separately produces a single resonance curve appropriate to the length of the loop ℓ. However, with the two loops following each other and separated by a distance L (L $\gg$ ℓ), there is an interference effect which modulates the single loop resonance to give a curve of the form shown in Fig. 6. The additonal pattern

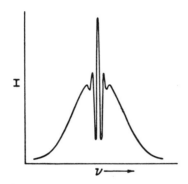

Fig. 6: Resonance curve for a Ramsey double loop.

is sharper than the single pattern and the width of the central peak is determined by the distance L between the two loops or $\Delta \nu = L/V$ where V is the velocity of the atom in the beam.

The importance of the Ramsey loop is that the peak of the resonance appears at the average of the energies involved in transit, i.e., $h\nu = (E_1 - E_2)_{AV} = (\Delta E)_{AV}$ where the average is taken over the region between the two loops. The Ramsey loop then has the important effect of averaging over perturbations between the loops.

The advantage of this technique is that one can perturb the energy of the atom while it is in the region between the loops and thus cause a shift in frequency even though the perturbation is not in the rf region. As an example, if the energy levels are perturbed by letting the atom pass through an electric field parallel to the magnetic field in the region between the Ramsey loops, the resonance will be shifted even though the electric field and the rf field nowhere overlap.

Many interesting experiments require the detection of very small shifts of the resonance. These shifts in frequency are conveniently detected by a modulation technique using the intensity at the detector. To a first approximation the intensity changes linearly either with oscillator frequency or with shift of the resonance. Thus a shift of the resonance by $\delta\nu$ leads to a proportional change in the intensity

$$\delta I = k \, \delta\nu_k \, . \tag{4}$$

The constant of proportionality can be readily found by changing the oscillator frequency a small amount and noting the change in intensity. By taking great pains to eliminate spurious effects, it is possible in practice to obtain a sensitivity given by

$$\delta\nu_k = \Delta\nu \times \frac{1}{\sqrt{N}} \tag{5}$$

where N is the number of atoms participating in the resonance and detected, and $\delta\nu$ is the half width of the Ramsey peak of the resonance. This technique has made possible observation of electric-field induced shifts of the resonance as small as 10^{-6} of the width of the resonance.

There are many experiments one can do with this sort of technique.

a. Electric Dipole Moments. First of all, one can search for a linear Stark effect, (Sandars and Lipworth, 1964), which implies that the atom has an electric dipole moment. Such an effect, is, of course, forbidden by both parity and time reversal invariance. However, parity is well known to be violated and there is growing evidence that time reversal is also violated. The results of such experiments on alkalies can be interpreted in several ways:

  i) It sets an upper limit to the electric dipole moment of the electron. This is a factor 10^6 smaller than has been obtained recently on the Stanford Linear Accelerator.

  ii) It puts a limit on the electric dipole moment of the proton. The proton moment is heavily shielded from the external field by the electrons so that it can not be observed except for the presence of hyperfine structure interactions.

   iii) It puts a limit on the magnetic quadrupole moment of the nucleus.

   b. <u>Quadratic Stark Effect.</u> In the quadratic Stark effect, one observes only differences in polarizabilities between hyperfine structure states. If the state has L as a good quantum number, then the shift of a level L, M_L, can be written in the form

$$\delta W = - \tfrac{1}{2}\, \alpha_{SC} E^2 - \tfrac{1}{2}\, \alpha_t \frac{\left(3M_L^2 - L(L+1)\,(3E_z^2 - E^2)\right)}{2L(2L-1)} \qquad (6)$$

Of the two parameters α_{SC} and α_t, only α_t, of course, can be observed with a hyperfine structure experiment. In the case of Al and Sm, where $L \neq 0$, the approximate magnitude of α_t is $\approx a_0^3$ although the polarization of Al and Sm differ by a factor of 10. This gives a shift of about 10 kc at 10^5 V/cm.

When $L = 0$, the polarizability vanishes since both terms vanish. However, fine structure effects can contribute and the differential polarizability depends on $3m_J^2 - J(J+1)$. In the case of the $^8S_{7/2}$ state of Eu, α_t is approximately $10^{-2}\, a_0^3$ which gives shift of 10 kc at 10^5 V/cm.

The polarizability also vanishes for $J = \tfrac{1}{2}$, but hyperfine structure effects can contribute and now the polarizability depends on a term proportional to $3 M_F^2 - F(F+1)$. For the alkalies then, the approximate magnitude of α_t is $10^{-6}\, a_0^3$ or about 10 cps at 10^5 V/cm. This turns out to be the most interesting case since there are three polarizabilities that can be measured due respectively to:

   1) contact hyperfine structure, $S \cdot I$

   2) the spin dipole hyperfine structure, $[SC^2]' \cdot I$

   3) the quadrupole hyperfine structure.

The orbital hyperfine structure interaction does not contribute.

Finally, we should remark, but will not discuss, that if the atom is placed in an inhomogeneous electric field, there will be an interaction between the field and the atomic quadrupole moment. Interactions of this type have recently been observed and give the possibility of determining the atomic quadrupole moment.

III. Theory of Atomic Hyperfine Structure

For an atom in zero external magnetic field, the interaction between the nucleus and the electrons is independent of the orientation of the atom as a whole. Therefore the hyperfine interaction is a scalar in the space of the atom as a whole and commutes with the total angular momentum of the atom, or:

$$[\mathbf{F}, \mathcal{K}_{hfs}] = 0 , \qquad \text{where} \qquad \mathbf{F} = \mathbf{I} + \mathbf{J}, \qquad (7)$$

I is the angular momentum of the nucleus and J is the electronic angular momentum. The scalar hfs operator can always be represented in terms of a multipole expansion:

$$\mathcal{K}_{hfs} = \sum_{k=0}^{\infty} \mathcal{K}_{hfs}^{k} , \qquad (8)$$

where $\mathcal{K}_{hfs}^{k}$ is the sum of terms of the form of scalar products $T(e)^k \cdot T(n)^k$, where

$$T(e)^k \cdot T(n)^k = \sum_{q}{}' (-1)^q T(e)_q^k T(n)_{-q}^k , \qquad (9)$$

As the arguments imply, T(e) operates only on the electrons and T(n) operates only on the nucleus.

The T^k's are spherical tensor operators, which means they transform like spherical harmonics of the same argument. Therefore

$$[J_{\pm}, T(e)_q^k] = \sqrt{(k \mp q)(k \pm q + 1)} \ T(e)_{q \pm 1}^k . \qquad (10)$$

since spherical harmonics of rank k and projection q satisfy

$$[J_{\pm}, Y_q^k] = \sqrt{(k \mp q)(k \pm q + 1)} \ Y_{q \pm 1}^k . \qquad (11)$$

Up to this point there have been no approximations other than the separability into electronic and nuclear factors, but now the assumption is made that I and J are good quantum numbers for the atom. The energy of the state of total angular momentum F is then

$$W(f) = \langle IJF | \sum_{k} \mathcal{K}_{hfs}^{k} | IJF \rangle . \qquad (12)$$

We now introduce parameters into the theory, using the stretched state where $\mathbf{F} = \mathbf{I} + \mathbf{J}$ and defining

$$A_k = \langle IIJJ| H_{hfs}^k | IIJJ \rangle \; . \tag{13}$$

The next step is to express the energy of arbitrary F in terms of the A_k's which represent physically different parts of the hyperfine structure. The energy can be expressed in terms of the A_k's in a unique way and the measured energy difference can be used to obtain values for the various interaction constants. We can write

$$W(F) = \sum_k M (IJ; F, k)A_k \; , \tag{14}$$

where the M values are tabulated by Schwartz (1955). The dipole term (k = 1) is given explicitly by

$$M(IJ; F, 1) = \frac{k}{2IJ} = \frac{F(F+1) - I(I+1) - J(J+1)}{2IJ} \; . \tag{15}$$

One can also reverse the argument and express the A_k in terms of the energies

$$A_k = F(I, J, k) \sum (2F+1) M (IJ; Fk) W(F) \cdot \tag{16}$$

If the quantum numbers are good, the maximum number of levels is equal to $2I+1$ (or $2J+1$, whichever is the lesser) and maximum k is equal to $2J$ or $2I$ (again the lesser of the two). However, even if I and J are not good quantum numbers, the same number of levels would occur and one would go through the same sort of analysis. The fact that we can fit the experimental spectra does not necessarily imply that I and J are good quantum numbers. This is unfortunate since we want to do two things, namely, (1) get physically useful numbers, i.e., the A_k's, and (2) check that the assumptions are correct. In other words, for the approach to be useful, one has to introduce some physics. We can do this by noting that the k = 1 (dipole) and k = 2 (quadrupole) terms are the large interactions since experience tells us that $A_1 \approx A_2 \gg A_3$, $A_4 \gg A_5$, A_6. We can try these and if they fit to within the experimental error, then we have a reasonable theory. It is amusing to note at this point that the close equality of dipole and quadrupole interactions is essentially a coincidence. Thus the ratio of the dipole interaction

$$\frac{\mu_0 \mu_N}{r_e^3} \sim \left(\frac{\alpha^2 e^2 a_0^2}{a_0^3} \right) \frac{m}{M} \sim \alpha^2 \frac{m}{M} \frac{e^2}{a_0} \tag{17}$$

to the quadrupole interaction

$$\frac{e^2 Q}{r_e^3} \sim \frac{e^2}{a_o} \times r_n^2$$

is

$$\frac{A_1}{A_2} \sim \alpha^2 \frac{m}{M} \frac{a_o^2}{r_n^2} \sim 1 \quad .$$

The next set of terms is smaller by the ratio $r_n^2/r_e^2 \sim 10^{-8}$. The term A_3, but not A_4, has been detected.

A. Breakdown of I or J

We now want to examine the breakdown of I or J via the hyperfine structure interaction. To second order, the interaction energy is

$$W(F)^{(2)} = \frac{\sum \langle I J F M | \mathcal{H}_{hfs}^{k_1} | I'J'FM \rangle \langle I'J'FM | \mathcal{H}^{k_2} | I J F M \rangle}{W - W'} + CC \cdot \quad (18)$$

Before interpretating the results in terms of higher multipoles, one must be sure they are not due to the breakdown of I or J, i.e., to $W(F)^{(2)}$. The interactions which can contribute to various A_k's through $W(F)^{(2)}$ are shown in Table II.

Table II: Second order contributions to A_k's.

Interaction	k_1	k_2	k
dipole-dipole	1	1	0, 1, 2
dipole-quadrupole	1	2	1, 2, 3
quadrupole-quadrupole	2	2	0, 1, 2, 3, 4

For A_3, second order perturbation can be important the the pseudo octupole contributions coming from the dipole-quadrupole and quadrupole-quadrupole terms must be considered.

B. Hfs Anomaly

Let us assume that the hyperfine structure Hamiltonian of rank k contains only a single term, i.e.,

$$\mathcal{H}_{hfs}^k = T(n)^k \cdot T(e)^k \quad , \quad (19)$$

If in addition we assume that the wavefunction is separable into atomic and nuclear parts, then we can write

$$A_k = \langle II | T(n)^k | II \rangle \, \langle JJ | T(e)^k | JJ \rangle \; . \tag{20}$$

We can then deduce that the ratio of A_k's in different J states for different isotopes should be equal since the nuclear part cancels out and

$$\frac{A_k(J)}{A_k(J')} = \frac{\langle JJ | T(e)^k | JJ \rangle}{\langle J'J' | T(e)^k | J'J' \rangle} = \frac{A'_k(J)}{A'_k(J')} \; , \tag{21}$$

for example, where the primed and unprimed A values refer to different isotopes of the same element. Comparing the ratio of the A factors in the two different J states, for the isotopes Lu^{175} and $Lu^{176}m$ we find

$$\frac{(A_1^{175}/A_1^{176\,m})_{J=\frac{5}{2}}}{(A_1^{175}/A_1^{176\,m})_{J=\frac{3}{2}}} = 1.003773\,(6).$$

One can also take the ratio of the quadrupole interaction constants A_2

$$\left(\frac{A_2^{175}}{A_2^{176\,m}} \right)_{\frac{5}{2}} \left(\frac{A_2^{176\,m}}{A_2^{175}} \right)_{\frac{3}{2}} = 1 + 0.000005\,(5) \; .$$

Experimentally, we see there is an anomaly in the dipole case but not in the quadrupole case. The anomaly could be due to any one of three causes:

   i) Breakdown of J or second order hyperfine effects (the second order effect of the dipole perturbation would contribute to the dipole constant).

  ii) Violation of $T(n)^k \cdot T(e)^k$ assumption. The hfs opera-tor cannot be written rigorously as a product of two terms. Physically, since the nucleus has a finite extension in space, one can no longer regard nuclear and electron coordinates independently when the elec-tron is inside the nucleus.

 iii) Breakdown of the assumption that the electronic wave-function is independent of the isotope. If the nucleus has a finite size, the wavefunction will depend on the nuclear volume and the electronic matrix element will not be independent of the isotope.

C. Hfs in SL Multiplet

The assumptions are now made that S and L are good quantum numbers and that relativistic effects are small. These assumptions are good, at least for the lighter atoms.

Using a very general notation, the hfs operator can be written in terms of S and L as

$$\mathcal{K}_{hfs}^{k} = \sum_{k_S k_L} \mathcal{K}_{hfs}^{(k_S k_L)k} . \tag{22}$$

The operator $\mathcal{K}_{hfs}^{(k_S k_L)k}$ is a sum over terms of the form of a tensor operator of rank k_S operating on the spin times a tensor of rank k_L and these are coupled to a tensor of rank k which is dotted into the nuclear operator, i.e.,

$$\mathcal{K}_{hfs}^{(k_S k_L)k} = \sum \left[S^{k_S} \times t^{k_L} \right]^k \cdot T(n)^k . \tag{23}$$

If we define

$$A_k^{k_S k_L} = \langle I I S S L L | \mathcal{K}_{hfs}^{(k_S k_L)k} | I I S S L L \rangle , \tag{24}$$

then the energies can be expressed in terms of $A_k^{k_S k_L}$. However, this is much too general and the number of possible values of k_S and k_L, and hence of the parameters $A^{k_S k_L}$, is too large to be useful. Restrictions must be included in some way.

First of all, we assume the hfs operator is a one electron operator. The spin matrix element will then be of the form $\langle \frac{1}{2} | S^{k_S} | \frac{1}{2} \rangle$. Spin $\frac{1}{2}$ can only have matrix elements with a scalar or vector operator and hence $k_S = 0, 1$ only. A second restriction which follows from the theory of angular momentum coupling is that $k_S k_L k$ must satisfy a triangular condition, i.e., $|k_S - k_L| \leq k \leq |k_S + k_L|$. A third restriction has to do with the hermiticity of the operator $\mathcal{K}_{hfs}^{k}$ (Eq. 21) and requires that $k_S + k_L + k$ be even. The possible values of k, k_S and k_L are listed in Table III.

We therefore have the important result that for a given k, all the constants A_k within an SL multiplet can be expressed in terms of three parameters $A^{(k_S k_L)k}$ which are properties of the given

Table III: Values of k_S and k_L for given k.

k	k_S	k_L
k	0	k
	1	k + 1
	1	k - 1
1	0	1
	1	2
	1	0
2	0	2
	1	3
	1	1

multiplet. It is often convenient to write this result in the form of an effective Hamiltonian operator within the multiplet. For example, the dipole effective operator takes the form

$$\mathcal{H}^{eff}_{dipole} = \frac{A_1^{1,0}}{SI}\, \mathbf{S} \cdot \mathbf{I} + \frac{A_1^{0,1}}{LI}\, \mathbf{L} \cdot \mathbf{I} + \frac{A_1^{1,2}}{ISL(2L-1)}$$
$$\times \left[\tfrac{3}{2}(\mathbf{L} \cdot \mathbf{S})(\mathbf{L} \cdot \mathbf{I}) + \tfrac{3}{2}(\mathbf{L} \cdot \mathbf{I})(\mathbf{L} \cdot \mathbf{S}) - L(L+1)\mathbf{S} \cdot \mathbf{I} \right]. \quad (25)$$

It is interesting to note that we would have obtained an identical result by considering the exact form of the interaction between the electrons and the nucleus, but our approach has been more general and has not required knowledge of the details of this interaction.

To check the three parameter fit, more than three A values must be measured. In the case of oxygen, four values of A have been measured using Eqs. (12), (13) and (25). The measured values may be expressed in terms of the parameters as follows:

$$A_1(J = 1) = \frac{A^{10} + A^{01}}{2} - \tfrac{5}{2} A^{12} \quad ;$$

$$A_1(J = 2) = A^{10} + A^{01} + A^{12} \quad ;$$

$$A_1(J = 0 \leftrightarrow J = 1) = \sqrt{2/3}[A^{10} - A^{01} + \tfrac{5}{2} A^{12}] \quad ;$$

$$A_1 (J = 1 \rightarrow J = 2) = \frac{A^{10} - A^{01}}{2} - A^{12} \; .$$

Using the experimental values, $A_1(1) = 11.84\,(8)$, $A_1(2) = -1092.845\,(20)$, $A_1(0, 1) = -229\,(20)$ and $A_1(1, 2) = -548\,(8)$, we may calculate A^{12} in two ways, from the diagonal elements ($A_1\,(J = 1$ and $A_1\,(J = 2)$) and from the off-diagonal elements ($A_1\,(0 \rightarrow 1)$ and $A_1\,(1 \rightarrow 2)$: $A_1{}^{12} = -186.09$ McS (diagonal terms); $A_1{}^{12} = -181 \pm 10$ McS (off-diagonal terms). The agreement to within experimental error implies the fit of the four measurements to the parameters.

In the quadrupole ($k = 2$) case we can make the additional physical assumption that the interaction should not depend on spin. Therefore $k_S = 0$ and $k_L = k$; there is only one term, $A^{0,2}$. There is evidence in many cases that this is not strictly correct which implies that relativistic effects are present; this violates the assumption of SL coupling.

D. Hfs in a Magnetic Field.

The usual assumption when dealing with an atom in a magnetic field is that the extra interactions can be expressed in terms of an effective Zeeman Hamiltonian of the form

$$H_z^{eff} = -\frac{\mu_J}{J} \; J \cdot H - \frac{\mu_I}{I} \; I \cdot H \; . \tag{26}$$

The two terms correspond to the separate interactions of the electrons and of the nucleus with the field. In many atomic states such a Hamiltonian is seriously in error since it does not take into account the breakdown of J by the hfs and by the magnetic field. There will in general be second order perturbations between the J states belonging to a given SL multiplet of the form

$$\frac{\langle J| \, hfs \, |J'\rangle \, \langle J'| \, H_z |J\rangle}{W_J - W_{J'}} \; . \tag{27}$$

A simple order of magnitude estimate shows that such terms are of the same order as the μ_I term in Eq. (26). Thus Eq. (27) is of order

$$\frac{hfs \times \mu_J H}{\text{fine structure splitting}} \sim \frac{\mu_I}{\mu_J} \, \mu_J H \sim \mu_I H \; ,$$

where we have used the fact that the ratio hfs/fine structure is of order μ_I/μ_J.

These breakdowns of J terms have two effects. First, the appropriate effective Hamiltonian to use within an IJ multiplet will contain terms in addition to those in Eq. (26). Second, the parameters obtained using the effective Hamiltonian must be interpreted with care. Thus a measurement of the magnitude of the $I \cdot H$ term is *not* a measurement of the true nuclear moment but of the true nuclear moment plus all contributions from the breakdown of J which look like $I \cdot H$. It is clear that a general theory of the second order effects of the breakdown of J is of some interest.

Such a theory has been given by Woodgate (1966a) who expressed the effects of the perturbations in terms of effective operators in spherical tensor form. With a slight change of notation, his expression for the general effective Hamiltonian within an IJ multiplet takes the form

$$
\begin{aligned}
H_z^{eff} = - &\frac{\mu_J}{J} J \cdot H - \frac{\mu_I}{I} I \cdot H \\
&+ \left[T(n)^1 U(e)^0 \right]^1 \cdot H + \left[T(n)^1 U(e)^2 \right]^1 \cdot H \\
&+ \left[T(n)^2 U(e)^1 \right]^1 \cdot H + \left[T(n)^2 U(e)^3 \right]^1 \cdot H \\
&+ Z^2(e) \cdot [HH]^2 .
\end{aligned}
\tag{28}
$$

The first two additional terms take into account the product of Zeeman and magnetic dipole terms, the next two, the product of Zeeman and electric quadrupole terms and the last one, the product of Zeeman and Zeeman terms. In these expressions the $T(n)^k$ are the nuclear moment operators as before. The $U(e)^k$ and $Z(e)^k$ are spherical tensors in the space of the total electronic angular momentum. Their magnitudes depend on the off-diagonal matrix elements of the hfs and the Zeeman interaction and on the energy differences between the J states.

Probably the most important term in Eq. (28) is $[T(n)^1 U(e)^0]^1 \cdot H$ since its matrix elements are all proportional to those of the true nuclear interaction $\mu_I/I \ I \cdot H$. It therefore constitutes a pseudo-moment interaction which cannot be experimentally separated from the true moment. It is convenient to lump them together and write the combined term as $\mu'_I/I \ I \cdot H$. The other hfs and Zeeman product term looks a little like a nuclear interaction since its matrix elements are proportional to M_I at high fields. However, it can readily be distinguished experimentally since its matrix elements also depend on M_J.

An analysis of these second order effects is of considerable importance when one considers the feasibility of measuring nuclear magnetic moments in paramagnetic atoms. One can distinguish a variety of situations. The simplest is when the hfs constants A^k are known from low field experiments. Then one can calculate the corrections due to the breakdown in J and determine the true nuclear moment from the measured effective moment μ'_I. The accuracy of the corrections will be of the same order as the fit of the zero field hfs measurements to the $A^{k_S k_L}$; the theoretical assumptions are the same. Thus, if we have a thorough understanding of the hfs at zero field, the breakdown of J corrections can be extremely reliable. A second simple situation occurs whenever J takes its maximum or minimum value. One finds then that the two hfs and Zeeman product terms depend on the hfs constants in the same combination. A measurement of the part which depends on M_I allows the calculation of the pseudo-nuclear moment part and hence the determination of the nuclear moment to the accuracy of the measurements. Other more complicated situations occur when the hfs constants are not completely determined from measurements at low field and additional information has to be obtained from the M_J dependent term in order that the pseudo-moment can be calculated. An example of this is given below.

Woodgate has applied his analysis to the $4f^6$, ^7F multiplet of Sm. From the hfs in Sm^{149} at zero field one finds after taking into account the breakdown of SL coupling that

$$A^{01} + A^{10} = -1428 \ (1) \quad McS$$
and
$$A^{12} = -167.0 \ (2) \quad McS$$

As in all states with S = L one cannot separate A^{10} and A^{01} by measurements diagonal in J. However, by analyzing the measurements at high field, Woodgate was able to separate A^{10} and A^{01} and hence to calculate the true nuclear moment from the measured moment term. The result for Sm^{149} is

$$\mu_I^{149} = -0.8074 \ (7) \text{ n. m.}$$

The error quoted is the experimental one. The error in the theory can only come from inaccuracy in the calculation of the effect of the breakdown of SL coupling. This error is a little difficult to estimate, but from the degree of fit of the zero field hfs one would expect it to be about one part in a thousand, i.e., of the same order as the quoted experimental error. The accuracy of this result is quite remarkable in view of the fact that the effective moment differs from the true moment by about 40%.

IV. The Central Field Approximation and Different $\langle r^{-3} \rangle$

We now turn to the most extreme approximation which we shall make — the central field model.* In this model we assume that the atomic electrons move in some sort of average potential from the nucleus and the other electrons. We also assume that the potential is central and spin-independent. Then we know that the wave-function for the atom can be expressed as a small number of determinantal products of single particle functions of the form

$$\varphi_{n\ell m \, m_s} = \frac{R_{n\ell}(r)}{r} \, Y_m^\ell (\theta, d) \, \chi_{m_s} \, , \tag{29}$$

where the radial functions are independent of the magnetic quantum numbers m and m_s.

In the usual non-relativistic approximation the magnetic dipole hfs interaction takes the form**

$$H_{dip} = \frac{2\mu_I \mu_0}{I} \, I \cdot \sum_i \left\{ \frac{\ell_i}{r_i^3} - \sqrt{10} \, \frac{[SC^2]^1 (i)}{r_i^3} \, + \right.$$

$$\left. \frac{8\pi}{3} \, \delta (r_i) \, S_i \right\} \, , \tag{30}$$

while the electric quadrupole interaction is

$$H_{quad} = - \frac{e^2}{2} \, Q_{op}^2 \cdot \sum_i \frac{C_i^2}{r_i^3} \, . \tag{31}$$

Here Q_{op}^2 is a tensor of rank 2 in the space of the nuclear coordinates; its magnitude is defined in terms of the nuclear electric quadrupole moment Q by

$$Q = \langle II | Q_{op}^2 | II \rangle \, . \tag{32}$$

The dipole and quadrupole hfs are given by the expectation

---

*See description by R.E. Watson and A.J. Freeman, Chap. 2.
**See Chap. 1 by B. Bleaney.

values of Eqs. (30) and (31) and taken over the determinantal atomic wave-functions. The expectation value readily reduces to matrix elements between single particle states. Because of spherical symmetry the sum of the contributions from the closed shells adds up to zero and we need consider only the open shells. For reasons of simplicity we shall confine ourselves to atomic states having only a single open shell.

A. Single Open Shell

Since the evaluation of the angular integrals is straightforward, the expectation value of the hfs operators reduces to a multiple of either $\langle r^{-3} \rangle = \int R_{n\ell}^2 \, 1/r^3 \, dr$ or $[R_{no}(r=0)]^2$, depending on the value of the open shell orbital momentum ℓ. If $\ell = 0$, we have the obvious result that $A^{01} = A^{12} = 0$. For $\ell \neq 0$ we have the important results $A^{10} = 0$ and $A^{01}/A^{12} = K$ where K is some known function of the quantum numbers and is independent of the radial integrals.

For $\ell \neq 0$ these results form specific predictions of the central field model which can be tested against experiment. Thus for fluorine in the $2p^5$, ^2P state one should have $A^{10} = 0$ and $A^{01}/A^{12} = -5$. From Harvey (1965) one finds

$$A^{10} = 101 \text{ McS}, \qquad A^{01}/A^{12} = -5 \times 0.905.$$

In both cases we have quite large deviations from the central field predictions indicating that these predictions have to be treated with care. Similar deviations have been found in other atoms where sufficient experimental data is available.

B. Different $\langle r^{-3} \rangle$

One way of describing these deviations from the central field model is in terms of the effective Hamiltonian in the open shell:

$$H_{dip}^{eff} = \frac{2\mu_I \mu_0}{I} \quad I \cdot \sum_i \left\{ \ell_i \langle r_\ell^{-3} \rangle - \sqrt{10}[SC^2]^1(i) \langle r_{sc}^{-3} \rangle \right.$$

$$\left. + S_i \langle r_S^{-3} \rangle \right\} . \tag{33}$$

We assign to each of the tensor operators in the dipole hfs Hamiltonian a separate radial integral.* The predictions of the central field model are now $\langle r_s^{-3} \rangle = 0$, $\langle r_\ell^{-3} \rangle = \langle r_{sC}^{-3} \rangle$. The convenience of this form of parameterization lies in the removal of any

*See also Chaps. 1 and 2.

dependence on either the particular nuclear moment or atomic state involved so that comparison between different elements can be made very readily. We give below some results expressed in this form (Bleaney, 1966; Woodgate, 1966b).

Table IV: Experimental $\langle r^{-3} \rangle$ values in a_0^{-3} units.

	O($2p^4$)	F($2p^5$)	Sm($4f^6$)	Eu($4f^7$)
$\langle r_\ell^{-3} \rangle$	4.58	7.35	6.390	–
$\langle r_{SC}^{-3} \rangle$	5.19	8.14	6.513	–
$\langle r_S^{-3} \rangle$	0.477	0.601	-0.208	-0.211

An important question concerning the use of different $\langle r^{-3} \rangle$ needs to be answered. What is the justification for this particular method of parameterization? It is clear that the results from any given SL multiplet can always be expressed in this way since the hfs depends on the three parameters A^{01}, A^{10} and A^{12} and these can always be expressed in terms of the different $\langle r^{-3} \rangle$. While obviously convenient as a test, it is not at all clear that this is a physically sensible way to express deviations from the central field model. In order to answer this question we have to consider more closely the different ways in which the central field model can break down.

C. Configuration Interaction

The most obvious cause for the breakdown of the central field model is the neglect of the residual two particle electrostatic interactions. We shall discuss the effect of this using perturbation theory. While convergence problems may make this an unsatisfactory method for getting accurate numerical results, it is often very convenient for seeing the form that various effects take. A particularly useful trick in this respect is to express the effect of the perturbations in terms of effective operators acting within the set of states belonging to a configuration of interest.

A fairly complete theory using diagrammatic techniques has been given elsewhere (Sandars, 1966). Here we shall just consider the simplest case of second order perturbations. The effect on the hfs of the configuration of interest can be expressed in terms of an effective hfs operator having matrix elements given by

$$\langle A | H_{hfs}^{eff} | B \rangle = \sum_{E} \left[\langle A | \frac{1}{2} \sum_{i \neq j} \frac{e^2}{r_{ij}} | E \rangle \langle E | H_{hfs} | B \rangle \right.$$

$$\left. + \langle A | H_{hfs} | E \rangle \langle E | \frac{1}{2} \sum_{i \neq j} \frac{e^2}{r_{ij}} | B \rangle \right] \frac{1}{\omega_o - \omega_E} \quad . \quad (34)$$

As usual the sum is taken over a complete set of central field states excluding, of course, the ones belonging to the configuration of interest.

The important question is: what form does H_{hfs}^{eff} take? To answer this we consider the ways in which $| E \rangle$ can differ from $| A \rangle$ and $| B \rangle$. We can distinguish two situations:

    i) An electron is promoted from the core to an unoccupied shell.

    ii) An electron is promoted into or out of the open shell.

These two types of perturbations have very different effective operators. Type (i) can always be written in terms of a single particle operator $H_{hfs}^{eff} = \sum_{i} h_{hfs}^{eff}$ (i); it then follows immediately from symmetry considerations that the effective operator can be written in the same form as Eq. (33). On the other hand, perturbations of type (ii) lead to an effective operator having both *one* and *two* particle terms which obviously cannot be written in the form of Eq. (33).

We therefore have the important result that the physical usefulness of the different $\langle r^{-3} \rangle$ parameterization depends on the dominance of core excitations over open shell excitations. There are reasons for thinking that in many atoms this dominance may exist so that to this extent the use of this parameterization is justified. Interestingly enough, the $2p^n$ shell for which this parameterization was originally devised is an exception. It is well known that open shell excitations play an important role in this shell and so in this case the validity of using different $\langle r^{-3} \rangle$ is not clear.

D. Relativistic Effects

A second possible cause of the deviations from the predictions of the central field model is the effect of relativity. We can distinguish two basic relativistic effects: (i) Breakdown of SL coupling by the admixture of other states from the same configuration. Effects of this type are well understood and can be taken into account with considerable accuracy. We shall not consider them further. (ii) Effects due to the difference between the relativistic and non-relativistic single particle hfs matrix elements. These are of more interest to us and we shall consider them in this section.

Sandars and Beck (1965) have considered these single particle relativistic effects in some detail. They find the interesting result that such effects can be entirely taken into account by means of a Hamiltonian of the form of Eq. (33). In other words the effect of relativity on the magnetic hfs is essentially the same as that of configuration interaction and the two cannot be separated by straightforward measurements of hfs interactions. Sandars and Beck give expressions for the different $\langle r^{-3} \rangle$ in terms of the relativistic hfs radial integrals.

We have then the important result that it is not possible to distinguish configuration interaction from relativity without additional information. Of course in the lightest elements we know that relativistic effects are likely to be small compared to configuration interaction. But for the medium and heavy elements such an assumption is not generally possible. The two effects are likely to be comparable in magnitude unless some particular near degeneracy makes configuration interaction effects abnormally large.

It is worth pointing out that in certain favourable cases it is possible to distinguish the two effects by means of the Bohr-Weisskopf anomaly which for an $\ell \neq 0$ configuration can occur only if $\ell = 0$ electrons are admixed by configuration interaction. In this way, or rather by its reverse, it was possible to show that the magnetic hfs in the $4f^7$, ^8S state of Eu must be relativistic in origin (Evans et al., 1965).

E. The Quadrupole Interaction

Thus far, we have concentrated our attention on the magnetic dipole interaction and have rather neglected the electric quadrupole interaction. The reason for this is that the nuclear magnetic dipole moment is normally known whereas the electric quadrupole moment is not. Thus atomic information free from uncertainties about the nuclear moments is much more readily available for the dipole than for the quadrupole interaction.

However, there is one important difference between the

dipole and quadrupole interactions which is worth noting here. We have pointed out that in the case of the dipole interaction it is not possible to differentiate between configuration interaction and relativistic effects. The situation is quite different for the quadrupole interaction. Single particle relativistic effects introduce quite different operators from configuration interaction effects and the two can be unambiguously distinguished in favorable cases. Thus the quadrupole interactions in the $3d^5$, ^6S and $4f^7$, ^8S states of manganese and europium cannot be ascribed to configuration interaction but must be due to relativistic effects. The breakdown of SL coupling gives predictions of the wrong sign whereas the single particle relativistic effects are in qualitative agreement with the experimental results (Evans et al. 1965).

References

Baker, J. M. and Williams, F. I. B. (1962). Proc. Roy. Soc. (London) A267, 283.

Bleaney, B. (1966). Colloques Internationaux du Centre National de la Recherche Scientifique (to be published).

Evans, L., Sandars, P. G. H. and Woodgate, G. K. (1965). Proc. Roy. Soc. A289, 108 and 114.

Harvey, J. S. M. (1965). Proc. Roy. Soc. A285 581.

Kopferman, H. (1958). Nuclear Moments (Academic Press, New York).

Marrus, R. and McColm, D. (1965). Phys. Rev. Letters 15, 813.

Ramsey, N. N. (1955). Molecular Beams (Oxford University Press).

Sandars, P. G. H. and Lipworth, E. (1964). Phys. Rev. Letters 13, 719.

Sandars, P. G. H. and Beck, J. (1965). Proc. Roy. Soc. A289, 97.

Sandars, P. G. H. (1966). Colloques Internationaux du Centre National de la Recherche Scientifique (to be published).

Schwarty, C. (1955). Phys. Rev. 97, 380.

Woodgate, G. K. and Sandars, P. G. H. (1958). Nature 181, 1395.

Woodgate, G. K. (1966a). Proc. Roy. Soc. A293, 117.

Woodgate, G. K. (1966b). Colloques Internationaux du Centre National de la Recherche Scientifique (to be published).

5.   OPTICAL HYPERFINE MEASUREMENTS

A. Steudel

*Technische   Hochschule
Hannover,   Germany*

Table of Contents

I. Introduction

The hyperfine structure (hfs) of atomic spectral lines emitted as electric dipole radiation in the visible and ultraviolet has been known nearly as long as interference spectroscopy itself. The high spectral resolution necessary to resolve the hfs of the lines is nearly always achieved by means of a Fabry-Perot (FP) interferometer. Three developments have given new life to optical hfs measurements: (i) the introduction of the photoelectric recording FP spectrometer by Jacquinot and Dufour in 1948; (ii) the introduction of dielectric multilayers as coatings for the FP plates; (iii) the recent availability of enriched isotopes.

A. Elementary Theory of Optical Hyperfine Structure Measurements

Let us recall what one does when we measure the hf splitting of a line. Figure 1 shows two fine structure energy-levels, one with total electronic angular momentum $J = 1/2$ and the other with $J = 3/2$; it is assumed that the parity of the two levels is different so that electric dipole transitions are possible. We further assume that there is a nuclear spin $I = 1/2$. Then each fine structure level splits up into two hf levels, labeled by the quantum numbers F, the total angular momentum of the atom; the allowed hf transitions for electric dipole radiation proceed according to the selection rule $\Delta F = 0, \pm 1$. The hfs observed in the line is shown schematically. There are three components corresponding to the three allowed hf transitions with intensity ratios given by the well known theoretical

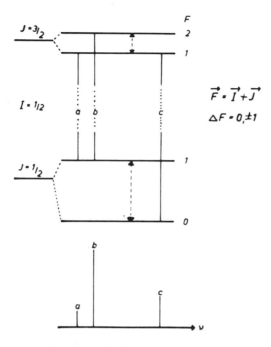

Fig. 1: Electronic levels split by magnetic hyperfine interactions and allowed dipole transitions.

intensity formulae (Kopfermann, 1958). The distance between the components a and b gives the hf splitting of the upper level and the distance between the components a and c gives the hf splitting of the lower level. The transitions indicated by the dashed lines are the magnetic dipole transitions one can observe by the methods of radio frequency spectroscopy.

Figure 2 shows the hf splitting in somewhat more detail. Here, a $^3P_1$ fine structure level and a nuclear spin of 5/2 is assumed. If there is only the magnetic interaction between the nuclear magnetic dipole moment and the magnetic field produced by the electron core at the nucleus, then the fine structure level splits up so that the Landé interval rule is fulfilled, which means that the ratio of the spacing between the F = 7/2 and F = 5/2 hf levels to the spacing between the F = 5/2 and F = 3/2 hf levels is 7 to 5. The absolute value of the splitting is given by the A factor which is defined as

$$A = \mu_I \overline{H(0)}/I \cdot J \qquad (1)$$

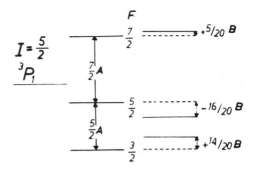

Fig. 2: $^3P_1$ fine structure
level and splittings due
to magnetic and electric
hyperfine interactions.

where μ_I is the nuclear magnetic moment and $\overline{H}(0)$ is the average
field due to the electrons at the nucleus.

If there also exists an electric interaction between the
nuclear electric quadrupole moment and the electric field gradient
(efg) produced by the electron core at the nucleus then the hf levels
are shifted (Fig. 2). The magnitude of this shift is determined by
the quadrupole coupling constant B;

$$B = e\, Q\, \overline{\rho_{JJ}(0)} \tag{2}$$

where e is the electronic charge, Q is the nuclear quadrupole
moment, and $\rho_{JJ}(0)$ is the average value of the efg at the
nucleus.

The energies of the hf levels are given by the well known
formula

$$W = W_I + A f_1 (IJF) + B f_2 (IJF) \tag{3}$$

where W_I is the energy of the fine structure level. The second
term is the magnetic interaction and the function f_1 is part of the
quantum mechanical expression for the cosine of the angle between
the directions of the vectors I and J. The third term is the electric interaction and the function f_2, first given by Casimir (1936),
corresponds to the quantum mechanical expression for the second
spherical harmonic of the angle between the directions of I and J.
As can easily be shown, the center of gravity of the hf splitting,
which is calculated taking into account the statistical weights of
the hf levels, coincides with the position of the unsplit fine structure level.

In optical hfs measurements one measures the distances between components in a line and the energy distances between
hyperfine levels in wave number units. The unit used is 10^{-3} cm^{-1},

abbreviated as 1 mK (milliKayser), which corresponds to 30 Mc/sec or 1.24×10^{-7} eV.

B. Determination of Nuclear Spins and Nuclear Magnetic Dipole Moments

Let us consider the determination of a nuclear spin and a nuclear magnetic dipole moment from optical hfs. In most cases, it is fairly easy to determine the nuclear spin as the spin can only be of integral or half-integral values. There are essentially three methods for the determination of a nuclear spin from optical hfs: (i) In many cases it is sufficient to count the number of the hf components of the corresponding isotope. This is, of course, only possible if the electronic angular momentum J of one of the levels is greater than the nuclear spin I. (ii) The nuclear spin can sometimes be determined from the ratios of the distances between hf components. (iii) The nuclear spin can sometimes be determined from the relative intensities of the hf components.

Apart from some special cases, no very high accuracy is required for the determination of nuclear spins. This is evident from the fact that about 80 percent of the known nuclear spins of the stable isotopes were first determined by optical hfs measurements.

There are two possible ways to determine the nuclear magnetic dipole moment from the hf splitting of a fine structure level. The first is the calculation of the nuclear magnetic moment from the measured A-factor; this means the magnetic field at the nucleus has to be calculated. To this end, it is necessary, of course, to know the exact electron configuration and the coupling of the electrons in the fine structure level. The accuracy under favorable circumstances with which the nuclear magnetic moment can be calculated from the A-factor is of the order of only a few percent. This is known from the comparison of the magnetic moments which were calculated in this way and from the values which have been measured very accurately, e. g. , by means of the nuclear induction method.

A second method can be used if there are two isotopes with hf splitting and if the nuclear g-factor is known for one of the isotopes from other measurements. It is then possible to calculate the nuclear g-factor for the second isotope from the ratio of the

A-factors of both isotopes since the A-factor is proportional to the nuclear g-factor. This method ignores a possible hf anomaly. *

II. The Fabry-Perot Spectrometer

A. Elementary Theory

Since the elementary theory of the FP interferometer is well known, it will be sufficient to recall the theory here only very briefly. The FP consists of two transparent plates with faces which are, in principle, perfectly plane and parallel and in the simple theory the surfaces of the plates are assumed infinite so that diffraction effects may be neglected. Each of these faces is covered by a reflecting coating of reflection coefficient R, transmission coefficient T and coefficient of absorption A, the three quantities being related by $R + T + A = 1$. (Of course, these are the coefficients for the intensities and not for the amplitudes.) An incident ray is divided by multiple transmissions and reflections into an infinity of rays transmitted parallel to each other which recombine at infinity and interfere. Thus at the focal plane of a lens one has interference fringes. If the FP is illuminated by an extended monochromatic light source one has the well-known system of concentric rings.

Between two successive transmitted rays there exists a path difference g. If the ratio of the path difference g to the wavelength λ is an integer, the transmitted rays interfere constructively and the incident energy is transmitted. If this condition is not fulfilled exactly, the multiple rays interfere destructively and the incident energy is reflected back to the source. The path difference has the value

$$g = 2 \, nt \cos \Phi \tag{4}$$

t being the geometric distance between the coated faces of the FP plates, n the index of refraction of the medium between the plates and Φ the angle of incidence of the beam. Since g depends on Φ, the different radiations of the spectrum are transmitted in different directions. Hence a photographic plate placed in the focal plane receives at each point the corresponding information. This is the application of the FP in the spectrographic method. As is usual in this method, the dispersion of the FP is crossed with the dispersion of a prism or a grating spectrograph giving the best

---

* *B. Bleaney, Chap. 1.*

exploitation of the photographic plate. This is the way in which the FP was used for a long time. In fact, up to 1948 nearly all optical hfs investigations of atomic spectra using high resolution were done by this method.

In 1948, Jaquinot and Dufour introduced the photoelectric recording FP spectrometer. Since then a great number of hfs investigations have been performed using this method. In principle the experimental setup is the following. From the atomic spectrum emitted by the light source, a premonochromator isolates the light of the fine structure line whose hfs is to be investigated. The FP interferometer is placed in the parallel light beam behind the premonochromator. In this application of the FP the photographic plate is replaced by a diaphragm, usually circular, which isolates part of the central order of the system of interference rings. FP and diaphragm together act as a filter or monochromator. To make a spectrometer it is sufficient to place a detector coupled to a recorder behind the isolating diaphragm and to vary continuously the wavelength transmitted by the FP in the direction of the optical axis. This is achieved by varying the optical thickness of the FP. An increase of the optical thickness expands the ring system in front of the diaphragm and thus the hfs of the line can be recorded.

For high resolution work in the visible and ultraviolet region, the variation of the optical thickness is normally achieved by changing the index of refraction of the gas between the FP plates while leaving the geometric distance of the plates constant; this is easily done by changing the pressure of the gas between the FP plates. One sees readily that in the FP spectrometer the FP acts as a wavelength filter with variable transmitted wavelength. The exploration of the line structure is done by the variation of the optical thickness while in the spectrographic application the angle of incidence is the variable used for the exploration. The decisive advantage of the FP spectrometer is that one measures the intensities immediately and exactly in a linear scale. This advantage enables hfs measurements to be done with much higher accuracy than was formerly possible with the photographic plate. This will be demonstrated quite clearly from the examples on hfs measurements which we give below. Another advantage is that the hfs is recorded in a linear wavelength scale if one changes the optical thickness linearly with time. This makes the measurements of distances between hfs components very simple.

B. The Real Fabry-Perot Interferometer

Before giving further experimental details of the spectrometer, we first make some general remarks on the FP interferometer itself.   Let us assume that we have an ideal FP, i. e. , the plates are perfectly plane and parallel and the diaphragm has a negligibly small width.   Let us further assume that the FP is illuminated by an exact monochromatic line; then the intensity distribution is given by the well-known Airy function and is shown in Fig. 3.   The successive orders of the interferometer are also shown.   The distance between two neighboring orders is called the free spectral range.   From the condition that the order k for a line with wave number $\nu + \Delta\nu$ just coincides with the order $k + 1$ for a line with wave number ν it is easily found that the free spectral range $\Delta\nu$ measured in wave numbers is given by

$$\Delta\nu = (1/2t) \qquad\qquad (5)$$

where t is the thickness of the FP $(n \approx 1)$.   The half-width a of each peak expressed as a fraction of the free spectral range turns out to be

$$\frac{a}{\Delta\nu} = \frac{1-R}{\pi\sqrt{R}} \; . \qquad\qquad (6)$$

One sees that the half-width measured as a fraction of the free spectral range depends only on the reflection coefficient R of the coating of the FP plates.   For a higher R, one has a smaller half-width.   By analogy with the diffraction grating, the reciprocal can be interpreted as the effective number of interfering beams

$$N_R = \frac{\pi\sqrt{R}}{1-R} \qquad\qquad (7)$$

where N_R is called the reflecting finesse.   The absolute half-width of a component is of course given by $a = (\Delta\nu/N_R)$.   Thus the larger the spacer of the FP, the smaller the half-width of the components.

Fig. 3: Intensity of light transmitted through the Fabry-Perot (see text).

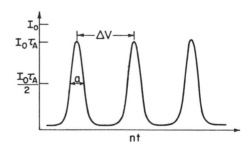

Consider the height of the maxima in Fig. 3. If the incident intensity is I_0, then the maxima of the transmitted light are given by $I_0 \tau_A$ where

$$\tau_A = \left(1 - \frac{A}{1-R}\right)^2 \tag{8}$$

One sees that this factor differs from unity only because the coatings have an absorption coefficient A. What one wants is to have coatings with an absorption coefficient A as small as possible.

We turn now to a more realistic FP. The surfaces of the plates are no longer perfectly plane; there are imperfections due to imperfect polishing. That means that the thickness of the FP is no longer a constant over the whole surface of the plate, but has a variation given by δt. We may describe this situation by saying we have now several small FP's all having a slightly different thickness. Of course this must result in a broadening of the lines observed.

For a more quantitative description, assume the hypothetical case in which $R = 1$; then the Airy function has infinitely sharp peaks, $a = 0$. If we illuminate the FP by a monochromatic line with wave length λ the observed intensity distribution, D, is caused only by the imperfections of the surfaces of the plates. Of course, the shape of the function D depends on the nature of the imperfections: for example, D is a Gaussian function in the case of randomly distributed micro-defects; it is a rectangular function if the circular plates have a slight spherical curvature. The shape of D can be deduced from experimental measurements on the plates. The half-width d of the function D is related to the variation δt of the thickness of the FP by

$$d \approx \Delta\nu \, \frac{2\,\delta t}{\lambda} \tag{9}$$

The ratio of $\Delta\nu$ to d is also a coefficient of finesse of the same nature as N_R defined in Eq. 7:

$$\frac{\Delta\nu}{d} = N_D = \frac{\lambda}{2\,\delta t} \quad . \tag{10}$$

It is usual to express δt in terms of the wavelength λ where λ equals 5000 Å. One says that the FP plates are flat to within $\delta t = \lambda/m$, then $N_D = m/2$. Good FP plates have $\delta t = \lambda/100$ over a diameter of 5 cm. This means $N_D = 50$. In this case it is impossible to observe lines with a half-width smaller than $\Delta\nu/50$. Therefore N_D is the most severe limitation for the resolving power obtained with the FP and for this reason N_D is often called the limiting finesse.

In the actual case, the instrumental function V of the FP is of course given by the convolution of the Airy function A and the function D describing the imperfections of the surfaces of the plates. We have

$$V(\nu) = \int A(\nu') \, D(\nu - \nu') \, d\nu' = A * D \qquad (11)$$

One can say that the Airy function is smeared out with the function D. Therefore the half-width v of the function V resulting from the convolution is greater than the half-width of the Airy function a and the half-width d of the function D. But the half-width v is always smaller than the sum $a+d$. If the intensity of the incident monochromatic line is I_0 then the maximum of the Airy function has the value $I_0 \tau_A$. The maximum of the function V has the value $I_0 \tau_A \tau_E$ with the factor τ_E, resulting from the convolution of the functions A and D, smaller than 1.

For our instrumental function V we can again define a finesse N_V by the ratio of the free spectral range to the half-width of the function V:

$$N_V = \frac{\Delta \nu}{v} . \qquad (12)$$

N_V is smaller than N_R and N_D. Our aim is to have as high a value of N_V as possible. Using dielectric multilayers as coatings on the FP plates, N_R can reach very high values (up to several hundreds, for example). On the other hand, the value of N_D is limited by the surface imperfections in the FP plates: in the visible region, N_D can hardly exceed 50; in the ultraviolet region, its value is still lower. This limitation of N_D to rather low values is actually the greatest disadvantage of the FP.

N_D is given by the FP plates used in the experiment. Let us choose a value for the reflecting power of our coatings so that $N_R = N_D$. For $N_D = 50$ this means $R = 0.94$. In the case $N_R = N_D$, we find from the convolution of the functions A and D the finesse $N_V \approx 0.7 \, N_D$ and $\tau_E \approx 0.8$. Let us compare these figures with the case $N_R = 3 \, N_D$. Here we have to choose a value of the reflecting power $R = 0.98$, again assuming $N_D = 50$. Now the effective finesse is approximately $N_V \approx 0.9 \, N_D$, but the transmission factor τ_E has decreased to about 0.3. These figures show that it is not always practical to have a reflecting power as high as possible. The increase of the reflecting power from 0.94 to 0.98 results in only a very small increase of the finesse N_V and hence in a very small increase of the resolving power. On the other hand, one has a serious loss of luminosity — the transmission factor τ_E decreases from 0.8 to 0.3. Moreover the transmission factor τ_A defined by the Airy function also decreases with increasing reflecting power because $1 - R$ appears in the denominator (Eq. 8). Therefore, one has to make a compromise between resolving power and luminosity. In many cases, it will be suitable to choose $N_R = N_D$. Then one has a finesse of about $N_V \approx 35$ assuming $N_D = 50$.

Up to now we have only discussed the FP interferometer itself assuming the width of the circular diaphragm (an essential part of the FP spectrometer) to be 0. To take the finite width of the circular diaphragm into account one has to evaluate the convolution of our function V with another function F which describes the diaphragm. In the case of the circular hole, F is a rectangular function whose width is determined by the diameter of the hole and the focal length of the lens forming the image of the interference rings on the diaphragm. The convolution $V*F = W$ gives the instrumental function W of our FP spectrometer. It is the convolution of the Airy function A, the function D describing the imperfections of the surfaces of the FP plates, and the rectangular function F describing the circular diaphragm. As there are no restrictions in choosing the width of the diaphragm, and therefore the width of the function F, we need not discuss the convolution with the function F in detail here. It may be sufficient to mention, that the convolution with the function F increases the line width only slightly. If the diameter of the circular hole is chosen in such a way that the half-width of the function F equals the half-width of the function D it turns out that in the case $N_R = N_D = 50$, the resulting finesse for the instrumental function W (defined by $N = (\Delta\nu/w)$ where w is the half-width of W) is $N = 30$. The resolving power is defined by $R = (\nu/\delta\nu)$, ν being the wave number of the monochromatic line, $\delta\nu$ the half-width of the line produced by the apparatus. For the FP spectrometer, $\delta\nu = w = (\Delta\nu/N)$ and therefore $R = (\nu N/\Delta\nu)$. Then for green light ($\nu = 20,000$ cm^{-1}) and a spacer $t = 10$ mm one has a resolving power of $R = 10^6$ for $N = 30$.

The instrumental function W just derived can only be observed if the FP is illuminated by a monochromatic light source such as a laser beam. The observed intensity distribution B′ in hfs investigations is of course the convolution of the instrumental function W with the intensity distribution B emitted by the light source, $B' = W*B$. The observed intensity distribution B′ approaches B as the width of the instrumental function W becomes smaller in comparison with the width of the emitted lines.

Let us mention briefly the coatings of the FP plates. Great progress has been made with the introduction of multi-layered dielectric coatings which have a very low absorption compared to the metallic layers used formerly (e. g. Hefft et al. , 1963). Therefore, the luminosity of the FP has been increased considerably. Moreover, in the ultraviolet region it is no problem to produce reflection coefficients of over 95 percent using dielectric multi-layers. Thus, especially in the ultraviolet region, a considerable gain in resolving power is achieved besides the increase in luminosity.

C.   The Spectrometer

We return to the FP spectrometer shown in Fig. 4. In many cases a hollow cathode is used as the light source. If isotope shift measurements are made, several light sources may be used where each light source contains one isotope; the light sources are exchanged during the recording. After the light source there is the premonochromator; in many cases a grating monochromator with plane grating is used.

The FP is enclosed in an air-tight box. Before starting a recording the box is evacuated to a few mm Hg. Then the pressure in the box is increased linearly with time up to a pressure of about 700 mm Hg; this can be achieved in a time varying between 10 minutes and several hours. A one atm change in pressure corresponds to an explored wavelength interval

$$\delta\lambda = \lambda(n-1) \ .$$ (13)

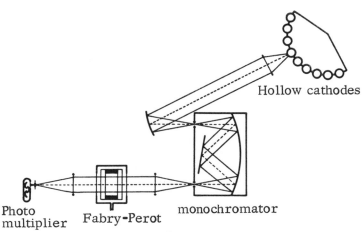

Fig. 4: Fabry-Perot spectrometer.

For air or N_2 the index of refraction at 1 atm is about $1+3 \times 10^{-4}$, which means that $\delta\lambda = 1.4 \,\text{Å}$ for $\lambda = 5000 \,\text{Å}$. The wavelength interval explored does not depend on the spacer used, but the number of orders which can be recorded does. With a spacer of 10 mm, 11 orders are recorded by a pressure variation of 1 atm if the wavelength is 5000 Å.

After the FP there is the circular diaphragm behind which is placed a photomultiplier. The photomultiplier is cooled by liquid air to reduce the dark current of the cathode.

The specimen material covers the sides or the base of the hollow cathode; it may be in the form of metal, oxide, nitrate, or another simple chemical compound. As carrier gas for the discharge, noble gases are used with a pressure of about 1 mm Hg. The positive column of the discharge is completely suppressed by bringing the anode close to the cathode. There is only the negative glow in the cathode space which yields an intense excitation of the atomic spectra. The material covering the walls of the cathode space is sputtered by ion bombardment. The cathode is partially submerged into liquid air and if small discharge currents, of the order of 5 mA, are used the temperature of the discharge is about 50° over that of liquid air. The line shape of the emitted lines is almost completely determined by the Doppler-effect corresponding to the temperature of the discharge.

The relative intensities of the hf components emitted by the hollow cathode agree well with the theoretical ones, since self-absorption in the lamp can be made negligibly small and since no electric field exists in the space of the cathode glow.

III. Nuclear Magnetic Moment of Os^{187}

The example we give for the determination of a nuclear magnetic moment concerns the stable isotope Os^{187} (Guthöhrlein et al., 1961). Up to 1961 no reliable data were available for the spin and magnetic moment of this isotope. One understands the reason for this when one looks at the natural abundance of the Os isotopes shown in Table I. There are essentially three even isotopes and an

Table I: Relative abundances of Os isotopes.

Mass No.	184	186	187	188	189	190	192
Relative Abundance in percent	0.018	1.586	1.643	13.27	16.14	26.38	40.96

abundant odd isotope, 189. The abundance of the Os^{187} is only
1.6 percent.

Figure 5 shows schematically what the hfs of an Os line
(4261 Å) looks like when natural Os is used. We see the three
most abundant even isotopes 192, 190, and 188 which have no hfs
because their nuclear ground states have zero spin. The lines of
these isotopes do not coincide because there is an isotope shift;
the relative intensities are given by the abundance of the isotopes
in the natural isotope mixture. The odd isotope with mass number
189 has a nuclear spin of 3/2 and the line splits into four components: 189 a, b, c, and d. The relative intensities of the four
components are determined by the relative intensities of the
different hf transitions. There is a weak component which belongs
to the isotope 186. Finally, there are two components belonging
to the isotope 187 which are labeled α and β. Of course the components cannot all be resolved when natural Os is used; the assignments are the result of many hfs investigations made with enriched
isotopes. When we record the hfs of this line with natural Os we
are able to resolve only the components of the three most abundant
even isotopes 192, 190, and 188, and the components a and d of
the 189. We see nothing of the components of the isotope 187
which are of interest here.

Fig. 5: Schematic repre-
   sentation of hfs of
   natural Os.

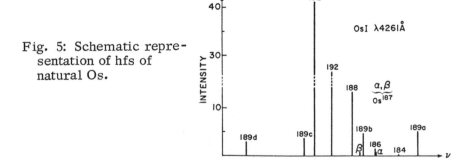

There is no possibility of detecting the weak components of
the isotope 187 using natural Os; obviously, the use of separated
isotopes would be the remedy. Normally, electromagnetically
enriched isotopes are used. In the case of Os^{187}, however,
nature itself has provided a pure Os 187 sample. As it is well
known, Re 187 decays by β-emission to Os 187 with a half-life τ
of about $5 \cdot 10^{10}$y. If one has a rhenium mineral available which
is not contaminated by natural osmium, the chemical separation of

Os from this rhenium mineral gives a pure Os 187 sample. In
this way a 5 mg sample of pure Os 187 was produced and the purity
of this sample (namely, the freedom of contamination by natural
Os) was checked by a mass spectrographic analysis.

Figure 6, which is part of a run, shows two orders of a
recording of the line and was made with the pure Os 187 sample.
One sees two well-resolved components, the more intense one
shifted to larger wave numbers; the distance between the components
turns out to be 52. 8 mK.

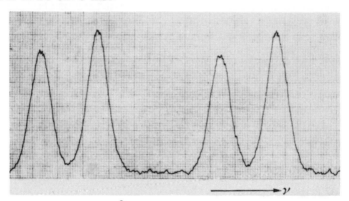

Fig. 6: Hfs of OsI (4261 Å) for a sample of pure Os^{187}. Two
orders are shown.

We studied three lines, and in all three lines a splitting of the
Os^{187} isotope into two components was found. The observed splitting in the three lines is caused by the splitting of the upper levels
belonging to the configuration $5d^6 6s\,6p$; the splitting of the lower
levels belonging to the configuration $5d^6\,6s^2$ is very small and
cannot be resolved. The fact that in all three lines just two components of Os^{187} are observed makes a spin I = 1/2 for this isotope very probable. It is also evident, however, that one can
assume a spin I = 3/2 and find a ratio of the magnetic splitting
factor A to the quadrupole splitting factor B such that just two
components are resolved and observed. However, since it does
not seem possible to do this for all the three lines the two observed
components are the first argument for a spin I = 1/2. The second
argument for I = 1/2 is the intensity-ratio. We measured this
ratio in all three lines for the two observed components, and the
results of the measurements are shown in Table II, with the theoretical intensity ratios for a spin of 1/2. The very good agreement leaves no doubt; the spin of Os^{187} is really 1/2.

Table II: Summary of Os^{187} hfs measurements.

λ [Å]	Ratio of Intensity		$\Delta\nu$[mK]	μ_I[n. m.]
	Theor.	Exp.		
4261	1. 200	1. 20 ± 0. 02	52. 8 ± 0. 1	0. 0652 ± 0. 0001
4420	1. 250	1. 25 ± 0. 03	35. 5 ± 0. 4	0. 0663 ± 0. 0007
4794	1. 333	1. 30 ± 0. 06	24. 0 ± 0. 4	0. 0656 ± 0. 0011

The measured values in mK for the splitting of Os^{187} are also given in Table II. All the three values derived from the measured splittings are in good agreement. The values for the magnetic moments have been calculated as follows. From the measurements on natural Os the structure of Os^{189} in these lines is known and therefore the A-factors of Os^{189} for these three lines are known. Furthermore, the magnetic dipole moment of Os^{189} has been measured by NMR. It is therefore possible to evaluate the magnetic dipole moment of Os^{187} by the relation g_I^{187} = $(A^{187}/A^{189})g_I^{189}$. As a summary result, we would give μ_I^{187} = (0. 0653 ± 0. 0010) n. m. The following uncertainties contributed the bulk of the error of about 2 percent (i) The hfs anomaly between Os^{189} and Os^{187} is apparently not known and therefore not considered in the calculations; (ii) The splitting of the levels of the configuration $6s^2$ is small, but not exactly known. We therefore chose our error for the magnetic moment so that these uncertainties were included. The contribution of the uncertainties of the measured splittings to this error of μ_I can almost be neglected.

Since the magnetic moment of Os^{187} is only about 0. 06 nuclear magnetons, there are unusually small interaction energies for this nucleus in an external magnetic field. Methods such as the nuclear induction method, which depend on this magnetic interaction energy, are therefore difficult to apply because the noise will usually exceed the signal. This is the reason why the magnetic moment of Os^{187} has only been measured by optical hfs investigations.

IV. Hyperfine Splitting of the Configuration $4f^7\,(^8S)\,6s\,6p$ in Eu

As our next example, we discuss the hf splitting of the configuration $4f^7(^8S)6s\,6p$ in the first spectrum of Eu. The lines corresponding to the transitions from this configuration to the ground state $4f^7\,6s^2$ lie in the visible region. By studying the hfs of these lines

Schüler and Schmidt (1935) established that the nuclear spin for the ground state of both stable isotopes of Eu (mass numbers 151 and 153) is 5/2. The neutron numbers are 88 and 90, and both isotopes have approximately the same natural abundance. However, the important point of Schüler and Schmidt's investigation was that they found deviations from the interval rule of the separation between hf levels. They concluded that the nuclei of both Eu isotopes are not perfectly spherical and this was the discovery of the existence of nuclear electric quadrupole moments.

The values for the quadrupole moments are about ~ 1.2 b for the isotope 151 and about ~ 2.5 b for the isotope 153, i. e., the moments of the two isotopes are very different. This strong change reflects the very striking increase in nuclear deformation as the number of neutrons increases from 88 to 90, as has been observed in the isotope shift and Coulomb excitation of the nuclei of Nd, Sm, and Gd with corresponding neutron numbers. This anomalous change in nuclear shape which results from the incorporation of the 45th neutron pair is understood in the light of Nilsson's (1955) model.

It is surprising that since the work of Schüler and Schmidt almost nothing was done to get more reliable and more accurate values for the quadrupole moments of the two Eu isotopes from hfs measurements. Thus, it seemed worthwhile to measure the hf splitting of levels of the configuration $4f^7(^8S)6s\,6p$ with improved accuracy using the recent advances in experimental technique mentioned above (Müller et al., 1965). Our experiments stimulated Prof. Judd and his co-workers (Bordarier et al., 1965) to attempt a fairly complete theoretical analysis of the configuration $4f^7\,6s\,6p$.

A. Experiment

To start with the experiment, we show in Fig. 7 the level diagram of the levels of the first spectrum Eu in which we are interested. The ground state belongs to the configuration $4f^7\,6s^2$ and is an $^8S_{7/2}$ state. There are 12 levels belonging to the configuration $4f^7(^8S)6s6p$ which has four multiplets: one ^{10}P multiplet, two ^8P multiplets, and one ^6P multiplet. The two ^8P multiplets are called z^8P and y^8P. Only those transitions between the levels of the configuration $4f^7\,6s\,6p$ and the ground state which have been investigated are shown. The level $^{10}P_{11/2}$ cannot combine with the ground state because a transition with $\Delta J = 2$ is forbidden for dipole radiation. However, it is of interest to measure the hf splitting of this level because it has the highest J value of this configuration. It is therefore independent of coupling and the probability of

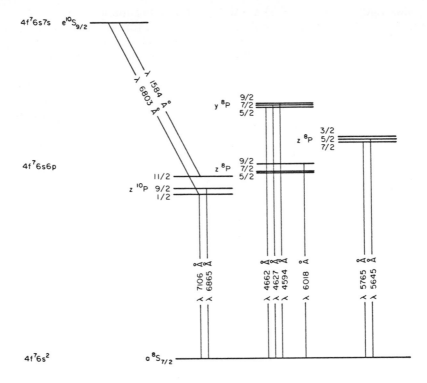

Fig. 7: Level diagram for EuI.

being perturbed by configuration interaction is small.

The usual way of finding the splitting of such a level in optical hfs investigations is shown in Fig. 7. The hf splitting of the $^{10}P_{7/2}$ level can be found from the transition ($\lambda = 7106$ Å) to the ground state. Then one investigates the hfs of the line $\lambda = 6803$ Å from which one can evaluate the hf splitting of the level $^{10}S_{9/2}$ belonging to the configuration $4f^7 6s\,7s$. This latter level also combines with the level $^{10}P_{11/2}$. Thus, the hfs of this transition enables us to find the splitting of the level $^{10}P_{11/2}$. Theoretically, one can find the splitting of both levels $^{10}P_{11/2}$ and $^{10}S_{9/2}$ by measuring only this transition. However, if the hfs of a line is somewhat complicated as it is in the case of this line, no high degree of accuracy would be achieved and so it is better to proceed by the way indicated.

Let us now consider the hfs of the lines corresponding to the transitions from the levels of the configuration $4f^7 6s\,6p$ to the ground state. We look first at the hf splitting of the ground state. There is the half-filled 4f-electron shell in which the 4f electrons are coupled to a $^8S_{7/2}$ state. In pure RS coupling neglecting relativistic effects the hf splitting of this state would be exactly zero. However, in all cases where a half-filled electron shell is coupled to an S-state, small hf splitting is found if the measurements are made with sufficient accuracy. The hf splitting of the ground state $^8S_{7/2}$ of Eu has been measured by Sandars and Woodgate (1960) by the method of magnetic resonance in an atomic beam. Therefore, the A and B values of the ground state are known with high accuracy for both Eu isotopes. The hf splitting of the isotope 151 in the ground state is of the order of 10 mK while the corresponding splitting of the isotope 153 is smaller because the ratio of the nuclear magnetic moments $(\mu_I^{151}/\mu_I^{153})$ is about 2.3.

This small hf splitting (10 mK) cannot be resolved by optical hfs investigation, if a hollow cathode is used as light source. Therefore, the hfs observed in a transition from a level of the configuration $4f^7 6s\, 6p$ to the ground state will be determined mainly by the hf splitting of the upper level containing an unpaired 6s-electron. The hfs to be expected for such a line for one isotope will be a flag pattern with $2I+1 = 6$ components if the nuclear spin I is smaller than or equal to the J value of the upper fine structure level. The intensities of the components are proportional to the statistical weights of the hf levels of the widely split fine structure level. This is shown in more detail in Fig. 8, where the splitting of the ground state and the splitting of the $^{10}P_{7/2}$ state of the configuration $4f^7 6s\, 6p$ are indicated. Of course, the energy scales are not the same for both states; the splitting of the upper state is about 70 times larger than the splitting

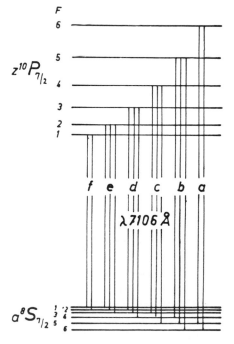

Fig. 8: Splitting of $z^{10}P_{7/2}$ and $a^8S_{7/2}$ level of EuI.

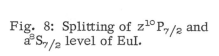

of the lower state.　Also indicated are the allowed hf transitions.
There are six groups of transitions labeled a, b, c, etc.　These
six groups correspond to the six components of the observed flag
pattern; each group consists of two or three transitions.　The wave
number difference between the transitions of one group is given by
the splitting of the ground state and therefore these distances are
too small to be resolved.

The investigations were done with highly enriched samples
of the Eu isotopes and the light source was a hollow cathode filled
with one or two mg of Eu_2O_3.　Figure 9a shows part of a recording
made with 151 sample with intensity shown as a function of wave
number.　The strongest component of the flag pattern is repeated
in the next order of the FP.　The two small components superposed
on the flag pattern are due to the remainder of the isotope 153 in
the sample 151.　There are four other still smaller components of
153 which are hidden by the components of 151.　The total hf splitting of 153 is about 2.3 times smaller than that of 151 and the
center of gravity of the 153 components is shifted with respect to
that of 151 by isotope shift.　The six components of the flag pattern
(Fig. 9a) are well resolved so that the five distances can be measured with a good accuracy.　Figure 9b shows part of a recording
of the same line, but now with the isotope 153.　Again there is a
flag pattern of six components, but the splitting is smaller.　The
free spectral range is only 357 mK in this recording compared to
833 mK in the 151 recording.

In both recordings the measured distances between the lines
are not exactly the splittings of the upper levels because of the
small (unresolved) splitting of the ground state.　In order to extract the values for the splitting of the upper level, the measured
distances must be corrected.　In order to do this one has to take
into account the small ground state splitting which is known from
measurements by the atomic beam method, the intensity ratios of
the hf transitions from the well-known intensity formulae and the
position of the components of the residuary isotope.　To do this
the splitting of the residuary isotope measured with the corresponding enriched sample, the known isotope shift and the ratio of
enriched to residuary isotope measured by mass spectroscopy
was used.

In order to calculate the corrections, one has to choose a
line profile.　As the corrections are very small, it is sufficient
to calculate the corrections using a Lorentzian or Gaussian line

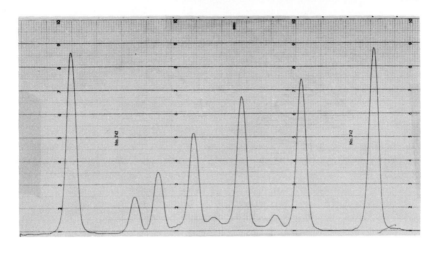

(a)

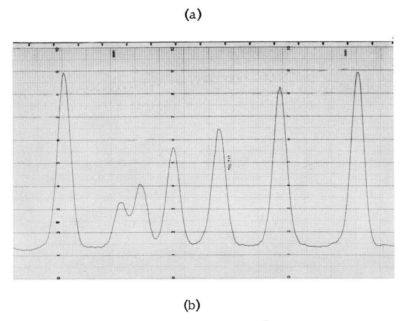

(b)

Fig. 9: Hfs spectrum of EuI (7106 Å). (a) Eu^{151} sample (free
spectral range 833 mK). (b) Eu^{153} sample (free
spectral range 357 mK).

shape. Both calculations were done and the results are nearly the same. The corrections are always smaller than 0.5 mK, corresponding to 2 percent of the linewidth. The distances between the hf levels can be determined with an accuracy of about 0.2 mK corresponding to three times the mean square error.

In order to calculate the A and B factors, two hf distances are necessary. Since more than two distances are available from the measurements it is possible to test the consistency of the results. Each hf distance between two neighboring levels F and F-1 called $\Delta W_{F-(F-1)}$ is given by A multipled by a function f depending on the quantum numbers I, J, and F, plus B multiplied by another function g of the quantum numbers I, J, and F.

$$\Delta W_{F-(F-1)} = Af(I, J, F) + Bg(I, J, F) \ . \tag{14}$$

The functions f and g are well known from theory. Therefore each measured hf distance ΔW defines a linear relation between A and B as shown in Fig. 10 for the level $^{10}P_{9/2}$. Each measured distance ΔW defines a straight line when B is plotted against A; the slope of each line is given by theory. Because of the uncertainty of the measurements each line can be shifted parallel to itself within the bars indicated which represent three times the mean

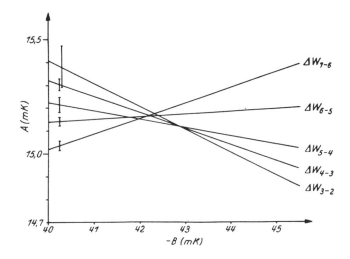

Fig. 10: A versus B, calculated for the level $^{10}P_{9/2}$. The experimental values are at the left (see text).

square error of the measurement. If the measurements are consistent, the five lines must intersect in one point, which they do, within the experimental error. In Table III we list the A and B values derived in this way. For three levels it was possible to measure A and B values for both isotopes, but in two levels the hf splitting is very small and it is only possible to give upper and lower limits for the A values.

Table III: Summary of hfs measurements in Eu^{151}, Eu^{153}.

Level	A(151)	B(151)	A(153)	B(153)
$z^{10}P_{11/2}$	31.13(10)	13.5 (15)		
$z^{10}P_{9/2}$	34.138(8)	-16.79(10)	15.16(2)	-42.13(12)
$z^{10}P_{7/2}$	32.32(2)	5.25(20)	14.38(1)	13.27(15)
$z^8P_{9/2}$	22.18(1)	9.65(15)	9.83(1)	24.62(15)
$z^6P_{5/2}$	-19.72(5)	-11.8(4)		
$y^8P_{9/2}$	-7.68(11)	8.6(12)		
$y^8P_{7/2}$	-7.1(2)	-15 (4)		
$z^6P_{7/2}$	$0<A<2.2$			
$y^8P_{5/2}$	$-5<A<0$			
$e^{10}S_{9/2}$	49.67(4)	0.3 (10)		

B. Analysis of A and B Values.

   1. Eigenfunctions

      For the discussion of the measured A and B values of Eu^{151} and Eu^{153} we need accurately coupled eigenfunctions for the 12 levels of $4f^7 6s 6p$ (Fig. 7). There is a large energy gap between the multiplet y^8P and the other multiplets of $4f^7 6s 6p$ (Table IV). The arrangement of the energies of the levels suggests taking, as basis for the calculations, the states in which the two electrons 6s6p are coupled either to ^1P or to ^3P. This means the states $| 4f^7 \, ^8S(6s6p) | \, ^{1\,3}P2S+1P \rangle$, i.e., $4f^7$ coupled to ^8S, 6s6p coupled to ^1P or ^3P, then ^8S and ^3P or ^1P coupled to the level $^{2S+1}P_J$. The multiplet y^8P which is separated from the other multiplets by an energy gap belongs in this approximation to the state in which 6s 6p is coupled to ^1P.

      These are only the basis states; the eigenfunctions for intermediate coupling have been derived by Bordarier et al. (1965). The energies of the levels depend on the spin-orbit coupling for the 6p

Table IV: Calculated and experimental values for the configuration
4f⁷6s6p of EuI (Bordarier et al., 1965).

Level	Experiment	Calculation α		Calculation β	
		Theory	Diff.	Theory	Diff.
$^{10}P_{11/2}$	15581.58	15588.5	- 6.9	15581.6	0.0
$^{10}P_{9/2}$	14563.57	14554.5	9.1	14559.8	3.8
$z^8P_{9/2}$	16611.79	16595.0	16.8	16600.3	11.5
$y^8P_{9/2}$	21761.26	21643.0	118.3	-	-
$^{10}P_{7/2}$	14067.86	14079.3	-11.4	14083.7	-15.8
$z^8P_{7/2}$	15952.31	15953.1	-0.8	15949.9	2.4
$y^8P_{7/2}$	21605.17	21602.5	2.7	21605.5	-0.3
$^6P_{7/2}$	17340.65	17324.8	15.9	17329.3	11.3
$z^8P_{5/2}$	15890.53	15886.8	3.7	15879.5	11.0
$y^8P_{5/2}$	21444.58	21564.2	-119.6	-	-
$^6P_{5/2}$	17707.42	17716.3	-8.9	17716.1	-8.7
$^6P_{3/2}$	17945.49	17964.4	-18.9	17960.6	-15.1

electron and on the Coulomb interactions between the nine electrons
4f⁷6s6p. Spin-spin and spin-other orbit interactions are expected
to amount to only a few cm^{-1}, and are therefore neglected. Using
adjustable parameters for the radial integrals, the calculated
energies of the levels were fitted to the experimental energies.
From the result of the least squares fit procedure shown in Table
IV, we immediately notice that the largest discrepancies between
theory and experiment appear in just two levels of the multiplet
y^8P — the highest multiplet of the configuration 4f⁷6s6p. Since
levels of another configuration, 4f⁷5d6p, lie only about 7000 cm^{-1}
above y^8P, configuration interaction may not be excluded and
as a configuration interaction is not included in the calculations we would expect the theoretical fit to be poorest for the
y^8P multiplet. To get an idea of the influence of a possible
configuration interaction a second least-squares fitting procedure
was carried out. This time, the two levels of y^8P that, in the
previous calculation, had shown the large discrepancies between

theory and experiment were rejected. The results of this second calculation, called calculation β, are also shown in Table IV. That there is an interconfiguration perturbation in the y^8P levels is also indicated by the results on the A-values and the B-values which will be discussed below. Furthermore, the measured isotope shifts for the y^8P levels show that these levels cannot be described by a pure $4f^7$ 6s6p configuration.

In addition to the energies of the levels, the corresponding eigenfunctions were also determined by the least squares fitting procedure. For example, the eigenfunction of the actual state $^6P_{7/2}$ is

$$| [^6P_{7/2}]) = 0.1177| ^8S, ^3P, ^{10}P_{7/2}\rangle + 0.5676| ^8S, ^3P, ^8P_{7/2}\rangle$$

$$+ 0.1100| ^8S, ^1P, ^8P_{7/2}\rangle + 0.8072| ^8S, ^3P, ^6P_{7/2}\rangle .$$

We see the mixture of the four RS states belonging to the J value 7/2; the actual state $^6P_{7/2}$ is only 65 percent pure. This demonstrates the importance of making allowance for deviations from perfect RS coupling. Actually the states of $4f^7$ 6s6p are best described in intermediate coupling.

2. Discussion of the A-factors of $4f^7$6s6p

A comparison between the measured and the calculated A-values may serve as a check on the eigenfunctions described above. Such a check will be possible since seven A-values were measured and only 2 or 3 parameters in the calculation of the A-values have to be adjusted. To explain this, we describe briefly the calculation of the A-factors.

The eigenfunctions were calculated by diagonalizing the matrix of the Coulomb and spin-orbit interactions, neglecting relativistic effects. However, the hyperfine interaction depends mainly on those parts of the electronic eigenfunctions lying close to the nucleus. The corresponding velocities of the electrons are not negligible compared to the velocity of light and therefore in calculating the hyperfine interaction, relativistic corrections have to be taken into account. To do this one normally has to transform all the eigenstates to jj coupling where one calculates matrix elements of single particle operators representing the hyperfine interactions of the single electrons using the relativistic Dirac eigenfunctions, a very cumbersome procedure. It would thus be extremely useful if one could construct an effective operator that would reproduce the correct relativistic results when acting between the ordinary, nonrelativistic states in LS-coupling. Such a method has been outlined by Sandars and Beck (1965).

Bordarier et al. (1965) have used the method of Sandars and Beck to calculate the A-factors of the levels of the Eu I configuration, $4f^7(^8S)6s6p$. Roughly speaking, each A-factor may be represented in the following form:

$$A = f_1 a_f + f_2 a_s + f_3 a_p , \tag{15}$$

where the constants a_f, a_s and a_p which include all relativistic corrections consist essentially of the product of the nuclear magnetic dipole moment μ_I and the expectation value of the magnetic field produced at the nucleus by the 4f electrons, the 6s-electron and the 6p-electron respectively. The factors f_1, f_2 and f_3 depend on the coupling of the electrons in the level concerned and can be calculated with the nonrelativistic eigenfunctions of this level. Hence, these factors are known quantities which depend on the level under consideration. We note that the 4f electrons are coupled to an ^8S term and therefore, in pure RS-coupling neglecting relativistic effects, a_f (non-rel.) = 0.

This is no longer the case if the 4f-electrons are treated relativistically. The reason for this is that the relativistic corrections are different for $f_{5/2}$ electrons and $f_{7/2}$ electrons and furthermore are different for the cross term between the $f_{5/2}$ and $f_{7/2}$ state. This means that the radial part of a $f_{5/2}$ electron is not exactly the same as the radial part of an $f_{7/2}$ electron. If one writes down the expression for a_f, we have something like this:

$$a_f \propto \mu_I \left\langle \frac{1}{r^3} \right\rangle_{4f} (12\ F' - 16\ F'' + 4\ F'''). \tag{16}$$

F', F'' and F''' are the well known relativistic correction factors calculated by Casimir (1936) where F' gives the correction for an $f_{5/2}$ electron, F'' the correction for an $f_{7/2}$ electron and F''' the correction for the cross term $f_{5/2,\ 7/2}$. In the non-relativistic limit the three corrections satisfy the relation F' = F'' = F''' = 1 and therefore the bracket and a_f vanishes. a_s is the a-factor for the 6s electron in the configuration $4f^7 6s6p$.

For a_p the situation is somewhat complicated because there are 3 contributions from the 6p electron to the magnetic hyperfine interaction, but we will not discuss the details here.*

*See Chap. 1 by B. Bleaney.

We will now attempt to fit the observed hyperfine structure constants A for the various levels of $4f^7(^8S)$ 6s6p using the states we have already calculated to determine the factors f_1, f_2 and f_3 of Eq. (15) and taking the quantities a_f, a_s and a_p as adjustable parameters. Two calculations have been carried out. In the first calculation a_s and a_f have been taken as adjustable parameters and a_p has been calculated from the spin-orbit coupling constant ξ_p and the nuclear magnetic moment. ξ_p has been accurately determined from the fine structure; the nuclear magnetic moment is very well known from atomic beam measurements. The relation between $\langle 1/r^3 \rangle_{6p}$ for the 6p electron entering the quantity a_p and the spin-orbit coupling constant ξ_p is given by the formula

$$\langle \frac{1}{r^3} \rangle_p = \frac{2m^2 c^2 \xi_p}{Z_{eff} H \hbar^2 e^2} . \tag{17}$$

H is a relativistic correction factor. One has to decide upon the value of the effective nuclear charge Z_{eff}; Bordarier et al. (1965) used $Z_{eff} = Z - 3$ which is a compromise between the traditional formula $Z - 4$ and $Z - 2.5$ which appears appropriate for a 6p electron in triply ionized rare-earth ions. On the other hand, Barnes and Smith (1954) proposed $Z_{eff} = Z - n$ where n is the principal quantum number of the p-electron; this means $Z - 6$ in our case. Using the value of $\xi_p = 1198$ cm^{-1} determined from the fine structure, the calculation of a_p gives, with $Z_{eff} = Z - 3$, $a_p = 17.4$ mK.

Let us now look at the comparison between observed and calculated A-values for Eu^{151} in Table V. A simple least-squares fit was carried out to determine a_s and a_f (method α). The discrepancies are of the order of 2% except for the two levels of the multiplet y^8P. This is not very surprising since in calculating the energy of the levels the largest discrepancies were also found for levels of the multiplet y^8P. This multiplet is the highest of the configuration $4f^7$ (^8S)6s6p and it lies near to levels of another configuration, so that an interconfiguration perturbation not included in the calculation may be possible. We note that in all cases the experimental errors are much smaller than the differences between experiment and theory and so it would be possible to check further refinements of the theory. The least-square squares fit carried out for 7 levels leads to A values for $^6P_{7/2}$ and $y^8P_{5/2}$ that lie within the bounds set for them by the experiment.

The fitting procedure gave for the 2 adjusted parameters: $a_s = 330.4$ mK; $a_f = -2.4$ mK. To get an idea of the sensitivity of the parameters to the conditions of the fitting procedure the calcu-

A. STEUDEL

Table V: Calculated and observed A-factor for Eu^{151}.

Level	Method	Calculated	Observed
$^{10}P_{11/2}$	α β	30.70 ⎤ 30.90 ⎦	31.13 ± 0.10
$^{10}P_{9/2}$	α β	34.35 ⎤ 34.62 ⎦	34.138 ± 0.008
$z^{8}P_{9/2}$	α β	22.16 ⎤ 21.69 ⎦	22.18 ± 0.01
$y^{8}P_{9/2}$	α β	-8.32 ⎤ -7.71 ⎦	-7.68 ± 0.11
$^{10}P_{7/2}$	α β	32.55 ⎤ 32.36 ⎦	32.32 ± 0.02
$z^{8}P_{7/2}$	α β	-10.23 ⎤ -10.44 ⎦	—
$y^{8}P_{7/2}$	α β	-7.57 ⎤ -6.95 ⎦	-7.1 ± 0.2
$^{6}P_{7/2}$	α β	1.09 ⎤ 0.54 ⎦	$0 < A < 2.2$
$z^{8}P_{5/2}$	α β	-24.20 ⎤ -25.44 ⎦	—
$y^{8}P_{5/2}$	α β	-4.68 ⎤ -4.11 ⎦	$-5 < A < 0$
$^{6}P_{5/2}$	α β	-18.98 ⎤ -19.74 ⎦	-19.72 ± 0.05
$^{6}P_{3/2}$	α β	-75.07 ⎤ -76.05 ⎦	—

lation was repeated with the eigenfunctions of calculation β. Furthermore a_p was taken as a variable parameter, in order to test the calculated value of a_p. Again a least-squares fit was carried out to determine the three parameters a_f, a_s and a_p. The agreement of the calculated A values with the experimental A-values is now slightly better. In particular, the large negative value of $^{6}P_{5/2}$ is accounted for. The parameters are now: $a_s = 332.5$ mK; $a_f = -2.5$ mK; $a_p = 18.3$ mK. The agreement between the results of the two methods of calculation is very satisfactory. It is the first time that such a comparison has been made for a large number of excited configuration A values which have been measured to high accuracy.

Another conclusion which may be drawn from these results concerns the good agreement between the a_p value derived from the fine structure and the a_p value derived from the hfs. The difference is only 5% and lies within the limits of uncertainty in the calculation. Theoretically, the two values for a_p need not be equal, because in the hfs the a_p value may be influenced by core polarization. Actually the two values of a_p are equal within the limits of error and we may conclude that the effect of core polarization on the a_p value is negligible.*

3. Core Polarization

We will now discuss the influence of core polarization on the hyperfine constants A. As is well known, core polarization means the polarization of the core s electrons by the electrons in unfilled shells. Let us consider, for example, the configuration of Eu III $\Psi = 4f^7 4s^2$, i.e., a closed 4s-shell and an unfilled 4f shell. From the point of view of perturbation theory it may be said that the Coulomb interaction admixes into the states of this configuration other states in which one 4s-electron has been excited to a vacant s-orbital, for instance of the configuration $\Psi' = 4s9s(^3S)4f^7$. In this configuration the two s-electrons give a contribution to the hyperfine splitting if they are coupled to a ^3S state. Then according to perturbation theory one should add to every matrix element of the normal hf interaction terms of the type:

$$\frac{\langle\psi\| \sum_i \frac{8\pi}{3}\, \delta\,(\mathbf{r}_i)\, \mathbf{S}_i\|\psi'\rangle\langle\psi'|\sum_{i\pm j} \frac{e^2}{r_{ij}}|\psi\rangle}{\Delta_{ss'}}\,, \tag{18}$$

where the first factor is the Fermi contact term, the second factor is the Coulomb interaction, and $\Delta_{ss'}$ is the energy difference between the two states. Of course, the admixture of this excited configuration is extremely small because the energy difference $\Delta_{ss'}$ is large; on the other hand the matrix elements of the hyperfine operator between 4s9s and $4s^2$ may be large thereby giving a significant effect. The total effect is the sum of all possible contributions, corresponding to the (virtual) excitation of every s-electron to all possible vacant s-electron orbitals, including those of the continuum.

*See Chap. 2 by R.E. Watson and A.J. Freeman.

Detailed calculation shows that for all levels of the configuration $4f^7$ we can allow for core polarization by replacing the a_f value by $a(4f) + a(s)_{c.p.}$ where $a(s)_{c.p.}$ is the part due to core polarization. When the normal contribution to the hfs from the valence electrons is small as is the case in the configuration $4f^7$, the effect of core polarization is particularly striking. We see this in comparing the A values of the ground states of Eu I and Eu III. Sandars and Woodgate (1960) measured the A values for the ground state of the first spectrum of Eu by the method of magnetic resonance in an atomic beam. For the isotope 151 the A value is $A^{151}(4f^7 6s^2) = -0.668$ mK. Baker and Williams (1962) measured the A-values of the ground state of the third spectrum of Eu by the method of electron nuclear double resonance (ENDOR). The measurements were done in a single crystal of calcium fluoride containing about 0.01% Eu^{2+}. For the A value of the isotope 151 they found $A^{151}(4f^7) = -3.430$ mK. Since the eigenfunctions of the 4f electrons are expected to be almost the same for the neutral atom ·as for the ion, the contribution to the A values coming from the 4f electrons must be almost the same in the neutral atom and in the ion. The difference between the two A values must be ascribed to different contributions of core polarization. The reason for these different contributions is that in Eu III inner s-electrons can be excited into the vacant 6s orbitals, i.e., $ns^2 \rightarrow (ns)(6s)$, with $n < 6$. In Eu I the 6s orbitals are occupied, but the 6s-electrons may be excited, i.e., $ns^2 6s^2 \rightarrow ns^2 (6s)(n's)$ with $n' > 6$. This makes all the difference. In both cases, of course, excitations like $ns^2 \rightarrow (ns)(n's)$ are possible.

Let us now return to our configuration in the first spectrum of Eu: $4f^7(^8S)6s6p$. We discuss only the core polarization produced by the 4f shell, and therefore will only discuss the a_f value. We found the for isotope 151 $a_f^{151}(4f^7 6s6p) = -2.4 \pm 0.1$ mK. If there were no core polarization the three values $A(4f^7 6s^2)$, $A(4f^7)$ and $a_f(4f^7 6s6p)$ would be almost equal because the eigenfunctions of the 4f-electrons are almost the same. Because the three values are different, we must take the core polarization into account. Detailed calculations of core polarization show that there is a simple connection between the three A values, i.e.,

$$a_f(4f^7 6s6p) = \tfrac{1}{2}[A(4f^7 6s^2) + A(4f^7)] \quad . \qquad (19)$$

This equation is only valid under the somewhat simplifying assumption that all s-electron eigenfunctions, all 4f-electron eigenfunctions, and all excitation energies are the same for the three electronic structures. In other words we may expect the equation to be only roughly fulfilled by the experimental data. Let us see now if this is the case: -2.4 mK $\approx \frac{1}{2}$ $(-0.668 -3.430)$mK $= -2.05$ mK. The agreement is very striking.

There is another simple relation between the a_f value of our configuration $4f^7 6s6p$ and another a_f value, namely the a_f value in configuration $4f^7 6s$ of the second spectrum of Eu:

$$a_f(4f^7 6s6p) = a_f(4f^7 6s) \qquad . \qquad (20)$$

As there are the same possibilities in the two configurations to excite inner s-electrons to vacant s-orbitals, the a_f values should be the same, again under the assumption that all s-electron eigenfunctions, all 4f-eigenfunctions and excitation energies are the same for the two electronic structures. The a_f value of the configuration $4f^7 6s$ in the second spectrum of Eu can be taken from the work of Krebs and Winkler (1960), who did optical hfs measurements on the resonance lines $4f^7 6s - 4f^7 6p$ in Eu II. From their measurements, the a_f of the configuration $4f^7 6s$ $a_f(4f^7 6s) = -2.4 \pm 0.2$ mK, in good agreement with Eq. (20) and the value of -2.4 ± 0.1 mK quoted above for $a_f(4f^7 6s6p)$.

4. Hyperfine Anomaly.

In discussing the A values of the ground states of Eu I and Eu III we have seen there is a different influence of c.p. but we could not decide how large the contribution from c.p. is. The consideration of the hf anomaly will enable us to do this.

For the two isotopes Eu[151] and Eu[153] the hf anomaly Δ of a level is given by

$$\Delta = \frac{A^{151}}{A^{153}} \cdot \frac{\mu_I^{153}}{\mu_I^{151}} - 1 \qquad . \qquad (21)$$

This expression will only be different from zero if two conditions are fulfilled: (i) the distribution of nuclear magnetism over the nuclear volume must be different for the two isotopes; (ii) the A value of the level under consideration must contain a contribution of an s-electron or a $p_{1/2}$ electron. As the influence of $p_{1/2}$ electrons is small, we will neglect it.

To calculate the hf anomaly we use the ratio of the nuclear magnetic dipole moments determined by Evans et al. (1965) by the method of triple resonance in an atomic beam:

$$\mu_I^{151}/\mu_I^{153} = 2.26505 \ (42) \qquad .$$

Let us first look at the ground state of Eu III for which Baker and Williams (1962) measured the A values of both isotopes by ENDOR. The hf anomaly turns out to be $\Delta(4f^7) = -0.53$ (2) %. This result means first, that the distribution of nuclear magnetism over the nuclear volume is different for the two isotopes; this was to be expected because the two nuclear magnetic dipole moments are very different. Second, there is a contribution from s-electrons to the A-values in the ground state of Eu III; therefore there is a contribution from core polarization.

Now let us look at the ground state of Eu I. Here the A-values of the two isotopes were measured by Sandars and Woodgate (1960). The hf anomaly turns out to be zero within the limits of error: $\Delta(4f^7 6s^2) = 0$. This means that there is no c.p. in the ground state of Eu I. Thus we can conclude that the A-values in the ground state of Eu I are caused only by the relativistic effects of the 4f-electrons.

If we assume that the contributions from the 4f-electrons a(4f) are approximately the same for the atom and the ion, we can easily calculate the contributions due to c.p. in the A-values of the ground state of Eu III. If we use only that part of the A-value, A(s), which is caused by s-electrons, we can define the hf anomaly due to s-electrons:

$$\Delta(s) = \frac{A(s)^{151}}{A(s)^{153}} \; \frac{\mu_I^{153}}{\mu_I^{151}} - 1 \; . \tag{22}$$

In the case of the ground state of Eu III we have to use for A(s) the contribution due to c.p., $a(s)_{c.p.}$. In this was we find: $\Delta(s) = -0.65\%$.

The hf anomaly is independent of the type of s-electrons chosen. This means the hf anomaly is independent of the principal quantum number of the s-electrons. Hence, we can compare this value from Eu III to the hf anomaly derived from our measurements in the configuration $4f^7 6s6p$ in Eu I, for which it was possible to measure the A-values for both isotopes in 3 levels. Therefore, the hf anomaly Δ could be derived for three levels. The values of Δ are given in Table VI. Of course, the values are different because the contribution from the 6s-electron to the A-values in the 3 levels is different. In the case of the configuration $4f^7 6s6p$ we deal only with the influence of the 6s-electron which gives the decisive contribution. Since we know the contribution from the 6s-electron to the measured A-values in the different levels from the theoretical analysis of the A-values we discussed

Table VI: Hyperfine anomalies for levels of EuI.

Level	$\Delta/\Delta(s)$(Theory)	Δ(Observed)	$\Delta(s)$(Calculated)
$1^{\circ}P_{9/2}$	0.88	$-0.57 \pm 0.12\%$	$-0.64 \pm 0.14\%$
$z^{8}P_{9/2}$	0.88	$-0.40 \pm 0.20\%$	$-0.45 \pm 0.23\%$
$1^{\circ}P_{7/2}$	1.18	$-0.75 \pm 0.12\%$	$-0.64 \pm 0.10\%$

above, we can easily deduce from the observed hf anomaly the values of the hf anomaly $\Delta(s)$ due to the 6s-electron. This is done simply by multiplying Δ by a factor given by the theory. These factors are listed in Table VI.

The 3 values for $\Delta(s)$ are in good agreement within their limits of error. Furthermore the mean value of about -0.6% is in good agreement with the figure of -0.65% derived from the resonance results in Eu III. We can conclude that the hf anomalies for Eu I and for Eu III that have so far been investigated fall into a consistent pattern.

5. Discussion of the B-values of $4f^{7}6s6p$

Now we come to the last point in our discussion of the measurements on the configuration $4f^{7}6s6p$, namely, the measured B-values. For 3 levels of the configuration $4f^{7}6s6p$ it was possible to measure the B values for both isotopes. The mean value of the ratio B^{151} to B^{153} is

$$\frac{B^{151}}{B^{153}} = 0.396 \,(9) = \frac{Q^{151}}{Q^{153}} \quad .$$

This ratio is equal to the ratio of the quadrupole moments Q^{151}/Q^{153} as the electric field gradient at the nucleus is the same for both isotopes.

Sandars and Woodgate (1960) measured the ratio of the B values in the ground state of the first spectrum of Eu by the method of magnetic resonance in an atomic beam. They found $B^{151}/B^{153} = 0.393\,(3)$. The two values are in good agreement. To get the absolute values of the quadrupole moments we have to calculate the electric field gradient at the nucleus. This is not possible in a reliable way for the ground state $4f^{7}6s^{2}$ but it may be done for the excited configuration $4f^{7}6s6p$.

be done for the excited configuration $4f^7 6s6p$.

In this configuration the electric field gradient at the nucleus is only caused by the 6p electron, the influence of the 4f-electrons being negligibly small. This is to be seen from the measured B value in the ground state. For the isotope 151 Sandars and Woodgate (1960) found B^{151} ($4f^7 6s^2$, $^8S_{7/2}$) = -0.02337 mK which is extremely small compared to the B values caused by the 6p electron, which are of the order of 10 mK. With the eigenfunctions for the levels of the configuration $4f^7 6s6p$ (which are well known, as we saw above), it is not difficult to calculate the electric field gradients for the different levels. As in the case of the A values the technique developed by Sandars and Beck (1965) was used to take relativistic effects into account.

The radial parameter one needs to calculate the electric field gradient is $\langle 1/r^3 \rangle_p$ for the 6p electron. There are two values available for this quantity: one from the spin-orbit coupling constant derived from the analysis of the fine structure, the other from the a_p value derived from the measured A values of the hfs. These two values agree satisfactorily. We used the mean value to determine the quadrupole moments, which are shown in Table VII.

Table VII: Quadrupole moment measurements.

Level	$Q(Eu^{151})$ [10^{-24} cm^2]	$Q(Eu^{153})$ [10^{-24} cm^2]
$z^{10}P_{11/2}$	1, 19 (4)[a] [7][b]	
$z^{10}P_{9/2}$	1, 18 (2) [5]	2, 95 (2) [10]
$z^{10} P_{7/2}$	1, 16 (6) [9]	2, 94 (4) [12]
$z^8 P_{9/2}$	1, 12 (2) [5]	2, 88 (2) [10]
$y^8 P_{9/2}$	0, 72 (10) [12]	
$y^8 P_{7/2}$	0, 97 (24) [27]	
$z^6 P_{5/2}$	1, 08 (5) [8]	

[a] Experimental errors.

[b] Errors introduced by theoretical evaluation.

The five values of Q derived from the multiplets $z^{10}P$, z^8P and $z^6 P$ are in excellent agreement. Only the two values derived from the two y^8P levels differ. This is not very astonishing, because in discussing the least squares fit of the energies of the levels and the A values we have seen that the y^8P levels are not very well described by our eigenfunctions.

The Eu^{153} nucleus is strongly deformed and its lowest excited energy levels are therefore rotational energy levels. For the less deformed Eu^{151} nucleus this is not the case. From measurements of the cross section for Coulomb excitation one can determine the intrinsic quadrupole moment Q_0 for Eu^{153}, as was done by Elbek (1963) who found the value $Q_0 = 7.00$ (35) b. The spectroscopic quadrupole moment Q is related to the intrinsic quadrupole moment Q_0 by the equation

$$Q = \frac{I(2I - 1)}{(I+1)(2I+3)} Q_0 .$$ (23)

With $I = \frac{5}{2}$, this leads to a value of $Q^{153} = 2.50$ (12) b. There is a discrepancy of 16% between the Q-value derived from hfs and the Q value derived from Coulomb excitation measurements. This discrepancy is not very surprising as one often finds discrepancies of this order of magnitude between the Q value derived from hfs measurements and the Q value derived from the reduced transition probability between rotational levels of the nucleus. It is assumed that the difference is due to the Sternheimer effect which we didn't apply to our results because there is no reliable calculation of the Sternheimer effect for Eu available at the present time. However, the Sternheimer antishielding factors normally applied are of the order of this 16% difference.*

V. Hyperfine Structure of Mn⁵⁵: Application of Atomic Beams to Optical HFS Investigations

After the theoretical discussion of the results on Eu let us now turn again to experimental problems. We have seen that there are two things which limit the resolving power achieved in optical hfs measurements: (i) the Doppler-width of the lines emitted by the light source; (ii) the instrumental width produced by the FP. We will discuss how these two widths can be reduced. Here we will deal with the problem of reducing the Doppler-width by the application of an atomic beam either in absorption or in emission.

This example concerns hfs measurements on Mn^{55}. Mn has only one stable isotope and the experiments were done to determine the nuclear electric quadrupole moment (Walther, 1962). Let us begin with a few remarks on the fine structure. The ground state of the first spectrum of Mn is $3d^5 4s^2$, $^6S_{5/2}$. As with Eu there is

*See Chap. 2 by Watson and Freeman and Chap. 11 by Mössbauer and Clauser.

a half-filled shell, in this case a half-filled 3d shell and as in Eu this state has a very small hf-splitting which has been studied by atomic beam resonance. The nuclear quadrupole moment cannot be determined from this splitting, but some levels of the first excited configuration 3d⁵4s4p are suitable for this purpose. In Fig. 11 we see part of the fine structure level diagram of the first

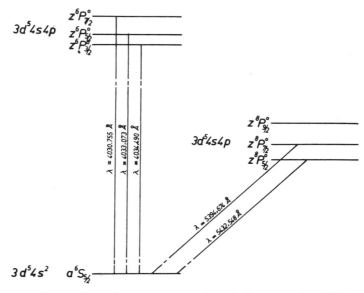

Fig. 11: Part of the fine structure level diagram for MnI.

spectrum of Mn. The configuration $3d^5 4s4p$ forms four multiplets, and contrary to Eu, the levels lie in good LS coupling. Consequently, the two transitions between the ^{8}P levels and the ^{6}S ground state which lie in the green region of the spectrum are typical intercombination lines; i.e., the ^{8}P levels have long lifetimes. In contrast, the three violet lines which connect the ^{6}P levels and the ground state are genuine resonance lines. The difference in lifetime between the ^{8}P and ^{6}P levels will be of importance later on.

Since the ground state has only a very small splitting while the excited states have a large splitting because of the unpaired 4s-electron, one expects a flag pattern for the hfs just as with Eu. The nuclear spin of Mn is $\frac{5}{2}$, so the flag pattern will consist of 6 components, as long as the J-value of the excited level is greater than or equal to $\frac{5}{2}$.

There are three difficulties which arise in the determination of the quadrupole moment of Mn in contrast to Eu: (i) the hfs splitting of the excited levels is only about half as wide as that of Eu, i.e., the splitting of the flag pattern is only half as large; (ii) the width of the lines for a hollow cathode light source is larger because the mass is smaller, i.e., the Doppler-width is larger; (iii) the effect to be measured, the deviation of the hfs-splitting from the Lande interval rule, is smaller by a factor of 4 than with Eu^{151}, since the quadrupole moment of Mn is only about 0.3b. From these three points one may conclude that the position of the components of the flag pattern for the determination of the quadrupole moment cannot be measured with sufficient accuracy, if a liquid air-cooled hollow cathod is used as light source. The line width would be too large and the components of the flag pattern would not be sufficiently well resolved. The difficulties can be avoided by reducing the Doppler width of the lines by using an atomic beam in emission or absorption. First let us discuss the investigation of the green intercombination lines $^8P_{5/2, 7/2} - {}^6S_{5/2}$ which have been carried out with an atomic beam in emission. The atomic beam arrangement consists of an oven and a collimator; the beam is observed vertically to its direction of flight. The Doppler width in this case is about 3.5 mK; with a hollow cathode the Doppler width would be about 20 mK.

When the heating coil of the beam oven is put at a negative potential with respect to the grounded collimator, an intensive discharge ignites in the Mn vapor between the collimator and the oven. The atoms excited in the discharge between the oven and the collimator fly through the collimator into the observation chamber; the flight time through the collimator is about 10^{-4} seconds. This means that during the flight time all excited states decay with the exception of the long-living ^8P states. Thus in the observation chamber the atomic beam emits the green intercombination lines only.* Figure 12 shows part of the fine structure spectrum of Mn which was taken with a small spectrograph with low dispersion. The lower spectrum is the emission spectrum of a hollow cathode. One sees the three strong violet resonance lines which are not resolved because of the low dispersion, and the weak green intercombination lines. The upper spectrum is that of the green atomic beam; the violet resonance lines are seen only very weakly.

*Precautions must be taken to exclude errors in the measurements that might arise from uncontrolled variations in the density or excitation of the beam. These will not be discussed here; for details, the reader is referred to Walther (1962).

Fig. 12: Fine structure spectrum of Mn.

Figure 13a shows part of a recording of one of the green intercombination lines. We see a flag pattern of 6 well resolved components, with one component repeated in the next order. The half width of the components is about 20 mK and is due essentially to the instrumental width. Looking closely, we see that the second and the third component are not symmetric because of the splitting of the ground state. With a hollow cathode source the half width is 2.2 times greater.

The violet resonance lines, of course cannot be detected in the same way, for the ^6P levels have a much shorter lifetime than the ^8P levels. For the investigation of the violet lines two methods have been employed: (i) the atomic beam has been used in absorption; (ii) the atomic beam has been excited by electron bombardment. In the absorption experiment, the light source was a high pressure Hg bulb or Mn in a water cooled hollow cathode.

Figure 13b shows a recording of one of the violet resonance lines from the beam in absorption (upper trace) compared to the same line recorded with a liquid air cooled hollow cathode (lower trace). The violet resonance lines were also observed in emission. For this purpose the atomic beam was excited by electron bombardment. Figure 13c shows part of a recording of violet resonance line with the 4 components (J of the upper level equals $\frac{3}{2}$) made with the atomic beam excited by electron bombardment. The asymmetry of the components is due to the splitting of the ground state. In the measurements with the atomic beam excited by electron bombardment, the photo-electric current of the multiplier was about ten times smaller than when investigating the green intercombination lines, which were excited by a discharge.

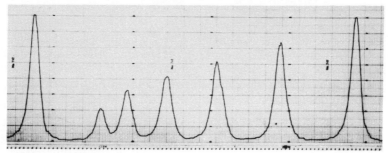

(a) Green intercombination line. (Free spectral range 500 mK).

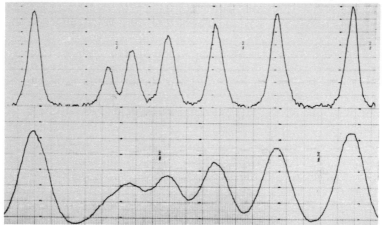

(b) Violet resonance line upper trace, absorption in an atomic beam; lower trace, hollow cathode source. (Free spectral range 417 mK).

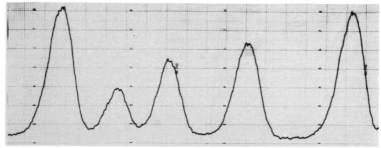

(c) Violet resonance line for atomic beam excited by electron bombardment. (Free spectral range 250 mK).

Fig. 13: Hfs spectra in Mn.

This means that the excitation of an atomic bean by a discharge is considerably more effective than the excitation of an atomic beam by electron bombardment. The excitation by a discharge, however, can be used only for investigation of long-lived states.

The distances of the components can be measured in the flag patterns in Fig.13. To derive the A and B factors of the excited levels from these distances, the splitting of the ground state has to be known; this has been discussed in detail in the example of Eu (Sec. IV). The splitting of the ground state has been measured with the atomic beam resonance method by Woodgate and Martin (1957), but only the absolute value of the splitting of the ground state and not the sign was determined at that time. However, the sign of the splitting of the ground state is absolutely necessary in order to derive the splitting of the excited states from our measurements. Therefore we now must discuss the question of how the sign of the splitting of the ground state can be determined optically.

For this purpose let us have a look at the hf levels of one of the green intercombination lines. The hf splitting of the $^8P_{5/2}$ level and the splitting of the ground state $^6S_{5/2}$ is drawn in Fig. 14. This has been done, assuming that the A factor of the ground state is positive, i.e., the level with the smallest F value lies lowest and assuming that the A factor of the ground state is negative, i.e., the level with the smallest F value lies highest. The effect of the sign of the splitting of the ground state on the hfs observed in the line may be seen in the strongest component of the observed flag pattern. As we see, this consists of a strong and a weak hf transition. If the A factor of the ground state is positive, the weak hf transition is on the side of greater wavenumbers; if the A factor of the ground state is negative, the weak component is on the side of smaller wavenumbers. The experiment has to determine which situation holds. On the recordings we have seen, indications of asymmetries in the components could be detected which are due to the ground state splitting. These minor asymmetries, however, are not enough to settle the question of the sign of the splitting of the ground state. For such a decision the instrumental width has to be reduced further. Principally this can be done by using a greater spacer in the FP, but this has the consequence of decreasing the free spectral range which results in an overlapping of neighboring orders and a complicated intensity distribution. Therefore a somewhat more complicated method has to be used.

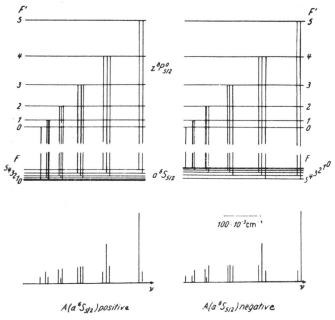

Fig. 14: Hf transitions assuming $A(a^6S_{5/2})$ positive and negative.

In the experiments described so far we used as premonochromator a grating monochromator which let pass a spectral range that
was greater than the entire hf splitting of the investigated line.
Now let us consider a pre-monochromator that lets pass only a
very narrow spectral range, namely, just the strongest component
of the flag pattern. Then we have only the light of the strongest
component available and this can, of course, be recorded with a
FP which has a large spacer without overlapping of neighboring
orders.

    The experimental set-up is shown in Fig. 15. The exit
slit of the grating monochromator lets pass as usual the light of
the fine structure to be investigated. Behind the grating monochromator there is a FP with a small spacer and the center of the
ring system of this FP is focused with the lens L_2 on the diaphragm. The pressure in this FP is chosen in such a way as to let
pass only the light of the strongest component of the flag pattern;
thus, the grating monochromator and the first FP together act as
the premonochromator. In this case the diaphragm represents
the exit slit of the premonochromator and the light can be recorded with a FP having a great spacer and thus a high resolving

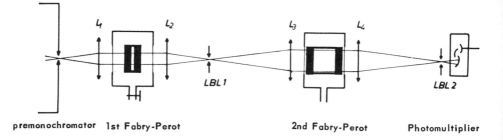

premonochromator   1st Fabry-Perot   2nd Fabry-Perot   Photomultiplier

Fig. 15: Set-up of the two FP in series.

power. Therefore only the second FP is pressure scanned during the recording. The interferences of the second FP are, as usual, focused on a diaphragm, behind which is a photomultiplier.

We see in Fig. 16 a recording of the strongest component of the green intercombination line, whose hf scheme we saw in Fig. 14. Here we clearly see the asymmetry caused by the weak hf

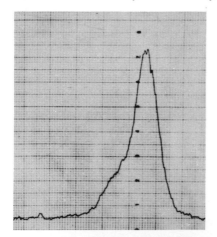

Fig. 16: Recording of strongest component of green intercombination line. (Goodman et al., 1962)

transition. Now it can be definitely decided that this weak transition is on the side of the smaller wavenumbers and consequently the A factor of the ground state has to be negative.

The recording we have just seen is a typical example of the progress achieved in optical hfs investigation using FP coatings of dielectric multi-layers with small absorption. Only a light source of low intensity in the form of the excited atomic beam was available and although the light had to pass two interferometers, it was not difficult to produce a recording with a good signal to noise ratio.

Having fixed the sign of the splitting of the ground state, the hf splittings of the levels of the configuration $3d^5 4s4p$ can be derived from the measured distances of the components of the flag pattern. This is done in the same way as described for Eu.

To conclude the discussion of the measurements on Mn let us discuss briefly the evaluation of the quadrupole moment from the measured B factors. To calculate the electric field gradient at the nucleus due to the 4p electron, eigenfunctions in RS coupling have been used; relativistic corrections have been taken into account. The value of ξ_p of the 4p electron, necessary for the evaluation, was derived, as usual, from empirical data. As with Eu, we can derive this value from the fine structure and from the measured A factors of the hfs. Table VIII summarizes the values of

Table VIII: Calculated electric field gradients for different Mn levels and values of $Q(Mn^{55})$ derived from the measured B-values.

Fine Structure Level	$z\,^8P_{\frac{7}{2}}^{\,o}$	$z\,^8P_{\frac{5}{2}}^{\,o}$	$z\,^6P_{\frac{7}{2}}^{\,o}$	$z\,^6P_{\frac{5}{2}}^{\,o}$	$z\,^6P_{\frac{3}{2}}^{\,o}$
$\text{e}\,\overline{\rho_{zz}(0)}$	-9, 18	2, 42	6, 88	-7, 85	1, 38
Q	$0,37 \pm 0,05$	$0,37 \pm 0,15$	$0,32 \pm 0,06$	$0,33 \pm 0,05$	$0,4 \pm 0,3$

the quadrupole moment of Mn calculated from the two ^8P and the three ^6P states. The five values are in excellent agreement within their errors. For the level $^6P_{3/2}$ the error is especially large, since here the measured distances depend only weakly on the B factor. The average value for the quadrupole moment of Mn is $Q(Mn^{55}) = 0.35$ (5) b. Again, Sternheimer corrections have not been taken into account in this evaluation.

VI. Hyperfine Structure of Re^{185,187}: Application of the Double Fabry-Perot

A. The Double Fabry-Perot

Now let us deal more generally with the problem of reducing the instrumental width and assume we have a line with a very large hf splitting, the total splitting being, for instance, of the order of 2000 mK. Since we want to avoid overlapping of neighboring orders, we have to choose a free spectral range larger than 2000 mK. But this would result in a large instrumental width of about 100 mK which gives a very insufficient resolution. In the case of Mn discussed above, it was sufficient to isolate part of the hfs by a grating monochromator and then to record only this part with high resolution. But now we want to record the whole hf splitting with high resolution. Our aim is to have a small instrumental width but at the same time a large free spectral range. For this purpose two recording FP's in series are used, the first one with a small spacer and the second one with a large spacer.

The principle is illustrated in Fig. 17. A fine structure line was recorded having no hf splitting and no isotope shift, that is, consisting of only one component. The upper recording was produced with a FP having a small spacer; there are two orders of the line. The middle recording was produced with a FP having a spacer six times as great. The wave number scale is the same in both recordings. Since the spacer in the middle recording is six times as great, the free spectral range is six times as small and one free spectral range of the upper recording contains six free spectral ranges of the middle recording. In addition, we see that in the middle recording the half-width of the lines is smaller than on the upper one, because of the greater spacer. The product of both intensity distributions is observed when both FP are used in series; this is shown on the lower recording. Now we have the large free spectral range given by the FP with the small spacer but the instrumental width is essentially determined by the FP with the large spacer (Fig. 18).

The resulting intensity distribution (Fig. 17) can only be obtained when each maximum of the upper recording just coincides with a maximum of the middle recording. That is, whenever the first FP with the small spacer has a maximum of transmission for a certain wavelength, the second FP with the greater spacer must have a maximum of transmission for this wavelength, too. This is only the case when the ratio of the spacers of both FP's is an integer. However, it is very hard to produce mechanically an exact integral ratio of the spacers. Therefore, to make the two FP simultaneously transparent for the same wavelength, one has to change slightly the optical path of one of them. The simplest way to do this is to set a constant pressure difference between the two interferometers. So the problem with the photoelectric recording with two FP in series may be stated as: in both interfer-

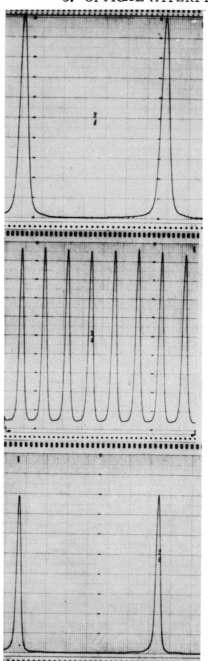

Fig. 17: Spectra illustrating the use of the Double Fabry Perot (see text).

ometers the pressure has to be increased linearly with time while the pre-set pressure difference between both interferometers is maintained. This is a complicated technical problem and the reader is referred to Kuhl et al. (1966) for details of the solution. It is possible to keep the preset pressure difference between the two FP constant to less than ± 0.03 mm Hg during the recording.

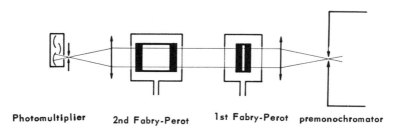

Photomultiplier   2nd Fabry-Perot   1st Fabry-Perot premonochromator

Fig. 18: Arrangement of the Double Fabry-Perot spectrometer.

This is sufficient for all practical purposes because in the realistic case the ratio t_2/t_1 of the spacers of the two FP is not exactly an integer k but $t_2/t_1 = k + \delta k$, which means that the values of maximum transmission of the two FP which coincide at the beginning of recording do not coincide after the pressure has increased to 1 atm. For example, for $k = 15$ a $\delta k \leq 2.10^{-3}$ can be achieved. It follows that after a pressure increase of about 1 atm the pressure difference begween the two FP should be changed by $\delta p = \delta k/k$ atm ≤ 0.1 mm Hg in order that the maxima of transmission of the FP still coincide, which means that the error resulting from δk is about 3 times larger than that of the pressure control.

B. Optical Hyperfine Measurements in Re

For an example of measurements made with the recording DFP interferometer let us look at the hf structure of the Re line $5d^5\ 6s^2\ ^6S_{5\ 2} - 5d^5\ 6s6p\ ^8P_{7\ 2}$. The ground state $^6S_{5\ 2}$ has a very small splitting which has not been measured in the natural Re isotopes with the atomic beam resonance method as yet. The upper level has a very wide splitting of the order of 2000 mK.

Our aim was to get information about the hf splitting of the ground state $^6S_{5/2}$ which is of the same order of magnitude as the Doppler width of the light source. Therefore the following conditions had to be satisfied as far as possible: (i) The instrumental width had to be kept small. This was achieved by using the DFP. (ii) The intensity values of the measured line structure had to be given out in digital form so that the analysis of unresolved hf transitions could be done easily and quickly on a computer.

The Re-spectrum was excited in liquid air cooled hollow cathodes filled with highly enriched samples of the two natural isotopes Re^{185} and Re^{187}. Figure 19 shows part of two recordings

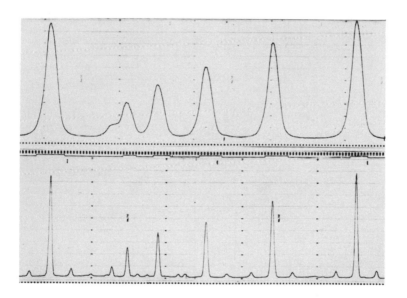

Fig. 19: Spectrum of Re^{187} hfs. Upper recording: Single FP; Lower recording: DFP.

of the hyperfine structure of Re^{187} obtained with one and with two FP interferometers. There is a flag pattern of 6 components because the nuclear spin is $\frac{5}{2}$. By the use of the double FP the line width of the components was reduced by a factor 5.5 whereas in the upper recording the linewidth is nearly purely instrumental that of the lower one is esentially determined by the Doppler width of the light source. The small components are "ghosts" of the double Fabry Perot which can always be observed if large spacer ratios are used because the intensity transmitted by the FP with the smaller spacer is not yet zero when the larger spaced FP is already transmitting in the next higher order.

Figure 20 shows the hyperfine level diagram for the line we

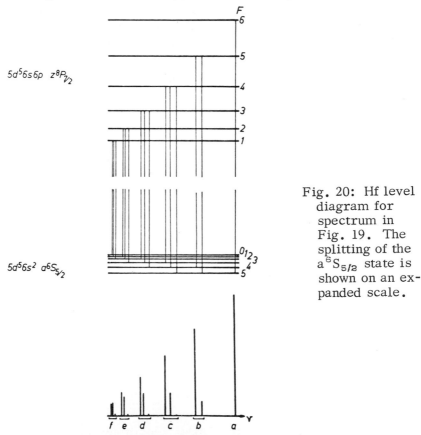

Fig. 20: Hf level diagram for spectrum in Fig. 19. The splitting of the $a\,^6S_{5/2}$ state is shown on an expanded scale.

saw in Fig. 19. The splitting of the $^8P_{7/2}$ level is about 50 times larger than that of the ground state and essentially determines the distances between the centers of gravity of the groups called a, b, etc., whereas the distances resulting from the splitting of the ground state are not resolved by the measurement. The component with the highest intensity consists of a single transition and makes it possible to evaluate the line shape of a single component which is necessary for the exact analysis of the composite components in order to get the ground state splitting.

The analysis of the groups of components was carried out separately for each measured order, i.e., for each measured order the profile of the component "a" which consists of a single transition was taken from the measurements anew and was only used for the evaluation of components in the same order. To get the line profile in a form usable for the analysis of the different groups of components a least square fit of the measured points of the single component "a" was made with a polynomial of 18th degree. In this way it was possible to reproduce the measured points to better than 0.3% of the maximum of the component. The analysis of the group of components was facilitated by the fact that the A-values of the ground state can be calculated because the A-values of the ground states for the radioactive isotopes Re^{186} and Re^{188} have been measured by the atomic beam method with high accuracy. Furthermore, the g_I values were known for the radioactive as well as for the natural isotopes. Therefore, the A-values for the ground state could be evaluated for the natural isotopes. In doing this, the hyperfine anomaly was not considered but it can be assumed that it is small enough so that it can be neglected. That means that we had only to determine the quadrupole coupling constant B for the ground state. Using the line shape of component a (Fig. 20), the theoretical ratios of the hyperfine intensities, and the calculated A-factors, the profiles for the groups of components were calculated by computer. B was varied and the sum of the squares of the residuals between the measured and the calculated profile was determined. For the groups of components b, d, and e, a minimum was always obtained. The result of the analysis is for both stable isotopes

$$B^{185, 187} \; (^6S_{5/2}) = (1.6 \pm 0.8) \; mK \quad .$$

This means that the completely unresolved distance between the two components in group b was determined with an error of only ± 0.5 mK, i.e., an accuracy of 5 percent.

Using the B factor for the ground state and the measured distances between the centers of gravity of the components a, b, c, etc., the quadrupole interaction constants for the excited $^8P_{7/2}$ level can be calculated for Re^{185} and Re^{187}. The same can be done for the $^8P_{5/2}$ level by investigating the transition $5d^5 6s^2 \; ^6S_{5\,2} - 5d^5 6s6p \; ^8P_{5/2}$. So far, no electronic eigenfunctions for the $^8P_{5/2}$ and $^8P_{7/2}$ level in intermediate coupling are available, and it is not possible to take advantage of the experimental accuracy to which B values of $^8P_{5/2}$ and $^8P_{7/2}$ are now determined in order to calculate the nuclear quadrupole moments of the natural isotopes.

The ReI energy scheme is very complex and indicates that the $5d^5$ electron configuration does not behave very much like a half-filled shell. To get reliable eigenfunctions for these states except for the other levels of d^5 (^6S) sp the interaction with the higher lying levels of d^5 dp must also be considered. Moreover the configuration interaction with the configurations d^6 p and d^4 s^2 p must be expected to be fairly large because the position of these levels is quite low. By the fit of the levels of $5d^5(^6S)6s6p$, excluding $x^6P_{7\,2}$, which seems to be mistakenly classified, a value of the spin orbit parameter of the 6p electron, $\xi_p = 3400$ cm^{-1} is obtained. To make a preliminary evaluation of the quadrupole moments from the B factors of the ^8P states we used this value and calculated the mean electric field gradient for LS coupling considering relativistic corrections. We find

$$Q(Re^{185}) = 2.30 \text{ b} \pm 0.9 \text{ b} \quad ,$$
$$Q(Re^{187}) = 2.20 \text{ b} \pm 0.9 \text{ b} \quad .$$

The quoted errors are nearly completely due to the errors of the theoretical evaluation. We see it would be extremely valuable to have better eigenfunctions for the states.

Now let us discuss the measurements on the ground states of the radioactive isotopes Re^{186} and Re^{188} in connection with our measurements on the stable isotopes. The splitting of the radioactive isotopes was measured by Schlecht et al.(1965) and by Armstrong and Marrus (1965) by the atomic beam resonance method. To explain the hf splitting Armstrong and Marrus carried out a theoretical analysis, the result of which is shown in Table IX. The smallest contribution to A and B is due to configuration interaction between $d^5 s^2$ and d^6 s. The two other more essential contributions are due to relativistic effects, namely, the break down of RS coupling by the spin orbit interaction within the d^5 configuration and by the fact that the radial integral $\langle 1/r^3 \rangle$ has to be replaced by three radial integrals in a relativistic treatment. For the A factors a comparison between the theoretical and the experimental values is possible because there exists an independent measurement of the magnetic dipole moment; satisfactory agreement is obtained. The calculation of B is more critical because two large contributions cancel each other. An exact comparison with theory is impossible because the quadrupole moment for Re^{186} or Re^{188} is not known independently but for the natural isotopes both the nuclear quadrupole moments and the ground state splitting could be evaluated independently. Therefore it is also possible to check the results for the quadrupole

Table IX: Contribution to the hyperfine constants A and B in rhenium (Armstrong and Marrus, 1965).

Source	Magnitude	
	A(Mc/sec)	B(Mc/sec)
Breakdown of L-S coupling within $(5d)^5(6s)^2$	$33.6\,\mu_I$ [a]	$+33.0\,Q$ [b]
Configuration mixing $(5d)^6(6s)$	$11.2\,\mu_I$	$-0.3\,Q$
Relativistic corrections	$-83.5\,\mu_I$	$-28.0\,Q$
Total calculated	$-38.7\,\mu_I$	$4.7\,Q$
Total experimental	$-46.0\,\mu_I$	8.0

[a] μ_I in nm

[b] Q in barns.

Table X: Comparison of theoretical and experimental results for Re^{187}.

Source	$A(10^{-3}\ cm^{-1})$	$B(10^{-3}\ cm^{-1})$
Breakdown of L-S coupling within $(5d)^5(6s)^2$	$+1.44$	$+2.42$
Configuration mixing $(5d)^6(6s)$	$+0.18$	-0.02
Relativistic corrections	-3.57	-2.05
Total calculated	-1.65	0.35
Total experimental	$-1.937\ (3)$	$1.6\ (8)$

interaction of the theoretical analysis of the ground state splitting by Armstrong and Marrus (1965). Table X shows the comparison of the theoretical and experimental results for Re^{187}. Whereas rather good agreement is obtained for the A-factors, the comparison of the B-factors shows a discrepancy by about a factor of four which cannot be explained by the moment. But it should be noted that the B-factor is the difference between nearly equal contributions which means that small inaccuracies in the matrix elements very much influence the result.

With B $(a^6S_{5/2})$ for the natural isotopes the ratio of B $(a^6S_{5/2})$ for the natural and radioactive isotopes can be derived and it is possible to calculate with $Q(Re^{185}, Re^{187})$ the nuclear quadrupole moments of Re^{186} and Re^{188}. The result is:

$$Q(Re^{186}, Re^{188}) = (0.4 \pm 0.2) \times 10^{-24} \text{ cm}^2.$$

No difference in the values for the nuclear quadrupole moments of Re^{186} and Re^{188} are to be expected because the error for $B(a^6S_{5/2})$ obtained for the natural isotopes is larger than the difference of the B-factors for the two radioactive isotopes. As Armstrong and Marrus (1965) pointed out, a value for the nuclear quadrupole moments of this magnitude would be in rather good agreement with the nuclear deformation which must be assumed to explain the magnetic moments of Re^{186} and Re^{188}, using the calculations of Mottelson and Nilsson (1955).

VII. Isotope Shifts

A. Theory

We saw in Sec. III, in discussing the optical spectrum of natural Os, that the fine structure lines of the various Os isotopes did not coincide in energy. This shift of the spectral lines between isotopes of the same element is known as the isotope shift and has two origins: (i) the mass effect, which is due to the fact that the atomic nucleus is not infinitely heavy and (ii) the volume effect, which is caused by the variation of the mean squared nuclear charge radius as one goes from one isotope to another one. Thus the volume effect depends on $\delta \langle r^2 \rangle$ where r^2 is to be averaged over the nuclear charge distribution.*

For elements with isotopes whose mass numbers are smaller than about 60 generally only the mass-dependent effect of the isotope shift is important, while for elements with isotopes whose mass numbers are greater than about 160, only the volume effect of the isotope shift plays a part. For the mass numbers between 60 and 160 both effects have to be taken into account, in general, with the mass effect prevailing with the lighter elements, the volume effect with the heavier ones.

1. Mass Effects

To describe the theory of the mass effect, we write the

See also discussion by Mössbauer and Clauser, Chap. 11.

non-relativistic Hamiltonian of an atom with N electrons whose centre of mass is at rest

$$H = \frac{1}{2m} \sum_{j=1}^{N} p_j^2 + \frac{1}{2M} P^2 + V \tag{24}$$

m being the electron mass, p_j the momentum of the jth electron, M the nuclear mass, P the momentum of the nucleus and V the potential energy. Because of momentum conservation

$$P = - \sum_{j=1}^{N} p_j \quad . \tag{25}$$

Substituting Eq. (25) into Eq. (24) and rearranging the terms,

$$H = \frac{1}{2} \left(\frac{1}{m} + \frac{1}{M} \right) \sum_{j} p_j^2 + \frac{1}{2M} \sum_{j \neq k} p_j \cdot p_k + V \quad . \tag{26}$$

If the nuclear mass were infinite both of the terms with the factor 1/M would disappear. Thus these two terms represent the influence of the finite mass of the nucleus. In the one electron-problem, i.e., for hydrogen-like spectra, the second term, which contains the scalar product of the momenta of two different electrons, disappears. The remaining term contains the electron mass and the nuclear mass and gives rise to the so-called normal mass effect.

The term value measured from the series limit of a hydrogen-like atom with nuclear-charge Z is given by

$$T_{\infty} = \frac{R_{\infty} Z^2}{n^2} \tag{27}$$

for an infinitely heavy nucleus; R_{∞} is the Rydberg constant for infinitely heavy nucleus and n is the principal quantum number. Taking into account the finite nuclear mass, the term value T is given by

$$T = T_{\infty} \left(1 - \frac{m}{M} \right) \quad . \tag{28}$$

Thus the term energy of a heavier isotope is shifted less towards the series limit than that of a lighter isotope (Fig. 21). If the mass numbers of the two isotopes are A_1 and A_2 $(A_2 > A_1)$, the

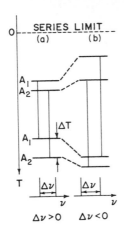

Fig. 21: Term energies for isotopes A_1, A_2 where $A_2 > A_1$.
(a) normal effect
(b) normal and specific effect.

term shift ΔT is given by

$$\Delta T = \frac{m}{m_p} \left(\frac{1}{A_1} - \frac{1}{A_2} \right) T_\infty \tag{29}$$

with m_p the proton mass (if we neglect mass defects). The shift is proportional to the term value and means that a lower term for the two isotopes with the mass numbers A_1 and A_2 has a larger splitting.

In the spectral line, the difference between the two isotope shifts in the terms is observed. The isotope shift in the line is

$$\Delta\nu = \frac{m}{m_p} \frac{A_2 - A_1}{A_1 A_2} \nu . \tag{30}$$

It is characteristic of the normal mass effect that the heavier isotope is shifted to larger wavenumbers; this is called a positive isotope shift.

The normal mass effect decreases with the mass number squared. For $A = 100$ and for lines in the visible region, the normal mass effect is about 2 mK for a mass number difference $\Delta A = 2$.

The second term in the Hamiltonian (Eq. (26)) no longer vanishes when there is more than one electron; it gives rise to an additional mass effect which is known as the specific mass effect or coupling effect. Roughly speaking, if the electrons mainly move in the same direction, the nucleus has to move strongly so that the centre of mass remains at rest. If the electrons, however mainly move in mutually opposite directions, the nuclear motion required to keep the center of mass of the whole system at rest is decreased. From this consideration it follows that the specific mass effect can both increase and decrease the normal mass effect, depending on the coupling of the electrons. As an example, let us assume that the specific effect increases the normal effect in the upper term of the level scheme but decreases it in the lower term. Then the sequence of isotopes in the line is inverted by the specific effect and the lighter isotope is shifted to larger wavenumbers, i.e., there is a negative isotope shift, $\Delta\nu < 0$.

Since for the lighter elements the volume effect can be neglected, the isotope shift observed in a line is the sum of the normal and specific mass effects. As the normal mass effect can be calculated easily, the specific effect can be found from the observed isotope shift. To calculate the specific effect the matrix elements of the product $p_i \cdot p_k$ have to be determined. Up to now the agreement of measured and calculated specific effects for atoms with more than 2 electrons has been extremely poor; the deviations often amount to more than a factor of 2. It can be hoped that with more exact eigenfunctions it will perhaps be possible to calculate the specific effects more exactly (Bauche, 1966). It will be seen to be of decisive significance for the evaluation of the volume effect from the measured isotope shifts to be able to calculate as exactly as possible the specific mass effect for atoms with many electrons.

The specific mass effect depends on the nuclear mass in the same way as the normal mass effect. Therefore the isotope shift $\Delta\nu$ observed in a line is proportional to $(A_2 - A_1)/A_2 A_1$ when only mass effects are present. If there are 3 isotopes with mass numbers A_1, A_2, and A_3 and $A_2 - A_1 = A_3 - A_2$ then $\Delta\nu_{12}/\Delta\nu_{23}$ equals A_3/A_1 where $\Delta\nu_{12}$ and $\Delta\nu_{23}$ are the isotope shifts between neighbouring isotopes. This relative isotope shift is characteristic for the mass effect and has to be constant, of course, for all spectral lines of an element. Within the experimental limits of error, the measurements verify this relationship for light elements.

For lighter elements, one finds specific effects whose sizes vary from -20 up to +16 times the normal effect. Especially large specific effects are observed in transitions of the type $d^{n-1} s^2$ to $d^n p$. If the level of the configuration $d^{n-1} s^2$ is the lower level, the specific effect is positive. Representative examples for this can be found in the first spectrum of copper and in the first spectrum of nickel. If the level of the configuration $d^{n-1} s^2$ is the upper level, very large negative specific effects are observed. For this the second spectrum of zinc is an example.

In the first spectrum of nickel large negative specific effects have been found in the transitions between the levels of the configuration $d^n s$, which are the lower ones and the levels of the configuration d^{n-1} sp. In alkali like s-p transitions, however, only small specific effects are found, as experiments with lighter elements show. These lies between -0.5 times and +2 times the normal effect. As the volume and mass effect cannot be separated experimentally, one is dependent on an empirical estimation of the mass effect, as long as it cannot be calculated reliably, to derive the volume effect from the measured isotope shifts.

2. Volume Effects

Figure 22 shows a nucleus with the nuclear charge radius, R. Outside the nucleus there is a Coulomb

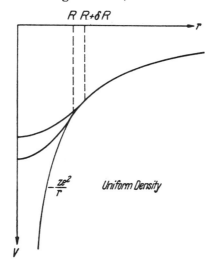

Fig. 22: Electronic potential for uniformly charged nuclei with radii R and R + δR, respectively.

potential, but inside the nucleus the potential differs from the Coulomb potential. If we look at a nucleus with the radius (R + δR), the deviation from the Coulomb potential starts at larger r and the potential in the nucleus corresponds to the upper curve of Fig. 22. This difference of potential in the nucleus can be seen by s-electrons and to a far lesser extent by $p_{\frac{1}{2}}$-electrons. For reasons of simplicity we will discuss s-electrons only. The s-electron is more strongly bound to the nucleus of the lighter isotope having a smaller nuclear radius than to the nucleus of the heavier isotope. This gives rise to an isotope shift known as nuclear volume effect or field effect.

An example is the isotope shift in the level $5d^{10}6s$ of the second spectrum of mercury, referred to the series limit $5d^{10}$. The level belonging to the lighter isotope A_1 lies a little lower in energy than the level belonging to the heavier isotope A_2. The level separation δT_s is given by

$$\delta T_s = |\psi_s(0)|^2 \frac{\pi a_H^3}{Z} C(Z, \langle r^2 \rangle, \delta\langle r^2 \rangle) \tag{31}$$

where $|\psi_s(0)|^2$ is the non-relativistically calculated charge density of the 6s-electron at the nucleus, and a_H the first Bohr radius. The remaining factor C is called the isotope shift constant and is given by

$$C = f(Z)\left(\frac{2Z\langle r^2 \rangle^{\frac{1}{2}}}{a_H}\right)^{2\sigma} \frac{\delta\langle r^2 \rangle}{\langle r^2 \rangle} \tag{32}$$

where f is a function depending only on Z, and σ is $\sqrt{1 - \alpha^2 Z^2}$. For the nuclear volume effect the sequence of the isotopes in a line depends on whether the upper or the lower level has the larger charge density at the nucleus. In the latter case, the lighter isotope is shifted to larger wavenumbers in the line, i.e., there is a negative isotope shift.

If several isotopes are present, the ratio of isotope shifts between neighbouring isotopes is given by the ratio of the $\delta\langle r^2 \rangle$ values, provided mass effects can be neglected, i.e., for heavy elements. Thus, the ratios of $\delta\langle r^2 \rangle$ can be determined with great accuracy for heavy elements from isotope shift measurements. As the ratio $\Delta\nu_{12}/\Delta\nu_{23}$ is not dependent on the electron core, the relative isotope shift in all lines of an element has to be constant if only the volume effect is present. This is also valid when the isotope shift is produced only by the mass effect. The difference is that the mass effect produces an almost equi-distant isotope position, while the volume effect causes a deviation from the equi-distant isotope position in many cases.

3. Combined Effects

If both mass and volume effects contribute to the observed isotope shift, the relative isotope shift in the different lines will not be constant as is the case if the volume effect produces a deviation from the equidistant isotope position and if the mass effect is of different size in different lines.

Figure 23 shows the situation schematically. The positions of four isotopes with mass numbers A, A+2, A+4 and A+6 are

represented, assuming that the
lighter isotope is shifted to greater
wavenumbers and that the isotopes do not lie equidistant. The
mass effect is plotted on the
ordinate in arbitrary units. Now
let us look at another spectral
line whose mass effect corresponds to a value on the ordinate; then almost the same mass
effect is added to every distance
between pairs of isotopes. Thus
the relative isotope position is
changed. In the diagram, the
relative isotope positions are
given by the points of intersection of the straight lines with the
horizontal line which corresponds
to the respective value of the

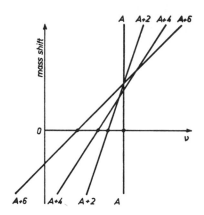

Fig. 23: Isotope shifts as a
function of the mass shift
(see text).

mass effect. We see that the sequence of the isotopes in the line
is changed if the mass effect is large enough. With very large
positive mass effects the sequence of the isotopes is reversed and
the relative isotope position gets closer to the equidistance corresponding to the pure mass effect. This is correspondingly true
for the lower part of the diagram where the mass effect is negative.

B. Isotope Shifts in Os

In the heavy element osmium, the isotope shift is due almost completely to the volume effect. Figure 5 showed the scheme
of the hyperfine structure in an Os-line. The line belongs to a
transition from the configuration s^2 to sp, where the level belonging to s^2 is lowest; therefore the lightest isotope in the line is
shifted to greater wave-numbers. The isotope shift between the
most abundant even isotopes 192, 190, and 188 can easily be
measured using the natural isotope mixture, but to determine the
position of the two components α and β of the odd isotope with the
mass number 187, one has to use an enriched sample. Two
hollow cathodes were used, one filled with natural Os, the other
one with pure Os 187 and the two hollow cathodes were alternately
placed in the light path of the spectrometer. In a similar way, the
isotope shift of the isotope 184 with natural abundance of 0.2% was
measured. The relative isotope shift was constant within the
limits of error in all investigated Os lines.

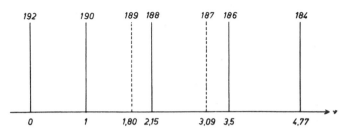

Fig. 24: Relative isotope positions in the Os spectrum. Dashed
          lines are centers of gravity of the hfs splitting for the odd
          mass isotopes. The distance between isotopes 190 and 192
          is normalized to 1.

Figure 24 shows the results of the relative isotope position
derived from isotope shift measurements in several Os lines. The
even isotopes deviate from equidistant spacing. It is characteristic
that the odd isotopes do not lie in the middle between the neighbouring even isotopes but are shifted toward the lighter even isotope.
This effect is often observed if the isotope shift is caused by the
nuclear volume effect and is usually referred to as odd-even staggering.

C. Isotope Shifts in Sr

It is known from the experiments on isotope shifts in cerium
and lead, i.e., in the neighbourhood of the closed neutron shells
with 82 and 126 neutrons, that the addition of neutrons to a closed
shell changes the nuclear volume effect suddenly from small to
large values. These observations led to the speculation that such
a discontinuity in nuclear volume effect should also appear near
50 neutrons, in the relative isotope positions of an element with
isotopes having more and less than 50 neutrons. The element
strontium is very suitable (Heilig, 1961) for such an investigation
because it has stable even isotopes with mass numbers 84 to 88
and neutron numbers 46 to 50 respectively, which fill the $g_{9/2}$
neutron shell. The long living radioactive isotope Sr^{90} has two
$d_{5/2}$ neutrons outside of the closed shell with 50 neutrons.

As the isotope shift expected in the Sr lines is smaller than
the Doppler width of the lines, separated isotopes were used in
the investigation. The dangerous properties of the radioactive
Sr^{90} enforced the construction of a special hollow cathode so that
the spark spectrum could be excited in very small quantities of
material — as little as one tenth of a microgram, or 5×10^{14} atoms.
A separate hollow cathode was used for each isotope; the measure-

ments were made by alternat-
ing the cathodes in the light
path of the spectrometer.
Figure 25 shows schematically
the results of the measurements
of the resonance lines of the
spark spectrum; within the limits of error the isotope shift
in both lines is the same. The
shift of the stable isotopes 84,
86, and 88 has the sign of the

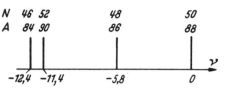

Fig. 25: Positions of Sr isotopes
in the spark spectrum.

normal mass effect (i. e. , the heavier isotope is shifted towards
larger wavenumbers) and these isotopes lie nearly equidistant,
but the distance 86 to 88 is slightly smaller than the distance 84
to 86, as one would expect from mass dependent effects. The isotope 90 does not lie where expected for a mass dependent effect,
but is shifted towards smaller wavenumbers compared with the
isotope 88.   These relative isotope positions signify that the
nuclear volume effect is smaller than the mass dependent effect
in the stable isotopes but in the isotope pair 88-90 the nuclear
volume effect is many times larger than the mass dependent effect.
This proves a discontinuity of the nuclear volume effect when one
passes the neutron number 50.

In order to obtain the nuclear volume effect from the measurements, the mass dependent effect has to be eliminated. It
may be roughly estimated by comparison with the measurements
in corresponding transitions in light elements, where only the
mass effect is of any significance.   Such an estimate yields values
shown in Table XI; most of the error reflects uncertainty in estimating the mass dependent effect.

Table XI: Nuclear volume effect between Sr isotopes.

Spectrum	Transition	84-86	86-88	88-90
Sr II	5s - 5p	0 to - 3	0 to - 3	-18. 4 ± 1. 9
Sr I	$5s^2$ - 5s5p	0 to - 1	0 to - 1	-12. 1 ± 0. 8

The nuclear volume effect is smaller for the transition
$5s^2, {}^1S_0$ - $5s5p, {}^1P_1$ in neutral Sr than for 5s-5p of the spark spectrum because of the mutual screening of the two 5s-electrons and
the screening of the 5s-electron by the 5p-electron.   The values
for the transition 5s-5p yield immediately the nuclear volume
effect of the 5s electron relative to the series limit, which is the
quantity δT_S needed to calculate the isotope shift constant defined

in Eqs. (31) and (32). However, it is also possible to calculate δT_S from the s^2-sp transition. In this connection, Table XII shows the measured nuclear volume effect in an s^2-sp transition divided by the effect of the s-electron referred to the series limit for different elements. This ratio is fairly constant and taking 0.66 as an average, one can calculate from the measurement of the s^2-sp transition in Sr $\delta T_S = 18 \pm 3$ mK. This value is in good agreement with the value obtained from the s-p transition which is $\delta T_S = 18.4 \pm 1.9$ mK.

Table XII

Element	$\Delta v(s^2\text{-sp})/\delta T_S$
Sm	0.60
Eu	0.64
Gd	0.63
Yb	0.72
Hg	0.73

D. Isotope Shift in Sm

In the rare-earths, the observed isotope shift is mainly due to the volume effect, the normal mass effect being of the order of 1 or 2 mK for $\delta A = 2$. Until about 1962 it was assumed that large specific mass effects observed in lighter elements play no role in the rare-earth region because the relative isotope shift seemed to be constant in all lines of the same element. However, this conclusion depended on the accuracy of measurements and we now know that large specific mass effects do exist. This result is of importance concerning the reliability of $\delta \langle r^2 \rangle$ derived from isotope shifts in the rare earths.

An element with relative isotope shifts which differ very much is especially suitable for the detection of a mass dependent shift. Such shifts are seen in the spectrum of Sm with isotopes of mass numbers 144, 148, 150, 152, and 154, corresponding to neutron numbers 82, 86, 88, 90, and 92 respectively. There is a large deviation from equidistance between the isotopes with neutron numbers 88 and 90. The reason for the large volume shift is the strong increase of the intrinsic nuclear quadrupole moment as the 45th neutron pair is incorporated into the nucleus and the corresponding increase of deformation which results in a large increase of $\delta \langle r^2 \rangle$.

Striganov et al. (1962) made an extensive sutdy of the isotope shift in the arc spectrum of Sm using enriched samples of the seven isotopes, and found that the relative isotope shift is different for lines with positive shift than for lines with negative shift. The lines with negative shift measured by these authors are supposed to be $4f^6 6s^2 - 4f^6 6s6p$ transitions and the lines with positive shift are supposed to be $4f^6 6s^2 - 4f^5 5d6s^2$ transitions; both cases are characterized by the same lower electron configuration $4f^6 6s^2$. In the first, the lower level has the larger s-electron charge density at the nucleus and therefore the lighter isotope is shifted towards larger wavenumbers, i.e., a negative shift. On the other hand in the second type of transitions the charge density at the nucleus is larger in the upper level than in the lower level because the s-electrons are screened by only five 4f-electrons in the upper level compared to six 4f-electrons in the lower level; therefore the observed isotope shift is positive. In both types of transition the absolute value of the isotope shift is of the same order of magnitude.

The fact that the relative isotope position is different in different lines of Sm can be explained by taking the mass dependent effect into account (King, 1963). It turns out that there are specific mass effects present in the investigated Sm-lines which are of the order of magnitude of 10 times the normal mass effect. Recent measurements (Hansen et al., 1965) carried out with high accuracy clearly demonstrated that the observed relative isotope positions can be described exactly by considering the mass effect. Although the specific effect amounts to less than 10 percent of the measured isotope shifts, even its small dependence on the mass number, which is of the form $1/A_1 \cdot A_2$, is shown up by the measurements.

Similar large specific effects have also been found in other rare-earth elements. This means one has to be careful in evaluating the change of the mean square charge radius from the measured isotope shifts because the specific mass effect cannot be calculated in a reliable way.

E. Isotope Shifts in Hg and Tl

When the relative isotope shifts in neighbouring elements referred to equal neutron numbers are compared, they turn out to be qualitatively the same for different elements. This is true for the majority of investigated cases and means that the volume effect in the isotope shift is primarily determined by the number of neutrons in the nucleus and is only slightly dependent on the number of protons.

A very good example are the measurements of the isotope shifts

Fig. 26: Relative shifts for Hg
and Tl isotopes, referred to
equal neutron numbers
(Tomlinson and Stroke,
1964).

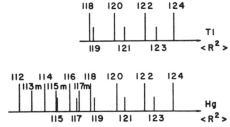

in radioactive and stable isotopes of the elements Hg and Tl (Z =
80 and 81, respectively). Figure 26 shows the relative isotope
shifts (Tomlinson and Stroke , 1964) to be almost the same in
both elements when referred to equal neutron numbers and means
that the $s_{1/2}$ odd proton in Tl produces little effect on the relative
isotope shifts. In the case of the Hg isotopes with the neutron
numbers 115 and 117, the isomeric states were measured in addition to the ground states; the shift between the ground and the
isomeric state is known as an isomeric shift.* For neutron
number 113, only the isomeric state shift was measured. The
most striking feature is that none of the isomers of Hg^{193}, Hg^{195},
and Hg^{197} are staggered. From the measured values of their
spin, I = 13/2, the shell-model assignment for the neutron orbits
is $i_{13/2}$. It is believed that the pairs of neutrons that are added
in going from one even isotope to the next in this region are also
in the $i_{13/2}$ state. It appears, therefore, that an $i_{13/2}$ neutron,
either singly or paired, always produces approximately the same
expansion of the mean-square charge radius. This conclusion,
however, is made uncertain by very recent measurements by
Davis et al. (1966) which indicate a staggering of Hg^{195} m and
Hg^{193} m which increases with decreasing mass numbers. In addition some calculations on the change of $\langle r^2 \rangle$ for the Hg isotopes
have been performed by Barret (1966) but so far the agreement
with the experimental data is still very poor.

In the case of the isotope 198 having the neutron number 118,
the $i_{13/2}$ shell is half filled. From the figure we see the conclusion drawn above applies for less than the half-filled shell. From
the measured ground-state spins, the shell-model assignments
for the odd-neutron orbits in the isotopes 195, 197, and 199, are
$p_{1/2}$ and in the isotopes 201 and 203 are $p_{3/2}$ and $f_{5/2}$ respectively.
The odd neutron seems to produce a smaller shift when it is in a
lower angular momentum state. On the other hand as we move
further away from the closed shell at 126 neutrons, the shift
appears to become equal to that for an $i_{13/2}$ neutron.

*See also R.L. Mössbauer and Clauser, Chap. 11.

A. STEUDEL

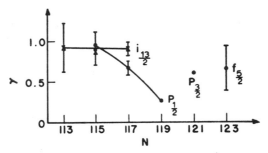

Fig. 27: Staggering parameter γ as a function of neutron number
for Hg isotopes (Tomlinson and Stoke, 1964).

Figure 27 shows the same results for the Hg isotopes in a
different way; an odd-even-staggering parameter γ is defined as:

$$\gamma = \frac{I.S.[(N+1) - (N)]}{\frac{1}{2} I.S.[(N+2)-(N)]}$$

where I.S. means isotope shift and (N) is an isotope with even
neutron number. γ equals 1 when no odd-even-staggering is present.

One can conclude that if the higher angular momentum particle produces a larger shift, we would expect to find an odd-even-
staggering of the type usually observed on the basis of the systematics of nucleon energy-level filling, i.e., for a pair of particles the competition between the lower single-particle energy and
the pairing energy is such that the two nucleons usually fill the
higher of two competing angular momentum states; for the single
particle, in the absence of pairing energy considerations, the
lower angular momentum orbit is usually filled. This, however,
is only a hypothetical statement; a quantitative explanation of the
observed odd-even-staggering has not been given to date.

In the case of Hg the incorporation of a single $i_{13/2}$ neutron
produces about half as great an isotope shift as the incorporation
of a pair of $i_{13/2}$ neutrons. It is of interest to examine whether
the same finding can be stated for other elements. For this purpose measurements of the odd-even-scattering in Nd and Sm are
appropriate (Hansen et al., 1967). Figure 28 shows γ for the odd
isotopes of Nd and Sm as a function of the neutron number. Nd^{143}
has one $f_{7/2}$ neutron outside of the closed neutron outside of the
closed neutron shell with 82 neutrons, Nd^{145} and Sm^{147} have
three $f_{7/2}$ neutrons and Sm^{149} has five $f_{7/2}$ neutrons. It is
believed that the pairs of neutrons that are added to go from

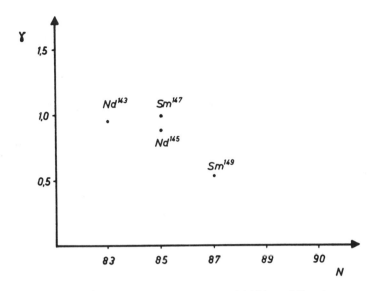

Fig. 28: Staggering parameter γ for odd Nd and Sm isotopes.

one even isotope to the next in this region are also in the $f_{7/2}$ state. One sees that the isotopes having respectively one to three $f_{7/2}$ neutrons show almost no odd-even-staggering, corresponding exactly to the situation for the isomers of the Hg isotopes. However Sm^{149} having one neutron more than the half-filled $f_{7/2}$ shell has an odd-even-staggering which cannot be compared with the measurements on the isomeric states of the Hg isotopes because in Hg, only those isomers were measured whose neutron number did not exceed the half-filled $i_{13/2}$ shell. Not even a qualitative theoretical explanation for the behaviour of the odd-even-staggering in Nd and Sm has been given. It seems that the odd-even-staggering depends sensitively on the admixture of nuclear states and the coupling scheme, making a separate detailed calculation necessary for each case. *

F. Screening Effects

    As an example of the evaluation of the isotope shift constant let us again look at the isotope shift in the configuration $5d^{10}6s$ of the spark spectrum of Hg referred to the series limit $5d^{10}$. If

*Odd-even-staggering has also been observed in the isotope shifts of μ-mesonic Sn atoms (Cohen et al., 1966).

in removing the 6s-electron the closed shell electronic core of the atom were rigid, then the isotope shift observed in this process would equal the shift δT_S. However, in removing the valence electron from the atom, the screening effect on the core electrons is removed also and consequently the core electrons move in toward the nucleus. Hence the measured isotope shift δT_{exp} differs from the pure contribution of the 6s valency electron δT_S. In reality the situation is still more complicated, for one can never exactly measure the isotope shift of a level referred to the series limit. What one measures, for example, is the isotope shift in a transition $5d^{10}6s-5d^{10}8p$ and one assumes that the isotope shift of the configuration $5d^{10}8p$ referred to the series limit $5d^{10}$ is negligibly small, which is not exactly true, because the 8p electron also produces a small screening of the closed s-electron shells of the electron core. The screening effects on the closed shells of the electron core are usually described by setting $\delta T_{exp} = \beta \delta T_S$. Hartree-Fock calculations and a semi-empirical estimate made for europium by Brix (1952) indicate that β is about 1. Recent calculations (Wolter, 1966) indicate, however, that β may be up to 10 percent smaller in many cases. The level to which the measured isotope shifts are referred is different for the different elements, and depends on the investigated lines. Therefore, there is an uncertainty in the comparison of the isotope-shifts of different elements because the values of β may be different.

Figure 29 shows some configurations of the first and second spectrum of Hg. Below the configurations, the measured isotope

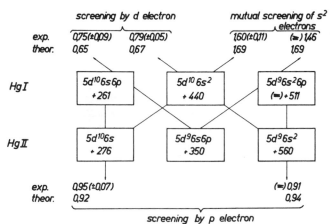

Fig. 29: Screening diagram for HgI and HgII.

shifts are given referred to the ground state of the third spectrum of Hg, namely the configuration $5d^{10}$. Because of the screening effects on the closed shells of the electron core, the values are not free of a certain uncertainty which has to be added to the experimental errors, but we will ignore this uncertainty. The isotope shift in the configuration $5d^{10}6s$ is 276 mK; the isotope shift in the configuration $5d^{10}6s^2$ is not twice this value but only 440 mK i. e., the ratio is 1. 60, and is a consequence of the mutual screening of the two 6s-electrons. The theoretical estimate, which was made with Hartree-Fock-Slater calculations using the eigenfunctions given by Herman and Skillman (Wolter, 1966), is in good agreement with the experimental value.

The isotope shift in the configuration $5d^9 6s^2$ is greater than in the configuration $5d^{10}6s^2$, because the s-electrons are less strongly screened by 9 d-electrons than by 10 d-electrons. The quotient of the shifts gives the screening caused by one d-electron; it is about 11 percent. Within the limits of error one finds the same value when comparing the isotope shifts in the configurations $5d^9 6s6p$ and $5d^{10}6s6p$ with each other. Here the theoretical value calculated by the Hartree-Fock method for the screening of the 6s-electrons due to one 5d-electron is again in good agreement with the experimental value. Comparing the isotope shifts in the configurations $5d^{10}6s$ and $5d^{10}6s6p$ it turns out that the screening of a 6s-electron caused by one 6p-electron is 5 percent. Within the accuracy of the measurements, one finds the same values for the mutual screening of two s-electrons or the screening of the outer s-electrons by a d- or a p-electron in other elements for which the isotope shifts have been measured in corresponding configurations. These screening numbers are often indispensable for evaluating the isotope shift due to one s-electron from the measured isotope shifts. For example, in some elements the isotope shift was measured only in s^2-sp transitions but taking the screening effects into account the isotope shift caused by an s-electron can be evaluated. Furthermore the screening factors are of great value for the discussion of the observed isotope shifts in complex spectra with configuration mixtures.

G. Systematics of Isotope Shifts

We define an experimental isotope shift constant βC_{exp}, by replacing $\beta \delta T_s$ by δT_{exp} in Eq. (31):

$$\beta C_{exp} = \frac{\delta T_{exp} Z}{|\psi_s(o)|^2 \pi a_H^3} \qquad (34)$$

There are two possibilities for the evaluation of $|\psi_s(o)|^2$: (i) If an alkali-like s-electron is present the Fermi-Goudsmit-Segré formula can be used, i. e. ,

$$|\psi_s(o)|^2 = \frac{Z_a^2}{n_a^3} \frac{dn_a}{dn} \times \frac{Z}{\pi a_H^3} \qquad (35)$$

where a equals 1 for the first spectrum, 2 for the second spectrum etc., n_a is the effective main quantum number and n the real main quantum number. (ii) If the fine structure level has one or more unpaired s-electrons and the hyperfine structure splitting of an odd isotope is measured, the a_s factor can then be taken from the measured A value. Then

$$|\psi_s(o)|^2 \frac{\pi a_H^3}{Z} = \frac{a_s}{G} , \quad \text{with } G = \frac{8}{3} R_\infty \alpha^2 Z \frac{m}{m_p} g_I F_r (1-\delta)(1-\epsilon) \qquad (36)$$

where δ takes account of the influence of the finite nuclear volume on the eigenfunction of the s-electron, ϵ takes account of the distribution of the nuclear magnetism over the nuclear volume, and F_r is a relativistic correction.

Usually, βC_{exp} is compared with a theoretical isotope-shift constant which one calculates for a given nuclear model. It is convenient to use the homogeneously charged nucleus as a standard model, with radius given by $R = r_0 A^{1/3}$; the isotope-shift constant calculated for the homogeneous charged nucleus is called C_{th}. Then,

$$\frac{\beta C_{exp}}{C_{th}} = \beta \left(\frac{R_{eq}}{r_0 A^{1/3}}\right)^{2\sigma-2} \frac{\delta\langle r^2\rangle}{\delta\langle r^2\rangle_{th}} \qquad (37)$$

where $R_{eq}^2 = 5/3 \langle r^2\rangle$ and $\delta\langle r^2\rangle_{th} = 2/5 r_0^2 A^{-1/3} \delta A$. The factor

$$\left(\frac{R_{eq}}{r_0 A^{1/3}}\right)^{2\sigma-2}$$

is 1 to good approximation and therefore Eq. (37) depends primarily on the change of the mean square charge radius as neutrons are added to the nucleus.

Figure 30 shows $\beta C_{exp}/C_{th}$ as a function of the neutron number; C_{th} is calculated with r_0 equal to 1. 20 fm. Plotted are the values for isotope pairs whose neutron number differs by 2 and the points are placed at the higher N-value for each pair of

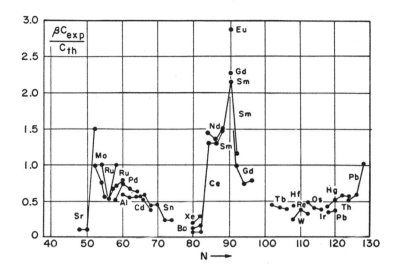

Fig. 30: Ratio of experimental and theoretical isotope shift constants as a function of neutron number (see text). (Heilig, 1960).

isotopes. If the mean square nuclear charge radius followed the $A^{1/3}$ law then all the values would lie on a horizontal straight line intersecting the ordinate at the value 1. This is not the case; the average value of the measured points is about 0.7. This is known as the isotope shift discrepancy and is supposed to have two causes: (i) The factor β which describes the screening of the inner s-electron shells by the valency-electrons is not exactly known. It may be only 0.9 instead of 1 in some cases (Wolter, 1966). However, the good agreement between the isotope shift effect observed in μ-mesonic atoms (Sn, Nd) (Cohen et al., 1966; Bardin et al., 1966) and the optically measured isotope shifts seems to indicate that β is not smaller than 0.9. (ii) Isotope shift measurements indicate that in adding neutrons to a nucleus the nuclear mean square charge radius changes less than according to the $A^{1/3}$ law. To explain this, nuclear compressibility is assumed (Bodmer, 1958). As a consequence, the incorporation of protons at constant neutron number should change the mean square nuclear charge radius more than required by the $A^{1/3}$ law. The data presently available seem to confirm this statement (Quitmann, 1966).

Recently, a qualitative explanation of the jumps in the nuclear volume effect at the closed neutron shells with 50, 82, and 126 neutrons has been given on the basis of the Fermi-liquid theory developed by Landau and Migdal. Also the isotope shift of nuclei adjacent to spherical nuclei has been explained on this basis (Bunatyan and Mikulinsky, 1965) but so far no quantitative agreement has been achieved.

In the rare-earth region, where the nuclei are strongly deformed, the behaviour of the volume effect was first explained by Brix and Kopfermann (1947) and later in somewhat more detail by Wilets et al. (1953). The change of the nuclear deformation upon going from one isotope to the next gives rise to a change in the mean square nuclear charge radius. In going from an isotope with 88 neutrons to an isotope with 90 neutrons the nuclear deformation parameter increases sharply and gives rise to the peak in the volume effect at $N = 90$. When the nuclear deformation has its maximum value and is therefore nearly constant when going from one isotope to the next, the volume shift has an average value. Going to higher neutron numbers ($N \geq 100$), the nuclear deformation parameter decreases and gives a negative contribution to the change of the mean square nuclear charge radius; therefore the volume-effect is smaller than its average value. However, taking the nuclear deformation parameters from measurements of the reduced transition probabilities for E2 radiation it turns out that the agreement between measured and calculated isotope shifts is still not satisfactory in some cases (Fradkin, 1962; Babuschkin, 1964).

If the nuclei have no static deformation, but a nuclear vibration exists, the change of the mean square amplitude of zero vibration of the quadrupole moment has to be taken into account instead of the change of the static deformation, but no satisfactory quantitative explanation of the observed volume shifts has been given.

VIII: Level Crossing

Here we consider another spectroscopic method which gives information about the hfs and the lifetime of excited atomic states with a high degree of precision namely, the level crossing method. This method is based on the fact that under certain conditions the crossing of two Zeeman levels of an excited state of an atom in a magnetic field is accompanied by a change of the angular distribution and the polarization of resonantly scattered light from these levels. A particular, simple case of this effect was investigated by Hanle (1924), i.e., the case of a zero-field level-crossing now often referred to as the Hanle effect.

A. Classical Theory

We consider a level with total angular momentum $J = 1$ (Fig. 31); this may be a fine structure level or a hf level. In a magnetic field this level splits up into its 3 Zeeman-levels with the quantum numbers m = +1, 0, -1; there is a crossing point at zero magnetic field. Assume a resonance transition from a ground state level with angular momentum zero ($J = 0$) to the excited $J = 1$ level. We will use a simple and somewhat restricted theory of the zero-field level crossing derived on classical grounds.

In a frame of reference x, y, z the magnetic field is along the z axis, and at the origin are the atoms to be investigated, either in the form of a free atomic beam, or in a closed evacuated container (a resonance cell). Let us send a beam of resonance radiation along the x-axis which we suppose is polarized with the electric field vector parallel to the y-direction. Classically one may consider the resonance light to excite electric dipoles oscillating along the direction of the y-axis; these dipoles then re-radiate energy with the usual dipole radiation pattern, producing maximum intensity perpendicular to the y-axis and zero intensity along the y-axis. However, if a magnetic field is present, directed along the z axis, the dipoles will precess about this field at their Larmor frequency given by:

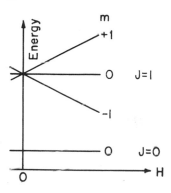

Fig. 31: Level diagram illustrating the Hanle effect.

$$\omega_L = \frac{g_J \mu_0}{\hbar} H \qquad (38)$$

where g_J is the electronic g-factor of the excited state, μ_0 the Bohr magneton. Consider a dipole in the x-y plane excited at time $t = 0$. Before re-radiating at a time t, the dipole has precessed about an angle $\omega_L t$ in the x-y plane and therefore an intensity I in the y-direction will be observed which is

$$I \propto \sin^2 \omega_L t \ . \qquad (39)$$

To account for the random finite excited state lifetimes over a large continuously excited collection of atoms, we have to multiply by an exponential damping factor $\exp(-\Gamma t)$ where Γ is the reciprocal of the mean lifetime τ of the excited state, and to integrate over all times. Then the intensity I observed along the y-axis is

$$I = C \int_0^\infty \exp(-\Gamma t) \sin^2 \omega_L t \, dt \tag{40}$$

where C is a constant related to the incident light intensity, the experimental geometry, and the number of scatters. The result of the integration is

$$I = \frac{C}{2} \left[1 - \frac{1}{1 + (2g_J\mu_0 H/\hbar\Gamma)^2} \right] \tag{41}$$

which is an inverted Lorentzian function of the magnetic field strength H. The full width at half maximum is determined by Γ or in other words by the mean lifetime τ. From the field value $H_{1/2}$ at half-maximum (I = C/4) one finds Γ from the relation

$$\Gamma = \frac{2g_J\mu_0}{\hbar} H_{1/2} \ . \tag{42}$$

Thus a simple determination of the value of the magnetic field $H_{1/2}$ serves in principle to determine the mean lifetime τ, if g_J is known. Also, from this picture it is evident that the half width of the resonance curve is larger the shorter the lifetime. To rotate a dipole within its mean lifetime through a given angle $\omega_L t$, ω_L and therefore the magnetic field H has to be larger if τ is smaller.

To observe the Hanle effect it is not necessary to have the incident light polarized. If the incident light is unpolarized we may describe the incoming light beam as an incoherent superposition of one light beam polarized with the electric field vector perpendicular to the direction of the applied magnetic field and another light beam polarized with the electric field vector parallel to the magnetic field. For the component polarized parallel to the y-axis (perpendicular to the magnetic field) the treatment is the same as just given. The component polarized parallel to the z-axis will excite a dipole oscillating parallel to H; such a dipole does not precess. Therefore, the scattered light from these dipoles is independent of the applied field. Thus, if the incident light is unpolarized, one observes the same resonance curve with an inverted Lorentzian line shape but with a constant background. This is true if, as in our treatment, the direction of the applied exciting light beam, the direction of the applied magnetic field and the direction of observation are mutually orthogonal.

If the exciting light beam is again along the x-axis, the applied magnetic field is again along the z axis, and if we are observing again in the x-y plane, but now with an angle of 45° between the direction of the incoming and outgoing light, then we will find the resonance signal is a dispersion curve. This is easily shown by a treatment analogous to that given above but qualitatively, one can see this at once. If the dipoles are rotating clockwise in the x-y plane, the observed intensity will first decrease and then, for large values of the magnetic field and therefore large values of the angle of precession, will again increase. For an inverted direction of the magnetic field, there is a precession of the dipole in the other direction and the observed intensity will first increase with increasing values of the magnetic field. It may be shown that in the general case of an arbitrary angle between incoming and outgoing light beam direction the observed signal always has a form which is a superposition of a Lorentz curve and a dispersion curve.

This simple classical explanation gives the exact result for a $J = 0 \rightarrow J = 1$ transition and was given in principle for the Hanle effect when it was discovered in 1924.

B. Quantum Theory

A complete quantum mechanical treatment of the effect of level crossing including crossings at finite values of the magnetic field was given by Breit in 1933. More recently, Colegrove et al. (1959) accidently rediscovered the interference effect for levels crossing in non-zero magnetic fields in the fine structure splitting $2^3P_1 - 2^3P_2$ in atomic helium. Since then the technique of level crossing has been applied to many other atoms. Franken (1961) as well as Rose and Carovillano (1961) have given a theoretical explanation of the effect which is based on the work of Breit on resonance fluorescence.

Let us reconsider the description of the Hanle effect given above in another way and look again at a $J = 0 \rightarrow J = 1$ transition, the directions of the incoming light beam, the applied magnetic field and the observation being mutually orthogonal. The component of the incoming light with electric field vector parallel to H only effects a π-transition, i.e., it only excites the Zeeman level with quantum number m = 0. On the other hand the component with electric field vector perpendicular to the magnetic field may be described as a superposition of σ^+ and σ^- light.

Therefore this light with electric field vector perpendicular to the magnetic field is able to excite an atom in a mixed state

$$\psi = \frac{1}{\sqrt{2}} (\psi_{+1} + \psi_{-1})$$ (43)

which is a coherent superposition of the pure states with quantum numbers +1 and -1, provided the spectrum of the incoming light is broad enough. Thus one has a coherent excitation of the two states which have quantum number difference $\Delta m = 2$.

As the two states are coherently excited, the angular distribution of the re-emitted light is the sum of the angular distribution of the light emitted from a $(+1 \rightarrow 0)$ transition plus the angular distribution from a $(-1 \rightarrow 0)$ transition, and in addition, interference terms which modify the angular distribution of the re-emitted light. In general, however, the coherence is not preserved during the lifetime τ of the excited state ψ. At the moment of excitation there is a fixed phase relation between ψ_{+1} and ψ_{-1} which is given by the matrix elements describing the excitation. The evolution of the phase of a state with energy E in time is given by $\exp[-i(E/\hbar)t]$; therefore after a time t a phase difference is introduced between the coherently excited states which is given by $\exp[-i(\Delta E/\hbar)t]$ where ΔE is the energy difference between the levels +1 and -1. It follows that coherence in the sample of atoms under consideration is preserved perfectly for $\Delta E = 0$, that is, at the crossing point of the levels and is destroyed completely for $(\Delta E/\hbar)\tau \gg 1$. Therefore interference effects in the re-emitted light will be observable only if

$$\frac{\Delta E}{\hbar} \tau \lesssim 1$$ (44)

that is, if the two levels +1 and -1 overlap within their natural widths and is the reason why the width of the observed signal measured in frequency units is of the order of $\Gamma = (1/\tau)$.

We have seen that excitation with pure π-light does not produce coherence because pure π-light can only excite one level. For the same reason, excitation with pure σ^+ or pure σ^- light will never produce a coherence. Only a polarization of the incoming light which is a coherent superposition of σ^+ and σ^- light or σ^+ and π light, etc. is able to introduce coherence in the sample of atoms.

If the incident light is unpolarized and perpendicular to the direction of the magnetic field, only states with $\Delta m = 2$ are excited coherently. To produce coherence between levels with

$\Delta m = 1$ (which is necessary in order to observe crossings between levels with $\Delta m = 1$), one has to excite with linearly polarized light neither parallel nor perpendicular to the direction of the magnetic field. For observing the interference effects there are, of course, analogous restrictions for the direction and polarization of the detected light.

For instance, if the exciting light and the detected light both are unpolarized and if the directions of incoming light, outgoing light and magnetic field are mutually orthogonal, only $\Delta m = 2$ level crossings are observed. In general, the selection rule for level-crossings which are observable is

$$0 < \Delta m \leq 2 \tag{45}$$

where the upper limit is given by the selection rules for dipole radiation, the lower limit by the fact that levels with the same quantum number m do not cross.

In the light of coherence the general scheme of a level crossing experiment is: (i) introduction of coherence into the sample of atoms by the excitation process; (ii) evolution in time in the excited state during which coherence is more or less lost; (iii) detection of the coherence. This description of the level crossing is, of course, also valid if two Zeeman-levels cross at finite values of the magnetic field.

To get a more quantitative description of the level crossing method, let us now consider for simplicity only two excited Zeeman-levels b and c which cross at a certain value of magnetic field. It is assumed that these excited states are connected to a ground state Zeeman level a by allowed electric dipole transition so that the phenomenon of resonance fluorescence can occur. The excitation of the states b, c is made by photons with specified direction and polarization. If the vector of polarization of the incoming photons is **f,** then we will call the matrix elements describing the excitation f_{ab} and f_{ac} respectively. Similarly the re-emission of photons with specified direction and polarization is described by matrix elements g_{ba} and g_{ca} where **g** is the vector of polarization for the outcoming photons. The rate $R(\mathbf{f}, \mathbf{g})$ at which photons of polarization **f** are absorbed and photons of polarization **g** are re-emitted is then easily given for two limiting cases: (i) The two levels b and c are completely resolved. Then

$$R(\mathbf{f}, \mathbf{g}) = k\left\{\left|f_{ab}g_{ba}\right|^2 + \left|f_{ac}g_{ca}\right|^2\right\} = R_0 \tag{46}$$

where k is a constant which depends on the photon density and the geometry. This is the well-known relation for the incoherent resonance fluorescence. (ii) The states b and c are exactly crossed. The rate $R(f, g)$ at which photons of polarization f are absorbed and photons of polarization g are re-emitted is given by

$$R(f, g) = k|f_{ab} g_{ba} + f_{ac} g_{ca}|^2 . \qquad (47)$$

Besides the term for the incoherent scattering R_o, we now have interference terms describing the coherent part of the resonance fluorescence. We can write

$$R = R_o + A + A^* \qquad (48)$$

with $A = k f_{ba} f_{ac} g_{ca} g_{ab}$. For the general case, we have a time-delayed scattering process. If an atom is excited at time 0 and re-radiates after a time t, then one has to take the excited state amplitudes at time t to calculate g_{ba} and g_{ca}. The time dependence of the excited state amplitude is given by:

$$|b_t\rangle = |b_o\rangle \exp\left[\left(-i \frac{E_b}{\hbar} - \frac{1}{2}\Gamma\right)t\right], \qquad (49)$$

where E_b is the energy of the state b and $\Gamma = 1/\tau$ describes the damping by the coupling to the radiation field. If the energy of the state b is different from the energy of state c, $E_b \neq E_c$, one has to take into account that at the decay time t the phase of the two states b and c is different, because the energies are different. This is of importance for the interference terms where one has the product $g_{ca} g_{ba}$. This effect cancels for the incoherent terms $|g_{ba}|^2$ and $|g_{ca}|^2$.

Of course, we have to integrate over all times t, and this brings the energy difference coming from the product $g_{ca} g_{ba}$ into the denominator and we have for the general case

$$R(f, g) = R_o + \frac{A}{1 - 2\pi i\tau\nu(bc)} + \frac{A^*}{1 + 2\pi i\tau\nu(bc)} = R_o + S . \qquad (50)$$

Here $\nu(bc)$ is the energy difference between the excited states measured in frequency units; at the crossing point ν disappears. For completely resolved levels, i.e., $2\pi\nu(bc) \gg 1/\tau$, the interference terms disappear and we have only the incoherent part of the resonance scattering. The coherent part or the signal S may be rearranged in the form:

$$S = \frac{A + A^*}{1 + 4\pi^2\tau^2 \nu^2(bc)} + \frac{(A - A^*)2\pi i\tau \nu(bc)}{1 + 4\pi^2 \tau^2 \nu^2 (bc)} . \qquad (51)$$

If the matrix product A is real, the second term disappears. Then the signal just has the well-known Lorentz lineshape with full half-width $\Delta\nu(bc) = 1/\pi\tau$. This width is just twice the natural width of each excited state. The linewidth when expressed in units of magnetic field, is dependent on the angle at which the levels cross as well as on the lifetime:

$$\Delta H = \left(\frac{dH}{d\nu(bc)}\right)_{H_c} \frac{1}{\pi\tau} \tag{52}$$

H_c being the magnetic field strength at the crossing points. For a pure imaginary matrix product A, the first term disappears and the signal becomes a dispersion curve. In the general case if A is complex, one has a mixture of the two pure forms. The conditions for which A is real, imaginary or complex depend on the direction and polarization of the incoming and outgoing beam of light. In general, all three cases can be realized experimentally.

The total absorption cross section of the two levels b and c for the resonance radiation is independent of whether the levels are crossed or not; therefore, the same amount of radiation is always re-emitted in the whole solid angle of 4π. The only effect of the crossing is to modify the angular distribution of the re-emitted radiation. This makes the level crossing phenomenon closely analogous to the classical phenomenon of double-slit interference patterns. In the double-slit experiment the same amount of light (the number of photons per second) goes through the slits whether they are close together or well resolved. The only effect produced when the slits are close is the modification of the distribution of light intensity on the display screen. It should be emphasized, too, that the level crossing is a precise counterpart of the angular correlation of a γ - γ - cascade. The replacement in the initial transition of an emission process in the γ - γ - cascade by an absorption process in level crossing does not change this equivalence.

If the Zeeman levels of the ground state are labeled by m and the Zeeman levels of the excited state by μ, then the rate at which photons of polarization **f** are absorbed and photons of polarization **g** are emitted is given by

$$R(\mathbf{f}, \mathbf{g}) = k \sum_{\substack{\mu\mu' \\ mm'}} \frac{f_{\mu m} f_{m\mu'} g_{\mu'm'} g_{m'\mu}}{\Gamma - i(E_\mu - E_{\mu'})/\hbar} \, . \tag{53}$$

Equation (50) is identical with this general expression if there are only two excited levels and one ground state level. This equation is derived with the following restrictions: (i) the incident light is uniform over the absorption region; (ii) the incident radiation field is weak, so that the number of excited atoms is small with respect to the number of atoms in the ground state; (iii) the atomic ground state population is initially random and remains so; (iv) multiple scattering effects are negligible.

C. Example: Level Crossing in Cd^{113}, Cd^{107}

As an example of the crossing of Zeeman levels at finite values of magnetic field, we take the $5s5p^3P_1$ level in the first spectrum of Cd. Figure 32 is for the stable isotope Cd^{113} which has the nuclear spin $I = 1/2$; therefore at zero magnetic field the fine structure level splits up into two hf-levels with quantum numbers $F = 3/2$ and $F = 1/2$. The Zeeman-levels ($F = 1/2$, $m_F = -1/2$) and ($F = 3/2$, $m_F = +1/2$) cross each other at the magnetic field value of 2055 gauss. In this example only this one crossing point exists; it is a $\Delta m = 2$ crossing and is sufficient to determine the A value of the hf-splitting. In this simple case the dependence of the Zeeman levels on the magnetic field strength is given by the Breit-Rabi formula. Using this formula the magnetic field H_C at which the levels cross turns out to be

$$H_c = \frac{A(^3P_1)}{(g_J + 1/2\, g_I)\mu_o} \quad \text{with} \quad g_I = \frac{\mu_I}{\mu_o I} \; . \tag{54}$$

Therefore the measurement of the magnetic field strength at the crossing point allows the calculation of the A-value if g_J and g_I are known. From this simple example it can be seen that the level-crossing method allows one to determine the ratio of the hf coupling constant A to g_J assuming that g_I is known from other measurements, for instance, by NMR. If there exists a B value, again only the ratio B/g_J is determined. Thus one compares hyperfine energy with magnetic energy. To get the absolute values of A and B, g_J and g_I must be determined by other methods. (For instance g_J can be determined with high accuracy by the $\Delta F = 0$ transitions of an optical double resonance experiment at low values of the magnetic field.)

The number of observable crossing points is always sufficient to determine all the hf interaction constants. Figure 33 shows an example for the radioactive isotope Cd^{107} whose nuclear spin is

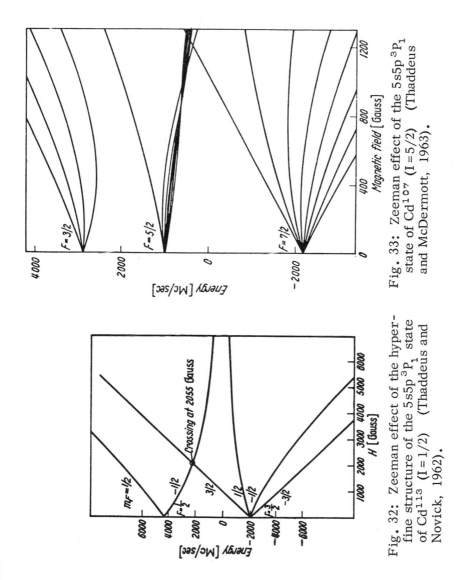

Fig. 33: Zeeman effect of the 5s5p $^3P_1$ state of Cd^{107} (I = 5/2) (Thaddeus and McDermott, 1963).

Fig. 32: Zeeman effect of the hyperfine structure of the 5s5p $^3P_1$ state of Cd^{113} (I = 1/2) (Thaddeus and Novick, 1962).

I = 5/2, for which we have three hyperfine levels with quantum numbers F = 3/2, 5/2, and 7/2. As we see, most of the crossings are "foldover" crossings, that is, crossings of sublevels which originate in the same F-level. There is only one observable crossing between sublevels belonging to different F-levels. Figure 34 shows a magnification of the interesting part of the level diagram. There are 4 crossing points with Δm = 1 and 4 crossing points with Δm = 2. Of course, the signals of the seven foldover crossings are very much broader than the signal of the ΔF = 1 crossing because of the smaller relative inclination of the crossing levels. All crossings with Δm = 1 and Δm = 2 have been measured in this case.

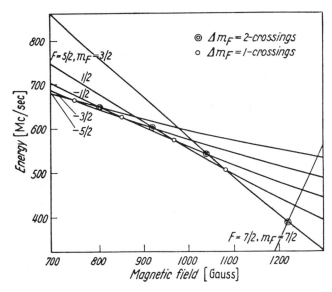

Fig. 34: Details of the level crossings in the (5s5p) $^3P_1$ state of Cd^{107}. (Thaddeus and McDermott, 1963).

D. Discussion: Advantages and Disadvantages

As a spectroscopic technique the level crossing method offers the advantages of experimental simplicity and high resolution. A change in resonance fluorescence is experienced only when the two excited state levels are separated by an energy of the order of their natural width and this is only a small fraction of the Doppler-width one has in the optical transition. Thus, one may determine A and B values of excited states with an accuracy of 10^{-4}. Of course, the accuracy achieved depends on the lifetime of the particular excited state. With the level crossing method one has just the same accuracy as in an optical double resonance experiment.

Against the simplicity and the advantages of the level crossing method must be opposed the computational difficulty of evaluating the hf constants from the observed crossings. At low fields the Zeeman interaction between hf levels can be treated by perturbation techniques. Level crossings occur, however, when the Zeeman and hf energies are comparable; this means the diagonal and the off-diagonal matrix elements of the Hamiltonian are of the same order of magnitude and the zero field splitting can be calculated only by solving the general secular equation. Fortunately, since this problem is amenable to high-speed computing techniques, the advantages of the level crossing method will considerably outweigh its disadvantages.

Now let us turn again to the zero field level crossing. We have seen that this particular case is suited for the determination of atomic excited state lifetimes. The determination of atomic transition probabilities is an old problem in physics, but the absolute values of lifetimes given in the literature often disagree by an order of magnitude. The reason for this is that most of the experimental methods applied to determine absolute values of the transition probabilities of spectral lines require a knowledge of the density of the scattering atoms, a requirement which causes a limitation of the precision of these methods. The zero field level crossing on the other hand does not suffer from this requirement in the limit of low vapour densities and is therefore much more reliable.

Many lifetime determinations have been carried out in the last few years using the zero field level crossing method; these are useful to determine the coupling constants of the electronic eigenfunctions in intermediate coupling. On the other hand, the results of lifetime measurements may be used as a good check on calculated eigenfunctions or as a test for approximation methods used to calculate oscillator strengths. Moreover lifetimes of excited atomic states are in many cases of great astrophysical interest.

References

Armstrong, Jr., L. and Marrus, R. (1965). Phys. Rev. 138, B310.

Babushkin, F. A. (1964). Soviet Phys. -JETP 18, 1022.

Baker, J. M. and Williams, F. I. B. (1962). Proc. Roy. Soc. (London) A267, 283.

Bardin, T. T., Barrett, C. R., Cohen, R. C., Devons, S., Hitlin, D., Macagno, E., Nissim-Sabat, C., Rainwater, J., Runge, K., and Wu, C. S. (1966). Progress Report, Columbia University.

Barnes, R. G. and Smith, W. V. (1954). Phys. Rev. 93, 95.

Barret, R. C. (1966). Nucl. Phys. 88, 128.

Bauche, J. (1966). (to be published).

Bodmer, A. R. (1958). Nucl. Phys. 9, 371.

Bordarier, Y., Judd, B. R., and Klapisch, M. (1965). Proc. Roy. Soc. (London) A289, 81.

Breit, G. (1933). Rev. Mod. Phys. 5, 91.

Brix, P. (1952). Z. Physik 132, 579.

Brix, P. and Kopfermann, H. (1947). Nachr., Akad. Wiss. Gottingen, Math. Phys. Kl., 31; (1949). Z. Physik 126, 344.

Bunatyan, G. G. and Mikulinsky, M. A. (1965). Soviet J. Nucl. Phys. 1, 26.

Casimir, H. B. G. (1936). Teylors Tweede Genootschap 11, 36 (trans. 1953, Freeman and Co., San Francisco).

Cohen, R. C., Devons, S., Kanaris, A. D., and Nissim-Sabat, C. (1966). Phys. Rev. 141, 48.

Colegrove, J. D., Franken, P. A., Lewis, R. R., and Sands, R.H. (1959). Phys. Rev. Letters 3, 420.

Davis, S. P., Aung, T., and Kleiman, H. (1966). Phys. Rev. 147, 861.

Elbek, B. (1963). "Determination of Nuclear Transition Probabilities by Coulomb Excitation" (Munksgaards Forlag, Copenhagen).

Evans, L., Sandars, P. G. H., and Woodgate, G. K. (1965). Proc. Roy. Soc. (London). A289, 114.

Fradkin, E. E. (1962). Soviet Phys. - JETP 15, 550.

Franken, P. A. (1961). Phys. Rev. 121, 508.

Goodman, L. S., Nöldeke, G., and Walther, H. (1962). Z. Physik 167, 26.

Guthöhrlein, G., Kopfermann, H., Nöldeke, G., and Steudel, A. (1961). Z. Physik 165, 356.

Hanle, W. (1924). Z. Physik 30, 93.

Hansen, J. E., Steudel, A. and Walther, H. (1965). Physics Letters 19, 565.

Hansen, J. E. Steudel, A. and Walther, H. (1967) (to be published lished).

Hefft, K., Kern, R., Nöldeke, G., and Steudel, A. (1963). Z. Physik 175, 391.

Heilig, K. (1961). Thesis, University of Heidelberg.

Heilig, K. (1961). Z. Physik 161, 252.

Jacquinot, P. and Dufour, Ch. (1948). J. Rech. CNRS 6, 91.

King, W. H. (1963). J. Opt. Soc. Am. 53, 638.

Kopfermann, H. (1958). Nuclear Moments (Academic Press, N.Y.).

Krebs, K. and Winkler, R. (1960). Z. Physik 160, 320.

Kuhl, J., Steudel, A. Walther, H. (1966). Z. Physik 196, 365.

Mottelson, B. R. and Nilsson, S. G. (1955). Phys. Rev. 99, 1615.

Müller, W., Steudel, A. and Walther, H. (1965). Z.Physik 183, 303.

Nilsson, S. G. (1955). Kgl. Danske Videnskab. Selskab, Mat. Fys. Medd 29, No. 16.

Quitmann, D. (1966) (to be published).

Rose, M. E. and Carovillano, R. L. (1961). Phys. Rev. 122, 1185.

Sandars, P. G. H. and Woodgate, G. K. (1960). Proc. Roy. Soc. (London) A257, 269.

Sandars, P. G. H. and Beck, J. (1965). Proc. Roy. Soc. (London) A289, 97.

Schlect, R. G., White, M. B., and McColm, D. W. (1965). Phys. Rev. 138, B306.

Schüler, H. and Schmidt, T. (1935). Z. Physik 94, 457.

Striganov, A. R., Katulin, V. A., and Eliseev, V. V. (1962). Optics and Spectroscopy 12, 91.

Thaddeus, P. and Novick, R. (1962). Phys. Rev. 126, 1774.

Thaddeus, P. and McDermott, M. N. (1963). Phys. Rev. 132, 1186.

Tomlinson, III, W. J. and Stroke, H. H. (1964). Nucl. Phys. 60, 614.

Walther, H. (1962). Z. Physik 170, 507.

Wilets, L., Hill, D. L., and Ford, K. W. (1953). Phys. Rev. 91, 1488.

Wolter, H. (1966). (unpublished).

Woodgate, G. K. and Martin, J. S. (1947). Proc. Roy. Soc. (London) A70, 458.

6. SPECIAL TOPICS IN HYPERFINE STRUCTURE IN EPR

S. Geschwind

Bell Telephone Laboratories
Murray Hill, New Jersey

Table of Contents

I. Electron-Nuclear Double Resonance (ENDOR)

A. Hyperfine Structure in EPR

As a point of departure for a discussion of ENDOR or electron-nuclear double resonance, let us examine closely the accuracy with which hyperfine interactions are measured via EPR. Consider a paramagnetic center such as Cu^{2+}, consisting of electron spin $S = \frac{1}{2}$ and nuclear spin $I = \frac{3}{2}$ in tetragonal symmetry. We will briefly review the main features of the hfs of the EPR spectrum as outlined earlier in Chap. 1 by Prof. Bleaney. The orbital angular momentum is quenched in the electronic ground state. The familiar spin Hamiltonian for this system is given by

$$\mathcal{H} = g_{||}\beta H_z S_z + g_{\perp}\beta(H_x S_x + H_y S_y) + A I_z S_z$$

$$+ B(I_x S_x + I_y S_y) + Q[I_z^2 - \tfrac{1}{3}I(I+1)] - g_I \mu_N \mathbf{H} \cdot \mathbf{I} \qquad (1)$$

The last term in Eq. (1) is the nuclear Zeeman energy in the external magnetic field. Q is the quadrupolar interaction energy given by

$$Q = \frac{3eQ'q}{4I(2I-1)} \qquad (2)$$

where q is the electric field gradient at the nucleus and Q' is the nuclear electric quadrupole moment. A and B are the magnetic hyperfine interaction terms.

With a magnetic field parallel to the c-axis, a microwave field at right angles to the c-axis induces transitions $\Delta m_S = \pm 1$; $\Delta m_I = 0$; ($m_S = \langle S_z \rangle$ and $m_I = \langle I_z \rangle$). For a fixed microwave frequency, this gives rise to a $(2I+1)$ or four line hyperfine structure pattern as the magnetic field is swept. There will also be "forbidden transitions," $\Delta m_S = \pm 1$, $\Delta m_I = \pm 1$ induced by a microwave field parallel to the dc field which will be down in intensity by $(B/g\beta H_0)^2 \ll 1$, which we will neglect. The allowed transitions are shown in Fig. 1 where the quadrupolar and nuclear Zeeman energies have been omitted from the energy level diagram for the sake of convenience. But note, of course, that these energies do not appear in the normal EPR spectrum because of the $\Delta m_I = 0$ selection rule in the $\Delta m_S = \pm 1$ microwave transition. Neglecting second order corrections of the order of $B^2/g\beta H$, one observes four equally spaced lines whose separation measures only the hyperfine interaction A, i.e. the product of nuclear moment and hyperfine field. This spectrum yields no information on the nuclear moment $g_I \mu_N I$, or the quadrupole coupling constant Q. If Q is comparable to A, then by applying H_0 at an angle to the c-axis, the m_I states are mixed since the hyperfine field tries to align the nuclei along its direction parallel to H_0, while the electric field gradient tries to align them along the c-axis. Thus, one obtains $\Delta m_I = \pm 1$, ± 2 transitions in the microwave spectrum from which one can determine Q (Bleaney, 1954; and Bleaney et al., 1955). In principle, these transitions also contain information on the nuclear Zeeman splitting. However, nuclear Zeeman splittings in external magnetic fields are typically of the order of 10 Mc/sec and therefore correspond to a shift of only a few gauss in the electronic spectrum which is of the order of the EPR linewidths. Thus in practice, nuclear moments *cannot* be determined by EPR with any significant accuracy. To a lesser degree similar restrictions apply to Q and even to A in those cases where they are of the order of an EPR linewidth. However, in the more typical cases such as the Cu^{2+} ion, $A/g\beta$ is about 100 gauss while ΔH may be several gauss. Thus A can typically be determined via EPR to an accuracy of a few percent which corresponds to the kind of accuracy realized in the Mössbauer effect.

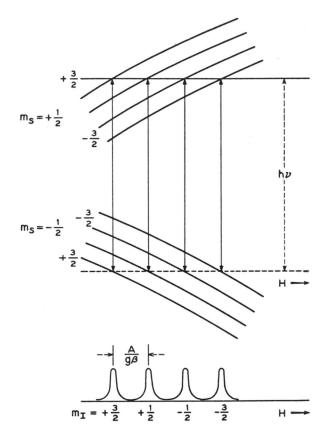

Fig. 1: Energy levels and EPR spectrum for an ion with S = 1/2,
I = 3/2 (i. e. , Cu^{2+} ground state) in a tetragonal environment with the external field along the c-axis.

B. How ENDOR Circumvents Problem of Inhomogeneous Line-width in EPR

The linewidths of a few gauss or more of the EPR spectrum
are generally due to inhomogeneous broadening of the electronic
states due to a spread of local fields at the different paramagnetic
centers. The ENDOR technique invented by Feher (1956a; Feher
and Gere, 1956b) overcomes this difficulty of inhomogeneous linewidth by allowing one to observe the very weak almost purely
nuclear transitions $\Delta m_s = 0$, $\Delta m_I = \pm 1$. By this method, even if
A is too small to be resolved in the EPR spectrum, one can still
measure A, Q, and g_I in dilute magnetic centers with the accuracy

characteristic of nuclear magnetic resonance (NMR).

Consider a simple $S = 1/2$, $I = 1/2$ system with an isotropic hf interaction whose Hamiltonian is

$$\mathcal{H} = g_e \beta H_0 S_z + A\mathbf{I} \cdot \mathbf{S} - g_I \mu_N I_z H_0 \ . \tag{3}$$

In the strong field region ($g_e \beta H_0 >> A$) the energy levels of the system are as shown in Fig. 2. The appropriate energy level diagram

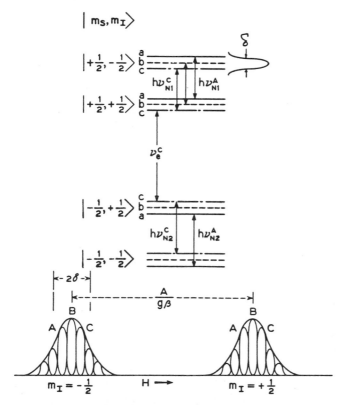

Fig. 2: Ion with $S = 1/2$, $I = 1/2$ and diagonal energy given by $W = g\beta Hm_S + Am_S m_I$. Levels A, B, C, etc. correspond to ions experiencing slightly different magnetic or electric fields (see text).

is shown for three species of centers which see slightly different local fields. These different local fields can correspond to variations in local magnetic field which may be due to random orientations of neighboring nuclei in the host crystal, for example. They may also be due to random strains and electric fields which produce slightly different electronic g-values at these centers. In either case, the net result is an inhomogeneous broadening of the electronic levels into a width δ comprising these different "spin packets." However, the variation of local fields has orders of magnitude smaller effect on the relative shift of the nuclear sub-levels within a given m_S level. The spread δ in electronic levels appears in $h\nu_N$ for the different centers, A, B, C, as a spread of something of the order of only

$$\delta' = \delta \times \frac{\text{nuclear magneton}}{\text{Bohr magneton}} \,. \tag{4}$$

Thus, if RF transitions or ENDOR transitions are made within a given m_S they will have the very small spread δ'. Note carefully, however, that the width of a given RF transition, for a given spin packet A, for example, is not to be confused with δ'. The width of the ENDOR transition is determined by other factors mentioned below and very often can be even much less than δ'.

The two RF frequencies ν_{N1} and ν_{N2} are given by

$$\nu_{N1} = 1/h \left[A/2 - g_I \mu_N H_o \right] \tag{5a}$$

$$\nu_{N2} = 1/h \left[A/2 + g_I \mu_N H_o \right] \tag{5b}$$

or

$$A/h = \nu_{N1} + \nu_{N2} \tag{6a}$$

$$g_I \mu_N H_o = \frac{\nu_{N1} - \nu_{N2}}{2} \tag{6b}$$

where the transverse terms in the hyperfine interaction have been neglected in Eqs. (5a) and (5b), $(g_e \beta H_o \gg A)$. Thus, if we measure the sum of the two RF frequencies, we determine A while their difference yields twice the nuclear Zeeman energy, $2g_I \mu_N H$. The procedure as just outlined gives no information on the signs of A and μ_I. For larger values of I or S, higher order corrections from off-diagonal terms containing A can usually give the signs as well.

We now examine how these ENDOR transitions are observed via the electron resonance in very dilute paramagnets. In Fig. 3a, the relative equilibrium populations in our $S = 1/2$, $I = 1/2$ system are shown, where $\epsilon = \beta H_o/2kT$. The equilibrium

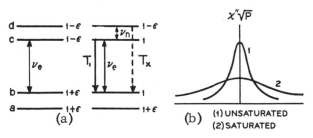

Fig. 3: Observation of ENDOR (ν_n) via electron resonance (ν_e) (see text).

Boltzmann factor for the nuclei within a given m_s level has been neglected as it is orders of magnitude smaller than ϵ. Microwave energy $h\nu_e$ is applied which tends to saturate the allowed transition and equalize the populations, as shown, and reduce the fractional absorbed microwave power. Assuming for the moment that the only relaxations in the system are $\Delta m_s = \pm 1$, $\Delta m_I = 0$, the resultant populations upon saturation of levels b and c are as shown. Note that one now has a difference in nuclear populations in each m_s state corresponding to ϵ, i.e. the electronic Boltzmann factor. One now induces RF transitions between levels c and d whose effect is to momentarily unsaturate levels b and c, giving a transient increase in the fractional absorbed microwave power. Thus, on a transient basis, one anticipates a change in the saturated electronic signal when the nuclei are resonated that is roughly comparable to the electronic signal itself. The linewidth of the ENDOR transition will, in a general way, be connected with the electronic relaxation time T_1. ENDOR signals can be as narrow as 10 kc/sec as compared with the Mc/sec linewidths of the normal EPR signals.

If we take as a typical favorable example a nuclear Zeeman interaction with the external field of 10 Mc/sec and a hyperfine interaction of 100 Mc/sec, then if the ENDOR frequencies are measured with an accuracy of a few kc/sec, the nuclear magnetic moment (uncorrected for shielding effects) is measured to a few parts in 10^4 and the hyperfine interaction to a few parts in 10^5. The main advantages of ENDOR are then: (i) It allows one to measure nuclear magnetic and electric hyperfine interactions and magnetic moments in magnetic ions present in extremely small dilution. (ii) This is done with the sensitivity of EPR. (iii) The accuracy, however, is comparable to that of NMR. ENDOR has also played a very important role in solid state physics by measuring hyperfine fields at neighboring nuclei in different shells

around a paramagnetic center such as donors in silicon and F-
centers. Such measurements provide information on the wavefunctions of these centers (Feher, 1958; Holton et al., 1960). Our
main interest in this chapter is, however, its role in measuring
hf fields at the nuclei of transition metal and rare-earth ions.

C. Mechanisms of ENDOR

In practice the actual *steady state* change in electronic
signal that is observed is usually only a few percent of the electron signal. This is due to the fact that other relaxation processes
are operative which give an equilibrium population difference
between c and d in the presence of microwave saturation of b
and c, that is, considerably less than ε (cf. Fig. 3).

The actual details of the ENDOR process are exceedingly
complex and many different mechanisms are separately and
jointly operative under different conditions. The complexity of
the process arises from the fact that one is dealing with a multi-
level system with different relaxation rates between the different
levels. Even for our simple system the populations must be
described by four coupled rate equations with many of the relaxation rates unknown. The performance of ENDOR is therefore
usually reduced to a knob twiddling exercise, albeit a relatively
easy one. We will, however, briefly describe three mechanisms
which have been discussed and refer the reader to the literature
for a more detailed discussion.

1. Change of Effective Electronic T_1

The peak microwave absorption signal seen in EPR
spectrometers with linear detection is proportional to $\chi''(P)^{\frac{1}{2}}$
where χ'' for a homogeneous line is given by

$$\chi'' = \frac{\chi_0 \, \omega_0 T_2}{1 + (\gamma H_1)^2 T_1 T_2} \tag{7}$$

and P, the incident power, is proportional to H_1^2, χ_0 is the dc
susceptibility, T_2 is the transverse relaxation time or reciprocal
of the *homogeneous* linewidth, γ is the electron gyromagnetic
ratio, T_1 the spin-lattice relaxation time between levels $\Delta m_S =
\pm 1$ and $\Delta m_I = 0$, and H_1 is the intensity of the microwave mag-
netic field (see Fig. 3b). Feher (1958) proposed that a steady state
change in χ'' upon application of ν_N results by effectively changing T_1 in Eq. (7); this is illustrated in Fig. 3a. There is a weak
"forbidden" relaxation shown by T_X. The effect of the ENDOR
power is to provide another relaxation path between levels b and

c via T_x by connecting c and d with the RF. In this picture one expects a change in electronic signal of the order T_1 / T_x. The treatment for an inhomogeneous line requires a modification of Eq. (7), but the essential feature, i.e. the change in effective T_1, still remains. Seidel (1961) has examined this problem in detail and has shown that after a fast transient a smaller steady state signal of a few percent is obtained in reasonable agreement with expectations.

    2. Packet Shifting Mechanism

       In the case of donors in silicon and F-centers in alkali halides, the inhomogeneous linewidth arises from the magnetic fields of neighboring nuclei, each spin packet in the microwave line corresponding to a class of electron centers experiencing the same local field from neighboring nuclei (Feher, 1958). ENDOR transitions which flip the neighboring nuclei change the local fields of the unsaturated packet at positions B_2 and B_3 in Fig. 4, thus

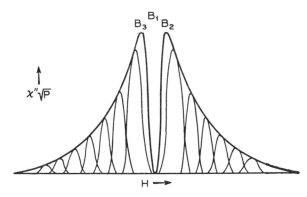

Fig. 4: Packet shifting mechanism of ENDOR (Feher, 1958).
      Flipping of nuclei in spin packet B_2 shifts this packet to
      B_1, and unsaturates the EPR signal.

filling up the "burned hole" at B_1 and giving an increased electron signal again.

    3. Distant ENDOR

       Lambe et al. (1961) found that when the Cr^{3+} EPR in Al_2O_3 was saturated, the flipping of Al nuclei far from the Cr^{3+} center changed the Cr^{3+} EPR signal. The recovery time of the changed electron signal when the RF power was removed was that of the Al spin-lattice relaxation. They also found that the ENDOR

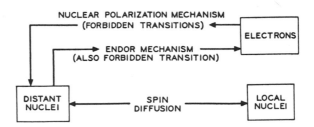

Fig. 5: Distant ENDOR mechanism in which bulk nuclei of sample
        act as a thermal reservoir for electronic signal via the
        "solid effect."

signal of the Cr nuclei also recovered with the same relaxation
time. They proposed that the saturation of the Cr^{3+} electron
resonance polarized the bulk Al nuclei by Abragam's "effet
solide"* as shown in Fig. 5. Flipping the Al nuclei unsaturated
the Cr^{3+} electron signal by the same connection. They also proposed that the Cr nuclei were connected to distant Al nuclei by
spin diffusion as shown in Fig. 5.

In considering these three mechanisms it should be recognized that both the packet-shifting mechanism and distant ENDOR
involve the host nuclei which must have magnetic moments.
Therefore, they would play no role in the ENDOR of Mn^{2+} in CaO,
for example, where there are no significant numbers of magnetic
host nuclei. In such a case the steady-state ENDOR mechanism
must involve an effective change in the electronic T_1 as described
in Sec. I. C. 1. above.

D.   Experimental Procedure

Experimentally, the modification needed on an EPR spectrometer to perform ENDOR is relatively trivial. One need
simply wind a small RF coil around the specimen in the microwave cavity in such a way as not to interfere with the microwaves
and apply the ENDOR frequency to this coil. The electron signal
is saturated and the RF oscillator is swept through a nuclear
transition, producing a change in the electronic signal. One such
scheme is shown in Fig. 6. More details involving this method
of winding the coil directly around the sample may be found in
Locher and Geschwind (1965). The advantage of this scheme is
that it concentrates the RF power at the sample. Many other
techniques of introducing the RF frequency to the sample may be

*See A. Abragam and J. Kirsch, Chap. 8.

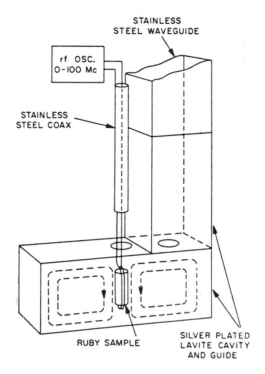

Fig. 6: ENDOR coil wound directly around sample (Lambe et al.).

found in the literature. Feher (1956; 1958) used a glass cavity coated with silver whose thickness was greater than a microwave skin depth but less than the RF skin depth. An RF coil was wound around the outside of the cavity as shown in Fig. 7. In Fig. 8 a scheme developed by Hyde (1965) for high power ENDOR is shown. Such high powers are needed in liquids where T_1's are short and for ENDOR on neighboring nuclei where the enhancement factor discussed in the next paragraph, is small. Hyde's microwave cavity is in effect a single turn RF coil.

E. RF Enhancement Factor

The amount of RF field, h_1, needed to saturate the ENDOR transitions will not be controlled by the nuclear spin-lattice relaxation but more nearly by the electronic T_1. Thus, $h_1 \propto 1/T_1^{elec}$. For relaxation times of 1 msec, this would mean an RF field of several gauss. In many problems this field could produce troublesome heating effects. This would be the case in combined RF-nuclear orientation experiments

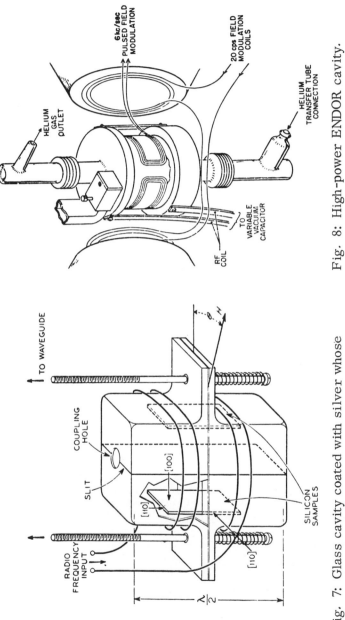

Fig. 8: High-power ENDOR cavity. Top and bottom plates of cavity are part of single turn RF coil (Hyde, 1965).

Fig. 7: Glass cavity coated with silver whose thickness is greater than microwave but less than RF skin depth. RF coil is wound on outside (Feher, 1958).

discussed by Dr. Matthias.* Fortunately, in many cases there is an *enhancement* of the RF via the hyperfine field which significantly reduces the size of the required h_1.

This enhancement can be very easily seen by a simple physical picture shown in Fig. 9. Imagine an isolated paramagnetic

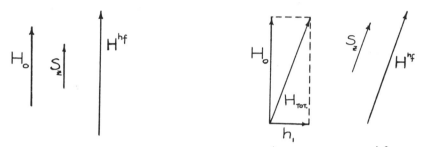

Fig. 9: Enhancement of RF field h_1, by hyperfine field, H^{hf}. Enhancement factor is approximately H^{hf}/H_o.

impurity in a given S_z state in an external magnetic field. The hyperfine field will be along S_z and therefore along H_0. When the RF field h_1 is applied at right angles to the dc field the total field seen by the electron is the vector sum of $\mathbf{H_0}$ and $\mathbf{h_1}$ Since the frequency $\mathbf{h_1}$ is much less than the Larmor precessional frequency of the electrons in the external field, the electronic motion will adiabatically follow $\mathbf{H}_{total}$ and so will the hyperfine field. Thus, H^{hf} will have a projection along h_1 given by $h_1 H^{hf}/H_0$ which oscillates at the frequency of h_1. The nucleus, however, cannot follow this rapid motion and so sees the RF field h_1 enhanced by the factor H^{hf}/H_0. For typical hf fields of several hundred kilogauss this enhancement factor is of the order of 10^3. This exact same enhancement is operative in NMR in *single domain* ferromagnets and is called domain rotation enhancement. Robert (1962) has quantitatively verified this enhancement in a single domain sphere of YIG, for example. It should be pointed out, however, that in ferromagnets there is a domain wall motion enhancement operative which usually is more important (Gossard and Portis, 1960).

This enhancement can also be seen quantum mechanically as pointed out by Abragam (1961). In the Hamiltonian of Eq. (3), the transverse terms of the hyperfine interaction, $A/2(S_+I_- + S_-I_+)$

*E. Matthias, Chap. 13.

produce admixtures of $|m_{s+1}, m_{I-1}\rangle$ and $|m_{s-1}, m_{I+1}\rangle$ states into each $|m_s, m_I\rangle$ state. If we let

$$p = \frac{A}{4\beta H_0} << 1 \tag{8}$$

and

$$\omega_{s,s-1} = \langle m_{s-1}|S_-|m_s\rangle$$

$$\omega_{s-1,s} = \langle m_s|S_+|m_{s-1}\rangle \tag{9}$$

and similarly for I_+ and I_- then two neighboring nuclear sub-states $|m_s, m_I\rangle'$ and $|m_s, m_{I-1}\rangle'$ become

$$|a\rangle = |m_s, m_I\rangle' = |m_s, m_I\rangle + \omega_{s,s-1}, \omega_{I,I+1} p |m_{s-1}, m_{I+1}\rangle$$

$$- \omega_{s,s+1}, \omega_{I,I-1} p |m_{s+1}, m_{I-1}\rangle \tag{10a}$$

$$|b\rangle = |m_s, m_{I-1}\rangle' = |m_s, m_{I-1}\rangle + \omega_{s,s-1}, \omega_{I-1,I} p |m_{s-1}, m_I\rangle$$

$$-\omega_{s,s+1}, \omega_{I-1,I-2} p |m_{s+1}, m_{I-2}\rangle \ . \tag{10b}$$

Now the RF field h_1, applied in the x-direction, produces a perturbation $\mathcal{H}'$ given by

$$\mathcal{H}' = g\beta h_1 S_x - g_I \mu_N h_1 I_x \tag{11a}$$

$$= \beta h_1 (S_+ + S_-) - \frac{g_I}{2} \mu_N h_1 (I_+ + I_-) \ . \tag{11b}$$

The transition rate will be proportional to

$$|\mathcal{H}'_{ba}|^2 = |\langle a|\mathcal{H}'|b\rangle|^2 \ . \tag{12}$$

If we neglect terms of order $p^2 << 1$, we find

$$\mathcal{H}' = h_1 \left[-\omega_{I-1,I} \frac{g_I \mu_N}{2} + \right.$$

$$\left. \left(\omega_{s,s-1}^2, \omega_{I-1,I} - \omega_{s,s+1}^2, \omega_{I,I-1} \right) p\beta \right] \tag{13}$$

or

$$\mathcal{H}'_{ba} = h_1 \omega_{I,I-1} \left[-\frac{g_I \mu_N}{2} + \frac{2m_s A}{4H_0} \right] \ , \tag{14}$$

$$\mathcal{H}'_{ba} = \frac{h_1}{2} \, g_I \mu_N \, \omega_{I,I-1} \left[-1 + \frac{H^{hf}}{H_o} \right] \tag{15}$$

where

$$H^{hf} = \frac{-A m_S}{g_I \mu_N} \, . \tag{16}$$

Thus, if $H^{hf} \gg H_o$, we see again that the RF field h_1 is enhanced by H^{hf}/H_o. Note that this enhancement factor is absent in an $m_S = 0$ state and is greatest for the largest values of m_S. This is borne out in all experiments where it is invariably found that the ENDOR signals are strongest in the higher m_S states.

II. Paramagnetic Shielding of Nuclear Moments

In view of the high experimental precision with which the nuclear Zeeman interaction can be determined by ENDOR, one is led to consider the magnetic shielding of the nuclear moment. The nucleus sees an effective field $H_o(1+\sigma)$ where σ is the shielding term which is independent of the magnitude of H_o. This is a problem common to the measurement of nuclear moments by NMR, Mössbauer effect, angular correlation, etc. We will not be concerned with the diamagnetic corrections, which are fully treated in Prof. Abragam's book (Abragam, 1961) and are usually quite small, but with the paramagnetic shielding corrections which even for *orbital singlet* ground states in crystals can be as large a *few percent*. One would very often like to know nuclear moment values to 0.1% as, for example, in studies of Knight shifts in metals.

The paramagnetic shielding correction has been briefly mentioned by Prof. Bleaney* who called it the pseudo-nuclear Zeeman effect and we wish to treat it in more detail and consider specific applications to certain transition metal ions. We wish to relate this paramagnetic shielding correction to some other observable such as an electronic g-shift or the Van Vleck temperature independent susceptibility. These quantities are also related to the orbital hyperfine field. Consider the full Hamiltonian of a transition metal ion such as Ni^{2+} in a cubic crystal field (Abragam and Pryce, 1951).

*B. Bleaney, Chap. 1.

$$\mathcal{H} = \underset{\substack{\text{crystal} \\ \text{field} \\ \text{energy}}}{\underbrace{V_{\text{cryst.}}}} + \underset{\substack{\text{spin} \\ \text{orbit}}}{\underbrace{\lambda \mathbf{L} \cdot \mathbf{S}}} + \underset{\substack{\text{electronic} \\ \text{Zeeman}}}{\underbrace{\beta \mathbf{H} \cdot (\mathbf{L} + 2\mathbf{S})}}$$

$$+ \left\{ \underset{\substack{\text{core} \\ \text{polariza-} \\ \text{tion}}}{\underbrace{A\mathbf{I} \cdot \mathbf{S}}} + \underset{\text{(orbital)}}{\underbrace{P\mathbf{L} \cdot \mathbf{I}}} \underset{\text{(dipolar)}}{\underbrace{-P\left[\frac{3}{2} \xi(\mathbf{L} \cdot \mathbf{S})(\mathbf{L} \cdot \mathbf{I}) - \frac{3}{2}(\mathbf{L} \cdot \mathbf{I})(\mathbf{L} \cdot \mathbf{S})\right]}} \right\}$$

$$\{ \longleftarrow \text{hyperfine interaction} \longrightarrow \}$$

$$- \underset{\text{(nuclear Zeeman)}}{\underbrace{g_I \mu_N \mathbf{I} \cdot \mathbf{H}}} \qquad . \tag{17}$$

Here

$$P = 2\beta g_I \mu_N \left\langle \frac{1}{r^3} \right\rangle \tag{18}$$

and

$$\xi = \frac{(2\ell + 1) - 4}{S(2\ell - 1)(2\ell + 3)(2L - 1)} \quad , \quad \ell = 2 \ . \tag{19}$$

Details of the derivation of these hyperfine terms may be found in the paper of Abragam and Pryce. We have omitted the quadrupolar interaction.

The electronic configuration of Ni^{2+} is $(3d)^8$ with a free ion ground term $L = 3$, $S = 1$, i.e., ^3F. In the cubic crystal field, the sevenfold orbital degeneracy is lifted into an orbital singlet, $^3A_2$ ground state and two excited state orbital triplets $^3T_2$ and $^3T_1$ at roughly 10,000 and 15,000 cm^{-1} respectively above the ground state. $V_{\text{cryst}} >>$ than all the other terms in the Hamiltonian. To first order then, the orbital angular momentum is quenched in the ground state, i.e., $\langle ^3A_2 | \mathbf{L} | ^3A_2 \rangle = 0$. However, the other terms will, in higher order, mix orbital angular momentum into the ground state, giving rise to the electronic g-shift, orbital hyperfine field, paramagnetic shielding of the nucleus and Van Vleck temperature independent susceptibility. We relate these to one another using the perturbation procedure of Abragam and Pryce (1951).

A. Electronic g-Shift

In second order, cross terms of $\lambda \mathbf{L} \cdot \mathbf{S}$ and $\mathbf{H} \cdot \mathbf{L}$ give an energy

$$W_{\Delta g} = \beta \sum_n \frac{\langle 0 | \lambda \mathbf{L} \cdot \mathbf{S} | n \rangle \langle n | \mathbf{H} \cdot \mathbf{L} | \rangle}{E_0 - E_n} + c.c \qquad (20)$$

where $\langle 0 |$ is the orbital singlet ground state and $| n \rangle$ are the excited states. Of course we can only do the perturbation theory this way, writing $\lambda \mathbf{L} \cdot \mathbf{S}$ instead of

$$\sum_i \xi \mathbf{l}_i \mathbf{s}_i,$$

etc., if the excited states are derived from the same free-ion state as the ground term. The generalization to other excited states is straightforward and may be found in Griffith's book (Griffith, 1961).

Let

$$W_{\Delta g}^{ij} = 2\beta \lambda \Lambda_{ij} S_i H_j \qquad (21)$$

where

$$\Lambda_{ij} = \sum_n \frac{\langle 0 | L_i | n \rangle \langle n | L_j | 0 \rangle}{E_0 - E_n} \quad .$$

The matrix Λ_{ij} can always be diagonalized and in cubic symmetry will be isotropic. Allowing for lower symmetry we may write a particular diagonal term as

$$W_{\Delta g}^{zz} = 2\beta \lambda \Lambda_{zz} S_z H_z \qquad (22)$$

which gives an electron g-shift

$$\Delta g_L^{zz} = 2\lambda \Lambda_{zz} \quad . \qquad (23)$$

We note that Λ_{zz} is negative so that

$$\Delta g < 0 \text{ for } \lambda > 0 , \text{ i.e., } d^n, n < 5$$
$$\Delta g > 0 \text{ for } \lambda < 0 , \text{ i.e., } d^n, n > 5 .$$

B. Orbital Hyperfine Field

Cross terms of $\lambda \mathbf{L} \cdot \mathbf{S}$ and $P \mathbf{L} \cdot \mathbf{I}$, in exact analogy to the procedure above, give

$$W_{orb}^{hf} = 2P \lambda \Lambda_{zz} S_z I_z \qquad (24)$$

and substituting for Λ_{zz} from Eq. (23), we have

$$W_{orb}^{hf} = \Delta g_L^{zz} \, P S_Z I_Z = A^{orb} S_Z I_Z \tag{25}$$

Since the hyperfine field H^{hf} per unit electron spin ($S = 1$) is

$$H^{hf} = -A/g_I \mu_N \tag{26}$$

and

$$P = 2\beta g_I \mu_N \left\langle \frac{1}{r^3} \right\rangle \, ,$$

$$H_{orb}^{hf} = +2\beta \left\langle \frac{1}{r^3} \right\rangle \Delta g_L \, . \tag{27}$$

This expression was first given by Abragam and Pryce. Equation (27) may be expressed numerically as

$$H_{orb}^{hf} = +125 \left\langle \frac{1}{r^3} \right\rangle_{\substack{atomic \\ units}} \cdot \Delta g_L \text{ kilogauss} \tag{28}$$

Δg has been written as Δg_L to emphasize that in applying this expression one must be certain that the g-shift is orbital in origin and does not arise from admixtures of other spin-substates as occurs when one uses an effective spin-Hamiltonian for orbitally degenerate ground states such as Co^{2+} (Abragam and Pryce, 1955).

If the excited states $|n\rangle$ are not derived from the same free-ion term as the ground state everything that has been done goes through, but instead we write

$$P L \cdot I \to P I \cdot \sum_j \boldsymbol{\ell}_j \, , \quad \beta L \cdot H \to \beta H \cdot \sum_j \boldsymbol{\ell}_j \, , \quad \lambda L \cdot S \to \sum_i \xi_i \boldsymbol{\ell}_i \cdot s_i \tag{29}$$

(see Griffith (1961) for details). It should also be noted that although Eq. (28) has been derived by perturbation theory it is good to any order and therefore exact. * This is so because one has simply made a correspondence between terms linear in $\mathbf{H}$ and $\mathbf{I}$ in which terms in L appear in exactly the same way. In this respect, our perturbation expression is only schematic for something more general. As an indication of how large the orbital hyperfine field may become for orbital singlet ground states with

*This will be exact only if $\sum_i \langle \ell_i / r_i^3 \rangle = \langle 1/r^3 \rangle \langle \sum_i \ell_i \rangle$, i.e., $\langle 1/r^3 \rangle$ is the same for all the orbitals, which will not be the case when covalency is taken into account.

ostensibly no orbital angular momentum consider the case of Ni^{2+}
in MgO, where $g = 2.2122$, $\Delta g = 0.2122$ and $\langle 1/r^3 \rangle = 7$. Substituting these values into Eq. (28) we find $H_{orb}^{hf} = +188$ Kg. The
field is opposite in sign and almost cancels the core polarization
hyperfine field of ~ -250 Kg. For Cr^{3+} in MgO $\Delta g = -0.02$ (Low,
1957) and $\langle 1/r^3 \rangle \sim 4$ so that H_{orb}^{hf} is only -10 Kg.

C. Paramagnetic Shielding

In analogous fashion to the procedure above, cross terms
of $\mathbf{PL \cdot I}$ and $\beta \mathbf{H \cdot L}$ give a term proportional to $\mathbf{H \cdot I}$, i.e., which
looks like a nuclear g-shift. This is sometimes called the para-
magnetic shielding, or the pseudo-nuclear Zeeman effect. Thus
the nucleus sees an effective field $H_z(1 + \sigma)$ where

$$\sigma = -\frac{2\beta P \Lambda}{g_I \mu_N} = -4\beta^2 \Lambda \langle 1/r^3 \rangle \tag{30}$$

$$= -\frac{2\beta^2 \Delta g_L}{\lambda} \langle 1/r^3 \rangle \tag{31}$$

or

$$\sigma = -5.84 \langle 1/r^3 \rangle_{a.u.} \frac{\Delta g_L}{\lambda(cm^{-1})}. \tag{32}$$

σ may also be expressed in terms of H_{orb}^{hf} as

$$\sigma = -\frac{\beta}{\lambda} H_{orb}^{hf} = \left| 0.0467 \frac{H_{orb}^{hf}(kilogauss)}{\lambda(cm^{-1})} \right|. \tag{33}$$

This equation contains the same number of unknowns as Eq. (32)
but may prove useful on occasion.

As an illustration of this correction for orbital singlets consider the case of Ni^{2+} in Al_2O_3 where the Ni substitutes for the Al
in sixfold oxygen coordination. The measured $\Delta g \approx +0.19$. Taking
$\lambda = -300$ cm^{-1} and $\langle 1/r^3 \rangle = 7$, one finds $\sigma = 2.8\%$ (Locher and
Geschwind, 1963). The combined uncertainty in λ and $\langle r^{-3} \rangle$ in
the solid may be as large as 30% so that it is very difficult to say
anything better than $\sigma = 2.8 \pm 1\%$. Therefore the accuracy in the
determination of $\mu_I(Ni^{61})$ is only about 1% (Locher and Geschwind, 1965). One could improve on this result by measuring
μ_I^{eff} in similar environments, i.e., six-fold oxygen coordination
such as CaO, MgO, Al_2O_3, etc. and then plotting μ_I^{eff} as a
function of Δg_L, as shown in the hypothetical plot in Fig. 10, and
extrapolating to $\Delta g_L = 0$.

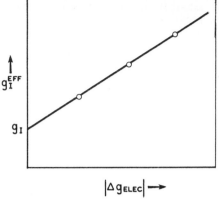

Fig. 10: Hypothetical plot of
   experimental determination
   of g_I^{eff} by ENDOR in similar
   hosts with different electronic g-shifts.

If the points lay on a straight line, the constancy in this series of
compounds of $\langle 1/r^3 \rangle / \lambda$ would be verified and one would be confident that the vertical intercept would give the correct unshielded
value of μ_I, to an accuracy of perhaps 0.2%. This experiment has
not been done as yet.

We have emphasized this correction for singlet states, because, albeit small, it is extremely important wherever one would
like to know μ_I to better than 1%. If the ion has low lying excited
states of the order of a few hundred cm^{-1} from the ground state,
such as one commonly finds in rare earths, this correction can
be as large as 100%. It should be emphasized that such large
shieldings can occur also for transition metal ions which can
equally well have low lying states. For example in Co^{2+} in MgO
this correction is as large as 40% (Fry, Llewellyn, and Pryce,
1962).

Therefore, if it is primarily a nuclear moment that one
wishes to measure with precision by ENDOR, one should choose
an ion with as small a Δg_L as possible. For example, in the
case of S-state ions such as Mn^{2+} and Fe^{3+} ($^6S_{5/2}$), whose g-
values are very close to the free-electron g-value this correction
is negligible, so that these ions would be particularly suitable for
a determination of the Mn or Fe moment (Locher and Geschwind,
1965).

D. Non-Magnetic Ground States and Van Vleck Temperature Independent Susceptibility

This very same nuclear shielding effect is present in ions
with a completely nonmagnetic ground state such as Co^{3+} ($3d^6$) in a

strong octahedral cubic crystal field. The crystal field energy is very much greater than the exchange energy between electrons so that Hund's rule is violated and we obtain a nonmagnetic ground state $S = 0$, $L = 0$ as shown in Fig. 11a. The shielding is again

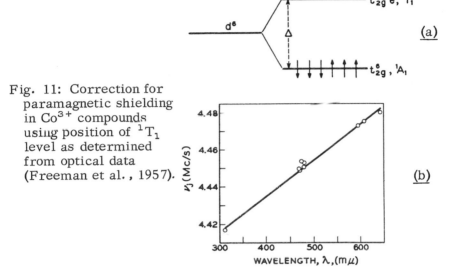

Fig. 11: Correction for paramagnetic shielding in Co^{3+} compounds using position of $^1T_1$ level as determined from optical data (Freeman et al., 1957).

given by Eq. (30) but cannot, of course, now be related to any electronic g-shift. Freeman et al. (1957) attempted to correct for σ in Co^{3+} by trying to evaluate Λ_{zz} in Eq. (30) directly. They reasoned that of the many excited states of the Co^{3+}, only $^1T_1$ had matrix elements of $\mathbf{L}$ connecting to the ground state. They measured by optical spectroscopy the separation Δ of the $^1T_1$ from the ground state for a host of different compounds. They assumed that the orbital matrix elements of Co^{3+} which appear in the numerator of Λ were the same in these compounds, i.e., they neglected the variation of covalent effects upon $\mathbf{L}$, i.e. orbital reduction, and also assumed that $\langle r^{-3} \rangle$ did not vary among these compounds. In this case $\sigma \sim 1/\Delta$ and would become zero as $1/\Delta \to 0$. They plotted the measured values of the NMR frequency of Co in the different compound vs $1/\Delta$ as shown in Fig. 11b. They then extrapolated to $1/\Delta \to 0$ to determine the correct unshielded nuclear moment. Note from Fig. 11b that the extrapolation amounts to a few percent and they estimated that the nuclear moment of Co^{59} was determined in this way to an accuracy of 0.1%.

Recent measurements of Knight shifts in Co doped metals and intermetallic compounds have led Jaccarino and Walstedt (1967) to believe that the Co^{59} moment as determined by Freeman et al. was off by many times their quoted error. They attribute this discrepancy to the assumption made by Freeman et al. regarding the constancy of $\langle 1/r^3 \rangle$ and the orbital matrix elements for the range of compounds used. This emphasizes the great care that must be exercised in measuring nuclear moments in transition metal compounds by NMR even when they have nonmagnetic ground states and raises questions about some other moment determinations, as will be seen below.

The paramagnetic shielding in nonmagnetic compounds can also be expressed in terms of the Van Vleck temperature independent susceptibility which comes from cross products of $\mathbf{H} \cdot \mathbf{L}$ with itself in the perturbation procedure outlined above, i.e.,

$$W_{VV} = \beta^2 \sum_n \frac{\langle 0|\mathbf{H} \cdot \mathbf{L}|n \rangle \langle n|\mathbf{H} \cdot \mathbf{L}|0 \rangle}{E_0 - E_n}$$

$$= \beta^2 \Lambda H^2 = -\tfrac{1}{2} \chi_{VV} H^2 \qquad (34)$$

or

$$\chi_{VV} = -2\Lambda\beta^2 \qquad (35)$$

so that using Eq. (30) we have

$$\sigma = +2 \chi_{VV} \langle 1/r^3 \rangle \qquad (36)$$

or expressed numerically

$$\sigma = 22.6 \langle 1/r^3 \rangle_{\substack{\text{atomic} \\ \text{units}}} \chi_{VV}(\text{emu/mole}) \ . \qquad (37)$$

Of course this equation also applies to the magnetic ions of a dilute paramagnet like Ni^{2+} in MgO but it would be ridiculous to try to measure σ this way, in such a case, rather than by the g-shift as in Eq. (32).

The Mn^{55} nuclear moment is given in the Varian Co. table of nuclear moments to five significant figures. Again, Jaccarino found reason to suspect the accepted value because of inconsistancies in studies of the Knight shift of Mn^{55} in a number of metals which could be resolved if the Mn^{55} nuclear moment were 0.7% smaller than the accepted value. The compounds in which the Mn^{55} moment had been measured were permanganates in which the Mn is in a seven plus oxidation state, i.e., all the d-electrons were stripped so that there should be little paramagnetism to worry about. Nevertheless, susceptibility measurements showed them to have positive temperature independent susceptibilities. Subtracting off a roughly estimated diamagnetic susceptibility, one arrived at a value of $\chi_{VV} \simeq +63 \times 10^{-6}$ emu/mole. It is of course, impossible to estimate a $\langle 1/r^3 \rangle$ for the electrons producing this χ_{VV} because of the very covalent nature of these compounds. It is more appropriate to say, however, that for a $\sigma = 0.7\%$, $\langle 1/r^3 \rangle$ in atomic units would have to be about five, which is not an unreasonable number.

In order to resolve this difficulty, Mims and Geschwind performed a series of ENDOR experiments on Mn^{2+} in several diamagnetic hosts. In view of the fact that the g-value is so close to the free electron g-value, the σ correction is completely negligible. For example, for Mn^{2+} in ZnS, g = 2.0024. It was found by Mims et al. (1967) that indeed the Mn^{55} nuclear moment was *significantly lower* from the point of view of Knight shifts than the old value determined by NMR in the perman ganates. Thus, here is a case where by proper choice of ion, the ENDOR measurement was able to yield a better value for the nuclear moment than the NMR measurement.

E. ENDOR Example: Ni^{2+}: Al_2O_3. Nature of EPR Inhomogeneity

As a concrete example of the application of ENDOR which will illustrate a number of the topics discussed above, let us examine the case of Ni^{2+} $(3d)^8$, present as a very small substitutional impurity for Al in Al_2O_3 (Locher and Geschwind, 1963). The predominant electric crystalline field at the Ni^{2+} site is cubic and splits the ^3F free ion configuration so as to give an orbital singlet ground state, $^3A_2$. Superimposed on the cubic field is a smaller trigonal field which in concert with the spin-orbit coupling removes the spin degeneracy by introducing a term in the spin Hamiltonian of the form DS_z^2. The spin Hamiltonian for the ground state with the external magnetic field along the c-axis of the crystal is given by

$$\mathcal{K} = D\left[S_z^2 - \tfrac{1}{3} S(S+1)\right] + g_{||} \beta H_o S_z + AS_z I_z$$

$$+ \tfrac{1}{2} B (S_+ I_- + S_- I_+) - g_I \mu_N H_o I_z + Q\left[I_z^2 - \tfrac{1}{3}I(I+1)\right]. \quad (38)$$

All terms other than D have the same definitions as in Eq. (1). The energy level diagram is shown in Fig. 12. The axial crystal

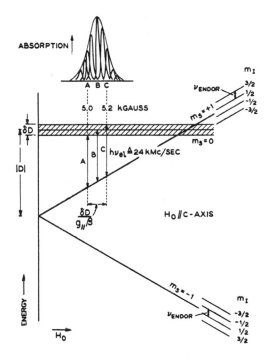

Fig. 12: Ground-state energy levels of a Ni^{2+} ion in Al_2O_3 for the
external dc magnetic field H_O parallel to the c-axis.
The spin packets (e.g., A, B, and C) correspond to different D values for these packets.

field splitting of the ground state is D = 39 kMc/sec. For a fixed
microwave frequency of 24 kMc/sec, an EPR absorption is observed at 5100 gauss corresponding to the m_S = +1 to m_S = 0 transition. This EPR line is observed to have a full width at half-
height of 180 gauss, due to inhomogeneous broadening associated
with a variation of the axial crystal field splitting from one Ni^{2+}
site to another, i.e. a variation δD around the mean value D as
shown in Fig. 12. This large inhomogeneous linewidth prevents
one from resolving the Ni^{61} hfs even when isotopically enriched
Ni is used.

If the external magnetic field is kept fixed at 5100 gauss,
corresponding to the m_S = 0 → +1 transition for spin packets in
the vicinity of B, and these packets are saturated, then one can
observe the ENDOR transitions among the m_I sublevels in the

$m_S = +1$ electronic level. However, in addition to these ENDOR frequencies one also observes weaker ENDOR transitions in the $m_S = -1$ level. The reason that these latter ENDOR lines can be observed as well, even though it is only the $m_S = 0 \rightarrow +1$ transition that is being saturated, is that the equilibrium population of the $m_S = -1$ level is disturbed via spin-lattice relaxation when the $m_S = 0 \rightarrow 1$ transition is saturated. It is this connection of the electronic levels with each other via spin-lattice relaxation, T_1, that often allows one to observe ENDOR transitions along an entire chain of m_S values even though only a particular pair are being saturated by microwaves. Again, the steady state ENDOR signals in our case must result from an effective modification of T_1 by the rf via T_x as illustrated in Fig. 3.

We indicated above that the 180 gauss linewidth in $Ni^{2+}:Al_2O_3$ was due to random axial crystal fields which give a spread in D values. Striking evidence for this origin of the inhomogeneity was found by observing the variation in frequency of a given ENDOR transition as the external magnetic field was swept through the inhomogeneously broadened line (i. e., from A to C in Fig. 12), keeping the microwave frequency constant. In this way, one is examining the same ENDOR transition in the different spin packets from A to C. One expects the shift in ENDOR frequencies to reflect a change in the nuclear Zeeman energy corresponding to the change in the external magnetic field, i. e. $\partial \nu_N / \partial H_0 = \pm g_I^{eff} \beta_N / h = \pm 0.39$ kc/sec gauss. g_I^{eff} had been determined in standard fashion by measuring the six ENDOR frequencies in the $m_S = +1$ and $m_S = -1$ levels at a fixed dc field corresponding to a particular spin packet, e. g., B. The expected variation $\partial \nu_N / \partial H_0$ is shown by the dashed lines in Fig. 13. Instead, Locher and Geschwind (1963) observed a variation given by the solid lines drawn through the experimental points, with slopes $\pm g_I^{eff} \beta_N / n + \partial |A| / \partial H_0$, implying a change in hyperfine field from those spin packets at A to those at C given by $\partial |A| / \partial H_0 = -0.26$ kc/sec (gauss). This implies a change in absolute value of the hyperfine field of 130 gauss from A to C, a distance in H_0 of 200 gauss. This variation of 130 gauss is, of course, a small fraction of the total hf field of $H_{tot}^{hf} = -97$ kG made up of $H_{orb}^{hf} = +171$ kG, $H_{core\ pol}^{hf} = -256$ kG, and $H_{dip}^{hf} = -12$ kG. Locher and Geschwind (1963) showed that this variation of 130 gauss was essentially due to a variation of H_{orb}^{hf} from A to C associated with the variation in D. The D splitting is given by (Abragam and Pryce, 1951)

$$D \simeq \frac{\lambda}{2} (g_{||} - g_\perp) \qquad \text{or} \qquad \delta D \simeq \frac{3\lambda}{4} \delta g_{||} \qquad (39)$$

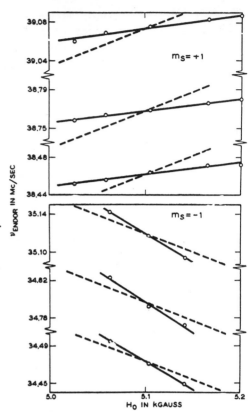

Fig. 13: the six ENDOR frequencies ν_{ENDOR} of Ni^{61} observed in Al_2O_3 corresponding for $H_0 \| c$ axis at the $m_S = 0 \to +1$ EPR line. H_0 was varied within the broad EPR line keeping the microwave frequency fixed. The points and the solid lines give the experimental results whereas the dashed lines indicate what would be expected for a constant hfs parameter, A, throughout the line (Locher and Geschwind, 1963).

since $\delta g_\perp \approx -g_\| /2$. Thus a variation in D implies a variation in g which in turn will give a variation in H_{orb}^{hf} via Eq. (28), i.e.

$$\delta D \to \delta g \to \delta H_{orb}^{hf} . \tag{40}$$

Equations (39) and (28) give for the variation of H_{orb}^{hf} from A to C

$$\delta H_{orb}^{hf} = 1.25 \times 10^5 \cdot \frac{4}{3\lambda} \cdot \delta D \langle 1/r^3 \rangle_{au} \text{ gauss} . \tag{41}$$

From Fig. 12 one finds δD from A to C to be $\delta D/g_\| \beta = -200$ gauss or $\delta D = -0.02$ cm^{-1}. Using $\lambda = -280$ cm^{-1} and $\langle 1/r^3 \rangle_{au} = 7$, one finds $\delta g \approx +1.0 \times 10^{-4}$ and $\delta H_{orb}^{hf} \approx +90$ gauss, or $\delta H_{tot}^{hf} = -90$ gauss compared to the observed value of -130 gauss. This agreement is quite satisfactory as small variations in $H_{c.p.}^{hf}$ may also be present. Thus we see how ENDOR has in effect probed

a g-value variation of *1 part in 10⁴* in an inhomogeneously
broadened line via its effect on the orbital hf field. In similar
fashion one can probe small changes in hf fields that result from
applied electric fields* (Reichert and Pershan, 1965) or from
axial pressure.

III. Higher Order Bleaney-Koster Terms in the Spin Hamiltonian

A. <u>Terms Allowed by Time Reversal Symmetry</u>

It was pointed out by both Bleaney (1959) and Koster and
Statz (1959a, b) that additional higher order terms could exist in
the spin Hamiltonian other than those normally considered. For
example, for an ion at a site of cubic symmetry, terms of the
type

$$(H_x S_x^3 + H_y S_y^3 + H_z S_z^3) \quad \text{and} \quad (I_x S_x^3 + I_y S_y^3 + I_z S_z^3) \qquad (42)$$

are cubically invariant and satisfy time reversal symmetry. **
In view of the high precision with which ENDOR measures nuclear
energies, it becomes important to consider such terms in attempting to fit the experimental data.

In general, such terms will be of the form

$$\mathcal{H} = \sum_{m_1, m_2, m_3} C(m_1, m_2, m_3) H^{m_1} S^{m_2} I^{m_3} \qquad (43)$$

where: (i) $m_1 + m_2 + m_3 = m =$ even integer to satisfy time reversal symmetry. (ii) The triangle rule for the addition of angular
momenta requires

$$m_2 \leq 2S \; ; \; m_3 \leq 2I \; . \qquad (45)$$

(iii) In principle, m_1 is unbounded. However, in practice only the
lowest powers of H need be considered as higher powers only
enter in higher-order perturbations.

Ray (1964) has indicated a general procedure for constructing the spin Hamiltonian containing all terms of the type appearing
in Eq. (43). Its essence is the following: each term in Eq. (43)
must be invariant with respect to all the operations of the point
group at the site of the ion, i. e. it must transform like the identity,

---

See J. Reichert, Chap. S.12.
**See B. Bleaney, Chap. 1, Appendix B.*

or Γ_1, representation of that point group. One then constructs irreducible tensor operators for each of I, S, and H belonging to the point group of the site and selects those combinations whose direct products transform as the Γ_1 representation. The coefficients of the different terms are the analogues for the point groups of the Clebsch-Gordon coefficients that appear in spherical symmetry. Full details may be found in Ray (1964). An example of this procedure will be given in Sec. C.

B. First Observation of Higher-Order Terms in Co^{2+} in Tetrahedral Coordination

It has been found necessary to include some particular terms in the nuclear spin Hamiltonian. In analogy to the familiar fine structure term in cubic symmetry

$$\frac{a}{6}\left\{S_x^4 + S_y^4 + S_z^4 - \frac{1}{5}\left[3S(S+1) - 1\right]S(S+1)\right\} \tag{46}$$

one has the additional hyperfine term

$$A'\left\{I_x S_x^3 + I_y S_y^3 + I_z S_z^3 - \frac{1}{5}\left[3S(S+1) - 1\right](I\cdot S)\right\} . \tag{47}$$

where $S \geq 2$ in (46) and $S \geq 3/2$ in (47). Such a term was first found by Ham, Ludwig, Watkins, and Woodbury (1960), for $Co^{2+}(d^7)$ in tetrahedral and eight-fold cubic coordinations whose level is analogous to $Cr^{3+}(d^3)$ in octahedral coordination. The free ion ^4F state is split in the cubic crystal field into the ground state orbital singlet, $^4A_2$, and the two excited state orbital triplets $^4T_2$ and $^4T_1$. In analogy to Eq. (24) one may consider still higher order perturbation terms in the orbital hf energy for example:

$$W_{IS^3} = \langle {}^4A_2 | \lambda L\cdot S | {}^4T_2\rangle\langle {}^4T_2 | \lambda L\cdot S | {}^4T_1\rangle\langle 4T_1 | PL\cdot I | {}^4T_2\rangle \ \times$$

$$\times \ \langle {}^4T_2 | \lambda L\cdot S | {}^4A_2\rangle \Big/ \left[W({}^4A_2) - W({}^4T_2)\right]^2 \left[W({}^4A_2) - W({}^4T_1)\right]. \tag{48}$$

If matrix elements of L are evaluated in analogy to the procedure in Sec. II, it is apparent that such an expression yields an IS^3 term. One can also get an IS^3 term in lower order by taking the spin-spin interaction $-\rho(L\cdot S)^2$ once instead of $(\lambda L\cdot S)$ twice as in Eq. (48). However, $\rho \sim 0.01\ \lambda$ so that using the spin-spin interaction gives something of the same order even though it occurs in one lower order of perturbation theory. Evaluation of Eq. (48) by

Ham et al. (1960) gives values of A' for Co^{2+} in tetrahedral and eight-fold environments of the order of 2.0 Mc/sec. These theoretical estimates agree in order of magnitude with the observed values, but in the cases of ZnTe and CdTe there is poor agreement; even the wrong signs are found. This is not too surprising, however, as these compounds are extremely covalent and the simple crystal field theory used to evaluate Eq. (28) should be inadequate in these cases.

C. Observation of Higher Order Nuclear hfs Terms in S-State Ions

1. $I S^3$ Terms

If one compares Eq. (48) with Eqs. (20) to (23),then one anticipates that A' will vary roughly as $(\Delta g)^3$. We do not propose to push this expectation towards a quantitative check as this would imply undue confidence in simple crystal field theory. However, in a qualitative way, one expects A' to vary monotonically with (Δg). For S-state ions whose g-shifts are far smaller than for the preceding example of Co^{2+}, one therefore expects far smaller values of A'. This is borne out by the size of A' (coefficient of Eq. (47)) for various S-state ions as listed in Table I where A' is measured in kc/sec. The experimentally observed value of A' given in Table I for Fe^{3+} is in reasonable agreement with a rough theoretical estimate (Locher and Geschwind, 1965).

2. $I^2 S^2$ Terms

a. Magnetic Type $I^2 S^2$ Term: If in the perturbation chain illustrated by Eq. (48), $PL \cdot I$ is taken twice and $\lambda L \cdot S$ twice, then one generates terms of the type $I^2 S^2$. These terms would be smaller than the IS^3 term just considered, by roughly $P/\lambda \sim 10^{-4}$. They would therefore be quite negligible even in ENDOR measurements in orbital singlet ground states, for which they would generally be less than 1 Kc. This type of term is also called the pseudo-quadrupolar interaction as it transforms the same way as the nuclear electric quadruple interaction. It is analogous to the term discussed by Bleaney* although in the example given there it would be much larger as very low lying excited states are involved.

b. $I^2 S^2$: Nuclear Electric Quadrupole Interaction: In addition to the $I^2 S^2$ terms just discussed, which are magnetic in origin, there will be the true electric quadrupole terms. These electric quadrupole terms are extremely significant even for some S-state ions in cubic symmetry. It is generally stated that the

*See B. Bleaney, Chap. 1, Eq. (101).

Table I: Coefficient A' of IS^3 term in Eq. (47) for S-state ions as measured by ENDOR.

Ion	Host	A'(kc/sec)	g-value
$Mn^{2+}(3d^5)$	ZnS	~ 0	2.0024[a]
$Fe^{3+}(3d^5)$	MgO	$+5.7 \pm 0.3$	2.0039[b]
$Eu^{2+}(4f^7)$	CaF_2	$+13.77 \pm 0.46\,(Eu^{151})$	1.9926[c]
$Eu^{2+}(4f^7)$	CaF_2	$+6.38 \pm 0.86\,(Eu^{153})$	1.9926[c]
$Gd^{3+}(4f^7)$	ThO_2	-9.9 ± 3.6	1.991[d]
$Tb^{4+}(4f^7)$	ThO_2	$+103.3 \pm 2.3$	2.0146[e]

(a) Mims et al. (1967).
(b) Locher and Geschwind (1965).
(c) Baker, J.M. and Williams, F.I.B. (1962).
(d) Hurrel, J. (1965).
(e) Baker, J.M. et al. (1965).

quadrupole interaction vanishes in *cubic* symmetry. This statement refers however, only to ions with no orbital angular momentum, but even S-state ions have some orbital angular momentum admixed by spin-orbit coupling from higher states. Given then that an ion has orbital angular momentum it can certainly have a quadrupole coupling in cubic symmetry, recalling that it has one in the even higher full rotational symmetry of free space. However, now in the crystal in cubic symmetry there may be more than one independent constant. While this was pointed out by Prof. Bleaney in Appendix IIC, we would like to formulate this in such a way as to give a simple illustration of the general procedure discussed by Ray (1964).

The quadrupole interaction in free space may be written as

$$H_Q = \sum_{m=-2}^{2} A_2^m B_2^{-m} \tag{49}$$

where A_2^m and B_2^m are second rank spherical tensors in the nuclear spin operators and electron angular momentum operators respectively,* i.e. they transform under rotation of coordinate axes as the $Y_2^m(\theta, \varphi)$. Alternatively stated, each set of A_2^m and B_2^m is a basis of the five-dimensional irreducible representation of the rotation group. H_Q is the appropriate direct product of

*See B. Bleaney, Chap. 1, Eqs. (49-51) and (55).

these representations which yields the identity representation of
the rotation group, i.e. a scalar. How is this modified in cubic
symmetry?

In cubic symmetry, a second rank spherical tensor is decomposed into the Γ_3 two-dimensional irreducible representation and the Γ_5 three-dimensional irreducible representation.
Reference to Ray's paper or any standard work on group theory
gives as a basis for the Γ_3 representation of rank two in the
angular momentum operators

$$\Gamma_3^{(1)}(S) = \sqrt{\frac{3}{2}}\left[S_z^2 - \frac{1}{3}S(S+1)\right]$$

or

$$\Gamma_3^{(1)}(I) = \sqrt{\frac{3}{2}}\left[I_z^2 - \frac{1}{3}I(I+1)\right]$$

$$\Gamma_3^2 = \frac{1}{\sqrt{2}}\left[S_x^2 - S_y^2\right]\cdots \tag{50}$$

and for the Γ_5 representation

$$\Gamma_5^{(1)} = \frac{\sqrt{3}}{2}(S_yS_z + S_zS_y)$$

$$\Gamma_5^{(2)} = \frac{\sqrt{3}}{2}(S_zS_x + S_xS_z)$$

$$\Gamma_5^{(3)} = \frac{\sqrt{3}}{2}(S_xS_y + S_yS_x)\ . \tag{51}$$

Matrix elements of the operators which form the bases of the
same representation are related to each other by the Wigner-
Eckart theorem, but those of different representations are not,
i.e. a separate independent constant describing the physical content of the problem, other than the symmetry of the problem, is
required for each representation. While this is true in principle
for the nuclear spin operators, it is of course completely unnecessary in practice as nuclear excited states are so far above
the ground state that $|I|$ still remains a very good quantum num-
ber in the crystal just as in the free atom, so that only a single
constant (the nuclear quadrupole moment) is needed.

We now wish to decompose the Γ_1 or identity representation
of the cubic group into direct products $\Gamma_3 \times \Gamma_3$, $\Gamma_5 \times \Gamma_5$ and
$\Gamma_3 \times \Gamma_5$, using the appropriate analogs of the Clebsch-Gordon
coefficients for the cubic group. These coefficients are given by

Tanabe and Sugano (1954) and Griffith* (1961). They are particularly simple in this case and one has

$$H_Q = a\frac{1}{\sqrt{3}}\left[\Gamma_5^{(1)}(S)\Gamma_5^{(1)}(I) + \Gamma_5^{(2)}(S)\Gamma_5^{(2)}(I) + \Gamma_5^{(3)}(S)\Gamma_5^{(3)}(I)\right]$$

$$+b\frac{1}{\sqrt{2}}\left[\Gamma_3^{(1)}(S)\Gamma_3^{(1)}(I) + \Gamma_3^{(2)}(S)\Gamma_3^{(2)}(I)\right]. \tag{52}$$

Two constants a and b are now in general needed to specify the quadrupole interaction in cubic symmetry as compared to the single constant, eqQ, in spherical symmetry.** Substitution of (50) and (51) into Eq. (52) gives the analogous expression for H_Q as (A.34) in Prof. Bleaney's lectures.

$$H_Q = a\Big\{(S_xS_y + S_yS_x)(I_xI_y + I_yI_x) + (S_yS_z + S_zS_y)(I_yI_z + I_zI_y)$$

$$+ (S_zS_x + S_xS_z)(I_zI_x + I_xI_z) + b\Big\{\left[3S_x^2 - S(S+1)\right]\left[3I_x^2 - I(I+1)\right]$$

$$+ \left[3S_y^2 - S(S+1)\right]\left[3I_y^2 - I(I+1)\right]$$

$$+ \left[3S_z^2 - S(S+1)\right]\left[3I_z^2 - I(I+1)\right]\Big\}. \tag{53}$$

In spherical symmetry, the constants a and b are related, namely $a = 9/2b$. In practice, the electronic Zeeman term $g\beta HS_z$ is so much greater than H_Q that only the diagonal term $[3S_z^2 - S(S+1)][3I_z^2 - I(I+1)]$ is the most important, and to this extent, again one constant is sufficient. However, one should bear in mind that in general there are off-diagonal correction terms of the order of $H_Q^2/g\beta HS_z$ which involve a second constant.

To bring the constant "b" into conformity with the expression used by Baker and Williams (1962) for H_Q, we write

$$b = \frac{B}{2I(2I-1)\,2S(2S-1)} \tag{54}$$

The values of B in Mc/sec found for the $^8S_{7/2}$ ground state of Eu^{2+}, Gd^{3+}, and Tb^{4+} are listed in Table II.

*See Appendix II, p. 396.
**The author is indebted to M. Blume for many clarifying remarks regarding this procedure.

Table II: Quadrupole coupling, B, in Mc/sec for different
S-state ions in cubic symmetry.

Ion	Host	B	g-value
Eu^{2+}	CaF_2	$-0.7855 \pm 0.0052(Eu^{151})$ $-2.0294 \pm 0.0068(Eu^{153})$	1.9926 ± 0.003 [a]
Gd^{3+}	CaF_2	-0.687 ± 0.018	1.991 ± 0.001 [b]
Tb^{4+}	ThO_2	6.194 Mc/sec	2.0146 [c]

(a) Baker, J.M. and Williams, F.I.B. (1962).
(b) Hurrell, S.P. (1965).
(c) Baker et al. (1965).

Note how large B is for the Tb^{4+}, again reflecting the large ad-mixture of orbital angular momentum as indicated by the very large g-shift. For the Tb^{4+}, $B^2/g\beta HS_z \sim$ few Kc/sec and one might perhaps obtain a better fit to the ENDOR data by using two quadrupolar constants, as in Eq. (53).

3. HSI^2 Term

In the ENDOR study of Tb^{4+} (^{159}Tb) referred to above, Baker et al. (1965) found an additional term $B'\beta HSI^2$ where β is the Bohr magneton and $B' = 1.02 \pm 0.14 \times 10^{-6}$. It should be stressed that this term is undoubtedly true nuclear electric quadrupole interaction where $\beta \Sigma_i \mathbf{H} \cdot \mathbf{l}_i$ has been used once instead of $\Sigma_i \zeta \mathbf{l}_i \cdot \mathbf{s}_i$ in the perturbation chain, i.e. the external magnetic field also acts to mix in orbital angular momentum into the ground state. The fact that $\mathbf{l}$ cannot connect ^8S to higher states of f^7 may be of no consequence as undoubtedly charge transfer states of the same multiplicity as the ^8S ground state are playing an important role in the case of the Tb^{4+} as indicated by the fact that $g > 2$.

In the better behaved Eu^{2+} and Gd^{3+}, $g < 2$, as it should be if the ^6P is the important admixed excited state. One anticipates that the HSI^2 term will be down from the S^2I^2 term by $\beta H/\zeta$ which is in fairly reasonable agreement with what is actually found.

In summary, these higher order terms in the nuclear hyperfine interaction that we have considered are important in accurately fitting ENDOR data to determine nuclear parameters. In addition, they are also interesting from a crystal field point of view, in that they can be at least qualitatively related to each other in terms of the higher order perturbations which give rise to them.

IV. Zero-Point Spin Deviation in Antiferromagnets and Some Systematics of Core Polarization Hyperfine Fields in $3d^n$ Ions

A. Ground State of Antiferromagnet is not the Néel State

The accuracy with which hf fields may be measured by ENDOR proves useful in looking for the zero-point spin deviation of the ground state of an antiferromagnet.* This search has been a particularly elusive one and the question of zero point spin deviation remains one of the incompletely resolved problems of antiferromagnetism.

Consider first the ground state of a ferromagnet, which for purposes of simple illustration is shown in Fig. 14a, for the case of a simple linear chain with $S = 1/2$. The ground state is the

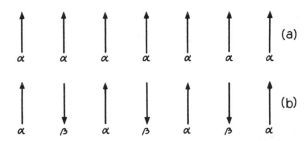

Fig. 14: (a) Ferromagnetic ground state. (b) Antiferromagnetic Néel state which is, however, not the ground state.

perfectly aligned state in which the individual spin state α for each ion corresponds to $\langle S_z \rangle = +S = +1/2$. The ground state wavefunction ψ_0 may then be written as

$$\psi_0^F = \alpha_1 \alpha_2 \alpha_3 \alpha \alpha \alpha_i \alpha_j \alpha \cdots \qquad (55)$$

where the subscripts label the sites. That the state given by Eq. (55) is indeed the ground state is seen as follows. The exchange Hamiltonian is given by

$$\mathcal{H}_{ex} = 2J \sum_{(i,j)} \mathbf{S}_i \cdot \mathbf{S}_j \qquad (56a)$$

*See also Chaps. 2 and 7.

where the sum is over all nearest pairs (i, j) and $J < 0$ for a ferromagnet. Equation (56) may be rewritten as

$$\mathcal{K}_{ex} = 2J \sum_{(i, j)} \mathbf{S}_i \cdot \mathbf{S}_j =$$

$$= 2J \sum_{(i, j)} \left[S_i^z S_j^z + \tfrac{1}{2} \left(S_i^+ S_j^- + S_i^- S_j^+ \right) \right] . \tag{56b}$$

The $S_i^z S_j^z$ term acting on ψ_o^F gives back the same state whereas $\left(S_i^+ S_j^- + S_i^- S_j^+ \right) \psi_o^F = 0$, since the S^+ terms cannot raise the spins any further. Therefore, Eq. (55) is an eigenstate of the exchange Hamiltonian, Eq. (56). The state is also one of minimum energy since turning any of the spins over increases the energy.

Now consider the corresponding aligned state, or Néel state, for the antiferromagnet shown in Fig. 14b whose wavefunction is given by

$$\psi_o^A = \alpha_1 \beta_2 \alpha_3 \ \beta \alpha \beta \ \alpha_i \beta_j \alpha \beta \ldots \tag{57}$$

where β corresponds to the state $\langle S_z \rangle = -1/2$. Equation (57) is not an eigenstate of the exchange since $S_i^+ S_j^- + S_i^- S_j^+$ acting on Eq. (4), gives

$$\alpha_1 \beta_2 \alpha_3 \ \beta \alpha \beta \ \beta_i \alpha_j \ \alpha \beta \ldots \tag{58}$$

which is orthogonal to Eq. (57). The

$$\sum_{(i, j)} \left(S_i^+ S_j^- + S_i^- S_j^+ \right)$$

term will generate wavefunctions such as Eq. (58), orthogonal to each other, and each of which is orthogonal to Eq. (57) so that Eq. (57) cannot be an eigenstate of $\mathcal{K}_{ex}$ and consequently it is not the ground state.

It should be pointed out that even the Néel state given in Eq. (55) is not the ferromagnetic ground state when magnetic dipolar forces are taken into account, i.e., the exchange does not commute with the dipolar Hamiltonian. Terms in the dipolar Hamiltonian of the type $S_i^z S_j^-$, i.e., the "stop-flop" terms operating on Eq. (55) do not give back Eq. (55). However, the departure of the ground state from the Néel state will be of the order of $(\mathcal{H}_{dip}/\mathcal{H}_{exchange})^2$, which will be quite small.

B. Bounds on Energy of Ground State

The calculation of the true ground state and its energy for an antiferromagnet is an exceedingly difficult problem and has only been done for a linear chain of $S = 1/2$ by Bethe (1931) and Hulthen (1938). Anderson (1951) has by a very simple, elegant argument put a lower bound on the ground state energy of an antiferromagnet which can be divided into two sublattices such that the nearest neighbors of atoms in lattice A are always in lattice B. This lower bound is $-NJS^2 Z(1+1/ZS)$ where N = total number atoms, and Z = number of nearest neighbors, so that we have for the energy of the ground state, E_g

$$-NJS^2 Z > E_g > - NJS^2 Z(1+1/ZS) \ . \qquad (59)$$
Néel
state

Spin wave calculations for a three-dimensional lattice (Anderson, 1952) place E_g almost midway between these limits. Thus, for $Z = 6$ and $S = 5/2$, the ground state energy is some 3% below the Néel energy. This ground state is reached by effecting spin reversals at the different sites in Eq. (57), i. e., the true ground state can be expanded in an orthonormal set of wavefunctions each corresponding to a spin reversal at a particular site or sites so that $|\langle S_z \rangle|$ at a site will now be less than S. The decrease in energy is brought about by these spin reversals, in spite of the fact that the diagonal part of the exchange energy is increased, because the correlation between the transverse components of the spins is increased so that the vector spins $\sqrt{S(S+1)}$ are aligned more nearly antiparallel.

Anderson (1952) has calculated this zero-point spin deviation for a number of lattices using spin wave theory and for a simple cubic lattice finds $(1 - \langle S_z \rangle/S) = 0.078/S$, so that for $S = 5/2$ one expects a deviation of about 3%.

C. Attempts to Observe Zero-Point Spin Deviation by Comparison of EPR in Dilute and NMR in Concentrated Crystals

One attempts to detect this zero-point spin deviation in antiferromagnets by measuring the hyperfine interaction $A_c \langle S_z \rangle$ by NMR in an antiferromagnet at sufficiently low temperatures so that thermal fluctuations in S_z are negligible. This is then compared with the hyperfine interaction $A_d S$ of the same magnetic ion present as a dilute impurity in an isomorphic diamagnetic crystal in the state $S_z = S$. The subscripts c and d refer to concentrated and dilute salt, respectively. Assuming that $A_c = A_d$, the difference between these two measurements will then give the zero-point spin deviation, $(S - \langle S_z \rangle)/S$.

One may rightfully question the assumption that $A_c = A_d$, i.e., that A does not change in going from the dilute to concentrated crystal. This change in A could come about, for example, because of the influence of lattice spacing upon the hyperfine field. However, the weight of empirical evidence shows that the core polarization hyperfine field (cphf) *(but only the cphf)* is constant to better than 1%, independent of lattice spacing for the same ion in similar chemical coordination, i.e., ligand number and type (Geschwind, 1965). If there is a sizeable orbital hyperfine field, H_{orb}^{hf}, for the magnetic ion in question, then H_{orb}^{hf} would indeed be sensitive to the lattice spacing as indicated by Locher and Geschwind (1963) for Ni^{2+} in Al_2O_3 and MgO. Thus, ions with large orbital hyperfine fields are unsuitable for the observation of this few percent zero-point spin deviation as the uncertainty in the variation of H_{orb}^{hf} for the same ion in different crystals will usually be greater than a few percent. However, for S-state ions, H_{orb}^{hf} is negligible so that they are very suitable for a study of the zero-point spin deviation. This is also true for d^3 ions (V^{2+}, Cr^{3+}, and Mn^{4+}) in octahedral symmetry where again the hyperfine field is predominantly cphf. This constancy of the cphf with lattice spacing is illustrated in Table III.

The constancy alluded to is indeed better than 1%. Similar results are found for fluorine coordination, etc. Note, however, that it is very important that the measurements be taken at, roughly, the *same* low temperature, as there are temperature effects which are greater than 1%. For example, $|A|$ in SrO decreases by more than 2% in going from 4.2°K to room temperature (Shuskus, 1964). We have also included in Table III, the cubic crystal field splitting parameter $\underline{a}$. Since $\underline{a}$ should vary as a very high inverse power of the metal-oxygen distance ($(1/r)^{10}$ for a point charge model), the rapid decrease of $\underline{a}$ in going from MgO to SrO can be taken as evidence that the Mn-O distance more nearly follows the host metal ion-oxygen distance. We have no theoretical understanding of this constancy of A, independent of ligand distance, but it must be accepted as a fairly strong experimental fact for the 3d ions. One may therefore safely rule out any objection to this comparison of the cphf field in the dilute and concentrated systems based upon a change in lattice parameter alone.

Table III: Hyperfine coupling of Mn^{2+} and Fe^{3+} in oxygen coordination.

Crystal	Metal-oxygen distance (A^b)	Crystal field parameter $a(10^{-4}cm^{-1})$	Temperature $(°K)$	$A(10^{-4}$ $cm^{-1})$ Mn^{55}
		Mn^{2+} (paramagnets)		
$MgO^{(a)}$	2.10	18.6	4.2	-81.5 ± 0.2 (EPR)
$CaO^{(b)}$	2.40	5.9	4.2	-81.640 ± 0.001 (ENDOR)
$SrO^{(c)}$	2.55	< 1	4.2	-80.9 ± 0.2 (EPR)
		Fe^{3+} (paramagnets)		
				$|A|/h$(sec)
$MgO^{(d)}$	2.10	~260	4.2	10.059 ± 0.001 (ENDOR)
$CaO^{(d)}$	2.40	65	4.2	10.05 ± 0.05 (EPR)
Al_2O_3 $^{(e)}$	1.98 1.85	380	4.2	10.09 ± 0.05 (Mössbauer data)
		Fe^{3+} (anti- and ferri-magnets)		
α-$Fe_2O_3^{(f)}$ (antiferromagnet)			4.2	9.92 ± 0.10 (Mössbauer data)
$YIG^{(g)}$ (ferrimagnet) octahedral site			4.2	10.083 ± 0.10 (NMR)

(a) Walsh et al. (1965).
(b) Mims and Geschwind (unpublished).
(c) Shuskus (1964).
(d) Locher and Geschwind (1965).
(e) Wertheim and Remeika (1964).
(f) Forrester (1965).
(g) Robert (1962).

If one now turns to an examination of the NMR of Fe^{57} in the antiferromagnet α-Fe_2O_3 and the ferrimagnet (uncompensated antiferromagnet) YIG as listed in Table III, we see that the hyperfine fields do not significantly differ by more than 1% from the paramagnetic case.

Along similar lines an upper limit of one-half percent was placed on any spin deviation of Mn^{2+} in MnF_2 by Jones and Jefferts (1964), and in $KMnF_3$ by Montgomery et al. (1962) and Witt and Portis (1964).

D. Super-Transferred Hyperfine Interaction

A possible clue to the failure to observe this zero-point spin deviation is provided by the situation in MnO (Lines and Jones, 1965) and MnS (Lines and Jones, 1966).

In these cases, not only is no zero-point spin deviation observed, but it is found that $\langle S \rangle / S > 1$. This observation is clearly anomalous and has led several authors to question the assumption that A is the same in both the dilute and concentrated material. Owen and Taylor (1966), and Huang et al. (1966), have suggested that $|A|$ is actually larger in the antiferromagnet due to the transfer of unpaired electron spin from one magnetic ion to the next. Namely, if one considers a $Mn(2)\downarrow - 0 - Mn(1)\uparrow$ pair then the hyperfine interaction for Mn(1) is $A_d S_1 \cdot I_1 + \alpha S_2 \cdot I_1$. Two mechanisms that can produce this extra term in α were considered. The pertinent atomic orbitals are shown in Fig. 15.

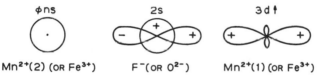

Fig. 15:   Atomic orbitals involved in constructing the antibonding molecular orbital at Mn(1) involving the ligand and Mn(2) orbitals. See text (Huang et al. , 1966).

(i) The $2p_z$ orbit on the ligand (F^- or O^{2-}) contains a certain fraction of unpaired spin density f_σ which has been transferred from a d_z^2 orbit on Mn(1) (the quantity f_σ can be determined experimentally from the fluorine NMR or from the fluorine super hfs in the EPR spectrum). This unpaired spin on the ligand orbits can be partly transferred to the s-orbitals on Mn(2) by orthogonalization, i.e., overlap $S_\sigma = \langle ns(Mn(2))| 2p_\sigma \rangle$, giving an unpaired spin density $f_\sigma S_\sigma^2$ in the occupied ns(Mn(2)) orbits. Huang et al (1966) also considered the 2s orbital of the ligand as well as the p_z. The net effect of Mn(1), therefore, is the creation of unpaired s-electron spin density at Mn(2) which has the same spin direction as the d_z^2 orbit of Mn(1), i.e., opposite to the spin direction of d_z^2 (Mn(2)). Since, by *negative* core polarization we mean that the hyperfine field produced by the d-electrons is opposite to that which would be produced by s-electrons with the *same* spin direction as the d-electrons, we see that the effect of this covalent transfer process is to increase the absolute value of the hyperfine field.

(ii) A second mechanism proposed by Huang et al. (1966) is illustrated in Fig. 16. An electron is transferred directly from the $3d_{z^2}^2$ of $Mn^{2+}(1)$, leaving it as Mn^{3+}, to an unoccupied 4s orbital on $Mn(2)$. The charge transfer Hamiltonian is spin independent, so that the spin of the electron transferred to the 4s orbital on $Mn(2)$ is the same as that on $Mn(1)$ or opposite to the d-orbitals on $Mn(2)$ since we are dealing with an antiferromagnet. Just as for mechanism (i) this again leads to an increase in the absolute value of the hyperfine field.

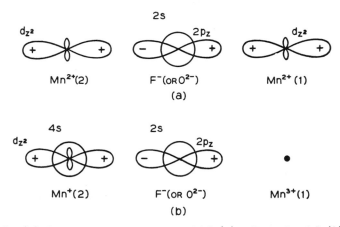

Fig. 16:   (a) Ground configuration of Mn(1) - ligand - Mn(2).
          (b) Excited configuration where an electron has been transferred from the $d_{z^2}^2$ orbital of Mn(1) to the unoccupied 4s orbital of the neighboring Mn(2).

If this effect is added for the six nearest Mn neighbors of a particular Mn, it is found that the absolute value of the hyperfine field is increased anywhere from 2 to 4 percent which therefore masks the sought for zero-point spin deviation. Owen and Taylor (1966) remark that this effect will be more marked in the oxides which are more covalent than the fluorides, which would account for Lines and Jones result that $A_c \langle S \rangle > A_d S$.

While these covalent effects undoubtedly play a most important role as indicated by the above authors, one may be justified in harboring a cautious reserve before accepting this as the complete explanation of the failure to observe the zero-point spin deviation. There are some difficulties in Fe^{3+} (Simanek et al., 1967) which are not completely resolved.

It would perhaps be appropriate to look for situations in which one on theoretical grounds expects larger zero-point spin deviations. For example, Lines (1967) has recently calculated that for the planar antiferromagnet $Ca_2 MnO_4$, the spin deviation for the Mn^{4+} should be some 13 percent.

E. Some Systematics of Core Polarization for $3d^n$ Ions

We saw above, in connection with the discussion of the zero-point spin deviation, that the cphf for a given $3d^5$ ion was, to an accuracy of roughly 1 percent, independent of ligand distance in the same chemical environment, i.e., same ligand number and same type of ligand. There is still a second constancy in the $3d^n$ series that is worth noting. This is the fact that the cphf is the same within an isoelectronic sequence in the same chemical environment. This second constancy is illustrated in Table IV for the $3d^3$ isoelectronic sequence V^{2+}, Cr^{3+}, and Mn^{4+}. Note that the small orbital hyperfine field has been taken into account in accordance with Eq. (28) in arriving at the cphf from the observed hyperfine field.

Table IV: cphf in $3d^3$ ions, per unit spin $(S = 1)$, in Al_2O_3.

	V^{2+}	Cr^{3+}	Mn^{4+}
H^{hf}_{total} (experimental)[a] ENDOR	-197.2 kG	-201.6	-197.9
$g_{\parallel}$[a]	1.991	1.984	1.993
Δg	-0.0113	-0.0183	-0.0093
$\langle 1/r^3 \rangle$[b]	2.75	3.96	5.34
H^{hf}_{orb}	-3.9 kG	-4.6	-6.3
H_{cp}	-193.3 kG	-192.0	-191.6

(a) *Laurence and Lambe (1963).*
(b) *Freeman and Watson (1965).*

In the $3d^5$ series, the cphf is found to be constant to roughly within 6 percent when the small orbital hyperfine fields are taken into account. Although this constancy is not as striking as for the $3d^3$ ions it is remarkable nonetheless, that it occurs to even this extent; for going from ligand coordination as ionic as fluorine to one as covalent as selenium (Estle and Holton, 1966) the cphf is reduced by 40%. A similar constancy is observed for $3d^8$ (Co^+, Ni^{2+}, and Cu^{3+}), i.e., $\sim$ -250 kG cphf in six-fold oxygen coordination (Locher and Geschwind, 1963) except that in this case the orbital hf field is quite large and so it is more difficult to establish this constancy with the same degree of accuracy as for $3d^3$ and $3d^5$. Again we wish to stress the surprising nature of this result as calculations for the *free ions* give for the cphf of V^{2+} = -236 kG and Mn^{4+} = -296 kG (Freeman and Watson, 1961 and 1965). One can speculate that the Mn^{4+}, being more covalent, would experience a greater reduction in its hf field in the crystal as compared to V^{2+} which would tend to make the hyperfine interactions equal. While qualitative arguments of this sort may be advanced, it would be interesting to see if one can provide a more quantitative explanation for these constancies.

V. Exchange Coupled Spectra

A. Nature of Exchange Coupled Spectra; Pairs and Higher Arrays

We wish to consider now the EPR spectra, and in particular the hfs, of exchange coupled similar ions. By extension of our analysis to a large number of exchange coupled ions, we will be led to a simi-classical picture of the reason for the absence of hfs in ferromagnetic resonance.

Let us consider a collection of N ions each with zero orbital angular momentum in the ground state so that we may write for the Hamiltonian of the system in an external magnetic field, H, along the z-axis

$$\mathcal{K} = g\beta H_z \sum_{i=1}^{N} S_{iz} + A \sum_{i=1}^{N} S_i \cdot I_i + \sum J_{ij} S_i \cdot S_j \; . \qquad (60)$$

Here A is the hf interaction constant for the individual ion and J_{ij} is an exchange integral and the $\Sigma J_{ij} S_i \cdot S_j$ is taken over all coupling ions. The nuclear Zeeman energy has been neglected as it will be assumed to be far smaller than $A I \cdot S$. The electronic Zeeman term commutes with the exchange term and hence both may be simultaneously diagonalized in a representation in which both $S_z = \Sigma_i S_{iz}$ and S^2 are diagonal. We assume that $|g\beta H| \gg |A|$ and $|J| \gg |A|$ so that we need only consider that part of the hyperfine interaction which is diagonal in S_z and S^2. Obviously the transverse terms $(S_{ix}I_{ix} + S_{iy}I_{iy})$ do not commute with S_z. While $\Sigma_i S_{iz}I_{iz}$ commutes with S_z, it does not commute with S^2. We therefore seek that part of $\Sigma_i S_{iz}I_{iz}$ which is diagonal in S_z and S^2. We assume that $\langle S_{iz} \rangle$ must be the same for all ions. This follows from the assumption of the indistinguishability of the sites, i.e., the wavefunction for the coupled angular momenta must be such as to express this symmetry. Therefore, since

$$\sum_{i=1}^{N} \langle S_{iz} \rangle = \langle S_z \rangle \ , \tag{61}$$

$$\langle S_{iz} \rangle = \frac{\langle S_z \rangle}{N} \ . \tag{62}$$

Thus the operator for the diagonal part of the hf interaction is given by

$$\text{diag part of} \sum S_{iz}I_{iz} = \frac{A}{N} S_z I_z \tag{63}$$

where

$$S_z = \Sigma_i S_{iz} \quad \text{and} \quad I_z = \Sigma_i I_{iz} \ .$$

The diagonal Hamiltonian is therefore

$$\mathcal{H} = g\beta H S_z + \frac{A}{N} S_z I_z + \sum J_{ij} \mathbf{S}_i \cdot \mathbf{S}_j \ . \tag{64}$$

The hyperfine term $A/N\, S_z I_z$, which is diagonal in the S_z, S^2 representation, may be physically interpreted as meaning that the electrons couple to form a total spin S, with projection S_z along the field such that the $\langle S_{iz} \rangle$ at each site is S_z/N so that each nucleus sees a hyperfine field proportional to $(A/N)S_z$. The total hyperfine interaction is then $(A/N)S_z \Sigma_i I_{iz} = (A/N)S_z I_z$. The neglected off-diagonal terms will be returned to later.

Let us apply Eq. (64) to the case of antiferromagnetically coupled Mn pairs in a crystal such as MgO. If one dopes MgO with 1 percent Mn, then in addition to the isolated single ions there will be a small percentage of ions (less than 0.1%) which have another Mn ion as a neighbor along the Mn-O line, i.e., a pair of the type Mn-O-Mn. The Mn^{2+} spin is $S_1 = S_2 = 5/2$ so

that the total spin of this exchange coupled pair can take on values
$S = 0, 1, 2, 3, 4, 5$ with the separation between adjacent states S and
$(S+1)$ given by $J(2S+1)$. With $J > 0$, (antiferromagnetic coupling)
the $S = 0$ ground state will be most heavily populated at low temperatures. As the temperature is raised the population of the
$S = 1$ level increases and by measuring the increase of intensity of
the $S = 1$ spectrum with temperature, Coles et al. (1960) and Owen
(1961) find $J/k = 28°K$, where k is Boltzmann's constant. (The
situation is far more complex for the case where J is the same
order as $g\beta H$; see for example, Birgeneau et al., 1966). The
magnetic dipole-dipole interaction between the Mn ions is different
in the different S states and adds a term to the Hamiltonian Eq.
(64) which looks like $D[S_z^2 - \frac{1}{3} S(S+1)]$. The effect of this term is
to displace the spectra corresponding to different regions of magnetic field. In particular, the $S = 1$ spectrum is displaced from the
isolated single ion spectrum of Mn^{2+} which is very much more
intense than the pair spectrum; this greatly helps in analyzing the
spectra.

However, since the observed microwave transitions in EPR
correspond to $\Delta S = 0$, $\Delta S_z = \pm 1$, $\Delta I_z = 0$, the resonance absorption lines for fixed microwave frequency, ν, according to Eq. (64)
will be given by

$$H = H_0 - \frac{A}{N} M_I \tag{65}$$

where $M_I = \langle I_z \rangle = \langle I_{z1} \rangle + \langle I_{z2} \rangle$ and $H_0 = h\nu/g\beta \pm D$ for $S = 1$. H_0
is parallel to the line joining the pair. Note that this hyperfine
pattern for the pair will be the same, independent of the particular
S-state or $S_z \rightarrow (S_z+1)$ transition being observed. Since $N = 2$ and
$I_1 = I_2 = 5/2$ for Mn^{55}, the total value of M_I will range from -5 to
+5, i.e., there will be eleven hfs lines separated by $A/2$ as shown
in Fig. 17. Note that the overall extension of the hyperfine pattern
is exactly the same as for the single ion, i.e., 5A. The intensities
of the individual components follow a binomial distribution and
correspond to the number of different ways the two nuclear spins
can be combined to give the same total M_I value. Further details
of this and other pair spectra may be found in the reviews by
Bagguley and Owen (1957) and Owen (1961).

B. Absence of hfs in Ferromagnetic Resonance

Let us extend the above considerations to the case $N > 2$.
Consider N strongly ferromagnetically exchange-coupled centers
each with $I = \frac{1}{2}$. Again the hyperfine structure pattern for such a
system in a state of total S is given by the factor $-(A/N)M_I$ of

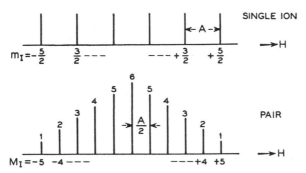

Fig. 17: (a) Hfs spectrum in EPR of Mn^{55} for single isolated Mn^{2+} ion (I = 5/2); (b) Hfs spectrum for exchange coupled pairs of Mn^{2+} ions.

Eq. (65) and is illustrated in Fig. 18 for values of N up to 8. It is seen that the overall extension of the hyperfine pattern *is always the same*, i.e., in this case A. However, since there are many more ways of forming the $M_I = 0$ state, the hyperfine pattern will be peaked in the center and will fall off rapidly as N increases with a binomial distribution. For example, for a ferromagnet with very large N, the intensity at a point A/4 from the center is down by $(0.26)^{-N}$ from the intensity at the center; i.e., the hfs is effectively washed out in ferromagnetic resonance. In this picture, we view ferromagnetic resonance as paramagnetic resonance for a large number of exchange coupled spins in which successive $\Delta S_z = -1$ transitions are induced.

The same result is expressed in the language of spin waves as follows. Normal ferromagnetic resonance is described by the excitation of k = 0 spin waves with the total nuclear orientation remaining unchanged. The spin deviation $\Delta S_z = 1$ in the k = 0 spin wave is not localized on any one site but uniformly distributed over all the spins in the crystal. It will, therefore, sample all the nuclei and so see the average value of M_I. This k = 0 spin wave with $\Delta M_I = 0$ will have a structure represented by the probability distribution of the different M_I values as outlined above and similarly will be washed out, in practice, for large N.

C. Observation of "Forbidden" hfs Line in Ferromagnetic Resonance

It should be recalled, however, that we have neglected those terms in the hf interaction which are nondiagonal in S_z and S^2, for example $A\Sigma_i(S_{ix}I_{ix}+S_{iy}I_{iy})$. In the case of an isolated single ion

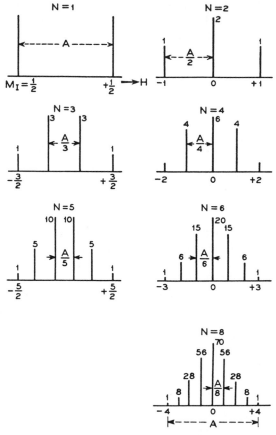

Fig. 18: EPR spectra of a ferromagnetically coupled ion with electronic spin $S = 1/2$ and nuclear spin $I = 1/2$ with hyperfine interaction $\mathbf{AI \cdot S}$, in strong field region. Note how maximum extension of hyperfine pattern is always A but that the intensity is crowded towards the center, so that for very large N the hfs is washed out.

it is well known that transverse terms of this nature mix states $|M_{S\pm1},\ M_{I\mp1}>$ into $|M_S,\ M_I>$ such that

$$|M_S,\ M_I> = |M_S,\ M_I> + \alpha|M_{S+1},\ M_{I-1}> +$$

$$+ \alpha|M_{S-1},\ M_{I+1}> \text{ etc.} \tag{66}$$

where $\alpha \sim A/g\beta H$. This gives rise in the microwave spectrum to $\Delta M_S = \pm 1$ $\Delta M_I = \mp 1$ transitions. These "forbidden" transitions are down in intensity from the normal $\Delta M_I = 0$ transitions by $(A/g\beta H)^2$. Ford and Jeffries (1966) have indicated that in a similar fashion one may observe $\Delta S_Z = +1, \Delta M_I = -1$ transitions in ferromagnetic resonance. On our semiclassical picture of ferromagnetic resonance as EPR for a very large value of S as represented by Eq. (64), the $\Delta S = 0$ $\Delta S_Z = +1$ transition is given by

$$W_a - W_b = g\beta H_z + \frac{A}{N} \left[S_Z^a I_Z^b - (S_Z^a - 1) I_Z^b \right]$$

$$= g\beta H_z + \frac{A}{N} S_Z^a (I_Z^a - I_Z^b) + \frac{A}{N} I_Z^b \qquad (67)$$

where a and b refer to initial and final states respectively of total S_Z and total I_Z. The case $(I_Z^a - I_Z^b) = 0$ corresponds to the $\Delta I_Z = 0$ case we have already considered, i.e., the normal ferromagnetic resonance with the structure factor $(A/N) I_Z^b$. However, if we allow $\Delta I_Z = -1$ transitions then we have an extra line displaced from the main one by $-(A/N) S_Z^a$, which also has the structure factor $(A/N) I_Z^b$ which in practice corresponds to an infinitely narrow line as outlined above. Since $S_Z^a \approx S$ at low temperatures, the extra line is displaced from the main line by $A(S/N) =$ spin of the individual ion. In other words, this extra line corresponds to exciting a $k = 0$ spin wave and simultaneously flipping a single nucleus by $\Delta I_Z = 1$ in the hyperfine field $A(S/N)$. Thus, it is by this "forbidden transition" that hyperfine field information might be obtained in ferromagnetic resonance. The only report of such an observation so far is by Ford and Jeffries (1966) in K_2CuCl_4 $2H_2O$. They indicate, however, that the intensity of this extra line has a completely wrong frequency dependence, going as ν^4 instead of $1/\nu^2$, i.e. as $1/H^2$. It would be interesting to understand this discrepancy and search for this forbidden line in other ferromagnets.

VI. Optical Detection of Excited State EPR

A. Three Methods of Optical Detection of Excited State EPR

The recent introduction of optical detection techniques makes it possible to study the excited states of magnetic impurity ions in crystals with the same high-resolution of EPR which has been so successfully applied to the study of ground states. The details of the new technique are given by Geschwind and others (1965), and by Imbusch and others (1967), and we briefly review some of the highlights in this section.

In the attempt to detect the microwave absorption in the excited states directly one is generally hampered by a leak of sensitivity. In effect, the number of ions that can be maintained in these excited states by the usual methods, such as optical excitation, is far too small. To do EPR, one needs approximately 10^{11} or so spins having $\Delta H \sim 1$ gauss and an integration time constant of about 1 sec. The combination of relevant factors such as available pumping power, optical absorption factor, and lifetime of the excited state are such as to generally yield a number of ions in the excited state well below the minimum required.

However, if the excited state in question is fluorescent, one can seek to monitor a change in the fluorescent light from this level when the microwave frequency coincides with its Zeeman splitting, rather than monitor the absorption of microwave power. The absorption of a microwave photon in the excited state will change some aspect of the fluorescence pattern by one optical photon. The observation of resonance is thus moved from the detection of microwave photons to the much more sensitive realm of detecting an equal number of optical photons. In favorable circumstances orders of magnitude increased sensitivity is thereby obtained, being roughly equal to the ratios of the energy of an optical to a microwave photon. This is the analog in solids of the optical rf double resonance techniques first suggested by Brossel and Kastler (1949) and widely used in gases.

Within the general framework of optical detection of microwave absorption in excited states in solids, three methods immediately suggest themselves and are illustrated by reference to Fig. 19. For the purposes of illustrating these different methods, consider a hypothetical excited state doublet which is maintained in a steady state by some continuous pumping means and which decays by fluorescence to a ground doublet. Assume that both doublets are split in a magnetic field and have selection rules as shown. Further assume that there is a thermalization of a certain degree or that if necessary, some selective means of filling levels a and b has been used so that the population of level a, n_a, is less than that of b, n_b.

Method 1. Use of High-Resolution Optical Spectrometer: This is a "brute force" method that requires a high resolution optical spectrometer. Assume that the Zeeman splitting between A and B can be resolved with the spectrometer. Then one may sit on line A and monitor its intensity with a photocell. If a microwave transition is induced between b and a, thereby increasing the population of a, one will observe an increase in the photocell output.

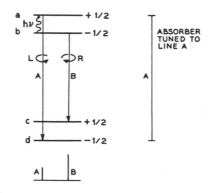

METHOD:

1. CIRCULAR POLARIZATION----DOES NOT REQUIRE
                          SHARP LINES

2. SELECTIVE REABSORPTION----REQUIRES SHARP
                           LINES

3. HIGH RESOLUTION
   RECORDING SPECTROMETER---REQUIRES SHARP
                          LINES

Fig. 19: Illustration of optical detection of EPR in an excited state doublet ab which fluoresces to the ground state doublet cd. It is assumed that the population of level b is greater than that of $\underline{a}$ as a result of either thermalization in the excited state or selective filling. $h\nu$ indicates an induced microwave transition which changes some aspect of the fluorescent light.

This method has been used by Geschwind et al. (1965) to study the EPR and spin-lattice relaxation time of the Zeeman components of the $\overline{E}(^2E)$ state of ruby (Cr^{3+} in $Al_2 O_3$).

   Method 2. Selective Reabsorption: Imagine that the *total* fluorescent light $A + B$ is viewed after being passed through a material that selectively absorbs line A. Then in effecting a microwave transition from b to a, light which was previously emitted in line B will now be emitted in line A which is more strongly attenuated by the absorber, so that the total light $A + B$ reaching the viewer will be decreased. The absorber in question need not be external to the fluorescent system. For example, lines A and B may have sufficient oscillator strength and enough centers may be present in the ground state so that A and B are internally reabsorbed in the sample. Reabsorption will decrease the intensity of emitted radiation from the sample as one may assume the existence of nonradiative decay to the ground state as well as the more probable decay by radiative transition. If, in addition, one is at sufficiently low temperature such that $n_d > n_c$, then A will be more strongly reabsorbed from b to a, then again the total light (A+B) viewed in a given direction will be found to decrease due to this selective reabsorption. This method was first used in solids for ruby (Geschwind et al., 1959). However, such large selective internal reabsorption is exceptional to ruby so that this method does not have wide applicability.

Method 3. Circular Polarization: If we look along the direction of magnetic field, the intensity of the left-circular component of light (line A) will be less than the right-circular component (line B) since $n_a < n_b$. If one, therefore, monitors light along the dc magnetic field with appropriate polarizers, one will observe an increase in left-circularly polarized light as microwave transitions are induced at the resonance between levels a and b, due to the increase in n_a and decrease in n_b.

Note that the Zeeman splitting need not be resolved at all in this method, i.e., the linewidths may be considerably greater than the splitting. This technique of monitoring circularly polarized light should have the widest application to the observation of magnetic resonance in the excited states of solids characterized by inhomogeneously broadened emission lines. Imbusch and Geschwind (1965) have used this method to study the excited $\bar{E}$ state of Mn^{4+} in Al_2O_3. In addition, Chase (1967) has made use of this method to study the ^2E state of V^{2+} and Cr^{3+} in the cubic sites of MgO.

The general experimental arrangement used for optical detection of excited state EPR is illustrated in Fig. 20. The crystal containing the paramagnetic impurity is mounted in a microwave cavity and continuously illuminated vertically through a small hole in the bottom of the cavity. This pumping light produces a small steady-state population in the excited state as will be illustrated in the next section. The fluorescent radiation from the excited state in question is viewed horizontally through slots cut in the cavity which do not interfere with the microwave current flow. In the case of the high-resolution technique, a particular Zeeman component in the fluorescent light is monitored using a high-resolution optical spectrometer. If the circular polarization technique is being used, the spectrometer is simply replaced by a quarter wave plate and linear polarizer placed in the liquid helium in the path of the fluorescent light. This latter combination acts as an analyzer for the circularly polarized light. The microwaves are square-wave modulated at some low audio frequency and the corresponding modulation in the fluorescent light as the external

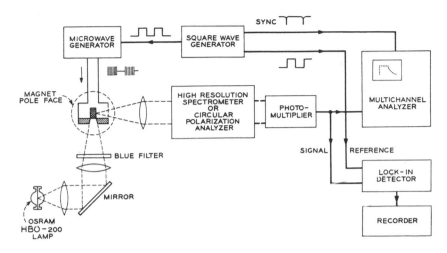

Fig. 20: Block diagram of system used for optical detection of excited state EPR.

magnetic field is slowly swept through resonance in the excited state is detected with a photomultiplier. The signal is then fed to a phase sensitive detector tuned to the modulation frequency and onto a pen recorder. For spin-lattice relaxation studies in the excited state, the external magnetic field is kept fixed at the peak of the resonance and the resultant signal is fed to a multi-channel analyzer to improve the signal-to-noise.

There are situations where excited state EPR can be seen by monitoring the microwave absorption. For example, the excited triplet states of organic molecules are so long-lived (one second or greater) that one can easily produce sufficient excited centers to observe directly the microwave absorption (Hutchison and Magnum, 1961). Even in the case of certain rare-earth impurity ions such as Dy^{2+} this can be done (Sabisky and Anderson, 1964). However, we believe that there is no advantage to be gained by doing direct microwave absorption and that in general orders of magnitude increased sensitivity may be had by using optical detection techniques.

B. Illustration with $\bar{E}$ (^2E) States of $(3d)^3$ Ions in Al_2O_3

We briefly review the very well known energy level scheme of a Cr^{3+} ion (V^{2+}, Mn^{4+} are analogous) in Al_2O_3 with the aid of Fig. 21. The free-ion ground state is ^4F with $L = 3$ and $S = 3/2$.

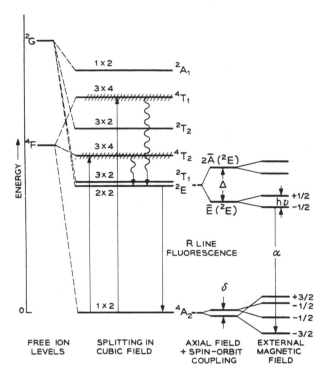

Fig. 21: Partial energy level diagram of d^3 ions (V^{2+}, Cr^{3+}, or Mn^{4+}) in Al_2O_3 in an external magnetic field.

The seven-fold orbital degeneracy is split in a cubic field into a $^4A_2$ orbital singlet and the $^4T_2$ and $^4T_1$ triplets which are shown cross-hatched and are the main absorption bands of ruby. The famous fluorescent ^2E state arises primarily from the free ion ^2G level but is, at the strength of the cubic crystal field in ruby an admixture of many of the free-ion doublet states, i.e., ^2G, ^2D, ^2H, ^2P. The splitting of the ^2G level in a cubic field is also shown. The strength of the cubic crystal field is such that the ^2E level falls below the $^4T_2$ and $^4T_1$ levels. The ^2E is populated by the ion-absorbing light in the green and blue, corresponding to the $^4A_2 \rightarrow {}^4T_2$ and $^4A_2 \rightarrow {}^4T_1$ transitions, and subsequent decay by radiationless transitions to the ^2E level. The quantum efficiency of this fluorescence is of order unity (anywhere from 50 to 90 percent for Cr^{3+}, but is less for V^{2+} and Mn^{4+}). In addition to the predominant cubic field there is also present a smaller trigonal field which in combination with the spin-orbit coupling splits the

$^4A^2$ ground state by 0.4 cm^{-1} for this isoelectronic sequence and the ^2E state into two Kramers doublets separated by approximately Δ. It is in the lower of these doublets, i.e., in the $\overline{E}(^2E)$ that EPR is performed. Δ is 12, 29, and 80 cm^{-1}, respectively for V^{2+}, Cr^{3+}, and Mn^{4+}.

In Fig. 22, we have extracted that portion of Fig. 21 most pertinent to the performance of optical detection of EPR in $\overline{E}$, illustrating in this case the use of the circular polarization techniques. The polarization and theoretical intensities of the fluorescent Zeeman components from $\overline{E} \rightarrow {}^4A_2$ are shown. The theoretical intensities are observed only if the populations of the -1/2 and

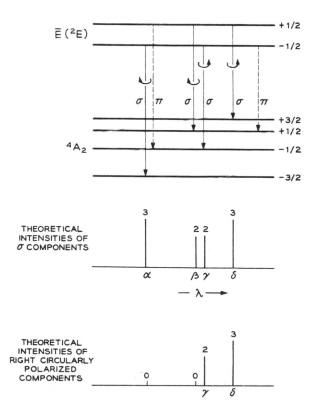

Fig. 22: Use of circular polarization of fluorescent light in detecting EPR in excited $\overline{E}(^2E)$ state.

+1/2 levels of $\overline{\mathrm{E}}$ are equal. Assuming, however, that the population of $-1/2(\overline{\mathrm{E}}) > +1/2(\overline{\mathrm{E}})$ as outlined in Sec. VI.A., then the intensity of the right circularly polarized components $(\gamma + \delta)$ will be weaker than the left circular components $(\alpha + \beta)$. Thus, when a microwave transition is induced between $-1/2(\overline{\mathrm{E}})$ and $+1/2(\overline{\mathrm{E}})$, resulting in a net transfer of ions from $-1/2(\overline{\mathrm{E}})$ to $+1/2(\overline{\mathrm{E}})$, the intensity of the right circularly polarized light $(\gamma + \delta)$ will increase.

C.   Spin-Lattice Relaxation

The measurement of the spin-lattice relaxation time, T_1, in the excited state is sketched in Fig. 23, where for purposes of illustration it is assumed that the high resolution optical spectrometer is being used. The sample is continuously illuminated with Hg light to maintain an equilibrium population in the Zeeman levels of $\overline{\mathrm{E}}$. At a fixed magnetic field, corresponding to resonance in $\overline{\mathrm{E}}$ for the microwave frequency used, a particular Zeeman component is monitored, for example, line A in Fig. 6(a), with a high resolution optical spectrometer and photomultiplier tube. As the microwaves are switched on, ions are transferred from (+1, -1/2) to the (-1, +1/2) level reducing the intensity of line A. When the microwaves are switched off, the (+1, -1/2) level will recover to

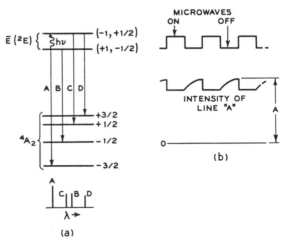

(a)

Fig. 23: (a) σ-components of fluorescent light with $H_0 \| c$. (b) Decrease of intensity of line A which is monitored with a high-resolution optical spectrometer as ions are transferred from $(+1, -1/2)$ to $(-1/2, +1/2)$ with microwaves and subsequent recovery due to spin-lattice relaxation and radiation to ground state. Sample is continuously irradiated with Hg light.

its initial population, as shown in Fig. 6(b). The recovery time τ is given by

$$1/\tau = 1/\tau_R + 1/T_1 , \tag{68}$$

where τ_R is the radiative lifetime and can be measured separately and T_1 is the spin-lattice relaxation time (Geschwind et al., 1965). The results of such a measurement on the $\bar{E}$ level of Cr^{3+} are illustrated in Fig. 24 (Geschwind et al., 1965). T_1 is found to be dominated by an Orbach process (Finn et al., 1961) in which the relaxation between the Zeeman components of $\bar{E}$ proceeds via the intermediate $2\bar{A}$ state 29 cm^{-1} above (see Fig. 21) and is given by

$$T_1 = 1/4 \ T_{(2\bar{A} \to \bar{E})} \ \exp(\Delta/kT) \tag{69}$$

where $T_{(2\bar{A} \to \bar{E})}$ is the time for spontaneous decay from $2\bar{A}$ to $\bar{E}$ with the emission of a phonon of energy Δ. This type of measurement of T_1 in the excited state indicates the maturity of this optical detection technique as it is quite comparable in accuracy and detail to similar studies in ground states.

D. Hyperfine Fields in the Excited State

The isoelectronic sequence V^{2+}, Cr^{3+}, and Mn^{4+} offers one an interesting series for the study of the hfs in excited states, and provides a good illustration of the different contributions to hf fields. The spin Hamiltonian for the $\bar{E}(^2E)$ level is given by

$$\mathcal{H} = g_{\|} \beta \ H_z S_z + g_\perp \beta (H_x S_x + H_y S_y) +$$

$$+ A_{\|} I_z S_z + A_\perp (I_x S_x + I_y S_y) \tag{70}$$

where $S = 1/2$. Due to the fact that $g_\perp$ in this state is very close to zero, only $A_{\|}$ can be determined.

In Fig. 25(a) is shown the hfs splitting for the $-1/2 \to +1/2$ transition of the $^4A_2$ ground state of an Al_2O_3 crystal containing 0.1% Cr enriched to 95% Cr^{53} (I = 3/2) (Geschwind et al., 1965). In Fig. 25(b) is shown the $(-1/2, +1) \to (+1/2, -1)$ in the $\bar{E}$ state, in the same crystal, with no apparent hfs. From the width of this line, we may put an upper limit of 25 kG on the hyperfine field per unit spin at the Cr^{53} nucleus in the excited $\bar{E}$ state in contrast approximately -200 kG in the ground state. This result is easily understood in terms of the accidental near cancellation of the core polarization hyperfine field (cphf) with the orbital hyperfine field in the excited state. The hyperfine field in the $^4A_2$ ground state is essentially a cphf field, i.e., $g_{\|}(^4A_2)$ is very close to 2.0, and as

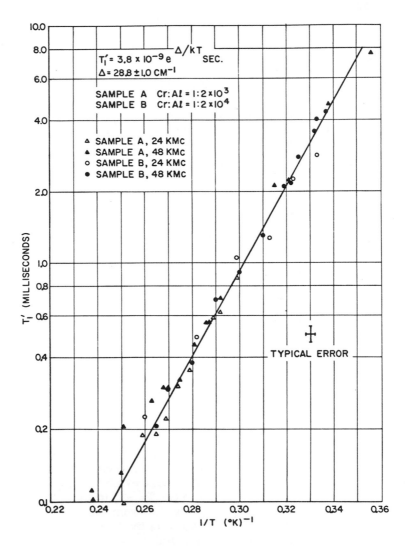

Fig. 24: Illustration of measurement of spin-lattice relaxation in excited state of ruby by optical detection technique.

92% ENRICHED Cr^{53} IN Al_2O_3 $(Cr:Al \sim 1:10^3)$

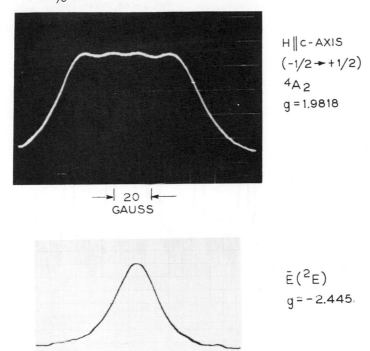

H ∥ c - AXIS
$(-1/2 \rightarrow +1/2)$
$^4A_2$
g = 1.9818

$\bar{E}(^2E)$
g = - 2.445.

Fig. 25: (a) EPR signal from $-1/2 \rightarrow +1/2$ electronic transition of
$^4A_2$ ground state in Al_2O_3:Cr with enriched Cr^{53}.
(b) Excited state EPR in same sample. Absence of observable hfs is due to near accidental cancellation of cphf field with orbital hyperfine field.

indicated in Table IV of Sec. IV. E. it is approximately -193 kG for $3d^3$ ions. As the electronic distribution in the ground and excited states are similar, (both have t_2^3 crystal field configurations), we expect the cphf to be the same in the ground and excited states. However, $g_{||} = 2.445$ in the excited state, and this departure of the g-value from 2.0 implies a significant orbital hf field, H_{orb}^{hf}, as given by Eq. (28), in contrast to the $^4A_2$ ground state. If we take $\langle 1/r^3 \rangle = 3.958$ (Freeman and Watson, 1965) and $\Delta g_{||} = 0.445$ in Eq. (28) we find $H_{orb}^{hf} \approx +219$ kG which almost cancels the -193 kG cphf field. In contrast, $g_{||}$ for V^{2+} and Mn^{4+} is respectively +2.22 and 3.10 so that assuming that the cphf remains the

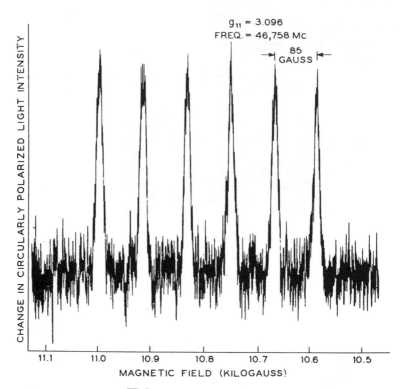

Fig. 26: EPR excited $\overline{E}\,(^2E)$ state of Mn^{4+} in Al_2O_3 showing hfs due to Mn^{4+}. Dominant hf field is orbital (Imbusch and Geschwind, 1965).

same, the near cancellation that occurred in Cr^{3+} should be absent and one should observe a well resolved hfs. This is shown in Fig. 26 for the excited $\overline{E}$ state of Mn^{4+} in Al_2O_3 (Imbusch and Geschwind, 1965). Similarly, a well resolved structure is observed for V^{2+} in $\overline{E}$ (Imbusch et al., 1965 and Imbusch et al., 1967). Note that the hfs pattern shown in Fig. 26 corresponds to a sensitivity of approximately 10^8 spins according to the usual criteria. In the case of Mn^{4+}, using $\langle 1/r^3 \rangle = 5.4$ and $\Delta g = 1.10$, one finds $H^{hf}_{orb} = +740$ kG, which completely swamps the -193 kG cphf field. This very large orbital hyperfine field for Mn^{4+} points up two difficulties. First, to the extent that it is large, a given percentage uncertainty in the value of $\langle 1/r^3 \rangle$ produces a larger absolute uncertainty in the calculated hyperfine field. Second, the dipolar hyperfine field will be more important and unfortunately

the calculation of H^{hf}_{dip} requires an exact knowledge of the excited
state wavefunction. For the E state of Mn^{4+}, Imbusch et al
(1967) calculate $H^{hf}_{total} = +459$ kG, whereas $H^{hf}_{exp} = +350$ kG.
Note that if $\langle 1/r^3 \rangle$ were taken 14% smaller, this would reduce
the calculated H^{hf}_{orb} by 100 kG and bring the experimentally observed and calculated hyperfine fields into coincidence. One certainly expects $\langle 1/r^3 \rangle$ to be smaller in the crystal and even more
so for the more covalent Mn^{4+} as compared to V^{2+} and Cr^{3+}. In
addition because of the covalent bonding to ligands, $\Sigma_i \langle \ell_i/r_i^3 \rangle \neq$
$\langle 1/r^3 \rangle \langle \Sigma_i \ell_i \rangle$ so that Eq. (28) is no longer exact. A detailed
analysis is to be found in Imbusch et al. (1967).

I should like to thank my colleagues, M. Blume, L. R. Walker and Y. Yafet for many illuminating and helpful discussions on
a variety of points covered in these lectures. In addition, I should
like to thank J. Asik for some helpful suggestions regarding some
points of presentation in these notes.

References

Abragam, A. and Pryce, M. H. L. (1951a). Proc. Roy. Soc.
A205, 135.

Abragam, A. and Pryce, M. H. L. (1951b). Proc. Roy. Soc.
A206, 173.

Abragam, A. (1961). Principles of Nuclear Magnetism (Oxford
University Press).

Anderson, P. W. (1951). Phys. Rev. 83, 1260.

Anderson, P. W. (1952). Phys. Rev. 86, 694.

Baker, J. M., Chardwick, J. R., Garton, G., and Hurrel, J. P.
(1965). Proc. Roy. Soc. A286, 352.

Baker, J. M. and Williams, F. I. B. (1962). Proc. Roy. Soc.
A267, 283.

Bagguley, D. M. S. and Owen, J. (1957). Reports Prog. Phys. 20,
304.

Bethe, H. (1931). Z. f. Phys. 71, 205.

Birgeneau, R. J., Hutchings, M. T. and Wolf, W. P. (1966). Phys.
Rev. Letters 4, 116.

Bleaney, B. (1951). Phil. Mag. [7], 42, 441.

Bleaney, B., Bowers, K. D., Ingram, D. J. E., Trenam, R. S. and Pryce, M. H. L. (1955). Proc. Roy. Soc. A228, 147, 157, and 166.

Bleaney, B. (1959). Proc. Phys. Soc. (London) 73, 389.

Brossel, J. and Kastler, A. (1949). Compt. Rend. 229, 1213.

Chase, L. (1966). Conf. on Optical Properties of Ions in Crystals, Johns Hopkins Univ., Sept. 1966, John Wiley.

Coles, B. A., Orton, J. W. and Owen, J. (1960). Phys. Rev. Letters 4, 116.

Estle, T. L. and Holton, W. C. (1966). Phys. Rev. 150, 159.

Feher, G. (1956). Phys. Rev. 103, 500.

Feher, G. and Gere, E. A. (1956). Phys. Rev. 103, 501.

Feher, G. (1959). Phys. Rev. 114, 1219.

Ford, N. C., Jr. and Jeffries, C. D. (1966). Phys. Rev. 141, 381.

Forrester, D. W. (1965). Oak Ridge National Laboratory Report ORNL (3705).

Freeman, A. J. and Watson, R. E. (1961). Phys. Rev. 123, 2027.

Freeman, A. J. and Watson, R. E. (1965). Magnetism, (edited by Suhl-Rado, Vol. IIA, p. 290, Appendix B).

Freeman, R., Murray, G. R. and Richards, R. E. (1957). Proc. Roy. Soc. A242, 455.

Fry, D. J. I., Llewellyn, P. M. and Pryce, M. H. L. (1962). Proc. Roy. Soc. A266, 84.

Geschwind, S., Devlin, G. E., Cohen, R. L. and Chinn, S. R. (1965). Phys. Rev. 137, A1087.

Gossard, A. C. and Portis, A. (1960). J. Appl. Phys. Suppl. 31, 205S.

Griffith, J. S. (1961). Theory of Transition Metal Ions (Cambridge University Press).

Ham, F. S., Ludwig, G. W., Watkins, G. D. and Woodbury, H. H. (1960). Phys. Rev. Letters 5, 468.

Holton, W. C., Blum, H. and Slichter, C. P. (1960). Phys. Rev. Letters 5, 197.

Huang, Nai Li, Orbach, R. and Simanek, E. (1966). Phys. Rev. Letters 17, 134.

Hulthen, L. (1936). Proc. Amst. Acad. Sci. 39, 190; Arkiv. Mat. Astron. Fysik 26A, Na 11.

Hurrel, J. (1965). Brit. J. Appl. Phys. 16, 755.

Hutchison, C. A. , Jr. and Mangum, B. W. (1961). J. Chem. Phys. 34, 908.

Hyde, J. S. (1965) J. Chem. Phys. 43, 1806.

Imbusch, G. F. and Geschwind, S. (1965). Physics Letters 18, 109.

Jaccarino, V. and Walstedt, R. E. (1967). Phys. Rev. (to be published).

Jones, E. D. and Jefferts, K. B. (1964). Phys. Rev. 135, A1277.

Koster, G. F. and Statz, H. (1959a). Phys. Rev. 113, 445.

Koster, G. F. and Statz, H. (1959b). Phys. Rev. 115, 1568.

Lambe, J. , Laurence, N. , Irvine, E. C. and Terhune, R. W. (1961). Phys. Rev. 122, 1161.

Laurence, N. and Lambe, J. (1963). Phys. Rev. 132, 1029.

Lines, M. E. and Jones, E. D. (1965). Phys. Rev. 139, A1313.

Lines, M. E. and Jones, E. D. (1966). Phys. Rev. 141, A525.

Lines, M. E. (1967). Phys. Rev. Letters (to be published).

Locher, P. R. and Geschwind, S. (1963). Phys. Rev. Letters 11, 333.

Locher, P. R. and Geschwind, S. (1965). Phys. Rev. 139, A1277.

Low, W. (1957). Phys. Rev. 105, 801.

Mims, W. B. , Jaccarino, V. and Geschwind, S. (1967). Phys. Rev. (to be published).

Montgomery, H. , Teaney, D. T. and Walsh, W. M. , Jr. (1962). Phys. Rev. 128, 80.

Owen, J. (1961). J. Appl. Phys. Suppl. 32, 214S.

Owen, J. and Taylor, D. R. (1966). Phys. Rev. Letters 17, 159.

Ray, T. (1964). Proc. Roy. Soc. A277, 76.

Reichert, J. F. and Pershan, P. S. (1965). Phys. Rev. Letters 15, 780.

Robert, C. (1962). Centre d'Etudes Nucleaires de Saclay Report No. 2213. (see also Aix Lectures).

Sabisky, E. S. and Anderson, C. H. (1964). Phys. Rev. Letters 13, 754.

Seidel, H. (1961). Zeit. Fur Physik 165, 239.

Shuskus, A. J., Jr. (1964). J. Chem. Phys. 41, 1885.

Tanabe, Y. and Sugano, S. (1954). J. Phys. Soc. Japan 9, 753.

Walsh, W. M., Jr., Jeener, J. and Bloembergen, N. (1965). Phys. Rev. 139, 1338.

Wertheim, G. K. and Remeika, J. P. (1964). Phys. Letters 10, 14.

Witt, G. L. and Portis, A. M. (1964). Phys. Rev. A135, 1616.

7. NUCLEAR MAGNETIC RESONANCE IN MAGNETIC AND METALLIC SOLIDS

Albert Narath

Sandia Laboratory
Albuquerque, New Mexico

Table of Contents

I. Introduction

In recent years nuclear magnetic resonance (NMR) has established itself as a powerful technique for the study of hyperfine interactions in a wide variety of materials and under diverse experimental conditions. The usefulness of this method depends on the large modifications in the frequency, line shape and relaxation behavior of the nuclear resonance which often arise from static as well as dynamic hyperfine effects. In the following discussion the term NMR will be restricted to experiments in which the nuclear resonance is detected directly by means of the electromagnetic coupling between the nuclear magnetization and an external electrical circuit. Because of the small magnitude of nuclear moments, the application of NMR is limited generally to the study of materials in which the resonant nuclear moments are present in relatively high abundance. The NMR technique is therefore especially useful for the study of hyperfine interactions in solids. Such studies have provided important information about the electronic properties of solids. The purpose of this chapter is to treat two important general areas of magnetic hyperfine studies, namely NMR in magnetic solids and in metals, together with a review of the necessary elementary magnetic resonance theory.

II. Magnetic Resonance Theory

A. Isolated Nuclear Spins

Consider a nucleus with total spin angular momentum $\mathbf{I}$, measured in units of $\hbar$. The proportionality of the matrix elements of $\mathbf{I}$ to those of the nuclear magnetic dipole moment μ leads to the definition of the gyromagnetic ratio γ_n

$$\mu = \gamma_n \hbar \mathbf{I} . \tag{1}$$

The Hamiltonian which describes the Zeeman interaction between μ and a magnetic field $\mathbf{H}$ can therefore be written as

$$\mathcal{K} = -\gamma_n \hbar \mathbf{I} \cdot \mathbf{H} . \tag{2}$$

The energies of the $2I+1$ eigenstates $|m\rangle$ of Eq. (2) are given by

$$E(m) = -\gamma_n \hbar H m , \tag{3}$$

where m are the eigenvalues of I^z, and z denotes the direction of $\mathbf{H}$. From Eqs. (1) and (2) we obtain immediately the equation of motion for μ since

$$\frac{d\mu}{dt} = \frac{i}{\hbar} \ [\mathcal{H}, \mu] \ . \tag{4}$$

Using the commutation relations of the angular momentum we find

$$\frac{d\mu}{dt} = \gamma_n \mu \times H \ , \tag{5}$$

which is just the classical equation of motion for a magnetic moment in a magnetic field. Thus, the expectation value of μ^z is time independent while those of μ^x and μ^y vary sinusoidally with Larmor frequencies $\omega_0 = \gamma_n H$. These frequencies correspond, of course, to the allowed magnetic dipole transitions ($\Delta m = \pm 1$) between the states of Eq. (3).

If H in Eq. (5) consists of a static component H_0 and a transverse, circularly polarized component of the form $H_1 (t) = H_1 \ (\hat{i} \cos \omega t + \hat{j} \sin \omega t)$ it is convenient to transform Eq. (5) to a new coordinate system x', y', z' in which $H_0 \parallel z'$; the x', y' axes rotate about z' with constant angular velocity ω, and H_1 is taken to lie along x'. The time derivative $\delta\mu/\delta t$ in the rotating system of coordinates is given by

$$\frac{\delta\mu}{\delta t} = \frac{d\mu}{dt} + \mu \times \omega \ , \tag{6}$$

which yields

$$\frac{\delta\mu}{\delta t} = \gamma_n \mu \times \left[\hat{x}' H_1 + \hat{z}'\left(H_0 + \frac{\omega}{\gamma_n}\right)\right], \tag{7}$$

where $\hat{x}'$ and $\hat{z}'$ denote unit vectors directed along the appropriate axes. The resulting precessional motion of μ, in the rotating frame, about an effective field H_{eff} given by the bracketed term in Eq. (7) is illustrated in Fig. 1. If μ is oriented initially along z' it will always return to that direction periodically. Thus, there is no net energy transfer, on the average, between the H_1 field and the magnetic moment. At resonance ($\omega = -\gamma_n H_0$) the effective field is simply H_1 and μ precesses about x' at a rate $\omega_1 = -\gamma_n H_1$.

The extension of the above arguments to a system of N identical, non-interacting spins in a volume V is straightforward. The eigenstates of the total system correspond to the product functions $|m_1, m_2, \ldots, m_N\rangle$ and the equation of motion for the total nuclear magnetization $M = V^{-1} \ \Sigma_i \ \mu_i$ ($i = 1, 2, \ldots, N$) is there-fore identical to that of μ in Eq. (7).

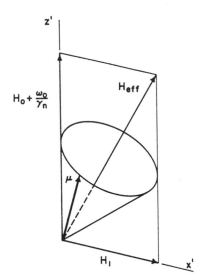

Fig. 1: Motion of the magnetic
moment μ in the ro-
tating coordinate system.

B. Interacting Nuclear Spins

In any real specimen the nuclear spins interact with their
environment. One can usually distinguish two types of interactions;
these are the spin-spin and spin-lattice interactions.

The spin-spin interactions (e. g. , the classical magnetic
dipolar coupling between the nuclear moments) tend to maintain
thermal equilibrium within the nuclear spin system and may be
characterized qualitatively by an effective spin-spin relaxation time
T_2. At equilibrium the system is described by a spin temperature
T_S defined by the Boltzmann distribution function

$$p_i = Z^{-1} \exp(-\beta_S E_i) \; ; \; \beta_S = (k_B T_S)^{-1} \; , \tag{8}$$

where p_i represents the probability that the system is in the i'th
eigenstate, and Z is the partition function

$$Z = \sum_i \exp(-\beta_S E_i) \; . \tag{9}$$

The equilibrium magnetization becomes

$$M_0 = \sum_i M_i^z p_i \; . \tag{10}$$

The sums in Eqs. (9) and (10) are extended over all the states of
the N-spin system. The Zeeman energies therefore range between
$\pm N \gamma_n \hbar I H_0$. However, in most NMR experiments the coupling
between the spins is quite weak compared to the Zeeman interaction

and of relatively short range. In that case only states for which $|E_i| << k_B T_S$ contribute significantly to the resonance behavior of the system provided, of course, that $k_B T_S >> |\gamma_n \hbar H_0|$. In this "high-temperature" approximation $Z \approx Z(\infty) = (2I+1)^N$ and the real system can be approximated by a system of isolated nuclear spins subjected to a strong external field, and a weak position-dependent local field representing the real spin-spin interactions. The local fields produce a non-zero resonance width $\Delta H \approx (\gamma_n T_2)^{-1}$.

The spin-lattice interactions provide contact between the nuclear spins and a "lattice" consisting of the other internal degrees of freedom of the specimen. Since the specific heat of the lattice is generally much greater than that of the nuclear spin system, the lattice serves as a heat reservoir of temperature T, and in the absence of external perturbations $T_S = T$. If the spin temperature (and hence M) is initially perturbed it will approach the lattice temperature, after removal of the perturbation, with a characteristic relaxation time T_1. In contrast to the spin-spin relaxation it is possible to assign a unique value to T_1 provided only that the spin-spin interactions can maintain thermal equilibrium among the spins during the thermal relaxation process. This is the so-called spin-temperature approximation. Consider a spin system whose total average energy

$$\overline{E} = \sum_i p_i E_i \tag{11}$$

can be related at any time to a unique β_S. For convenience, we define a zero of energy such that $\mathrm{Tr}(E_i) = 0$, where Tr denotes a trace over the spin eigenstates. The time dependence of β_S can be derived from

$$\frac{d\beta_S}{dt} = \frac{d\overline{E}}{dt} \bigg/ \frac{d\overline{E}}{d\beta_S} . \tag{12}$$

We assume that the p_i's obey linear rate equations of the form

$$\frac{dp_i}{dt} = \sum_j (p_j W_{ji} - p_i W_{ij}) . \tag{13}$$

The transition probabilities W_{ij} and W_{ji} are related by the principle of detailed balance according to which each term in the sum in Eq. (13) vanishes when $dp_i/dt = 0$ (i.e., when $\beta_S = \beta$). Hence

$$W_{ij} = W_{ji} \exp\left[-\beta(E_j - E_i)\right] . \tag{14}$$

Combining Eqs. (11), (13), and (14) with Eq. (12) yields in the high-temperature approximation

$$\frac{d\beta_s}{dt} = \frac{(\beta - \beta_s)}{T_1} ,$$ (15)

where

$$\frac{1}{T_1} = \frac{1}{2} \sum_{ij} (E_i - E_j)^2 W_{ij} \Big/ \sum_i E_i^2 .$$ (16)

The transition probability in Eq. (16) can be calculated using time-dependent perturbation theory since the asymmetry between W_{ij} and W_{ji} in Eq. (14) is small in the present case and can therefore be ignored in Eq. (16). Hence

$$W_{ij} = \frac{2\pi}{\hbar} \sum_{ab} |\langle bj|\mathcal{H}_1|ia\rangle|^2 \delta(\Delta E) ,$$ (17)

where a, b are the lattice quantum numbers and $\mathcal{H}_1$ is the Hamiltonian of the perturbation. It is often more convenient to calculate the transition probability from the correlation function $G_{ij}(\tau)$ of $\mathcal{H}_1$, in which case

$$W_{ij} = \frac{1}{\hbar^2} \int_{-\infty}^{+\infty} d\tau\, G_{ij}(\tau) \exp[-(i/\hbar)(E_i - E_j)\tau] .$$ (18)

For a stationary perturbation

$$G_{ij}(\tau) \equiv \langle \mathcal{H}_1(\tau)\mathcal{H}_1(0)\rangle = \overline{\langle i|\mathcal{H}_1(\tau)|j\rangle \langle j|\mathcal{H}_1(0)|i\rangle} ,$$ (19)

where the bar denotes an ensemble average. The correlation function $G_{ij}(\tau)$ is also related to the spectral density function $J_{ij}(\omega)$ as

$$G_{ij}(\tau) = \frac{1}{2\pi} \int_{-\infty}^{+\infty} d\omega\, J_{ij}(\omega) \exp(i\omega\tau) .$$ (20)

In most cases it is possible to carry out the summations over the nuclear spin states in Eq. (16). For example, if the most important contribution to E_i arises from the Zeeman interaction and if $\mathcal{H}_1$ is a linear function of I one obtains for any spin

$$1/T_1 = 2W ,$$ (21)

where W is evaluated for $I = \frac{1}{2}$. In other words, the relaxation rate is independent of I. It must be emphasized again, however, that Eqs. (16) and (21) are only valid if the spin system can be described by a spin temperature.

C. Nuclear Susceptibilities

The relaxation forces which were introduced in the preceding section to describe the interactions between the nuclear moments and their surroundings have a profound effect on the response of the spin system to an external time-dependent magnetic perturbation. Since there is now a mechanism whereby thermodynamic equilibrium can be established within the spin system, a net absorption of energy can take place. We assume that the response of the system to a transverse field

$$H(t) = H^X \exp(i\omega t) \tag{22}$$

can be described by a complex susceptibility

$$\chi = \chi' - i\chi'' . \tag{23}$$

The observable magnetization produced by the perturbation is given by the real part of the complex magnetization $[\chi] \cdot H(t)$. Hence

$$M^X = H^X(\chi' \cos \omega t + \chi'' \sin \omega t) . \tag{24}$$

The establishment of a transverse magnetization corresponds to an average power dissipation

$$\overline{P} = \frac{\omega}{2\pi} \int_{t=0}^{t = 2\pi/\omega} H(t) \cdot dM = \tfrac{1}{2}\omega\chi'' (H^X)^2 . \tag{25}$$

We note that $H^X = 2H_1$ is defined as the peak value of a linearly polarized field while H_1 is the magnitude of the two counterrotating fields into which $H(t)$ can be decomposed.

We can use perturbation theory to calculate χ''. The power absorbed by the system per unit volume is

$$\overline{P} = \hbar\omega V^{-1} \sum_{ij} (p_i - p_j) W_{ij} ,$$

$$= \frac{\pi\omega(\gamma_n \hbar H^X)^2}{2V} \sum_{ij} (p_i - p_j) |\langle j|I^X|i\rangle|^2$$

$$\times \delta (E_i - E_j + \hbar\omega) . \tag{26}$$

Since $|E_i - E_j| << \beta_s^{-1}$ in most experiments we have

$$(p_i - p_j) = \hbar\omega\beta_s Z^{-1} \exp(-\beta_s E_j) . \tag{27}$$

Substituting Eq. (27) into Eq. (26) and comparing the resulting expression with Eq. (25) yields

$$\chi'' = \pi \hbar \omega \beta_S \, f(\omega) \; , \tag{28}$$

where $f(\omega)$ is the shape function

$$f(\omega) = (\gamma_n \hbar)^2 \, (ZV)^{-1}$$
$$\sum_{ij} |\langle j | I^x | i \rangle|^2 \, \exp(-\beta_S E_j) \, \delta(E_i - E_j + \hbar \omega) \, . \tag{29}$$

In the high temperature approximation the exponential can be replaced by unity. The real part of χ can be obtained from Eq. (28) by means of the Kramers-Kronig relation

$$\chi'(\omega) = \frac{1}{\pi} \mathcal{P} \int_{-\infty}^{+\infty} \frac{d\omega' \, \chi''(\omega')}{\omega' - \omega} \; , \tag{30}$$

where $\mathcal{P}$ means the principal part.

The shape function Eq. (29) leads to the selection rule $\Delta m = \pm 1$. Unfortunately, it is usually impossible to calculate $f(\omega)$ from Eq. (29) since the eigenstates of an interacting many-spin system are not known exactly. However, the moments

$$\langle \omega^n \rangle \equiv \int_0^\infty d\omega \, \omega^n \, f(\omega) \Big/ \int_0^\infty d\omega \, f(\omega)$$

$$\langle \Delta \omega^n \rangle = \int_0^\infty d\omega \, (\omega - \langle \omega \rangle)^n \, f(\omega) \Big/ \int_0^\infty d\omega \, f(\omega) \tag{31}$$

can be evaluated since they involve only traces and are thus independent of the choice of representation. Consider the trivial example

$$\int_0^\infty d\omega \, f(\omega) = \frac{(\gamma_n \hbar)^2}{2ZV} \int_{-\infty}^{+\infty} d\omega \sum_{ij} |\langle j | I^x | i \rangle|^2$$

$$\times \exp(-\beta_S E_j) \, \delta(E_i - E_j + \hbar \omega) \, . \tag{32}$$

In the high-temperature approximation we obtain

$$\int_0^\infty d\omega \, f(\omega) = \frac{(\gamma_n \hbar)^2}{2\hbar(2I+1)NV} \, \mathrm{Tr}(I^x)^2$$

$$= \frac{N\gamma_n^2 \hbar}{6V} \, I(I+1) \, . \tag{33}$$

A phenomenological solution to the problem of the NMR response of a many-spin system is provided by the Bloch formulation. In this formulation the equation of motion of the macroscopic magnetization $(dM/dt = \gamma_n M \times H)$ is modified by the addition of damping terms of the form $-M^x/T_2$, $-M^y/T_2$, and $(M_0-M^z)/T_1$, where M_0 is the thermal equilibrium magnitude of M. The solution to the resulting equations is given by the Bloch susceptibilities

$$\chi'(\omega) = \tfrac{1}{2} \chi_0 \omega_0 T_2 \frac{T_2(\omega_0 - \omega)}{1 + T_2^2(\omega_0 - \omega)^2 + \gamma_n^2 H_1^2 T_1 T_2} \quad , \qquad (34)$$

$$\chi''(\omega) = \tfrac{1}{2} \chi_0 \omega_0 T_2 \frac{1}{1 + T_2^2(\omega_0 - \omega)^2 + \gamma_n^2 H_1^2 T_1 T_2} \quad , \qquad (35)$$

where χ_0 is the static nuclear susceptibility and $\omega_0 = \gamma_n H_0$ is the resonance frequency. These equations have only qualitative significance for solids since the assumption of an exponential decay for the transverse magnetization is only valid in special cases. The deviations from the predicted behavior become especially pronounced in solids at very high power levels. In particular, χ' does not saturate as quickly as predicted (Redfield, 1955). Despite their shortcomings the Bloch equations are quite useful since they give an indication of the general shape of the NMR absorption (χ'') and dispersion (χ') curves and predict correctly the onset of saturation $(\gamma_n^2 H_1^2 T_1 T_2 \approx 1)$.

The absorption rate calculated in Eqs. (25) and (26) is time independent. This differs from the conclusion reached for a system of non-interacting spins. In order to examine this difference we use the following intuitive argument. We suppose that spin-spin interactions produce a resonance width $\Delta\omega \approx T_2^{-1}$. If a perturbation of magnitude $\langle \mathcal{H}_1 \rangle$ is applied, an appreciable population change will have occurred after a time $\tau \approx \hbar/\langle \mathcal{H}_1 \rangle$. Thus

$$\frac{T_2}{\tau} \approx \frac{\langle \mathcal{H}_1 \rangle}{\hbar \Delta\omega} \quad . \qquad (36)$$

If $\langle \mathcal{H}_1 \rangle \ll \hbar \Delta\omega$, then $T_2 < \tau$ and internal equilibrium will be maintained resulting in a time dependent rate process. On the other hand when $T_2 > \tau$ the system responds to the perturbation like a system of free spins.

D. Detection Methods

The domain of nuclear magnetic resonance spectroscopy encompasses an extremely broad frequency spectrum. Although experiments in typical laboratory electromagnets usually fall in the range 10^6 - 10^8 Hz, important experiments have been carried out at frequencies as low as ~10^3 Hz (e. g., ^{1}H and ^{3}He in the earth's magnetic field) and as high as ~10^9 - 10^{10} Hz (e. g., ^{159}Tb, ^{161}Dy, ^{163}Dy in the hyperfine fields of the corresponding metals). Linewidths as small as $\Delta\omega/\omega \approx 10^{-8}$ are common in liquids, whereas resonances with relative widths approaching unity have been observed in some ferromagnetic alloys. The impressive versatility of the NMR method which is indicated by these examples can only be achieved, of course, by the correct application of a number of instrumental techniques. Although the observation of NMR results in every case from the coupling of the nuclear magnetization to an inductive circuit element (either lumped or distributed) the manner in which this interaction is detected varies greatly. In this section we shall discuss very briefly a few of the more general methods. For convenience we distinguish between steady state and transient methods. The former are most useful for studying line shapes, positions, and intensities. The latter are particularly useful for the investigation of relaxation times.

1. Steady-State Methods ($T_2 < \tau$)

The simplest steady-state detector is the marginal oscillator. This device is essentially a Q-meter whose oscillator tank coil (or cavity) contains the sample. The nuclear resonance produces a decrease in the Q of the coil and hence a reduction in the level of oscillation. The circuit therefore measures χ''. This type of detector is usually operated as a variable frequency spectrometer.

Another type of steady-state spectrometer makes use of a balanced bridge circuit in which one arm contains a resonant inductor surrounding the sample, while the other arm contains a dummy resonant circuit. The bridge is excited by an external oscillator. The bridge is balanced in order to protect the receiver from overload and to reduce the oscillator noise at the receiver input. Balance is usually achieved by introducing a 180° phase shift in one of the arms. By unbalancing the bridge very slightly, either χ' or χ'' can be detected when sweeping through resonance, depending on whether the residual unbalance is produced by a small phase or amplitude difference, respectively, between the two arms.

The crossed-coil induction spectrometer is closely related to the bridge circuit. As the name suggests, the induction spectrometer utilizes separate, orthogonal transmitter and receiver coils.

The transmitter coil excites the nuclear resonance. The resulting precessing magnetization is detected by the receiver coil. Isolation is achieved by geometrical balancing of the coils. Again, either χ' or χ'' can be selected by adjusting the phase of a small leakage component.

Since the signal level at the receiver input is often of the order of microvolts or less it is usually necessary to employ narrow-band detection schemes in order to achieve useful signal-noise levels. It has therefore become almost standard practice to field- or frequency-modulate the resonant absorption in the audio frequency range and to employ narrow band amplification and synchronous detection of the modulation products. In this way spectrometer bandwidths of less than one Hz are easily attained. Further increases in sensitivity are possible by using time-averaging techniques in which the results of repetitive sweeps through the region of interest are added (and thus averaged) by a multichannel analyzer.

2. Transient Methods ($T_2 > \tau$)

We have seen that a spin system exhibits free-spin behavior for a time T_2 provided that H_1 exceeds the linewidth. For example the magnetization $M^z = M_0$ can be tipped into the transverse plane by an rf pulse of frequency ω_0 and duration $t(<T_2)$ if $\gamma_n H_1 t = \pi/2$. Following the $\pi/2$ pulse the precessing magnetization, which can be detected by means of a receiver coil, decays in a time $\sim T_2$. The resulting signal envelope is called the free-precession decay and is the Fourier transform of the steady-state line shape. The longitudinal magnetization recovers in a time T_1 following a $\pi/2$ pulse. A reliable method for measuring T_1 consists of saturating the resonance with a series of short pulses and utilizing the free-precession amplitude following a subsequent $\pi/2$ pulse to measure the magnitude of M^z at different times following the saturating "comb." This method has the advantage that the system can always be prepared in an initial state of definite spin temperature ($T_S = \infty$). The recovery of M^z then follows a time dependence

$$M^z(t) = M_0[1 - \exp(-t/T_1)] , \tag{36}$$

where T_1 is given by Eq. (21).

The above example is only intended to illustrate the general usefulness of transient measurements. Many transient experiments involve far more complex pulse sequences. However, a discussion of these techniques falls outside the scope of this review.

E. Hyperfine Interactions

   1. Magnetic Dipole

        We now turn our attention to the hyperfine coupling be-
tween the nuclear magnetic dipole moment and the electronic spin
and orbital magnetic moments. These interactions may be represented by a magnetic hyperfine field H_{hfs}. The total magnetic
interaction is then given by the dipole Hamiltonian

$$\mathcal{H}_D = -\gamma_n \hbar \mathbf{I} \cdot (\mathbf{H}_0 + \mathbf{H}_{hfs}) \ . \tag{37}$$

The important contributions to H_{hfs} are the following:

   (i) Fermi contact: $(8/3)\, \pi \gamma_e \hbar \, |\psi(0)|^2 \, \mathbf{s}$;

   (ii) Dipolar: $\gamma_e \hbar \, [r^2 \, \mathbf{s} - 3(\mathbf{r} \cdot \mathbf{s})\mathbf{r}]\, r^{-5}$;

   (iii) Orbital: $-\gamma_e \hbar\, r^{-3}\, \boldsymbol{\ell}$,

where γ_e is the electronic gyromagnetic ratio, $|\psi(0)|^2$ is the spin
density at the nucleus, and $\mathbf{s}$ and $\boldsymbol{\ell}$ are the electronic spin and
orbital angular momentum operators, respectively.

   2. Electric Quadrupole

        Nuclei with spin greater than $1/2$ possess electric quad-
rupole moments and therefore interact with electric field gradients
produced by the surrounding charge distribution. The resulting
changes in the NMR spectrum are often quite large and can provide
valuable information in favorable cases about the electronic structure of solids.

        The quadrupole Hamiltonian may be written

$$\mathcal{H}_Q = [Q] \cdot [\nabla\epsilon] \ , \tag{38}$$

where $[Q]$ is the nuclear electric quadrupole tensor and $[\nabla\epsilon]$ is
the electric field gradient tensor.

        The Cartesian elements of $-[\nabla\epsilon]$ are

$$-[\nabla\epsilon]^{ij} = \frac{\partial^2 V}{\partial x^i \partial x^j} \ ; \quad (x^i, x^j = x, y, z) \ , \tag{39}$$

where V is the potential at the nucleus due to the external charge
distribution. We let $|V^{XX}| < |V^{YY}| < |V^{ZZ}|$, where X, Y, Z are
the principal axes of $[\nabla\epsilon]$. Defining

$$eq = V^{ZZ} \ , \tag{40}$$

$$\eta = (V^{XX} - V^{YY})/V^{ZZ} \ , \tag{41}$$

where η is the asymmetry parameter, we find

$$\mathcal{H}_Q = \frac{e^2 qQ}{4I(2I-1)} \left\{ 3(I^Z)^2 - I(I+1) + \frac{\eta}{2} \left[(I^+)^2 + (I^-)^2 \right] \right\} , \quad (42)$$

where Q is the nuclear electric quadrupole moment. According to Laplace's equation

$$\sum_i V^{ii} = 0 , \quad (43)$$

and therefore $eq = \eta = 0$ for nuclei occupying positions of cubic symmetry in a crystal. The static effects of $[\nabla \epsilon]$ also vanish in fluids because of the rapid reorientation of the charge distribution.

3. Combined Electric and Magnetic Interactions

In many practical situations both magnetic and electric hyperfine effects are encountered, i.e., $\mathcal{H} = \mathcal{H}_D + \mathcal{H}_Q$. The eigenvalues of $\mathcal{H}$ are easily found if $\eta = 0$ and $(\mathbf{H}_0 + \mathbf{H}_{hfs}) \| \mathbf{Z}$. In that case $\mathcal{H}$ and I^Z commute and hence,

$$E(m) = -\gamma_n \hbar H m + \frac{3e^2 qQ}{4I(2I-1)} m^2 . \quad (44)$$

The selection rules for I^X are the same as in the pure dipole case. If the dipole term is larger than the quadrupole term the spectrum consists of $2I$ equally spaced lines, arranged symmetrically about the dipole frequency $\omega_0 = \gamma_n |H_0 + H_{hfs}|$. If the quadrupole term dominates, the spectrum for integral spin consists of I lines, each split into a doublet by the dipole interaction; for half integral spin there are $I-\frac{1}{2}$ doublets as well as a line at ω_0 corresponding to the $\frac{1}{2} \leftrightarrow -\frac{1}{2}$ transition.

For non-zero η and general orientation of magnetic and electric hyperfine tensors the eigenvalue problem becomes much more complicated and must usually be treated by perturbation or numerical techniques. Furthermore, additional transitions may become observable because of the mixing of $\Delta m = \pm 1$ levels by the $I^{\pm}$ terms in $\mathcal{H}_Q$.

III. NMR in Non-Metallic Magnetic Solids

A. General Considerations

The Hamiltonian of a nuclear spin $\mathbf{I}$ and an electronic spin $\mathbf{S}$ in a magnetic field $\mathbf{H}_0$ can be written *

*See also B. Bleaney, Chap. 1.

$$\mathcal{K} = -\gamma_n \hbar \mathbf{I} \cdot \mathbf{H}_0 - \gamma_e \hbar \mathbf{S} \cdot \mathbf{H}_0 + \mathbf{I} \cdot [A] \cdot \mathbf{S} \quad , \tag{45}$$

where $[A]$ is a symmetric second rank tensor. In addition one must often consider orbital hyperfine and electric quadrupole interactions in complex systems. The strength of typical electron-nuclear interactions $(A/\gamma_n\hbar)$ varies between 10^3 and 10^7 Oe. This range may be subdivided since one can usually distinguish three types of lattice sites in magnetic crystals:

(1) non-magnetic ions (dipolar fields $\sim 10^3 - 10^4$ Oe)

(2) partially magnetic ions (transferred hyperfine fields $\sim 10^4 - 10^5$ Oe)

(3) magnetic ions (direct hyperfine fields $\sim 10^5 - 10^7$ Oe).

Examples of these three cases are ^{1}H in $CuCl_2 \cdot 2H_2O$ (Poulis et al., 1958), ^{19}F in MnF_2 (Shulman and Jaccarino, 1957) and ^{55}Mn in MnF_2 (Jones and Jefferts, 1964).

If $[A]$ is isotropic, Eq. (45) simplifies to

$$\mathcal{K} = \mathcal{K}_0 + \tfrac{1}{2} A \, (I^+ S^- + I^- S^+), \tag{46}$$

$$\mathcal{K}_0 = -H_0 \, (\gamma_n \hbar I^Z + \gamma_e \hbar S^Z) + A I^Z S^Z \quad . \tag{47}$$

The eigenstates of $\mathcal{K}_0$ are simply $|m_S m_I \rangle$ since I^Z and S^Z commute with $\mathcal{K}_0$. For $I = \tfrac{1}{2}$, $S = \tfrac{1}{2}$ the second order correction due to the transverse hyperfine terms in Eq. (45) yields states

$$|++\rangle = |\tfrac{1}{2}, \tfrac{1}{2}\rangle$$
$$|+-\rangle = a|\tfrac{1}{2}, -\tfrac{1}{2}\rangle + b|-\tfrac{1}{2}, \tfrac{1}{2}\rangle$$
$$|-+\rangle = -b|\tfrac{1}{2}, -\tfrac{1}{2}\rangle + a|-\tfrac{1}{2}, \tfrac{1}{2}\rangle$$
$$|--\rangle = |-\tfrac{1}{2}, -\tfrac{1}{2}\rangle \quad ,$$

where $b = A(A - 2\gamma_e\hbar H_0)^{-1} \approx -A(2\gamma_e\hbar H_0)^{-1}$ and $a = (1-b^2)^{\frac{1}{2}} \approx 1$. For sufficiently small $A/\gamma_e\hbar H_0$ a perturbation

$$\mathcal{K}_1(t) = (\gamma_e \hbar S^+ + \gamma_n \hbar I^+) H_0^- \cos \omega t \tag{48}$$

induces transitions whose frequencies can be calculated from the zeroth-order energies.

$$|\pm \pm\rangle \leftrightarrow |\pm \mp\rangle \; : \; \hbar\omega_n = |\gamma_n\hbar H_0 \mp \tfrac{1}{2}A|$$
$$|\pm \pm\rangle \leftrightarrow |\mp \pm\rangle : \; \hbar\omega_e = |\gamma_e\hbar H_0 \mp \tfrac{1}{2}A| \quad .$$

The nuclear transition probabilities, on the other hand, are strongly enhanced by the transverse terms provided that $|A/\gamma_n \hbar H_o| > 1$, since

$$W(\omega_n) \propto (\gamma_n \hbar a)^2 + (\gamma_e \hbar b)^2 = [\tfrac{1}{4}A^2 + (\gamma_n \hbar)^2 H_o^2] H_o^{-2}. \quad (49)$$

The spin Hamiltonian Eq. (45) is not very useful for predicting NMR frequencies in solids since it ignores interactions which lead to spin relaxation effects. In practice the correlation time τ_c of the electron spin fluctuations is shorter than the nuclear Larmor period in the electronic field (i.e., $\tau_c^{-1} > |AS/h|$). The nuclear magnetization therefore responds only to an average electronic field, which in turn is proportional to the average value of the spin $\langle S \rangle$. The effective nuclear Hamiltonian is therefore

$$\mathcal{H}_n = -\gamma_n \hbar \, \mathbf{I} \cdot \mathbf{H}_o + \mathbf{I} \cdot [A] \cdot \langle \mathbf{S} \rangle. \quad (50)$$

For an isotropic $[A]$ the resonance frequency becomes $\omega_o = |\gamma_n H_o - (A/\hbar)\langle S^z \rangle|$, which is often much smaller than ω_n. The study of NMR in magnetic systems consequently affords an opportunity to measure $[A] \cdot \langle \mathbf{S} \rangle$. It should also be noted that the enhancement of the transition probability as predicted by Eq. (49) becomes negligible when $\langle \mathbf{S} \rangle \ll S$, i.e., when $\omega_o \ll \omega_n$.

B. Paramagnetic State

In the paramagnetic state $\langle \mathbf{S} \rangle / S \ll 1$ for values of $\gamma_e \hbar H_o / k_B T$ encountered in most experiments. The hyperfine interaction therefore manifests itself in a field-induced shift of the NMR frequency relative to the undisplaced frequency $\gamma_n H$. For S-state ions $\langle S^z \rangle$ is proportional to χH_o, where χ is the magnetic susceptibility (corrected for diamagnetic contributions). Hence if $[A]$ is isotropic, a plot of the frequency

$$\omega_o = \gamma_n H_o [1 - (A\chi/\gamma_e \gamma_n \hbar^2)], \quad (51)$$

as a function of the measured susceptibility (with temperature the implicit variable) leads to a determination of A. The variation of ω_o with χ yields A even in the presence of field-induced orbital paramagnetism, provided that the orbital contribution to the susceptibility can be treated as a temperature independent Van Vleck term.

Since $\langle \mathbf{S} \rangle$ is usually quite small compared to the instantaneous magnitude of $\mathbf{S}$, the amplitude of the spin fluctuations $\delta \mathbf{S} = \mathbf{S} - \langle \mathbf{S} \rangle$ is very large. The direct observation of NMR is only feasible, however, if the field seen by the nuclear spins has a sufficiently sharp value. Thus it is necessary that the spectral intensity $J(\omega)$ of the spin fluctuations at the nuclear frequency ω_0 be sufficiently small. We note that the highest frequency for which $J(\omega)$ has an appreciable magnitude is given by the cut-off frequency $\omega_c \approx \tau_c^{-1}$. According to Eq. (20), however, the integrated intensity is independent of τ_c since

$$\int_{-\infty}^{+\infty} d\omega \, J(\omega) = G(0) = \langle (\delta S)^2 \rangle \approx \tfrac{1}{3} S(S+1) \quad . \tag{52}$$

It follows that $J(\omega_0)$ becomes smaller as τ_c decreases because the fluctuations are distributed over a wider frequency range. If $|A| \gtrsim |\gamma_n \hbar H_0|$, as is usually the case for hyperfine interactions, we therefore require that $\tau_c^{-1} \gg \omega_n$.

In dilute paramagnetic crystals τ_c is usually not sufficiently short to satisfy the above requirement. In concentrated crystals, on the other hand, exchange interactions between electron spins

$$\mathcal{H}_E = - \sum_{ij} J_{ij} \, \mathbf{S}_i \cdot \mathbf{S}_j \tag{53}$$

may greatly decrease the electronic correlation time and thus narrow the nuclear resonance. For nearest neighbor interactions (J) we find an exchange frequency

$$\omega_E = [\, 8J^2 \, zS(S+1)/3\hbar^2 \,]^{\frac{1}{2}} \quad , \tag{54}$$

where z denotes the number of nearest neighbors which are exchange coupled to a given spin. Crudely speaking the exchange frequency corresponds to the rate at which the electron spins are reversed by the flip-flop terms ($S^+ S^-$) in Eq. (53). At sufficiently high temperatures the exchange interaction yields a Gaussian distribution of fluctuations, centered at $\omega = 0$. The corresponding spin auto-correlation functions are

$$\langle \{ \delta S^i(\tau) \, \delta S^i(0) \} \rangle = \tfrac{1}{3} S(S+1) \, \exp(-\tfrac{1}{2} \omega_E^2 \tau^2) \quad , \tag{55}$$

where $i = x$, y, z and the curly brackets denote a symmetrized product $\{AB\} = \tfrac{1}{2}(AB + BA)$. We can use Eq. (55) to define a correlation time $\tau_c = \sqrt{2} \, \omega_E^{-1}$. In practice τ_c can be extremely short (e.g., $\sim 10^{-13}$ sec). Combining Eqs. (18), (19) and (21) we find a suitable expression for the nuclear spin-lattice relaxation rate

$$T_1^{-1} = (A/\hbar)^2 \int_0^\infty d\tau \, \langle \{ \delta S^+(\tau) \, \delta S^-(0) \} \rangle \quad , \tag{56}$$

where use has been made of the relation $\tau_c \ll \omega_0$ in order to eliminate the exponential in Eq. (18). Because of the rapid reorientation of **S** the transverse nuclear magnetization also decays exponentially, and the absorption is therefore characterized by a Lorentzian lineshape. The rate constant is given by the sum of secular $(T_2')^{-1}$ and nonsecular $(T_1')^{-1} = (2T_1)^{-1}$ contributions;

$$T_2^{-1} = (T_2')^{-1} + (2T_1)^{-1} . \tag{57}$$

The secular term is identical to Eq. (56) except for the substitution of δS^Z for δS^+ and δS^-. Finally we obtain

$$T_1^{-1} = T_2^{-1} = (2\pi)^{\frac{1}{2}} (A/\hbar)^2 (3\omega_E)^{-1} S(S+1) , \tag{58}$$

which shows that the linewidth is proportional to the square of the hyperfine coupling constant and inversely proportional to the exchange frequency. The equality of T_1 and T_2 only holds, of course, if $[A]$ is isotropic.

In summary, we have shown that direct observability of the nuclear resonance requires that $|(AS/\hbar)| \tau_c \ll 1$ and $(AS/\hbar)^2 \tau_c \ll |\gamma_n H_0|$. It is interesting to note that the hyperfine-induced shift of the nuclear resonance is proportional to A whereas the linewidth is proportional to A^2. For this reason the accuracy with which the hyperfine constant can be determined by NMR measurements in the paramagnetic state is proportional to A^{-1}.

In the following we discuss a few illustrative examples of NMR experiments on paramagnetic crystals.

i. Magnetic Ions: Because of the requirement of a high exchange frequency, NMR experiments involving magnetic ions have only been successful for substances with relatively high magnetic ordering temperatures. To date the NMR has been observed for ^{59}Co in CoO and $KCoF_3$ (Shulman, 1959), and for ^{55}Mn in MnO, MnS and MnSe (Jones, 1966a). The observed linewidths are in qualitative agreement with predictions based on Eq. (58). For example, in CoO the observed half width $T_2^{-1} = 3 \times 10^6$ sec^{-1} compares with a calulcated value of 0.86×10^6 sec^{-1} based on $\omega_E = 1.5 \times 10^{13}$ sec^{-1}.

ii. Partially Magnetic Ions: Since transferred hyperfine fields are generally smaller than the direct hyperfine fields, the requirement of a high exchange frequency is often greatly relaxed. A large body of experimental results has therefore accumulated which includes many cases involving non-cubic site symmetries. As an example of the complications which are introduced by a non-isotropic hyperfine tensor we consider briefly the ^{19}F NMR in

K_2NaCrF_6, $KMnF_3$, and $KNiF_3$ (Shulman and Knox, 1960). Each fluorine ion has two nearest-neighbor paramagnetic ions situated along a four-fold symmetry axis (e.g., Cr-F-Cr) which we shall denote as the Z axis. The paramagnetic ions have octahedral site symmetry. The elements of the interaction tensor [A] were determined by measuring the NMR shifts in single crystals as a function of external field orientation and relating them to the experimental magnetic susceptibilities. The dipole field at the fluorine sites in these compounds due to the magnetic cations is comparable in magnitude to the transferred hyperfine field. The dipole-field tensor can be computed by carrying out the necessary lattice sums over the magnetic sites

$$A^{ij}_{dip} = \gamma_n \gamma_e \hbar^2 \sum (3r^i r^j - r^2 \delta_{ij}) r^{-5}; \quad i, j = x, y, z. \quad (59)$$

The difference between [A] and $[A_{dip}]$ represents the transferred hyperfine tensor $[A_{hfs}]$ which has axial symmetry about the Z axis and which can be decomposed into isotropic and anisotropic contributions.* The isotropic part arises from contact interactions with spin-polarized F^- s orbitals. The anisotropic part arises from dipolar interactions with spin-polarized F^- p(x), p(y) and p(z) orbitals. The principal elements of $[A_{hfs}]$ can be written

$$A^{ii}_{hfs} = A_s + \sum_{j=x,y,z} A_{p(j)} (3 \cos^2 \theta_{ij} - 1). \quad (60)$$

The individual contributions of the three p orbitals cannot be determined, of course, because the dipole tensor is traceless and consequently has only two independent principal elements. Thus, only the contact interaction A_s and pairwise differences between the three p-dipolar hyperfine interactions $A_{p(i)}$ can be deduced from the NMR measurements. The four-fold rotation symmetry about the Z axis requires that $A_{p(X)} - A_{p(Y)} = 0$. We can therefore write

$$A^{ii}_{hfs} = A_s + (A_\sigma - A_\pi)(3 \cos^2 \theta_{iZ} - 1), \quad (61)$$

where σ and π denote the p(z) and p(x), p(y) interactions, respectively. It follows that

$$A_s = \tfrac{1}{3} \sum_i A^{ii}_{hfs}, \quad A_\sigma - A_\pi = \tfrac{1}{3}(A^{zz}_{hfs} - A^{xx}_{hfs}) \quad . \quad (62)$$

*
$See\ R.E.\ Watson\ and\ A.J.\ Freeman,\ Chap.\ 2.$

The coupling constants can be used to estimate the effective fractions (f_s and $f_\sigma - f_\pi$) of unpaired spins in the fluorine s and p orbitals by comparing the observed values with the corresponding free ion 2s and 2p hyperfine constants. The fluorine σ and π orbitals can only be admixed into the cation e_g and t_{2g} orbitals, respectively. One expects therefore a strong correlation between the sign of $f_\sigma - f_\pi$ and the occupation numbers of the 3d orbitals. This is indeed the case, as is shown in Table I which summarizes the experimental results.

Table I: Transferred hyperfine constants (in 10^{-4} cm^{-1}) and fractional unpairing coefficients for ^{19}F in K_2NaCrF_6, $KMnF_3$, and $KNiF_3$.

	Cr^{3+}	Mn^{2+}	Ni^{2+}
t_{2g}	3	3	6
e_g	0	2	2
A_s	-1.1 ± 0.5	16.3 ± 0.5	39 ± 4
$A_\sigma - A_\pi$	-7.2 ± 1.2	0.2 ± 0.1	10.9 ± 1.4
f_s	~0%	0.52 ± 0.02%	0.50 ± 0.05%
$f_\sigma - f_\pi$	-4.9 ± 0.8%	0.2 ± 0.1%	4.9 ± 0.6%

iii. Non-Magnetic Ions: In this case the shift of the resonance is due to the classical dipolar field, which is usually small since the separation between the non-magnetic and magnetic ions is generally large.

C. Ordered Magnetic State

1. Resonance Conditions

The magnetic ordering temperature is marked by the appearance of long-range order in the electronic spin system. As a consequence, the time averaged magnitude of $\mathbf{S}$ at a given magnetic lattice site becomes non-zero even in the absence of an applied magnetic field. Since $\langle \mathbf{S} \rangle$ approaches S at low temperatures, the observed hyperfine effects may become extremely large. In the absence of quadrupolar interactions the nuclear Hamiltonian may be written

$$\mathcal{H}_n = - \gamma_n \hbar \mathbf{I} \cdot \mathbf{H}_{eff} , \qquad (63)$$

where

$$|H_{eff}| = \left[\sum_{i=x,y,z} \left(H_o^i + H_{dip}^i + H_{hfs}^i \right)^2 \right]^{\frac{1}{2}} . \qquad (64)$$

The dipolar and hyperfine fields in Eq. (64) are proportional to the thermal average values of the electronic magnetic moments. The NMR frequency therefore gives a measure of the average magnetization at specific lattice sites. For this reason, the nuclear resonance technique provides a powerful method for studying the relationships between the sublattice magnetization and variables such as temperature, pressure and magnetic field strength. This is particularly useful in antiferromagnetic systems since the macroscopic magnetization in that case vanishes in zero external field. In the interpretation of experiments of this type, care must be taken, of course, to take account of possible changes in the hyperfine coupling constants.

2. Intensity Enhancement

The detection of NMR in the ordered state is often facilitated by large enhancements of the transverse driving field which are associated with the large magnitude of $\langle S \rangle$. The origin of the enhancement is identical to that which gives rise to the large nuclear transition probabilities in free paramagnetic ions (Eq. (49)). In both cases the nuclear resonance is driven indirectly via the nuclear-electron hyperfine coupling. The enhancement factor is directly proportional to the angle through which $\langle S \rangle$ (and thus H_{hfs}) is turned by a given transverse field H^x. In magnetic crystals the magnitude of the enhancement is consequently strongly influenced by the detailed properties of the exchange-coupled electron spin system.

a. Ferromagnets: We consider the excitation of the nuclear resonance in a single domain particle in which the nuclear spins are quantized along a z axis which is defined by the direction of the electronic magnetization, M. We assume that this direction coincides with the orientation of a magnetizing field H which is composed of an effective anisotropy field H_A and an external field H_o. We also assume that the electronic resonance frequency lies far above the nuclear frequency. A weak transverse field H^x then produces an angular displacement of H_{hfs}

$$\theta \equiv \tan^{-1}(H^x/H) \approx H^x/H \qquad . \qquad (65)$$

The resulting transverse hyperfine field H_{hfs}^x, and the total effective driving field $H^x(\text{eff})$ are given by

$$H^x_{hfs} = H_{hfs} \sin \theta \approx H^x H_{hfs}/H \quad , \tag{66}$$

$$H^x(\text{eff}) = H^x + H^x_{hfs} = H^x(1 + \eta) \quad . \tag{67}$$

The driving field is therefore enhanced by a factor η which is directly proportional to the hyperfine field and inversely proportional to the field which provides the restoring torque. Since $H_{hfs} \gg H_A$ in many cases, η can be extremely large (e.g., ~ 200 in Co metal) (Gossard and Portis, 1959).

The steady-state detection of NMR in magnetic materials is usually accomplished with marginal oscillators. The signal intensity is proportional to the power absorption which in turn, according to Eq. (25), should be proportional to $\chi''[H^x(\text{eff})]^2$ and thus to $\chi'' \eta^2$. The spin-lattice relaxation times T_1 are often very short in magnetic crystals. In such cases it is possible to maintain reasonable values of χ'' even in the presence of large enhancements, as can be seen by inspecting Eq. (35). Actually, the power absorption at resonance is not simply proportional to χ'' in the present case, because of the hyperfine coupling between electronic and nuclear magnetizations. Following Eq. (25), we find an absorption rate for the combined electron-nuclear system

$$\overline{P} = \tfrac{1}{2} \text{Re} \{i\omega(H_n m^x + H_e M^x)\} \quad , \tag{68}$$

where H_n and H_e are the effective transverse fields seen by the transverse components of the nuclear and electronic magnetizations m^x and M^x, respectively. The effective fields are

$$H_n = H^x(1 + \eta) = H^x + H_{hfs}(M^x/|M|) \quad , \tag{69}$$

$$H_e = H^x + H_{hfs}(m^x/|M|) \approx H^x \quad . \tag{70}$$

The magnetizations are related to the appropriate complex transverse susceptibilities χ_n and χ_e.

$$m^x = \chi_n H_n \quad , \qquad M^x = \chi_e H_e \quad . \tag{71}$$

Combining Eqs. (68-71) we find

$$\overline{P} = \tfrac{1}{2} \omega \, (H^X)^2 \left\{ \chi_n'' + \chi_e'' + \left(\frac{H_{hfs}}{|M|}\right)^2 \right.$$
$$\left. \times \left[\chi_n'' \, (\chi_e')^2 + \chi_e'' \, (2\chi_n' \chi_e' + \chi_n'' \chi_e'') \right] \right\} . \tag{72}$$

Since the nuclear resonance frequency ω_0 is generally far removed from the electronic frequency we need only retain terms of lowest order in χ_e''.

$$\overline{P} = \tfrac{1}{2} \omega_0 \, (H^X)^2 \left\{ \chi_n'' \left[1 + \left(\frac{H_{hfs}}{|M|}\right)^2 (\chi_e')^2 \right] \right.$$
$$+ \chi_e'' \left[1 + 2 \left(\frac{H_{hfs}}{|M|}\right)^2 \chi_n' \chi_e' \right] \Big\}$$
$$= \tfrac{1}{2} \omega_0 \, (H^X)^2 \left\{ \chi_n'' \left[1 + \eta^2 \right] + \chi_e'' \left[1 + 2 (\chi_n'/\chi_e') \eta^2 \right] \right\} .$$
$$\tag{73}$$

The absorption rate at ω_0 therefore consists of two parts. The first is the ordinary nuclear absorption χ_n'', enhanced by the hyperfine coupling. The second part consists of the electronic losses χ_e'' which are modulated by the real part of the nuclear susceptibility χ_n'. At high power levels the nuclear resonance therefore has the dispersion shape since χ_n'' saturates more easily than χ_n'.

In pulsed NMR experiments the enhancement has two effects. In the first place, the magnitude of the required driving field is reduced by the factor $(1 + \eta)$; in the second place, after removal of the excitation the precessing nuclear magnetization induces through the hyperfine interaction a coherent precession of the electronic magnetization. The total transverse magnetization is $m^X(1 + \eta)$ and the enhancement of the induced signal in the receiver coil is therefore also given by $(1 + \eta)$.

In multidomain particles the response of the macroscopic magnetization to weak external magnetic fields involves domain wall displacements rather than domain rotations. For this reason the zero-field nuclear resonance in such particles is usually due to nuclei situated within domain walls. The wall resonance is strongly enhanced as a result of periodic wall translations which are induced by the H^X field. This motion produces a rotation of the electronic spins in the wall and hence a transverse hyperfine field at the nuclei. The spin rotation angle is proportional to the amplitude of the wall displacement and inversely proportional to the thickness of the wall. In typical cases the signal from multidomain particles is one to two orders of magnitude stronger than the corresponding single domain signal despite the fact that the walls only constitute a small fraction of the total sample volume. The reason for this behavior can be found in the much smaller magnitude of wall anisotropies compared to domain anisotropies. The enhancement factor associated with wall displacements is therefore correspondingly larger (Portis and Gossard, 1960).

The enormous intensity enhancement of the wall resonance is of great advantage when searching for unknown resonances. Indeed, from an instrumental standpoint the zero-field NMR in ferromagnetic materials undoubtedly represents the least difficult of all nuclear resonance experiments. Unfortunately, the continuous variation of the direction of magnetization within the domain walls introduces complications in the interpretation of the resonance data. For example, it is difficult to obtain accurate values of hyperfine constants because the contribution of long range dipolar interactions to the measured frequencies cannot be estimated reliably. It is also obvious that the domain wall NMR yields little quantitative information about anisotropies in the hyperfine interaction.

The intensity of the wall resonance decreases sharply with increasing external field because of the loss of wall volume. Above the coercive field the domain rotation mechanism becomes dominant, decreasing only as $|H_A + H_0|^{-1}$.

The above discussion applies not only to ferromagnets but to all magnetic systems which possess a spontaneous magnetic moment such as ferrimagnets and canted antiferromagnets with weak ferromagnetic moments.

b. Antiferromagnets: In most antiferromagnetic crystals weak external magnetic fields produce only small changes in the directions of sublattice magnetization since such changes can only be induced at the expense of exchange energy. Significant enhancement effects are therefore not expected. An exception occurs when the exchange and anisotropy interactions are relatively weak. The energy of an antiferromagnetic spin system with uniaxial anisotropy in an external magnetic field H_0 can be expressed in terms of the perpendicular and parallel susceptibilities

$$E = -\tfrac{1}{2}\chi_{\perp}H_0^2 \sin^2(\alpha+\theta) - \tfrac{1}{2}\chi_{\parallel}H_0^2 \cos^2(\alpha+\theta) - 2K\cos\theta,$$

$$(74)$$

where α is the angle between $\mathbf{H}_0$ and the easy axis, θ is the field-induced displacement in the direction of sublattice magnetization from the easy axis, and K is the anisotropy constant. We have assumed that the canting of the sublattices is small compared to θ. The displacement θ can be calculated by minimizing the energy

$$\partial E/\partial\theta = 0 = -H_0^2(\chi_{\perp}-\chi_{\parallel})\sin 2(\alpha+\theta) + 2K\sin\theta. \quad (75)$$

If the driving field $\mathbf{H}_1$ is applied at right angles to $\mathbf{H}_0$ (and in the plane formed by $\mathbf{H}_0$ and the easy axis) the effective transverse field seen by the nuclear spins is

$$H^x(\text{eff}) = H^x(H_{hfs}/H_0)\,(\partial\theta/\partial\alpha) \equiv \eta H^x \quad . \qquad (76)$$

Using Eq. (75) to calculate the variation of θ with α we find, for $\alpha + \theta = \pi/2$

$$|\eta| = \frac{H_{hfs}H_0(\chi_{\perp}-\chi_{\parallel})}{K + H_0^2(\chi_{\perp}-\chi_{\parallel})} \quad . \qquad (77)$$

In weak fields the enhancement is a linear function of H_0, reaches a maximum when $H_0^2 = K/(\chi_{\perp} - \chi_{\parallel})$, and decreases as H_0^{-1} in high fields. The maximum enhancement $\eta(\text{max}) = \tfrac{1}{2}H_{hfs}(\chi_{\perp} - \chi_{\parallel})^{\tfrac{1}{2}}K^{-\tfrac{1}{2}}$ can be large provided that $\chi_{\perp}/K$ is sufficiently large. This type of behavior has been observed for example in $CrCl_3$ (Narath, 1963), where enhancement factors of several hundred were observed.

3. Elementary Spin-Wave (Magnon) Theory

At low temperatures the exchange interactions produce almost complete ordering of the electronic spins. We are interested in the elementary excitations of such a system and how they manifest themselves in the static and dynamic properties of the nuclear resonance. We consider a system of identical spins which can be described by the Hamiltonian

$$\mathcal{H}_e = -\sum_{ij} J_{ij}\,\mathbf{S}_i \cdot \mathbf{S}_j - \gamma_e \hbar H_A \sum_i S_i^z , \qquad (78)$$

where J_{ij} are exchange constants (which are assumed to be sufficiently large to permit the neglect of dipolar couplings) and H_A

is an effective anisotropy field whose direction is assumed to coincide with the *negative* z axis. (It is convenient to define directions in such a way that the spins tend to align along the *positive* z axis. This requires that $\gamma_e H_A > 0$.) A useful representation for the spin operators is provided by the Bose creation ($a^\dagger$) and annihilation (a) operators (Holstein and Primakoff, 1940).

$$S_i^+ = (2S)^{\frac{1}{2}} [1 - (2S)^{-1} a_i^\dagger a_i]^{\frac{1}{2}} a_i \quad , \tag{79}$$

$$S_i^- = (2S)^{\frac{1}{2}} a_i^\dagger [1 - (2S)^{-1} a_i^\dagger a_i]^{\frac{1}{2}} \quad , \tag{80}$$

$$S_i^z = S - a_i^\dagger a_i \quad . \tag{81}$$

The Bose operators are defined by the commutation relations

$$[a_i, a_j^\dagger] = \delta_{ij}, \ [a_i^\dagger, a_j^\dagger] = [a_i, a_j] = 0 \quad , \tag{82}$$

and have the properties

$$a_i^\dagger \, |\, n_i \rangle = (n_i + 1)^{\frac{1}{2}} \, |\, n_i + 1 \rangle \quad , \tag{83}$$

$$a_i |\, n_i \rangle = n_i^{\frac{1}{2}} |\, n_i - 1 \rangle \quad , \tag{84}$$

$$a_i^\dagger a_i |\, n_i \rangle = n_i |\, n_i \rangle \quad , \qquad n_i = 0, 1, 2, \ldots \tag{85}$$

where $|\, n_i \rangle$ is a state with n_i spin deviations at the ith site. At low temperatures $\langle n_i \rangle$ is small and the spin operators may therefore be linearized by letting $a_i^\dagger a_i = 0$ in Eq. (79) and Eq. (80). This is the basic assumption of the non-interacting spin-wave approximation.

a. Ferromagnetic Spin Waves: We restrict ourselves to nearest neighbor exchange interactions, $J > 0$. Transforming Eq. (78) according to Eqs. (79-81) and retaining only bilinear terms we obtain

$$\mathcal{H}_e = E_o - 2JS \sum_{ij} (a_i^\dagger a_j - a_i^\dagger a_i) \delta(\mathbf{r}_i - \mathbf{r}_j - \rho) + \gamma_e \hbar H_A \sum_i a_i^\dagger a_i \quad , \tag{86}$$

where ρ denotes vectors from a given site to its nearest neighbors. The ground state energy (i.e., the energy of the fully aligned state) is

$$E_o = -NJzS^2 - N\gamma_e \hbar H_A S \quad , \tag{87}$$

where z is the number of nearest neighbors surrounding each spin. The coupling between different lattice sites in Eq. (86) can be removed by a Fourier transformation to reciprocal lattice coordinates

$$a_i^\dagger = N^{-\frac{1}{2}} \sum_k a_k^\dagger \exp(i\mathbf{k} \cdot \mathbf{r}_i) \quad , \tag{88}$$

$$a_i = N^{-\frac{1}{2}} \sum_k a_k \exp(-i\mathbf{k} \cdot \mathbf{r}_i) \quad , \tag{89}$$

which yields the diagonal expression

$$\mathcal{H}_e = E_o + \sum_k \hbar\omega_k a_k^\dagger a_k \quad , \tag{90}$$

in terms of the spin-wave (magnon) energies

$$\hbar\omega_k = [2JzS(1-\gamma_k) + \gamma_e \hbar H_A] \quad , \tag{91}$$

where

$$\gamma_k = z^{-1} \sum_\rho \exp(-i\mathbf{k} \cdot \rho) \quad , \tag{92}$$

It is apparent that the anisotropy field not only introduces a gap at k = 0 ($\hbar\omega_G = \gamma_e \hbar H_A$), but also shifts the entire spectrum uniformly to higher energies by the same amount. The effect of an external field is simply to add an additional term $\gamma_e \hbar H_o$ to the spin-wave energies. The small-k modes can be approximated by expanding γ_k for a given lattice to order k^2. In the long-wave limit the energies therefore have the form

$$\hbar\omega_k \approx \hbar\omega_G + Dk^2 \quad . \tag{93}$$

    b. <u>Antiferromagnetic Spin Waves:</u> We consider a primitive crystal lattice in which J < 0, forcing the spins to arrange themselves in two sublattices of opposite spin orientation. In the absence of intrasublattice interactions the Hamiltonian for this system is

$$\mathcal{H} = -2J \sum_{ij} \hat{\mathbf{S}}_i \cdot \hat{\mathbf{S}}_j \delta(\mathbf{r}_i - \mathbf{r}_j - \rho) - \gamma_e \hbar H_A \left[\sum_i S_i^z - \sum_j S_j^z \right] ,$$
$$\tag{94}$$

where i and j identify spins belonging to the two sublattices and ρ

represents vectors from a given sublattice site to nearest neighbors on the other sublattice. The creation and annihilation operators for the two sublattices are defined in the linear spin-wave approximation by

$$S_i^+ = (2S)^{\frac{1}{2}} a_i \quad , \qquad\qquad S_j^+ = (2S)^{\frac{1}{2}} b_j^{\dagger} \quad , \qquad (95)$$

$$S_i^- = (2S)^{\frac{1}{2}} a_i^{\dagger} \quad , \qquad\qquad S_j^- = (2S)^{\frac{1}{2}} b_j \quad , \qquad (96)$$

$$S_i^z = S - a_i^{\dagger} a_i \quad , \qquad\qquad S_j^z = -S + b_j^{\dagger} b_j \quad . \qquad (97)$$

Carrying out the indicated transformation, followed by a Fourier transformation as in the ferromagnetic case, we obtain

$$\mathcal{K} = E_o + (-2JzS + \gamma_e \hbar H_A) \sum_k (a_k^{\dagger} a_k + b_k^{\dagger} b_k)$$

$$- 2JzS \sum_k \gamma_k (a_k^{\dagger} b_k^{\dagger} + a_k b_k) \quad , \qquad (98)$$

$$E_o = NJzS^2 - N\gamma_e \hbar H_A S \qquad , \qquad (99)$$

where N is the total number of spins. The coupling terms between the two branches are removed by the transformation

$$a_k^{\dagger} = u_k \alpha_k^{\dagger} + v_k \beta_k \quad , \qquad\qquad b_k^{\dagger} = u_k \beta_k^{\dagger} + v_k \alpha_k \quad , \qquad (100)$$

$$a_k = u_k \alpha_k + v_k \beta_k^{\dagger} \quad , \qquad\qquad b_k = u_k \beta_k + v_k \alpha_k^{\dagger} \quad , \qquad (101)$$

where the u_k and v_k are real and $u_k^2 - v_k^2 = 1$ in order that the new operators satisfy Bose commutation relations. These requirements can be satisfied if we make the substitution

$$u_k = \cosh x_k \quad , \qquad\qquad v_k = \sinh x_k \quad , \qquad (102)$$

The off-diagonal terms in Eq. (98) vanish if

$$\tanh 2x_k = -2JzS\gamma_k (2JzS - \gamma_e \hbar H_A)^{-1} \quad . \qquad (103)$$

The Hamiltonian in diagonal form is

$$\mathcal{K}_e = E_o' + \sum_k \hbar \omega_k (\alpha_k^{\dagger} \alpha_k + \beta_k^{\dagger} \beta_k) \quad , \qquad (104)$$

$$E_0' = E_0 + \tfrac{1}{2}N(2JzS - \gamma_e \hbar H_A) + \sum_{k} \hbar w_k \quad . \tag{105}$$

The sum over magnon energies in Eq. (105) represents a contribution to the ground-state energy which arises from the fact that the simple "up-down" state is degenerate with the "down-up" state. The two states are connected by the $S_i^+ S_j^-$ operator and therefore cannot represent the true ground state. The spin-wave spectrum is doubly degenerate, with

$$\hbar w_k = -2JzS \left[(1 + \alpha)^2 - \gamma_k^2 \right]^{\frac{1}{2}} \quad , \tag{106}$$

$$\alpha = - \gamma_e \hbar H_A / 2JzS \quad .$$

The antiferromagnetic spin-wave energies differ significantly in their functional dependence on k and H_A from the ferromagnetic energies [Eq. (91)]. The antiferromagnetic spin-wave gap, for example, depends strongly on the exchange energy because the precession of the sublattice magnetizations about their respective anisotropy fields produces a periodic canting of the sublattices.

$$\hbar w_G = -2JzS \left[\alpha^2 + 2\alpha \right]^{\frac{1}{2}} \approx - \gamma_e \hbar \left[2H_A H_E \right]^{\frac{1}{2}} \tag{107}$$

for small α, where $H_E = (\gamma_e \hbar)^{-1} (2JzS)$. For a given H_A the gap ($k = 0$) is therefore much larger for the antiferromagnet than for the ferromagnet. For large k on the other hand the anisotropy has relatively little effect on $\hbar w_k$ in the antiferromagnetic case. Furthermore, for $H_A = 0$ the small-k spectrum is linear in k, instead of quadratic as in the ferromagnet. These differences are illustrated in Fig. 2.

An external field splits the degeneracy of the spin-wave states. The new energies become $\hbar w_k \pm \gamma_e \hbar H_0$.

4. The Sublattice Magnetization at Low Temperatures

One of the important types of NMR experiments on ordered magnetic crystals involves measurements of the temperature dependence of the zero-field frequency. In many cases the hyperfine coupling constants are independent of temperature over the range of interest. The measured frequencies are then proportional to the sublattice magnetization, and can therefore be compared directly at low temperatures with predictions of the spin-wave theory since

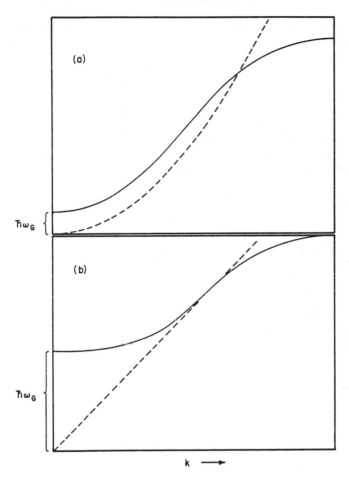

$$\hbar\omega_G$$

$$\hbar\omega_G$$

k ⟶

Fig. 2: Schematic representation of magnon energies between
k = 0 and the zone boundary: (a) ferromagnet, (b) antiferromagnet.

$$\nu(T) = \nu(0) \left[1 - (\langle n \rangle / \langle S \rangle_{T=0}) \right] \quad , \qquad (108)$$

where $\langle n \rangle$ is the thermal average value of the spin deviation. In
cases where the constancy of $[A]$ cannot be assumed because of
significant thermal expansion effects it is desirable to combine
measurements of $\nu(T)$ with pressure dependence measurements
of the NMR frequencies (Benedek and Kushida, 1960).

   a. Ferromagnets: In this case the spins are completely
aligned in the ground state (in the absence of significant dipolar

interactions) and hence $\langle S \rangle_{T=0} \equiv S$. The spin-wave excitations obey Bose statistics

$$\langle n \rangle = \langle a_i^\dagger a_i \rangle = N^{-1} \sum_k \langle n_k \rangle = N^{-1} \sum_k [\exp(\hbar\omega_k/k_B T) - 1]^{-1},$$

(109)

where the sum is extended over all states in the first Brillouin zone. At sufficiently low temperatures only the small-k modes contribute to Eq. (109) and we can therefore use the approximate dispersion relation (Eq. (93)). We obtain

$$\langle n \rangle = N^{-1} \sum_{n=1}^{\infty} [\exp(-n\hbar\omega_G/k_B T) \sum_k \exp(-nDk^2/k_B T)] .$$

(110)

The sum on k can be replaced by an integration. The upper limit can be extended to infinity because of the rapid convergence of the integrand at low temperatures. The results for two- and three-dimensional spin configurations are given (for a magnetic unit cell volume V_0) by

$$\langle n \rangle = \pi(2\pi)^{-2} \left(\frac{k_B T}{D}\right) V_0 \sum_{n=1}^{\infty} n^{-1} \exp(-n\hbar\omega_G/k_B T)$$

(111)

for two dimensions and

$$\langle n \rangle = \pi^{\frac{3}{2}} (2\pi)^{-3} \left(\frac{k_B T}{D}\right)^{\frac{3}{2}} V_0 \sum_{n=1}^{\infty} n^{-\frac{3}{2}} \exp(-n\hbar\omega_G/k_B T)$$

(112)

for three dimensions.

An interesting example of a relatively simple ferromagnet is provided by EuS ($T_C = 16.5°$K) which has the NaCl structure. Charap and Boyd (1964) studied the [151] Eu and [153] Eu NMR and observed the expected $T^{3/2}$ variation (Eq. (112)) in the range $1-4°$K. Applying spin-wave theory to NMR as well as specific heat data, they were able to obtain values for the nearest-neighbor and next-nearest-neighbor exchange constants and the effective anisotropy field H_A.

The linear temperature dependence (Eq. (111)) has been observed between $2°$K and $4°$K in the hexagonal layer compound $CrCl_3$ (Narath, 1961). In this structure ($T_N = 16.8°$K) the intralayer exchange interaction (J_T) is ferromagnetic. The interlayer interaction (J_L), although antiferromagnetic, is sufficiently weak ($J_T/J_L \approx$ -400) that it can be considered to a first approximation as part of a weak anisotropy field ($H_A \approx 1.6$ kOe). The observed temperature dependence of the ^{53}Cr NMR is shown in Fig. 3.

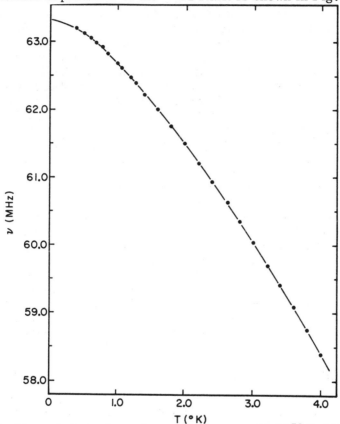

Fig. 3: Temperature dependence of the zero-field ^{53}Cr NMR in antiferromagnetic $CrCl_3$. Only the variation of the central component of the quadrupole triplet is shown.

The rapid decrease of $\nu(T)$ with increasing temperature is related to the small value of H_A. According to Eq. (111) the average spin deviation $\langle n \rangle$ diverges in a two-dimensional ferromagnet for $H_A = 0$ since $\sum n^{-1} = \infty$. The sublattice magnetization of a two-dimensional ferromagnet is therefore expected to be strongly field dependent. This has been demonstrated in $CrCl_3$ on the basis of detailed ^{53}Cr NMR measurements (Narath and Davis, 1965).

The compounds $CrBr_3$ ($T_C = 32.5\,^\circ K$) and CrI_3 ($T_C = 68\,^\circ K$) are structurally isomorphous to $CrCl_3$ but have ferromagnetic interlayer exchange constants. Since $J_L < J_T$ in both cases, the spin-wave dispersion relations are highly anisotropic. For example, the zone-boundary energy in $CrBr_3$ for spin waves propagating in a direction perpendicular to the hexagonal layers is only 6.0 k_B. For this reason *large*-k_L excitations become very important even at temperatures far below T_C. The sublattice magnetization therefore deviates markedly from the $T^{3/2}$ prediction of the simple spin-wave model, as was first observed by Gossard, et al. (1961). These authors obtained reasonably accurate values of J_T and J_L for $CrBr_3$ by fitting their 1-4°K ^{53}Cr resonance data to an expression for the magnetization which included a $T^{5/2}$ correction for zone-boundary effects. Another interesting feature of the ^{53}Cr NMR in $CrBr_3$ is the zero-field observation of two distinct signals with different $0\,^\circ K$ frequencies and different temperature dependences (Gossard, et al., 1962). The high-frequency signal is due to nuclei within the domains and consists of a well resolved quadrupole triplet; the low-frequency signal is due to nuclei within domain walls and is extremely broad, presumably because of the variation of the quadrupole splitting across the wall. The frequency difference at $0\,^\circ K$ is interpreted to arise from differences in dipole fields and a small anisotropy in the hyperfine interaction. The domain-wall resonance has a stronger temperature dependence than the domain resonance. This reflects the reduction in the wall magnetization resulting from thermally driven wall motions. This effect is very important in $CrBr_3$ because of the small width of its walls (i.e., $J_L/\gamma_e \hbar H_A$ is small). Similar observations were made subsequently in CrI_3 (Narath, 1965) as shown in Fig. 4.

b. <u>Antiferromagnets</u>: The calculation of $\langle n \rangle$ is somewhat more difficult than in the ferromagnet because of the complicated form of the transformations leading to the spin-wave states. We find

$$n_i \equiv a_i^\dagger a_i = 2N^{-1} \sum_{kk'} \exp\left[-i(\mathbf{k}-\mathbf{k'})\cdot\mathbf{r}_i\right] a_k^\dagger a_{k'}$$

$$= 2N^{-1} \sum_{kk'} \exp\left[-i(\mathbf{k}-\mathbf{k'})\cdot\mathbf{r}_i\right](u_k \alpha_k^\dagger + v_k \beta_k)$$

$$\times(\mu_{k'}\alpha_{k'} + v_{k'}\beta_{k'}^\dagger) \quad . \tag{113}$$

Averaging Eq. (113) over all lattice sites gives

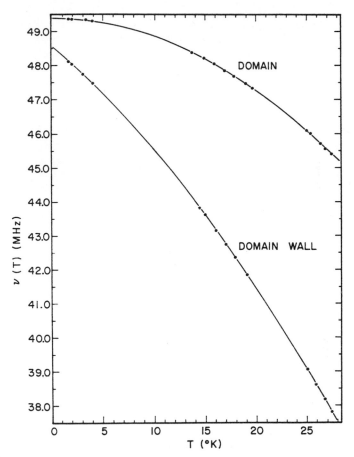

Fig. 4: Comparison of zero-field domain and domain-wall NMR frequencies of ^{53}Cr in ferromagnetic CrI_3 .

$$n = 2N^{-1} \sum_k [(u_k^2 \alpha_k^\dagger \alpha_k + v_k^2 \beta_k \beta_k^\dagger) + u_k v_k (\alpha_k^\dagger \beta_k^\dagger + \alpha_k \beta_k)] .$$

$$(114)$$

The diagonal part of Eq. (114) corresponds to the average spin deviation, while the off-diagonal part represents fluctuations about the statistical average which are associated with the fact that the sublattice moment operator does not commute with the antiferromagnetic exchange Hamiltonian. Since $\beta\beta^\dagger = \beta^\dagger\beta + 1$, we can write, using Eqs. (102) and (103)

$$\langle n \rangle = 2N^{-1} \sum_k \langle n_k \rangle \, F_k + N^{-1} \sum_k (F_k - 1) \quad , \tag{115}$$

where

$$F_k = \{1 - [\gamma_k/(1 + \alpha)]^2\}^{-\frac{1}{2}} \quad . \tag{116}$$

The first term in Eq. (115) is the spin deviation resulting from the thermal excitation of spin waves. The second term is due to zero-point fluctuations in the spin system. The resulting zero-point spin deviation $\Delta S/S$ decreases with increasing S and H_A. Representative values of $\Delta S/S$ predicted by spin-wave theory for zero anisotropy are compared in Table II with values obtained by Davis (1960) from a perturbation calculation. Numerous experimental

Table II: Comparison of spin-wave derived values of the zero-point spin deviation in antiferromagnets ($H_A = 0$) with the more accurate perturbation results of Davis (1960).

Lattice	Spin-Wave		Davis	
	$S = 1/2$	$S = 5/2$	$S = 1/2$	$S = 5/2$
Quadratic Layer	0.394	0.078	0.236	0.043
Simple Cubic	0.156	0.031	0.127	0.024
BCC	0.118	0.023	0.095	0.018

attempts have been made to detect the zero-point spin deviation by comparing hyperfine constants derived from electron-spin resonance measurements in dilute paramagnetic salts with low temperature NMR frequencies in the antiferromagnetic state. These attempts have failed so far because the effect has been obscured by slight differences between the hyperfine constants in the dilute and concentrated salts. Such differences can arise, for example, from cation-cation transferred hyperfine interactions which are only present, of course, in the concentrated salt (Heeger and Houston, 1964a; Owen and Taylor, 1966; Huang et al., 1966).

Until recently, the measured temperature dependence of the sublattice magnetization in typical antiferromagnets has also proved difficult to explain by means of the spin-wave theory. Early attempts consisted of expanding ω_k (Eq. (106)) in powers of k as in the ferromagnetic case. For zero anisotropy the leading term in the resulting expansion of $\langle n \rangle$ in powers of T was found to be proportional to T^2. Such a dependence has never been observed at temperatures where the spin-wave theory is believed to

be valid. The reason for this lies in the large gap which is characteristic of antiferromagnets even for small H_A and which dominates the small-k spin-wave spectrum. Even when the gap is very
small, the T^2 dependence of $\langle n \rangle$ is probably unobservable because
the power series expansion of ω_k converges rather slowly as a
result of the square root in Eq. (106).

To date the best understood antiferromagnet is MnF_2 (T_N =
66.9°K). Although its anisotropy energy ($H_A \approx 8.8$ kOe) is quite
small compared to $k_B T_N$, the small-k spin-wave approximation
(including corrections for a finite gap) can reproduce the resonance
data only up to ~ 6°K where $\langle n \rangle / S \approx 3 \times 10^{-5}$ (Jaccarino and
Walker, 1959). However, by evaluating the magnetization exactly
using numerical methods and taking into account next-nearest-
neighbor interactions in addition to the nearest-neighbor interactions, Lines (1965) was able to extend the agreement to almost
30°K, as shown in Fig. 5.

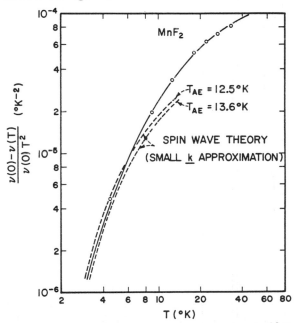

Fig. 5: Temperature dependence of the zero-field ^{19}F NMR in
antiferromagnetic MnF_2. The data are represented by
the solid curve. The small-k spin-wave prediction is
shown for two different values of $T_{AE} = \hbar \omega_G / k_B$. The
open circles represent a numerical fit of the complete
linear spin-wave theory to the data.

5. The Sublattice Magnetization at High Temperatures

Nuclear resonance experiments covering a wide range of temperatures have been carried out on many ordered magnetic materials. In most cases the variation of the measured frequencies with temperature have been compared, with varying degrees of success, against predictions of the molecular field model. In this approximation all spin correlations are ignored and each spin is assumed to interact with a constant exchange field H_E whose strength is proportional to the magnetization. The resulting temperature dependence of the magnetization is described by the Brillouin function $B_S(\gamma_e \hbar H_E/k_B T)$ and is, at best, only qualitatively correct.

Since the molecular field model rarely does justice to the high accuracy which is achieved in most NMR measurements of $\nu(T)$ vs T, it is more useful to correlate the NMR data with predictions based on more sophisticated quantum-statistical treatments of the exchange problem. We have already discussed the application of spin-wave theory to low temperature resonance data. With increasing temperature the spin-wave approximation becomes progressively poorer because of interactions among thermally excited spin waves. This interaction is a consequence of the non-linear relationship between the spin operators and the Bose creation and annihilation operators (Eqs. 79-81). The physical reason for this interaction is simply that less energy is required to reverse a given spin if a neighboring spin is already partially reversed. Each spin wave therefore experiences an exchange field which is proportional to $\cos \theta_E$, where θ_E is the average angle between adjacent spin directions. The decrease in the exchange field implies a corresponding decrease in the spin-wave energies. The magnetization is therefore expected to fall more rapidly with increasing temperature than predicted by the linear theory. Fortunately the contribution to θ_E from long-wavelength (small k) spin waves is small. The breakdown of the spin-wave approximation only becomes significant therefore at temperatures which are sufficiently high to produce appreciable numbers of short-wavelength spin waves. The excitation energies decrease only in proportion to the total spin-wave energy and not to the magnetization as the molecular field model would predict.

It is possible to take account of spin-wave interactions in an approximate way by renormalization of the spin-wave energies. This can be accomplished by retaining all diagonal fourth-order terms during the initial transformation of the exchange

Hamiltonian. The effect of these terms on $\mathcal{K}_e$ is then approximated by letting $a_k^\dagger a_k a_{k'}^\dagger a_{k'} = 2a_k^\dagger a_k \langle n_{k'} \rangle$. The determination of the renormalized spectrum therefore requires, in general, an iterative numerical solution for the temperature dependent renormalization corrections. The validity of this approach has been demonstrated for the ferromagnets $CrBr_3$ (Davis and Narath, 1964) and CrI_3 (Narath, 1965) and the antiferromagnet $CrCl_3$ (Narath and Davis, 1965) to temperatures of about $T_C/2$. In the case of antiferromagnetic MnF_2 the theory has been remarkably successful in explaining the sublattice magnetization behavior to temperatures approaching T_N (Low, 1963).

A number of very precise measurements have been carried out very near the transition temperature. A notable example is the temperature dependence of the ^{19}F NMR in antiferromagnetic MnF_2 (Heller and Benedek, 1962; Heller, 1966). These experiments have demonstrated the usefulness of NMR for the study of critical point phenomena.

6. Non-Magnetic Ions

The zero-field NMR frequency of nuclei belonging to nonmagnetic lattice sites is determined by the dipolar interaction with the ordered magnetic moments and is therefore just as useful for studying variations in the sublattice magnetization as the NMR of magnetic ions. The long-range nature of dipolar interactions makes the NMR of non-magnetic ions particularly useful, however, for the elucidation of complex magnetic structures. In the presence of an external field H_0 the frequency is given by

$$\omega_0 = \gamma_n |H_0 + H_{dip}| , \qquad (117)$$

where

$$H_{dip} = -(\gamma_n \hbar)^{-1} [A_{dip}] \cdot \langle S \rangle , \qquad (118)$$

and $[A_{dip}]$ is defined by Eq. (59). For a sufficiently weak external field one may assume that the orientation of $\langle S \rangle$ is independent of H_0. The components of the dipole field tensor can therefore be determined with great accuracy in single crystals by varying the orientation of H_0 and measuring the resulting variation of ω_0. From the number of independent resonance patterns and their symmetry relationships a considerable amount of information about the magnetic space group can be deduced provided, of course, that the crystal structure is known. In ideal cases, a comparison between the measured elements of $[A_{dip}]$ with values based on lattice sum calculations can lead to an unambiguous determination of the magnetic structure. This technique has been applied successfully to the proton NMR in a number of hydrated transition metal salts, such as $CuCl_2 \cdot 2H_2O$ (Poulis and Hardeman, 1952), $CoCl_2 \cdot 2H_2O$ (Narath, 1964), and $MnCl_2 \cdot 4H_2O$ (Spence and Nagarajan, 1966).

An interesting application of proton NMR is provided by the sublattice-switching experiment on antiferromagnetic $CuCl_2 \cdot 2H_2O$ by O'Sullivan, et al. (1962). The purpose of the experiment was to test the stability of a given antiferromagnetic spin configuration with respect to an interchange of the two sublattice directions. The protons in $CuCl_2 \cdot 2H_2O$ belong to two sets. Each set bears the same spatial relationship to the lattice sites of one sublattice as the other set bears to the sites belonging to the other sublattice. The degeneracy of the respective frequencies was removed by a 230 Oe magnetic field. One of the resonances was saturated while the other resonance was continuously monitored at low power levels. A switching of the sublattices would have transferred the saturation to the monitored frequency resulting in a momentary loss of signal intensity. No transition was observed during a 10-hour vigil.

7. Nuclear Spin-Lattice Relaxation

One expects, on general grounds, that the large static hyperfine effects in ordered magnetic materials be accompanied by dynamic effects of similar importance. In this section we examine contributions to the nuclear spin-lattice relaxation rate which arise from the hyperfine interactions. The relevant operator is

$$\mathcal{H}^+ = \tfrac{1}{2} I^+ ([A] \cdot S)^-$$

(119)

where

$$([A] \cdot S)^- = S^- [\tfrac{1}{2}(A^{xx} + A^{yy}) - iA^{xy}] + S^+ [\tfrac{1}{2}(A^{xx} - A^{yy})]$$

$$+ S^z (A^{xz} - iA^{yz}) .$$

(120)

The z axis is chosen to coincide with the nuclear axis of quantization. The relaxation rate can now be calculated from Eqs. (17) and (21) if the normal modes of the electronic spin system are known. At low temperatures the electron spin operators must therefore be transformed into spin-wave variables. The relaxation process involves the inelastic scattering of spin waves due to the hyperfine interaction. We consider several possible cases.

a. Isotropic Hyperfine Interaction: The only non-vanishing term in Eq. (119) is

$$\tfrac{1}{2} I^+ S^- [\tfrac{1}{2}(A^{xx} + A^{yy})] = \tfrac{1}{2} A I^+ S^- .$$

(121)

The most general transformation of S^- involves a series expansion
of Eq. (80) in powers of $(2S)^{-1}$ which yields

$$\tfrac{1}{2} AI^+ S^- \to \tfrac{1}{2}(2S)^{\frac{1}{2}} AI^+ \left[a^\dagger + (4S)^{-1} a^\dagger a^\dagger a + \ldots \right] . \quad (122)$$

An isotropic hyperfine interaction therefore leads to scattering
processes involving only odd numbers of spin waves. However,
energy conservation requirements severely restrict the importance
of odd-magnon contributions to nuclear spin-lattice relaxation.
For example in all real magnetic materials the electronic and
nuclear frequencies are always sufficiently separated that the
creation of a single spin wave requires more energy than is
available from a nuclear spin transition. The higher order terms
are also ineffective unless the magnetic spin-wave spectrum is
very dispersive. For example, the three-magnon process cannot
occur if $2\omega_G > \omega_{max}$ since only one magnon is annihilated while
two new magnons are created. The three-magnon process is
therefore only of importance if the magnetic anisotropy is sufficiently small. This condition is satisfied in $CrCl_3$ where the three-
magnon relaxation mechanism appears to dominate in the range
$2°-4°K$ (Narath and Fromhold, 1966).

   The calculation of the three-magnon rate is complicated by
the existence of a second order process which interferes constructively with the direct three-magnon process as shown in Fig.
6 (Pincus, 1966). The interfering process involves the creation

Fig. 6: Three-magnon
   scattering processes:
   (a) direct three-magnon
   process, (b) second-
   order exchange scat-
   tering process.

$$\vec{k} - \vec{k}' - \vec{k}'' + \vec{k}''' = 0$$

(a)   (b)

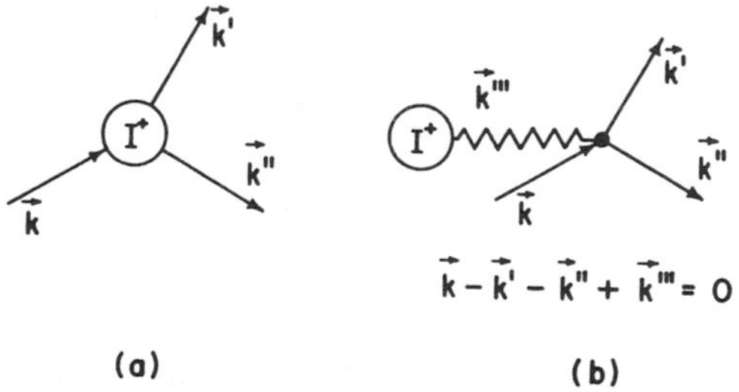

of a virtual magnon by the $AI^+ a^\dagger$ interaction which is annihilated in
a four-magnon exchange scattering process. The latter arises from
quartic terms in the exchange Hamiltonian which have the following form for a ferromagnet:

$$Jz a_{k'}^\dagger a_{k''}^\dagger a_k a_{k'''} \left[\gamma_{k'''-k''} - \tfrac{1}{2} (\gamma_{k'} + \gamma_{k''}) \right] \delta(k - k' - k'' + k'''). \quad (123)$$

The total three-magnon nuclear relaxation rate for a simple ferromagnet is therefore given by

$$1/T_1 = 2W = \frac{4\pi A^2}{32\hbar SN^3} \sum_{kk'k''} \langle n_k \rangle \left(\langle n_{k'} \rangle + 1 \right) \left(\langle n_{k''} \rangle + 1 \right)$$

$$\times \, \delta(\Delta E) \left[1 + \frac{Jz(2\gamma_{k'''} - k'' - \gamma_{k'} - \gamma_{k'''})}{\hbar\omega_{k'''}} \right]^2$$

$$\times \, \delta(k - k' - k'' + k''') \, , \tag{124}$$

where the first term inside the square brackets represents the
direct three-magnon contribution, while the second term represents
the exchange scattering contribution. In the limit of a large gap
the exchange term approaches unity when averaged over all angles;
for small gaps it exceeds unity. It is interesting to note that the
three-magnon process is a direct consequence of the intrinsic nonlinearity of the transverse spin operators. This nonlinearity can
therefore be detected at much lower temperatures by means of
dynamic hyperfine interactions than is the case for the static interactions.

The above discussion applies also to antiferromagnets although
the expression for T_1 [Eq. (124)] is, of course, different.

It often happens that the nuclear and electronic spins are
quantized along different directions. This can occur, for example,
if the nucleus is subjected to a quadrupole interaction with an electric field gradient whose major axis does not coincide with the
direction of the magnetic hyperfine field. (This differs from the
case where the magnetic hyperfine interaction is anisotropic.) If
the electronic spins are quantized along a Z axis, we find that

$$W \propto |\langle |S^-| \rangle|^2 = \sin^2 \theta_{zZ} |\langle |S^Z| \rangle|^2 \, . \tag{125}$$

However, $S^Z \propto a^\dagger a$ and the nuclear relaxation process therefore
results from Raman scattering of thermal spin waves. This two-
magnon process is clearly important even if the spin-wave gap is
large as it is in most antiferromagnets.

b. Anisotropic Hyperfine Interaction: If the net hyperfine
interaction contains anisotropic contributions the relaxation mechanism may be dominated by two-magnon processes resulting from the
S^Z term in Eq. (120) (Moriya, 1956). This has been clearly demonstrated for the ^{19}F spin-lattice relaxation in antiferromagnetic
MnF_2 (Kaplan et al., 1966a). In this compound each fluorine
nucleus is coupled to the spins of three Mn^{2+} neighbors through
the transferred hyperfine interaction as shown in the insert of

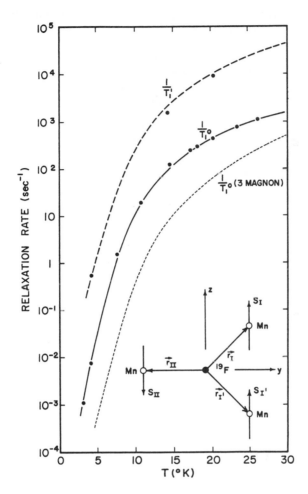

Fig. 7: Nuclear spin-lattice relaxation rates $(T_1)^{-1} = (T_1^0)^{-1} +$ $(T_1')^{-1} \sin^2 \theta_{zZ}$ for ^{19}F in antiferromagnetic MnF_2 as a function of temperature. The solid curve $(T_1^0)^{-1}$ represents the best fit of the two-magnon theory to the zero-field experimental points. The heavy dashed curve $(1/T_1')^{-1}$ is the coefficient of the $\sin^2 \theta_{zZ}$ term, where θ_{zZ} is the angle between the nuclear and electronic spin directions. The light dashed curve is a theoretical estimate of the three-magnon relaxation rate.

Fig. 7. The only nonvanishing off-diagonal elements of the three hyperfine tensors are $A_I^{yz} = A_I^{zy} = -A_{I'}^{yz} = -A_{I'}^{zy}$. The ^{19}F spins are quantized along the z axis since the static contributions of A_I^{yz} and $A_{I'}^{yz}$ exactly cancel. The dynamic effects, however, do not vanish and are described by the perturbing Hamiltonian

$$\mathcal{H}^+ = -\tfrac{1}{2}iI^+(A_I^{yz}S_I^z + A_{I'}^{yz}S_{I'}^z) = -\tfrac{1}{2}iA^{yz}I^+(S_I^z - S_{I'}^z) \quad . \quad (126)$$

Since MnF_2 is a two-sublattice antiferromagnet, we transform Eq. (126) according to Eqs. (97), (100) and (101).

$$\mathcal{H}^+ = -(i/N)A^{yz}I^+\sum_{kk'}\left[u_ku_{k'}\alpha_k^\dagger\alpha_{k'} + v_kv_{k'}\beta_{k'}^\dagger\beta_k\right.$$

$$+ u_kv_{k'}\alpha_k^\dagger\beta_{k'}^\dagger + u_{k'}v_k\alpha_{k'}\alpha_k + v_kv_{k'}\Big]$$

$$\times \left[\exp[-i(k-k')\cdot r_I] - \exp[-i(k-k')\cdot r_{I'}]\right]\delta(\Delta E) \quad .$$
$$(127)$$

Only the $\alpha^\dagger\alpha$ and $\beta^\dagger\beta$ terms contribute to relaxation since the others violate energy conservation requirements. We note that $\alpha^\dagger$ and $\beta^\dagger$ create different spin waves. Thus, there are no interference terms between the two spin-wave branches. The exponential terms in Eq. (127) can be simplified using simple trigonometric identies. The resulting relaxation rate becomes

$$1/T_1 = 2W = (16\pi/\hbar N^2)(A^{yz})^2\sum_{kk'}$$

$$(u_k^2u_{k'}^2 + v_k^2v_{k'}^2)(\langle n_k\rangle + 1)\langle n_{k'}\rangle$$

$$\times \sin^2[\tfrac{1}{2}(k-k')\cdot(r_I - r_{I'})]\delta(\Delta E) \quad , \quad (128)$$

where $\langle n_k\rangle = \langle n_{k'}\rangle$ because energy conservation requires that the initial and final magnon energies be identical (i.e., the nuclear Zeeman energy can be neglected in $\delta(\Delta E)$). The experimental results for MnF_2 are in excellent agreement with predictions based on Eq. (128) as indicated in Fig. 7. The fit to the data was obtained for $|A^{yz}| = 5.4 \times 10^{-4}$ cm^{-1} which compares with a measured value of $(4.4 \pm 0.4) \times 10^{-4}$ cm^{-1} for Mn^{2+} in ZnF_2. Also shown in Fig. 7 are results of experiments in which the axis of quantization of the ^{19}F spins was turned slightly by application of an external magnetic field. The observed increase in $1/T_1$ was explained quantitatively on the basis of two-magnon scattering contributions from I^+S^- terms in $\mathcal{H}^+$ (Eq. (125)).

The examples presented above suggest that intrinsic magnon-induced processes play an important role in nuclear spin-lattice relaxation in many magnetic insulators. In principle, spin-wave theory provides the necessary theoretical apparatus for explaining the observed rates, provided that the dispersion relations are known. Finally, it should be pointed out that in many instances the dominant relaxation mechanism involves interactions with paramagnetic impurities (de Gennes and Hartmann-Boutron, 1961). Such processes become particularly important at very low temperatures where the number of thermal magnons becomes extremely small.

8. Indirect Nuclear Spin-Spin Interactions.

It is a general observation that linewidths in the ordered state, even at extremely low temperatures, are much greater than one would expect from direct dipolar interactions among the nuclear moments. It is natural to seek an explanation for the broadening in the fluctuations of the longitudinal and transverse electronic spin components. We have seen that such fluctuations can result from the Raman scattering of spin waves. In practice, however, the contribution of direct spin-wave scattering processes to the transverse relaxation is much too small at low temperatures to account for the observed linewidths. This follows from the fact that the number of thermally excited spin waves is relatively small in this temperature range. What is required therefore is a higher order scattering process in which magnons appear only as virtual excitations and therefore do not introduce any statistical factors. In crystals in which the nuclear moments are present in high concentration this requirement is satisfied by indirect nuclear spin-spin interactions via virtual excitation of magnons (Suhl, 1958; Nakamura, 1958).

a. Suhl-Nakamura Interaction: The Hamiltonian for a system of nuclear spins subjected to both external and hyperfine fields is given by

$$\mathcal{K} = \sum_i \left(A_i I_i \cdot S_i - \gamma_n \hbar I_i \cdot H_o \right) . \tag{129}$$

The process in which a magnon is created by a nuclear spin flip at one site and absorbed by a spin flop at another site can be obtained from the second-order matrix element

$$\mathcal{K}_{ij} = -\tfrac{1}{4} A_i A_j I_i^+ I_j^- \sum_k w_{e,k}^{-1} \Big[\langle n_k | S_j^+ | n_k + 1 \rangle \langle n_k + 1 | S_i^- | n_k \rangle$$

$$- \langle n_k | S_i^- | n_k - 1 \rangle \langle n_k - 1 | S_j^+ | n_k \rangle \Big] \delta(\Delta E) \qquad , \qquad (130)$$

where the $w_{e,k}$ are electronic spin-wave energies. Because of energy conservations requirements, Eq. (130) vanishes unless the two nuclear transition energies are identical. This implies, in general, identical nuclear moments. Transforming the spin operators in Eq. (130) into appropriate magnon operators we obtain a total nuclear Hamiltonian for the *ferromagnet*

$$\mathcal{K}_n = (A\langle S^z \rangle - \gamma_n \hbar H_0) \sum_i I_i^z + \sum_{ii'} U_{ii'} I_i^+ I_{i'}^- \quad . \qquad (131)$$

Here $U_{ii'}$ is the coefficient of the Suhl-Nakamura interaction

$$U_{ii'} = -(A^2 S/2N) \sum_k w_{e,k}^{-1} \exp[ik \cdot R_{ii'}] \qquad , \qquad (132)$$

where $R_{ii'} = r_i - r_{i'}$. The terms $i = i'$ represent self-energy contributions which shift the energy by a small amount. The resulting shift in the NMR frequency is usually negligible. It is apparent from Eq. (132) that the Suhl-Nakamura interaction is temperature independent as long as the linear spin-wave theory is valid. We also note that the interaction leads to a broadening of the NMR since $I_i^+ I_{i'}^-$ does not commute with the transverse moment operator $\gamma_n \hbar (I_i^+ + I_{i'}^+)$.

The range of the Suhl-Nakamura interaction can be very large. This can be seen by evaluating $U_{ii'}$ in the long-wavelength approximation.

$$U_{ii'} \approx -\frac{A^2 S V_0}{2(2\pi)^3} \int_0^\infty dk \, \frac{\exp[ik \cdot R_{ii'}]}{\hbar w_G + Dk^2}$$

$$\approx -\frac{A^2 S \hat{a}^3}{8\pi D R_{ii'}} \exp[-(\hbar w_G/D)^{\frac{1}{2}} R_{ii'}] \qquad . \qquad (133)$$

Thus the range of the interaction is of the order

$$R_{max} = (D/\hbar w_G)^{\frac{1}{2}} \quad , \qquad (134)$$

which is typically 10-100 lattice spacings.

For the *antiferromagnet* a similar calculation gives

$$U_{ii'} = -(A^2 S/2N) \sum_k w_{e,k}^{-1} (u_k^2 + v_k^2) \exp[i\mathbf{k} \cdot \mathbf{R}_{ii'}] , \qquad (135)$$

which vanishes unless both sites belong to the same sublattice. The range function is identical to Eq. (134) except that $\hbar w_G$ is replaced by $\gamma_e \hbar H_A$.

The Suhl-Nakamura interaction yields a Gaussian line whose second moment, aside from some constant factors, is

$$\langle \Delta w^2 \rangle \propto \hbar^{-2} I(I+1)(A^2 S/\hbar w_E)^2 (w_E/w_A)^{\frac{1}{2}} , \qquad (136)$$

where $w_E = \gamma_e H_E$ and $w_A = \gamma_e H_A$. This expression applies to both ferromagnetic and antiferromagnetic cases. The predicted linewidth $\Delta w \approx \langle \Delta w^2 \rangle^{\frac{1}{2}}$ is independent of temperature, directly proportional to the square of the hyperfine coupling constant, and only weakly dependent on the anisotropy. In general Eq. (136) is in satisfactory agreement with observed linewidths. There are a few disturbing cases, however, where the observed widths are considerably smaller than the predicted values (e.g., ^{55}Mn in RbMnF$_3$ (Heeger and Teaney, 1964)).

b. Nuclear Spin Waves; Frequency Pulling: The best evidence for the existence of a long-range nuclear spin-spin interaction is provided by the observation of temperature dependent frequency-pulling effects in the NMR of low-anisotropy magnetic materials. We notice that the nuclear Hamiltonian (Eq. (131)) resembles the electronic exchange Hamiltonian. Although the nuclear spin system is highly disordered at ordinary low temperatures the long range of $U_{ii'}$ suggests that strong correlations should exist among the nuclear spins. It should therefore be possible to define a set of normal modes for the nuclear magnetization. We assume that the nuclear spins are 100% abundant and introduce the Fourier transforms

$$I_i^{\pm} = N^{-\frac{1}{2}} \sum_k I_k^{+} \exp(\mp i\mathbf{k} \cdot \mathbf{r}_i) \qquad (137)$$

in Eq. (131) and find for the *ferromagnet*

$$\mathcal{H}_n = (A\langle S^z \rangle - \gamma_n \hbar H_o) \sum_k I_k^z - \frac{1}{2}A^2 S \sum_k w_{e,k}^{-1} I_k^+ I_k^- . \qquad (138)$$

The equation of motion of I_k^+ is

$$\frac{dI_k^+}{dt} = -i[I_k^+, \mathcal{K}_n] = iI_k^+\left\{(A\langle S^z\rangle - \gamma_n\hbar H_0) + (A^2 S/\omega_{e,k})I_k^z\right\} .$$
$$(139)$$

At very low temperatures $\langle S^z\rangle = S$. We also assume that the motion of I_k^+ is a small oscillation relative to the thermal average value of I^z. This has been justified in detail by de Gennes et al. (1963). We therefore substitute $I_k^+(t) = I_k^+\exp(i\omega_{n,k}t)$ into Eq. (139) and obtain immediately the nuclear spin-wave spectrum

$$\omega_{n,k} = \gamma_n H_0 - \hbar^{-1}AS[1 + (A/\omega_{e,k})\langle I^z\rangle] .$$
$$(140)$$

The last term inside the brackets represents the frequency pulling effect which is important for large A, small $\omega_{e,k}$ and relatively large nuclear polarizations. The effect is very large when $A\langle I^z\rangle$ becomes comparable to the unperturbed electronic spin-wave gap. One can also show that the hyperfine interaction simultaneously shifts the electronic spectrum by an amount $-A\langle I^z\rangle$. It is clear that the predicted resonance shifts are not only a sensitive function of temperature, but also of rf power level since the nuclear polarization $\langle I^z\rangle$ vanishes in the limit of complete saturation of the nuclear resonance. The range of the nuclear pulling effect in k space depends on the value of k for which the exchange contribution to ω_k becomes larger than the gap. This occurs for $k \sim (\hbar\omega_G/D)^{\frac{1}{2}}$. In other words the range is simply the reciprocal of the Suhl-Nakamura range (Eq. (134)). For shorter wavelengths the indirect nuclear spin-spin interaction cannot shift the nuclear frequency coherently.

The direct excitation of the nuclear resonance requires k=0 because

$$\mathcal{K}_1 = -\gamma_n\hbar H_1 N^{-\frac{1}{2}}\sum_i\sum_k I_k^+\exp(-ik\cdot r_i) = -\gamma_n\hbar H_1 N^{\frac{1}{2}}I_0^+ .$$
$$(141)$$

Furthermore,

$$(A/\omega_{e,o})\langle I^z\rangle = -\gamma_n\hbar H_{hfs}\langle I^z\rangle(\gamma_e\hbar H\langle S^z\rangle)^{-1} = -\eta(m/M) ,$$
$$(142)$$

where m and M are the absolute average magnitudes of the nuclear and electronic magnetizations, respectively, and η is the enhancement factor which is defined in Eq. (67). The nuclear resonance frequency may therefore be written as

$$\omega_{n,o} = \gamma_n H_o - \hbar^{-1} AS[1 - \eta (m/M)] , \qquad (143)$$

which shows that the effective hyperfine field is reduced in proportion to the enhancement factor. Since η is usually much larger within domain walls than within bulk domains, one expects particularly large frequency pulling effects for the domain-wall enhanced NMR. A marked difference between wall and domain pulling has indeed been observed in ferrimagnetic $MnFe_2O_4$ (Heeger and Houston, 1964b).

Frequency pulling effects are also important in *antiferromagnets* in which the anisotropy is very small. This follows directly from the large enhancement factors (Eq. (77)) which apply in such cases. For the configuration which was used in deriving Eq. (77) the nuclear resonance frequency is given by

$$\omega_{n,o} = \hbar^{-1} AS[1 - (\Omega_e/\omega_{e,o})^2]^{\frac{1}{2}} , \qquad (144)$$

where Ω_e is the electronic frequency in the nuclear anisotropy field

$$\Omega_e = \hbar^{-1}[4JzSA \langle I^z \rangle]^{\frac{1}{2}} , \qquad (145)$$

and $\omega_{e,o}$ is the transverse antiferromagnetic resonance frequency, which is strongly field dependent. Whereas the fractional pulling of $\omega_{n,o}$ is proportional to $\langle I^z \rangle$ in the ferromagnet, it is proportional to $\langle I^z \rangle^{\frac{1}{2}}$ in the antiferromagnet. Figure 8 shows [55] Mn frequency pulling data for antiferromagnetic $RbMnF_3$ which illustrate the expected variations of $\omega_{n,o}$ with temperature and magnetic field strength (Heeger and Teaney, 1964).

It should be emphasized that frequency-pulling is a general phenomenon associated with ordered magnetic systems in which the nuclei are present in high abundance and the hyperfine interactions are reasonably large. In many systems the effects may not be as dramatic as for [55] Mn in the perovskite antiferromagnets ($KMnF_3$, $RbMnF_3$, etc.); they may nevertheless be significant if accurate measurements of the sublattice magnetization are desired. Fortunately, the presence of frequency-pulling can always be detected by observing the NMR frequency as a function of saturation level.

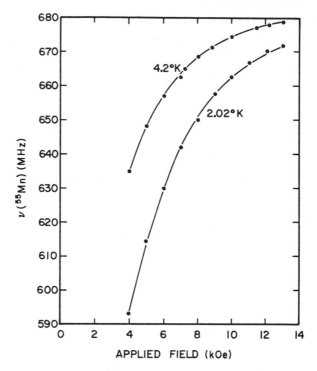

Fig. 8: Variation of the ^{55}Mn NMR in antiferromagnetic RbMnF$_3$ with temperature and external magnetic field strength.

IV. NMR in Metallic Solids

A. Simple Metals

1. Physical Properties

For purposes of the present discussion the term "simple" refers to metals whose conduction electrons can be treated in the nearly-free-electron (NFE) approximation. In general, this implies the absence of partially filled d bands. Typical examples of such metals are the alkali metals Li, Na, K, Rb, Cs and the noble metals Cu, Ag, Au.

The conduction electron states are easily obtained in the independent particle approximation in which each electron is assumed to move in an average static potential arising from the nuclear and electronic charge distribution of the crystal. The motion of the electrons is described by the Bloch functions

$$\psi_k(\mathbf{r}) = u_k(\mathbf{r}) \exp\,(i\mathbf{k}\cdot\mathbf{r}) \qquad , \tag{146}$$

where $\mathbf{k}$ is the wave vector and $u_k(\mathbf{r})$ is a function which has the periodicity of the lattice. The total wave function for each electron is then

$$\psi_k(\mathbf{r},\,\sigma) = \psi_k(\mathbf{r})\,\Phi_\sigma \qquad , \tag{147}$$

where Φ_σ is a spin function. In the following, E_k and $E_{k\sigma}$ will denote the eigenenergies of $\psi_k(\mathbf{r})$ and $\psi_k(\mathbf{r},\,\sigma)$, respectively. Since the electron-electron interactions have been approximated by a static potential, the electronic wave function of an N-electron metal is therefore an antisymmetrized product function constructed from the one-electron functions (Eq. (147)). The corresponding energies for a cubic lattice are

$$E_k = (\hbar k)^2\,/2m^* \tag{148}$$

where m^* is an effective mass defined by

$$m^* = \hbar^2 \left[\frac{\partial^2 E_k}{\partial k^2}\right]^{-1}. \tag{149}$$

One of the bulk electronic properties which plays a central role in the interpretation of many nuclear resonance experiments in metals is the Fermi energy E_F which is defined by the Fermi-Dirac distribution function

$$f_{k\sigma} = [\,\exp\,(E_{k\sigma} - E_F)\beta + 1]^{-1}. \tag{150}$$

The total number of electrons in a given band with spin σ is therefore

$$n_\sigma = \int_0^\infty dE_k\,N(E_k)\,f_{k\sigma} \qquad , \tag{151}$$

where $N(E_k)$ is the density of electronic states per unit energy interval, for one direction of the spin, at the energy E_k. In the absence of many-body effects the density of electronic states at the Fermi energy can be obtained from the low-temperature electronic specific heat C_e

$$N(E_F) = \tfrac{3}{2}\gamma\,(\pi k_B)^{-2} \qquad , \qquad \gamma = C_e/T \qquad , \tag{152}$$

which compares with the NFE prediction

$$N(E_F) = (2\pi m^*/\hbar^2)(3nV^2/\pi \mathscr{n}^2)^{\frac{1}{3}} \quad , \tag{153}$$

where n is the total number of electrons in the band, V is the molar volume, and $\mathscr{n}$ is Avogadro's number. The Pauli paramagnetic susceptibility (per atom) can be calculated from

$$\chi = \sum_k \chi_k = \tfrac{1}{2}(\gamma_e \hbar)^2 \, N(E_F) \quad . \tag{154}$$

The susceptibilities χ_k are nonzero only in the immediate vicinity of the Fermi level because of the complete spin pairing in all momentum states with energy appreciably lower than E_F.

2. Knight Shift

In simple metals the dominant coupling mechanism between nuclear and electronic spins is the Fermi contact interaction

$$\mathcal{H} = \tfrac{8}{3}\pi\gamma_n\gamma_e \hbar^2 \mathbf{I} \cdot \sum_i \mathbf{S}_i \, \delta(\mathbf{r}_i) \quad , \tag{155}$$

where the summation is over all conduction electrons and $\mathbf{r}_i$ is the position coordinate of the i'th electron. Using Eqs. (146) and (147) the static part of the hyperfine interaction is given by

$$\begin{aligned}
\mathcal{H}_0 &= \tfrac{8}{3}\pi\gamma_n\gamma_e \hbar^2 I^z \sum_{k,\sigma} |u_k(0)|^2 \, S^z f_{k\sigma} \\
&= -\tfrac{8}{3}\pi\gamma_n \hbar I^z H_0 \sum_k |u_k(0)|^2 \, \chi_k \quad .
\end{aligned} \tag{156}$$

However, we may assume that $|u_k(0)|$ and χ_k are essentially constant near E_F. Hence, the nucleus sees an effective hyperfine field

$$\Delta H = \tfrac{8}{3}\pi\langle |u(0)|^2 \rangle\chi H_0 \quad , \tag{157}$$

where the average is taken over all states at the Fermi level. The nuclear resonance frequency is therefore

$$\omega_0 = \gamma_n H_0 \, (1+K) \quad , \tag{158}$$

where K is the Knight shift parameter

$$K = \tfrac{8}{3}\pi \langle |u(0)|^2 \rangle \, \chi \equiv -(2/\gamma_e \hbar)H_{hfs}^{(s)}\chi \quad , \tag{159}$$

and $H_{hfs}^{(s)}$ is the average contact hyperfine field per electron at the

Fermi level. The Knight shift K has the following well-known properties: It is positive, independent of H_0, essentially independent of T, and increases with increasing atomic number.

3. Spin-Lattice Relaxation

The transverse part of the hyperfine interaction (Eq. (155)) induces transitions between states of the nuclear spin system. This process may be viewed as a spin-flip scattering of a conduction electron due to the contact interaction. The relevant transition matrix element is

$$\langle m'k'\sigma'|\mathcal{H}^{\pm}|mk\sigma\rangle = \tfrac{4}{3}\pi\gamma_e\gamma_n\hbar^2 \langle m'|I^{\mp}|m\rangle\langle k'\sigma'|S^{\mp}\delta(\mathbf{r})|k\sigma\rangle$$

$$= \tfrac{4}{3}\pi\gamma_e\gamma_n\hbar^2 \langle m'|I^{\pm}|m\rangle\langle\sigma'|S^{\mp}|\sigma\rangle u_{k'}^*(0)u_k(0) \quad .$$

$$(160)$$

The spin-lattice relaxation rate can now be calculated by combining Eqs. (17), (21) and (160).

$$1/T_1 = 2W = \frac{4\pi}{\hbar}\left(\frac{4\pi\gamma_e\gamma_n\hbar^2}{3}\right)^2 \sum_{kk'}\sum_{\sigma\sigma'} |u_k(0)|^2|u_{k'}(0)|^2$$

$$\times f_{k\sigma}(1 - f_{k'\sigma'})\,\delta(\Delta E) \quad . \tag{161}$$

At this point we can introduce two simplifications. In the first place the electronic and nuclear Zeeman energies can ordinarily be ignored in the delta function $\delta(\Delta E)$ since they are small compared to the kinetic energy of the electrons. It is therefore possible to let

$$f_{k\sigma}(1 - f_{k'\sigma'}) = -k_BT\frac{\partial f_k}{\partial E_k} = k_BT\,\delta(E_k - E_F) \quad . \tag{162}$$

In the second place we may assume that the electronic densities at the nucleus $|u_k(0)|^2$ are slowly varying functions of the energy. The sums in Eq. (161) can therefore be replaced by integrations over the energies E_k and $E_{k'}$. The result is

$$1/T_1 = \tfrac{64}{9}\pi^3\hbar^3\gamma_e^2\gamma_n^2 k_BT\left[N(E_F)\langle|u(0)|^2\rangle\right]^2$$

$$= 4\pi\gamma_n^2\hbar k_BT\left[N(E_F)H_{hfs}^{(s)}\right]^2 \quad . \tag{163}$$

The relaxation rate is seen to be directly proportional to the absolute temperature, i.e., the product $T_1 T$ is a constant. Moreover, at ordinary temperatures the conduction electron relaxation mechansim is far more effective than mechanisms involving other degrees of freedom of the "lattice".

4. Indirect Nuclear Spin-Spin Interactions

In addition to the single scatttering process which was discussed above one may have to consider higher order processes involving multiple scatterings. Consider, for example, the effect of a hyperfine-induced spin-flip scattering of a conduction electron at the i'th nucleus, followed by a second scattering at the j'th nucleus which returns the electron to its original state. This process leaves the total nuclear spin moment unchanged and hence does not contribute to spin-lattice relaxation; it does however contribute to the spin-spin relaxation and thus influences directly the NMR linewidth.(Ruderman and Kittel, 1954; Bloembergen and Rowland, 1955). The matrix element of Eq. (155) which connects the states $|k\rangle$ and $|k'\rangle$ is

$$A_{kk',i} I_i \cdot s \exp[i(k - k') \cdot r_i] \quad , \tag{164}$$

where

$$A_{kk',i} = \tfrac{8}{3} \pi \gamma_n \gamma_e \hbar^2 u_{k',i}^*(0) u_{k,i}(0) \quad . \tag{165}$$

The second order Hamiltonian which describes the double scattering is therefore given by

$$\mathcal{K}_{ij} = 4 J_{ij} (I_i \cdot s)(I_j \cdot s) \quad , \tag{166}$$

where

$$J_{ij} = \tfrac{1}{4} \sum_{kk'} \left\{ \frac{f_k A_{kk',i} A_{k'k,j} \exp[i(k - k') \cdot R_{ij}]}{E_k - E_{k'}} + C.C. \right\} . \tag{167}$$

The statistical factor f_k appears because only states which are initially occupied contribute to the indirect spin-spin interaction. In the NFE approximation (Eq. (148)) we obtain the usual Ruderman-Kittel coupling constant*

$$J_{ij} = (2/9\pi)\hbar^2 \gamma_{n,i} \gamma_{n,j} \gamma_e^2 m^* \langle |u_i(0)|^2 \rangle \langle |u_j(0)|^2 \rangle R_{ij}^{-4}$$

$$\times (x \cos x - \sin x) \quad , \tag{168}$$

*See Chap. 9 by R.E. Watson.

where $x = 2k_F R_{ij}$. For large separations R_{ij} the interaction is therefore proportional to $R_{ij}^{-3} \cos x$. Finally, we can eliminate the electronic spin operators in Eq. (166) by summing over all possible initial and final spin states (σ, σ'). The result is

$$\mathcal{K}_{ij} = J_{ij} \, \mathbf{I}_i \cdot \mathbf{I}_j \quad , \tag{169}$$

which has the form of an exchange interaction. We note that the exchange constant J_{ij} is directly proportional to the product of the average hyperfine coupling constants of the two nuclei. Hence, J_{ij} is expected to increase strongly with increasing atomic number. For example, in silver ($Z = 47$) the strength of the indirect interaction is slightly smaller than that of the direct dipolar interaction. In thallium ($Z = 81$), on the other hand, the indirect coupling is much stronger than the dipolar coupling.

The effect of the indirect spin-spin interaction on the observed NMR lineshape depends on whether the interacting nuclear spins have like or unlike resonance frequencies. If the frequencies are all identical, the linewidth is decreased (exchange narrowed) approximately in the ratio of the dipolar to indirect exchange interactions. Indirect couplings between unlike nuclear spins lead to a broadening of the line since the $I^+ I^-$ terms do not conserve energy in this case. It follows that broadening can also result from the indirect exchange coupling between like nuclear spins provided that the resonance is inhomogeneously broadened.

The magnitude of the Ruderman-Kittel indirect exchange constant is usually inferred from lineshape measurements. A direct determination is possible, however, if the inhomogeneous width of the NMR is sufficiently large that the difference between the resonance frequencies of nearest-neighbor nuclear spins exceeds J/h. Froidevaux and Weger (1964) showed that the decay of the spin-echo amplitude as a function of time separation τ between two exciting rf pulses is characterized in this case by a strong modulation. If the dipolar interaction is weak compared to the indirect interaction, the modulation is periodic in $J\tau$. In this way the nearest-neighbor exchange constant was measured for platinum in which the inhomogeneous broadening was produced by alloying with gold or iridium.

Indirect nuclear spin-spin interactions can also arise from anisotropic hyperfine interactions. The resulting pseudodipolar interactions always broaden the nuclear resonance.

5. Korringa Relation

We now return to an examination of the relationship

between the fractional resonance shift and spin-lattice relaxation rate. Combining Eqs. (159) and (163) we find an expression for the so-called Korringa product

$$K^2 T_1 T = (\pi \hbar^3 \gamma_n^2 \gamma_e^2 k_B)^{-1} [\chi/N(E_F)]^2 \quad . \tag{170}$$

In the independent particle approximation the spin susceptibility is given by Eq. (154). Therefore Eq. (170) reduces to

$$K^2 T_1 T = \hbar \gamma_e^2 (4\pi \gamma_n^2 k_B)^{-1} \quad , \tag{171}$$

which is clearly independent of the electronic structure of the metal. According to the above model it should be possible to calculate the spin-lattice relaxation rate if the Knight shift is known. Table III illustrates the degree to which the Korringa relation is

Table III. Comparison of experimental spin-lattice relaxation times for the alkali and noble metals with values calculated from the measured Knight shifts using the Korringa relation.

Metal	K(%)	$T_1 T$ (exp.) (sec °K)	$T_1 T$ (Korringa) (sec °K)
^{7} Li	0.0263	45 ± 2	26
^{23} Na	0.112	4.8 ± 0.1	3.1
^{85} Rb	0.650	0.81 ± 0.08	0.63
^{133} Cs	1.47	0.13 ± 0.01	0.069
^{63} Cu	0.232	0.9 ± 0.2	0.7
^{109} Ag	0.522	9 ± 1	4.5
^{197} Au	1.4	4.0 ± 0.5	4.5

obeyed in metals where the neglect of non-contact interactions should be most valid. The observed relaxation times are appreciably longer than predicted by the Korringa relation (except in gold where the nuclear moment, however, is not known with sufficent accuracy to permit any definite conclusions). If non-contact interactions were important (which is unlikely) the agreement would become even poorer, since such interactions would contribute primarily to the relaxation and not to the Knight shift in these cubic metals.

6. Collective Electron Effects.

The above discrepancies are believed to arise from electron-electron interactions which affect both the Knight shift (Pines, 1954) and the relaxation rate (Moriya, 1963). Electron-phonon interactions, on the other hand, have no direct effect on the Korringa product since they enhance the total quasi particle density at E_F (and thus the "electronic" specific heat) but have little influence on the magnetic susceptibility. The density of states which appears in the theory of nuclear spin-lattice relaxation (Eq. (163)), however, refers to the "bare" electronic density. Electron-phonon effects are therefore only of importance in the present case when attempts are made to evaluate the enhancement of the spin susceptibility by comparing calculated susceptibilities with values obtained from the specific heat (Eq. (154)).

a. Magnetic Susceptibility: We wish to evaluate the linear response function for a system of conduction electrons for a general wave number (q) and frequency (w) dependent magnetic perturbation. We assume that the screening radius is sufficiently small that the interelectronic Coulomb potential may be approximated by a delta function. Hence, the Fourier coefficients of the potential are simply $V(q) = v \equiv$ constant. In the random phase approximation the weak-field susceptibility is isotropic and is given by

$$\chi(q, w) = \chi_0(q, w) \left[1 - \zeta \chi_0 (q, w) \right]^{-1} \quad . \tag{172}$$

In this approximation the enhancement of the independent particle susceptibility $\chi_0(q, w)$ due to the opposing effects of exchange and correlation is described by a single parameter

$$\zeta = (v/\gamma_e^2 \hbar^2) \quad . \tag{173}$$

In general $\chi(q, w)$ is complex since $\chi_0(q, w) = \chi_0'(q, w) - i\chi_0''(q, w)$. Substituting this form into Eq. (172) yields

$$\chi'(q, w) = \chi_0'(q, w) \left\{ \frac{[1 - \zeta\chi_0'(q, w)] - \zeta[\chi_0''(q, w)]^2}{[1 - \zeta\chi_0'(q, w)]^2 + [\zeta\chi_0''(q, w)]^2} \right\}, \tag{174}$$

$$\chi''(q, w) = \chi_0''(q, w) \left\{ \frac{1}{[1 - \zeta\chi_0'(q, w)]^2 + [\zeta\chi_0''(q, w)]^2} \right\} . \tag{175}$$

Moreover, according to first order perturbation theory

$$\chi_0'(q, \omega) = \tfrac{1}{2}(\gamma_e \hbar)^2 \, \mathcal{P} \sum_k (f_{k+q} - f_k)(E_k - E_{k+q} + \hbar\omega)^{-1}, \quad (176)$$

$$\chi_0''(q, \omega) = \frac{\pi}{2} (\gamma_e \hbar)^2 \sum_k (f_{k+q} - f_k) \, \delta \, (E_k - E_{k+q} + \hbar\omega). \quad (177)$$

The above results may be simplified since we are interested only in nuclear resonance frequencies. Since the NMR frequencies are far below the characteristic resonance frequencies of the electronic spin system, the quantities inside the curly brackets of Eqs. (174) and (175) may be evaluated in the limit $\omega \to 0$. From Eqs. (176) and (177) we find

$$\lim_{\omega \to 0} \chi_0'(q, \omega) = \chi_0(0, 0) \, F(q) \quad , \quad\quad\quad (178)$$

$$\lim_{\omega \to 0} \chi_0''(q, \omega) = 0 \quad , \quad\quad\quad (179)$$

where $F(q)$ is the linear dielectric function which for a spherical Fermi surface has the form*

$$F(q) = \tfrac{1}{2} \left[1 + \frac{4k_F^2 - q^2}{4k_F q} \ln \left| \frac{2k_F + q}{2k_F - q} \right| \right] . \quad (180)$$

Thus, for low frequencies Eqs. (174) and (175) reduce to

$$\chi'(q, \omega) \approx \chi_0(0, 0) \, F(q) \, [\, 1 - \alpha F(q)]^{-1} \quad , \quad\quad (181)$$

$$\chi''(q, \omega) \approx \chi_0''(q, \omega) \, [\, 1 - \alpha F(q)]^{-2} \quad , \quad\quad (182)$$

where

$$\alpha = \zeta \chi_0(0, 0) \quad\quad\quad\quad (183)$$

    b. <u>Knight Shift</u>: The resonance shift is proportional to the static susceptibility $\chi(0, 0)$. Substituting Eq. (178) into (159) yields (since $F(0) = 1$)

$$K = -(2/\gamma_e \hbar) \, H_{hfs}^{(s)} \, \chi_0(0, 0) \, (1 - \alpha)^{-1} = K_0 (1 - \alpha)^{-1}, \quad (184)$$

where K_0 is the shift for $\zeta = 0$.

    c. <u>Spin-Lattice Relaxation</u>: Although the influence of electron-electron interactions on the Knight shift has long been recognized, their effect on the relaxation rate has been largely

*

ignored. In the presence of electron-electron interactions Eq. (163) is no longer valid since its derivation was based on the one-electron Bloch states (Eq. (146)). We can make use of the susceptibilities calculated above by basing the calculation of the transition probability on Eq. (19) instead of the first-order time-dependent perturbation result (Eq. (18). In this way an explicit knowledge of the eigenstates of the many-electron system is not required. In the present case $G_{ij}(\tau)$ is an even function and Eq. (19) may therefore be written as

$$W = \frac{1}{\hbar^2} \int_{-\infty}^{+\infty} d\tau \, \langle \{ \mathcal{H}^+(\tau)\mathcal{H}^-(0) \} \rangle \, \cos(\omega_0 \tau) \quad . \quad (185)$$

The transition probability is therefore proportional to the fluctuation density of the electron-nuclear coupling at the nuclear resonance frequency ω_0. Using Eqs. (155) and (165) we find

$$1/T_1 = \tfrac{1}{2}\gamma_n^2 \sum_q |A_q|^2 \int_{-\infty}^{+\infty} d\tau \, \langle \{ S_q^+(\tau)S_{-q}^-(0) \} \rangle \, \cos(\omega_0 \tau) , \quad (186)$$

where S_q is the Fourier transform of S_i and $A_q = A_{k, k+q}$ is assumed to depend on q but not on k. The latter is a reasonable assumption since only q's which span the Fermi surface are expected to contribute significantly to the relaxation. We can now use the fluctuation-dissipation theorem to express the spin correlation function in Eq. (186) in terms of the imaginary part of the transverse magnetic susceptibility. A general statement of this theorem is

$$J(q, \omega) = \frac{\hbar \chi''(q, \omega)}{2\omega} \left[\frac{\exp(-\beta\hbar\omega) + 1}{\exp(-\beta\hbar\omega) - 1} \right] , \quad (187)$$

which relates the spectral density $J(q, \omega)$ of the equilibrium fluctuations of a system to its linear response $\chi''(q, \omega)$ to an external perturbation. Since the susceptibility is assumed to be isotropic. Eqs. (186) and (187) yield in the high temperature limit $(\hbar\omega_0 \ll k_B T)$

$$1/T_1 = 2\gamma_n^2 k_B T \, (\gamma_e \hbar)^{-2} \sum_q |A_q|^2 \omega_0^{-1} \chi''(q, \omega_0) \quad . \quad (188)$$

Substituting Eq. (177) and (182) in Eq. (188) gives, after a straight forward calculation

$$1/T_1 = 4\pi\gamma_n^2 \hbar k_B T \left[N(E_F) H_{hfs}^{(s)} \right]^2 \langle [1 - \alpha F(q)]^{-2} \rangle$$

$$= (T_1^{-1})_0 \langle [1 - \alpha F(q)]^{-2} \rangle \qquad . \tag{189}$$

The average is taken over all q's which connect states at the Fermi level (i.e., for a spherical Fermi surface $0 \le q \le 2k_F$). The enhancement of the relaxation rate $(T_1^{-1})_0$ is generally smaller than that of K_0^2 because F(q) decreases for free electrons with increasing q.

d. <u>Korringa Relation</u>: According to Eqs. (184) and (189) the corrected Korringa product is

$$K^2 T_1 T = \hbar\gamma_e^2 (4\pi\gamma_n^2 k_B)^{-1} [K(\alpha)]^{-1} \qquad , \tag{190}$$

where

$$K(\alpha) = (1 - \alpha)^2 \langle [1 - \alpha F(q)]^{-2} \rangle \qquad . \tag{191}$$

For a spherical Fermi surface

$$K(\alpha) = 2(1 - \alpha)^2 \int_0^1 dx\, x[1 - \alpha F(x)]^{-2} \quad , \tag{192}$$

where $x = q/2k_F$ and F(x) is defined by Eq. (180). The functional dependence of $K(\alpha)$ on α for the spherical case is shown in Fig. 9.

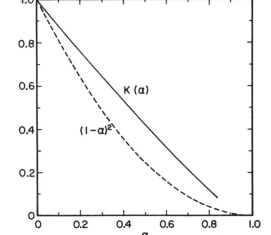

Fig. 9: Plot of $(1 - \alpha)^2$ and $K(\alpha)$ as a function of the enhancement factor α.

The magnitude of α can be estimated by comparing experimental values of $K^2 T_1 T$ with the collective electron expressions derived above. The usual approach has consisted of considering only the static effect of α. In this case the modification of the Korringa product is given by the factor $(1 - \alpha)^{-2}$. If the dynamic effects are also included, somewhat larger values of α are required to obtain agreement between calculated and observed Korringa products since $1 < K(\alpha)^{-1} < (1 - \alpha)^{-2}$ for metals with spherical Fermi surfaces. This difference is illustrated for representative metals in Table IV. Also listed are values of α_P and α_E obtained from a comparison of theoretical (Pines, 1955) and experimental (Schumacher and Slichter, 1956) spin susceptibilities,

Table IV: Summary of enhancement factors (α) associated with collective electron effects. The first two columns list enhancement factors which were obtained by fitting $(1 - \alpha)^2$ and $K(\alpha)$ to the experimental Korringa products, respectively.

Metal	α_K		α_P	α_E
	$(1 - \alpha)^2$	$K(\alpha)$		
^{7}Li	0.24	0.36	0.37	0.44
^{23}Na	0.20	0.30	0.24	0.3
^{85}Rb	0.12	0.19	0.15	
^{109}Ag	0.29	0.43	0.32	

respectively, with the corresponding NFE susceptibilities (Eqs. (153) and (154)). The latter were based on effective masses computed by the quantum defect method. The experimental spin susceptibilities were obtained from a comparison of the areas under the conduction-electron and nuclear spin resonances. Both measurements were carried out at the same frequency w_0. According to Eq. (30) the area under the resonance is given for a narrow line by

$$\int_0^\infty dw \chi''(0, w) = \tfrac{1}{2} \pi w_0 \chi'(0, w_0) \approx \tfrac{1}{2} \pi w_0 \chi(0, 0) . \qquad (193)$$

Since the nuclear susceptibility is easily calculated using Boltzmann statistics, the ratio of the areas gives an absolute measure of the static electron spin susceptibility. A direct determination of the spin susceptibility in simple metals is not feasible, of course, because of interference from diamagnetic contributions to the bulk susceptibility which are of comparable magnitude.

The over-all agreement shown in Table IV is quite

encouraging and suggests that the Korringa derived values of α can be used together with Eq. (184) to obtain reasonably reliable values of $H_{hfs}^{(s)}$ from the experimental Knight shift. Thus, if the free-atom hyperfine fields are known, the ratio $\xi = \langle |u(0)|^2 \rangle_{metal} / \langle |u|(0)|^2 \rangle_{atom}$ can be computed. For example for lithium we obtain $\xi = 0.49$. This is in satisfactory agreement with the result of a direct measurement $\xi = 0.442 \pm 0.015$ based on the hyperfine induced shift of the conduction electron resonance (Ryter, 1960).

B. Transition Metals.

1. Physical Properties.

Transition metals are characterized by partially filled d bands which are usually quite narrow and therefore have a high density of states at the Fermi level. The d bands usually overlap with a much wider s band. Since the d electrons are quite localized compared to free electrons, a useful description of the conduction band states of transition metals is provided by the tight-binding approximation in which the Bloch functions are constructed from atomic orbitals.

$$\psi_{\mu k \sigma}(\mathbf{r}) = N^{-\frac{1}{2}} \sum_{\mathbf{R}} \exp{(i\mathbf{k} \cdot \mathbf{R})} \, a_{\mu k}(\mathbf{r} - \mathbf{R}) \, \Phi_\sigma \quad , \tag{194}$$

where μ is a band index, $\mathbf{R}$ denotes the atomic coordinates and $a_{\mu k}(\mathbf{r} - \mathbf{R})$ are LCAO functions defined by

$$a_{\mu k}(\mathbf{r} - \mathbf{R}) = \sum_{m} c_{\mu m k} \, \Phi_m(\mathbf{r} - \mathbf{R}) \quad , \tag{195}$$

where $\Phi_m(\mathbf{r} - \mathbf{R})$ are atomic functions which form bases for irreducible representations of the appropriate crystal point group. The $c_{\mu m k}$ are elements of a unitary transformation. Hence

$$\sum_{\mu} c_{\mu m k} c_{\mu m' k} = \delta_{mm'} \tag{196}$$

$$\sum_{m} c_{\mu m k} \, c_{\mu' m k} = \delta_{\mu \mu'} \quad . \tag{197}$$

The advantage of the tight-binding model lies in the fact that it leads to analytical expressions for the nuclear resonance shifts and relaxation rates. Of course, one might question the validity of the tight-binding model for the interpretation of nuclear resonance data since this model is usually not capable of yielding accurate band structures. Fortunately, hyperfine interactions depend most strongly on the behavior of the wave function near the nucleus. In this region the conduction-electron wave functions are expected to resemble the free-atom functions. For this reason the tight-binding model provides a reasonably reliable method for parameterizing the dependence of the hyperfine interaction on the conduction electron properties.

The simplest model of transition metals assumes that the s and d bands are distinguishable at the Fermi level. Since the variation with energy of the density of states of an s band (i.e., the NFE band) is much slower than that of a narrow d band, it has been common practice to assume that the number of electrons (n_s) in the s band lies in the range $\sim 0.2 - 1$. The contribution of the s band to the total hyperfine interaction can then be estimated by means of the free-electron density of states using Eq. (153) with $m^* = m$ and $n = n_s$. In most cases, however, this is a dangerous approximation because the crystal potential may produce strong s-d mixing in regions of k space where the bands overlap. If the s-d mixing is significant, it is useful to characterize the states at the Fermi level by their average fractional s and d character. Correspondingly, one may define fractional s and d densities such that

$$N(E_F) = N_s(E_F) + N_d(E_F) \quad . \tag{198}$$

The ratio $N_s(E_F)/N_d(E_F)$ will depend, in general, on the details of the band structure.

If spin-orbit interactions are not too important, the total magnetic susceptibility of a transition metal can be partitioned into spin and orbital contributions.

$$\chi = \chi_s + \chi_d + \chi_{VV} + \chi_L + \chi_{dia} \quad . \tag{199}$$

The first two terms in Eq. (199) are the s- and d-spin susceptibilities, respectively, which can be related by means of Eq. (154) to the corresponding effective state densities $N_s(E_F)$ and $N_d(E_F)$. The third term (χ_{VV}) is the field-induced orbital paramagnetic susceptibility which arises from the orbital degeneracy of the atomic d states. This term is analogous to the temperature independent Van Vleck susceptibility in magnetic insulators and is given in the tight-binding approximation by

$$\chi_{VV} = \tfrac{1}{4}(\gamma_e \hbar)^2 \sum_k \sum_{\mu\mu'} \left[\frac{f_{\mu k} - f_{\mu'k}}{E_{\mu'k} - E_{\mu k}} \right] |\langle \mu'k| L |\mu k\rangle|^2 \, . \tag{200}$$

Finally, we need to consider the Landau diamagnetic susceptibility of the conduction electrons

$$\chi_L = -\tfrac{1}{2}(\gamma_e \hbar)^2 \, N(E_F) \, (m^2/3m^{*2}) \quad , \tag{201}$$

and the diamagnetic susceptibility due to the ion cores

$$\chi_{dia} = -(e^2/6mc^2) \sum_i \langle r_i^2 \rangle \, . \tag{202}$$

Because of the high density of states at the Fermi level, the paramagnetic contributions to χ in transition metals are much larger than $\chi_L + \chi_{dia}$. This is in contrast to the situation in simple metals where the diamagnetic terms usually dominate. In practice, the individual contributions to χ cannot be calculated from first principles because of insufficient knowledge about the conduction electron states. One of the important applications of nuclear resonance in transition metals therefore involves the partitioning of χ into its various parts on the basis of the measured resonance shifts and relaxation times.

In the above discussion no mention was made of possible p contributions to the conduction electron wave function near E_F. This omission is justified because p hyperfine interactions in metals are weak in comparison to s and d interactions. It is convenient therefore to treat the p admixture as part of an effective s density of states. The s-electron contact hyperfine field is consequently reduced in proportion to the fractional p character.

2. Knight Shift

The important contributions to the total resonance shift (K) are associated with the three paramagnetic contributions to the magnetic susceptibility. The hyperfine Hamiltonian may be written as

$$\mathcal{K} = \gamma_n \gamma_e \hbar^2 \, \mathbf{I} \cdot \theta \quad , \tag{203}$$

where θ operates on the one-electron spin (s) and orbital angular momentum (ℓ) coordinates. Using an obvious notation

$$\theta = \theta_s + \theta_d + \theta_{orb} \quad , \tag{204}$$

where

$$\theta_s = (2/\gamma_e \hbar)\, H_{hfs}^{(s)}\, s_s \quad , \tag{205}$$

$$\theta_d = (2/\gamma_e \hbar)\, H_{hfs}^{(d)}\, s_d \quad , \tag{206}$$

$$\theta_{orb} = \langle r^{-3} \rangle \ell = (\gamma_e \hbar)^{-1}\, H_{hfs}^{(orb)}\, \ell \quad . \tag{207}$$

The Knight shift therefore becomes

$$K = K_s + K_d + K_{orb}$$

$$= -(2/\gamma_e \hbar) \left[H_{hfs}^{(s)} \chi_s + H_{hfs}^{(d)} \chi_d + H_{hfs}^{(orb)} \chi_{VV} \right], \tag{208}$$

where $H_{hfs}^{(s)}$ and $H_{hfs}^{(d)}$ are the effective s-contact and d-spin (core-polarization) hyperfine fields per electron, respectively, and $H_{hfs}^{(orb)}$ is the orbital hyperfine field per unit orbital angular momentum. Since $H_{hfs}^{(d)}$ is negative while $H_{hfs}^{(s)}$ and $H_{hfs}^{(orb)}$ are positive, the total shift in transition metals may be of either sign.

3. Spin-Lattice Relaxation

The three hyperfine interactions which determine the Knight shift also contribute separately to spin-lattice relaxation (Korringa, 1950; Yafet and Jaccarino, 1964; Obata, 1963). In exceptional cases magnetic dipole and electric quadrupole interactions with conduction electrons may also contribute measurably to the relaxation (Obata, 1963, 1964; Narath and Alderman, 1966). In the absence of many-body effects, the magnetic interactions yield

$$1/T_1 = (\pi/\hbar)(\gamma_n \gamma_e \hbar^2)^2 \sum_{\mu\mu'} \sum_{kk'} \sum_{\sigma\sigma'} |\langle \mu'k'\sigma'|\,\theta\,|\mu k\sigma\rangle|^2$$

$$\times f_{\mu k\sigma}(1 - f_{\mu'k'\sigma'})\,\delta(\Delta E) \quad . \tag{209}$$

The matrix elements in Eq. (209) can be evaluated in the tight-binding approximation (Eq. (194)). Retaining only matrix elements for which $R = R'$, and neglecting the Zeeman terms in $\delta(\Delta E)$ as before, Eq. (209) becomes

$$1/T_1 = (\pi/\hbar N^2)(\gamma_n \gamma_e \hbar^2)^2 k_B T \sum_{\mu\mu'} \sum_{kk'} \sum_{\sigma\sigma'} \delta(E_{\mu k} - E_{\mu' k'})$$

$$\times \quad \delta(E_{\mu k} - E_F)$$

$$\times \sum_{m_1 m_2 m_3 m_4} c_{\mu m_1 k}{}^{c*} c_{\mu m_3 k}{}^{c} c_{\mu' m_2 k'}{}^{c*} c_{\mu' m_4 k'}$$

$$\times \langle m_2 \sigma' | \theta^- | m_1 \sigma \rangle \langle m_4 \sigma' | \theta^+ | m_3 \sigma \rangle \qquad . \qquad (210)$$

This expression can be simplified using straight-forward group-theoretical arguments. Since the $|m\rangle$ form bases of irreducible representations of the crystal point group, one can show that

$$c_{\mu m(Gk)} = \sum_{m'=\Gamma(m)} c_{\mu m' k} D^{\Gamma}_{m'm}(G) \qquad , \qquad (211)$$

where G is an operation of the point group, $m' = \Gamma(m)$ means all m' belonging to the same irreducible representation Γ as m, and $D^{\Gamma}_{m'm}(G)$ are elements of the appropriate transformation matrix. Since k vectors which are related by the operations of the point-group correspond to identical energies, we can use Eq. (211) together with the standard orthogonality relation

$$\sum_G D^{\Gamma}_{m'_1 m_1}(G) D^{\Gamma}_{m'_2 m_2}(G) = \delta_{m_1 m_2} \delta_{m'_1 m'_2} (\ell/\ell(\Gamma)) \quad , \quad (212)$$

where ℓ is the order of the group and $\ell(\Gamma)$ is the dimensionality of the representation, to obtain

$$1/T_1 = (\pi/\hbar N^2)(\gamma_n \gamma_e \hbar^2)^2 k_B T \sum_{\mu\mu'} \sum_{kk'} \sum_{\sigma\sigma'} \delta(E_{\mu k} - E_{\mu' k'})$$

$$\times \quad \delta(E_{\mu k} - E_F)$$

$$\times \sum_{m_1 m_2} F_{\mu k}[\Gamma(m_1)] F_{\mu' k'}[\Gamma(m_2)]$$

$$\times \quad |\langle m_2 \sigma' | \theta^- | m_1 \sigma \rangle|^2 \quad . \qquad (213)$$

Here $F_{\mu k}[\Gamma(m)] \equiv |c_{\mu m k}|^2$ are fractional admixture coefficients which have the same value for all m belonging to a given representation $\Gamma(m)$. By defining average values of $F_{\mu k}[\Gamma(m)]$

according to

$$F[\Gamma(m)] = \left[\sum_{\mu k} F_{\mu k}[\Gamma(m)] \, \delta(E_{\mu k} - E_F)\right] N(E_F)^{-1} , \quad (214)$$

we can write Eq. (213) in the form

$$1/T_1 = (\pi/\hbar N^2)(\gamma_n \gamma_e \hbar^2)^2 \, k_B T [N(E_F)]^2$$

$$\times \sum_{m_1 m_2} \sum_{\sigma \sigma'} F[\Gamma(m_1)] \, F[\Gamma(m_2)] |\langle m_2 \sigma' | \theta^- | m_1 \sigma \rangle|^2 . \quad (215)$$

Comparing Eq. (215) with Eq. (163) we note that the $F[\Gamma(m)]$ factors (which are normalized to unity) tend to inhibit relaxation. For a given static hyperfine interaction the d electron relaxation processes are therefore less effective than the s electron process. The density of states in Eq. (215) refers to the bare-electron density, which may be significantly smaller than the density computed from the electronic specific heat if electron-phonon effects are important. Finally, we need to evaluate the matrix elements of θ^- in the atomic basis $|m \sigma\rangle$. Since spin-orbit interactions were assumed to be negligible, there are no interference terms between spin and orbital contributions to the relaxation.

a. <u>Cubic Symmetry</u>: For this case Eq. (215) reduces to

$$1/T_1 = 4\pi \gamma_n^2 \hbar \, k_B T [N(E_F)]^2 \left\{ \left[\rho H_{hfs}^{(s)}\right]^2 + \left[(1-\rho)H_{hfs}^{(d)}\right]^2 q \right.$$

$$\left. + \left[(1-\rho)H_{hfs}^{(orb)}\right]^2 p \right\} , \quad (216)$$

where

$$\rho = N_s(E_F)/N(E_F) , \quad (217)$$

and q and p are reduction factors which depend only on the relative weights at the Fermi level of the irreducible representations of the atomic d functions. Since the s functions transform as the Γ_1 representation ($\ell(\Gamma) = 1$) while the d functions transform as the Γ_3 ($\ell(\Gamma) = 2$) and Γ_5 ($\ell(\Gamma) = 3$) representations of the cubic point group (O) there are no interference terms between s and d relaxation mechanisms even in the presence of s-d mixing. The factors inhibiting d-spin and orbital relaxation processes are found to be

$$q = \tfrac{1}{3} [f(\Gamma_5)]^2 + \tfrac{1}{2}[1 - f(\Gamma_5)]^2 , \quad (218)$$

$$p = \tfrac{2}{3} f(\Gamma_5)[\, 2 - \tfrac{5}{3} f(\Gamma_5)] \qquad , \qquad (219)$$

where $f(\Gamma_5)$ is the relative weight of the Γ_5 representation

$$f(\Gamma_5) = \ell^{\Gamma_5} [\, 1 - \rho]^{-1} F[\Gamma_5] = 3[\, 1 - \rho]^{-1} F[\Gamma_5] \quad . \quad (220)$$

The strong dependence of q and p on $f(\Gamma_5)$ is illustrated in Fig. 10.

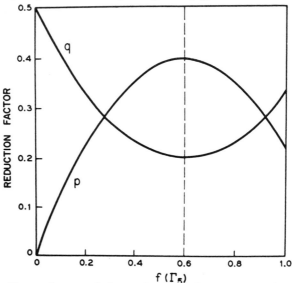

Fig. 10: Dependence of the reduction factors p and q on the average fractional admixture $f(\Gamma_5)$ of the Γ_5 d orbitals at
the Fermi level. An equal contribution from all five
orbitals corresponds to $f(\Gamma_5) = \tfrac{3}{5}$.

Fortunately the sum of d-spin and orbital relaxation rates is not
strongly dependent on $f(\Gamma_5)$ because the two hyperfine fields are
usually of approximately equal magnitude so that the effects of
variations in p and q compensate each other.

It should be pointed out that the orbital hyperfine field in
Eq. (216) represents an average over the Fermi surface, while
the corresponding field in Eq. (208) is a weighted average over
all states which contribute to χ_{VV}. Hence, the two fields need
not be identical. In practice, of course, this difference is always
neglected. We have also assumed that the hyperfine coupling
constant is the same for all d orbitals, regardless to which symmetry type they belong. These approximations are necessary in
order to keep the number of unknown parameters at a reasonable
level.

b. Hexagonal Symmetry: The appropriate point group for this case is D_6 which splits the orbital degeneracy of the d functions into $\Gamma_1(\ell^{\Gamma}=1)$, $\Gamma_5(\ell\,\Gamma=2)$, and $\Gamma_6(\ell^{\Gamma}=2)$ representations. If s-d mixing can be neglected, the relaxation rate is again given by Eq. (216) but with

$$q = \left\{1 - 2[\,f(\Gamma_5) + f(\Gamma_6)] + \tfrac{3}{2}\,[\,f(\Gamma_5)^2 + f(\Gamma_6)^2\,] + 2f(\Gamma_5)f(\Gamma_6)\right\} ,$$
(221)

$$p = \left\{3f(\Gamma_6)[\,1 - f(\Gamma_6) - \tfrac{2}{3}f(\Gamma_5)]\right\} ,$$
(222)

where the $f(\Gamma)$ factors are defined by Eq. (220) with $\ell^{\Gamma}=2$. If the five d functions are equally represented at the Fermi level, we find $q = 0.2$ and $p = 0.4$ as in the cubic case. If s-d mixing occurs for the Γ_1 functions, we must consider an additional contribution

$$(1/T_1)_{s-d} = 8\pi \gamma_n^2\,\hbar k_B T[\,N(E_F)]^2\,H_{hfs}^{(s)}\,H_{hfs}^{(d)}$$
$$\times \langle \rho(1-\rho)[\,1 - f(\Gamma_5) - f(\Gamma_6)]\rangle$$
(223)

which interferes destructively with Eq. (216) provided that $H_{hfs}^{(d)}$ is negative.

4. Comparison with Experiment

In this section we illustrate briefly some of the complexities which are encountered in the interpretation of Knight shift and spin-lattice relaxation data for transition metals. It is obvious that no Korringa-like relation exists between the Knight shift and the relaxation rate. In other words, the product $K^2 T_1 T$ is not independent of the details of the total hyperfine interaction, even if collective electron effects are ignored, as can be seen by comparing Eqs. (208) and (216).

a. Molybdenum, Tungsten: These metals have six valence electrons $(n=6)$ per atom and are characterized by unusually small electronic specific heat coefficients and nearly temperature independent magnetic susceptibilities which are about four times larger than predicted by the measured specific heat. Because of the small magnitude of $N(E_F)$ many-body effects are expected to be relatively unimportant. The transition metal character of these metals is strikingly evidenced by the observation of very large values of $K^2 T_1 T$. For example, the measured Knight shift of $+1.06\%$ in tungsten leads to a Korringa prediction of $T_1 T = 1.3$ sec$^\circ$K, while the observed value is 37 ± 2 sec$^\circ$K (Narath and Fromhold, 1965). The various contributions to K and

$T_1 T$ have been determined by applying the formalism derived above to the NMR data using independent estimates of the relevant hyperfine fields. The results for molybdenum are shown in Table V for two possible values of $f(\Gamma_5)$ (Narath and Alderman, 1966).

Table V: Summary of conduction-electron contributions to the ^{95}Mo hyperfine fields, spin-lattice relaxation rates, and Knight shifts in molybdenum metal.

	$H_{hfs}(10^6 \text{ Oe})$	$(T_1 T)^{-1}$ $[\,10^{-2}(\sec {}^{\circ})^{-1}\,]$		$K(\%)$
		$f(\Gamma_5) = 1$	$f(\Gamma_5) = \frac{3}{5}$	
Contact	$+2.72$	1.56	1.36	0.09
Core-Polarization	-0.27	0.68	0.41	-0.11
Orbital	$+0.30$	0.56	1.03	$+0.59$
$N_s(E_F)(10^{11} \text{ erg}^{-1} \text{ atom}^{-1}) =$		0.20	0.18	
$N_d(E_F)(10^{11} \text{ erg}^{-1} \text{ atom}^{-1}) =$		2.25	2.27	

A fit to the observed relaxation rate was achieved by treating ρ in Eq. (216) as an adjustable parameter and using the specific heat derived value of $N(E_F)$. Agreement with the observed Knight shift was then obtained by adjusting χ_{VV}. The required orbital susceptibility has a magnitude which is about 80% of the experimental susceptibility. The nuclear resonance measurements therefore yield an explanation for the apparent discrepancy between χ (specific heat) and χ (observed). The NMR derived values of ρ and χ_{VV} are insensitive to the exact choice of $f(\Gamma_5)$. It is interesting to note that the largest contribution to the relaxation arises from the contact interaction, which is unusual in transition metals. The Knight shift on the other hand is dominated by the orbital interaction. The s density of states obtained from this analysis corresponds to an extremely small effective number of s electrons, $n_s = 0.013$. This result demonstrates the importance of s-d mixing in these metals.

The results for tungsten are very similar to those for molybdenum.

b. Vanadium-Chromium Alloys: These alloys demonstrate the variation of K and $T_1 T$ with changes in Fermi level in a system which can be described to a first approximation by a rigid band model (Drain, 1962; Butterworth, 1964). The experimental results for the ^{51}V resonance are compared in Fig. 11

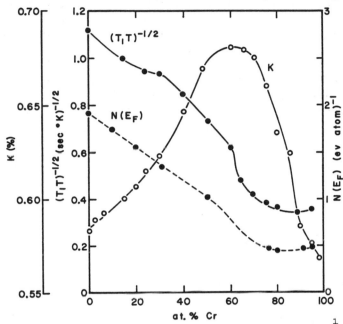

Fig. 11: Plot of the experimental values of K and $(T_1 T)^{-\frac{1}{2}}$ for ^{51}V and $N(E_F)$ calculated from the specific heat as a function of composition in the vanadium-chromium alloy system.

against the variation of $N(E_F)$ with composition. The experimental values of $(T_1 T)^{-\frac{1}{2}}$ track the density of states as would be expected if the d interactions dominate the relaxation. The Knight shift, however, exhibits a more complex behavior because the orbital magnetic susceptibility, and hence K_{orb}, is not related to $N(E_F)$. The initial increase of K on addition of chromium (n = 6) to vanadium (n = 5) is undoubtedly associated with a reduction in the negative core-polarization interaction. As $N(E_F)$ becomes small, however, the core-polarization shift loses importance and the orbital interaction becomes the dominant contributor to the total shift.

c. Palladium, Platinum: These metals (n = 10) have a nearly filled d band which is well separated from the s band at the Fermi level. The density of d states $N_d(E_F)$, as inferred from the specific heat, is very large in both metals. The magnetic susceptibilities are strongly enhanced by exchange effects and are temperature dependent due to a peak in N(E) near E_F. The temperature dependence is exaggerated by the exchange and is particularly large in palladium. Because of the large d-spin susceptibilities the Knight shifts are dominated by the core-polarization interaction and are consequently negative and temperature dependent. Furthermore, $dK/d\chi$ is negative as expected. Since s-d mixing is probably unimportant the slope of K vs. χ measures directly the d-spin hyperfine field. The results of a diagramatic analysis of the Knight shift data for palladium are illustrated in Fig. 12 (Seitchik et al., 1964) and are similar to those for platinum

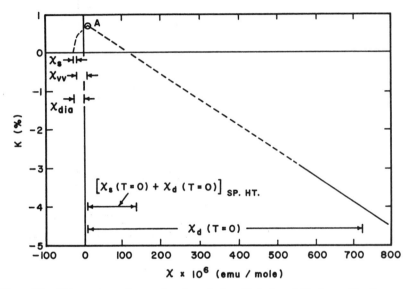

Fig. 12: Diagramatic analysis of the Knight shift in palladium
          metal. The solid portion of the diagram represents the
          experimental data (Clogston et al., 1964).

(Clogston et al., 1964). In this analysis the s-contact and d-orbital hyperfine fields were estimated. The s-band spin susceptibility χ_s was calculated in the free-electron approximation. (The number of electrons in the s band of palladium is known to be ~ 0.32.) The d-band susceptibility was then separated into spin and orbital contributions by extrapolating the experimental K vs. χ plot. Its intersection with the K_{orb} vs. χ portion of the diagram (marked A in Fig. 12) determines χ_d and χ_{vv}. This type of analysis is applicable when the d-spin susceptibility is the only temperature dependent term in χ and the s-electron contribution is either known or can be ignored. These conditions are unfortunately seldom satisfied. For example, in the hexagonal metals scandium, yttrium, and lanthanum the sign of $dK/d\chi$ is positive, indicating strong s-d mixing effects and/or a temperature dependent orbital susceptibility.

A comparison of observed and calculated spin-lattice relaxation rates for palladium and platinum, based on hyperfine fields determined from the Knight shift analysis and values of $N(E_F)$ obtained from the specific heat is shown in Table VI (Yafet and Jaccarino, 1964; Narath et al., 1966). The agreement for platinum

Table VI: Comparison of calculated and observed spin-lattice relaxation rates $(T_1 T)^{-1}$ in palladium and platinum metals. The rates in parenthesis correspond to $f(\Gamma_5) = \frac{3}{5}$, those without parenthesis to $f(\Gamma_5) = 1$. The units are $(\sec {}^{\circ}K)^{-1}$. Inclusion of the d-spin dipolar mechanism would increase the calculated rates by a small amount: $(T_1 T)^{-1}_{dip} = (T_1 T)^{-1}_{orb} \{ \frac{3}{98} [6(6f(\Gamma_5)^2 - 5f(\Gamma_5)^2)^{-1} - 1] \}$.

	^{105}Pd		^{195}Pt	
Contact	0.12		17.5	
Core-Polarization	0.15	(0.09)	18.1	(10.8)
Orbital	0.37	(0.66)	10.5	(19.0)
Predicted	0.64	(0.87)	46.1	(47.3)
Observed	9.1		34	

is quite good, particularly in view of the possible enhancement of the specific heat due to electron-phonon interactions. In the case of palladium, however, the agreement is very poor. It is possible that this discrepancy is associated with the enormous exchange enhancement of χ_d. The corresponding enhancement of the d-spin induced nuclear relaxation rate (Eq. (189)) may also be very large because of the cylindrical geometry of the major portion of the d band Fermi surface. This geometry leads to a much more gradual decrease in $F(q)$ for $|q| \leq 2k_F$ than is the case for a spherical surface. If $F(q) \approx 1$ throughout this range, the relaxation rate is enhanced by the factor $(1 - \alpha)^{-2}$ (Moriya, 1966).

d. Ferromagnetic Metals: In the ordered state the static hyperfine interaction can be extremely large as in the case of magnetic insulators. The spin-lattice relaxation, on the other hand, is determined at sufficiently low temperatures by the scattering of conduction electrons as in non-magnetic metals and is therefore not unusually rapid. This behavior is a consequence of the small number of thermal magnons at low temperatures. The collective excitations of the ordered spin system therefore contribute to the relaxation only at temperatures for which T/T_c is reasonably large. The resulting deviation from a constant $T_1 T$ behavior has been observed for dilute ^{55}Mn in iron (Kaplan et al., 1966b).

C. Rare-Earth Intermetallic Compounds

The interest in these compounds arises in part from the fact that the f electrons of rare-earth ions are highly localized. In the metallic state the localized f spins are exchange coupled to the conduction electron spins. This interaction leads to a coupling mechanism between the rare-earth ion spins S_j and the nuclear spins I_i of non-magnetic ions in the crystal which is analogous to the Ruderman-Kittel indirect exchange coupling between two nuclear spins. Using Eqs. (169) and (167) we can therefore write

$$\mathcal{H}_{ij} = -(4N)^{-1} I_i \cdot S_j \sum_{kk'} \left\{ {}_k^f A_{kk'}, {}_i^{} J_{k'k, j} \frac{\exp[i(k - k') \cdot R_{ij}]}{E_k - E_{k'}} \right.$$

$$\left. + \text{C.C.} \right\} \quad , \tag{224}$$

where $J_{k'k, j}$ are matrix elements of the exchange potential. In the following we assume that $A_{kk', i}$ is a constant and that $J_{kk', j}$ depends at most on* $q = k' - k$. We also assume that the rare-earth ions form a primitive lattice. Since the average value of S_j is the same at all rare-earth sites, we can calculate the total static effect on the nuclear spin by performing a sum over all S_j.

$$\mathcal{H}_i = \sum_j \mathcal{H}_{ij} = -A I^z \langle S^z \rangle \not{j}(r_i) \quad , \tag{225}$$

where

$$\not{j}(r_i) = \sum_G F(G) J(G) \cos (G \cdot r_i) \quad , \tag{226}$$

$\langle S^z \rangle$ is the average value of each rare-earth spin, G are reciprocal lattice vectors, and $F(G)$ is the dielectric function defined by Eqs. (176) and (178). The sign of $\not{j}(r_i)$ is therefore determined by the behavior of the product $F(G)J(G)$ for non-zero G. The interaction (Eq. (225)) is equivalent to an effective field acting on the nucleus

$$H(\mathbf{r}_i) = A(\gamma_n \hbar)^{-1} \langle S^z \rangle \, \mathcal{f}(\mathbf{r}_i) \quad . \tag{227}$$

The average value of S^z can be related to that of J^z ($J = L + S$) and therefore to the magnetic susceptibility χ of the rare-earth ions (in the paramagnetic state).

$$\langle S^z \rangle = \langle J^z \rangle \frac{\langle | \, S \cdot J | \rangle}{J(J+1)} = - \frac{H_0 \chi \langle | \, S \cdot J | \rangle}{\gamma_e \hbar J(J+1)} \quad . \tag{228}$$

According to Eqs. (227) and (228) the nuclear resonance is shifted by an amount which is a linear function of the external field. The fractional shift is

$$K_i = -A(\gamma_n \gamma_e \hbar^2)^{-1} \, \mathcal{f}(\mathbf{r}_i) \langle | \, S \cdot J | \rangle [J(J+1)]^{-1} \quad . \tag{229}$$

In the uniform polarization model only the $G = 0$ term is retained in $\mathcal{f}(\mathbf{r}_i)$. The interaction then becomes position independent. Except for the obvious convenience which it introduces, the only justification for this simplification is the experimental observation that the NMR shifts in rare-earth intermetallic compounds are always positive for less than half-filled f shells and negative for more than half-filled f shells. Since these two cases correspond to $\langle | \, S \cdot J | \rangle < 0$ and $\langle | \, S \cdot J | \rangle > 0$, respectively, the experimental values of $\mathcal{f}(\mathbf{r}_i)$ are therefore always negative (i.e., antiferromagnetic) which is somewhat surprising.*

Because of the linear dependence of K_i on χ the resonance shift exhibits a strong temperature dependence. For this reason measurements of the resonance shift provide a convenient method for determining the temperature dependence of the susceptibility. The advantage of this method lies in its lack of sensitivity to magnetic impurities which often interfere with direct bulk measurements. The ordinary Knight shift due to the Pauli spin susceptibility of the conduction electrons is usually very much smaller than the indirect shift and therefore introduces no uncertainty in the interpretation of the resonance data. A typical example of this approach is provided by the binary rare-earth phosphides, in which the variation of the ^{31}P shift K^{31} with temperature was found to obey a Curie-Weiss law, as shown in Fig. 13 (Jones, 1966b).

D. Superconductors

The transition from the normal metallic to the

*See also discussion by R.E. Watson in Chap. 9.

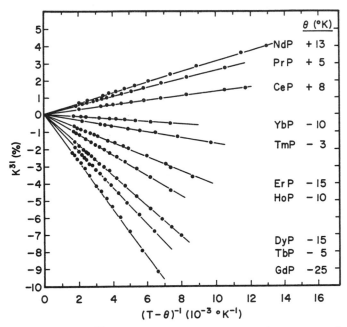

Fig. 13: Plot of the ^{31}P Knight shift for several rare-earth phosphides as a function of $(T - \theta)^{-1}$. The Curie-Weiss
constants θ were determined from a fit to the nuclear
resonance data.

superconducting state is accompanied by profound changes in the
nuclear resonance. In the first place the spin-induced Knight
shift is expected to be zero at T = 0 since the spin susceptibility
vanishes in the superconducting state at T = 0 as a result of spin
pairing in the superconducting ground state. Although the extremely small rf penetration depth makes Knight shift measurements in superconductors extremely difficult, this prediction
appears to be correct. The orbital Knight shift need not vanish,
of course.

The nuclear spin-lattice relaxation rate vanishes exponentially near T = 0 because the energy gap (2Δ) inhibits thermal
excitations from the ground state. The most interesting behavior
of the relaxation, however, occurs immediately below T_c. As
the temperature falls below T_c, the relaxation rate increases
quite sharply before falling as $\exp(-\Delta\beta)$ at low temperatures.
This striking behavior is a direct consequence of the coherence
between $k\sigma \rightarrow k'\sigma'$ and $-k-\sigma \rightarrow -k'-\sigma'$ scattering processes

predicted by the BCS theory. In the case of nuclear relaxation these two processes interfere constructively; i.e., the corresponding transition matrix elements must be added before squaring (Hebel and Slichter, 1959).

References

Benedek, G. B. and Kushida, T. (1960). Phys. Rev. 118, 46.

Bloembergen, N. and Rowland, T. J. (1955). Phys. Rev. 97, 1679.

Butterworth, J. (1964). Proc. Phys. Soc. (London) 83, 71.

Charap, S. H. and Boyd, E. L. (1964). Phys. Rev. 133, A811.

Clogston, A. M., Jaccarino, V., and Yafet, Y. (1964). Phys. Rev. 134, A650.

Davis, H. L. (1960). Phys. Rev. 120, 789.

Davis, H. L. and Narath, A. (1964). Phys. Rev. 134, A433.

Drain, L. E. (1962). J. Phys. Radium. 23, 745.

Froidevaux, C. and Weger, M. (1964). Phys. Rev. Letters 12, 123.

de Gennes, P. G. and Hartmann-Boutron, F. (1961). Compt. Rend. 253, 2922.

Gossard, A. C. and Portis, A. M. (1959). Phys. Rev. Letters 3, 164.

Gossard, A. C. and Portis, A. M. (1959). Phys. Rev. Letters 3, 164.

Gossard, A. C., Jaccarino, V., and Remeika, J. P. (1961). Phys. Rev. Letters 7, 122.

Gossard, A. C., Jaccarino, V., and Remeika, J. P. (1962). J. Appl. Phys. 33, 1187.

Hebel, L. C. and Slichter, C. P. (1959). Phys. Rev. 113, 1504.

Heeger, A. J. and Houston, T. W. (1964a). Proceedings of the International Conference on Magnetism, Nottingham, 395.

Heeger, A. J. and Houston T. W. (1964b). Phys. Rev. 135, A661.

Heeger, A. J. and Teaney, D. T. (1964). J. Appl. Phys. 35, 846.

Heller, P. and Benedek, G. B. (1962). Phys. Rev. Letters 8, 428.

Heller, P. (1966). Phys. Rev. 146, 403.

Holstein, T. and Primakoff, H. (1940). Phys. Rev. 58, 1098.

Huang, N. L., Orbach, R., and Simanek, E. (1966). Phys. Rev. Letters 17, 343.

Jaccarino, V. and Walker, L. R. (1959). quoted by Jaccarino, V. (1965). Magnetism, V. IIA, Academic Press, Inc., 307.

Jones, E. D. and Jefferts, K. (1964). Phys. Rev. 135, A1277.

Jones, E. D. (1966a). Phys. Rev. 151, 315.

Jones, E. D. (1966b). to be published, private communication.

Kaplan, N., Loudon, R., Jaccarino, V., Guggenheim, H. J., Beeman, D., and Pincus, P. A. (1966a). Phys. Rev. Letters 17, 357.

Kaplan, N., Jaccarino, V., and Wernick, J. H. (1966b). Phys. Rev. Letters 16, 1142.

Korringa, J. (1950). Physica 16, 601.

Lines, M. E., quoted by Jaccarino, V. (1965). Magnetism, V. IIA, Academic Press, Inc., 307.

Low, G. G. (1963). Proc. Phys. Soc. (London) 82, 992.

Moriya, T. (1956). Prog. Theoret. Phys. (Kyoto) 16, 23; ibid. 16, 641.

Moriya, T. (1963). J. Phys. Soc. Japan 18, 516.

Moriya, T. (1966). private communication.

Nakamura, T. (1958). Progr. Theoret. Phys. (Kyoto) 20, 542.

Narath, A. (1961). Phys. Rev. Letters 7, 410.

Narath, A. (1963). Phys. Rev. 131, 1929.

Narath, A. (1964). Phys. Rev. 136, A766.

Narath, A. (1965). Phys. Rev. 140, A854.

Narath, A. and Davis, H. L. (1965). Phys. Rev. 137, A163.

Narath, A. and Fromhold, Jr., A. T. (1965). Phys. Rev. 139, A794.

Narath, A. and Alderman, D. W. (1966). Phys. Rev. 143, 328.

Narath, A. and Fromhold, Jr., A. T. (1966). Phys. Rev. Letters 17, 354.

Narath, A., Fromhold, Jr., A. T., and Jones, E. D. (1966). Phys. Rev. 144, 428.

Obata, Y. (1963). J. Phys. Soc. Japan 18, 1020.

Obata, Y. (1964). J. Phys. Soc. Japan 19, 2348.

O'Sullivan, W. J., Robinson, W. A., and Simmons, W. W. (1961). Phys. Rev. 124, 1317.

Owen, J. and Taylor, D. R. (1966). Phys. Rev. Letters 16, 1164.

Pincus, P. (1966). Phys. Rev. Letters 16, 398.

Pines, D. (1954). Phys. Rev. 92, 626.

Pines, D. (1955). Solid State Physics, V. 1, Academic Press, Inc. 367.

Portis, A. M. and Gossard, A. C. (1960). J. Appl. Phys. 31, 205S.

Poulis, N. J. and Hardeman, G. E. G. (1952). Physica 18, 201; ibid. 18, 315.

Poulis, N. J., Hardeman, G. E. G., Van der Lugt, W., and Haas, W. P. A. (1958). Physica 24, 280.

Redfield, A. G. (1955). Phys. Rev. 98, 1787.

Ruderman, M. A. and Kittel, C. (1954). Phys. Rev. 96, 99.

Ryter, C. (1960). Phys. Rev. Letters 5, 10.

Seitchik, J. A., Gossard, A. C., and Jaccarino, V. (1964). Phys. Rev. 136, A1119.

Schumacher, R. T. and Slichter, C. P. (1956). Phys. Rev. 101, 58.

Shulman, R. G. and Jaccarino, V. (1957). Phys. Rev. 108, 1219.

Shulman, R. G. (1959). Phys. Rev. Letters 2, 459.

Shulman, R. G., and Knox, K. (1960). Phys. Rev. Letters 4, 603.

Spence, R. D. and Nagarajan, V. (1966). Phys. Rev. 149, 191.

Suhl, H. (1958). Phys. Rev. 109, 606.

Yafet, Y. and Jaccarino, V. (1964). Phys. Rev. 133, A1630.

8. RELAXATION AND DYNAMIC POLARIZATION BY PARAMAGNETIC IMPURITIES

Lectures by A. Abragam

*Collège de France and
Commissariat à L'Energie Atomique
France*

Prepared by J. Kirsch*

*Bell Telephone Laboratories
Murray Hill, New Jersey*

Table of Contents

From the unedited lecture notes of A. Abragam.

I. Quantum Statistical Mechanics

Nuclear resonance in solids differs greatly from that performed in liquids. In the former case, dipolar coupling between nuclear spins leads to linewidths of several gauss. In liquids, however, this dipolar coupling is modulated by the rapid Brownian motion leading to linewidths which, in the first approximation, are infinitely sharp. The fact that the spins are decoupled in liquids also leads to a much simpler theoretical situation. In rigid solids, because of the tight coupling between nuclear spins, the correct approach to nuclear magnetism is a collective one, where a single large spin system with many degrees of freedom is considered, rather than a collection of individual spins. A spin temperature, distinct from the lattice temperature, can be defined for such a system.

For the purposes of this discussion we will consider conduction electrons in metals as impurities even though typical densities are of the order of 10^{22} per cm^3. This is justified because the electrons obey Fermi statistics and thus only a small fraction, given approximately by $kT/E_F \approx 10^{-4}$ or 10^{-5}, are effective.

We consider a spin system described by states $|s)$, a lattice system of states $|f)$ and a coupling between them due to an interaction Hamiltonian $\mathcal{H}_1$ which has matrix elements $(f, s|\mathcal{H}_1|f', s')$. Conservation of energy requires

$$E_f + E_s = E_{f'} + E_{s'} . \tag{1}$$

We assume that the lattice is in thermal equilibrium with itself and that the lattice has a heat capacity which is very much larger than that of the spin system (this latter assumption is not always justified at low temperatures where a phenomenon known as the "phonon bottleneck" in electron relaxation can take place).

The transition probability between two well-defined spin states $|s)$ and $|s')$ can be written as the sum

$$W_{s \to s'} = \sum_{f, f'} P_f W_{f, s \to f', s'} \tag{2}$$

where $|f)$ and $|f')$ are all the states of the lattice such that (1) is satisfied. P_f is the normalized Boltzmann factor $\exp(-E_f/kT)$ giving the probability of finding the lattice in the state f. One can thus deduce the relation

$$\frac{W_{s \to s'}}{W_{s' \to s}} = \exp\{(E_s - E_{s'})/kT\} , \tag{3}$$

which, from the principle of detailed balancing, $N_s W_{s \to s'} = N_{s'} W_{s' \to s}$, leads to a Boltzmann distribution for the populations of the spin system.

A. Density Matrix

We introduce the concept of the density matrix, ρ, with matrix elements $\langle sf|\rho|s'f'\rangle$. The theory of the density matrix can be found in any book on quantum statistics and we will only briefly review some of the important properties. The density matrix contains all the information necessary for the description of a statistical ensemble of identical systems. In particular, the expectation value of any observable Q (the operator Q may act on spin variables or lattice variables or both) is given by

$$\langle Q \rangle = \text{trace}\{\rho Q\} . \tag{4}$$

The variation of ρ with time is given by

$$i \frac{d\rho}{dt} = + [\mathcal{K}, \rho] , \tag{5}$$

where $\mathcal{K}$ is the Hamiltonian of an individual system; $\rho(t)$ is related to $\rho(0)$ through

$$\rho(t) = U(t) \rho(0) U^{-1}(t) , \tag{6}$$

where $U(t)$ is a unitary operator. In the case of a time-independent Hamiltonian $\mathcal{K}, U$ can be written

$$U = \exp\left\{-i \frac{\mathcal{K}}{\hbar} t\right\} . \tag{7}$$

Any operator which does not specifically involve s is diagonal with respect to s. We can then define another density matrix σ such that

$$\sigma = \underset{\substack{\left(\text{over lattice} \atop \text{variables}\right)}}{\text{trace}} \{p\} \ .$$

This justifies the more approximate treatment,

$$i \frac{d\sigma}{dt} = [\mathcal{H}_0(t) + \mathcal{H}_1(t), \sigma \,] \ . \tag{8}$$

We may consider, for example, an interaction Hamiltonian $\mathcal{H}_1(t)$ given by

$$\mathcal{H}_1(t) = \mathbf{I} \cdot \gamma \hbar \mathbf{H}_1(t) \tag{9}$$

where $H_1(t)$ is a random classical vector. First, however, we must specify what we mean by a random function. Let $y(t)$ be a function of a parameter t. We shall say that it is a random function if the value y which it takes at any instant t is a random variable subject to a law of probability $p(y, t)$ depending on the parameter t. The average value of the random function at an instant t, represented by $\langle y(t) \rangle$, is defined by

$$\langle y(t) \rangle = \int y(t)\, p(y, t) dy \ . \tag{10}$$

If $f(y)$ is a given function of y, f will also be a random function of t and we shall have

$$\langle f(t) \rangle = \int p(y, t)\, f(y)\, dy \ . \tag{11}$$

We define the function $p(y_1, t_1; y_2, t_2)$ as the probability of y taking the value y_1 at time t_1 and y_2 at time t_2.

B. Correlation Functions

We shall call the function $G(t_1, t_2)$ defined by

$$G(t_1, t_2) = \langle f^*(t_1) f(t_2) \rangle$$

$$= \int \int f^*(y_1) f(y_2) p(y_1, t_1; y_2, t_2) dy_1\, dy_2 \tag{12}$$

the correlation function of the random function $f(y)$ relative to the times t_1 and t_2. Often the correlation function $G(t_1, t_2)$ is a function only of the difference $|t_1 - t_2| = \tau$. We will consider only these functions $G(\tau)$. Other useful quantities are the spectral densities which are the Fourier transforms of the correlation function:

$$j(\omega) = \int_0^\infty G(\tau) \exp(-i\omega\tau)\, d\tau$$

$$J(\omega) = 2\int_0^\infty G(\tau)\cos(\omega\tau)\, d\tau = \int_{-\infty}^\infty G(\tau)\exp(-i\omega\tau)\, d\tau$$

$$k(\omega) = \int_0^\infty G(\tau)\sin(\omega\tau)\, d\tau \; . \tag{13}$$

A correlation time τ_c is defined somewhat loosely by the condition that $G(\tau)$ is very small for $|\tau| \gg \tau_c$.

C.   Master Equation for the Density Matrix

We shall try to obtain a master equation for the average density matrix starting from Eq. (8). In the interaction representation with

$$\sigma^* = \exp(i\mathcal{H}_0 t)\,\sigma\,\exp(-i\mathcal{H}_0\tau)$$

$$\mathcal{H}_1^*(t) = \exp(i\mathcal{H}_0 t)\,\mathcal{H}_1(t)\,\exp(-i\mathcal{H}_0 t) \; , \tag{14}$$

the Eq. (8) becomes

$$i\frac{d\sigma^*}{dt} = \left[\mathcal{H}_1^*(t), \sigma\right] \; . \tag{15}$$

This can be integrated by successive approximations to give

$$\sigma^*(t) = \sigma^*(0) - i\int_0^t \mathcal{H}_1^*(t'), \sigma^*(0)\Big] dt'$$

$$- \int_0^t dt' \int_0^{t'} dt''\left[\mathcal{H}_1^*(t'), [\mathcal{H}_1^*(t''), \sigma^*(0)]\right] \; . \tag{16}$$

By taking the time derivative of (16) and then introducing the new variable $\tau = t - t'$ we get

$$\frac{d\sigma^*}{dt} = -i[\mathcal{H}_1^*(t), \sigma^*(0)]$$

$$- \int_0^t d\tau\left[\mathcal{H}_1^*(t), [\mathcal{H}_1^*(t-\tau), \sigma^*(0)]\right] \; . \tag{17}$$

We now take the average of this equation making the following important assumptions:

    (i) it is permissible to neglect the correlation between $\mathcal{H}_1^*(t)$ and $\sigma^*(0)$ and average over them separately;

    (ii) it is then permissible to replace $\sigma^*(0)$ by $\sigma^*(t)$ on the right-hand side of (17);

    (iii) it is permissible to extend the upper limit of the integral in (17) to $+\infty$;

    (iv) it is permissible to neglect all unwritten higher-order terms on the right-hand side of (17). Thus omitting the symbols denoting average quantities we obtain the result

$$\frac{d\sigma^*}{dt} = -\int_0^\infty \left[\mathcal{H}_1^*(t), \left[\mathcal{H}_1^*(t-\tau), \sigma^*(t) \right] \right] d\tau \ . \tag{18}$$

D. Relaxation Matrix

We transcribe this into a matrix notation (Redfield, 1957; 1965),

$$\left(\alpha \left| \mathcal{H}_1^*(t)\sigma^*(t)\mathcal{H}_1^*(t-\tau) \right| \alpha' \right)$$

$$= \sum_{\beta\beta'} \left(\alpha \left| \mathcal{H}_1^*(t) \right| \beta \right)\left(\beta \left| \sigma^* \right| \beta' \right)\left(\beta' \left| \mathcal{H}_1^*(t-\tau) \right| \alpha' \right) \ . \tag{19}$$

Let us consider the variation of $\sigma^*_{\alpha\alpha'}$, due to the term

$$\left(\alpha \left| \mathcal{H}_1^*(t) \right| \beta \right)\left(\beta \left| \sigma^* \right| \beta' \right)\left(\beta' \left| \mathcal{H}_1^*(t-\tau) \right| \alpha' \right) \ .$$

Since $\sigma^*(t)$ is independent of τ we can take it out of the integral:

$$\frac{d\sigma^*_{\alpha\alpha'}}{dt} = \sigma^*_{\beta\beta'}(t) \int_0^\infty \langle \alpha | \exp(i\mathcal{H}_0 t)\, \mathcal{H}_1(t)\, \exp(-i\mathcal{H}_0 t | \beta \rangle$$

$$\times \langle \beta' | \exp(i\mathcal{H}_0(t-\tau))\mathcal{H}_1(t-\tau)\exp(-i\mathcal{H}_0(t-\tau))|\alpha'\rangle\, d\tau \tag{20}$$

where we have used the definition of the interaction representation $\mathcal{H}_1^*(t) = \exp(i\mathcal{H}_0 t)\mathcal{H}_1(t)\exp(-i\mathcal{H}_0 t)$. Here α, α', β, and β' are eigenfunctions of $\mathcal{H}_0$ and we can write:

$$\frac{d\sigma^*_{\alpha\alpha'}}{dt} = \exp\{i[(\alpha-\alpha')-(\beta-\beta')]t\}\,\sigma^*_{\beta\beta'}$$

$$\times \left[\int_0^\infty \exp[i(\alpha'-\beta')\tau]\,\langle\alpha|\mathcal{K}_1(t)|\beta\rangle \right.$$

$$\left. \times \langle\beta'|\mathcal{K}_1(t-\tau)|\alpha'\rangle\,d\tau \right]. \tag{21}$$

The integral is just a number. Summing up the contribution of all terms we get a master equation:

$$\frac{d\sigma^*_{\alpha\alpha'}}{dt} = \exp\{i[(\alpha-\alpha')-(\beta-\beta')]t\}\sum_{\beta,\,\beta'}\sigma^*_{\beta\beta'}R_{\alpha\alpha',\,\beta\beta'} \tag{22}$$

where the coefficients $R_{\alpha\alpha',\,\beta\beta'}$ are numbers. We will restrict our interest to only those cases for which the exponential = 1, i.e., the summation $\Sigma_{\beta\beta'}$ is restricted to states of energy $\hbar\beta$ and $\hbar\beta'$ such that $\beta-\beta'=\alpha-\alpha'$, because the influence of all other terms will be negligible since they will be fast-modulated. We will hereafter use a prime on the summation to signify this restriction,

$$\frac{d\sigma^*_{\alpha\alpha'}}{dt} = \sum_{\beta\beta'}{}'\,\sigma^*_{\beta\beta'}R_{\alpha\alpha',\,\beta\beta'}. \tag{23}$$

We have shown that the influence of the lattice can be described by a random Hamiltonian (that is, a Hamiltonian with random matrix elements) and that this gives us a relaxation matrix. This master equation is just a generalization of a more usual equation for the populations:

$$\frac{dP_\alpha}{dt} = -\sum_\beta W_{\alpha\beta}P_\beta. \tag{24}$$

For the statistical description of a system (of spins) which can be prepared in an initial **coherent** state, we must, in addition to defining the diagonal elements $P_\alpha = \sigma_{\alpha\alpha}$, also define the off-diagonal elements $\sigma_{\alpha\beta}$.

To reiterate, we have shown that for a simple spin system with an unperturbed Hamiltonian $\mathcal{K}_0 = \omega_I I_z$, where $\omega_I = -\gamma H_0$, and a lattice which is described by an ensemble of fluctuating random functions, the statistical behavior of the system is completely known if we know the matrix elements $\sigma^*_{\alpha\alpha'}$. Using these matrix elements we can find the expectation value of any operator

$$\langle Q \rangle = \text{Trace } \{\sigma Q\} = \sum_{\alpha\alpha'} \sigma_{\alpha\alpha'} Q_{\alpha\alpha'} . \qquad (25)$$

This is just a generalization of the case where the operator commutes with the Hamiltonian. For instance, if the operator Q has only diagonal matrix elements and no off-diagonal elements,

$$\langle Q \rangle = \sum_{\alpha} Q_{\alpha} P_{\alpha} \qquad (26)$$

where Q_{α} are eigenvalues of Q.

E. Extreme Narrowing

Let us consider the extreme narrowing case. Specifically, $|\tau_c \omega_{\alpha\alpha'}| \ll 1$ where $\omega_{\alpha\alpha'}$ represent the fastest frequencies encountered in the problem. This is the situation encountered in most nonviscous liquids and is even more valid for conduction electrons. Under these circumstances, we can write for the correlation function of $\mathcal{H}_1^*$ (t): $G(\tau) \propto 2\tau_c \delta(\tau)$. Substituting this into the master equation:

$$\frac{d\sigma^*}{dt} = -\int_0^\infty \left[\mathcal{H}_1^*(t), [\mathcal{H}_1^*(t-\tau), \sigma^*(t)] \right] d\tau \qquad (18)$$

we get a much simpler master equation

$$\frac{d\sigma^*}{dt} = -\tau_c \left[\mathcal{H}_1^*(t), [\mathcal{H}_1^*(t), \sigma^*(t)] \right]. \qquad (27)$$

Now, in the case considered (τ_c infinitely short), it may be worthwhile to go back from the interaction representation to the normal representation, i.e., $\mathcal{H}_1^* \rightarrow \mathcal{H}_1$, $\sigma^* \rightarrow \sigma$. Remember that σ in the normal representation varies very quickly because it interacts with the Hamiltonian $\mathcal{H}_0$, and that σ^* in the interaction representation varies much more slowly because the fast interaction with $\mathcal{H}_0$ has already been taken out. All that is left is the much slower relaxation motion due to the coupling with the lattice:

$$\frac{d\sigma}{dt} = -i[\mathcal{H}_0, \sigma] - \tau_c \left[\mathcal{H}_1(t), [\mathcal{H}_1(t), \sigma] \right]. \qquad (28)$$

Although this equation looks very much like the last equation [Eq. (27)] with the * removed, it is derived from Eq. (27) only in the case of infinitely short τ.

There is one point which must be discussed here, which demonstrates the inadequacy of the classical approach. If we have two levels of the spin system s and s', the probabilities of lattice induced transitions $s \rightarrow s'$ and transitions $s' \rightarrow s$ are not equal. This would appear properly if we used the quantum-mechanical approach. But if we treat our Hamiltonian as a classical field, it does not appear and we must make an ad hoc modification replacing σ by $\sigma - \sigma_0$ in all the equations where σ_0 is the equilibrium Boltzmann distribution.

The random Hamiltonian $\mathcal{H}_1(t)$ can be expanded

$$\mathcal{H}_1(t) = \sum_q F^{(q)} A^{(q)} \tag{29}$$

where the $F^{(q)}$ are random functions of time and the $A^{(q)}$ are operators. Let us take the example of a random field:

$$\gamma \mathbf{H}_1(t) \cdot \mathbf{I} = \gamma H_{1z}(t) I_z + \tfrac{\gamma}{2} H_1^-(t) I_+ + \tfrac{\gamma}{2} H_1^+(t) I_- \tag{30}$$

where

$$H_1^-(t) = H_{1x} - iH_{1y}, \quad H_1^+(t) = H_{1x} + iH_{1y}, \quad \text{and} \quad I_\pm = I_x \pm iI_y.$$

Here we make the identification:

$$F^{(0)}(t) \rightarrow \gamma H_{1z}(t) \; ; \; A^{(0)} \rightarrow I_z;$$

$$F^{(+)}(t) \rightarrow (\gamma/2) H_1^-(t) \; ; \; A^{(+)} \rightarrow I_+ \; ;$$

$$F^{(-)}(t) \rightarrow (\gamma/2) H_1^+(t) \; ; \; A^{(-)} \rightarrow I_- \; .$$

We must transform this to the interaction representation which we do using the definition:

$$\exp(i\mathcal{H}_0 t) A^{(q)} \exp(-i\mathcal{H}_0 t) = \sum_p A_p^q \exp(i\omega_p^q t) \; . \tag{31}$$

(1) Example: Dipole-Dipole Hamiltonian between Spins I and S.

Consider the special case of one spin in a dc magnetic field; $\mathcal{H}_0 = \omega_I I_z$. $I_z \rightarrow \exp(i\mathcal{H}_0 t) I_z \exp(-i\mathcal{H}_0 t) = I_z$ because I_z commutes with the $\exp(-i\omega_I I_z t)$, but $I_+ \rightarrow I_+ \exp(i\omega_I t)$.

Assume the correlation functions $F_q^*(t) \, F_{q'}(t-\tau) \propto \delta_{q-q'}$, i.e., H_x and H_y and H_z are uncorrelated with each other. We end up with the formula:

$$\frac{d\sigma^*}{dt} = -\tfrac{1}{2} \sum_{q,p} J_q \left(\omega_p^{(q)} \right) \left[A_p^{(-q)} \left[A_p^{(q)}, \sigma^* \right] \right] . \tag{32}$$

As an example, we will expand the dipole-dipole Hamiltonian between spins I and S

$$\sum_q F^{(q)} A^{(q)} = \frac{\gamma_I \, \gamma_S \hbar}{r^3} \, \{ \mathbf{I} \cdot \mathbf{S} + 3(\mathbf{I} \cdot \hat{n})(\mathbf{S} \cdot \hat{n}) \} \tag{33}$$

where $\hat{n}$ is the unit vector between I and S. We can expand the random part in terms of (unnormalized) spherical harmonics:

$$F^{(0)} = \frac{1 - 3 \cos^2 \theta}{r^3} \; ;$$

$$F^{(1)} = \frac{\sin \theta \, \cos \theta \, \exp(-i\varphi)}{r^3} \; ;$$

$$F^{(2)} = \frac{\sin^2 \theta \, \exp(-2i\varphi)}{r^3} \; ; \tag{34}$$

$$A^{(0)} = \alpha \left\{ -\tfrac{2}{3} \, I_z \, S_z + \tfrac{1}{6} \, (I_+ S_- + I_- S_+) \right\} \; ;$$

$$A^{(1)} = \alpha \, \{ I_z S_+ + S_z I_+ \} \; ;$$

$$A^{(2)} = \tfrac{1}{2} \, \alpha \, I_+ S_+ \; ;$$

$$\alpha = -\frac{3}{2} \, \gamma_I \, \gamma_S \hbar \; . \tag{35}$$

Now we can transform from $A^{(q)}$ to $A_p^{(q)}$ and substitute into the master equation above. The foregoing was just meant to demonstrate the method. We will not go into the calculation at this time.

(2) Example: The Bloch Equations

We will now try to show how we can derive the Bloch equations using this formulation. Bloch wrote the equations:

$$\frac{dI_z}{dt} = -\frac{I_z - I_0}{T_1} \quad ; \quad \frac{dI}{dt} = -\frac{I_x}{T_2} \tag{36}$$

from intuition (Bloch, 1946) and then derived them (over a period of years) from a microscopic viewpoint (Wangness and Bloch, 1953; Bloch, 1956).

Let us start with our master equation, multiply both sides by I_z (or any spin operator, Q, for that matter) and take the trace;

$$\frac{d\langle Q \rangle}{dt} = -\text{trace}\left\{ \sigma^* \int_0^\infty \left[\mathcal{H}_1^*(t-\tau), [\mathcal{H}_1(t), Q] d\tau \right] \right\} . \tag{37}$$

The interesting point is the σ^* may be taken out of the integral. The integral represents a certain operator B and therefore the brackets represent the expectation value of B

$$\frac{d\langle Q \rangle}{dt} = \langle B \rangle . \tag{38}$$

We will have derived the Bloch equation if the B that we find is proportional to Q and the reciprocal of the proportionality constant will be the relaxation rate. To demonstrate this we will take a simple example of relaxation by a random field choosing as our perturbing Hamiltonian:

$$\mathcal{H}_1(t) = \gamma H_1(t) \cdot I . \tag{39}$$

Consider the extreme narrowing case

$$\frac{d\sigma}{dt} = -i[\mathcal{H}_0, \sigma] - \tau_c \left[\mathcal{H}_1, [\mathcal{H}_1, \sigma] \right]. \tag{28}$$

Multiply both sides by I_z and take the trace:

$$\frac{d\langle I_z \rangle}{dt} = i\left[I_z, [\omega_I I_z, \sigma] \right] - \tau_c \, \text{trace}\left[\sigma[\mathcal{H}_1, [\mathcal{H}_1, I_z]] \right]. \tag{40}$$

Consider for simplicity $I = \frac{1}{2}$. Then we know from elementary quantum mechanics that

$$[(A \cdot I), (B \cdot I)] = \frac{1}{2} A \cdot B + iI \cdot [A \times B] . \tag{41}$$

For example, if we take as A the unit vector along x, $\hat{n}_x$, and $B = \hat{n}_y$

$$[I_x, I_y] = \frac{1}{2} \hat{n}_x \cdot \hat{n}_y + iI \cdot [\hat{n}_x \times \hat{n}_y] , \tag{42}$$

but because n_x, n_y, and n_z are mutually orthogonal, the scalar product vanishes and the vector product $= \hat{n}_z$ so we get the elementary result:

$$[I_x, I_y] = i I_z .\tag{43}$$

Let $A = \gamma H_1$ and $B = \hat{n}_z$, $I_z = \hat{n}_z \cdot I$

$$[(\gamma H_1 \cdot I), (\hat{n}_z \cdot I)] = \tfrac{1}{2} \gamma H_1 \cdot \hat{n}_z + i I \cdot (\gamma H_1 \times \hat{n}_z)\tag{44}$$

Now we take the second commutator once more:

$$\Big[(\gamma H_1 \cdot I), [(\gamma H_1 \cdot I), (\hat{n}_z \cdot I)] \Big]$$

$$= 0 + i \Big[\big(\gamma H_1 \cdot I \big), \big(I \cdot (\gamma H_1 \times \hat{n}_z) \big) \Big]$$

$$= I \cdot [\gamma H_1 \times (\gamma H_1 \times \hat{n}_z)] .\tag{45}$$

The first term is zero because $\tfrac{1}{2} \gamma H_1 \cdot n_z$ is a classical quantity. The remaining term, Eq. (45) is a double cross product and from elementary mathematics we get

$$\Big[(\gamma H_1 \cdot I), [(\gamma H_1 \cdot I), (\hat{n}_z \cdot I)] \Big]$$

$$= - I \cdot [(\gamma H_1 \cdot \hat{n}_z) \gamma H_1 - (\gamma H_1)^2 \hat{n}_z] .\tag{46}$$

The first parentheses just equals γH_{1z} and this is multiplied by $\gamma(H_{1x} + H_{1y} + H_{1z})$. But there is no correlation between H_{1z} and either H_{1x} or H_{1y} and $H_{1z}^2 = \tfrac{1}{3} H_1^2$ so the square brackets become $-\tfrac{2}{3}(\gamma H_1)^2 \hat{n}_z$ and we end up with

$$\frac{d\langle I_z \rangle}{dt} = -\tfrac{2}{3}(\gamma H_1)^2 \tau_c \langle I_z \rangle .\tag{47}$$

We have derived the Bloch equation by a random field method where

$$\frac{1}{T_1} = -\tfrac{2}{3}(\gamma H_1)^2 \tau_c\tag{48}$$

II. Relaxation and Dynamic Polarization in Liquids

Now we come back to the subject of the lecture which is re-laxation and dynamic polarization of nuclei by paramagnetic im-purities in liquids. It has been remarked by Felix Bloch that if you put paramagnetic impurities in liquids, then because of their large moments and fast relaxation times, their interaction with the nuclear moments modulated by the Brownian motion should be a very important mechanism for nuclear relaxation.

We can use the same formalism as we have just used except that instead of the classical field Hamiltonian $\gamma H_1 \cdot I$ we use the dipolar interaction Hamiltonian. The unperturbed Hamiltonian for one nuclear spin and one electron spin is $\mathcal{H}_0 = \omega_I I_z + \omega_S S_z$.

The equation for the expectation value of I_z is:

$$\frac{d\langle I_z \rangle}{dt} = -\frac{1}{T_1} \left\{ \left[\langle I_z \rangle - I_0 \right] + \xi \left[\langle S_z \rangle - S_0 \right] \right\} , \qquad (49)$$

where the $-I_0$ and $-S_0$ are required because this is a classical treatment and where ξ is a numerical coefficient. We see that if the magnetization of one species of spin is changed, this will have an effect upon the other because the spins are coupled. For example, we may *dynamically polarize* the I spins by saturating the S resonance (reducing S_z to zero) obtaining an enhanced nuclear polarization $I_z = \xi S_0$. Under conditions of extreme narrowing and purely dipolar coupling, the coefficient ξ is exactly $\frac{1}{2}$. Actually, the coupling between a nuclear and electronic spin is really a tensor interaction and this can always be broken down into a traceless part of which the dipole-dipole interaction is a special case, and a scalar or isotropic part. A molecule of water may stick to a paramagnetic center for a time which is long compared to the correlation time (for example, correlation times in nonviscous liquids may be of the order of 10^{-12} sec. while sticking times are of the order of 10^{-6} sec.). Under these circumstances, the dipole-dipole interaction is more or less averaged out by rotation and one is left with the scalar part which cannot be averaged out by rotation because it is isotropic. Thus, on top of the dipolar interaction one has a scalar interaction which can only lead to relaxation if it is modulated in time.

There are two ways in which $AI \cdot S$ can be modulated in time; either A is a function of t due to the nucleus sticking to different centers (called relaxation of the first kind) or, because of the fast electronic relaxation, S flips in times of the order of 10^{-9} sec., leading to relaxation of the second kind. In the first case $\xi = -1$. Under these circumstances, if we do a dynamic polarization experiment, instead of getting $I_z = +\frac{1}{2} S_0$ we will get $I_z = -S_0$. Thus we have a striking way of telling whether the relaxation is dipolar or scalar. For example, Bloembergen (1957) has dissolved Mn^{++} in water and saturated the electronic resonance and he got a *positive* enhancement (since $S_0 < 0$) showing therefore that the dominant mechanism is a scalar one. Another example is sodium metal dissolved in liquid ammonia. If we saturate the very sharp electronic line we find a positive enhancement for all the nuclei present including protons, nitrogen and sodium demonstrating that the relaxation is the result of a scalar interaction.

Now what happens if we kill S_z by saturating the electron resonance in the case of a dipolar coupling? Under steady-state conditions we get

$$\langle I_z \rangle = I_0 + \tfrac{1}{2} S_0 . \tag{50}$$

The interesting point, of course, is that S_0 is very much larger than I_0 (660 times larger for electrons and protons) so we have transferred the large electron polarization to the protons, i. e., we have a dynamic polarization phenomenon. This came a short time after the Overhauser (1953) effect which is a similar phenomenon in metals. It is quite significant that since S_0 is negative (the electron moment and the proton moment have different signs) as one applies the microwave field, the polarized proton signal, instead of growing as in the Overhauser effect, actually shrinks to zero and then grows to a large but negative value (sometimes called the Underhauser effect).

This negative polarization corresponds to the upper proton level being populated while the lower one is not and so you have the possibility of a maser (Allais, 1958). If our sample is in an rf coil with a quality factor Q we know that at resonance the energy losses are given by $\omega H_1^2 / 8\pi Q$. The maser condition is

$$\frac{V_C \omega H_1^2}{8\pi Q} < \frac{\gamma H_1^2}{\Delta H} \hbar\omega (n_- - n_+) V_S$$

where V_S is the volume of the sample, V_C is the volume of the coil, and ΔH is the linewidth. Defining the filling factor $\eta = V_S / V_C$ we get for the maser condition $2\pi\eta Q M > \Delta H$ when M equals nuclear magnetization. The free radical used had a nitrogen nucleus and the electron had a hyperfine coupling with this nucleus and so, in the EPR spectrum, there were three equally spaced lines separated by about 13 gauss, which is the field seen by the electron due to the nitrogen nucleus. Thus, as one scans the microwave frequency through these three lines, he sees three proton "maser" signals (Fig. 1).

This type of dynamic polarization has also been done using a signal from the protons in water in the earth's magnetic field (Abragam et al., 1958). Here the enhancement seen was of the order of 2000 rather than the maximum enhancement expected which was $\tfrac{1}{2} (\gamma_e H / \gamma_n H) = \tfrac{1}{2} \times 660 = 330$. The maximum enhancement would be 330 if the electron and proton saw the same field.

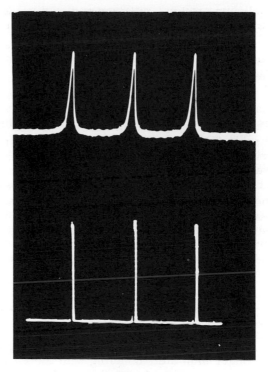

Fig. 1: The upper photo-
graph shows the electronic
spectrum of peroxylamine
disulphonate in an aqueous
solution, observed in a
field of 3000 gauss. The
lower photograph shows
the proton maser signal,
observed when the cor-
responding electronic
line of the upper photo-
graph is saturated.

Actually, the proton sees only the earth's field while the electron
sees also the 13 gauss due to the nitrogen nucleus.

We now pass on to the subject of the interaction between
paramagnetic impurities and nuclear spins in solids. The difficulty
here is that in a solid, nuclear spins are strongly coupled together.

III. Spin Temperature

The concept of a spin temperature distinct from the lattice
temperature is often used in nuclear magnetism for a pictorial
description of a saturation experiment. An analogy can be drawn
between a system of nuclear spins in a large magnetic field coupled
to a lattice and exposed to an rf field inducing transitions between
their Zeeman levels, and a wire with an electric current flowing
through it, immersed in a bath. The establishment of an equilibrium temperature of the wire, higher than that of the bath, represents
a balance between two competing processes: the input of heat dissipated in the wire by the electric current and the heat transfer

from the wire to the bath. Similarly, the heat dissipated inside the
spin system (the wire) by the rf field (the electric current) is
transferred to the lattice (the bath) by a spin-lattice relaxation
mechanism and the idea of a spin temperature higher than the lattice temperature follows naturally from this analogy.

Similarly, if after an equilibrium magnetization $M_O = \chi_O H_O$
has been established in a field H_O at a temperature θ, this field
is lowered adiabatically to a smaller value H_O' in a time short
compared to the spin-lattice relaxation time T_1, the existence of
the *same* magnetization M_O in a *lower* field H_O' can be described
by assigning to the spins a *lower* temperature $\theta' = \theta (H_O'/H_O)$.

Finally, if the magnetization is reversed either by a 180°
pulse or an adiabatic passage, or by dynamic polarization, a
negative temperature can be assigned to the spins. As the energy
spectrum of the spin system has an upper bound, there is no contradiction in considering negative temperature, a concept meaning-
less for systems with kinetic energy.

However, all this is nothing more than a way of speaking;
convenient perhaps, but so far without any deep physical significance. In order for the concept of spin-temperature to be useful,
two things are required:

First, there must be a tight coupling between the spins, much
stronger than their coupling with the lattice. Thus the spin system
reaches an internal equilibrium described by a temperature. Its
subsequent trend towards an equilibrium with the lattice can then be
described by the variation of a single constant, the spin temperature. This definitely restricts the usefulness of the concept of
spin-temperature to solids.

Secondly, there must exist a low magnetic field regime. For
normal Zeeman systems in high fields (much higher than the local
field) the concept of spin temperature is neither very useful nor
necessarily valid. It is not useful because for most purposes the
dipolar spin-spin energy can be neglected in comparison with the
Zeeman energy, and the description of the system by the populations of its energy levels is straightforward. It is not valid because in high fields the exchange of energy between Zeeman and
dipolar parts is exceedingly slow. As Van Vleck puts it: These
two systems are not on speaking terms, and can only come into
equilibrium with each other through the lattice. On the other
hand, in low fields that are comparable to the local fields, the
concept of spin temperature is vital. When the dipolar energy
becomes comparable to the Zeeman energy, it is not possible to

find the eigenstates and eigenvalues of a very complicated Hamiltonian and its statistical description by a spin temperature is a great simplification. Also, as investigated first by Abragam and Proctor (1957, 1958a) and in greater detail by Bloembergen et al. (1959), the flow of energy between dipolar and Zeeman systems becomes very fast for applied fields only a few times the local field and the assumption that the spins come into internal equilibrium much faster than with the lattice is legitimate.

Since straight resonance experiments in solids are hardly practicable in such fields one may well ask what is the incentive for studying the low-field situations. Three different motivations could be assigned originally to these studies (many more have appeared since):

(i) One wished to verify whether the concept of spin temperature (positive or negative) had really all the properties of thermodynamic temperature. After the pioneer experiments of Purcell and Pound (1951), this was the purpose of the investigations of Abragam and Proctor (1957) and their first experiments of nuclear calorimetry in low fields. These were pursued by Jeener and his collaborators (1965) and a deeper understanding of the thermodynamic processes involved was reached.

(ii) The interest in nuclear relaxation in superconducting materials where a small magnetic field destroyed the superconductivity has led Hebel and Slichter (1959) and independently Anderson and Redfield (1959) to study what happened to nuclear spins in vanishingly low applied fields.

(iii) By far the more widespread use of the concept of spin temperature is its extension by Redfield (1955) to the rotating frame in order to describe the saturation behavior of nuclear spins in solids in strong rf fields. Redfield has shown that the Hamiltonian of a system of nuclear spins in the presence of an rf field of frequency ω could be made time independent by means of a canonical transformation provided nonsecular terms varying at the frequencies ω or 2ω were discarded. In the process the applied field was replaced by a much smaller effective field thus bringing about a low field situation. He then made the far reaching assumption that the statistical behavior of the system with its time independent effective Hamiltonian $\mathcal{K}^*$ could be described by a unique spin temperature in the rotating frame, widely different from that of the lattice. The condition postulated for the validity of this assumption was that the transition probability induced by the rf field and calculated by the classical BPP method (Bloembergen et al., 1948) be much greater than the spin-lattice relaxation rate $(1/T_1)$.

We shall treat on the same footing the problem of the spin temperature in the laboratory frame and the rotating frame. In the first case the Hamiltonian is:

$$\mathcal{K} = \omega_0 I_z + \sum_{i<j} b_{ij} \left\{ I_i I_j - 3(\mathbf{n}_{ij} I_i)(\mathbf{n}_{ij} I_j) \right\} \tag{51}$$

with

$$b_{ij} = \frac{\gamma^2 \hbar}{r_{ij}^3} .$$

In the second case:

$$\mathcal{K} = (\omega_0 - \omega) I_z + \sum_{i<j} B_{ij} \left\{ I_{iz} I_{jz} - \tfrac{1}{3} I_i I_j \right\} \tag{52}$$

$$B_{ij} = \frac{3}{2} \frac{\gamma^2 \hbar}{r_{ij}^3} (1 - 3\cos^2 \theta_{ij}) .$$

In either case we shall write $\mathcal{K} = Z + \mathcal{K}_d$.

The assumption of spin temperature is that however the spin system has been prepared, after a time of order T_2 its density matrix becomes of the form

$$\rho = A \exp(-\beta\mathcal{K}) \text{ where } A^{-1} = \text{Trace} \exp\{-\beta\mathcal{K}\} . \tag{53}$$

The exact meaning of this assumption, usually made for thermodynamic systems, warrants some scrutiny.

The form (53) implies that the eigenvalues of the operator ρ are $A \exp - (\beta E_i)$. However, if the system of spins is isolated (as we assume) its density matrix obeys the equation

$$\frac{i d\rho}{dt} = [\mathcal{K}, \rho] \tag{54}$$

and its eigenvalues *do not* change with time. There seems to be a contradiction in the statement that ρ tends asymptotically to the form (53), whatever its initial form which may have arbitrary eigenvalues. We cannot discuss here this delicate problem of the theory of irreversible processes. In any case the off-diagonal part does not, strictly speaking, go to zero but rather its matrix elements get out of phase in such a manner that the expectation value $\langle Q \rangle$ = Trace $\{Q\rho\}$ of any off-diagonal operator goes to zero. The decay of the transverse magnetization after a 90° pulse is a case in point.

Except in very special cases to be discussed later the temperatures are "high" and a first order expansion of $\exp - \{\beta \mathcal{H}\}$ into $1 - \beta \mathcal{H}$, where 1 is the unit matrix, is permissible.

Let us calculate the entropy of the system. The partition function is:

$$Z = \sum_n \exp\{-\beta E_n\} \tag{55}$$

$$Z = \text{trace}\{\exp - \beta \mathcal{H}\} \tag{56}$$

$$\approx \text{tr}\left\{1 - \beta \mathcal{H} + \frac{\beta^2 \mathcal{H}^2}{2}\right\}; \ \text{tr}\{\mathcal{H}\} = 0 \tag{57}$$

$$\approx \text{tr}\{1\}\left\{1 + \frac{\beta^2}{2} \frac{\text{tr } \mathcal{H}^2}{\text{tr }\{1\}}\right\} \ ; \tag{58}$$

$$\log Z \approx \log \text{tr}\{1\} + \log\left\{1 + \frac{\beta^2}{2} \frac{\text{tr }\{\mathcal{H}^2\}}{\text{tr }\{1\}}\right\} \tag{59}$$

$$\approx \log \text{tr}\{1\} + \frac{\beta^2}{2} \frac{\text{tr }\{\mathcal{H}^2\}}{\text{tr }\{1\}} \ ; \tag{60}$$

$$S = -\frac{\partial F}{\partial T} = \frac{\partial}{\partial T} T \log Z \tag{61}$$

$$= \log Z + \frac{T \partial \log Z}{\partial T} = \log Z - \frac{\beta \partial \log Z}{\partial \beta} \tag{62}$$

$$S = \log \text{tr}\{1\} - \frac{\beta^2}{2} \langle \mathcal{H}^2 \rangle \tag{63}$$

where we have defined

$$\langle \mathcal{H}^2 \rangle = \frac{\text{tr}\{\mathcal{H}^2\}}{\text{tr}\{1\}} . \tag{64}$$

$$S = \log \text{tr}\{1\} - \frac{N\beta^2}{2} \frac{I(I+1)}{3} \{\omega_e^2 + \omega_L^2\} \tag{65}$$

where

$$\omega_e^2 = \omega_1^2 + (\omega_0 - \omega)^2 \quad \text{(in the rotating frame)}$$

$$\omega_e^2 = \omega_0^2 \quad\quad\quad \text{(in the laboratory frame)} . \tag{66}$$

ω_e is the effective field (in frequency units) and is the vector resultant of ω_1, the applied rf field perpendicular to H_0 and $\Delta = \omega_0 - \omega$ along H_0; ω_L is a local field given by

$$\omega_L^2 = \frac{\text{tr}\{H_d^2\}}{\text{tr}\{I_z^2\}} . \tag{67}$$

Its calculation is straightforward and if the spin-spin interaction is purely dipolar it is related to the Van Vleck second moment $M_2 = \Delta\omega^2$ by the following relations:

$$\left(\omega_{\text{Local}}^{\text{Rotating}}\right)^2 = \tfrac{1}{3} M_2 \tag{68}$$

$$\left(\omega_{\text{Local}}^{\text{Laboratory}}\right)^2 = 5\left(\omega_{\text{Local}}^{\text{Rotating}}\right)^2 = \frac{5}{3} M_2 . \tag{69}$$

We know that when we vary any external parameter adiabatically the entropy will remain constant. Thus we may vary Δ (by changing frequency or applied field), we may vary ω_1 (by changing amplitude of applied rf field), or we may even vary ω_L (by changing the orientation); β will vary in such a way that

$$S = -\frac{N}{2} \beta^2 \frac{I(I+1)}{3} \{\omega_e^2 + \omega_L^2\} \tag{65}$$

will remain constant, and once we know how β varies, we can, by going back to the density matrix, calculate everything.

In all this we have forgotten about the lattice. But in a steady-state experiment eventually the lattice will make itself felt.

Let us calculate the spin-lattice relaxation in the rotating frame assuming that the relaxation Hamiltonian has an infinitely short correlation time. We define two coordinate systems in the rotating frame: the xyz system with $\omega_1 \| x$ and ω_0 (and also Δ) $\| z$, and the XYZ system with $\omega_e \| Z$; θ is the angle between ω_e and Δ so that $\cos \theta = \Delta/\omega_e$ and $\sin \theta = \omega_1/\omega_e$. Then

$$\frac{\partial \langle I_z \rangle}{\partial t} = -\frac{1}{T_1} \{ \langle I_z \rangle - I_0 \} , \tag{70}$$

$$\frac{\partial \langle I_x \rangle}{\partial t} = -\frac{1}{T_1} \langle I_x \rangle . \tag{71}$$

The Boltzmann distribution I_0 does not enter into Eq. (70) because the equilibrium value of $I_X = 0$. We can convert from the xyz coordinate systems to the XYZ system by multiplying both sides of Eq. (69) by $\cos \theta$ and both sides of Eq. (70) by $\sin \theta$:

$$\frac{\partial \langle I_Z \rangle}{\partial t} = -\frac{1}{T_1} \{ \langle I_Z \rangle - I_0 \cos \theta \} . \tag{72}$$

Recalling that $\langle Z \rangle = \omega_e I_Z$ we get

$$\frac{\partial \langle Z \rangle}{\partial t} = -\frac{1}{T_1} \{ \langle Z \rangle - \Delta I_0 \} ,$$

$$\frac{\partial \langle \mathcal{H}_d^* \rangle}{\partial t} = -\frac{\delta}{T_1} \langle \mathcal{H}_d^* \rangle . \tag{73}$$

There is no a priori reason to assume that the dipole-dipole energy relaxes at the same rate as the Zeeman energy. The first guess might be that perhaps the dipolar energy would relax twice as fast, since the spin-spin energy is bilinear and therefore to relax a system of two spins it is enough to flip only one. Unfortunately it is not as simple as this. Take for example the relaxation by the random magnetic field produced by the conduction electrons in a metal. How will a homogeneous coherent field seen by two neighboring spins relax the $I \cdot I$ scalar interaction between them? Since the two interactions commute, it will have no effect. On the other hand, if the field is completely incoherent, $\delta = 2$. Experiment shows that δ is not exactly two so there is some coherence. Now, since we are assuming temperature equilibrium between the Zeeman and dipolar systems

$$\frac{\langle Z^* \rangle}{\omega_e^2} = \frac{\langle \mathcal{H}_d^* \rangle}{\omega_L^2} = \frac{\langle \mathcal{H}^* \rangle}{\omega_e^2 + \omega_L^2} , \tag{74}$$

we get

$$\frac{d\langle \mathcal{H} \rangle}{dt} = -\frac{1}{T_1} \langle \mathcal{H} \rangle \left\{ \frac{\omega_e^2 + \delta\omega_L^2}{\omega_e^2 + \omega_L^2} \right\} + \text{constant terms.} \qquad (75)$$

Recalling Eq. (66) which defined the effective field, ω_e, we can write

$$\frac{1}{T_1} = \frac{1}{T_{1\infty}} \left\{ \frac{H_0^2 + \delta H_L^2}{H_0^2 + H_L^2} \right\} \text{(in the laboratory frame)} \qquad (76)$$

or

$$\frac{1}{T_1} = \frac{1}{T_{1\infty}} \frac{\Delta^2 + H_1^2 + \delta H_L^2}{\Delta^2 + H_1^2 + H_L^2} \text{ (in the rotating frame).} \qquad (77)$$

Δ has been previously defined as $\omega_0 - \omega$ and $T_{1\infty}$ is just the usual longitudinal relaxation time describing the variation of I_Z (the ∞ subscript signifies that $T_{1\infty}$ is the relaxation time observed when $H_0 >> H_L$). δ is the ratio of the time constant $T_{1\infty}$, describing the relaxation of the Zeeman energy to that describing the relaxation of the nuclear spin-spin interaction energy. The local field, H_L, is defined by Eq. (67) and

$$H_L = \omega_L / \gamma . \qquad (78)$$

The δ factor is related to the correlation between the fluctuating magnetic fields due to the electrons and seen by neighboring nuclei, and gives information about the electronic wave functions and the structure of the metal. δ may vary between two (if the spins relax completely independently) and three (for complete spatial correlation).

Anderson and Redfield (1959) were the first to measure δ. They measured T_1 in Al^{27}, Cu^{63}, Li^7, and Na^{23} as a function of field between 0 and 1000 gauss, using a method involving adiabatic fast passages due to Hebel and Slichter (1959). A typical field dependence is shown in Fig. 2 where the solid curve is Eq. (76). Their results for lithium and sodium are shown in Table I.

Galleron and Jerome (1963) measured δ for sodium by polarizing the nuclei via the Overhauser effect and then observing the Overhauser shift (also called the Day shift) when the rf field was cut off. The experiment was performed at a field of 2.88 gauss corresponding to an electronic resonance frequency of 8050 kc/sec. Their results fit the curve (Fig. 3)

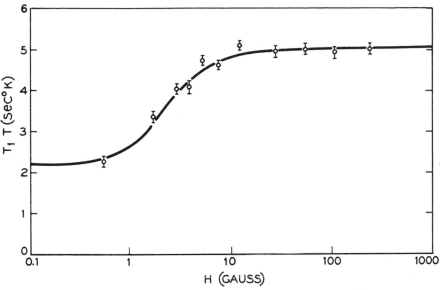

Fig. 2: Field dependence of the relaxation time of Na^{23} at $1.1°K$.

Table I

Method	δ for Na^{23}	δ for Li^7
Adiabatic Fast Passage[a]	2. 28	2. 2
Overhauser Shift[b]	2. 15 ± 0. 06	
Rotating Frame[c]	2. 12 ± 0. 03	2. 31 ± 0. 05
(a) Anderson and Redfield, 1959. (b) Jerome and Galleron, 1963. (c) Poitrenaud and Winter, 1965.		

$$T_1 T = 5.08 \, \frac{H^2 + H_L^2}{H^2 + (2.15)H_L^2} \tag{79}$$

giving a value of $δ = 2.15$.

Poitrenaud and Winter (1964) have recently measured T_1 in the rotating frame [see Eq. (77)] as a function of $Δ$ for several different values of H_1 and have thereby been able to deduce quite accurate values of $δ$ for Na^{23} and Li^7. Their results appear in Table I.

A. ABRAGAM AND J. KIRSCH

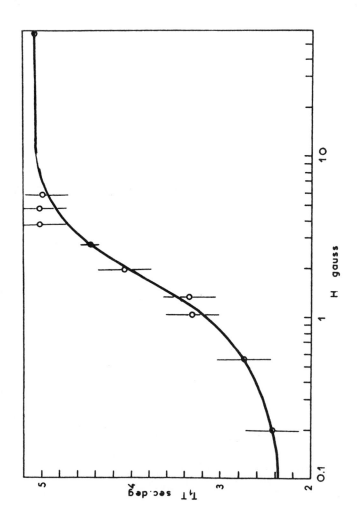

Fig. 3: Field dependence of the relaxation time of Na²³ at 1.5°K. The value of δ = 2.15 was obtained by fitting the curve at H = 2.88 g and at a field large compared with the local field.

IV. Electron-Nuclear Interaction in Metals

The contact part of the hyperfine interaction has several important consequences which we will discuss now. The first is the so-called Knight shift (Townes et al., 1950) which is the shift of the nuclear resonant field due to the addition of the field produced by the conduction electrons in a metal. This field H is an ensemble average over all the conduction electrons:

$$H_e = \frac{8\pi}{3} \gamma_e \hbar \langle |\psi(0)|^2 \rangle_F \langle S_z \rangle , \tag{80}$$

where F signifies that the average is taken over the Fermi surface. Since S_z is proportional to H_0, the applied field, the shift is also proportional to the applied field.

In the same way, naturally, the electrons also see a field due to the nuclei and the electron resonance is shifted. This shift is sometimes referred to as the Day shift, H_n and

$$H_n = \frac{8\pi}{3} \gamma_n \hbar \langle |\psi(0)|^2 \rangle_F \langle I_z \rangle . \tag{81}$$

I_z is usually very small, but when one polarizes the nuclei dynamically (as will be described in Sec. VI), $\langle I_z \rangle$ can be very large. In Na (I = 3/2) for example, when one makes $I_z = I$, one comes up with about 200 gauss as was first noticed by Overhauser.

Another important consequence of the electron-nuclear interaction is the effect it has on the relaxation. We have already shown that the electron contribution to the relaxation time can be written

$$\frac{1}{T_1} \sim \frac{2}{3} \gamma_n^2 |H_e|^2 \tau_c . \tag{82}$$

Using a simple dimensionality argument one can replace τ_c by $\hbar/E_F$ where E_F is the Fermi energy. We must also multiply on the right by a factor kT/E_F which gives the fraction of electrons which are not paired.

A final important consequence of the electron-nuclear coupling taken to the second order is the Ruderman-Kittel (1954) interaction which is an indirect nucleon-nucleon coupling.

It would be interesting to measure $\langle |\psi(0)|^2 \rangle_F$ and in principle, this could be obtained either from the Knight shift or from the Day shift. The latter would be easier because nuclei obey Boltzmann statistics and their susceptibility should be easier to calculate. In order to measure accurately the Day shift, we need metals which give narrow electronic lines and until very recently, the only likely candidates were Na and Li.

In a simple-minded picture of electron resonance in metals we might expect the width of the line to be of the order of $1/\tau$ where τ is the mean time that an electron spends in the skin depth. This picture would lead to absurdly broad lines. The argument is obviously wrong because the electron continues to feel the dc magnetic field even after leaving the skin depth. Thus, in the interior of the metal the electron continues to precess coherently and when it returns to the skin depth, the forced precession takes over again with a motion coherent with its earlier motion. The real width will be given by the reciprocal of the spin-lattice relaxation time.

Another erroneous argument led people to believe that it would be impossible to saturate the resonance of the electrons in the center of the sample and that, in fact, if it takes a field of H_1 to saturate an electron on the surface, it would take a field of $H_1 \exp(d/\delta)$ to saturate an electron in the center of the metal, where d is the dimension of the sample and δ is the skin depth. This is incorrect because the electrons themselves carry the information about the saturating field from the skin depth into the center of the metal. The actual field necessary to saturate the electrons in the center of the sample is $H_1(d/\delta)$ which is much smaller than $H_1 \exp(d/\delta)$. This result can be derived more rigorously from the Bloch equations including the diffusion term.

In Fig. 4 we see the results of an experiment (Gueron and Ryter, 1959) on the Overhauser effect in lithium. At lower powers the line shape of the electron resonance in lithium metal is independent of the direction of sweep of the magnetic field. At higher powers however, the width and the shape of the line change considerably and depend on the direction of sweep. This is a result of the narrowness of the EPR line in lithium metal and the fact that the sample contains particles of varying grain sizes. For grains of dimensions $d > \delta$, it can be expected because of electron spin diffusion, that the saturation parameter will be uniform within the grain but reduced by a factor of the order of $(\delta/d)^2$, resulting in a spread of the observed electron spin resonance shifts (Day shifts).

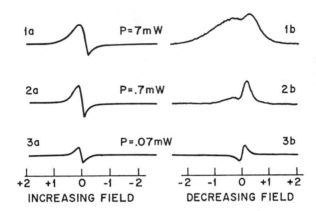

Fig. 4: Recorded electron spin resonance absorption derivative in neutron-irradiated LiH for various power levels P at 4.2°K and 10 Gc/scc. One division on the horizontal axis corresponds to one gauss; the sweep is 0.4 gauss/min.

As one approaches the electron line from above, the nuclear enhancement increases resulting in an added magnetic field which tends to repel the line. Thus, the line is broadened.

The further that one displaces the electron line by the Overhauser effect, the smaller the line becomes (because of saturation) and so in order to get the total Day shift one must plot inverse displacement against inverse microwave power and then extrapolate to infinite power. From the displacement of the EPR line in Li at 4.2°K extrapolated to complete saturation, Ryter (1960) measured the important parameter

$$\xi = \frac{\langle |\psi^2(0)| \rangle_F}{\langle |\psi^2(0)| \rangle_{atomic}} = 0.44 \pm 0.015 . \tag{83}$$

After the removal of the microwave power, the EPR line, displaced by the nuclear field, returns to its original position at the rate of the nuclear relaxation. Figure 5 shows the exponential

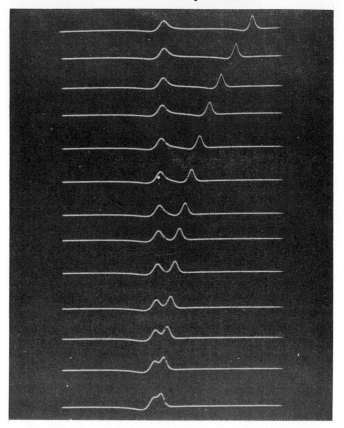

Fig. 5: Exponential decay of the dynamic nuclear polarization in Li metal at 4.2°K carrying the shifted EPR line back to its normal position. Overall length of the trace is 8.7 gauss, duration of the sweeps 0.02 sec., repetition time 2 sec. The undisplaced line on the left originates in metal grains too large to be saturated and therefore to be displaced by the nuclear field.

decay of the dynamic nuclear polarization carrying the shifted EPR line back to its normal position. The overall length of the trace is 8.7 gauss, duration of sweeps 0.02 sec., repetition time 2 sec. The undisplaced line on the left originates in metal grains too large for the metal grains to be saturated and therefore to be displaced by the nuclear field. The nuclear relaxation time of 9.8 sec. found in this manner at 4.2°K is in good agreement with that found using the fast passage technique.

Of course, even without the Overhauser enhancement there is a Day shift due to the natural, thermal equilibrium, nuclear polarization. Even at 4.2°K this natural polarization is very small and in sodium the Day shift has been measured to be only 38 milli-gauss (Ryter, 1963). By applying an rf field sufficiently strong to saturate the sodium nuclear resonance and thus eliminating the "nuclear field" Ryter was able to measure the displacement of the sodium EPR line. He used a spectrometer which automatically plotted the separation (~3 gauss) between the sodium EPR line and that of a sample of lithium which was placed in the same spectro-graph.

The metallic sodium particles used in this experiment are formed spontaneously in a sample of NaH. The NMR line due to the nuclei in the sodium metal is distinguished from those in the NaH by its higher frequency (due to the Knight shift), its narrow-ness at 300°K due to self-diffusion and by its width of 0.7 gauss at 1.2°K corresponding to a value of $T_1 T = 5.08$ sec. °K, in agree-ment with previous results.

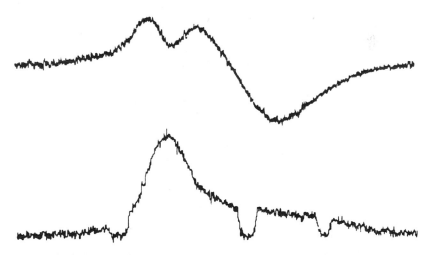

Fig. 6: Upper trace: derivative of nuclear resonance signal of NaH containing particles of metallic sodium at 1.2°K. Lower trace: displacement of the metallic sodium ESR line produced by the saturation of the nuclear resonance. Notice the shoulder due to the coupling, described in the text, between nuclei in the metallic sodium and nuclei in the NaH. The stability of the base line has been checked at three points by stopping the rf.

This method has demonstrated an appreciable coupling between the nuclear spins in the metallic sodium and those in the NaH. When the rf frequency is slowly varied, the magnetization $\langle I_Z \rangle$ of the nuclei in the metal (which is the only part of the magnetization which enters into the expression for the "nuclear field") is reduced in the entire region of the NaH resonance. This effect is quite visible in Fig. 6 where the derivative of the NMR signal from all the sodium nuclei is reproduced on top and the variation of the "nuclear field" H_n is reproduced below, both as a function of the applied rf frequency.

V. Fixed Paramagnetic Impurities

Until now, we have been dealing mostly with relaxation by paramagnetic impurities in liquids and in metals. The main feature of the relaxation mechanisms was that these impurities, either free radicals and paramagnetic salts dissolved in liquids or conduction electrons in metals, were highly mobile. This motion has two effects. First, there is a *dynamic* effect. The motion provides the reservoir of energy which is required for the relaxation mechanism. There is also the *kinematical* effect. The motion enables the electron, or paramagnetic ion, to come near each nucleus and inform it of the relaxation.

Now we are coming to the subject of relaxation by *fixed* paramagnetic impurities such as, for instance, paramagnetic ions dilutely imbedded in an otherwise diamagnetic crystal. Here the paramagnetic impurities are not in motion and they are far away from most of the nuclei. The first problem is where will the energy, or the fluctuating character of the magnetic field seen by the nucleus come from. The second problem is how will the information be transported from the fixed impurities to the distant nuclei.

A. Direct Interaction

We shall mainly be concerned with the dipolar coupling between the electron and the nucleus and this can be written $S \cdot A \cdot I$ where A is a known traceless tensor. In liquids it is A which fluctuates in time, because $\langle 1/r^3 \rangle$ or terms like $1 - 3\cos^2\theta$ will vary with time. In solids A is fixed in time, and it is S which fluctuates, a fluctuation caused by the electronic relaxation. The correlation time of the fluctuating magnetic field seen by the nucleus is the electronic relaxation time.

If we write out the matrix elements for the dipole Hamiltonian we will have several terms corresponding to the various processes: flip-flop, flip-flip, etc. But for the calculation of the nuclear relaxation time, we are interested only in those terms containing either I_+ or I_-. These are the terms which make the nucleus flip. As far as the electron is concerned we can have S_z, S_+, or S_-. Now consider terms such as S_+I_+ or S_-I_- corresponding to simultaneous flips of both electron and nucleus. S_+I_+ requires energies of the order of $\omega_e + \omega_n$ which is a large energy which must be provided by the fluctuation of the electronic spin itself. In the continuous spectrum of the relaxation of the electronic spin we have to find this frequency. This will be very difficult as seen by looking at the usual form for the correlation function:

$$G(\tau) = \exp(-\tau/\tau_e) , \tag{84}$$

where τ_e = electronic relaxation time. The spectral density of this function is of the form $1/1 + \omega_e^2 \tau_e^2$ and will be very small unless $\omega_e \tau_e \ll 1$. In other words, one would want the electronic frequency to be smaller than the electronic linewidth meaning that the electronic resonance would be unobservable. The only term that will not lead to similar difficulties will be the $S_z I_-$ (stop-flop) because then we will have in the denominator $1 + \omega_e^2 \tau_e^2$. Thus, we need only consider one term in the dipole-dipole Hamiltonian, $S_z I_+$ and we can write for the transition probability:

$$\frac{1}{T_1'} = \frac{9}{2} \gamma_S^2 \gamma_I^2 \frac{\hbar^2 \sin^2\theta \cos^2\theta}{r^6}$$

$$\int_{-\infty}^{\infty} S_z(0) S_z(t) \exp(-i\omega_n t)\, dt \tag{85}$$

Averaging over the angles, we end up with:

$$\frac{1}{T_1'} = Cr^{-6} \quad \text{where} \quad C = \frac{2}{5} \gamma_S^2 \gamma_I^2 \hbar^2 S(S+1) \frac{\tau_e}{1 + \omega_n^2 \tau_e^2} . \tag{86}$$

This approximate expression can be written in another form if we neglect the factor 1 with respect to $\omega_n^2 \tau_e^2$. We get

$$\frac{1}{T_1'} = \frac{1}{\tau_e} \left(\frac{H_e}{H_0}\right)^2 \tag{87}$$

where the electronic magnetic field, H_e, is defined as $H_e = \gamma_S \hbar/r^3$. The relaxation rate of the nuclei is equal to the relaxation rate of the electrons reduced by the square of the ratio of $H_{(electronic)}$ to $H_{(applied)}$.

We draw the usual four-level scheme (Fig. 7), where the terms involving the α's signify that the static part of the dipole Hamiltonian mixes the states $++$ and $+-$ by a fraction α where $\alpha = (H_e/H_0)$. Thus, the rate for transitions between the two upper electronic states is α^2 times slower than the rate for the allowed electronic transitions.

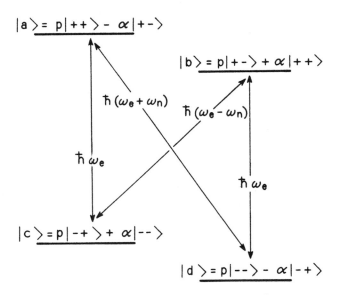

Fig. 7: Energy levels of an electronic spin $S = \frac{1}{2}$ coupled to a nuclear spin $I = \frac{1}{2}$, at a distance r, by a dipole-dipole interaction, in a strong magnetic field H. The admixture coefficients are $\alpha = \gamma_S \hbar/r^3 H = H_e/H_0 \ll 1$; $p = (1 - \alpha^2)^{1/2} \approx 1$.

B. Spin Diffusion

We have shown that as far as its *dynamic* effects are concerned, the translational motion of paramagnetic impurities in liquids can be replaced in solids by electron relaxation. But what of the kinematical effect of the motion? That is to say, what about those nuclei which are far from the paramagnetic impurity? Another question is, how can we explain the observation of a single relaxation rate rather than a distribution of relaxation rates depending on the distance from the paramagnetic impurity?

Bloembergen (1949) has shown that spin diffusion can provide the answer to these questions. As we know, spin diffusion is not a bodily diffusion of matter. Rather, it is a diffusion of the orientation of spins. We can write a diffusion equation for the diffusion of the nuclear polarization p with a diffusion constant $D \approx Wa^2$ where a is the lattice spacing, the distance between two neighboring nuclei and W is the probability of mutual flip-flops between two neighboring nuclei:

$$\frac{\partial p}{\partial t} = D\nabla^2 p - C \sum_n \frac{1}{|r - r_n|^6} (p - p_0) . \tag{88}$$

Typical values of D are of the order of 10^{-13} cm^2/sec. C has previously been defined [Eq. (86)] and p_0 is the nuclear polarization for thermal equilibrium.

This problem has been solved with fairly sophisticated mathematics by Khutsishvili (1956) and independently by De Gennes (1958). Their result is

$$\frac{1}{T_1} \simeq 4\pi NbD , \tag{89}$$

where N is the number of paramagnetic impurities per unit volume and b is a length defined by

$$b = 0.68 \left(\frac{C}{D}\right)^{\frac{1}{4}} . \tag{90}$$

From the expression (86) for C and the value $D \simeq Wa^2$,

$$b \sim a \left(H_e^0/H_0\right)^{\frac{1}{2}} \left(W\tau_e\right)^{-\frac{1}{4}} \tag{91}$$

where we define $H_e^0 = \gamma_s \hbar/a^3$, the electronic field at a distance of one lattice spacing. $(W\tau_e)^{1/4}$ will not be very different from unity and H_e^0 is typically of the order of one kilogauss, so b = constant × a where the constant is of the order of a few units at most.

One of the most interesting features of the model is the dependence of T_1 on $H^{1/2}$ rather than the much faster dependence on H^2 which we found for the direct case without spin diffusion. Another interesting feature is the very weak dependence of the nuclear relaxation time on the electronic relaxation time.

Blumberg (1960) has derived essentially the same result by the following argument. Nuclei near to the paramagnetic center get the relaxation information directly in a time C/r^6 where C is

defined by Eq. (86) and r is the distance from the paramagnetic
center. Nuclei far from the center receive the information by spin
diffusion in a time D/r^2. There will then be some distance,
which we will call b', at which information coming via both routes
arrives at the same time:

$$\frac{C}{(b')^6} = \frac{D}{(b')^2} \; , \tag{92}$$

$$\therefore \; b' = \left(\frac{C}{D}\right)^{\frac{1}{4}} . \tag{93}$$

We can assume that all nuclei beyond b' are in thermal equilibrium
(as indeed demonstrated by the existence of a single relaxation
rate, single exponential). We can thus surround each impurity by
its sphere of influence of radius R such that $(4/3) \pi R^3 N = 1$ where
N, as we have stated, is the number of impurities per unit volume.
If ρ is the number of nuclei per unit volume, all nuclei outside b'
have the same relaxation rate given by:

$$\frac{4}{3} \pi R^3 \rho \frac{1}{T_1} = \int_{b'}^{R} \frac{C}{r^6} 4 \pi \rho r^2 \, dr \tag{94}$$

$$\frac{1}{T_1} = \frac{4 \pi NC}{3b'} = \frac{4 \pi N}{3} b'D = 4 \pi NbD \tag{95}$$

leading to $b = \frac{1}{3}(C/D)^{1/4}$ rather than $b = 0.68\,(C/D)^{1/4}$. Considering the crudeness of the calculations, these results are equivalent.

1. Diffusion Barrier

There is however, a strong condition for the validity of
this theory, namely, that spin diffusion actually does take place as
near as b (or b') to the impurity. There is indeed a diffusion
barrier which prevents nuclei seeing too large an electronic magnetic field, H_e, from being on "speaking terms" with the "normal"
nuclei.

One could define another radius, d, which is the distance at
which nuclei become on "speaking terms" with the nuclei far from
the impurity. If the electronic spin does not flip too fast (usually
the case at low temperatures) the condition is

$$\frac{\gamma_e \hbar}{d^3} = \frac{z \hbar \gamma_n}{a^3} \; , \tag{96}$$

$$d \sim \left(\frac{\gamma_e}{z\gamma_n} \right)^{\frac{1}{3}} a \qquad (97)$$

where z is a small integer; d may be either smaller or greater than b.

If $d > b$ then we should replace b' with d as the lower limit of the integral in Eq. (94). If we do so, we find that

$$\frac{1}{T_1} \approx \frac{4\pi NC}{3d^3} . \qquad (98)$$

In that case $1/T_1 \propto 1/\tau_e H_0^2$, a quite different result from the case without a diffusion barrier where, we recall

$$\frac{1}{T_1} \propto \frac{1}{\tau_e^{\frac{1}{4}} H_0^{\frac{1}{2}}} . \qquad (99)$$

A striking example has been given by Goldman (1965) who has found both kinds of behavior in a single sample. Since $b \sim (C/D)^{1/4} \propto H_0^{-1/2}$, for low fields $b > d$ and we have the $H_0^{1/2}$ dependence for T_1 while at higher fields $b < d$ and we find the H_0^2 dependence for T_1. His results are shown in Fig. (8).

C. Nuclear Relaxation When the Electron Spins Are Highly Polarized

Two other remarks are in order. At very low temperatures and in high fields in the thermal equilibrium value of $\langle S_z \rangle = S_0$ may be quite large. ($\langle S_z \rangle = S$ for completely polarized spins.) The correlation function $\langle S_z(0), S_z(t) \rangle$, which is correct at high temperatures, must be replaced at low temperatures by

$$\langle (S_z(t) - S_0), (S_z(0) - S_0) \rangle = \exp(-\tau/\tau_e) \langle S_z(t) - S_0 \rangle^2 . \qquad (100)$$

For spin 1/2,

$$\langle (S_z - S_0)^2 \rangle = 1 - p_e^2 \qquad (101)$$

where p_e is the electronic polarization. In the formula for $1/T_1$, $1/\tau_e$ must be replaced by $1/\tau_e(1 - p_e^2)$, which represents a sizable decrease.

D. NMR in Heavily Doped Silicon

Recently an interesting experiment (Jerome et al., 1965) has been performed at 4.2°K in a sample of silicon doped with phosphorus (Fig. 9). P is a donor and it goes easily into a lattice site

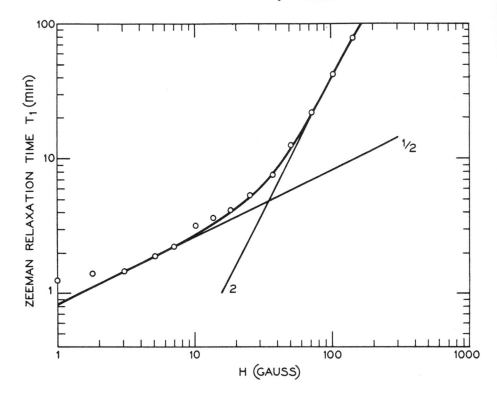

Fig. 8: Proton Zeeman spin-lattice relaxation time as a function of magnetic field in paradibromobenzene at 4.2°K.

conserving one electron so it is rather like a large hydrogen atom, but one with a very much smaller hfs. The separation of peaks in the top trace of Fig. 9 is 42 gauss rather than 500 gauss in hydrogen. The single line in the middle appears as the concentration is increased and is due to clusters of impurities. For still larger concentrations further lines appear, representative of clusters of more than two atoms which grow at the expense of the two initial lines until at a concentration of about 2×10^{18} cm^{-3} a single line appears very similar in appearance, width and relaxation to the conduction electron line observable at 77°K. All hfs has disappeared and we have the beginning of what are known as impurity bands, a single band formed by the overlap of these electrons.

It was originally thought that in heavily doped silicon the wave functions of the electrons would be uniformly spread and the

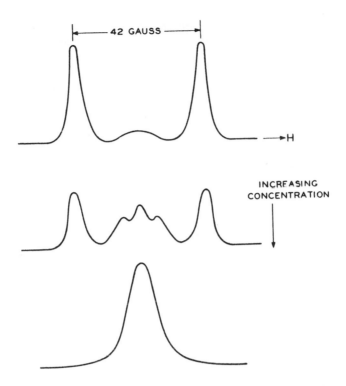

Fig. 9: Electron resonance spectrum of phosphorus-doped silicon at 4.2°K. Concentration of phosphorus atoms in the top trace is 5×10^{16}/cm^3. Concentration in bottom trace is 2×10^{18}/cm^3. Concentration in middle trace is inter-mediate between these two.

electrons would behave like conduction electrons in metals. We were able to show that this was not so. When we observed the Overhauser effect, we noticed that the nuclear relaxation time increased with field. With the power available we obtained an enhancement of ~900. By extrapolating to infinite power, one could expect the full enhancement of

$$\mu_{electron}/\mu_{Si^{29}} = 3300 \; .$$

The polarization time and the relaxation time were different. The explanation is as follows. Although the radii of these hydrogen-like atoms are 20-30 Å, the direct contact between electron and nucleus is still not sufficient, so there must be a certain amount of spin diffusion. The diffusion barrier is proportional to the electronic field which in turn is proportional to the applied field:

$$d \propto H_e \propto S_z \propto H_o \ .$$

This explains why T_1 increases as the applied field is raised; the diffusion barrier grows and impedes diffusion.

When one performs the Overhauser effect, one saturates S_z reducing it to zero, thus also reducing the diffusion barrier. This is why in the presence of saturation the relaxation time, which is equal to the polarization time, is shorter than in the absence of saturation.

VI. Dynamic Polarization

We now discuss dynamic polarization and its application to polarized nuclear targets. It has been said that there are about one hundred different methods of dynamic polarization. This is not quite true. There are many fewer but each method has been invented by about ten different people and each inventor gives it a different name, usually his own. The one we are going to describe, we have named the "solid effect" (Abragam and Proctor, 1958b).

We have already written the dipolar Hamiltonian, and its matrix elements and we know the various processes it can induce. The static dipole interaction mixes states $|++)$ and $|+-)$ in the ratio $\alpha^2 = (H_e/H_0)^2$ so that a flip-flop (simultaneous electron and nuclear transitions in opposite directions) or a flip-flip (simultaneous electron and nuclear transitions in the same direction) are no longer completely forbidden. Such a process will not occur spontaneously in the rigid lattice because it does not conserve energy. The flip-flop will require the energy $\hbar(\omega_e - \omega_n)$ and the flip-flip will require $\hbar(\omega_e + \omega_n)$. We shall assume that the electronic linewidth $\Delta\omega_e$ is smaller than ω_n (this is not always the case but let's just make that assumption). This requires using dilute paramagnetic impurities in diamagnetic crystals. The impurities must be sufficiently dilute so as not to broaden the electronic line. We can induce these processes by supplying microwave energy at either the frequency $\omega_e - \omega_n$ or $\omega_e + \omega_n$. The method is based on the fact that the electronic relaxation time is much shorter than the nuclear relaxation time. For simplicity we will make the approximating assumptions that the electrons are 100 percent polarized and the natural nuclear polarization is very small. (At 1°K and 18 kG the electrons are 94 percent polarized and the nuclear polarization is a fraction of a percent.) Suppose the electrons are all pointing up and we set our microwave frequency to induce flip-flops. The nuclei, because they are completely unpolarized, will be pointing half up and half down. (For simplicity we consider $I = \frac{1}{2}$.) Consider the nucleus that points up. It is surrounded by electrons which all point up, so it cannot do a flip-flop. Thus, nothing happens to the nuclei which point up. They might do a flip-flip but this does not conserve energy because we have set our microwave frequency to $\omega_e - \omega_n$. Now consider a nucleus pointing down surrounded by electrons pointing up. It is quite eager to make a flip-flop with one of these electrons because this is energetically favorable. One might ask, "Once it has flip-flopped, why doesn't it flip-flop back?" It does not because it has not time for it. The electronic relaxation time is fast and as soon as the flip-flop has occurred, the electron goes back to its original polarized state and the nucleus is left locked in the spin-up position. And so we pump all the nuclei with the wrong direction into the right direction. Once they are there they stay there. * Of course, if we had applied the frequency $\omega_e + \omega_n$ instead of $\omega_e - \omega_n$ we would have driven all the nuclei antiparallel to the electrons. This is one of the advantages of this method, the one that is mostly appreciated by nuclear physicists. Without touching the magnetic field and just by shifting the microwave frequency by a fraction of a percent, we can reverse the nuclear polarization.

A. LiF Experiment

Figure 10 shows the results of the first experiment using this method (Abragam and Proctor, 1958b). We used LiF which contains Li^6, Li^7, and F^{19}. All we need is two different spins, one of which has a higher gyromagnetic ratio than the other. It need not necessarily be an electron. The F^{19} played the role of the electronic spin and Li^6 was the nuclear spin. The gyromagnetic ratio of F^{19} is about six times that of Li^6.

*We might compare the situation of an electronic spin surrounded by all the nuclear spins with that of King Solomon surrounded by his 1000 wives. This electronic spin has to please them all. As soon as it has flipped with one nucleus it must go back again and be ready for the next nucleus. This naturally asks for some qualities (of fast relaxation) which means that not all paramagnetic ions can qualify. Rare earths are very good in that respect.

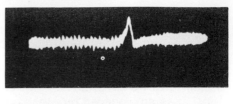

Fig. 10: (1) Normal signal of Li^6 after polarization in a field of 12,000 gauss. (2) Signal of Li^6 after dynamic polarization in a field of 2800 gauss irradiating at a frequency $\Omega \approx \omega(F^{19}) - \omega(Li^6) \approx 9.4$ mc/sec. (3) Signal of Li^6 after dynamic polarization in a field of 2000 gauss while irradiating at a frequency $\Omega = \omega(F^{19}) + \omega(Li^6) \approx 9.4$ mc/sec.

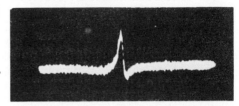

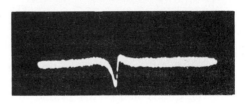

The top line in Fig. 10 is just the natural signal of Li^6 in a field of 12 kG. Skipping to the bottom line we have the Li^6 resonance at a field of 2 kG. One sees that the size of the signal is about the same as the 12 kG resonance although it should be six times smaller. This is because during the measurement we were irradiating the sample with a frequency which is the sum of the frequencies of Li^6 and F^{19}. We see that the polarization is reversed. The middle line was made at 2800 gauss and the irradiating frequency was the difference of the Li^6 and the F^{19} frequencies. The signal has the same polarization and is about 1.4 times greater than that of the natural signal as predicted.

B. Polarized Protons

In Fig. 11 we see a natural signal of protons in the water of hydration of a crystal of lanthanum magnesium nitrate in which one percent of the lanthanum was replaced by paramagnetic neodymium. There are two things to notice. The first is that the signal-to-noise is poor and the second is that the signal is symmetrical. Van Vleck has shown that in an absorption signal in an insulator, all the odd moments of the line vanish.) In Fig. 12 we have an enhanced signal where the protons are polarized to about 60 percent corresponding to an enhancement of about 350. We notice that the signal-to-noise is vastly improved but what is more important we

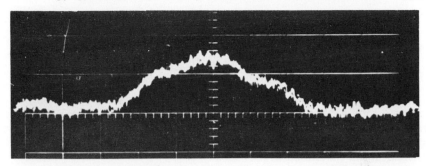

Fig. 11: Normal signal of protons in the water of hydration of a
         $La_2 Mg_3 (NO_3)_{12} \cdot 24H_2O$ doped with 1 percent Nd.

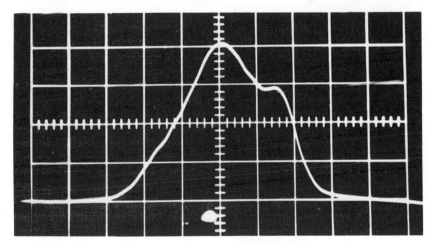

Fig. 12: Signal of dynamically polarized protons in the water of
         hydration of a crystal of $La_2 Mg_3 (NO_3)_{12} \cdot 24H_2O$ doped
         with 1 percent Nd.

also notice that the line is now highly asymmetrical. One can
theoretically derive this asymmetry showing for instance that the
first moment of the line will be quadratic in the polarization, but
more simply one can consider the following physical picture. Consider one nuclear spin. At low polarization its neighbors are just
as likely to have spin-up as spin-down. So that for any environment where the local field seen by a nuclear spin has one orientation we can find another spin which sees a local field of the opposite orientation. Therefore, because the linewidth is due to the
distribution of the local fields, the line will be symmetric.

On the other hand, when the polarization is of the order of 50 percent or more, there are definitely more nuclear spins pointing up than pointing down and it is no longer true that it is likely to find a local field of one sign as of the other.

This asymmetry is actually very useful because it can be used as a measure of the polarization. The more classical method for measuring the enhancement consists of measuring the ratio of the area under the enhanced signal to that under the natural signal. But when one works with very small samples, it is possible that the natural signal be unobservable because of signal-to-noise considerations.

C. Sign of the Quadrupole Constant

Before moving on to the subject of nuclear targets we will discuss another nice experiment which shows the usefulness of high polarization. In Fig. 13 we show the levels of a spin 7/2 both with a quadrupole interaction and without. We have assumed a positive quadrupole constant, ν_Q. We see that the unperturbed levels are equally spaced resulting in a single line. To first order the quadrupole splitting leaves the central frequency unchanged with three equally spaced satellites on each side. At high-temperaratures, that is temperatures at which the linear approximation $\exp(-h\nu_L/kT) \approx 1 - h\nu_L/kT$ is valid, the difference

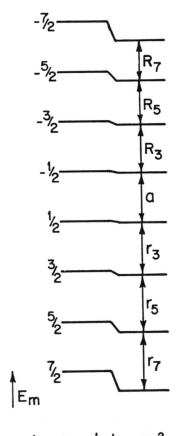

$$-h\nu_L m - \tfrac{1}{2} h\nu_Q m^2$$

$$\nu_L > 0 \quad \nu_Q > 0$$

Fig. 13: Energy levels of a spin 7/2 system without quadrupole interaction (left) and with quadrupole interaction (right). ν_L and ν_Q are both assumed positive.

in population between successive levels is the same for all the levels. Thus all the satellites will have equal intensities. The line pattern obtained for a positive quadrupole constant will be identical to that obtained for a negative constant. It is in fact a general theorem that no experiment performed at high temperatures can provide the sign of the quadrupole constant. This theorem is proved in "Principles of Nuclear Magnetism," p. 262 (Abragam, 1961).

However, with dynamic polarization we can get to spin temperatures such that the upper levels are distinctly less populated than the lower ones. For the case of a positive quadrupole constant we see from Fig. 13 that this would result in the higher frequency satellites being more intense than the lower frequency ones. One need only compare the intensities of r_3 and R_3 (Fig. 13) to get the sign of ν_Q. In this way, Abragam and Chapellier (1964) have recently been able to measure the sign of the quadrupole constant of La^{139} in $La_2 Mg_3 (NO_3)_{12} \cdot 24H_2O$. Their results are reproduced in Figs. 14a, 14b showing that $\nu_Q > 0$. Furthermore, they showed that one can reverse the inequality in satellite intensity by reversing the polarization (Figs. 14c and 14d).

VII. Polarized Targets

Finally, we come to the subject of the application of these methods of dynamic polarization to actual polarized targets used in nuclear physics experiments. The experimental restrictions imposed by the nuclear physicists are often quite severe. This is demonstrated by the fact that although we first got useful polarization of 20 percent in 1960, the first nuclear physics experiment using a dynamically polarized target was performed in 1962 after two years of hard work. The nuclear physicists often do not understand the fact that the sample must have a coil around it to measure the nuclear polarization, that it has to be placed in a microwave cavity, be cooled by liquid helium often without being in contact with the helium, that the cavity must be placed in a dewar and the dewar in a magnetic field.

The first experiment using polarized targets was performed at Saclay in 1962 (Abragam et al., 1962). One thing that is absolutely essential in this experiment is to record both the scattered and the recoil proton. This is because although these targets contain as much hydrogen as pure hydrogen (in terms of nuclei per cm^3) they also contain La, Mg, N, O and these all contribute spurious scattering. One of the problems in low energy scattering

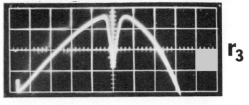

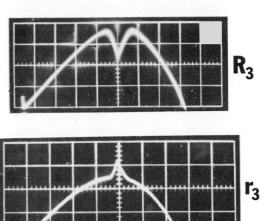

Fig. 14: The top two
traces show the La^{139}
satellite lines dynami-
cally polarized positively.
The bottom two traces
show the same satellites
negatively polarized. The
parabolic base line re-
sults from the frequency
response of the Q-meter.

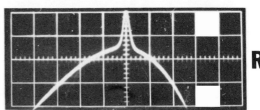

experiments is that the crystal thickness must be very small
(~ 0.1 mm) and there can be no liquid helium in direct contact
with the target (because this would attenuate the beam). This
problem was solved by using a cavity with thick walls through
which liquid helium was flowing. The crystal was cooled by having
its edges in contact with the cavity walls.

For the analysis of the scattering data it is very important
to measure the polarization. As we have already discussed, the
most straightforward way is to compare the area under the natural
signal with that under the enhanced signal. However, in this case
the natural signal was well below the level of noise so this method
was impossible. Instead, we took advantage of the fact that the
electronic signal was quite good. The electron spin sees an added

magnetic field which is due to the surrounding nuclei. This field is not of the contact type as in metals but rather of the long range dipolar type. It's just a Lorentz field plus a demagnetizing field depending on the shape of the sample. As a rough estimate of the size of this field we consider that in water when all the protons are polarized the magnetization is about one gauss. In these samples the magnetization is about the same. If you can neglect the demagnetizing factor and have cubic symmetry, this contributes a Lorentz field $4\pi M/3 \approx 4$ gauss. There was a coil which did not enable us to see the nuclear signal but did enable us to saturate it. By observing the derivative of the electronic signal at the center of the line and then suddenly turning on the rf field to saturate the nuclear polarization we observed a displacement of the electronic signal. Finally, by slightly changing the applied magnetic field by a measured amount so as to return to the center of the line, we can calibrate the displacement directly in terms of nuclear polarization.

This has been a description of experiments performed with thin targets which are necessary for low-energy nuclear physics (up to 28 MeV) experiments. For high energy experiments, one uses thick targets.

VIII. Possible New Target Materials

Considering that polarizations of better than 80 percent are now rather routinely obtained in targets of LMN by the solid effect, one might suspect that there is very little room left for improvement. However, as we have already pointed out the La, Mg, N, and O nuclei all provide spurious background scattering. Much of the present target research is directed toward finding materials which are relatively richer in protons.

One of the most promising of such substances is frozen toluene in which polarizations of 30 percent have already been obtained. This material may well supersede others but there is not much physics in it and it will not be discussed here.

An obvious possibility is solid hydrogen. One might irradiate it, creating a few hydrogen atoms thus providing the paramagnetic impurities. The trouble with H_2 is due to the fact that protons are fermions of spin 1/2. We also know that the hydrogen molecule in the solid is very loosely bound so that to a first approximation it is just a gas. The rotational angular momentum J is a good quantum number. The total spin I is also a good quantum number.

The lowest state is $J = 0$ $I = 0$ which is obviously unpolarizable. The first excited state is $J = 1$ $I = 1$. The para-ortho conversion is very slow (of the order of days) so if you want $I = 1$ you are stuck with $J = 1$ and the molecule rotates. Because it rotates, the fluctuating field produced by one proton and seen by the other proton causes relaxation with relaxation times ~ 1 msec. This is far too short.

One is also led to try HD. This is nice because there are no constraints on symmetry and one can have states with $J = 0$ with protons having $I = 1/2$. Hardy (1966) has succeeded in getting proton relaxation times as long as 10,000 sec. Unfortunately the impurities have relaxation times ~ 100 sec and since the ratio of impurity atoms to protons is of the order of 10^{-5} this is still not good enough. *

Time does not permit discussion of the rotating crystal method of dynamic polarization (Jeffries, 1963; Abragam, 1963).

References

Abragam, A. and Proctor, W. (1957). Phys. Rev. <u>106</u>, 160.

Abragam, A., Combrisson, J., and Solomon, I. (1958). C. R. Acad. Sci. <u>245</u>, 157.

Abragam, A. and Proctor, W. (1958a). Phys. Rev. <u>109</u>, 1441.

Abragam, A. and Proctor, W. (1958b). C. R. Acad. Sci. <u>246</u>, 2253.

Abragam, A. (1961). Principles of Nuclear Magnetism, (Oxford University Press).

Abragam, A., Borghini, M., Catillon, P., Coustham, J., Roubeau, P., and Thirion, J. (1962). Phys. Letters <u>2</u>, 310.

Abragam, A. (1963). Cryogenics <u>3</u>, 42.

Abragam, A. and Chapellier, M. (1964). Phys. Letters <u>11</u>, 207.

Allais, E. (1958). C. R. Acad. Sci. <u>246</u>, 2123.

Anderson, A. G. and Redfield, A. G. (1959). Phys. Rev. <u>116</u>, 583.

*In terms of the footnote in Sec. VI, the poor king has 10^3 wives and he is only good for 100 of them. Oxygen may help (since the addition of a small amount may short-in the impurity relaxation time).

Bloch, F. (1946). Phys. Rev. 70, 460.

Bloch, F. (1956). Phys. Rev. 102, 104

Bloembergen, N., Purcell, E. M., and Pound, R. V. (1948). Phys. Rev. 73, 679.

Bloembergen, N. (1949). Physica 15, 386.

Bloembergen, N. (1957). J. Chem. Phys. 27, 572.

Bloembergen, N., Shapiro, S., Pershan, P. S., and Artman, J. O. (1959). Phys. Rev. 114, 445.

Blumberg, W. E. (1960). Phys. Rev. 119, 79.

De Gennes, P. G. (1958). J. Phys. Chem. Solids 3, 345.

Goldman, M. (1965). Phys. Rev. 138, A1675.

Gueron, M. and Ryter, C. (1959). Phys. Rev. Letters 3, 338.

Hardy, W. (1966). to be published.

Hebel, L. C. and Slichter, C. P. (1959). Phys. Rev. 113, 1504.

Jeener, J., DuBois, R., and Broekaert, P. (1965). Phys. Rev. 139, A1959.

Jeffries, C. D. (1963). Cryogenics 3, 41.

Jerome, D. and Galleron, G. (1963). J. Phys. Chem. Solids 24, 1557.

Jerome, D., Ryter, C. and Winter, J. M. (1965). Physics 2, 81.

Kutsischvili, G. R. (1956). Publ. Georgian Inst. Sci. 4, 3.

Overhauser, A. W. (1953). Phys. Rev. 92, 411.

Poitrenaud, J. and Winter, J. M. (1965). Phys. Letters 17, 199.

Purcell, E. M. and Pound, R. V. (1951). Phys. Rev. 81, 279.

Redfield, A. G. (1955). Phys. Rev. 98, 1787.

Redfield, A. G. (1957). IBM J. Res. and Dev. 1, 19.

Redfield, A. G. (1965). Advances in Magnetic Resonance, Vol. I, J. S. Waugh editor (Academic Press, N. Y.).

Ruderman, M. A. and Kittel, C. (1954). Phys. Rev. 96, 99.

Ryter, C. (1960). Phys. Rev. Letters 5, 10.

Ryter, C. (1963). Phys. Letters 4, 69.

Townes, C. H., Herring, C., and Knight, W. D. (1950). Phys. Rev. 77, 852.

Wangness, R. K. and Bloch, F. (1953). Phys. Rev. 89, 728.

9. CONDUCTION ELECTRON CHARGE AND SPIN DENSITY EFFECTS DUE TO IMPURITIES AND LOCAL MOMENTS IN METALS

R.E. Watson

Brookhaven National Laboratory *
Upton, New-York

Table of Contents

Supported by the U.S. Atomic Energy Commission.

413

I. Introduction

In this chapter, we inspect the perturbation of conduction electron charge and spin densities due to local magnetic moments and charge impurities in metals. In the charge case we concentrate on Knight shifts in solid and liquid alloys and only briefly inspect the associated quadrupole interaction problem. The spin density perturbations have magnetic hyperfine fields directly associated with them and the information gained by Mössbauer effect and other means will be discussed. The charge and spin density problems are normally considered separately in the literature. There is strong similarity in the formal features of the two and much can be gained by considering them simultaneously. The theories employ simplifying assumptions which introduce difficulties when one attempts to relate theory and experiment and the difficulties on one front often have relevance for the other. In the course of this chapter we will employ the traditional simple models and in so doing we will attempt, on one hand, to be alert to the implications of the simplifications and will attempt, on the other, to gain information pertinent to real metals which, as a general rule, are more complicated than the models employed. *

II. Charge Oscillation Effects

Consider an impurity in a metal which provides a perturbing potential

$$\Phi(r) \equiv V_{\text{impurity}}(r) - V_{\text{normal}}(r) \tag{1}$$

which is assumed to be spherical and is centered about the impurity site. There are three ways to account for the effect of $\Phi(r)$ on the conduction electrons: First is the method of partial wave scattering and phase shifts commonly known as Friedel theory (Friedel, 1952, 1954, and 1958). This has been most frequently employed semi-empirically and has supplied great intuitive insight into the problem. Second, is the direct application of perturbation theory, mixing excited orbital character into the occupied Bloch electron states. Third, is dielectric response theory, the most elegant and concise description of the physics involved — but also the least satisfactory, when asking quantitative questions.

*Time will not allow consideration of the interesting problem of the occurrence of local charge or magnetic moments. Some aspects of the latter case are briefly considered elsewhere (Chaps. S.9 and S.10.

A. Friedel Phase Shift Approach

In the Friedel phase shift approach, one starts with simple unperturbed Bloch electron states,

$$\psi_k^0(r) = U_k(r) \exp(i\mathbf{k} \cdot \mathbf{r}) \tag{2}$$

where the $U_k(r)$ display the periodicity of the lattice. These ψ^0 are scattered by the impurity into the states

$$\psi_k(r) = U_k(r) \left\{ \exp(i\mathbf{k} \cdot \mathbf{r}) + \chi_k(r) \right\} . \tag{3}$$

Utilizing the plane wave expansion

$$\exp(i\mathbf{k} \cdot \mathbf{r}) = \sum_\ell i^\ell \left[2(2\ell+1) \right]^{\frac{1}{2}} j_\ell(k\,r) \, P_\ell(\cos\theta) \tag{4}$$

and

$$\exp(i\mathbf{k} \cdot \mathbf{r}) + \chi_k(r) = \sum_\ell i^\ell \exp(i\eta_\ell) \left[2(2\ell+1) \right]^{\frac{1}{2}} P_\ell(\cos\theta)$$

$$\times \left[j_\ell(kr) \cos \eta_\ell - n_\ell(kr) \sin \eta_\ell \right] \tag{5}$$

a result appropriate for a spherical $\Phi(r)$ (Schiff, 1949), where $j_\ell(r)$ and $n_\ell(r)$ are the spherical Bessel and Neumann functions, the fractional change in density at some radial distance r is, on substitution

$$\frac{\Delta \rho_k(r)}{\rho_k^0(r)} = \frac{|\psi_k|^2 - |\psi_k^0|^2}{|\psi_k^0|^2}$$

$$= \sum_{\ell=0}^{\infty} (2\ell+1) \left\{ \sin^2 \eta_\ell \left[n_\ell^2(kr) - j_\ell^2(kr) \right] - \sin 2\eta_\ell j_\ell(kr) n_\ell(kr) \right\} \tag{6}$$

a result involving a directional average or sum over a sphere of fixed $|\mathbf{k}|$ in k space (thus anticipating a spherical, essentially free-electron, energy band structure). The form of the potential $\Phi(r)$ fixes the relative phase shifts, η_ℓ. Schiff (1949) has developed the problem for the square well potential which has been heavily employed by Friedel and associates. For these η_ℓ's Friedel derived the important sum rule

$$\Delta Z = (2/\pi) \sum_\ell (2\ell+1) \, \eta_\ell \tag{7}$$

where ΔZ is the difference in valency, or charge, of the impurity with respect to the host. For each scattered partial wave of oscillatory character, the phase shift indicates the extent to which the charge in the partial wave is shifted either onto or off of the impurity site. Physically, the Friedel sum rule says that at some distance from the impurity the excess charge of the impurity is exactly shielded (neutralized) by the perturbed (i. e. , phase shifted) conduction electrons.

As r approaches infinity

$$j_\ell(kr) \rightarrow \frac{1}{kr} \cos\left[kr - \frac{\pi(\ell+1)}{2} \right] \tag{8}$$

and

$$n_\ell(kr) \rightarrow \frac{1}{kr} \sin\left[kr - \frac{\pi(\ell+1)}{2} \right] \tag{9}$$

Employing these limiting values gives the relative charge shift

$$\frac{\Delta\rho_k(r)}{\rho_k^o(r)}\bigg|_{r\rightarrow\infty} = \sum_\ell (-1)^\ell (2\ell+1) \sin \eta_\ell \frac{\sin(2kr + \eta_\ell)}{(kr)^2} \tag{10}$$

$$\sim \sin(2kr + \theta)/(kr)^2$$

appropriate (along with the set of η_ℓ or θ) to a particular $|k|$ value; it is oscillatory and of long range because of the low power of r in the denominator.

The total charge requires a summation over k values (the direction of **k** having already been summed) up to the Fermi momentum, k_F. Upon taking the asymptotic limit for free electrons

$$\Delta\rho_{tot}(r)\bigg|_{r\rightarrow\infty} = -\sum_\ell (-1)^\ell \frac{(2\ell+1) \sin \eta_\ell^F \cos(2k_F + \eta_\ell^F)}{2\pi^2 r^3} \tag{11}$$

$$= -\frac{\alpha}{2\pi^2 r^3} \cos(2k_F r + \theta)$$

where

$$\tan \theta = \frac{\Sigma (2\ell+1) \sin \eta_\ell^F \cos(\eta_\ell^F - \ell\pi)}{\Sigma (2\ell+1) \sin \eta_\ell^F \sin(\eta_\ell^F - \ell\pi)} , \tag{12}$$

and where the η_ℓ^F are defined for orbitals at the Fermi energy. These expressions are normally employed, along with the Friedel sum rule, in semi-empirical fits to experiment. These asymptotic results are, of course, only rigorously justified for large r and we must emphasize that experiment *never* significantly samples this region in space. We should hasten to add that the $\Delta\rho$, inside this region may, and often does, display the character predicted by equations such as (10) and (11). Employment of such expressions may, in other words, be justified, but only with suitable caution.

B. Perturbation Theory Approach

Consider a conduction electron band, represented by orbitals ψ_k^0, filled with electrons up to a Fermi energy ϵ_F. Turning on a perturbing potential $\Phi(r)$, centered at the origin, will in lowest order in perturbation theory cause an occupied orbital to become

$$\psi_k(r) \to \psi_k(r) + \sum_{\substack{k+q \\ \text{outside} \\ \text{Fermi} \\ \text{surface}}} \frac{\langle k|\Phi|k+q\rangle}{\epsilon_k - \epsilon_{k+q}} \psi_{k+q}(r) \tag{13}$$

The sum is limited to unoccupied orbitals because, as described in an earlier chapter* the only mixing of physical significance is that between *unoccupied* and *occupied* orbitals but *not* between occupied orbitals. ** At this point we make the traditional assumption of free-electron bands where

$$\psi_k(r) = \frac{1}{\sqrt{V}} \exp(ik \cdot r) \; ; \; \epsilon_k = k^2 \text{ (in units } \hbar^2/2m = 1) \tag{14}$$

and the Fermi surface is spherical with wave vector k_F; $1/\sqrt{V}$ is a normalization factor. Our perturbed Bloch function then becomes

$$\psi_k(r) = \frac{1}{\sqrt{V}} \left\{ \exp(ik \cdot r) + \sum_{|k+q|>k_F} \frac{\Phi(q) \exp[i(k+q) \cdot r]}{k^2 - (k+q)^2} \right\} \tag{15}$$

Chapter 2 by R.E. Watson and A.J. Freeman.
**The mixing of one occupied orbital into another by Eq. (13) will, of course, be exactly compensated by the mixing of the latter into the first when their combined density is considered. This fact is exploited shortly.*

where, apart from a $1/V$ factor $\Phi(q)$ is just the Fourier transform* of (the spherical) $\Phi(r)$. The total change in conduction electron charge density, to first order in Φ is obtained by squaring
Eq. (15), retaining appropriate terms, and summing k up to k_F.
This yields

$$\Delta\rho(r) = \frac{1}{V} \sum_{k<k_F} \sum_{|k+q|>k_F} \frac{\Phi(q)\{\exp(iq\cdot r)+\exp(-iq\cdot r)\}}{k^2 - |k+q|^2} \qquad (16)$$

One may extend the $|k+q|$ sum from zero to infinity since

$$\sum_{k<k_F} \sum_{|k+q|<k_F} \frac{\Phi(q)\{\exp(iq\cdot r)+\exp(-iq\cdot r)\}}{k^2 - |k+q|^2} = 0 \qquad (17)$$

because the denominator is odd in k and $k+q$. Doing this, replac-
ing the $|k+q|$ summation coordinate by q and doing the k summa-
tion one obtains

$$\Delta\rho(r) = \frac{1}{V} \sum_q \Phi(q)\{\exp(iq\cdot r)+\exp(-iq\cdot r)\}$$

$$\times \sum_{k<k_F} \frac{1}{k^2 - |k+q|^2}$$

$$= \sum_q F(q)\Phi(q)\{\exp(iq\cdot r)+\exp(-iq\cdot r)\} \ . \qquad (18)$$

The simplicity of this result follows from potential matrix elements
which depend only on q. We have then, a distortion, $\Delta\rho$, which is
the Fourier transform of a driving term, $\Phi(q)$, times a response
or susceptibility function, $F(q)$, which has the form

$$F(q) \equiv 2 \times \frac{k_F}{16\,\pi^2} \left\{1 + \frac{4k_F^2 - q^2}{4k_F q} \ln\left(\frac{2k_F + q}{2k_F - q}\right)\right\} \qquad (19)$$

*Since $\int_0^\infty dr\, \frac{1}{r}\, exp(-iQ.r) = \frac{4\pi}{Q^2}$ then a potential $\Phi(r) = \int \frac{\rho(R)}{|r-R|}\, dR$
where $\rho(R)$ is the charge density, has a Fourier transform
$\Phi(Q) = \int dr\, exp(iQ\cdot r) \int [dR\,\rho(R)/(r-R)]$ which, letting $x = r-R$
can be written as
$\Phi(Q) = \int dx\, [exp(-iQ\cdot x)/x] \int dR\,\rho(R)\, exp(-iQ\cdot R) = (4\pi/Q^2)\,\rho(Q)$.
This simple reliance of the Fourier transform of the poten-
tial on the transform of the density suggests the convenience of operating in reciprocal space.

where the factor of two, in front, accounts for the occurrence of electrons of both spins.

The F(q) function, plotted in Fig. 1, has a singularity at $q = 2k_F$ (overemphasized in the plot) which is the source of the Friedel oscillations — as can be seen if we evaluate Eq. (18) in the asymptotic limit of large r. Transforming the q sum to an integral, the exponentials then oscillate rapidly with q, making the integral zero valued except for that q where $\Phi(q) F(q)$ is singular — namely at $2k_F$. The result,

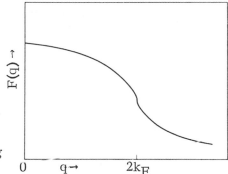

Fig. 1: The susceptibility func-tions, $F(q)$, as a function of $\mathbf{q}$.

$$\Delta\rho(r)_{asymptotic} \sim \frac{\cos (2k_F r)}{r^3} , \tag{20}$$

is of the same form as Eq. (11). (The singularity in our suscepti-bility, or response, function is also the source of Kohn anomalies in phonon dispersion curves.)

The appearance of the singularity in F(q) is readily under-stood. It arises from the integration of the energy denominator $1/(\epsilon_k - \epsilon_{k+q})$. Consider the spherical Fermi surface, shown in Fig. 2; one sees that for $q \leq 2k_F$, one has one or more q vectors

Fig. 2: The q vector yielding the minimum denominator in Eqs. (15)-(18), for given $|q|$, for free electron Fermi surfaces and $|q|$ values less and greater than $2k_F$.

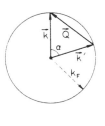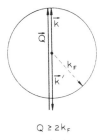

such that $\mathbf{k}$ just touches the inside, and $\mathbf{k} + \mathbf{q}$ the outside, of the Fermi surface. These cases have an essentially *zero* valued denominator associated with them. When $q > 2k_F$, $\mathbf{k+q}$ *must* leave the Fermi surface and a zero valued denominator cannot occur. The singularity in F(q) appears at that point where this zero denom-inator is first lost, i.e., at the extremal caliper $q = 2k_F$.

The form of the singularity is a function of the topology of the bands and the associated Fermi surface and is not unique. Figure 3 displays F(q) behavior for the cases where **k**+**q** leaves normal to a Fermi surface segment which is one of a pair (**k** touching the other segment) of either infinite parallel planes (I), or infinitely long parallel lines (II) or points (III) — the result in Fig. 1). These three curves are what one derives for one, two, and three dimensional free electron metals respectively. In other words, if one had a Fermi surface with two segments which were parallel planes, F(**q**), for **q** normal to these planes, would display the peaked character shown in the figure. Overhauser has considered this matter in detail and, contrary to arguments occasionally made in the literature, he concludes that such a singularity requires truly parallel planar Fermi surface segments, that "very flat" or "almost parallel" segments are not sufficient and that in such cases, Fig. 1 displays the essential q dependence of F(q).

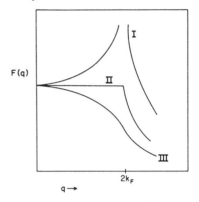

Fig. 3: F(q) for one (I), two (II), and three (III) dimensional free electron metals.

Before going on, we might note what is to be expected when we abandon our over-simplified parabolic bands with their spherical Fermi surface. Figure 4 shows an ellipsoidal Fermi surface and the **q** corresponding to that extremal caliper at which one loses the zero valued denominator for the off axis **q** (and **r**) direction of interest. The extension to still more complicated band structures and Fermi surfaces can be made readily and it is distinctly possible that a given **q** direction could involve *several* extremal calipers implying *several* singularities in the susceptibility function.

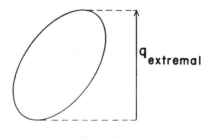

Fig. 4

C. Dielectric Response Theory

The formal features of the perturbation theory result could have been obtained more concisely with dielectric response theory (Pines, 1963). Here one employs the macroscopic Poisson equations, which, Fourier transformed (in space and time), are

$$i\mathbf{k} \cdot \mathbf{D}(\mathbf{k}, \omega) = 4\pi \rho_{ext}(\mathbf{k}, \omega) \tag{21}$$

$$i\mathbf{k} \cdot \mathbf{E}(\mathbf{k}, \omega) = 4\pi \left[-\rho_{ind}(\mathbf{k}, \omega) + \rho_{ext}(\mathbf{k}, \omega) \right] \tag{22}$$

and

$$\mathbf{D}(\mathbf{k}, \omega) = \mathcal{E}(\mathbf{k}, \omega) \mathbf{E}(\mathbf{k}, \omega) \tag{23}$$

where $\mathcal{E}(\mathbf{k}, \omega)$ is the Fourier transformed dielectric constant, ρ_{ext} is an external charge perturbing the system and ρ_{ind} is the induced charge.* The relation of the dielectric constant to $F(q)$, the static susceptibility function, is

$$\mathcal{E}(q, o) = 1 + \frac{4\pi}{q^2}(F(q) \tag{24}$$

in units where $e = 1$. The factor $4\pi/q^2$ comes from dealing with equations in terms of fields and is the Fourier transform** of $1/r_{12}$.

D. Conduction Electron-Conduction Electron Effects

The sum rule associated with the phase shift treatment arose from self-consistency arguments but the perturbation expressions omit conduction electron-conduction electron effects. The role of such self-consistent terms is trivially obtained for the charge case in terms of the dielectric function approach (Pines, 1963). Given the Fourier transformed Poisson equations [Eqs. (21) - (23)] and an externally applied potential

$$\Phi_{ext}(\mathbf{k}, \omega) = \frac{4\pi}{k^2} \rho_{ext}(\mathbf{k}, \omega) \tag{25}$$

we can define a total scalar potential Φ_{tot} by

$$\mathbf{E}(\mathbf{k}, \omega) \equiv -i\mathbf{k}\Phi_{tot}(\mathbf{k}, \omega) = -i\mathbf{k}\left[\frac{4\pi}{k^2} \left\{ \rho_{ext}(\mathbf{k}, \omega) - \rho_{ind}(\mathbf{k}, \omega) \right\} \right]$$

We then can obtain, algebraically, the useful relations

---

*The minus sign multiplying it reflects the repulsive character of like charge.
** See the footnote on page 418.

$$\Phi_{tot}(\mathbf{k}, \omega) = \frac{\Phi_{ext}(\mathbf{k}, \omega)}{\varepsilon(\mathbf{k}, \omega)} \tag{27}$$

and

$$\rho_{ind}(\mathbf{k}, \omega) = \frac{k^2}{4\pi} \Phi_{tot}(\mathbf{k}, \omega) [\varepsilon(\mathbf{k}, \omega) - 1] \tag{28}$$

which is the response to the total self-consistent potential. The induced density, omitting self-consistent terms, is obtained with Eq. (21) yielding

$$\langle \rho_{ind}(\mathbf{k}, \omega) \rangle_{non\ sc} = \frac{k^2}{4\pi} \Phi_{ext}(\mathbf{k}, \omega) [\varepsilon(\mathbf{k}, \omega) - 1] \tag{29a}$$

and for $\omega = 0$

$$\langle \rho_{ind}(\mathbf{k}, 0) \rangle_{non\ sc} = F(k) \Phi_{ext}(ko) \tag{29b}$$

which is the same static result obtained in Eq. (18). In the self-consistent case we want the response to the total potential Φ_{tot}, i.e. we want to solve Eq. (28) for ρ_{ind} in terms of Φ_{ext}. Inserting (26) in the right-hand side of (28) and solving explicitly for ρ_{ind}

$$\langle \rho_{ind}(\mathbf{k}, \omega) \rangle_{sc} = \frac{\varepsilon(\mathbf{k}, \omega) - 1}{\varepsilon(\mathbf{k}, \omega)} \frac{4\pi}{k^2} \Phi_{ext}(\mathbf{k}, \omega) \tag{30a}$$

and in the static limit, $\omega = 0$

$$\langle \rho_{ind}(\mathbf{k}, 0) \rangle_{sc} = \frac{F(k)}{1 + \frac{4\pi}{k^2} F(k)} \Phi_{ext}(\mathbf{k}, 0) . \tag{30b}$$

Here we have the density induced by Φ_{ext} plus the density's own average effective potential. This is commonly known as a random phase, and by a few as a Hartree-Fock,* result. The appearance of a denominator is characteristic of all self-consistent linear response theories. Here it reduces the strength of the response by shielding the perturbing potential.** In first approximation this leads to a simple scaling of the charge response in the asymptotic region.

---

*Equations (29) have sometimes been called the "Hartree-Fock" result but, not being self-consistent, we think this terminology violates the spirit of traditional Hartree-Fock theory which is self-consistent.
**It is possible that high ω components are, in fact, enhanced.

E. Perturbed Charge Density Contributions to Knight Shifts and Electric Field Gradients

A charge density distortion due to an impurity can contribute to a Knight shift and to a quadrupole field gradient at a nuclear site $\mathbf{R}$ away from the impurity. In the latter case the resultant gradient is

$$\Delta q(\mathbf{R}) = \int \Delta \rho(\mathbf{R}+\mathbf{r}') \, 3\, \frac{\cos^2 \theta' - 1}{(r'^3)} \, [1 - \gamma(r')] \, d\mathbf{r}' \qquad (31)$$

where $\gamma(r')$ is an r' dependent Sternheimer antishielding factor. * An asymptotic result can be obtained (Kohn and Vosko, 1960; Blandin and Friedel, 1960) by exploiting the fact that (1) one may take $R >> r'$ because of the local, $1/(r')^3$, character of the quadrupole operator and (2) the oscillatory $q(= 2k_F)$ vector is parallel to $\mathbf{R}$. With these, and ignoring the $[1-\gamma(r')]$ factor and any local atomic character built into $\Delta\rho$, one has

$$\Delta q(R) \sim \frac{\cos(2k_F R + \theta)}{R^3} \qquad (32)$$

which again has the same spatial form as the $\Delta\rho$ of Eq. (11).

The Knight shift contribution is no more difficult to deal with, but as it is of more immediate interest, we consider it in somewhat greater detail. By a Knight shift we mean the constant

$$K = \frac{\Delta H}{H} \qquad (33)$$

designating the additional hyperfine field per unit applied magnetic field, caused by application of a magnetic field to a metal. Low order Knight shift contributions arise in two ways. First, the magnetic field populates conduction electron states, of spin parallel to the field, and energy just above the Fermi energy and depopulates antiparallel spin states just below ϵ_F. This causes a net conduction electron spin $H\chi_p$, where χ_p is the Pauli spin susceptibility. Its density distribution is, of course, characteristic of orbitals at the Fermi energy, and this in turn produces a hyperfine field. Secondly, the magnetic field can induce changes in orbital character, in much the same way as $\Phi(q)$ perturbed the orbitals, which then give rise to a hyperfine field. The orbital Knight shift is an example of this type and is discussed by Narath in Chap. 7.

*See R.E. Watson and A. J. Freeman, Chap. 2.

The spin density associated with the first type of Knight shift produces a hyperfine field either directly via the Fermi contact term (or spin dipolar effects if the crystal is of low enough symmetry), or indirectly via core polarization or some other mechanism. Whatever the coupling, the Knight shift samples Fermi surface wave function character and any perturbation by a charge impurity of this character may affect K. Now the charge impurity formalism described above is most applicable and most commonly applied to nearly free electron-like metals. For these metals, which have a large share of "s"-like conduction electrons, the Fermi contact term tends to dominate. Let us therefore inspect the impurity induced Knight shift arising from this source.

The total contact Knight shift seen by a nucleus at position R with respect to an impurity is

$$K(R) + \Delta K(R) = \chi_p [\rho_F(R) + \Delta \rho_F(R)] , \qquad (34)$$

i.e. the susceptibility times the original plus impurity induced density per electron associated with Fermi surface electrons. Equations (16) - (19) are not appropriate since they pertain to the *total* density but a similar result is readily obtained. Let us separately consider the $\Delta \rho$ spin density contribution from the populated and depopulated orbitals. Considering the populated ones first, utilizing integrals rather than sums and writing the analog of Eq. (16) we have

$$(+)(+) \frac{1}{(2\pi)^3} \int_{FS} dk \int_{k'>k_F} dk' \frac{\Phi(q) \{\exp(iq \cdot r) + \exp(-iq \cdot r)\}}{k^2 - (k')^2} \qquad (35)$$

where $k' = k + q$. The first (+) indicates that these are populated states, the second that the states are of plus spin. The k sum (or integral) is now restricted to the Fermi surface and the k' sum to unoccupied orbital states external to *the Fermi surface* since we are dealing with the impurity distortion of the density of *occupied* orbitals. The depopulated states have a density

$$(-)(-) \frac{1}{(2\pi)^3} \int_{FS} dk \int_{k'<k_F} dk' \frac{\Phi(q) \{\exp(iq \cdot r) + \exp(-iq \cdot r)\}}{k^2 - k'^2} \qquad (36)$$

the first (-) because these are hole states, the second because they are of spin down and now the k' integration is limited to *occupied* states since the mixing is into *unoccupied* ψ_k. Summing Eqs. (29) and (30), the k' integration spans all reciprocal space and we can immediately change the k' integration variable to q. Doing this and performing the k integration over the spherical Fermi surface one obtains an impurity Knight shift:

$$\frac{\Delta K(R)}{K(R)} \sim \int dq\ \Phi(q)\ \frac{q}{k_F}\ \ell n\ \left| \frac{2k_F + q}{2k_F - q} \right|\ \left\{ \exp(i q \cdot R) + \exp(-i q \cdot R) \right\}$$
(37)

a result similar but not identical to Eq. (18). We again have an effect whose Fourier transform is simply $\Phi(q)$ times a q (and k_F) dependent response function.

Since $\Delta K(R)$ varies with R, it produces a line shift and a line width. Assuming a random alloy, the impurity shift is of the form

$$\frac{\Delta K}{K} = c \sum_{R_i} \frac{\Delta K(R_i)}{K}$$
(38)

where c is the impurity concentration and the sum* is over lattice sites R_i. Such an equation assumes additivity in the effect of impurities, namely that one impurity doesn't alter, or scatter, the $\Delta \rho_F(r)$ of another. We have also assumed that the addition of impurities has not appreciably perturbed the band structure and Fermi surface — an assumption one might hope "works" for very dilute alloys but is obviously dangerous as c increases.

Whether it be the ΔK of Eq. (38), in turn involving Eq. (37), or the charge density of Eq. (19), one frequently requires a sum over lattice sites. This makes it particularly convenient to work in reciprocal space. Inserting Eq. (37) into (38) and performing the lattice sum for the case of one atom per unit cell one obtains:

$$\Delta K \sim c \sum_{Q} \Phi(Q)\ \frac{Q}{2k_F}\ \ell n\ \left| \frac{2k_F + Q}{2k_F - Q} \right|$$
(39a)

where the sum is over reciprocal lattice vectors, Q. Given more than one atom per unit cell

*Some workers have replaced the lattice sum by an integral over all space when dealing with such expressions. This is an obviously dangerous practice, when dealing with Knight shift or other magnetic hyperfine predictions, a practice which could even yield an incorrect sign, much less magnitude, for the result.

$$\Delta K \sim c \sum_{Q} \left[\Phi(Q) \frac{Q}{2k_F} \ln \left| \frac{2k_F + Q}{2k_F - Q} \right| \times \right.$$

$$\left. \times \sum_{\delta r} \left\{ \exp(iQ \cdot \delta r) + \exp(-iQ \cdot \delta r) \right\} \right] \qquad (39b)$$

where the extra term (the structure factor familiar from x-ray scattering) is a sum over atomic positions, δr, within a unit cell. It is obviously computationally desirable to deal directly with the Q sum rather than with $\int dq$ and in turn Σ_R. In practice the sum is not rapidly convergent and its greatest virtue may well be, that in using it, one has a painfully clear indication of how difficult it is to obtain a numerically accurate result for an impurity ΔK or $\Delta \rho$.

Impurities have as pronounced an effect on line width and shape as on line shift. From a moments analysis one expects a line width

$$(\delta K)^2 \sim c(1 - c) \sum_{R_i} \left[\Delta \rho(R_i)/\rho(R_i) \right]^2 . \qquad (40)$$

Given the spatial character of $\Delta \rho$, one would expect a distorted line shape.

F.   Charge Polarization Knight Shifts: Experiment vs Theory

We believe it reasonable to say that the original Friedel charge approach has been shown to yield the physics, essential to observed Knight shift and quadrupole effects, for alloys of largely free electron character. This assertion rests on inspection of shifts, line widths and line shapes. The relevance of the approach to the transition metal alloys is masked by magnetic effects, multiple d bands, complicated Fermi surfaces and densities of states with structure (this structure encourages temperature dependent and nonlinear "saturation" effects). For such alloys one normally invokes rigid band, or alternatively *atomic* d charge occupancy arguments. Narath touches on the transition metal case in Chap. 7 and we will make a few comments concerning it in the next section. Here we will attempt to convey the basis and necessary qualifications to our assertion concerning the Friedel picture for the nontransition metal alloys. In much of this section we will inspect Knight shifts in liquid alloys — an area of considerable current activity and one which has provoked thinking relevant to the case of solids as well.

1.   Solid Alloys
The majority of Knight shift data in solid alloys have been

interpreted semi-empirically in terms of phase shifts. The problem largely reduces to making a *choice* of the set of phase shifts to be dealt with. Residual resistivities due to impurities have often been employed, via the relation

$$\Delta \rho_{resist} \sim \frac{1}{k_F} \sum_{\ell} \ell \sin^2 (\eta_{\ell-1} - \eta_{\ell}) \tag{41}$$

to supply further information concerning the η_{ℓ}'s. For example Kohn and Vosko (1960) employed this and the Friedel sum rule to obtain η_0 and η_1 *alone* for an array of alloys, which they then applied to the quadrupole problem and others applied to Knight shifts. Friedel and associates on the other hand, employed a square well analysis (Schiff, 1949), to obtain larger sets of η_{ℓ}'s. In addition to following different routes to obtain sets of η_{ℓ}, workers have considered modifications of the Friedel sum [Eq. (7)] utilized in obtaining the sets. The work of Blatt (1957) deserves particular mention. He introduced an effective ΔZ_{eff}, related to the charge difference ΔZ by

$$\Delta Z_{eff} = \Delta Z - \frac{\delta V}{\Omega} \tag{42}$$

where the second term is the fractional change in size of the atomic cell due to the impurity, thus accounting for impurity size effects. The introduction of such a term is intuitively desirable but in practice it has not improved numerical agreement between theory and experiment. Such failures are typical of most improvements which have been made.

The classic study of charge polarization Knight shifts is that of Rowland (1962) where he inspected his and Drain's data for Ag alloys. The results appear in Fig. 5 and, within the scatter, the shifts vary linearly out to quite large concentrations. This linear dependence is characteristic of charge impurity ΔK's in alloys and is in marked contrast with the spin density case (to be discussed in the next section) where "saturation" effects set in relatively rapidly. Rowland employed the phase shift approach to inspect these data. While quantitative fits were not obtained with shifts and widths, it is fair to say that this work established the importance and essential correctness of the Friedel view. One of the strongest pieces of evidence was the strongly asymmetric line shape which could not be rationalized in other ways. Little has been learned from the temperature dependence of the effects (associated with the smearing of the Fermi surface) because experimentally

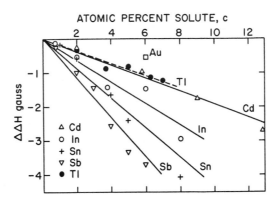

Fig. 5a

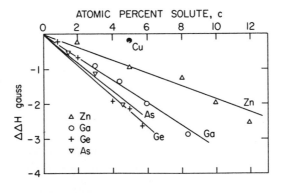

Fig. 5b

Ag alloy Knight shifts (Rowland, 1962) as a function of impurity concentration.

and theoretically the dependence is slight. *

The results of Fig. 5 correlate quite well with the Friedel sum rule, i.e. with ΔZ. In Fig. 5a, we see Knight shifts plotted for the fifth row impurities Cd, In, Sn, and Sb whose ΔZ vary from +1 to +4. The shifts display slopes which vary roughly with ΔZ. The sixth row impurities Au ($\Delta Z = 0$) and Tl($\Delta Z = +2$) also appear. The Au data shows a small rather than zero effect but this is not surprising considering matters such as Eq. (42). What is more damaging is that Tl shows no indication to conform with In, both being $\Delta Z = 2$ impurities. Rowland's fourth row impurity results appear in Fig. 5b ranging from Cu to As ($\Delta Z = 0$ to $+4$). Zn, Ga, and Ge lines are drawn with the *same* slopes as those for their fifth row counterparts but As is definitely out of line. From all of this one concludes that Knight shifts generally correlate well with ΔZ except when ΔZ becomes too large. This correlation is even more strikingly seen, for positive and negative ΔZ, in the Knight shift results for Pb alloys of Snodgrass and Bennett (1964).

When endeavoring to guage the adequacy of the phase shift approach one encounters the usual problem of a semi-empirical theory, namely that several uniquely different parametrizations yield equally good or poor (depending on one's view) fits of experiment. The Pb results are an example of this where Odle and Flynn (1966) and Snodgrass and Howard (unpublished) have separately produced fair fits, employing significantly different fitting schemes.

2. Liquid Metal Alloys

Liquid metals and alloys are currently the object of extensive and fascinating investigations and we would like to turn to their Knight shift results now. This is necessary, not simply because they are interesting, but because some of the most recent thinking, relevant to both solids and liquids, has been done here.

Crudely speaking, a metal maintains its metallic character going through the melting point, although long-range order is

*In one sense this is to be expected because the approach is being applied to metals whose densities of states at ε_F have little structure. One might expect significant temperature dependence in, for example, a transition metal but this is just where the simple impurity charge picture has little applicability.

destroyed. * This affects the band structure and, as a general
rule, transport properties and NMR are observably perturbed.
Typically, liquid alloy Knight shifts vary linearly with concentration out to at least 10 percent and sometimes over the full, 0 to 100
percent, range of concentration! A correlation time of $\sim 10^{-11}$ sec
associated with atomic motion is sufficiently short to average out
Knight shift line broadening and electric quadrupole effects, leaving only the impurity shift itself. Since we are no longer dealing
with an ordered metal, we must abandon the lattice sum estimate
of $\Delta K/K$ of Eq. (38) and instead employ

$$\frac{\Delta K}{K} = c \int \frac{\Delta K(r)}{K} P(\mathbf{r}) \, d\mathbf{r} \tag{43}$$

where $P(\mathbf{r})$ is the atomic pair correlation function of the liquid;
i. e. the probability, given an atom at the origin, of a second being
at $\mathbf{r}$.

Odle and Flynn(1966) studied an array of liquid Cu alloys, all
of which display linear behavior over the ranges concentration
inspected. These results appear in Fig. 6 and, for common impurities, the slopes are in striking agreement with the silver

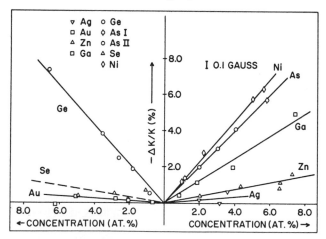

Fig. 6: Liquid Cu alloy Knight shifts (Odle and Flynn, 1966) as a
function of impurity concentrations.

*The question of the extent and nature of the local order is
one of great current interest. Paskin (1966), for example,
asserts that small groups of atoms show less of a tendency
to display crude crystalline order, than has been traditionally assumed.

results of Fig. 5. Zn, Ga, and Ge again show concentration dependences reflecting their ΔZ's and As is out of line in the same way again. In their paper, Odle and Flynn made one of the most complete recent inspections of Knight shifts employing phase shift analyses (including the Pb alloys already discussed). In the course of this they noted that the $\Delta\rho(\mathbf{r})$, and in turn $\Delta K(\mathbf{r})$, for *small* $\mathbf{r}$, largely determine the shift of Eq. (43). In this region asymptotic theories are very dangerous and "rigorous, accurate" estimates of $\rho(\mathbf{r})$ are very difficult. This observation bodes ill for *a priori* estimates of Eqs. (38) and (43).

3. Pseudopotentials

At this point it is useful to insert the perturbation expression for $\Delta K(\mathbf{r})$, i.e. Eq. (37) into (43), do the d$\mathbf{r}$ integration and obtain

$$\frac{\Delta K}{K} \sim \int \Phi(q) \, [1 - a(q)] \frac{q}{k_F^2} \, \ell n \left| \frac{1 + q/2k_F}{1 - q/2k_F} \right| \, dq \qquad (44)$$

where $[1 - a(q)]$ is the Fourier transform of the pair correlation function, $P(\mathbf{r})$. In principle this holds no more physical information than a phase shift analysis (where $\Phi(q)$ would be employed to relate different η_ℓ to one another, thus allowing a large number of ℓ values in the scheme). In practice, it is more directly amenable to improvement. This and Eqs. (16), (18), and (31) were derived assuming free electron orbitals and bands. The $\exp(i\mathbf{k}\cdot\mathbf{r})$ orbital character led to the matrix element, $\Phi(q)$, being the simple transform of $\Phi(r)$. Deviations from pure free electron orbital and band character can be, in large part, accounted for by making $\Phi(q)$ an *effective* q dependent function — a pseudopotential. Pseudopotentials have been very satisfactorily employed in energy band and transport theory [for a review see Harrison (1966)] and information gained there can, in principle, then be utilized in evaluating Eq. (44).

Equation (44) was employed by Seymour and co-workers when analyzing the Knight shifts of binary liquid alloys involving constituents (Ga, In, Tl) of common valency. These and some of their other results are notable in varying linearly over the *full* range of concentration.* The three components of Eq. (44) appropriate

Such a tendency is not terribly surprising for alloys made up of constituents of similar valency where each pure metal is free electron-like. Marked deviations from this tendency have been attributed to incipient local intermetallic compound order in the liquids.

to the In-Tl system appear in Fig. 7, h_{In} - h_{Tl} being the difference in their pseudopotentials. The atoms, having common valency, cause this difference to be zero for q = 0. Inspecting the figure, it is conceivable that one could have difficulty obtaining the sign, much less the magnitude, of $\Delta K/K$. Note, by the way, the distinct suggestion that one must integrate accurately out to large q values, well off of the plot, in order to obtain any sort of convergence. Inspection of pseudopotential differences provided a rationalization of the difference in sign and magnitude of the shifts seen for two alloys but full quantitative estimates were impossible because of inadequate knowledge of the components of Eq. (44) (and perhaps of the equation itself). It was stated that cases, where $\Delta Z \neq 0$, would be even more difficult.

A pseudopotential estimate employing Eq. (39) or (44) has yet to produce significantly better results than the generally poor ones available via phase shift treatments. If one attributes this to inadequate knowledge of the pseudopotentials, one might hope to utilize the Knight shift data to refine our knowledge of the $\Phi(q)$. We are not optimistic about this for reasons quite aside from the numerical difficulties suggested in Fig. 7. We believe that these

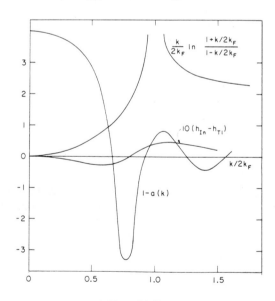

Fig. 7: The components of Eq. (44) for the In-Tl alloy system.

(after Moulson, et al., (1965)).

hyperfine effects provide a particularly difficult case for pseudo-potential theory, which is, after all, approximate, to deal with. A similar situation will be encountered in the next section where it will be difficult to make quantitative contact between magnetic hyperfine effects and overall spin density behavior (much less the basic theory). Refinement of the response function for self-consistency, non-free electron character and perhaps correlation, as well as refinement of the associated hyperfine interaction matrix element (which here is simply the Fermi contact term for plane wave functions) is needed. This might be crudely incorporated into a q dependent term appropriate for insertion into Eqs. (39) or (44) but ultimately we must acknowledge that a q dependent theory is an approximation* and ask what, if any, effect this has on our predictions. As we have already indicated, we believe these Knight shifts provide a particularly difficult test for the pseudo-potential approach.

We might note, in closing, that the theory for various properties of liquid alloys, while qualitatively satisfactory, has been quantitatively poor and not amenable to easy, unique, numerical improvement. Knight shift studies may well provide information helping us refine these theories but this information involves more than simple improvements of pseudopotentials.

III. Spin Density Effects

A. Ruderman-Kittel-Kasuya-Yosida Theory

Here, one is interested in the effect of a local electronic magnetic moment on the conduction electron spin distribution — the Ruderman-Kittel-Kasuya-Yosida (RKKY) problem. The wave function distortion effects, such as we have seen in the charge impurity case, contribute to the distribution of spin density but *not* to the net conduction electron spin. There are, in addition, re-population effects which do contribute a net spin and which are intimately related to the Pauli spin susceptibility.

The local moment will interact with the conduction electrons via an exchange coupling, the leading term of which involves an exchange integral

N.H. March informs us that pseudopotential theory appears to be in quantitative difficulty for other observables.

$$J(\mathbf{k}, \mathbf{k}') \equiv N \langle \iint \psi^*_{\mathbf{k}'}(\mathbf{r}_1) \, \psi^*_{loc}(\mathbf{r}_2) \frac{1}{r_{12}} \psi_{loc}(\mathbf{r}_1)$$

$$\psi_{\mathbf{k}}(\mathbf{r}_2) \, d\tau_1 d\tau_2 \rangle \qquad (45)$$

where the $\langle \, \rangle$ indicates an average over local orbitals, ψ_{loc}, which contribute to the moment; N, the number of lattice sites, is included in the definition so that $J(\mathbf{k}, \mathbf{k})$ is of the order of an atomic exchange integral. Diagonal, $\mathbf{k} = \mathbf{k}'$, integrals contribute to repopulation and $\mathbf{k} \neq \mathbf{k}'$ terms contribute to density redistribution. Let us consider the repopulation or Zener term first. The exchange integral interaction occurs between electrons of like spin;[*] the net energy gained by conduction electrons of spin parallel to the local moment is

$$E_{ex} = -\frac{2S}{N} J(\mathbf{k}, \mathbf{k}) \qquad (46)$$

where S is the spin of the local moment (2S is the number of unpaired electrons contributing to the moment and in turn to the exchange energy). We should note that such a diagonal (i. e., $\mathbf{k} = \mathbf{k}'$) exchange integral is inevitably positive,[**] implying that this exchange term always lowers the energy of conduction electrons of spin parallel to the moment with respect to those which are antiparallel. Equation (46) can be conveniently rewritten as

$$E_{ex} = -\frac{2}{N} \, \mathbf{s} \cdot \mathbf{S} \, J(\mathbf{k}, \mathbf{k}) + K \, J(\mathbf{k}, \mathbf{k}) \qquad (46a)$$

an expression appropriate to conduction electrons of either spin $\mathbf{s}$. The constant K is a function of $|S|$ and this term, which is effectively a change in the zero of energy, acts on electrons independently of spin. As such, it will not affect the spin distribution but may be added to any purely Coulomb impurity effects of the local moment and will contribute to an impurity charge polarization after the manner of the preceding section. The separation of charge and spin density effects occurs in a theory linear in the impurity potential.

The effect of the exchange term on a pair of previously nonmagnetic bands is seen in Fig. 8 for free-electron-like bands where $\epsilon = k^2$. Since the exchange lowers the energy of parallel

*For a discussion of exchange and the associated Fermi hole see Chap. 2 by Watson and Freeman.

**This is best seen by inspecting Eq. (45) and noting that we are dealing with the Coulomb interaction of an overlap charge density with itself.

Fig. 8: Zener or Pauli repopulation of conduction bands under the influence of a local moment's exchange field.

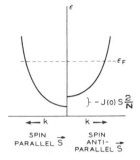

(+) spin electrons, antiparallel (-) spin electrons near the Fermi surface flip their spin and occupy the lower energy (+) spin states. The number of conduction electrons, per atom, of either spin becomes

$$n_{\pm} = n_0 \pm \frac{3n_0 \, J(k_F k_F)S}{2N\epsilon_F}$$

$$= n_0 \pm \frac{V J(k_F, k_F)S}{(2\pi)^3 N} \qquad (47)$$

where n_0 was the number of electrons of either spin prior to polarization and V is the volume of the metal. The resultant polarization is positive, in the sense of producing a net spin which is parallel to that of the local moment, because the exchange integral is positive. This implies, among other things, that if a local magnetic moment induces an antiparallel spin density in a medium, then some other mechanism is responsible. The net spin induced here, is exactly the Pauli spin susceptibility term except that an exchange rather than a magnetic field drives it. Taken alone it yields an infinitely ranged-constant spin density distribution in the metal.

Mixing effects analogous to the orbital Knight shift and to the charge impurity case redistribute the spin density. Again, using perturbation theory but with exchange, the source of the off-diagonal matrix element, we have for an occupied Bloch orbital

$$\psi_{k,\pm} = \psi^0_{k,\pm} - \frac{1}{N} \sum_{k'>k_F} \frac{J(k,k')}{\epsilon_k - \epsilon_{k'}} \left\{ \pm S^z \, \psi^0_{k'\pm} + S^{\mp} \psi^0_{k'\mp} \right\} \quad (48)$$

where S^- and S^+ are the step down and step up spin operators acting on the local moment. Concentrating on a spin density, rather than relaxation effects, we will ignore the $S^{\pm}$ terms. At this point it is traditional to assume free electron bands [Eq. (14)] from which one obtains, as in Eq. (16), the total (±) density linear in J,

$$\Delta \rho_{\pm}^{S}(r) = \mp \frac{S^{Z}}{NV} \sum_{k<k_F} \sum_{k'>k_F} \frac{J(k, k')}{k^2 - (k')^2}$$

$$\times \left\{ e^{i(k-k')\cdot r} + e^{-i(k-k')\cdot r} \right\} . \tag{49}$$

The charge densities of (+) and (-) spin are equal but opposite in sign implying that there is *no* associated charge density distortion. As was discussed for the second term of Eq. (46a), exchange matrix elements emanating from the local moment may contribute to the charge distortion but what is important to us here (and is to be expected), is that charge and spin density effects are decoupled in terms linear in the perturbation.

In order to obtain analytic results and to make contact with normal linear response theory, it has been traditional to assume the exchange coupling to be a function only of $q(=|k-k'|)$, i.e., to set

$$J(k, k') = J(q) , \tag{50}$$

yielding a J which is effectively the Fourier transform of some quantity. One then obtains, as in Sec. II, a total spin density

$$\Delta \rho^{S}(r) \equiv \Delta \rho_{+}^{S}(r) - \Delta \rho_{-}^{S}(r) = \frac{S^{Z}}{N} \sum_{q} F(q)J(q) \left\{ e^{iq\cdot r} + e^{-q\cdot r} \right\} , \tag{51}$$

the same result as for the charge density [cf. Eq. (18)] except that $\Phi(q)$ has been replaced by $S^{Z}J(q)/N$. Ruderman and Kittel (1954) pointed out that the $q=0$ term in the sum is the Zener or Pauli repopulation term determining the net spin induced in the conduction bands, while the $q \neq 0$ terms affect the distribution but not the net spin.

1. Approximate J(q)

The original investigations of Ruderman and Kittel assumed J(q) constant. This choice let them obtain an analytic result, an important factor in itself, and seemed reasonable because they were considering the case of a nuclear local moment as the source of the polarization. A delta function interaction between the nucleus and the conduction electrons would, of course, yield a constant $J(q)$. This resulted in a spin density

$$\rho_{RK}(r) \sim \frac{1}{k_F} \frac{2k_F r \cos(2k_F r) - \sin(2k_F r)}{r^4} \tag{52}$$

which has the asymptotic form [cf. Eq. (11)]

$$\rho_{RF}(r)_{r \to \infty} \sim \frac{\cos 2k_F r}{r^3} \tag{53}$$

Unfortunately, ρ_{RK} goes to infinity as $r \to 0$, due to keeping $J(q)$ a constant as $q \to \infty$. This nonphysical result implies that even a nuclear moment, interacting via the Fermi contact term, does not provide a δ function perturbation for the purpose of estimating conduction electron polarization.

Yosida considered the problem of a local electronic moment as the source of the polarization and made another approximation for $J(q)$ which also yields analytic results. He took

$$J(q) = \text{constant} \qquad q \le 2k_F$$

$$J(q) = 0 \qquad q \ge 2k_F \tag{54}$$

and obtained

$$\rho_Y(r) = k_F r \, \rho_{RK}(r) \tag{55}$$

which avoids the infinity at $r = 0$ but falls off as $\cos(2k_F r)/r^2$ for large r, a slower rate than one would expect for the density.

Overhauser obtained a more reasonable approximation for $J(q)$ but at the price of abandoning an analytic result for the density. He employed the standard assumption that the Coulomb $1/r_{12}$ interaction is strongly shielded and replaced the $1/r_{12}$ of the exchange integral [Eq. (45)] by a delta function obtaining

$$J_{FF}(q) = \text{const} \times \int |\psi_{loc}(r)|^2 \, e^{iq \cdot r} \, dr \tag{56}$$

which is simply ψ_{loc}'s form factor.

2. $J(q)$ Versus Exact $J(k, k')$ Behavior

The advantage of dealing with an equation such as (51) is that $F(q)$ is, apart from constants, the static magnetic susceptibility appropriate to the conduction electron polarization due to the qth Fourier component of a magnetic field, $H(q)$. This lets us employ our knowledge of the effect of conduction electron-conduction electron interactions on the susceptibility (a matter to be inspected shortly); most recent developments of RKKY theory have been in this direction.

Unfortunately, the exchange integral is not simply a function of q. For a spherical local moment

$$J_{spher}(\mathbf{k}, \mathbf{k'}) = \sum_{\ell} P_{\ell}(\cos \omega)\, \mathscr{Y}_{\ell}(k, k') \tag{57}$$

where ω is the angle between $\mathbf{k}$ and $\mathbf{k'}$ and $\mathscr{Y}$ is a function only of the magnitudes k and k'. Only by sheer accident will such a function be even crudely approximated by a J(q). While Eq. (57) is intuitively obvious, let us sketch its derivation which involves inserting ψ_k and ψ_{loc} into Eq. (45). The spatial part of ψ_{loc} will be taken as

$$\psi_{loc}(\mathbf{r}) = R(r) Y_L^M(\theta, \varphi) \tag{58}$$

where R is a radial function, presumably atomic in its essential character.* The ψ_k will be expanding at the local moment site in the general form

$$\psi_k(\mathbf{r}) = \sum_{\ell, m} (i)^{\ell} Y_{\ell}^m(\theta, \varphi)\, Y_{\ell}^{-m}(\theta_k, \varphi_k)\, \Xi_{\ell, m}^k(r) \tag{59}$$

where φ_k and θ_k are the direction angles of $\mathbf{k}$ with respect to a chozen z axis and Ξ is a general radial function (incorporating in it the necessary normalization of ψ_k) which (apart from normalization) would be a spherical Bessel function if ψ_k were a plane wave. Inserting these into Eq. (45) and doing the angular integrals

$$J(\mathbf{k}, \mathbf{k'}) = \Big\langle \sum_{\substack{\ell, \ell', m \\ \mathscr{L}\, m}} (i)^{\ell - \ell'}(2L+1)[(2\ell+1)(2\ell'+1)]^{\frac{1}{2}}$$

$$\times Y_{\ell}^{-m}(\theta_k \varphi_k)\, Y_{\ell'}^m(\theta_{k'} \varphi_{k'})$$

$$\times \begin{pmatrix} \ell & \mathscr{L} & L \\ 0 & 0 & 0 \end{pmatrix}\begin{pmatrix} \ell' & \mathscr{L} & L \\ 0 & 0 & 0 \end{pmatrix}\begin{pmatrix} \ell' & \mathscr{L} & L \\ m & -m & -M \end{pmatrix}\begin{pmatrix} \ell' & \mathscr{L} & L \\ -m & m & M \end{pmatrix} \mathscr{F}^{\mathscr{L}}(k, k') \Big\rangle \tag{60}$$

where the brackets ( ) denote 3j coefficients** and

Restriction of ψ_{loc} to a single L is normally reasonable and not important to the essential result. Restriction to a single M is not significant since an average will be taken over a spherical moment.

**For their definition and properties which lead from Eq. (60) to (63), see Edmonds (1957).*

$$\mathscr{F}^{\mathscr{L}}(k, k') \equiv \int \int R_L(r) R_L(r') \, \Xi_{\ell m}^k(r) \, \Xi_{\ell' m}^{k'}(r') \, \frac{r_<^{\mathscr{L}}}{r_>^{\mathscr{L}+1}} \, r^2 \, dr \, r'^2 \, dr' \tag{61}$$

Performing the $\mathscr{M}$ summation and averaging over a spherical local moment (i.e., over M) one obtains

$$J(k, k') = \sum_{\ell, m} \frac{4\pi}{2\ell+1} \, Y_\ell^m(\theta_k \varphi_k) \, Y_\ell^{-m}(\theta_{k'} \varphi_{k'}) \, \mathscr{J}_\ell(k, k') \tag{62}$$

where

$$\mathscr{J}_\ell(k, k') \equiv \frac{2\ell+1}{4\pi} \sum_{\mathscr{L}} \mathscr{F}^{\mathscr{L}}(k, k') \begin{pmatrix} \ell & \mathscr{L} & L \\ 0 & 0 & 0 \end{pmatrix}^2 \tag{63}$$

Equation (62) is the same as Eq. (57) providing that the $\mathscr{F}^{\mathscr{L}}$, hence the $\mathscr{J}_\ell$, are independent of m — a quite good assumption.* Note that since the ℓth component of the exchange integral is associated with the ℓth spherical harmonic component of both ψ_k and $\psi_{k'}$, any opinions concerning the ℓ character of the conduction electron orbitals at the site of the moment have immediate consequences for the k, k' dependence of J.† All other factors being equal, the term involving ℓ equal to the L of the local moment orbitals will dominate. This follows from the $\mathscr{F}^{\mathscr{L}}$'s which tend to be larger, the smaller the $\mathscr{L}$ value. Since

$$|L - \ell| \le \mathscr{L} \le L + \ell \tag{64}$$

[coming from the 3j coefficients of Eq. (63)], the $\ell = L$ term is the one case where $\mathscr{L}$ may equal zero, encouraging $\mathscr{J}_L$ to be of largest magnitude.

Examples of the calculated exchange integral are plotted in Fig. 9 for an Fe ($3d^5$) and a Gd ($4f^7$) local moment and for ψ_k which are single plane waves orthogonalized to the ion cores [for further details, see Watson and Freeman (1966) and (1967)]. The

*This is a better assumption than simply assuming that the $\Xi(r)$ are independent of m because the $\mathscr{F}$ integrals sample conduction electron orbital behavior at the site of the spherical moment and in that region (of small r) the $\Xi(r)$ tend to be most strongly independent of m.

†For a nonspherical moment there will, of course, be contributions to $J(k, k')$ from ψ_k and $\psi_{k'}$ components of differing ℓ. These will be relatively unimportant but what is of immediate concern here is that their contributions will normally not encourage $J(k, k')$ to conform with Eq. (50).

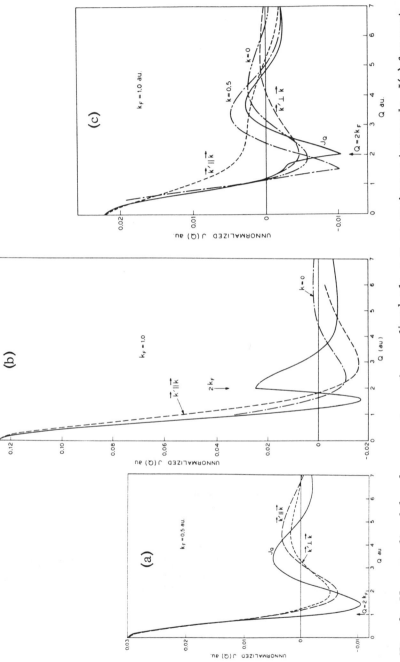

Fig. 9: Unnormalized local moment - orthoganalized plane wave exchange integrals, J(q) for various cores of **k** and **k'** for (a) Gd 4f⁷ k_F = 0.5 a.u., (b) Fe 3d⁵ k_F = 1.0 a.u., (c) Gd 4f⁷ k_F = 1.0 a.u.

J's are plotted as a function of q for a variety of choices of the magnitudes and relative orientation of $\mathbf{k}$ and $\mathbf{k}'$ as indicated on the figures. Unless otherwise indicated, $|\mathbf{k}| = k_F$. The solid curves, J_Q, conform to the q choice of Fig. 2, namely that $\mathbf{k}$ and $\mathbf{k}'$ each trace the Fermi surface for $q < 2k_F$ and are antiparallel for $q > 2k_F$. This choice is associated with the minimum energy denominator, for given $|q|$ in our perturbation theory expressions, such as Eq. (49). For any given case one wishes to decide whether a $J(\mathbf{k}, \mathbf{k}')$ can be reasonably approximated by a suitably chosen $J(q)$. From the figures one would conclude that this cannot be done for Fe (Fig. 9b) but can for Gd when $k_F = 0.5$ (Fig. 9a). Part of the trouble for the Fe case is the occurrence of a significant $\ell = 2$ term in $J(\mathbf{k}, \mathbf{k}')$.

The Overhauser $J_{FF}(q)$ approximation and the solid curve $J_Q(q)$ of Fig. 9a appear in Fig. 10 where $J_{FF}(q)$ has been scaled so that integrals match at $q = 0$. The disagreement is significant and, in part, rests on the question of whether one expects substantial Coulomb shielding over distances short with respect to a local moment's dimensions. While there is considerable evidence

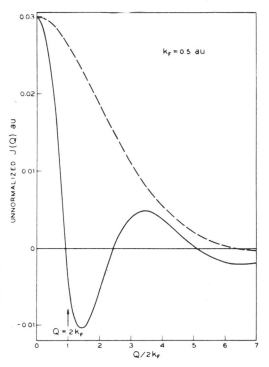

Fig. 10: The form factor $J_{FF}(q)$ and minimum energy denominator $J_Q(q)$ for a local Gd $4f^7$ moment and $k_F = 0.5$ a.u.

for strong shielding over distances as short as interatomic lattice spacings in metals [Herring (1966)], we do not expect such on an *intra*-atomic scale.

3. Computed Spin Densities: Gd Local Moments

Dealing explicitly with $J(\mathbf{k}, \mathbf{k'})$, in a spin density estimate, involves a double integration with an unpleasant denominator. Rather little is known (and nothing published) of what it yields and how and when it differs significantly from $J(q)$ predictions. We will concentrate on $J(q)$ predictions throughout the remainder of this chapter.

Spin density results for Gd obtained with J_Q and with J_{FF} appear in Fig. 11. All display the characteristic Friedel oscillations in their outer reaches with periods proportional to $[2k_F]^{-1}$.

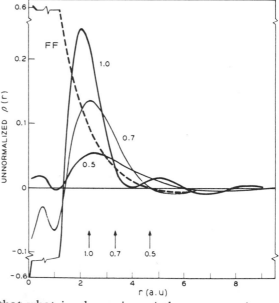

Fig. 11: Unnormalized spin density predictions employing the unenhanced susceptibility $F(q)$ with J_Q for $k_F = 0.5, 0.7,$ and 1.0 a.u. and with J_{FF} for $k_F = 0.5$ a.u.

It is to be emphasized that what is shown is *not* the asymptotic region. All the plotted results have a positive net spin associated with positive $J(0)$'s. The *same* net spin, i.e., $\int \rho(r) r^2 \, dr$, occurs for the form factor and $k_F = 0.5$ a.u. result. The J_Q results show an outward shift of the region where the spin density is concentrated and indicate that the spin at the origin may be parallel or antiparallel to the net spin. We also see that $\rho(0)$ may be larger or smaller in magnitude than the density at near neighbor

distances (typically 5 a.u.). These facts will be of interest when
we later attempt to relate theory with experiment. The peaking of
$\rho(0)$, obtained with J_{FF}, becomes more pronounced in the Yosida
and, of course, in the Ruderman-Kittel approximations.

The results of Fig. 11 are striking in certain similarities
with the atomic exchange polarization results seen for Gd^{3+} in
Chap. 2. Having neither a Fermi surface, nor Bloch orbital character, the atomic results do not display Friedel oscillations. Instead, they show a pile up of majority spin density in the vicinity
of the local moment (the open 4f shell) and exactly the same tendency is seen for the conduction electrons here. Having a Fermi
energy and allowing repopulation effects, the conduction electron
density has a net spin which the atomic case of course does not.

B. Interband Mixing

As discussed, the electrostatic exchange *integral* $J(0)$ is
positive, implying an induced net spin parallel to that of the local
moment. Antiparallel net spins are known to occur experimentally
for example for Gd as an impurity in a Pd host metal. There
exists an *effective* exchange mechanism which will produce such
an antiparallel spin arrangement. While familiar since the 1930's
its significance to the problem at hand was emphasized more recently by Anderson and Clogston. This is interband mixing. Let
us consider the simple case of parabolic bands and a Gd $4f^7$ local
moment shown in Fig. 12. We start with a simple unmagnetized

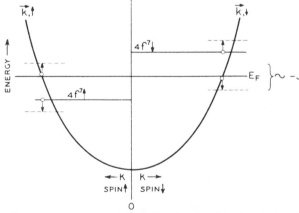

Fig. 12: A schematic representation of interband mixing for a
          $4f^7$ local moment and its contribution to a $J'[0]$ defined
          for Fermi surface electrons.

conduction band of either spin, occupied up to the Fermi energy and a half-filled 4f shell of, say, spin ↑. Being highly localized, these 4f electrons form a very narrow band which lies below the Fermi surface; associated with the 4f ↓ orbitals there exists another narrow band of unoccupied virtual states lying above the Fermi surface. A conduction-electron state ψ_k of spin ↑ which lies just above the Fermi surface will, in general, have a nonzero matrix element $\langle \psi_{4f} | \mathcal{H} | \psi_k \rangle$, with an occupied 4f ↑ orbital causing the two functions to mix. This mixing will raise the energy of the state at the Fermi surface as is indicated in the figure. Such mixing occurs almost inevitably if only because the nonmagnetized bands, which represent our starting point, are not exact eigenstates of the magnetized system with its Hamiltonian $\mathcal{H}$. This particular mixing will be termed an "emission" process since an occupied 4f state has conduction-electron character part of the time. There is a similar "absorption" process which involves the 4f ↓ virtual states and an occupied conduction-electron orbital (also of minority spin). In this case, the state with predominantly conduction-electron character will have its energy lowered. The combined effect of absorption and emission processes is to lower the minority spin (↓) conduction-electron energies with respect to those of majority spin (↑), in opposition to the effect of the exchange *integral* between the $4f^7$ ↑ shell and the conduction electrons (which, of course, involves only conduction electrons of ↑ spin). These interband mixing effects may be characterized by a parameter $J'(k, k')$ of the form

$$ J'(k, k') \sim -\frac{1}{S} \sum_i \frac{\langle k | \mathcal{H} | 4f_i \rangle \, \langle 4f_i | \mathcal{H} | k' \rangle}{|\,\epsilon_{4f_i} - \epsilon_k\,|} \tag{65} $$

where the sum spans occupied and unoccupied 4f levels and only the *magnitude* of the energy difference appears in the denominator.*

Two spin density contributions arise from this effect. First, the mixing of conduction electron ↑ into the occupied 4f ↑ states and of unoccupied 4f ↓ into the ↓ conduction states, redistributes the local moment's spin. No net change in the system's spin occurs and as Anderson and Clogston pointed out, the density falls off very rapidly (roughly as $1/r^4$), limiting the effect of this term to the impurity site. It is thus a minor distortion of the impurity moment, which, by the way, produces little or no spin density at the impurity nucleus — a matter touched on shortly. Secondly, and

The signs of the denominators have already been combined with signs of numerators to yield the minus appearing outside the sum.

of greater interest, the effective exchange, which can be rewritten

$$J'(k, k') = \sum_{\ell} P_{\ell} (\cos \omega) \, \Omega_{\ell} (k, k') \tag{66}$$

contributes to the RKKY mixing. It is added to the exchange integral when Eq. (49) is to be evaluated. Here, as in Eq. (57), the ℓth component is associated with the ℓth component of the Bloch orbitals but, in addition and quite aside from the character of the Bloch orbitals, there is a strong tendency for the term with ℓ in common with the L of the local moment orbitals, to dominate to the almost complete exclusion of other terms. This is due to the $\hbar$ matrix elements of Eq. (65) which are zero valued or small when $\ell \neq L$ [Watson, Koide, Peter and Freeman (1965)]. To a good first approximation we thus have:

$$J'(k, k') \simeq P_{L} (\cos \omega) \, \Omega_{L} (k, k') \tag{66a}$$

where Ω is a function only of the magnitudes of k and k'. Such a J' is a particularly bad candidate for the assumed q dependence of exchange necessary if one wishes to employ Eq. (51) to estimate the spin density.

There is one important feature of a coupling of the form of Eq. (57) or (66), namely, when inserted into Eq. (49), the ℓth component of the coupling projects out the ℓth spherical harmonic component of the exponential products. (This will also occur when the exponentials are replaced by $\psi_k^* \psi_{k'}$ products which are more realistic than the plane wave character of the exponentials.) Now the $\ell = 0$ density component is the one which is nonzero at the origin and of the $\mathscr{L}_0$ and Ω_0 terms which may drive it, the Ω_0 term is normally zero or almost zero valued. As a result, interband mixing may be important in determining the net spin induced in the conduction bands and in determining the character of the spin distribution off the local moment site but it will contribute little or nothing to the spin density sampled, via the Fermi contact term, by the local moment's own nucleus. This is of some significance when one tries to relate a local moment's hyperfine field to other spin dependent experimental data.

C. Conduction Electron-Conduction Electron Effects

Very different things happen in the spin problem then was seen to occur in the charge case treated in Sec. II-D. In the original treatment, Wolff (1960, 1963) assumed a delta function conduction electron-conduction electron exchange interaction whose Fourier transform is a constant v and, crudely speaking, obtained

$$\rho_\pm^{sc}(q) = \pm \frac{S^z}{2N} \frac{F(q)}{1 - vF(q)} J(q) \equiv \pm \frac{S^z}{2N} \chi(q) J(q). \qquad (67)$$

Self-consistency again appears as a term in the denominator and its minus sign is associated with the negative sign of electrostatic exchange coupling (v being positive). It therefore leads to an *enhancement* of the spin response. Energetically this is to be expected. For example, as spins are flipped, the induced spin produces an exchange field encouraging still more spins to flip, hence enhancing the response. [It is just this type of argument which underlies the traditional Slater band theory picture of ferromagnetism.]

Experimentally, we know that the exchange enhancement is significant. Comparing the static susceptibility with that predicted for a density of states deduced from a specific heat measurement, or an energy band calculation, yields the q = 0 ratio, $\chi(0)/F(0)$. For most metals the ratio is less than 7 but for Pd it is roughly 15.* Inspecting the q dependence of $F(q)$ (see Fig. 1), we see that the enhancement is nonlinear and falls off with increasing q. For example, for a factor of 10, or greater, enhancement of $F(0)$, there is but a factor of ~ 2 enhancement of $F(2k_F)$. The effect of this is to lift the spin density like a rug and examples of this are shown in Fig. 13 for a Gd local moment. The enhanced results are for $\chi(0)/F(0) = 7$ and we see the rug lifting at work with the first negative oscillation going positive for the $k_F = 0.5$ result. The first, $k_F = 1.0$, oscillation had already been driven positive by the exchange coupling and the second, in both cases, remains

---

A factor of ~15 is suggested by comparison with the band calculations (Freeman et al., 1966) and by inspection of the electronic specific heat, γ, if one assumes the latter undergoes a factor of two enhancement due to electron-phonon (and any other) effects. Recently Berk and Schrieffer (1966, 1967) have inspected a spin fluxuation term which may introduce a stronger enhancement of the specific heat, implying a larger χ(0)/F(0) ratio as well. If this is true, the band calculations have <u>overestimated</u> the density of states to an extent greater than reasonably expected. This matter remains to be resolved, but in any case, a χ(0)/F(0) ratio of 15 or greater appears to hold for Pd.

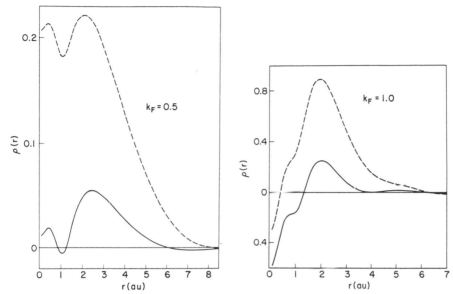

Fig. 13: Unnormalized spin density predictions with the unenhanced (solid line) and seven-fold enhanced (dashed line)
susceptibility for k_F values equal to a) 0.5 a.u. and
b) 1.0 a.u.

negative. It would take an enhancement ratio of the order of 15 or
20 to wash out the second negative region in either case. Note
that $\rho(0)$, for $k_F = 1.0$, has remained negative, although it has become smaller in magnitude. Exchange enhancement of form factor
or other traditional predictions enhances the maximum density at
$r = 0$ most violently, an inconvenience when trying to relate theory
to experiment, as will be discussed shortly.

D. Relation to Experiment

A comprehensive review of spin density experiments and
their relation to theory could occupy this entire volume. We therefore limit ourselves to the inspection of two general features of
experimental results and two examples. We must first note two
features of the theory of the preceding subsections, which have yet
to be adequately acknowledged.

First, the treatment is physically equivalent to the Hartree-
Fock exchange polarization of ion cores discussed in Chap. 2 and
all the uncertainties of principle, seen there, apply here. In particular,
there is the question of how correlation effects between local moment and conduction electrons perturb the conduction electrons'

response. Little is known concerning this [Herring (1966) has inspected some of the physics relevant to this matter].

Secondly, the derivation assumed free electron bands and much, though not all, of the experimental data pertains to transition metal hosts. Energy band results for Pd (see Fig. 14), a typical and particularly interesting case, show multiple, non free electron-like bands and several pieces of Fermi surface. This

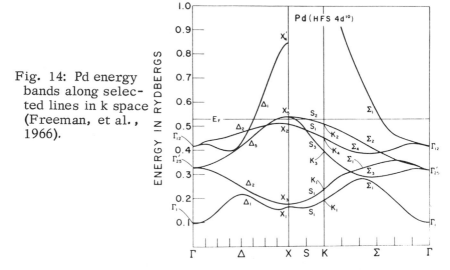

Fig. 14: Pd energy bands along selected lines in k space (Freeman, et al., 1966).

raises the question of interband contributions to a $\Delta\rho^S$ [or charge $\Delta\rho$]. Ignoring these, one expects any one extremal Fermi surface caliper to produce characteristic Friedel oscillations in the asymptotic region. But questions arise as to how relevant our free electron experience is to the inner non-asymptotic region most heavily explored by experiment. For example, the deviations of band and orbital character, from that of free-electrons, will cause changes in the shape of $J(q)$ and $F(q)$ [quite aside from its behavior at the singularity]. These should visibly affect the nonasymptotic predictions of the simple theory employing Eq. (51), with or without the enhanced $\chi(q)$. (Such refinements will undoubtably appear in the future.) The question of going, or not going, from the q to a more rigorous k, k' dependent theory will become as important as the refinements.

The discussion of experiment, below, employs the inexact q dependent picture.

1. General Observations

The metallic spin density problem is complicated by the fact that our richest source of information — magnetic hyperfine interactions — usually involve several contributions *of the same magnitude.* Hyperfine fields at local moment sites provide a direct measure of $\Delta\rho^S(0)$, but unfortunately the contact interaction of the conduction bands with the nucleus is but one of a number of such hyperfine field terms. Knowledge of $\Delta\rho^S(0)$ therefore involves assumptions and crude estimates of the other terms, but it appears reasonable to say that the vast body of experimental data for various alloys is most easily understood if the ratio of the magnitude of the spin density at the origin to that at a typical near neighbor distance is between 1 and 10. (This range of ratios reflects different alloys and different workers' estimates of the various contributions.) Spin density calculations, employing F(q) and traditional assumptions for the exchange coupling, yield ratios of 500 or larger — in poor agreement with experiment. Introduction of the exchange enhanced susceptibility, $\chi(q)$, rapidly makes the situation worse since the "rug lifting" is greatest for the maximum in the spin density, i.e., $\Delta\rho^S(0)$. Figure 14 suggests that improved treatment of the exchange coupling significantly reduces the ratio, bringing theory and experiment into at least qualitative agreement. An even more accurate evaluation of RKKY theory is required before we know to what, if any, extent it disagrees with experiment on $\Delta\rho^S(0)$ behavior.

Charge impurity Knight shift and electric quadrupole effects tend to show a linear dependence on impurity concentration over a surprising concentration range. As discussed, this implies additivity, without interference, of individual impurity contributions. While a similar additivity of magnetic effects sometimes occurs out to mild impurity concentrations (we will consider an example shortly), an outstanding difference between the spin and charge density perturbations is that linearity disappears with comparative rapidity in the spin case. An example of this is seen in Fig. 15 which displays Fe hyperfine fields as a function of Fe impurity concentration in Pd metal. A distinct suggestion of curvature has appeared by the time five or ten percent iron is reached. Non-linear or "saturation" effects may arise in a variety of ways, the simplest being the perturbation of the host metal's bands and Fermi surface character causing them to respond differently with varying impurity concentration. In the spin case, unlike that for charge, repopulation effects occur and increased concentration involves repopulation of states further

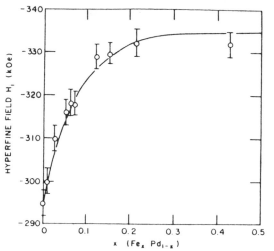

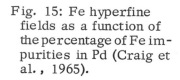

Fig. 15: Fe hyperfine fields as a function of the percentage of Fe impurities in Pd (Craig et al., 1965).

and further from the Fermi surface [orbital distortion, i.e., the $q \neq 0$ terms, will also be affected]. This, we suspect, is the main source of curvature seen in Fig. 15 because on one hand, Pd has considerable structure in both the bands and density of states near ϵ_F and on the other, exchange enhancement causes it to respond strongly to a magnetic perturbation. The situation is severe; the experiments of Vuillemin and Priestley (1965) and the band calculations of Freeman et al., (1965) indicate ~ 0.18 holes per spin per atom in the unmagnetized pure metal's 4d bands (seen in the vicinity of points X and K in Fig. 14). Invoking simple repopulation of these bands alone, full magnetic saturation is then reached with $0.36 \mu_B$ per atom. The Fe-Pd alloys are ferromagnetic and a moment of ~ $0.25 \mu_B$ per atom appears [Cable et al., (1965)] in the Pd matrix for the five percent alloy. This is a large perturbation in itself and approaches the crude estimate of the 4d saturation limit.*

Another nonlinear effect is simply the scattering of the perturbed density due to one impurity by another. Unlike most of the

*The estimate of $0.36 \mu_B$ is a lower limit since it omits contributions from the "s" band (seen midway out from Γ to X and K in Fig. 14) and the possibility that the iron impurities deplete the charge, per atom, at Pd sites. The neutron diffraction results of Cable et al. (1965) suggest that the Pd matrix becomes fully saturated at 0.35-0.4 μ_B per atom, in surprising agreement with the value of 0.36.

other nonlinear terms, this is amenable to simple treatment,
de Gennes (1962) has investigated this for the case of Ruderman-
Kittel coupling [J(q) is a constant] where he has introduced a scattering length, ℓ (which is $\sim 1/c$). Some of his results appear in
Fig. 16 and we see a phase shift and a damping which increase

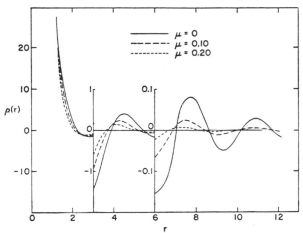

Fig. 16: Ruderman-Kittel spin density polarization as obtained by
         de Gennes (1962) for varying $\mu^{-1} = 2k_F \ell$ where the scatter-
         ing length ℓ measures the effect of one impurity on the
         polarization due to another.

with decreasing ℓ. Ignoring the phase shift, the resulting asymptotic spin density is crudely

$$\rho(r) \underset{r \to \infty}{\sim} \frac{\cos 2k_F r}{r^3} e^{-r/\ell} \tag{68}$$

i.e., the unscattered density of Eq. (53) multiplied by a damping
exponential. One would expect this effect to be most important in
nontransition metals where the other saturation effects are relatively unimportant. Recently, Heeger and associates (1966) investigated a $Cu_{0.9995}Mn_{0.0005}$ alloy, monitoring the effect of the Mn
polarization on the Cu Knight shift line width, as a function of
adding nonmagnetic Al to scatter the polarization. The results
were consistent with an exponential damping of the Mn spin density
perturbations. The experiment sampled "asymptotic" spin density
behavior since Cu's near a Mn have their resonances shifted well
outside the main Knight shift peak. It is then plausible to employ
an equation such as (68) when reducing the data. There arises the

question of the value of a Mn-Cu cut-off radius, r_c, inside of
which a Mn shift does not contribute to the broadening but instead
to a signal outside the main resonance line. Heeger et al., obtained an r_c/ℓ value of 0.12, from which they argued an ℓ equal to
forty lattice spacings, for the alloy with one percent Al.

2. An Example: Iron Alloys

For our first example, let us consider hyperfine effects
in iron alloys. We will inspect Stearns' Mössbauer results (1966)
to see what one can encounter and what difficulties there are in interpretation. Space does not allow complete inspection of the experimental data appropriate to this alloy system.*

There is rather little detailed knowledge, experimental or
computational, of the iron metal bands and Fermi surface. The
crude qualitative features of interest are suggested by Fig. 15 if
one mentally lowers the Fermi energy to ~ 0.4 Ryd. The Fermi
energy then falls in a region where bands are not simply s-like *or*
d-like in nature, but are of strongly admixed character.** There
will be multiple volumes surrounded by Fermi surface with one
probably resembling a severely distorted sphere centered at Γ,
the others being of more complicated shape. This introduces a
variety of intra *and* interband extremal k_F vectors which may
contribute Friedel oscillations and *these will vary with direction in k space.*   Matters will be further complicated by the
fact that iron, being ferromagnetic, will have different Fermi surfaces, and different band behavior in the vicinity of ε_F, for the two
different spins.

The Mössbauer experiments involve the observation of Fe^{57}
spectra as a function of impurity concentration in iron. The experimental spectra are superpositions of sets of magnetically
split hyperfine lines associated with different configurations of impurities in the vicinity of a given Fe site. It has been common
practice to assume that the effect of impurities is additive. Assuming this, an Fe with an N_n near neighbor, N_{nn} next near neighbor, etc, impurities would have a hyperfine field

$$H(N_n, N_{nn} \ldots) = H'(1 + N_n \Delta_n + N_{nn} \Delta_{nn} \ldots) \qquad (69)$$

*See also Budnick and Skalski, Chap. S.10.
**Such behavior is typical of all transition metals, including
the rare earths, to the left of Ni, Pd, and Pt in the periodic table.

where a Δ_i is the fractional field shift associated with an impurity
in the ith shell of neighbors and H' is the pure metal hyperfine
field modified by any effects of truncating of the series at a finite
number of neighboring shells. One then averages Eq. (69) over
all appropriate configurations of neighboring impurities, assuming
a random alloy of the concentration of interest, and then fits this
to the observed Mössbauer spectrum, obtaining H' and the Δ's as
empirical parameters. The apparent success of the method and
its approximations lies in the fact that one gets a common set of
Δ's for different alloy concentrations up to eight percent — a tendency seen in Fig. 17. Conservative fits obtain H' plus the first
two Δ's, but if one is optimistic and careful with one's computer
fits, one will obtain Δ's out to the fifth shell of neighbors as Stearns
has done here for Mn. Such fits are not trivial and occasionally
there arises the question of the uniqueness of a given set of parameters — a matter which does not concern us here.

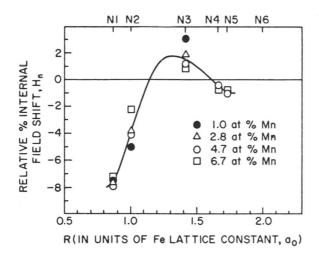

Fig. 17: Fe-Mn alloy hyperfine field shifts, Δ_i,
         plotted vs. a function of neighbor distance
         R_i (Stearns, 1966).

Stearns plotted the Δ's as a function of neighbor distance obtaining the highly suggestive results seen in Fig. 17. We see oscillations which, if of the Friedel type in origin, correspond to a k_F of ~ 0.6 a.u. The results are almost identical for the ions Al, Si, V and somewhat less so for the case of Cr. As originally emphasized by Wertheim, this has been the outstanding feature for all impurities (transition metal *and* otherwise) to the left of Fe in the periodic table — namely, their Δ's are surprisingly alike. Impurities to the right of Fe in the table generally display reverse shifts. It is as if there is an effective magnetic ΔZ, after the manner of the charge problem, which has one value for one region of the periodic table and reverses sign for the other. This behavior is as yet not understood.

Now, since different shells of neighbors are in different directions with respect to an Fe site, one is justified in placing the Δ's on a common radial plot only if the disturbances arise from a spherical band and Fermi surface — something which we have indicated is not to be expected. The first and fourth neighbors are the only two along common lines of those plotted. The clear suggestion of oscillations is, in every case, associated with Δ_3, raising the question of whether the spin response along (112) third neighbor directions is pathological or appropriate for comparison with other directions. Inspection of Δ_1, Δ_4 pairs alone suggests, but by no means clearly indicates, the occurrence of oscillations — oscillations which need not have the period plotted on the figure. Granted the uncertainties, it is quite possible that the oscillations shown are of the Friedel type because, as we have discussed, we expect at least one segment of Fermi surface to have the form of a distorted sphere (with k_F's of the order of $\frac{1}{2}$ a.u.). If, by chance, this dominated in producing the observed hyperfine shifts, then plots such as those of the figure (perhaps with R values adjusted, so as to account for variations in extremal k_F's) have considerable justification. Of course, since the results are associated with the region *close* to an impurity, any oscillation seen is still not inevitably of the asymptotic Friedel type.

Low and Collins have obtained neutron form factors for the $\Delta\rho^S(r)$ induced by impurities for some of the same alloy systems. Some of their results appear in Fig. 18. These are the Fourier transforms of the spin densities and the tendency to rise, before falling off with increasing wave vector, implies a sign reversal[*] in the spin density — evidence consistent with, but not proof of,

Note that the Fe-Mn system as well as other systems shows this trend.

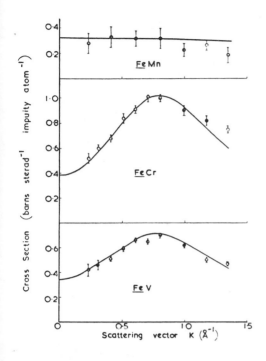

Fig. 18: Fe alloy impurity form factors (Low and Collins, 1963; Collins and Low, 1964, 1965).

Friedel type spin density oscillations. These data have been obtained with powder samples making it impossible to infer anything concerning aspherical effects. If one compares the trends seen in Figs. 17 and 18, one can obtain agreement or inconsistency, depending on one's inclinations. Campbell (1966) has considered this matter in detail and obtains crude agreement in the trends. As we will shortly discuss, it is not obvious that we should want or expect detailed consistency between the two sets of plots.

Neutron diffraction has supplied one other item of information for these alloys which deserves comment. The spin density difference induced in the host metal by an impurity is less for these alloys than the Fe–Pd system of Fig. 15, suggesting that saturation effects will not be felt as soon and that the assumption of hyperfine field additivity might well work out to 8% concentration for the Fe alloys. This seems to be the case.

Often it is assumed that hyperfine effects, such as the Δ's, arise directly from the contact interaction of the perturbed conduction band spin density, $\Delta\rho^S(r)$, with the nucleus. The Δ_i and $\Delta\rho^S(R_i)$ are then, of course, linearly related. In turn, it is often assumed that these samplings, taken at nuclear sites, are characteristic of spin density behavior in the entire region off of the impurity site, in other words that the curves of Fig. 17 are, apart from scale, spin density plots. Assuming this, the observed concentration dependence of the average internal field and that predicted from magnetization data disagree. Stearns argues that this disagreement arises because the latter involves a static sampling of moment behavior, the former, a dynamic one, involving times of the order of a nuclear precession (10^{-8} sec). Wertheim has suggested after inspection of these and other data, that the Δ_1's should not be placed on what is thought to be a spin density plot common with the other Δ_i's – that the near neighbor site is "chemically" special. (We might note that on a number of occasions workers have found it necessary to consider near neighbor alloy spin impurity effects as special and apart.)

Hyperfine field shifts need not be linearly related to $\Delta\rho^s$ sampled over atomic sites for a variety of reasons. Of greatest immediacy to the iron alloys is that there is more than one contribution to the shifts. While the perturbed bands, and in turn $\Delta\rho^s$, are of mixed 3d-4s character, one expects the 3d to predominate. The lesser 4s character becomes more important to hyperfine effects since the contact term of an unpaired 4s electron is roughly an order of magnitude greater (and opposite in sign) to the core polarization hyperfine field produced by an unpaired 3d. A set of hyperfine field shifts will then *only* be linearly related to spin density behavior if the *relative* weight of 3d versus 4s character in $\Delta\rho^s$ remains *constant* throughout the metal lattice. We do not expect this situation to hold.

We have inspected these iron Mössbauer results in order to sample a few of the complications one can encounter in attempting to analyze such results. We will not inspect the physical conclusions one might be tempted to draw concerning the ferromagnetism of iron as such conclusions are largely a function of the model chosen (and would also require inspection of an array of additional experimental data). We have suggested that the relation between hyperfine and overall spin density perturbations in such a metal need not be straightforward. The comparisons of experiment by Campbell (1966) and by others display considerable, though crude, common behavior for the two. The implications of this are not yet understood.

3. An Example: Pd Alloys

As a second example we would like to inspect an equally complicated situation but emphasize a few of its "simple" features.

This is Pd metal* with and without paramagnetic impurities such as Fe.

Pd becomes ferromagnetic on the introduction of traces of Fe impurities. Fe sites are coupled ferromagnetically presumably by the RKKY interaction. The coupling, as derived first by Kasuya for a free electron conduction band, has the form

$$S_1 \cdot S_2 J_{12} \sim S_1 \cdot S_2 \int [J(q)]^2 \, F(q) \, e^{iq \cdot R_{12}} \, dq \qquad (70)$$

where R_{12} is the vector connecting local moment sites 1 and 2 with spins S_1 and S_2 respectively. Here we see the q th Fourier component of the disturbance induced at the first site being picked up by a $J(q)$, of *same* q, at the second site, multiplied by the exponential phase factor. Kim (1966) has recently transformed the Hamiltonian into an effective one in terms of conduction electron operators where the local moment-conduction electron coupling introduces an *effective* conduction electron-conduction electron matrix element tending to drive the bands ferromagnetic. Whether employing this view or explicitly including local moment terms, as in Eq. (70), the RKKY disturbance of the Pd matrix appears to be the key feature of the magnetic properties of these alloys.

The spin density disturbance has been inferred from hyperfine, neutron diffraction and spin resonance work. The essential feature of the $\Delta \rho^s$ distribution, first suggested by spin resonance and subsequently bourne out by neutron diffraction, is that its first node occurs at 15 to 20 a.u. (and any negative region external to this has yet to be seen). This is a large radius (compare with Fig. 11) and assuming traditional RKKY theory, and an unenhanced $F(q)$, this would imply a k_F appropriate to an occupancy of $\sim$ 1/100th of an electron per atom in the conduction bands. When first obtained, such results seemed disastrous to RKKY theory. Actually, as we will now suggest, RKKY theory is quite capable of yielding such a spin distribution if one invokes the exchange enhanced susceptibility and the *actual* band structure of Pd metal.

In the calculated Pd energy bands (see Fig. 14) the Fermi level was found to cross near the top of the 4d bands and the bands in its vicinity can be quite reasonably described as either 4d *or* 5s, i.e., we are above the region of strong interband mixing (Freeman et al., 1966). The large density of states and exchange enhanced

Budnick and Skalski, Chap. S.10, consider this case and Watson and Freeman, Chap. 2, inspect the role and magnitude of its 4d core polarization hyperfine field.

susceptibility are presumably due almost entirely to the rather flat d bands crossing the Fermi surface. The principal pieces of Fermi surface consist of an s electron band surface in the shape of a distorted sphere familiar from inspection of Ni, Cu and Ag, and a d hole surface, of almost equal volume, which is a "jungle gym" of rods lying along the x, y and z axes at the faces of the Brillouin zone. There are additional small d band ellipsoids lying inside the rods which are small in volume, contain very few electron (hole) states, and may, in first approximation be ignored.* The jungle gym surface has the unusual property of providing small extremal k_F calipers** (for most directions in k space) while having a significant volume. These small calipers, taken with an exchange enhancement of $\sim$ 15, yield a theoretical first node in $\Delta\rho^S(r)$ in the vicinity where it is seen experimentally. The net spin sitting in the region out to this first node is several orders of magnitude greater than that in the first negative, or antiparallel, region outside, a possible explanation as to why antiparallel spin density character has yet to be seen experimentally.†

The Mössbauer spectra, leading to the results plotted in Fig. 15 were the simple six line magnetic spectra for Fe^{57} — each line broadened by a few kilogauss but otherwise displaying no structure such as is seen in the iron alloy case described by Eq. (69). In other words, the effect of varying configurations of surrounding impurities on a given Fe's hyperfine field is a variation of but a few kilogauss in that field. This is not surprising providing 1) that $\Delta\rho^S$ has the same sign and magnitude over a large number of lattice sites (and is significantly smaller outside) and 2) that the hyperfine field shift at one Fe, due to one other is small. Given these, the statistics of taking an average over a large sample leads to a small broadening. The spin density distribution inferred from spin resonance and neutron diffraction meets the first requirement and, given it and the concentration dependence of Fig. 15, one concludes that the effect of one iron on another's hyperfine field is a fraction of a kilogauss, meeting the second requirement. The Fe hyperfine field behavior is therefore

---

*If quantitatively of any significance, most likely it would be via interband mixing effects with the bands giving rise to to the rods.
**For example inspect its intercept on the X-Γ line in Fig.14.
†Graham and Schreiber (1966) report observing such an oscillation in the similar Pt-Co alloy system.

consistent with the $\Delta\rho^S$ picture. The hyperfine fields at Pd sites have also been observed and are much more complicated, displaying a distribution of fields (as discussed by Budnick and Skalski in Chap. S. 10). In this case the neighboring Fe's are responsible for the entire hyperfine field whereas they cause but a ten percent shift (with 15% saturation concentration) in the Fe fields of Fig. 15.

In the above, we have attempted to convey the suggestion that certain elementary features of the experimental data for Pd alloy systems are readily understood in terms of the RKKY picture.* We would, in fact, argue that this is one of the outstanding qualitative successes of theory.** There are many complications when one inspects matters further; one of these deserves mention here since it is connected with the band structure and the Fermi surfaces.

The $\Delta\rho^S$ we have discussed has been associated with the d band jungle gym Fermi surface. One expects the induced net spin to be almost entirely associated with it. There will, of course, also be a density $\Delta\rho^S_{(s)}$, associated with the s band and its Fermi surface, and it may be of experimental significance to hyperfine effects at Pd or similar sites (e.g., Ag in Pd). Its net spin will be small but the hyperfine field associated with it, coming via its contact term, will be relatively large for such a spin. We expect that the application of an external magnetic field or the introduction of a local impurity moment would have its greatest effect of $\Delta\rho^S_{(s)}$ *indirectly via* exchange coupling with the polarized d bands. Enhancement effects would be primarily associated with the magnitude and distribution of the d band spin providing the exchange field driving $\Delta\rho^S_{(s)}$ and the s band susceptibility would be essentially the unenhanced $F(q)$. The resulting $\Delta\rho^S_{(s)}$, measured with respect to a particular Pd site whose d distribution is causing the polarization, would look much more like a normal RKKY function than does the d band counterpart we have been discussing. Its

*Detailed computations remain to be done, the structure of the 4d bands of interest is quite convenient, as band structures go, for the necessary estimate of F(q) and, in turn, the density. The greatest difficulty would be an adequate estimate of the local impurity moment-conduction electron coupling.
**RKKY theory does not necessarily provide the unique best description. Clogston (to be reported) is developing a description based on Koster-Slater (1954) impurity theory (with which he obtains, among other things, a "saturation" moment of ~1μ_B). When ultimately refined, the two approaches will likely be physically equivalent.

first node would fall in the vicinity of a near neighbor radius. This spin density, summed over nuclear sites for the purpose of estimating a hyperfine field could then vary in magnitude, and even in *sign* dependent on whether the r = 0 contribution, $\Delta\rho^S_{(s)}(0)$ was included. Comparison, for example, of Knight shifts observed for Ag in Pd with those appropriate to pure Pd could thus be severely affected since a Ag nucleus would sample a lattice sum which included a *different* $\Delta\rho^S_{(s)}(0)$ than that sampled by a Pd nucleus. There have been recent efforts to determine the relative roles of d band core polarization and s band contact contributions to the pure Pd Knight shift by inspection of the Ag impurity Knight shift. Factors such as the potential role of $\Delta\rho^S_{(s)}$ and whether there are or are not holes in the Ag d shell makes this difficult and dangerous.

When discussing the effect of impurities in iron it was suggested that hyperfine effects need not be linearly related to local (atomic scale) spin density behavior. We see the same situation here for Pd, now caused by two distinct sets of bands, Fermi surfaces and associated $\Delta\rho^S$ distributions. One set is almost entirely responsible for spin density behavior, while the second is of increased importance for hyperfine fields and is of spatially different character than the first.

IV. Conclusion

In the above, we have inspected some features and complications of the spin density problem which, at this point, may seem more complex than the charge case. In some cases the complexity is merely more apparent and in other cases its increase is real. While the important fact of the charge and spin density problems is their similarity, it is perhaps appropriate to close the chapter by relisting four significant differences. First, dealing with polarization arising from exchange effects, there is a serious question of how correlation may modify the coupling which produces the polarization. The situation is presumably less serious in the charge case. Secondly, it is clear that the exchange coupling is at best crudely approximated by a q dependent $J(q)$. The similar assumption of a $\Phi(q)$ for the charge case has *much* better basis (though, as we have suggested, deviations from this may be significant). Thirdly, when dealing with spins, we are forced by experiment to consider higher order interband effects which can induce antiparallel net densities. To our knowledge, the charge problem has yet to be forced to higher order. Finally, the theory in its simple form is more directly applicable to the free electron-like metals where charge effects appear, than to the transition metals normally encountered in the spin problem. The transition metals, with multiple extremal calipers and multiple bands of differing or strongly admixed character, offer real complications — particularly if one wishes to formally relate hyperfine results to overall spin density behavior.

Acknowledgements

I am indebted to many people for discussion and correspondence and of these I would particularly like to thank L. H. Bennett, M. Blume, J. I. Budnick, T. A. Kitchens, S. Koide, A. Narath, M. Peter, L. R. Walker and my longstanding collaborator, A. J. Freeman.

References

Berk. N. F. and Schrieffer, J. R. (1967). Proc. 10th Internl. Low Temp. Phys. Conf. (Moscow, 1966) and J. Appl. Phys. (to be published, 1967).

Blandin, A. and Friedel, J. (1960). J. Phys. Rad. 21, 689.

Blatt, F. J. (1957). Phys. Rev. 108, 285.

Cable, J. W. , Wollan, E. O. and Koehler, W. C. (1965). Phys. Rev. 138, A755.

Collins, M. F. and Low G. G. (1964). J. Phys. 25, 596.

Collins, M. F. and Low, G. G. (1965). Proc. Phys. Soc. 86, 535.

Craig, P. P. , Mozer, B. and Segnan, R. (1965). Phys. Rev. Letters 14, 895.

De Gennes, P. G. (1962). J. Phys. Rad. 23, 630.

Edmonds, A. R. (1957). Angular Momentum in Quantum Mechanics (Princeton University Press).

Freeman, A. J., Furdyna, A. M. and Dimmock, J. O. (1966). J. Appl. Phys. 37, 1256.

Friedel, J. (1952). Phil. Mag. 43, 153.

Friedel, J. (1954). Advances Phys. 3, 466.

Friedel, J. (1958). Nuovo Cimento 2, 287.

Graham, L. D. and Schreiber, D. S. (1966). Phys. Rev. Letters 17, 650.

Harrison, W. (1966). Pseudopotentials in the Theory of Metals, (Benjamin).

Heeger, A. J., Klein, A. P. and Tu, P. (1966). Phys. Rev. Letters 17, 803.

Herring, C. (1966). Treatise on Magnetism (Academic Press, Suhl-Rado, eds.) Vols. IIB and IV.

Kohn, W. and Vosko, S. H. (1960). Phys. Rev. 119, 912.

Koster, G. F. and Slater, J. C. (1954). Phys. Rev. 95, 1167; ibid, 96, 1208.

Odle, R. L. and Flynn, C. P. (1966). Phil. Mag. 13, 699.

Paskin, A. (1966). Proc. of the Conf. on the Properties of Liquid Metals, Brookhaven, New York.

Pines, D. (1963). Elementary Excitations in Solids (Benjamin).

Rowland, T. J. (1962). Phys. Rev. 125, 459.

Ruderman, M. A. and Kittel, C. (1954). Phys. Rev. 96, 99.

Schiff, L. I. (1949). Quantum Mechanics (McGraw-Hill).

Snodgrass, R. J. and Bennett, L. H. (1964). Phys. Rev. 134, A1294.

Stearns, M. B. (1966). Phys. Rev. 147, 439.

Watson, R. E. and Freeman, A. J. (1967). Phys. Rev. (to be published).

Watson, R. E., Koide, S., Peter, M., and Freeman, A. J. (1965). Phys. Rev. 139, A167.

Wolff, P. A. (1960), Phys. Rev. 120, 814.

Wolff, P. A. (1963). Phys. Rev. 129 84.

Bibliography

The purpose of this is to augment the references, providing adequate, but by no means complete, access to the spin and charge density polarization literature.

Original charge oscillation papers: Friedel (1952, 1954, 1958).

Square well analysis: Daniel, E. (1959). Doctor's thesis, University of Paris.

Charge oscillation Knight shift: Blandin, A. and Daniel, E. (1959). J. Phys. Chem. Sol. 10, 126; Blandin, A., Daniel, E., and Friedel, J. (1960). Phil. Mag. 4, 180; and Rowland (1962).

Charge oscillation electric quadrupole effects: Kohn and Vosko (1960): Blandin, A. and Friedel, J. (1960). J. Phys. Radium 21, 689; Rowland, T. J. (1960). Phys. Rev. 119, 900.

Dielectric response theory: Pines (1963) and Lindhard, J. (1954). Kgl. Danske Vid Sel Mat Phys 28, No. 8.

Sets of phase shifts heavily relied on elsewhere: Blatt (1957); Kohn and Vosko (1960) and the work of Blandin, Daniel and Friedel.

Temperature dependence of impurity effects: Kohn and Vosko (1960); March, N. H. and Murray, A. M. (1962). Proc. Phys. Soc. 79, 1001; Flynn, C. P. and Odle, R. L. (1963). Proc. Phys. Soc. 81, 412.

The Zener spin polarization term: Zener, C. (1951). Phys. Rev. 81, 440; ibid. (1951). 83, 299.

Early RKKY theory: Vonsovski, S. (1946). JETP 16, 981; ibid. (1953). 24, 419; Ruderman and Kittel (1954); Kasuya, T. (1956). Prog. Theoret. Phys. 16, 45; Mitchell, A. H. (1957). Phys. Rev. 105, 1439; Yosida, K. (1957). Phys. Rev. 106, 893.

Form Factor Exchange Coupling, $J_{ff}(q)$: Overhauser, A. W. (1963). J. Appl. Phys. 34, 1019S.

Exact $J(k, k')$ behavior: Watson, R. E. and Freeman, A. J. (1965). Phys. Rev. Letters 14, 695; Watson and Freeman (1967).

Interband mixing and effective exchange coupling: Anderson, P. W. and Clogston, A. M. (1961). Bull. Am. Phys. Soc. 2, 124; Kondo, J. (1962). Prog. Theoret. Phys. 28, 846; Koide, S. and Peter, M. (1964). Rev. Mod. Phys. 36, 160; Watson, Koide, Peter, Freeman (1965).

Connection of partial wave and dielectric response treatments: Blandin, A. (1961). J. Phys. Rad. 22, 507.

Conduction electron enhancement of susceptibility: Wolff, P. A. (1960, 1963); Giovannini, Peter and Schrieffer, (1964). Phys. Rev. Letters 12, 7361; Moriya, T. (1965). Prog. Theoret. Phys. 34, 329

Blandin, Gousseland, Overhauser, Kaplan, Kasuya, Keffer, and many others have considered various aspects of going away from the strict free-electron picture, occasionally with conflicting conclusions.

Early Thomas Fermi estimate of charge redistribution: Huang, K. (1948). Proc. Phys. Soc. 60, 161.

Charge impurity Knight shift data: Rowland (1962); Snodgrass and Bennett (1964); Drain, L. E. (1959). Phil. Mag. 4, 484.

Liquid metal Knight shifts: Flynn, C. P. and Seymour, E. F. W. (1959). Proc. Phys. Soc. 73, 945 and (1960). 76, 301; Hewitt, R. R. and Williams, B. F. (1964). Phys. Rev. Letters 12, 216; Seymour, E. F. W. and Styles, G. A. (1964). Phys. Letters 10, 269.

Pseudopotential theory: Harrison (1966) and Heine, V. and Abarenkov, I. (1964). Phil. Mag. 9, 451.

Liquid alloy Knight shifts: Seymour, E. F. W. and Styles, G. A. (1966). Proc. Phys. Soc. 87, 473; Moulson, D. J., Place, C. M. and Seymour, E. F. W. (1965). Proc. "Magnetic Resonance in Metals" Leeds; Odle, R. L. and Flynn, C. P. (1966).

Transport properties in liquid alloys using pseudopotentials: Faber, T. E. and Ziman, J. M. (1965). Phil. Mag. 11, 153.

A recent and interesting application of the Friedel Sum rule — resonant scattering of conduction electron by impurities: Ferrell, R. A. and Prange, R. E. (1966). Phys. Rev. Letters 17, 163.

Liquid alloys with magnetic impurities: Gardner, A. and Flynn, C. P. (1966). Phys. Rev. Letters 17, 579.

Spin echo NMR of Fe alloys: Budnick, J. I. (this volume); Budnick, J. I., Skalski, S. and Burch, T. J. (to be published) J. Appl. Phys.; Rubenstein, M., Stauss, G. H. and Stearns, M. B. (1966). J. Appl. Phys. 37, 1334S.

Mössbauer effect in Fe alloys: Stearns (1966); Wertheim, G. K. (unpublished APS talks); Wertheim, G. K., Jaccarino, V, Wernick, J. H. and Buchanan, D. N. E. (1964). Phys. Rev. Letters 12, 24.

Hyperfine fields at impurities in transition metals hosts: Johnson, C. E., Ridout, M. S. and Cranshaw, T. E. (1963). Proc. Phys. Soc. 81, 1079; Asayama, K., Kotani, M., Itoh, J., (1964). J. Phys. Soc. Japan 19, 1984; Ho, J. C. and Phillips, N. E. (1965). Phys. Rev. 140, A648; Shirley, D. A. and Westenberger, G. A.

(1965). Phys. Rev. 138, A170; Daniel, E. (elsewhere in this volume).

Neutron diffraction of impurities in Fe and Ni: Collins and Low (1964, 1965); Low, G. G. and Collins, M. F. (1963). J. Appl. Phys. 34, 1195S; and Arrott, A., Collins, M. F., Holden, T. M., Low, G. G., and Nathans, R. (1966). J. Appl. Phys. 37, 1194S.

Relation of iron alloy neutron diffraction and hyperfine field data: Campbell, I. A. (1966). Proc. Phys. Soc. 89, 71.

Neutron diffraction of Pd alloys: Cable et al. (1965); Low, G. G. and Holden, T. M. (1966). Proc. Phys. Soc. 89, 119.

Fe-Pd hyperfine effects: Craig et al. (1965); Kitchens, T. A. and Craig, P. P. (1966). J. Appl. Phys. 37, 1187; Trousdale, W. L. Kitchens, T. A. and Longworth, G. (to be published 1967). J. Appl. Phys.; Budnick, J. I., Lechaton, J. and Skalski, S. (to be published, 1967). J. Appl. Phys.; Kobayashi, S. and Itoh, J. (to be published).

Pd alloy electron spin resonance: Shaltiel, D., Wernick, J. H., Williams, H. J. and Peter, M. (1964). Phys. Rev. 135, A1346.

Dynamical exchange polarization effects: Hasegawa, H. (1959). Prog. Theoret. Phys. 21, 483; Giovannini, B. and Koide, S. (1965). Prog. Theoret. Phys. 34, 705; Giovannini, B., Peter, M. and Koide, S. (to be published). Phys. Rev.

10. NUCLEAR SPECIFIC HEATS IN METALS AND ALLOYS

O.V. Lounasmaa

*Technical University of Helsinki
Otaniemi, Finland*

Table of Contents

I. Introduction

One of the important methods for investigating hyperfine interactions in ferro- and antiferromagnetic metals and alloys involves measurements of the so-called nuclear or hyperfine specific heat C_N. These experiments, their interpretation, and some of the results obtained will be the subject of this chapter. We shall begin by discussing the theory involved and by writing down the relevant formulae for C_N, then examine the components of the measured total specific heat C_p and the separation of C_N. Next we shall discuss briefly experimental techniques and compare specific heat measurements with other methods for investigating hyperfine interactions. In later sections, we shall present and discuss experimental results, first on transition metals and their alloys and then on rare earth metals.

II. General Considerations

A. Theoretical Expression for the Nuclear Specific Heat C_N

Let us first find the formula which gives the temperature dependence of the nuclear specific heat as a function of the positions of the nuclear Zeeman levels.

In an external magnetic field a nucleus with a spin I will have $2I+1$ energy levels. Let the potential energies of these levels be W_i, where $i = -I, -I+1, \ldots, +I$. Statistical mechanics tells us that the average energy of one system is

$$\langle W \rangle = -d(\ln Z)/d(1/kT) , \tag{1}$$

where Z, the partition function, is

$$Z = \sum_{i=-I}^{I} \exp(-W_i/kT) . \tag{2}$$

Thus

$$\langle W \rangle = -\frac{\sum\limits_{i=-I}^{I} -W_i \exp(-W_i/kT)}{\sum\limits_{i=-I}^{I} \exp(-W_i/kT)} \tag{3}$$

The average energy of a system of N nuclei is $\langle E \rangle = N\langle W \rangle$ and, consequently, the nuclear specific heat is $C_N = d\langle E \rangle /dT$. By carrying out the differentiation and by observing that $Nk = R$, we find, after some manipulations,

$$C_N = \frac{R}{(kT)^2} \frac{\displaystyle\sum_{i=-I}^{I} \sum_{j=-I}^{I} (W_i^2 - W_i W_j) \exp\left[-(W_i + W_j)/kT\right]}{\displaystyle\sum_{i=-I}^{I} \sum_{j=-I}^{I} \exp\left[-(W_i + W_j)/kT\right]} \cdot (4)$$

This is the exact expression for the nuclear specific heat and the resulting curve has been plotted in Fig. 1. At low temperatures the increase in C_N is exponential, at high temperatures the decrease is proportional to T^{-2}; the maximum occurs approximately at $T_{max} = (W_{i+1} - W_i)/kI$. In practice, $T_{max} < 0.1°K$ for all metals except holmium (cf. Fig. 1 and Sec. IV. B. 8). The specific heat curve is called a Schottky anomaly; such an anomaly is, in general, observed when a system has a definite (usually small) number of

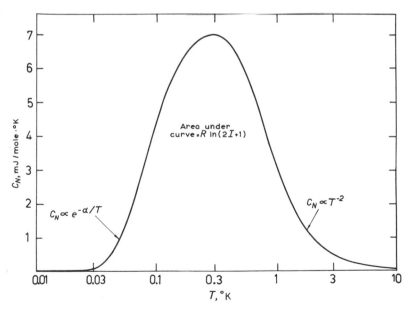

Fig. 1: The nuclear Schottky anomaly in the specific heat of holmium metal.

energy levels and when the level spacing does not change with temperature.

B. Calculation of the Energy Levels W_i

In order to calculate C_N from Eq. (4) the positions of the W_i's must be known. The hyperfine interaction between electrons and the nucleus arises from two sources: the magnetic interaction, proportional to μH_{eff}, and the quadrupole interaction proportional to Qq. Here μ is the nuclear magnetic moment, H_{eff} the effective magnetic field at the nucleus, Q the nuclear quadrupole moment, and q the electric field gradient at the nucleus. The former interaction, which is of dipole character, is linear in I, whereas the latter is quadratic in I.

The relative positions of the W_i's are determined by the magnetic and quadrupole interaction Hamiltonians (Freeman and Watson, 1965). * The magnetic term may be expressed by an interaction between the nuclear magnetic moment and an effective magnetic field, proportional to the electronic magnetization $\langle J_z \rangle$:

$$\mathcal{H}_D = -\overline{\mu} \cdot \overline{H}_{eff} = -(\mu H_{eff}/I)I_z \ , \tag{5}$$

where $\overline{\mu} = g_I \mu_N \overline{I}$ is the nuclear magnetic moment and $\overline{H}_{eff}$ is assumed to be in the z-direction. The components of the field are the orbital contribution, proportional to $\langle \overline{L}/r^3 \rangle$, the dipolar contribution, proportional to $\langle 3(\overline{S} \cdot \overline{r})\overline{r}/r^5 - \overline{S}/r^3 \rangle$, and the contribution due to the Fermi contact interaction, which is proportional to $\langle \overline{S} \rangle |\psi_s(0)|^2$.

For the quadrupole interaction one obtains, by first choosing a suitable set of orthogonal axes, the following Hamiltonian

$$\mathcal{H}_Q = \frac{3e^2 Qq}{4I(2I-1)} \left[I_z^2 - \tfrac{1}{3} I(I+1) + \tfrac{\eta}{3} (I_x^2 - I_y^2) \right] . \tag{6}$$

The three orthogonal axes are x, y, and z and the two parameters are the z-component of the gradient eq, assumed to be larger than the x- and y-components, and the asymmetry parameter η, which is zero if the field is axially symmetric. For cubic and spherical symmetry all components of the gradient vanish and the quadrupole interaction is zero. In the case of strong spin-orbit coupling eq and $\overline{H}_{eff}$ are both parallel to $\langle \overline{J} \rangle$ and thus parallel to each other. The z-direction is then the same in Eqs. (5) and (6).

*See also Bleaney, Chap. 1.

The Hamiltonians in Eqs. (5) and (6) are in agreement with the so-called one-electron theory of hyperfine interactions. According to this theory, if the atom has several electrons outside closed shells, the total Hamiltonian is simply taken as the sum of individual contributions. This theory is by no means adequate for describing hyperfine interactions. For instance it has been observed that, contrary to the one-electron theory, all closed shells contribute significantly both to the magnetic and electric parts of hyperfine interaction.

To explain the discrepancies Sternheimer (1954) has emphasized contributions to the magnetic dipole and electric quadrupole interactions arising from the distortion of otherwise spherical closed electronic shells. An example is the polarization induced by electric field gradients in solids. Sternheimer considers two contributions: first, the gradient coming from the outer valence electrons q_V, and second, the gradient due to the crystalline field, q_c. The induced field gradients are proportional to their sources and thus the quadrupole Hamiltonian in Eq. (6) must be modified by replacing q with $[q_V(1 - R_q) + q_c(1 - \gamma_\infty)]$ for the two contributions. R_q and γ_∞ are commonly called Sternheimer anti-shielding factors; computed values for $|R_q|$ are < 1.0 whereas γ_∞ ranges from -10 to -100. The induced field gradients can thus be two orders of magnitude larger than the source gradients. For more complete discussions of Eqs. (5) and (6) refer to Freeman and Watson (1965) and to Chap. 2.

By writing

$$a' = \mu H_{eff}/kI \text{ (magnetic interaction parameter)}, \qquad (7)$$

$$P = 3e^2 Qq/4kI(2I - 1) \text{ (quadrupole coupling constant)}, \qquad (8)$$

we find, after combining the two Hamiltonians in Eqs. (5) and (6), the energy levels of the system:

$$W_i/k = -a'i + P[i^2 - \tfrac{1}{3}I(I+1)] ,$$

$$i = -I, -I+1, \ldots, +I , \qquad (9)$$

where the asymmetry term in $\mathcal{H}_Q$ has been ignored, i.e. we assume $\eta = 0$. The magnetic interaction would separate the hyperfine levels evenly but the quadrupole term distorts this even spacing. As an example, Fig. 2 shows the nuclear Zeeman levels of Tb^{159} (cf. Sec. IV. B. 6).

We should again point out that the magnetic interaction involves the product μH_{eff} and, similarly, the quadrupole interaction

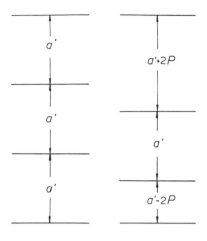

Fig. 2: The hyperfine levels of
    Tb^{159} (I = 3/2) with and without
    quadrupole coupling.

the product Qq. Thus there is always one nuclear and one electronic parameter involved. Consequently, the determination of
the nuclear quadrupole moment Q from an experiment involving
hyperfine interactions requires an independent determination of q,
either theoretically or from some other type of experiment. In
the magnetic case the situation is more favorable as external fields
of the same order of magnitude as H_{eff} can sometimes be produced, allowing the separation of μ and H_{eff}. On the other hand,
appreciable electric field gradients cannot be obtained by external
means.

C.   Calculation of Interaction Parameters from C_N

       The magnetic hyperfine constant a$'$ should vary as $\langle J_z \rangle$,
which measures the electronic magnetization, and the quadrupole
coupling constant P as $\langle J_z^2 - \frac{1}{3} J(J+1) \rangle$, which is a measure of
the average value of the electronic quadrupole moment. Here J_z
refers to the electronic ground state of the ion. Below a few
degrees Kelvin the electronic system in a ferro- or antiferromagnetic metal has reached saturation and thus J_z may be replaced by J. We thus find

$$a' \propto J , \quad P \propto J(2J-1) . \tag{10}$$

The parameters a$'$ and P are, therefore, temperature independent constants. The orbital momentum $\overline{L}$ is quenched in the
iron group metals and thus J ($\overline{J} = |\overline{L} \pm \overline{S}|$) must be replaced by S
in Eq. (10). In a paramagnetic metal $\langle J_z \rangle = 0$ and, consequently,
a$'$ = 0 also.

According to Eqs. (4) and (9) C_N depends on T and on three constants a', P, and I, of which I is normally known. Consequently, by experimentally measuring C_N as a function of temperature and by fitting the data to Eq. (4) with a' and P as adjustable parameters, these interaction constants can be determined quite accurately.

In practice measurements are most often made well above the maximum in C_N (because temperatures $T < T_{max}$ are difficult to reach). In such cases it is convenient to expand the nuclear specific heat in power series with inverse powers of T, i.e.,

$$C_N = c_2 T^{-2} + c_3 T^{-3} + \ldots \quad . \tag{11}$$

It might be useful to write down the coefficients of the first few terms:

$$c_2/R = (1/3)a'^2 I(I+1) + (1/45)P^2 I(I+1)(2I-1)(2I+3) , \tag{12}$$

$$c_3/R = -(1/15)a'^2 PI(I+1)(2I-1)(2I+3) , \tag{13}$$

$$c_4/R = -(1/30)a'^4 I(I+1)(2I^2 + 2I +1) . \tag{14}$$

Some higher order terms have been omitted in c_3 and c_4. If the quadrupole interaction is zero (P = 0), all odd powers disappear from Eq. (11). Often just the first term is sufficient for fitting the experimental data, i.e. we may frequently write $C_N = c_2 T^{-2}$.

D. The Measured C_p and the Separation of C_N

As the experimentally observed heat capacity always refers to the total specific heat of the system, it is impossible to investigate only one component of C_p. Thus, after the measurements are completed, it becomes necessary to analyze the specific heat into its component parts. The following contributions of C_p are relevant in magnetic metals:

i. The lattice specific heat C_L. At $T < \theta/50$, $C_L = AT^3$. Here A is a constant and θ is the Debye characteristic temperature of the metal (usually θ is between 100° and 400°K). At higher temperatures the behavior of C_L cannot be predicted theoretically with accuracy.

ii. The electronic specific heat $C_E = \gamma T$. This contribution is due mainly to the conduction electrons and, because of the degeneracy of the electron gas, the linear temperature dependence of C_E is valid up to 1000°K at least. The coefficient γ is proportional to the density of states at the Fermi level if one excludes the contribution of the electron-phonon interactions* which also give rise to a term linear in T.

iii. The magnetic specific heat C_M. This term is caused by exchange interactions between the localized electronic spins of neighboring ions. According to the simple spin-wave theory (van Kranendonk and van Vleck, 1958) $C_M \propto T^{3/2}$ in a ferromagnet and $C_M \propto T^3$ in an antiferromagnet. Exponential factors exp(-E_g/kT) appear with magnetic anisotropy (Cooper, 1962). Here E_g is the energy gap at the bottom of the spin-wave spectrum, i. e. the minimum energy required to excite a long wave length spin wave.

iv. The nuclear specific heat C_N which we have already discussed.

v. Impurities might further complicate the picture. An entropy $S_i = xR \ln(2J+1)$ is associated with a magnetic transformation from an ordered to a disordered state in the impurity phase. This amount of entropy is large by low temperature standards even when the impurity concentration x is quite low, e. g. ≈ 0.001. Very high purity samples are a necessity in order to exclude this source of trouble but often such specimens are not available.

We are thus dealing with at least four components of C_p of which we are here only interested in C_N.

Generally, the biggest drawback of specific heat data is that C_p is an integrated quantity over all degrees of freedom in the system and it is often difficult or impossible to separate the individual contributions accurately. Only when precise C_p measurements are available over a sufficiently wide range and when we also know the temperature dependencies of the different contributions, a suitable analytical method (such as the method of least squares) may be employed with success. These conditions are rarely satisfied in practice. As a compensation, however, specific heat measurements are very useful for "detective" work in finding new and unsuspected processes. All these involve a change in the internal energy E of the system and thus are observable in $C_V = \partial E/\partial T$.

On the basis of the previous paragraph specific heat measurements do not appear to be very good for our task of determining

*See for example discussions by Narath in Chap. 7.

hyperfine interactions with precision. However, when we study the nuclear specific heat we are in a very favorable position. The interactions between nuclei and their own electrons are such that the interaction energy W is of the same order of magnitude as the thermal energy only at very low temperatures, i.e. $W \approx kT$ at $T << 1°K$. This immediately implies that changes in the internal energy, due to hyperfine interaction, take place in the system only below $1°K$. Thus, for investigating C_N, measurements must also be made below $1°K$. In this range C_M is effectively zero because the electronic spin system has reached saturation and no longer contributes to C_p. Similarly, $C_L = AT^3$ is negligible and $C_E = \gamma T$ is small and normally sufficiently well known from measurements at higher temperatures. The result is that C_N is the dominant contribution to C_p below $1°K$ and can be determined with precision.

If we assume $C_N = C_2 T^{-2}$ and put $C_M = 0$ (i.e., the Curie or Néel point is at a sufficiently high temperature), we get

$$C_p = AT^3 + \gamma T + c_2 T^{-2} \quad , \tag{15}$$

where AT^3 is almost negligible below $1°K$ and the nuclear term is small above $1°K$. If experimental C_p data are available in both temperature ranges (say, between 0.4 and $4°K$) the coefficients in Eq. (15) can be determined as follows:

    i.   First assume $C_p = \gamma T + c_2 T^{-2}$ and plot the experimental points below $1°K$ as $C_p T^2$ vs. T^3 to determine γ and c_2 provisionally.

    ii. Assume Eq. (15) and plot points above $1°K$ as $(C_p - c_2 T^{-2})/T$ vs. T^2 to determine A and γ.

    iii. Plot points below $1°K$ as $(C_p - AT^3)T^2$ vs. T^3 to determine final values of γ and c_2.

Of course, if $C_N = c_2 T^{-2}$ is assumed, a' and P cannot be separated (cf. Eq. (12)).

E. Experimental Techniques

    The experimental procedure most commonly employed for measuring nuclear specific heats is the standard "almost adiabatic" method. The specimen is thermally isolated by high vacuum, by suspending it from a thread of poorly conducting material such as nylon, by preventing all kinds of radiation (including that from radio and TV stations) from reaching it, and by stopping harmful mechanical vibrations. During heat capacity measurements energy is supplied electrically to the sample and the corresponding increase in temperature is measured with the thermometer.

Since temperatures below 1°K are usually necessary for successful investigations of C_N, the experimentalist has three methods of cooling to choose from. The simplest one is to use a He^3 cryostat. By pumping on a liquid of this isotope, temperatures in the neighborhood of 0. 3°K can be reached and maintained rather easily. Such a cryostat is relatively simple to operate; its chief drawback is that ~0. 3°K is the lowest temperature attainable.

The second method is to use adiabatic demagnetization techniques. The apparatus becomes considerably more complicated but, as a compensation, temperatures in the vicinity of 0. 01°K can be reached. Additional drawbacks of this method are that its cooling capacity is relatively small and that continuous refrigeration cannot be obtained.

The third procedure for attaining temperatures below 1°K, the He^3/He^4 mixture cryostat, has recently caused much interest (Hall et al. , 1966). This type of apparatus is relatively simple in principle but sufficient "know how" appears to be lacking at the present time to guarantee proper operation of any given refrigerator. Once the design problems have been worked out it is expected that this method will largely replace adiabatic demagnetization techniques. The He^3/He^4 cryostat provides continuous cooling and is capable of removing relatively large heat loads; temperatures well below 0. 1°K can be reached with this method.

Before the specific heat measurements can be started, the sample is cooled to the lowest experimental temperature by a suitable heat switch. Its construction can be either mechanical or based on the fact that a metal in its superconducting state below 1°K is a much poorer heat conductor than the same metal in its normal state. Exchange gas should never by used as a heat switch; the specimen will absorb a considerable quantity of the gas and when it is subsequently warmed during heat capacity measurements a large error, which cannot be corrected for, is caused by the heat of desorption.

Securing a reliable calibration for the thermometer is one of the biggest difficulties in heat capacity measurements at low temperatures. This is because we need not only the relation between the thermometric parameter (usually the electrical resistance of the thermometer) and the absolute temperature but the derivative of this relation also enters directly into the calculations. The actual heat capacity measurements are made by using either carbon or preferably germanium resistance thermometers, which must be calibrated against the vapor pressures of He^4 and He^3 and against a magnetic thermometer. Suitably constructed germanium resistors, which keep their calibration between experiments, have helped in making calorimetric work less tedious than before.

The inner parts of a He^3 cryostat used by the author (Lounasmaa and Guenther, 1962) are shown in Fig. 3. The apparatus has a platform type heat switch onto which the specimen is lowered when contact is desired. A magnetic thermometer is located inside the He^3 pot.

A non-adiabatic method for measurements of C_N down to about 50 m°K has been successfully employed by van Kempen et al. (1964). In their apparatus the specimen is connected by a brass strip to the cooling salt. The thermal conductivity of the strip can be calculated from measurements of its electrical

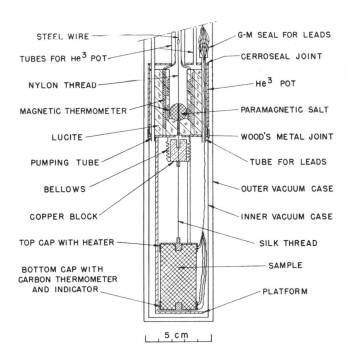

Fig. 3: The inner parts of a He^3 cryostat (Lounasmaa and Guenther, 1962).

resistivity above 1°K. After adiabatic demagnetization, the sample is cooled via the brass strip, and the heat capacity is calculated from observations of the cooling rate.

For more complete descriptions of experimental techniques we refer to papers cited in Secs. III and IV.

F. Comparison with Other Experimental Methods

The following methods are important for experimental investigations of hyperfine interactions in magnetic materials: (i) nuclear magnetic resonance, (ii) electron spin resonance, (iii) Mössbauer-effect, (iv) angular correlation of successive γ-rays, (v) interaction of polarized neutrons with polarized nuclei, (vi) nuclear orientation, and (vii) nuclear specific heats. Each of these methods has its advantages and drawbacks; we shall briefly discuss all of them from the point of view of nuclear specific heat experiments.

Measurements of C_N can be made, in principle and usually in practice, on every metal and alloy. This is an advantage as compared with Mössbauer and angular correlation methods requiring nuclei with special properties. A second advantage is that C_N is easily identifiable and can be interpreted without difficulty; this favorable situation should be compared with the need in NMR to search for the resonance, which sometimes can be quite difficult. In fact, measurements of C_N have often helped NMR workers to find the resonant frequency. A side advantage of C_N experiments is that usually investigations can be extended up to 4°K with very little extra effort and thus important information is obtained about C_L, C_E, and C_M as well.

Nuclear specific heat measurements have several disadvantages. The first drawback is the necessity to work below 1°K, which creates special experimental problems. These were discussed in Sec. II. E. Further, the temperature dependence of the magnetization cannot be investigated (cf. Sec. II. C) because below 1°K H_{eff} has already reached its saturation value and at higher temperatures, where changes in H_{eff} are expected, C_N vanishes.

Most metals are a mixture of isotopes with different nuclear magnetic and quadrupole moments. Sometimes all stable isotopes of an element have $\mu = Q = 0$, and thus H_{eff} and q in the lattice cannot be investigated. The measured C_N in any case referes to the average properties of the metal in its natural isotopic composition. Isotopically separated specimens could be used, but gram quantities are required for successful investigations of C_N. Finally, a disadvantage is that insulators are normally unsuitable for the heat capacity method because thermal equilibrium is reached too slowly in them at low temperatures.

Since a fair amount of useful information about hyperfine interactions has been obtained from measurements of C_N, advantages apparently outweigh disadvantages in many cases.

III. Transition Metals and Their Alloys

A. Theoretical Considerations

Most of the information about hyperfine interactions in transition metals and their alloys has been obtained through the use of Mössbauer techniques with Fe^{57} as a probe. One of the important discoveries by this method was made by Hanna et al. (1960) who observed that for iron H_{eff} is negative, i.e. antiparallel to the direction of magnetization. This fact, surprising at first, was the impetus for a great deal of fruitful theoretical work on the subject. Even though Mössbauer measurements have provided the bulk of information in this field there is, nevertheless, a sufficient amount of specific heat data available to warrant a brief discussion on transition metals in this article. We shall first consider the various terms causing the observed H_{eff}, referring to Sec. II.B. and, for a more complete discussion, to Marshall and Johnson (1962) and Freeman and Watson (1965).

In the iron group ions the orbital angular momentum $\bar{L}$ is quenched by the strong crystal field but a small orbital moment is still present due to the spin-orbit coupling. This produces a positive contribution to H_{eff}, estimated theoretically as +70 kOe for iron.

The dipolar interaction is zero for cubic metals such as iron, and estimates show that it is only a few kilo-oersteds for hexagonal cobalt. We may thus ignore this term.

The observed H_{eff} in iron is -340 kOe and it then follows that a hyperfine field of -410 kOe is caused by the Fermi contact interaction between the s-electrons and the nucleus. Ordinarily the charge densities of spin-up (s↑) and spin-down (s↓) electrons have an equal distribution in space for closed shells but if the atom has a partially filled shell (3d in the iron series metals) the balance is upset. This is because the interaction between a d↑ electron and an s↑ electron is attractive whereas that between d↑ and s↓ electrons is repulsive. As a result the radial wave functions of s↑ electrons expand and those of s↓ electrons contract. Hence the charge density due to $s\downarrow$ electrons wins at the nucleus and this produces, through the Fermi contact interaction, a magnetic field opposite to $\bar{S}$. For a description of the Hartree-Fock calculations used for theoretical investigations of H_{eff} we refer to Freeman and Watson (1965).*

Although the polarization of the 1s, 2s, and 3s electrons is probably responsible for the bulk of the contact interaction, a further contribution is caused by the 4s conduction electrons. These are polarized both by exchange interaction with the 3d electrons and by the complicated effects of mixing with the 3d band which occurs in a solid. This contribution is difficult to calculate but it appears to be negative for iron.

We have thus seen that the effective field in transition metals is caused, through the mechanism of the Fermi contact interaction, mainly by the polarization of the core s electrons. We shall next present some experimental data on the nuclear specific heat of these metals and their alloys.

B. Experimental Results

On the basis of nuclear orientation experiments Heer and Erickson (1956) suggested that the hyperfine contribution to the specific heat of cobalt metal should be observable below $1°K$. Subsequently (1957) they carried out measurements between 0.6 and $3°K$ and found $C_N = 3.3\ T^{-2}$ mJ/mole·$°K$. A little later Arp et al. (1957) investigated cobalt down to $0.3°K$ and obtained $C_N = 5.2\ T^{-2}$ in the same units. The results correspond to an effective field of 180 and 230 kOe, respectively. These were the first experiments which demonstrated the existence of a nuclear specific heat.

The naturally occuring isotopes of iron and nickel have zero nuclear magnetic moment and thus the effective field in the lattices of these elements must be determined by using other atoms as a probe. Of course, the concentration of these probe atoms must be sufficiently high so that a reasonable nuclear contribution is observed. The first investigations of this type were made by Arp et al. (1959) with the alloys Co-Fe and Co-Ni. As may be seen from Table I, H_{eff} acting on the cobalt nuclei decreases approximately linearly with decreasing iron concentration. No discontinuities in H_{eff} were found as might be expected if the electronic configuration were to change suddenly in a narrow concentration range. Such a rapid change, coming from an increase in the number of 3d electrons localized around iron atoms, had been theoretically postulated at 35% Co in Fe. Neither were there

*Also see Chap. 2.

Table I: H_{eff} at Co in Co-Ni and Co-Fe alloys[a]

Alloy (atomic %)	H_{eff} (kOe)
$Co_{0.600}Ni_{0.400}$	121
$Co_{1.00}$	219
$Co_{0.915}Fe_{0.085}$	223
$Co_{0.587}Fe_{0.413}$	256
$Co_{0.172}Fe_{0.828}$	293
$Co_{0.048}Fe_{0.952}$	314
$Fe_{1.000}$	325[b]

(a) *From Arp et al. (1959).*
(b) *Extrapolated value.*

discontinuities in H_{eff} at the hcp ↔ fcc phase transition in Co-Ni, showing that the dipolar term in H_{eff}, zero in a cubic lattice, was negligible in the hcp phase as well.

Wei et al. (1961) have measured the specific heat of the alloys $Co_{0.3}Fe_{0.7}$ and $V_{0.33}Fe_{0.67}$ between 1.6 and 4.2°K. Both of these specimens are ferromagnetic and have an fcc structure. The results gave H_{eff} at the cobalt and vanadium nuclei as 312 and 61 kOe respectively. This large difference in the effective field was interpreted as resulting from the fact that in $Co_{0.3}Fe_{0.7}$ the cobalt nucleus is located in an atom with polarized 3d electrons, while in $V_{0.33}Fe_{0.67}$ no atomic moment is connected with the vanadium atom. Since in ferromagnetic alloys the polarization of core s electrons is expected to be much stronger in those atoms which have polarized d electrons than in adjacent atoms which do not, the data suggest that the dominant contribution to H_{eff} arises through the Fermi contact interaction from the polarization of core s electrons (cf.Secs. II.B. and III.A.) Nikitin et al. (1965) found for $V_{0.044}Fe_{0.956}$ and $V_{0.138}Fe_{0.862}$ alloys H_{eff} = 78 and 58 kOe, respectively.

Lounasmaa et al. (1962) have measured the specific heat of $Re_{0.10}Fe_{0.90}$ and $Sb_{0.054}Fe_{0.946}$ alloys; the observed effective fields were 610 and 169 kOe, respectively. Kogan et al. (1963)

found 670 kOe for H_{eff} at Re and 1350 kOe at Ir in several Re-Fe and Ir-Fe alloys.

Ho and Phillips (1965) have investigated the iron alloys $Os_{0.0075}Fe_{0.9925}$ and $Pt_{0.0321}Fe_{0.9679}$ between 0.08 and 1.15°K. These extremely low temperatures were needed for determining C_N because of the smallness of the nuclear contribution. Their data on the Pt-Fe alloy are shown in Fig. 4; the relation

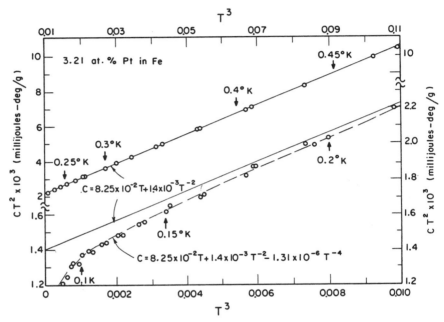

Fig. 4: The specific heat of $Pt_{0.0321}Fe_{0.9679}$ (Ho and Phillips, 1965). Observe the importance of the T^{-4} term below 0.2°K.

$C_N = c_2 T^{-2} - c_4 T^{-4}$ was used in fitting the results (cf. Sec. II.C). The effective fields found were 1400 and 1390 kOe, respectively; the same, within experimental error, for both Os and Pt. Considering the electronic structures of these metals such a result is to be expected.

H_{eff} depends on the crystal structure, e.g., in γ-manganese the hyperfine field is 65 kOe (Ho and Phillips, 1964, cf. Fig. 5) and in α-manganese 90 kOe (Scurlock and Stevens, 1965). Stetsenko and Avksentiev (1965) found H_{eff} = 150 kOe for chromium. Thus manganese and chromium, the only antiferromagnetic transition elements in the iron group, both exhibit considerable hyperfine interactions.

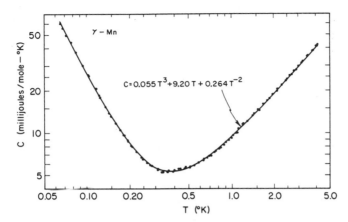

Fig. 5: The specific heat of γ-manganese
(Ho and Phillips, 1964).

Spatial ordering in the specimen can also cause large changes in the observed hyperfine field. Stetsenko and Avksentiev (1966) found that H_{eff} at Mn nuclei in $MnNi_3$ increased from 340 to 490 kOe after 120 hours of heat treatment. This enhancement may be due to an increase of the local and mean magnetic moments of the ordered alloy with a contribution from the polarized 4s electrons.

Nuclear specific heats entirely due to quadrupole interactions have been observed by Keesom and Bryant (1959) and by Seidel and Keesom (1959) for rhenium, gallium, and zinc. The measurements were carried out down to $0.3°$ K, but still lower temperatures are necessary for accurate values of the quadrupole coupling constant P.

IV. Rare Earth Metals

A. Theoretical Considerations

The bulk of information about hyperfine interactions in rare earth metals has been obtained from measurements of the nuclear specific heat. This type of investigation has been made by several groups of people, notably by Dreyfus, Goodman, Trolliet, and Weil (Trolliet, 1964) at Grenoble and by Lounasmaa (1962-64) at Argonne. More recently Mössbauer experiments have provided additional data.

The outer electronic structure of rare-earth atoms is $(4f^n, 5s^2, 5p^6, 6s^2, 5d^1)$ where the value of n increases from 0 for lanthanum to 14 for lutetium. The atoms are normally trivalent with the 6s and 5d electrons in the conduction band. Europium and ytterbium are exceptions to be discussed later. The magnetic electrons are thus buried relatively deep in the 4f shell, which maintains much of its free ion character. This fact has been very useful for a theoretical understanding of hyperfine interactions in these elements. The situation is different in transition metals with exposed magnetic 3d electrons. Orbital and spin dipolar terms are unquenched in the rare earths and, consequently, the relative and absolute magnitudes of the various components of H_{eff} are very different in the 4f and 3d elements.

By far the largest contribution to H_{eff} in the rare earths comes from the unquenched orbital angular momentum of the 4f electrons. This field is of the order of several mega-oersteds. The spin angular momentum contributes a term which is about one tenth of that produced by the orbital interaction.

A further contribution to H_{eff} is due to the core and conduction s electrons, which are polarized by an interaction with the 4f electrons. This causes, owing to the Fermi contact term in Eq. (5), a field of the order of several hundred kOe.

Since the hyperfine interactions are thus mainly due to the orbital and spin angular momenta of the 4f electrons, which have largely retained their free ion wave functions, it is expected and found (cf. Sec. IV. C.) that the interaction parameters in the rare earth metals and their salts are approximately equal. Calculations, which demonstrate this convincingly and which are based on experimental EPR data on salts, have been made by Kondo (1961) and by Bleaney (1963).

Quadrupole interactions are often fairly sizeable in these metals and may sometimes (cf. Sec. IV.B.) be separated from the magnetic term.

After these brief comments we shall next give experimental results on the nuclear specific heat of the rare earth metals.

B. Experimental Results

1. Lanthanum and Cerium

In both of these metals $C_N = 0$. For lanthanum this is caused by lack of magnetic 4f electrons and for cerium the result is due to the fact that all stable isotopes of this element are even-even nuclei, i.e., $\mu = Q = 0$.

2. Praseodymium

By analyzing his experimental C_p data between 0.4 and $4°K$ Lounasmaa (1964a) found $C_N = 20.9 \, T^{-2}$ mJ/mole $\cdot °K$. A calculation by Bleaney (1963), assuming complete electronic magnetization (cf. Eq. (10)), gave a much larger value, $C_N = 1070 \, T^{-2} - \ldots$. Neutron diffraction measurements by Cable et al. (1964) show, however, that $\langle J_z \rangle$ in praseodymium does not approach J at low temperatures, but rather tends to a much smaller limiting value. Using Cable's data we get $C_N = 25 \, T^{-2}$ mJ/mole $\cdot °K$, in reasonable agreement with the specific heat result.

According to Bleaney's (1963) calculations, the main difficulty in trying to explain the nuclear specific heat of praseodymium is not why the experimental C_N is so small, but why it is so large. Heat capacity measurements by Parkinson et al. (1951) between 2 and $180°K$ show that the entropy associated with C_M is close to R ln 9 (the ground state of Pr^{3+} ion is $^3H_4$), indicating that the degeneracy of the J = 4 state is completely lifted by the crystal field, i.e., the only electronic level populated at liquid helium temperatures is a singlet state. This is in agreement with the constant magnetic susceptibility of praseodymium below $4°K$ as observed by Lock (1957). With an electronic singlet state the metal is, according to the van Vleck (1932) theory, nonmagnetic in zeroth order and the magnetic hyperfine interaction should thus be zero. The quadrupole term is also very small and it seems difficult to find large enough internuclear exchange interactions (cf. Bleaney, 1963).

A possible explanation for this dilemma would be the s-f exchange interaction described by Chevalier and Baltensperger (1961); they predicted antiferromagnetic ordering for praseodymium at low temperatures. The calculation is in agreement with the neutron diffraction data of Cable et al. (1964). Another explanation for the observed C_N is based on small magnetically ordered clusters in the metal (cf. Lounasmaa, 1964a).

Dreyfus et al. (1963) have measured the specific heat of a $Pr_{0.27}Gd_{0.63}$ alloy, for which the nuclear contribution was $C_N = 228 \, T^{-2}$ mJ/mole $\cdot °K$. This corresponds to $C_N = 850 \, T^{-2}$ per mole of praseodymium, relatively close to the value calculated by Bleaney (1963).

3. Neodymium

In neodymium a transition to the antiferromagnetic state occurs at $7°K$ and thus C_M is large even below $1°K$. As a result the nuclear contribution has not been determined very accurately, but Lounasmaa (1964a) found $C_N = 7 \ T^{-2}$ mJ/mole $\cdot °K$. By assuming full electronic magnetization Bleaney (1963) obtains $C_N = 14 \ T^{-2}$. However, the crystal field splittings are large in neodymium and one cannot expect $\langle J_z \rangle$ in the cooperative state to tend to $J = 9/2$ (ground state of Nd^{3+} is $^4I_{9/2}$). The disagreement seems reasonable, but a precise calculation is difficult. For obtaining more accurate values on C_N and for separating the magnetic and quadrupole terms measurements at temperatures below $0.4°K$ are needed.

4. Samarium

Since promethium has no stable isotopes the next element in the rare earth series, for which heat capacity data are available, is samarium. For this metal Lounasmaa (1962a) found $C_N = 8.63 \ T^{-2} - 0.021 \ T^{-4}$ mJ/mole $\cdot °K$; since the T^{-3}-term is missing, the quadrupole interaction is too small to be detected. Bleaney (1963) obtains $C_N = 8.9 \ T^{-2}$. Because the effect of crystal field admixtures from the excited $J = 7/2$ state (the ground state of Sm^{3+} is $^6H_{5/2}$) is quite large in samarium, this value is uncertain up to 10% but, nevertheless, agrees with the calorimetric C_N.

5. Europium and Gadolinium

The outer electronic configuration of europium is somewhat different from the majority of the rare earths: one of the conduction electrons is moved to the 4f shell which thereby becomes half full. Consequently, we have Eu^{2+} ions in a $^8S_{7/2}$ ground state. In the next element gadolinium, Gd^{3+} ions have the same ground electronic state. The orbital angular momentum is thus zero and only a small field, caused mainly by core polarization, is expected at the nucleus. For europium the observed (Lounasmaa, 1964c) $C_N = 2.36 \ T^{-2}$ mJ/mole $\cdot °K$ which, indeed, corresponds to a field about an order of magnitude smaller than is found for the rare earths with $L \neq 0$ (cf. Table III, Sec. IV.C.).

Due to unfortunate impurity effects it has so far been impossible to measure the specific heat of gadolinium metal at low temperatures. According to Bleaney's (1963) calculations a very small C_N is expected. Using polarized neutrons and polarized nuclei Shore et al. (1965) found $H_{eff} = 350$ kOe for gadolinium metal, which corresponds to $C_N = 0.027 \ T^{-2}$ mJ/mole $\cdot °K$.

6. Terbium

Figure 6 shows specific heat data on terbium below 4°K. Filled squares are by Kurti and Safrata (1958), filled triangles by Stanton et al. (1960), filled circles by Heltemes and Swenson

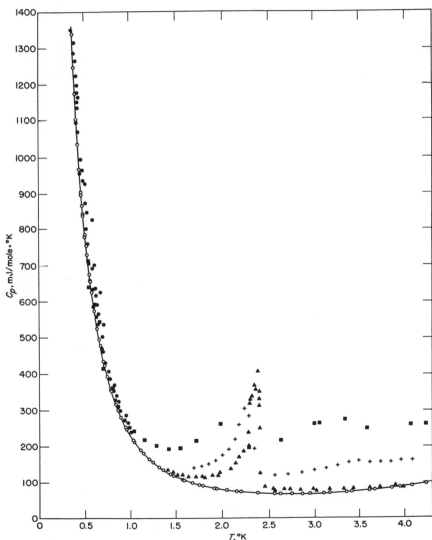

Fig. 6: The specific heat of terbium metal. For references see text.

(1961), crosses by Bailey (1962), and open circles by Lounasmaa and Roach (1962). In general, there is reasonable agreement below 1°K, but at higher temperatures there is no agreement at all. It is likely that the differences are caused by Tb_2O_3 impurity which undergoes a magnetic transformation (Gerstein et al., 1962) from an antiferromagnetic to a paramagnetic state at 2.3°K (cf. Sec. II.D.).

In terbium the huge nuclear contribution in C_p is mainly caused by the large magnetic moment, $\mu = 1.52$ nuclear magnetons, of Tb^{159}, but there is also a sizeable quadrupole interaction present. The two contributions can be separated as is shown in Fig. 7 (Lounasmaa and Roach, 1962), where C_NT^2 has been

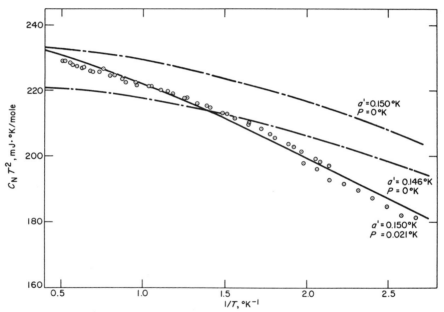

Fig. 7: Quadrupole interaction in the nuclear specific heat of terbium (see text).

plotted against $1/T$. Two lines have been calculated using Eq. (4) and by assuming magnetic interactions only ($P = 0$), the third by assuming both magnetic and quadrupole interactions. It is clear from the figure that a quadrupole term is necessary to explain the experimental results. The interaction parameters can be determined as was explained in Sec. II.C; the best fit to the measured

points is obtained with a' = 0.150°K and P = 0.021°K. The hyperfine levels calculated from Eq. (9) by using these numbers were
shown in Fig. 2. The result is in reasonable agreement with specific heat data of van Kempen et al. (1964) who found a' = 0.152°K
and P = 0.013°K, and with Bleaney's (1963) calculations which
gave a' = 0.152°K and P = 0.029°K.

7. Dysprosium

This metal has also been studied by a number of inves-
tigators and again the results show large discrepancies above
1°K. There is, however, reasonable agreement below 1°K and
thus also in the size of the nuclear contribution. Lounasmaa and
Guenther (1962) found $C_N = 26.4\ T^{-2} - 1.32\ T^{-3}$ mJ/mole·°K.
For more accurate data on the quadrupole term, measurements
should be extended well below 0.4°K.

8. Holmium

In holmium the nuclear specific heat is even larger than
in terbium; already at 4°K, C_N is over 50% of the total C_p. Experimental points by van Kempen et al. (1964) below 0.7°K are
shown in Fig. 8. The full curve is the best fit to the data

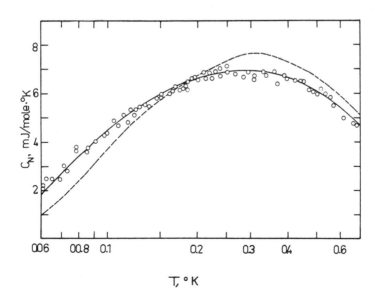

Fig. 8: The nuclear specific heat of holmium (van Kempen et al.,
1964). For an explanation see text.

assuming both magnetic and quadrupole interactions; the dashed curve is the best fit assuming magnetic interaction only. The need for a quadrupole term is again clearly demonstrated and the following values were obtained for the parameters: $a' = 0.320°$ K, $P = 0.008°$ K. These numbers are in excellent agreement with the measurements by Lounasmaa (1962b) who found $a' = 0.320°$ K and $P = 0.007°$ K. Bleaney's (1963) calculations gave $a' = 0.311°$ K and $P = 0.001°$ K. His quadrupole term, in particular, is considerably different from that obtained from specific heat data. The nuclear Schottky anomaly for holmium is shown in Fig. 1.

9. Erbium

Specific heat measurements on this metal have been made by Parks (1962) and by Trolliet (1964). The former found $C_N = 22\ T^{-2}$ and the latter $C_N = 30\ T^{-2}$, both in mJ/mole $\cdot °$ K.

10. Thulium

According to Lounasmaa (1964d) the nuclear specific heat of thulium can be expressed by $C_N = 23.4\ T^{-2} - 1.79\ T^{-3} - 0.066\ T^{-4}$ mJ/mole $\cdot °$ K. An analysis of the data clearly shows the need for a T^{-3} term. The trouble with this is that the only stable thulium isotope, Tm^{169}, has a nuclear spin $I = \frac{1}{2}$ and thus has no quadrupole moment. Various possibilities can, of course, be put forward to explain the "wrong" temperature dependence, but measurements below $0.4°$ K are needed before a thorough discussion is attempted.

11. Ytterbium and Lutetium

These last two metals in the rare earth series both have a full 4f shell, ytterbium is divalent and lutetium trivalent. There are thus no magnetic electrons and as a result $H_{eff} = 0$. The crystal structure of ytterbium is fcc and, consequently, the quadrupole interaction is also zero for this metal, i.e., $C_N = 0$. Lutetium, however, has a hcp structure and thus a quadrupole term, due to crystalline field effects, is a possibility. A small nuclear specific heat, $C_N = 0.094\ T^{-2}$ mJ/mole $\cdot °$ K, was, indeed, found by Lounasmaa (1964b). This value corresponds, if de Wette's (1961) calculations are used for estimating q_c (cf. Sec. II.B.), to a Sternheimer antishielding factor of -140, in reasonable agreement with theoretical predictions.

C. Summary and Comparison with Other Measurements

In Fig. 9 specific heat data on most of the rare earths are shown together. It should be noted that at $0.4°$ K the difference

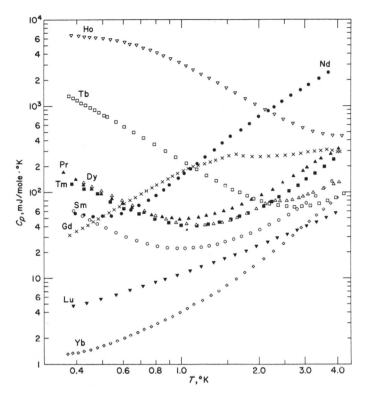

Fig. 9: The specific heat of most of the rare earth metals at low temperatures.

between the C_p of holmium and of ytterbium is almost four orders of magnitude.

In Table II the coefficient c_2 (cf. Eq. (11)), calculated from specific heat measurements on metals and from ESR work on salts, is listed for rare earth elements. In general, there is good agreement between specific heat and ESR data, and where discrepancies exist, they have mostly been explained. The difference in ytterbium is caused by the fact that Yb ions are di valent in the metal (full 4f shell) and trivalent in salts.

In Table III we list H_{eff} at the nucleus in rare earth metals, calculated from specific heat and Mössbauer measurements on the metals and from ESR data on the salts. The values show that H_{eff} is several maga-oersteds provided that maximum electronic mag- netization is reached and that the orbital angular momentum of the

Table II: Coefficient c_2 (mJ/mole$\cdot^\circ$K; cf. Eq. (11)) calculated from specific heat and ESR data.

	Sp.ht.[a]	ESR[b]		Sp.ht.[a]	ESR[b]
Pr	20.9	1070	Dy	26.4	26.6
	20[c]			30[c]	
	37.5[d]		Ho	4470	4220
Nd	7	14		4470[e]	
Sm	8.6	8.9		3980[c]	
	11[c]		Er	30[c]	-
Eu	2.4	4.2	Tm	23.4	23
Gd	-	0.02		27[c]	
Tb	238	250	Yb	0	16
	241[e]		Lu	0.09	--

(a) Lounasmaa (1962-64).   *(d) Dempesy et al. (1962).*
(b) Bleaney (1963).   *(e) van Kempen et al. (1963).*
(c) Trolliet (1964).

Table III: H_{eff} (mega-oersteds) at the rare earth nuclei.

	Sp.ht.[a]	Möss-bauer	ESR[b]		Sp.ht.[a]	Möss-bauer	ESR[b]
Pr	0.49	-	3.4	Tb	4.1	-	4.1
Nd	2.9	-	4.1	Dy	7.1	5.9[e]	7.4
Sm	3.3	-	-	Ho	9.3	-	9.0
Eu	0.260	0.264[c]		Er	9.3[f]	7.6[g]	7.7
Gd	-	0.350[d]		Tm	6.8	7.0[h]	6.9

(a) Lounasmaa (1962-64).
(b) Kondo (1961) (H_{eff} recal-
culated using current
values of μ).
(c) Barrett and Shirley
(1963).

(d) Shore et al. (1965) (polar-
ized neutrons).
(e) Ofer et al. (1964).
(f) Trolliet (1964).
(g) Hufner et al. (1965).
(h) Kalvius et al. (1963).

4f electrons is not zero. When L = 0, as in europium and gadolinium, the field is at least an order of magnitude smaller.

V. Conclusions

In this chapter we have given an account of the nuclear contribution to the specific heat of metals and alloys, together with
a selection of experimental results. The data presented are
reasonably complete on the rare earths, much less so for the
transition metals and their alloys.

It is likely that in the future more specific heat measurements
will be made, particularly on alloy systems with transition metal
or rare earth components. New efforts for determining the quadrupole coupling constant in hexagonal metals also will probably be
made.

The discussion of experimental results indicate, without a
doubt, that specific heat measurements at low temperatures are
a useful tool for investigating hyperfine interactions in metals and
alloys. For reliable separation of the magnetic and quadrupole
terms and for studying other finer details, experiments should be
extended to the lowest temperatures possible.

Acknowledgements

The author wishes to thank Pertti Reivari for help in the
preparation of this manuscript.

References

Arp, V., Kurti, N., and Petersen, R. (1957). Bull. Am. Phys.
Soc. 2, 388.

Arp, V., Edmonds, D., and Petersen, R. (1959). Phys. Rev. Letters 3, 212.

Bailey, C.A. (1962). Private communication (Clarendon Laboratory, Oxford).

Barrett, P.H. and Shirley, D.A. (1963). Phys. Rev. 131, 123.

Bleaney, B. (1963). J. Appl. Phys. 34, 1024.

Cable, J.W., Moon, R.M., Koehler, W.C., and Wollan, E.O. (1964). Phys. Rev. Letters 12, 553.

Chevalier, J. and Baltensperger, W. (1961). Helv. Phys. Acta 34, 859.

Cooper, B.R. (1962). Proc. Phys. Soc. (London) 80, 1225.

Dempesy, C.W., Gordon, J.E., and Soller, T. (1962). Bull. Am. Phys. Soc. 7, 309.

De Wette, F.W. (1961). Phys. Rev. 123, 103.

Dreyfus, B., Lacaze, A., and Michel, J.-C. (1963). Compt. rend. 257, 3355.

Freeman, A.J. and Watson, R.E. (1965). Magnetism IIA (G.T. Rado and H. Suhl, Eds.), pp. 168-306. Academic Press, New York.

Gerstein, B.C., Jelinek, F.J., and Spedding, F.H. (1962). Phys. Rev. Letters 8, 425.

Hall, H.E., Ford, P.J. and Thompson, K. (1966). Cryogenics 6, 80.

Hanna, S.S., Heberle, J., Littlejohn, C., Perlow, G.J., Preston, R.S. and Vincent, D.H. (1960). Phys. Rev. Letters 4, 177.

Heer, C.V. and Erickson, R.A. (1956). Bull. Am. Phys. Soc. 1, 217.

Heer, C.V. and Erickson, R.A. (1957). Phys. Rev. 108, 896.

Heltemes, E.C. and Swenson, C.A. (1961). J. Chem. Phys. 35, 1264.

Ho, J.C. and Phillips, N.E. (1964). Phys. Letters 10, 34.

Ho, J.C. and Phillips, N.E. (1965). Phys. Rev. 140, A648.

Hüfner, S., Kienle, P., Wiedemann, W., and Eicher, H. (1964). Z. Physik 182, 499.

Kalvius, M., Kienle, P., Eicher, H., Wiedemann, W., and Schüler, C. (1963). Z. Physik 172, 231.

Keeson, P.H. and Bryant, C.A. (1959). Phys. Rev. Letters 2, 260.

Kogan, A.V., Kulkov, V.D., Nikitin, L.P., Reinov, N.M., and Stelmakh, M.F. (1963). J. Exptl. Theoret. Phys. (USSR) 45, 1; (English transl.: Soviet Phys.-JETP 18, 1).

Kondo, J. (1961). J. Phys. Soc. Japan 16, 1690.

Kurti, N. and Safrata, R. S. (1958). Phil. Mag. 3, 780.

Lock, J. M. (1957). Proc. Phys. Soc. (London) B70, 566.

Lounasmaa, O. V. (1962a). Phys. Rev. 126, 1352.

Lounasmaa, O. V. (1962b). Phys. Rev. 128, 1136.

Lounasmaa, O. V. (1964a). Phys. Rev. 134, A1620, and other
papers listed in this reference.

Lounasmaa, O. V. (1964b). Phys. Rev. 133, A211.

Lounasmaa, O. V. (1964c). Phys. Rev. 133, A502.

Lounasmaa, O. V. (1964d). Phys. Rev. 133, A219.

Lounasmaa, O. V., Cheng, C. H., and Beck, P. A. (1962). Phys.
Rev. 128, 2153.

Lounasmaa, O. V. and Guenther, R. A. (1962). Phys. Rev. 126,
1357.

Lounasmaa, O. V. and Roach, P. R. (1962). Phys. Rev. 128, 622.

Marshall, W. and Johnson, C. E. (1962). J. Phys. Radium 23, 733.

Nikitin, L. P., Kogan, A. V., Kulkov, V. D., and Shiryapov, I. P.
(1965). J. Exptl. Theoret. Phys. (USSR) 49, 1028; (English
transl.: Soviet Phys. -JETP 22, 714).

Ofer, S., Rakavy, M., Segal, E., and Khurgin, B. (1964). Phys.
Rev. 138, A241.

Parkinson, D. H., Simon, F. E., and Spedding, F. H. (1951). Proc.
Roy. Soc. (London) 207, 137.

Parks, R. D. (1962). Rare Earth Research (J. F. Nachman and C. E.
Lundin, Eds.), p. 225. Gordon and Breach, N. Y.

Scurlock, R. G. and Stevens, W. N. R. (1965). Proc. Phys. Soc.
(London) 86, 331.

Seidel, G. and Keesom, P. H. (1959). Phys. Rev. Letters 2, 261.

Shore, F. J., Reynolds, C. A., Sailor, V. L., and Brunhart, G.
(1965). Phys. Rev. 138, B1361.

Stetsenko, P. and Avksentiev, Yu. (1965). Proc. Intl. Conf. on
Magnetism (The Inst. of Phys. and the Phys. Soc., London),
p. 217.

Stetsenko, P. and Avksentiev, Yu. (1966). Proc. of the 1966 Low Temp. Calorimetry Conf., Ann. Acad. Sci. Fennicae AVI, No. 210, p. 226.

Sternheimer, R.M. (1954). Phys. Rev. 95, 736.

Trolliet, G. (1964). Thesis (Univ. of Grenoble) and other papers of the Grenoble group listed in this reference.

Van Kempen, H., Miedema, A.R., and Huiskamp., W.J. (1964). Physica 30, 229.

Van Kranendonk, J. and Van Vleck, J.H. (1958). Rev. Mod. Phys. 30, 1.

Van Vleck, J.H. (1932). Electronic and Magnetic Susceptibilities. p. 232 et seq. Oxford University Press.

Wei, C.T., Cheng, C.H., and Beck, P.A. (1961). Phys. Rev. 122, 1129.

11. RECOILLESS ABSORPTION OF GAMMA RAYS AND STUDIES OF NUCLEAR HYPERFINE INTERACTIONS IN SOLIDS

Lectures by R.L. Mössbauer

Prepared* by M.J. Clauser †

Physik Department
Technische Hochschule
Munich, Germany

Table of Contents

*From the unedited lecture notes of R.L. Mössbauer.
†U.S. Natl. Science Foundation Postdoctoral Fellow.

I. Introduction

The phenomenon of resonant absorption has been known in optics since early in the century. The nuclear analogue was predicted in 1929 (Kuhn, 1929) but was not observed until 1951 (Moon, 1951). In 1958 the phenomenon of recoilless nuclear resonance was discovered (Mössbauer, 1958). The essence of this discovery was that both the energy loss due to nuclear recoil and the Doppler broadening due to thermal motion are eliminated under certain circumstances. The result was that very narrow gamma lines were observed, lines which can be used in many fields of physics, chemistry, and biology because of the high energy resolution.

II. Principles of Recoilless Nuclear Resonance Absorption

The phenomenon of photon emission is a well-known quantum effect in which a system emits a photon while making a transition from one state to another state of lower energy. The reverse transition can also take place (see Fig. 1). Here a photon is absorbed and a transition to a higher energy state is made. This latter process is called resonant absorption because the photon must have just the right energy to cause the transition. In optical resonance the transitions take place between electronic levels, while in nuclear resonance, nuclear levels are involved. In principle, sources and absorbers must be made of identical atoms or nuclei so that the resonance condition is met.

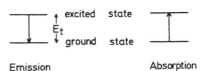

Fig. 1: Photon emission and resonance absorption processes.

Emission and absorption spectra are shown in Fig. 2. The transition energy E_t is just the difference in energy of the two levels. However, the energy of the emitted photon usually differs

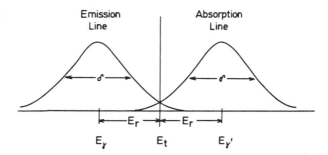

Fig. 2: Emission and absorption spectra in a gas of free atoms.
Due to the recoil energies Er, the spectrum lines overlap
poorly. δ is the thermal Doppler width; E_t is the transition
energy.

slightly in energy from the transition energy because the emitting
nucleus recoils in the opposite direction from the photon in order
to conserve momentum. The transition energy is divided between
both the photon energy E_γ and the recoil kinetic energy E_r;

$$E_t = E_\gamma + E_r \, ,$$

or   (1)

$$E_\gamma = E_t - E_r \, .$$

This recoil energy is inconsequential in optical spectroscopy but
is very important for nuclear resonance spectroscopy. On the
other hand, for resonance *absorption,* the incoming photon must
provide both the transition energy and the recoil energy in order
for resonance to take place;

$$E_\gamma' = E_t + E_r \, .$$ (2)

As can be seen, there is a deficit in energy of $2\,E_r$ between the
emission and absorption lines. In the optical case this is typically
small compared to the line width, but in the nuclear case it is large
compared to the line widths. In the optical case this means that
the emission and absorption lines overlap nearly perfectly and there
is a good chance that a photon will be resonantly absorbed in the
experiment illustrated in Fig. 3. In the typical nuclear case there
is very little chance of resonant absorption because the overlap of
the two lines is very small.

Table I gives some typical numbers for a free (gaseous) atom.
The Doppler width δ is just the line broadening caused by the

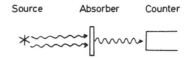

Fig. 3: Optical resonance experiment. When the atoms of the source and absorber are identical, photons emitted by the source may be resonantly absorbed by the absorber, producing a decrease in the number of photons reaching the counter.

Table I: Typical parameters for a low energy nuclear transition in a free atom.

Atomic Weight	A	$=$	100
Transition Energy	E_t	$=$	10^5 eV
Recoil Energy	E_r	$=$	0.1 eV
Doppler Width	δ	$=$	0.1 eV
At the temperature	T	$=$	$300\,°K$

thermal motion of the atoms,

$$\delta = \frac{\overline{v}}{c} E_t \tag{3}$$

where $\overline{v}$ is an rms thermal velocity. As can be seen, there should be little overlap of the two lines. The transition energy of 10^5 eV is rather low for a gamma transition but the situation becomes worse for larger transition energies, since, as can easily be shown,

$$E_r \approx \frac{E_t^{\,2}}{2mc^2} \tag{4}$$

where m is the atomic mass, c the velocity of light. The recoil energy increases as the square of the transition energy, while the Doppler widths increase linearly. Since optical transitions have a much lower energy, it is easy to see why the recoil energy is unimportant for optical spectroscopy.

This deficit in energy, $2\,E_r$, was an obstacle to the observation of gamma absorption for several decades until 1951 when the British physicist P. B. Moon successfully demonstrated the existence of the nuclear resonance effect. To overcome the recoil energy, he mounted the source on an ultra-centrifuge which he then rotated with such high speeds that the energy of the emission line was increased due to the linear Doppler effect (see Fig. 4). Sufficiently high speeds were obtained so that perfect overlap of the emission and absorption lines was obtained. He used a gamma transition of relatively low energy, 411 keV.

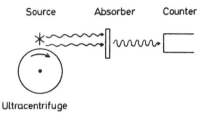

Source   Absorber   Counter

Ultracentrifuge

Fig. 4:   Nuclear resonance experiment.   This is similar to the optical experiment in Fig. 3 except that the ultracentrifuge is needed to compensate for the recoil energy loss.

Up to this point, only freely recoiling nuclei have been considered for which the Doppler widths are typically in the range 10^{-2} eV to 10^{2} eV.   Now, nuclei bound in solids will be considered. These may be thought of as nuclei connected with springs.   Momentum conservation must be considered again for the solid.   The means of conservation is basically the same as for the free atom, i.e., by recoil.   The main question then is what is the *energy* associated with this recoil?   Irrespective of the detailed mechanism of momentum transfer, the recoil momentum must eventually be taken up by the solid as a whole through center of mass motion. The *energy* associated with the motion of the solid as whole is very much smaller than for a single nucleus.   The mass of the atom, m, in Eq. (4) must now be replaced by the mass of the solid, which is some 10^{22} times larger.   Consequently the recoil *energy* of the solid as a whole can be completely neglected.

There are, however, other ways in which a nucleus can transfer energy to the solid in which it is bound.   There is for example, the possibility of creating all kinds of elementary excitations, primarily, vibrations within the solid, that is, of creating or destroying phonons. The question then becomes: what is the probability of creating or destroying a phonon during the gamma transition?   It should perhaps be emphasized that, in contrast to the free atom case, one can speak only of the probability of transferring a given amount of energy to the lattice. That is, when the initial state of the lattice, $|i>$, is operated on by the momentum transfer operator, $e^{-ik\cdot r}|i>$, an eigenfunction will not generally be produced. Consequently only a probability distribution may be obtained for the creation and/or destruction of various combinations of phonons. This leads directly to a probability distribution for the energy transferred to the lattice when the gamma quantum is emitted. The emission and absorption spectra for a solid are shown in Fig. 5. These spectra

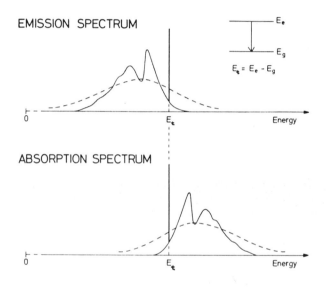

Fig. 5: Structure of gamma emission and absorption lines of
nuclei bound in solids;
(1) the case of very high recoil energy where multiphonon
processes dominate (dashed lines), and
(2) the case of very low recoil energy, where few phonons
participate (solid lines).

(solid lines) would be obtained for either low gamma transition energies or low temperatures. The very sharp line at $E = E_t$ is due to gamma transitions which produce no phonons; it has a "natural" linewidth determined by the nuclear lifetime. As either the temperature or gamma energy becomes larger, each spectrum becomes transformed into the free atom spectrum (dashed lines). Independent of the structure of the phonon spectrum, it can be shown that the *average* recoil energy of a bound nucleus is equal to the recoil energy of a nucleus free to recoil:

$$E_{r_{bound}} = E_{r_{free}} \quad . \tag{5}$$

Of course nothing has been said about the recoil energy of a particular transition; only probabilities for different recoil energies can be given. Hence the above result applies only to the average energy transferred to the lattice. This result gives a hint that the average recoil energy must be comparable to or smaller than a typical phonon excitation energy in order to have an appreciable fraction of zero-phonon (recoilless) transitions. As a typical phonon energy, $k\theta$ may be used, where θ is the Debye temperature of the crystal, or in frequency units, $\hbar\omega = k\theta$. Now if $k\theta \gg E_r$, only a few gamma transitions will produce phonon excitations; the remainder will be recoilless. If $E_r \gg k\theta$, then each gamma transition will produce many phonon excitations and very few will be recoilless. At higher temperatures there are more phonons in the lattice and the probability of phonon excitation is correspondingly increased.

The main point of interest is the fraction of zero phonon transitions. A rigorous treatment of this question will not be given here; we give only an outline of the physical processes which are relevant. Whenever the uncertainty in the momentum of the lattice Δp is large compared to the recoil momentum $\hbar k$, a large recoil-free fraction can be expected since it can no longer be easily distinguished whether or not the momentum has been transferred to the lattice. Using the uncertainty relation for the momentum and position coordinates of the lattice,

$$\Delta p \cdot \Delta x \approx \hbar \ , \tag{6}$$

the condition for a large recoil-free fraction becomes

$$\Delta x \cdot \hbar k \ll \hbar \ ,$$

$$(\Delta x)^2 k^2 \approx \langle u^2 \rangle k^2 \ll 1 \tag{7}$$

or finally,

$$\langle u^2 \rangle \ll \lambdabar^2$$

Here k is the gamma wave vector, λ is the wave length, and $<u^2>$ is the mean square displacement of the nucleus.

For simplicity only two possibilities will be considered: zero-phonon transitions or one-phonon transitions where a phonon of energy $\hbar\omega$ is excited. This situation is most appropriate at low temperatures. The average energy transferred to the lattice is then $\hbar\omega(1 - f)$ where f is defined as the fraction of zero phonon transitions. This is equal to the average recoil energy,

$$E_r = \frac{\hbar^2 k^2}{2m} \, . \tag{8}$$

Then

$$f = 1 - \frac{\hbar^2 k^2}{2m\hbar\omega} \approx \exp\left(-\frac{\hbar^2 k^2}{2m\hbar\omega}\right) \tag{9}$$

For an oscillator the energy $\hbar\omega$ is also given by $2m\omega^2 <u^2>$. The factor of 2 comes from the fact that half of the energy is kinetic, half potential, on the average. Using this, the recoilless fraction becomes

$$f = \exp\left[-k^2 <u^2>\right] \tag{10}$$

This result is in fact more general than the derivation would imply. For a rigid body there will be no vibrations so that $<u^2> = 0$ and $f = 1$. For any real crystal f will always be smaller than unity, even at zero temperature, because there will always be zero point motion of the atoms, or, equivalently, phonons can always be excited. At higher temperatures $<u^2>$ increases so that the recoil-free fraction decreases.

Figure 6 shows the recoil-free fraction for two different gamma transition energies as a function of temperature. The upper curve is for the 6.2 keV transition in Ta-181. This is the lowest energy yet observed in gamma resonance measurements. The other curve is for the 134 keV transition in Re-187. This is one of the highest energy transitions that has been observed in gamma resonance absorption measurements. For the low energy transition f is relatively large over a wide range of temperatures until $<u^2>$ becomes large. In the high energy case only a few of the transitions are recoilless, even at low temperatures. This means that with low energy gamma transitions a wide range of temperatures may be used with little worry, while for high energy transitions very low temperatures must be used and even then only a few percent of the transitions will be zero-phonon transitions.

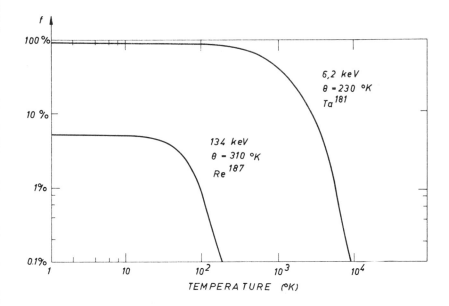

Fig. 6:   Temperature dependence of the f factor for the
gamma transitions of the lowest energy and one of
the highest energies which have yet been observed
in measurements of recoilless resonance absorption.

The recoil-free fraction f is similar to the Debye-Waller
factor which is familiar from x-ray scattering. In x-ray diffraction, the Debye-Waller factor gives the fraction of x-rays which
are scattered without creating any excitations in the crystal. The
f factor has the same origin in gamma resonance scattering, but
not quite the same form. For scattering (i.e., absorption and re-
emission) f becomes:

$$f_\gamma = \exp\left[- k_i^2 <u^2> \right] \exp\left[- k_f^2 <u^2> \right] \qquad (11)$$

whereas for x-ray scattering the Debye-Waller factor is

$$f_x = \exp\left[- (\mathbf{k}_i - \mathbf{k}_f)^2 <u^2> \right] \qquad (12)$$

In both cases k_i and k_f are the initial and final wave-vectors, respectively. The reason for the difference is that for gamma resonance scattering, the lifetime of the intermediate nuclear state is
long ($\approx 10^{-9}$ sec) compared with typical lattice periods ($\approx 10^{-13}$ sec),
but for the x-ray case, the intermediate states are in the optical
continuum and have short lifetimes compared with the lattice

periods. Other than this difference, the physics of the two processes is the same.

III. Experimental Technique

The apparatus used for observing the existence of recoilless
nuclear resonance is relatively simple. The discussion here will
be limited to resonant absorption experiments since scattering experiments, while they are important in some areas of research,
have not been generally used in studies of hyperfine interactions.
The basic equipment consists of a radioactive source, a resonant
absorber and a radiation detector. The detector is used to observe
the radiation which passes through the absorber. In order to observe the resonance, the source is mounted on a carriage which is
moved with velocity v with respect to the absorber (Fig. 7).

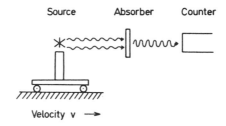

Fig. 7: Recoilless nuclear resonance
experiment.

Due to the Doppler effect, the spectrum line of the source is shifted
in energy with respect to the absorber line. When the source is at
rest with respect to the absorber, the source and absorber lines
overlap perfectly, and a maximum absorption is obtained so that
the transmitted intensity is a minimum. When the source moves
with respect to the absorber, the overlap of the two lines is smaller
so that less radiation is absorbed, more is transmitted. This is
illustrated in Fig. 8. As a function of velocity, the transmitted
intensity looks like a resonance line with twice the width Γ of the
source and absorber. When a line with width Γ is moved over
another line of width Γ, the fold of the two lines is a line with width
2Γ.

A word should be said here about the sources. The excited
nuclear state is usually produced as the result of a radioactive decay from a parent nucleus to an excited state of a daughter nucleus.

The gamma transition in the daughter nucleus is then used in the experiment. As an example, the decay scheme of Co^{57} is illustrated in Fig. 9. The Co^{57} decays to successive levels of Fe^{57} with a half-life of 270 days. The gamma transition which is used in experiments is the 14.4 keV transition which has a half life of 1.4×10^{-7} sec. The natural line width associated with this half life is $\Gamma = 4.6 \times 10^{-9}$ eV. This should be compared with the Doppler width $\delta \approx 0.1$ eV.

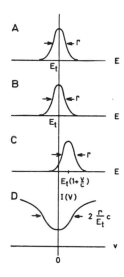

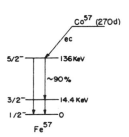

Fig. 8: A. Absorption spectrum. B. Source emission spectrum, $v = 0$. C. Source emission spectrum, $v \neq 0$. D. Transmitted intensity as a function of velocity.

Fig. 9: Decay scheme of Co^{57}. The 14.4 keV gamma transition is used for recoilless nuclear resonance experiments.

For iron, the recoil free fraction at $T = 0°K$ is about 0.9 so that there are about ten times as many recoilless transitions as there are transitions which produce recoil. Consequently, the height of the recoilless line is about 10^8 larger than the broad peak associated with the phonon-producing transitions, and the effects of the phonon peaks on the resonance spectrum are completely negligible.

The formula for the absorption cross section as a function of energy is given by

$$\sigma(E) = \frac{\lambda^2}{2\pi} \cdot \frac{2I+1}{2I_o+1} \cdot \frac{1}{1+\alpha} \, f \, h \cdot \frac{(\Gamma/2)^2}{(E-E_t)^2+(\Gamma/2)^2} \tag{13}$$

where λ is the gamma quantum wave length, I is the spin of the nuclear excited state, I_o is the spin of the ground state, α is the conversion coefficient, f is the recoil free fraction, and h is the relative abundance of the isotope in question. For natural iron the relative abundance of Fe^{57} is $h = 2.2\%$; however, this can be enriched to nearly 100%. At 0°K the recoil free fraction $f = 0.9$, while at room temperature, 300°K, $f = 0.8$. The maximum absorption cross section at $E = E_t$ is $\sigma(E_t) = 3.6 \times 10^{-20}$ cm². For comparison, the cross section for all other non-resonant processes is about 10^{-20} cm². It should be pointed out that the non-resonant absorption is essentially independent of velocity so that there is no trouble distinguishing the two types of absorption.

The resonant cross section given above is really an overestimate since the intensity is usually split up into several lines by hyperfine interactions. The magnetic hyperfine interaction in Fe^{57} splits the nuclear ground state into two levels and the excited state into four levels (Fig. 10). The transition is essentially pure M1 so that only $\Delta m_I = 0, \pm 1$ transitions are observed. The resulting spectrum has six lines, as shown in Fig. 11. These lines can

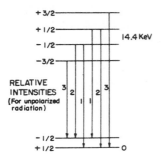

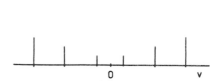

Fig. 10: Magnetic hyperfine splittings in Fe^{57}.

Fig. 11: Magnetic hyperfine spectrum lines of Fe^{57}.

be observed because the splitting is larger than the line width of the recoilless gamma lines. If both the source and the absorber have a hyperfine splitting, then a complicated pattern of lines will be the result when the source spectrum is moved over the absorber spectrum. Consequently, it is preferable to have either the source or the absorber, usually the source, free from hyperfine interactions. This can usually be accomplished by using a paramagnetic material with high crystallographic symmetry. In the paramagnetic region the magnetic hyperfine interaction usually vanishes due to electronic relaxation, and the high symmetry usually eliminates the electric quadrupole interaction. In Fe^{57} the quadrupole interaction would split the nuclear excited state into two levels in the absence of magnetic interactions.

There are many different versions of velocity spectrometers, the name given to the apparatus needed to perform an experiment; however, two basic types may be distinguished. One is the "constant speed" type where the source (or absorber) moves back and forth at a constant speed ($+v$, $-v$; see Fig. 12). This type of drive is useful if only one part of the spectrum is to be measured. For instance it may be necessary to measure only the position of one peak. If several points in the spectrum are to be measured, the drive must be successively adjusted to different speeds. There is one main disadvantage with this method. The electronic system used to count the gamma rays is subject to long term drifts. The spectrum that is picked up by the detector usually has several lines due to different gamma transitions, x-ray transitions, etc. The pulses from the detector are amplified and then analyzed by a single channel analyzer (SCA) so that only the desired portion of the spectrum is counted. Due to drifts in the gain of the amplifier and in the window settings of the SCA the counting rate may change during the time that the different points of the spectrum are being measured. Consequently, a change in the counting rate occurs not only because of the change in resonance absorption, but also because of changes in the electronics.

The usual way to avoid the problem of drift is to sweep through a series of velocities quickly and repeatedly. It should be done quickly so that there is no drift in the electronics and repeatedly so that the spectrum peaks are larger than the statistical fluctuations in counting rate. It is usually desirable that the switching of speeds be done continuously. To accomplish this, an electromechanical transducer, for instance a loudspeaker, is commonly used. The transducer consists of a coil connected rigidly to a rod on which the source is mounted (See Fig. 13). The coil is mounted

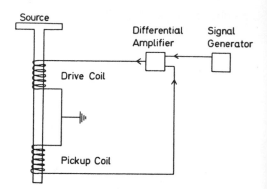

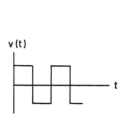

Fig. 12: Velocity as a function of time for a "constant speed" velocity spectrometer.

Fig. 13: Schematic of an electro-mechanical transducer system.

inside a magnetic field so that the source is moved when a voltage is applied to the coil. Due to the complicated response of the transducer, the motion of the source does not duplicate the wave-form of the applied voltage. To ensure that the source has the proper velocity, an ordinary feedback system is used. A second transducer which is used to measure the velocity is connected rigidly to the rod of the first transducer. The output voltage of this transducer is directly proportional to the velocity of the source. This voltage is compared with the reference signal; the difference is amplified and then fed to the drive coil. The reference signal can be any one several waveforms, depending on the requirements of the experiment. The two simples ones are the sine wave and the triangular wave, shown in Fig. 14. In order to record the gamma rays as a function of velocity, a multichannel analyzer is usually used. One method is to modulate the output

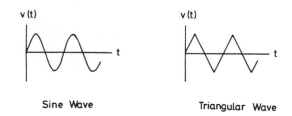

Sine Wave

Triangular Wave

Fig. 14: Typical waveforms used as reference signals for electromechanical transducers.

pulses of the SCA with the velocity pickup signal so that the pulse
height is proportional to the velocity. These pulses are then fed
into the multichannel pulse height analyzer. The CRT of the analyzer then displays directly the spectrum as a function of velocity.
This method has several problems, some of which are associated
with the dead time of the analyzer. A more common method is to
use the analyzer in a multiscaler mode where the channels are
swept through at a clock controlled rate. The clock in the analyzer
must be synchronized with the signal generator so that each channel
will be open at the correct velocity interval. This can be done by
triggering the analyzer clock with the signal generator. Once each
cycle, when the reference signal passes through zero, the signal
generator also produces a synchronization signal which is used to
start the clock running at the first channel. An alternative method
is to let the analyzer clock run free and use the analyzer as a
square wave signal generator. For example, if two hundred channels are used, the analyzer produces a signal which is, say, positive during the first hundred channels, and negative during the second hundred channels. This square wave can then be integrated to
provide a triangular wave reference signal.

One final remark should be made concerning these drive
systems. Since the source is moving back and forth, the solid
angle seen by the detector will be different for different velocities,
so that the counting rate will also
be different, quite aside from the
resonance absorption. To lowest
order this geometrical effect is
proportional to the displacement of
the source. The counting rate is
greater when the source is close to
the detector, smaller when the
source is away from the detector.
The reference signal will pass
through each velocity interval
twice during each cycle, once
accelerating, the other time de-
celerating. Thus two different
channels will correspond to the
same velocity interval. For the
commonly used reference signals

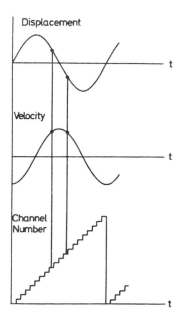

Fig. 15: Relationship between displacement, velocity, and channel
number when the analyzer is used
as a signal generator.

these two channels correspond to *displacements* of the same magnitude, but of opposite sign. This is illustrated for a sinusoidal displacement in Fig. 15. Consequently, by folding the two halves of the spectra together, adding each pair of corresponding channels together, the geometric effect is cancelled to lowest order.

IV. Observations of Recoilless Nuclear Resonance

Fig. 16 shows the elements in which recoilless nuclear resonances have been observed to date. They are shown on the background of the periodic system primarily to show in which ranges of the periodic system experiments can be performed. In particular, experiments can be performed in all the transition element series. There are elements in the 3d, 4d, 5d, and 4f series; there is even one element in the Actinide (5f) series. There are a number of other qualified members in the Actinide series and elsewhere in which experiments can be performed. The largest number of elements lies in the 4f series. In fact there are several elements with more than one isotope in which experiments can be performed.

I	II	III	IV	V	VI	VII	VIII
19 K							26 Fe 28 Ni
	30 Zn		32 Ge				36 Kr
							44 Ru
			50 Sn	51 Sb	52 Te	53 I	54 Xe
55 Cs		58-71	72 Hf	73 Ta	74 W	75 Re	76 Os 77 Ir 78 Pt
79 Au							
		90-103					

			62 Sm	63 Eu	64 Gd	65 Tb	66 Dy	68 Er	69 Tm	70 Yb	
		93 Np									

Fig. 16: Summary of elements with observed recoilless gamma transitions. In some cases, transitions have been observed in several isotopes of the same element.

Fig. 17 summarizes the types of information which can be obtained from gamma resonance spectra. The first spectrum, a), shows a simple splitting caused by hyperfine magnetic dipole or electric quadrupole interactions. In the spectrum shown there is only one parameter, the splitting ΔE. Of course more complicated patterns may occur in which there are several lines and several splitting parameters. From these parameters information may be obtained on both the magnetic dipole and electric quadrupole coupling coefficients in both the nuclear ground and excited states. This situation should be contrasted to other techniques such as NMR where only the nuclear ground state is involved.

A second type of information which can be obtained from spectra are shifts of the center of the spectrum in Fig. 17b away from zero velocity. There are several causes of such shifts. The most important is the isomer shift, about which more will be said later. Another cause is the second order Doppler shift, which is a relativistic effect due to the thermal motion of the nuclei (Pound and Rebka, 1960). As has already been shown, the first order Doppler effect vanishes because the average velocity of the nucleus is zero. The second order doppler effect does not vanish, since the mean square velocity is not zero. This effect is generally quite small and will not be considered further here.

A third type of information which may be obtained from spectra is an intensity difference in the lines (cf Fig. 17c). These differences may arise for a variety of reasons. One trivial reason may be that the relative transition probabilities (Clebsch-Gordan coefficients) of the various hyperfine components are different. A less trivial difference arises from the fact that the angular dependence of radiation intensity is different for different hyperfine components. Consequently, when single crystals are used, the intensities of the spectrum peaks will depend on the angle between the emitted quantum and the crystal axes in the source, the angle of the absorbed quantum and the crystal axes in the absorber, etc. However, if polycrystalline materials are used, all these angles are averaged over and the angular dependence vanishes. Intensity differences may also arise even for polycrystalline materials in case there is an anisotropy in the f-factors (Kagan, 1961; Karyagin, 1963; Gol'danskii, et al, 1963).

A fourth type of information can be obtained from spectra which exhibit complicated structure with lines of different shapes or widths. These spectra (cf. Fig. 17d) are quite different from spectra discussed previously, where all the lines had essentially twice the natural width. Such spectra can occur in cases where

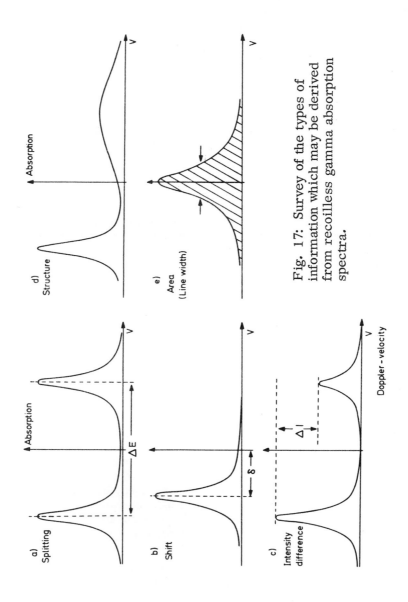

Fig. 17: Survey of the types of information which may be derived from recoilless gamma absorption spectra.

electronic relaxation effects are important, that is, when the relaxation times are roughly comparable to nuclear precession times. Spectra of this type can reveal much concerning the mutual interactions in the crystal, such as spin-spin and spin-lattice interactions. A specific example of such structure in spectra will be discussed later.

A fifth type of information may be obtained from the areas or widths of the spectrum lines. For instance, information about the recoil free fraction f may be obtained from the area. As was mentioned earlier, the total absorption cross section is proportional to f, and the area in the spectrum line is a measure of this. Of course these measurements of f are complicated by the fact that not all of the radiation counted by the detector comes from the desired gamma transition. For instance, due to the Compton effect in a sodium iodide detector, radiation from higher energy transitions is registered in the window of the desired line. So, the amount of nonresonant background must be known in order to make accurate measurements of f. The width of the lines may also provide information. Under ideal circumstances the width is just twice the natural width. However, there are many things that may cause the lines to be broadened. There may be statistically distributed hyperfine interactions when the surroundings of the nuclei are not all identical. A more important cause of broadening is due to the finite thickness of the absorbers. The transmitted spectrum is not simply a Lorentzian but rather $\exp\left[-\sigma(E)\rho\tau\right]$ folded with the source spectrum, where $\sigma(E)$ is the (Lorentzian) absorption cross section of a single nucleus, ρ is the density, and τ is the thickness of the absorber. The effect of the exponential is to flatten the peak, causing the peak to appear broader (Fig. 18). For relatively thin absorbers with $\tau < \left(\sigma(E_T)\rho\right)^{-1}$ the resulting spectrum can be closely approximated by a Lorentzian with a greater-than-natural width.

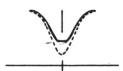

Fig. 18: Broadening of an absorption peak due to absorber thickness. The dashed line represents the unbroadened natural line.

V. The Isomer Shift

The remainder of the chapter will be spent on hyperfine interactions themselves. The first topic will be the isomer shift (Kistner and Sunyar, 1960) which measures the charge density at the nucleus. Considerable attention will be devoted to this subject since gamma resonance is the only technique in solids which can measure some of the quantities involved. Optical measurements of *isotope* shifts* can be made in some cases, but these are done in free atoms and involve nuclear ground states only. Gamma resonance is the only technique at present which can measure changes in charge densities in solids. In this context, it should be stressed that the Knight shift measures *spin* density, not *charge* density.

A. Theory

The derivation of the isomer shift will be outlined here primarily to show what assumptions are made and what quantities enter into the expression. The following three assumptions will be made:

i) The derivation will be nonrelativistic. This assumption is most serious in the heavy atoms where corrections can be as high as 30 percent.

ii) The electron charge will be considered to be constant over the nuclear region. This means, in effect, that only s electrons contribute, since they are the only nonrelativistic electrons which have finite density at the nucleus.

iii) A perturbation treatment will be used. It will be assumed that the size of the nucleus does not affect the electronic wave functions.

The Coulomb interaction energy between the electrons and the nucleus is

$$W_e = - e^2 \iint \frac{\rho_n(r_n)\,\rho_e(r_e)}{|r_e - r_n|} \, d\tau_e d\tau_n \tag{14}$$

where the subscripts n and e refer to the nucleus and electrons, respectively; $\rho_e(r_e)$ and $\rho_n(r_n)$ are the charge distributions, and $d\tau_e$ and $d\tau_n$ are volume elements. The usual multipole expansion of $1/|r_e - r_n|$ is used:

*See Chap. 5 by A. Steudel.

$$\frac{1}{|r_e - r_n|} = 4\pi \sum_{\ell=0}^{\infty} \sum_{m=-\ell}^{\ell} \frac{1}{2\ell+1}$$

(15)

$$\cdot \frac{r_<^\ell}{r_>^{\ell+1}} \, Y_{\ell m}^*(\theta_n \Phi_n) \, Y_{\ell m}(\theta_e, \Phi_e)$$

where the symbol $r_<$ means the lesser of r_e and r_n, and $r_>$ is similarly defined. $Y_{\ell m}(\theta, \Phi)$ is the usual spherical harmonic. The monopole interaction, which is the one of interest here, is the term with $\ell=0$ (the $\ell=2$ terms, for example, give rise to the electric quadrupole interaction). Then,

$$(W_e)_{\ell=0} = -e^2 \iint \frac{\rho_n(r_n)\,\rho_e(r_e)\,d\tau_e\,d\tau_n}{r_>}$$

(16)

The integration over angular coordinates can be done immediately to obtain

$$(W_e)_{\ell=0} =$$

$$- (4\pi e)^2 \iint \frac{\rho'_n(r_n)\,\rho'_e(r_e)\,r_e^2\,dr_e\,r_n^2\,dr_n}{r_>}$$

(17)

where $\rho'(r)$ is an average charge density, averaged over a sphere of radius r

$$\rho'(r) = \frac{1}{4\pi} \int \rho(r)\,\sin\theta\,d\theta\,d\Phi$$

(18)

The expression for W_e can then be broken up into a sum of two integrals which can be more readily handled:

$$(W_e)_{\ell=0} = -(4\pi e)^2 \left[\int_{r_n=0}^{\infty} \left\{ \int_{r_e=0}^{r_n} \frac{\rho'_e(r_e)}{r_n} r_e^2\,dr_e \right.\right.$$

$$\left.\left. \int_{r_e=r_n}^{\infty} \frac{\rho'_e(r_e)}{r_e} r_e^2\,dr_e \right\} \rho'_n(r_n)r_n^2\,dr_n \right] .$$

(19)

The integral over r_e in the second term may be rewritten

$$\int\limits_{r_e=r_n}^{\infty} = \int\limits_{r_e=0}^{\infty} - \int\limits_{r_e=0}^{r_n} \tag{20}$$

so that

$$(W_e)_{\ell=0} = -(4\pi e)^2 \int\limits_0^{\infty} \int\limits_0^{r_n} \left(\frac{1}{r_n} - \frac{1}{r_e}\right) \rho'_e(r_e)\rho'_n(r_n)r_e^2 \, dr_e \, r_n^2 \, dr_n + W_0 \tag{21}$$

where

$$W_0 = -e^2 \left[\int \rho_n(r_n) d\tau_n\right]\left[\int \frac{\rho_e(r_e)}{r_e} \, d\tau_e\right]$$

$$= -Ze^2 \int \frac{\rho_e(r_e)}{r_e} d\tau_e \tag{22}$$

which is just the Coulomb energy for a point nucleus. Now since the value of the integral over r_e in Eq. (21) is of interest only in the nuclear region, $\rho'_e(r_e)$ is replaced by a constant:

$$\rho'_e(r_e) \rightarrow \rho'_e(0) = |\Psi(0)|^2 \tag{23}$$

and defining

$$\delta = (W_e)_{\ell=0} - W_0 , \tag{24}$$

the shift then becomes

$$\delta = \frac{2}{3}\pi e^2 Z |\Psi(0)|^2 \langle r_n^2 \rangle \tag{25}$$

where

$$Z\langle r_n^2 \rangle = \int r_n^2 \rho_n(r_n) d\tau_n$$

$$= 4\pi \int\limits_0^{\infty} r_n^4 \rho'_n(r_n) \, dr_n . \tag{26}$$

The two principal factors in the energy difference δ are the solid state factor, i.e., the electronic charge density at the nucleus, and the nuclear factor, i.e., the mean square nuclear radius.

The derivation up to this point applies equally well to the gamma resonance isomer shift and the optical isotope shift*. In the optical case, the shift of an optical line is observed, that is to say the *difference* in δ for two electronic levels is observed:

$$\delta_b - \delta_a = C <r_n^2 > \left[|\Psi_b(0)|^2 - |\Psi_a(0)|^2 \right]$$

$$C = \frac{2\pi}{3} Ze^2 \qquad\qquad (27)$$

where a and b refer to the two different electronic levels. Since the optical transition energy for a point nucleus is not usually known, a comparison can only be made between two different isotopes of the same element - hence the name "isotope shift." So, one measures the frequency of a given optical transition in two different isotopes. The difference in energy of these two transitions is then

$$\Delta = C \left[<r_n^2>_1 - <r_n^2>_2 \right] \left[|\Psi_b(0)|^2 - |\Psi_a(0)|^2 \right] \qquad (28)$$

where the 1 and 2 refer to the two isotopes.

In the gamma resonance case the situation is similar, but the quantities have different meanings; the shift of the absorption line is just the difference of the shifts of the nuclear ground state, δ_g, and the nuclear excited state, δ_e,

$$\delta_e - \delta_g = C|\Psi(0)|^2 \left[<r_n^2>_e - <r_n^2>_g \right] . \qquad (29)$$

The expression for the source is similar. If both source and absorber lines are shifted the same amount, no shift of the absorption spectrum will be observed in an experiment. Consequently it is the difference between source and absorber which is measured;

$$\Delta = C \left[<r_n^2>_e - <r_n^2>_g \right] \left[|\Psi_a(0)|^2 - |\Psi_s(0)|^2 \right] \qquad (30)$$

where s and a refer to source and absorber. As can be seen the expression here is essentially the same as for the isotope shift. From the above equation it can be seen that there are two conditions for the observation of an isomer shift:

*See Chap. 5 by A. Steudel.

i) The chemical makeup in the source and absorber must be different. For example two different valence states may be used so that the electron density at the nucleus is different in source and absorber.

ii) The mean square radius of the nuclear ground state must be different from that of the nuclear excited state.

A little should be said concerning the nuclear mean square radius, since there is some confusion on this point in the literature. If one assumes a particular nuclear model, for example constant charge density inside a sphere of radius R and zero outside, then one obtains

$$\rho'_n(r_n) = \frac{3Z}{4\pi R^3} \quad , \quad r_n < R \tag{31}$$

$$<r_n^2> = \frac{4\pi}{Z} \int_0^R r_n^4 \, \frac{3Z}{4\pi R^3} \, dr_n \tag{32}$$

$$<r_n^2> = 3/5 \; R^2 \tag{33}$$

and Eq. (30) becomes

$$\Delta = \frac{2\pi}{5} \; Ze^2 \left[|\Psi_a(0)|^2 - |\Psi_s(0)|^2 \right] (R_e^2 - R_g^2)$$

or

$$\Delta = \frac{4\pi}{5} \; Ze^2 \left[|\Psi_a(0)|^2 - |\Psi_s(0)|^2 \right] R^2 \; \frac{\delta R}{R} \tag{34}$$

where $R = (R_1 + R_2)/2$. The main difference between these expressions is the numerical factors. It should also be pointed out that for a distorted (ellipsoidal) nucleus the value of $<r_n^2>$ will be different than for a spherical nucleus with the same charge density.

In order to account for two of the assumptions that were made in the beginning, it is necessary to multiply the expressions above by a correction factor $S'(Z)$. This corrects for relativistic effects and for the fact that a finite nucleus modifies the electronic wave functions in the vicinity of the nucleus. These correction factors are given as a function of Z by Shirley (1964).

Gamma resonance can only measure the product of the nuclear and the electronic properties. There is no experimental technique at present which can measure either property individually. Consequently one of the factors must be calculated theoretically if the other factor is to be determined. From nuclear wavefunctions the difference of the mean square radii can be calculated, but these calculations are not very reliable. One advantage, however, is that for a given isotope there is only one nuclear factor, while the electronic factor can be changed by using different chemical compounds. Once the nuclear factor has been determined, a large number of compounds may be studied. This problem of determining the nuclear radius difference is referred to as the isomer shift calibration problem. That is, one must calibrate the velocity scale of the isomer shift in terms of the electron densities, and this is a serious problem.

From a naive point of view one would expect that the outer electrons would be most affected by changes in chemical surroundings and consequently that the changes in the outer s electron densities would contribute most to the isomer shift. Consequently the isomer shift should provide important information concerning the nature of the chemical bond.

It should be emphasized again that the isomer shift measures the total charge density at the nucleus, that is, the *sum* of the spin up and the spin down electrons, while the Fermi contact term in e. g. , the Knight shift, measures the spin density, the *difference* between spin up and spin down electrons.

B.   Measurements in Iron Compounds

Table II shows an older collection of data (Walker, et al. , 1961). (There have been many more measurements since then.) Divalent iron has the configuration $3d^6$ and trivalent iron has the configuration $3d^5$. As can be seen, the divalent compounds and the trivalent compounds form two separate groups, so that there seems to be a more or less unique shift associated with trivalent iron compounds and with divalent iron compounds. This might appear strange at first since no s electrons are removed in going from divalent to trivalent iron. However, this is explained by shielding effects. When a 3d electron is removed, the shielding of the nuclear potential is reduced so that the s electrons move inward, particularly the 3s electrons. Consequently, when a 3d electron is removed the net charge density at the nucleus increases. Using calculated values of the s electron density (Watson, 1959) the change in the nuclear radius can be derived from the difference in the isomer shifts. It is found that $\delta R/R = -1.8 \times 10^{-3}$, with the nuclear ground state radius *larger* than the excited state radius. This change is rather a large one, considering that the change in radius caused by adding one particle is not much larger: $\delta R/R = 1/3 \ \delta A/A = 5.9 \times 10^{-3}$. It should be mentioned that the isomer shifts are measured relative to stainless steel; the zero point of the isomer shifts is more or less arbitrary.

Table II: Isomer shifts in iron (Walker et al. , 1961).

		Shift (cm/sec)
$3d^6$	FeF_2 (single crystal)	0.140 ± 5
$3d^6$	$KFeF_3$	0.139 ± 5
$3d^6$	$FeSO_4 \cdot 7H_2O$	0.140 ± 5
$3d^6$	$FeCl_2 \cdot 4H_2O$	0.130 ± 5
$3d^6$	FeS	$\sim 0.11 \pm 1$
$3d^5$	$Fe_2(SO_4)_3 \cdot 6H_2O$	0.052 ± 5
$3d^5$	Fe_2O_3	0.047 ± 5
$3d^5$	Yttrium-iron garnet, octahedral	0.057 ± 5
$3d^5$	Yttrium-iron garnet, tetrahedral	0.026 ± 5
	FeS_2 (pyrites)	0.048 ± 5
	FeS_2 (marcasite)	0.048 ± 5
Metals	Fe	0.015 ± 5
	Co	0.012 ± 5
	Ni	0.015 ± 5
	Mn	-0.008 ± 2
	Cr	-0.005 ± 2
	Mo	-0.001 ± 2
Cyanides	$K_4Fe(CN)_6 \cdot 3H_2O$	0.0083 ± 10
	$K_3Fe(CN)_6$	0.0000 ± 10

Figure 19 (Walker et al., 1961) shows a plot of isomer shifts for different electronic configurations. The isomer shift was calibrated in terms of s-electron density by assuming that the difference of the isomer shifts of the most divalent and trivalent compounds correspond to the difference in Watson's (1959) calculated values of electron densities. In order to explain the isomer shifts of the other compounds, one assumes a certain amount of covalency. This covalency has the effect of adding part of a 4s electron. The

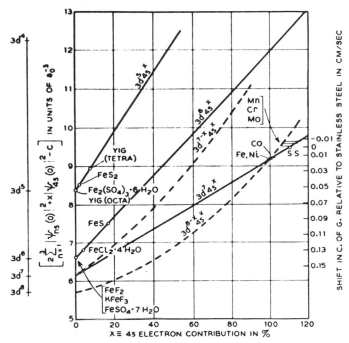

Fig. 19:   A possible interpretation of the Fe^{57} isomer shifts in various solids. The total s-electron density is plotted as a function of the percentage of 4s character for various d-electron configurations. (Walker, et al., 1961).

effects of the additional 4s electron were calculated using the Fermi-Segré-Goudsmit formula, the results of which are shown by the solid lines. The slope of the lines is different because the greater number of electrons in the $3d^7$ configuration, for instance, provide a greater shielding of the 4s electrons from the nuclear attraction. One particular point should be noted: The isomer shifts for the two different lattice sites in YIG (Yttrium Iron Garnet) are different, indicating that the two sites have different degrees of covalency. Finally, in metals, the 3d electrons are partly converted into conduction electrons, where they appear primarily as s-electrons. The dashed lines represent this situation. For Fe in Fe metal, there are eight electrons to be accounted for, so that the isomer shift points strongly to a $3d^7 4s$ configuration. From this illustration it can be seen what sort of detailed information may be extracted from isomer shifts.

C. Measurements in the Alkali Iodides

An interesting series of measurements have been made in alkali iodides (Hafemeister, et al., 1964). These have been chosen because they illustrate some of the complexities in the interpretation of isomer shifts. The 26.8 keV, M1 transition in I^{129} is used. The ground state spin is 1/2; the excited state spin is 5/2. The electronic configuration of neutral iodine is $5s^2 5p^5$. In the alkali iodides one would expect this to become $5s^2 5p^6$ (a xenon core) as a first approximation. In fact, what happens is that the configuration appears to be $5s^2 5p^y$ with $5.8 < y < 6.0$, as will be seen. If the iodide had a perfect xenon core, then the isomer shift in all the alkali iodides from LiI to CsI would be identical. As can be seen in Fig. 20, this is not the case. In fact, in the series from Li to Cs the isomer shift goes through a maximum. This means that the perfect xenon core is not there; instead there are some holes in the p shell. As in the iron case, an increase in p electrons increases the shielding and results in a decrease in the charge density at the nucleus. The p-hole interpretation seems to be quite successful. Since the number of p-holes is small, 0.0-0.2, one expects that the isomer shift will bear a linear relationship to the number of holes. Data concerning the number of holes can be obtained from the chemical shift in NMR and from quadrupole resonance. The Fermi-Segré formula can then be used to calculate the electron density at the nucleus. In this way the isomer shift scale can be calibrated.

The concept of electronegativity is often used in the interpretation of isomer shifts, but as

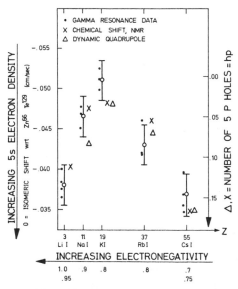

Fig. 20: The isomeric shifts and the number of p-holes versus alkali atomic number for the alkali iodides. The data points for each alkali are spread horizontally for the sake of clarity. (deWaard, et al., 1964; Bloembergen and Sookin, 1958; Menes and Bolef, 1961).

will be seen this can sometimes be dangerous. The electronegativity is defined as

$$X = 0.18 (i + e) \tag{35}$$

where i is the ionization energy of the atom, and e is the electron affinity, both measured in electron volts. Both of these quantities can be taken from tables. Since Cs is less electronegative than Li, the Cs should have a smaller tendency to pull electrons towards itself than Li. Consequently CsI should have the smallest number of p-holes in the iodide series. This picture seems to hold for Li, Na, and K, but breaks down for Rb and Cs. The reason for the breakdown is due to the polarizability of the alkali ions, which increases by a factor of a hundred or so from Li to Cs. The electronegativity model does not take this into account. The effect of the polarizability is to distort the iodide ion. This essentially transfers 5p electrons into higher orbitals, creating a larger p hole and reducing the shielding. This effect more than counteracts the decreased electronegativity of Cs. The main point of this illustration is that one has to be extremely careful about using such concepts as electronegativity in interpreting isomer shifts. It is really necessary to consider all possible effects which may be important. For example, if only KI, RbI and CsI had been measured, then using the electronegativity interpretation, the wrong *sign* of δR/R would have been obtained.

D. Measurements in Tin Compounds

This is an area in which considerable confusion still exists. The nuclear transition used is the 24 keV transition in Sn^{119}. The neutral atom has the configuration $4d^{10}5s^25p^2$. Divalent tin, if it exists, has a configuration $4d^{10}5s^2$, tetravalent tin has the configuration $4d^{10}$. Covalent compounds such as alpha tin (gray tin) have hybridized orbitals $4d^{10}5SP^3$ which share in the four bonds. Each of these hybridized orbitals is usually assumed to contribute one quarter of a 5s electron, so that the net density is that of one 5s electron. This provides three sets of materials in which measurements can be made: Tetravalent tin with no 5s electron, covalent tin with effectively one 5s electron, and divalent tin with two 5s electrons. One can then use the Fermi-Segré formula to calculate the difference in 5s electron densities for these ions assuming that the inner s electrons remain unchanged. Doing this in a naive way, one concludes from the experimental data that δR/R > 0.

Figure 21 shows an older compilation by Gol'danskii (1964) of data on Sn^{4+}. Also plotted is the ionicity of the bond (found by other means). The degree of ionicity is the degree to which the electrons are pulled away from the tin. This means in the case of

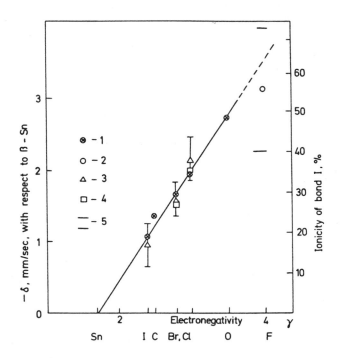

Fig. 21: Chemical shifts in SnX_4 compounds as a function of the electronegativity of X and the degree of ionicity (Gol'danskii, 1964).

the fluoride that the electrons remain about 40 percent covalent, so that roughly 40 percent of a 5s electron is present from the $5SP^3$ configuration. (A purely ionic compound would have no 5s electron.) Going left from the fluoride to the iodide the ionicity decreases, so that one expects the s electron density at the tin to increase. As can be seen, the isomer shift also increases (the *negative* isomer shift is plotted) leading to the conclusion that $\delta R/R > 0$.

The experimental situation in divalent tin is more confused than for tetravalent tin. Different laboratories find different isomer shifts for the same compound, sometimes even differing in the sign of the isomer shift. The reason is probably that the chemical compounds are difficult to produce. Figure 22 shows a set of data collected by Lees and Flinn (1965) on divalent tin compounds. The idea behind the plot is the following: If there is a mixture of covalent and ionic bonding, the covalent bonds provide a certain

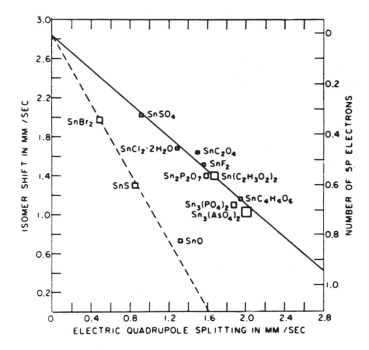

Fig. 22:   The relation between isomer shift and quadrupole splitting for stannous compounds. (Lees and Flinn, 1965).

amount of p electrons. The p electrons give rise to a quadrupole interaction, the strength of which should be a measure of the amount of covalent bonding. As can be seen, the data lie along two different lines, which are associated with two types of covalent bonds, one with p_z character, the other with a p_x, p_y character. By extrapolating these lines to zero quadrupole splitting, one obtains the isomer shift for a purely ionic bond.

From these sets of data it can be seen that the isomer shift increases with the number of 5s electrons. At first glance, one would conclude that $\delta R/R > 0$ since one assumes that increasing the number of 5s electrons leads to an increase of the electron density at the nucleus. However, this is not necessarily the case. As 5s electrons are taken away, the shielding of the inner electrons changes, the ion as a whole contracts, leading to an increase in the density of inner electrons that may more than compensate for the loss of the 5s electrons. For this reason it is possible that $\delta R/R < 0$. One set of calculations by Flinn and Lees, using free ion wavefunctions supports the first view that adding 5s electrons increases the electron density at the nucleus. Another set of calculations by Bersuker, et al., (1966) using molecular orbital theory combined with the Fermi Segré formula come to the opposite conclusion. Consequently the present state is quite confused.*

E. Measurements in Rare Earth Compounds

Here there is not very much experimental data. The main reason is that the divalent compounds are generally difficult to prepare. Fairly large isomer shifts have been observed in divalent and trivalent europium compounds and europium metal. The interpretation of these data was done by relying heavily on isotope shift data. There is also data on isomer shifts between trivalent dysprosium compounds and dysprosium metal. These are the only data which presently exist. Many laboratories are presently working on further experiments.

F. Measurements Under High Pressure

In addition to varying the chemical surroundings, one may hope to change the electron density by applying a large hydrostatic pressure. Several experiments of this type have been performed. In addition to pressure-induced isomer shifts, pressure induced changes in hyperfine interactions may also be observed. However, the latter can generally be observed with greater sensitivity by other techniques such as NMR. Most pressure experiments have been performed in Fe^{57} compounds for a very simple reason: in addition to the difficulty of producing high pressures in the first place, it is even more difficult to produce high pressures at anything but room temperatures. Consequently a low energy nuclear transition such as that in Fe^{57} is most convenient. In addition to an isomer shift, the pressure may induce a second order Doppler shift due to increased lattice kinetic energies. However, this effect is usually a small correction. In most experiments the results were relatively trivial. The s-electron density increases in inverse proportion to the volume change of the solid.

*Ed. Note: A very recent measurement of the chemical effect on the outer shell internal conversion of the 23.9-keV MI transition in Sn^{119} by J.P. Bocquet, Y.Y. Chu, O.C. Kistner, M.L. Perlman, and G.T. Emery (1966). Phys. Rev. Letters 17, 809, shows that the s-electron density at the nucleus is higher in white Sn than in SnO_2. From the magnitude of the effect and from the sign and magnitude of the isomer shift in Sn metal relative to SnO_2, they conclude that $\Delta R/R = +3.3 \times 10^{-4}$, i.e., the excited state is larger than the ground state.

Experiments have also been performed in beta tin (white tin). The isomer shift was found to decrease with increasing pressure. The interpretation of these results, however, have the same problem as with other tin measurements. If one assumes that the increasing pressure forces the outer 5s electron inward, one still does not know what the effects on the inner electrons will be, whether the net electron density at the nucleus increases or decreases. This is just the same question that arises in the other measurements on tin. *

VI. Hyperfine Interactions

A. Measurements in Paramagnetic States

The interaction of the electrons with the Crystalline Electrical Field (CEF) is large compared to the interaction with the nuclear spin. Therefore the electronic and nuclear spins may be regarded as precessing independently around a common axis of quantization with the electronic precession rates large compared to nuclear precession rates. Thus the nucleus may be considered as being exposed to fields which undergo fluctuations due to the fluctuating electronic spins. The effective fields seen by the nucleus are then time averages of the instantaneous fields produced by the electrons. These time averages are taken over times of the order of the nuclear precession time. Three regions will be discussed: electronic relaxation (i.e., fluctuation) rates that are fast, slow, or comparable with the nuclear precession rate. **

1. Fast Electronic Relaxation

When the fluctuations are fast, the hyperfine magnetic field averages to zero in the absence of an external magnetic field. This occurs because the electronic spin is "up" as often as "down," and the fluctuation between these states is very rapid due to the interactions with the surrounding ions. Consequently no magnetic hyperfine interaction will be observed in paramagnetic crystals with fast relaxation. This leaves only the electric field gradient, the average of which is not zero.

In the free ion, the spin-orbit interaction couples the electronic spin and orbital angular momenta together to produce sets

*See Ed. Note on page 528.
**See Chap. S.6 by A.J. Dekker for a detailed discussion of
relaxation effects on Y-resonance spectra of Fe⁵⁷.

of degenerate "J multiplets" for which J, the total angular momentum, is a good quantum number. When ions with partially filled 3d shells are put into crystals this coupling is often broken by the CEF interaction with the orbital angular momentum. In rare earths the CEF interaction is not very strong so that the J-multiplets are each split into a series of levels for which J is still a good quantum number in most cases. A simple reason for this difference is that in the iron transition series the 3d electrons are the outermost electrons and are directly exposed to the surrounding ions while in the rare earths, the 4f electrons are shielded by the surrounding $5s^2 5p^6$ closed shell. In the rare earths, the overall CEF splitting of a J-multiplet is typically about 300°K (see Fig. 23).

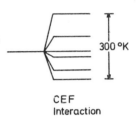

CEF
Interaction

Fig. 23: Typical splitting of a 4f J-multiplet in a crystalline electric field.

The CEF interaction does not necessarily remove the degeneracy of the electronic levels completely. Two essentially different cases must be considered: 1) where there are an odd number of electrons, and 2) where there are an even number of electrons. In the first case all the levels will have at least a two-fold Kramer's degeneracy. This can be most easily seen in the case of a single s state electron where an electrical interaction can never remove the degeneracy between the spin-up and the spin-down states. Since the Hamiltonian is invariant under time reversal, and since time-reversal of the spin-up state produces the spin-down state, both states must be solutions of the Hamiltonian for the same energy eigenvalue, i.e., they must be degenerate. This argument does not apply to ions with an even number of electrons since the spins can be paired off so that each state is the time reversal of itself. This means that for crystals of very low symmetry, ions with an odd number of electrons will have all levels doubly degenerate, while ions with an even number of electrons will have all levels non-degenerate. For crystals of higher symmetry the degree of degeneracy increases. Non-degenerate levels in the absence of an external magnetic field have no magnetic dipole moment, i.e., $< \upsilon / \mu / \upsilon > = 0$. Again this is due to time reversal symmetry: the non-degenerate states are unchanged by time reversal, and applying time reversal to $< \mu >$ produces $- < \mu >$, which must equal $+ < \mu >$.

a. Electric Quadrupole Hyperfine Interaction in Thulium Salts. Thulium-169, which is the only stable isotope of thulium, has an 8.4 keV gamma transition which is excellent for gamma resonance. The excited nuclear state has spin I = 3/2, the

ground state, $I_0 = 1/2$.   The lowest lying J-multiplet of the Tm^{3+}
ion has $J = 6$, so that there are at most 13 electronic levels, which
typically span about 300°K.   Each electronic level produces a different electric field gradient at the nucleus, however the relaxation
time between the electronic levels is generally fast so that only the
thermal average of the electric field gradients is observed. As
the temperature is raised from helium temperature to room temperature or above, the populations of the levels change considerably, so that the effective field gradient at the nucleus will vary
with the temperature. The CEF levels of Tm_2O_3 and thulium
ethyl sulfate (TmES) are shown in Fig. 24, as obtained from optical spectroscopy measurements. The Tm_2O_3 has a rather low
symmetry (C_2) so that all the levels are non-degenerate. The
TmES has a higher symmetry (C_{3h}) so that some of the levels are
two-fold degenerate. The electric field gradient splits the nuclear
excited state $I = 3/2$ into two levels but does not split the ground
state ($I_0 = 1/2$).   Consequently two spectrum lines are observed.

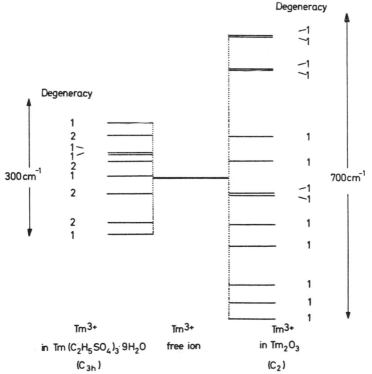

Fig. 24:   Crystalline electrical fields of thulium ethyl sulfate and
thulium oxide (Barnes, et al., 1964).

The quadrupole splitting is shown in Fig. 25 for TmES at several temperatures (Barnes et al., 1964). As can be seen, the quadrupole splitting decreases as the temperature increases so that at room temperature the splitting has virtually vanished. This can be explained by a fairly simple picture. At higher temperatures all the electronic levels of the lowest J-multiplet are roughly equally populated. In such a case, the average charge density is roughly spherical — like a closed shell— and the quadrupole interaction vanishes on the average.

However, this is not the general trend, as can be seen in Fig. 26. For Tm_2O_3 the low temperature behavior is similar to TmES. At higher temperatures the splitting reaches a minimum, then turns back up and reaches a saturation

Fig. 25: Quadrupole splitting of the 8.4 keV level of Tm^{169} in an absorber of thulium ethyl sulfate at various temperatures (Barnes et al., 1964).

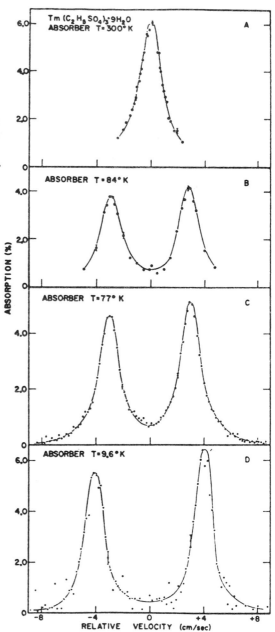

value. The reason for this is that there are several contribu-tions to the electric field grad-ient. Each component of the field gradient tensor is given by

$$q_{ij} = <q_{ij}^{4f}>_T (1-R_Q)$$

$$+ q_{ij}^{(Lat)} (1-\gamma_\infty) \qquad (36)$$

whereby four contributions may be distinguished.* The first, the direct contribution from the 4f electrons, has already been mentioned. The 4f electrons also introduce a distortion in the closed electron shells, which in effect produces a shielding of the direct 4f field gradient. This "atomic" Sternheimer effect is accoun-ted for by the factor R_Q.

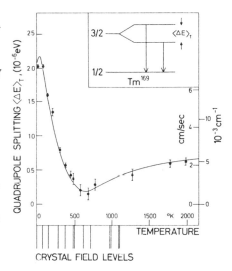

Fig. 26: Temperature dependence of the nuclear quadrupole inter-action of Tm^{169} in $Tm_2 O_3$ (Barnes, et al., 1964).

This is roughly a ten percent effect.

In addition to these two temperature dependent contributions, there are also two contributions which are more or less tempera-ture independent. The surrounding ions produce a field gradient which acts on the nucleus. This field gradient is also shielded (or in this case, antishielded) by the closed shell electrons. This "lattice" Sternheimer effect is accounted for by the factor γ_∞. The direct contribution from the lattice is quite small, but γ_∞ is quite large. For Tm, $\gamma_\infty = -74$ (Sternheimer, 1963). The sources of these contributions are illustrated graphically in Fig. 27.

From these contributions the behavior of the quadrupole splitting in the oxide can be explained. At low temperatures the behavior is predominantly due to the 4f electrons. The minimum around 600°K arises because the 4f contribution and the lattice contribution have different signs. At higher temperatures the 4f contribution dies out and the "saturation" value is due to the lat-tice contribution. One other feature of Fig. 26 should be noted: measurements were made up to nearly 2000°K. This was possible

*See Chap. 2 by R.E. Watson and A.J. Freeman.

because of the low energy of the gamma transition. The recoil free fraction is not greatly reduced at these temperatures.

b. Magnetic Interactions in Thulium. As was discussed previously, fast relaxation wipes out magnetic interactions in the absence of external fields. However, when an external magnetic field is applied, magnetic interactions can be observed, as shown in Fig. 28 (Snively, 1965). The angular portions of the electronic wave functions

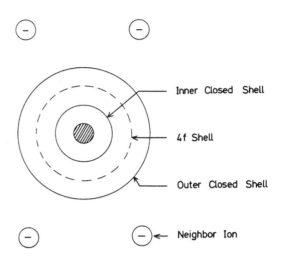

Inner Closed Shell

4f Shell

Outer Closed Shell

Neighbor Ion

Fig. 27: Arrangement of the various electron shells in a rare earth ion, illustrating the sources and the shielding of the electric field gradient.

for TmES are shown in Table III, as calculated from crystal field theory (Barnes et al., 1964). The measurements were done at $6.5°K$ so that only the electronic ground state was appreciably occupied. This state is a singlet and consequently has no magnetic moment. Applying a magnetic field changes this by mixing in the excited states. The matrix elements are such that a field parallel to the crystal symmetry axis has virtually no effect, while a perpendicular field has a large effect. The reason for this is simple: For the parallel field the magnetic interaction is $g_J\beta H_z J_z$. The excited states that can be mixed into the ground state by this perturbation are merely the singlets at 215 and 221 cm^{-1}. On the other hand, for the perpendicular field the interaction is $1/2\ g_J\beta H_x (J_+ + J_-)$, which can mix the doublet at 31 cm^{-1} into the ground state. Due to both the energy denominators and the size of the matrix elements, the perpendicular field produces a much larger effect. For the parallel field, the spectrum (top of Fig. 28) shows only the quadrupole interaction. The difference in intensity of the two peaks is due to the use of a single crystal absorber. This will be treated in more detail later. Applying a magnetic field perpendicular to the symmetry axis strongly mixes in the excited states. The external magnetic field is then strongly enhanced (by a factor of ≈ 75 for TmES) by the 4f electrons.

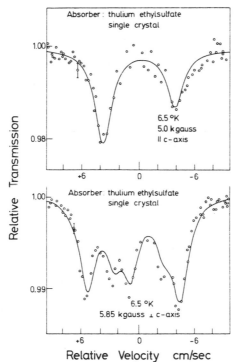

Fig. 28: Absorption spectra of Tm^{169} in thulium ethyl sulfate at 6.5°K with magnetic fields parallel and perpendicular to the c axis (symmetry axis) of the crystal. The gamma-ray direction was perpendicular to the c axis and to the magnetic field (Snively, 1965).

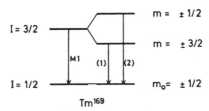

Fig. 29: Nuclear levels and gamma transitions of Tm^{169} in the presence of an electric quadrupole interaction.

Table III: Wavefunctions of the $^3H_6$ term of thulium ethyl sulfate
(Barnes, et al. , 1964)

Energy (cm^{-1})	Degeneracy	Wavefunction
300. 1	1	$-0.707\|-3>+0.707\|+3>$
273. 6	2	$-0.446\|-2>+0.895\|+4>$
		$0.895\|-4>-0.446\|+2>$
221. 1	1	$0.697\|-6>-0.168\| 0>$
		$+0.697\|+6>$
214. 8	1	$-0.707\|-6>+0.707\|+6>$
198. 1	2	$-0.305\|-1>+0.953\|+5>$
		$-0.953\|-5>+0.305\|+1>$
157. 1	1	$0.707\|-3>+0.707\|+3>$
110. 0	2	$0.895\|-2>+0.446\|+4>$
		$0.446\|-4>+0.895\|+2>$
31. 3	2	$0.305\|-5>+0.953\|+1>$
		$0.953\|-1>+0.305\|+5>$
0	1	$0.119\|-6>+0.986\| 0>$
		$+0.119\|+6>$

*The wavefunctions are written in the form $\sum_m a_m |m_J>$ where
$|m_J>$ is an abbreviation of $|LSJ\ m_J>$ with $L = 5$, $S = 1$,
and $J = 6$ in Russel-Saunders coupling.*

The bottom spectrum in Fig. 28 shows the combined quadrupole
and magnetic interactions. The only undetermined parameter is
$\langle r^{-3}\rangle_M$ (M for Magnetic) so that this experiment can serve as a
measure of this quantity. This experiment has not yet been completed.

c. Intensities of Spectrum Lines. A simple example is
given here showing how information may be obtained from the
relative intensities of spectrum lines. The case of an axially
symmetric quadrupole interaction in Tm^{169} will be used (Fig. 29).
The relative transition probabilities for the M1 transitions may be
written as

$$P_{m, m_0} = (C_{m, m_0})^2\ F_1^M (\theta) \tag{37}$$

where

$$F_1^0(\theta) = \sin^2\theta \; , \tag{38}$$
$$F_1^{\pm 1}(\theta) = 1/2(1+\cos^2\theta) \; ,$$

$$M = \Delta m = m - m_0 \; , \tag{39}$$

C_{m,m_0} is a Clebsch-Gordan coefficient, and θ is the angle between the gamma ray and the symmetry axis. Aside from common inconvenient numerical factors, the Clebsch-Gordan coefficients are given in Table IV. For line (1) in Fig. 29 there are two possible transitions: $-3/2 \rightarrow -1/2$ and $+3/2 \rightarrow +1/2$. The transitions $-3/2 \rightarrow +1/2$ and $+3/2 \rightarrow -1/2$ are forbidden since they would require $\Delta m = 2$. Consequently the intensity of line (1) is given by

$$P_{(1)}(\theta) = (3 + 3) \, F_1^1(\theta) = 3 + 3\cos^2\theta \; . \tag{40}$$

For line (2) there are four transitions possible: $-1/2 \rightarrow -1/2$, $+1/2 \rightarrow +1/2$, $-1/2 \rightarrow +1/2$, and $+1/2 \rightarrow -1/2$. Consequently the intensity is given by

$$P_{(2)}(\theta) = (2 + 2) \, F_1^0(\theta) + (1 + 1) \, F_1^1(\theta)$$

$$= 5 - 3\cos^2\theta \; . \tag{41}$$

Table V shows the relative intensities for several special cases.

Table IV: $(C_{m,m_0})^2$

m_0 \ m	-3/2	-1/2	1/2	3/2
-1/2	3	2	1	0
1/2	0	1	2	3

Table V: Relative intensities for special cases.

Sample	θ	Relative Intensities		
		Line 1	Line 2	Ratio
Polycrystalline	-	4	4	1:1
Single Crystal	0	6	2	3:1
	90°	3	5	3:5

Spectra of a polycrystalline absorber are shown in Fig. 25; as can be seen, the two lines are of about equal intensity. A single crystal with $\theta = 90°$ can be seen in the first spectrum of Fig. 28.

In this case the intensities are in the ratio of about 3:5. This illustrates an important use of single crystals. In the polycrystalline case it cannot be determined whether the m = ± 3/2 level lies above or below the m = ± 1/2 level. In the single crystal spectrum, the smaller line is clearly the m = ± 3/2 line so that the sign of the quadrupole coupling constant can be determined. In transitions for which I is larger, there will be more lines which have different intensities, even for polycrystalline samples, so that for these cases it may not be necessary to use a single crystal.

If there is a magnetic field instead of a quadrupole field, the degeneracy of the nuclear states is completely removed, and six spectrum lines are observed. By observing the gamma rays parallel to the magnetic field (θ = 0), the Δm = 0 transitions (+1/2 → +1/2, -1/2 → -1/2) vanish and only four lines will be observed. This can be done either in a single crystal or by applying a magnetic field to a ferromagnetic material and lining up the domains. This can be useful in interpreting complex, partially resolved spectra. By removing some of the lines, the resolution of the spectrum may improve. The cases treated here have been quite simple; Abragam (1964) gives an excellent treatment of the more general case.

2. Slow Electronic Relaxation

When the electronic relaxation rates are slow compared with the nuclear frequencies, the hyperfine interactions of the individual electronic states are observed. This condition is fulfilled in $ErCl_3 \cdot 6H_2O$, $YbCl_3 \cdot 6H_2O$, and Dy_2O_3. In each of these paramagnetic salts a magnetic hyperfine interaction is observed, although in some cases it is only partially resolved. The slow relaxation rate in these salts is due to a highly anisotropic electronic g factor which causes the spin-spin relaxation to be very slow. The spin lattice relaxation is slowed down by cooling to low temperatures. Aside from the very interesting features concerning the relaxation rates, these experiments show ordinary magnetic hyperfine interactions, which will be dealt with in more detail later.

3. Intermediate Relaxation Rates

The most complicated of the three cases is the one where the electronic relaxation rates are within an order of magnitude of the nuclear frequencies. Such a case is shown in Fig. 30 (Clauser, 1966).

If the relaxation rates were fast, as in the case of TmES, two identical peaks would be observed at approximately ± 7 cm/sec.

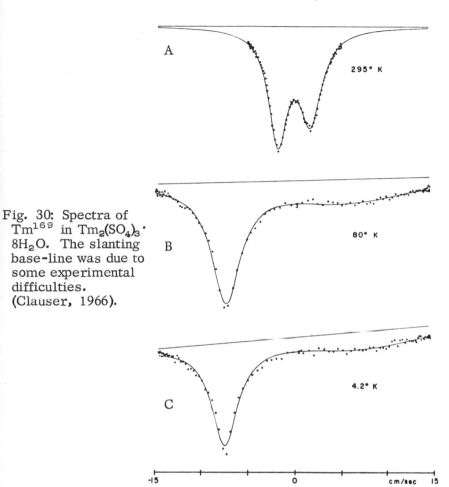

Fig. 30: Spectra of Tm^{169} in Tm$_2$(SO$_4$)$_3$· 8H$_2$O. The slanting base-line was due to some experimental difficulties. (Clauser, 1966).

Obviously this is not the case. To understand such spectra, two things must be explained; the effect of a second order magnetic hyperfine interaction, or "psuedo-quadrupole" interaction, and the effect of the electronic relaxation.

This type of spectrum has been observed in both TmCl$_3$· 6H$_2$O and Tm$_2$(SO$_4$)$_3$· 8H$_2$O. In both of these salts the ground state and first excited state lie unusually close to each other; they are separated by only about 1 cm^{-1}. Neither of these states is degenerate, so they have no magnetic moments. Nevertheless the magnetic hyperfine interaction is important since the second order term is appreciable. Writing the hyperfine interaction as A**I·J**,

a) Nuclear level scheme

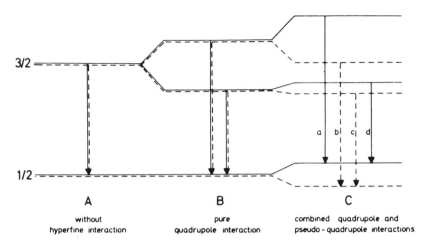

b) Line pattern

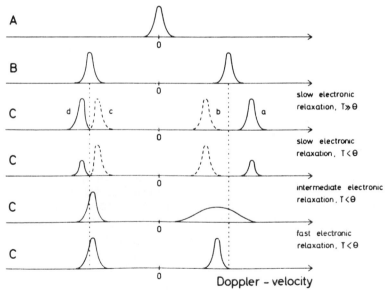

Fig. 31: Nuclear levels, gamma transitions, and hypothetical gamma spectra of Tm^{169} in the presence of the pseudo-quadrupole interaction.

one may use second order perturbation theory to find the energy levels:

$$E_{mag} = <g|A\mathbf{I} \cdot \mathbf{J}|g> - \frac{|<g|A\mathbf{I} \cdot \mathbf{J}|e>|^2}{E_e - E_g} + \ldots \qquad (42)$$

for the electronic ground state. Here e and g refer to the electronic excited and ground states, respectively. The first term, as has been said, is zero. The second term is not zero, and for the two salts mentioned above, it is appreciable. This term is called the "pseudo-quadrupole" term* because it is proportional to the square of the nuclear magnetic quantum number, m_I.

The effect of the pseudo-quadrupole interaction on the gamma resonance spectra can be explained with the help of Fig. 31. The true quadrupole interaction splits the nuclear excited state into two levels and leaves the nuclear ground state unaffected. The dashed lines refer to the electronic ground state, the solid lines to the electronic excited state. It may be assumed that the two electronic states produce the same quadrupole interaction, as shown. When the pseudo-quadrupole interaction is included, the pairs of levels "repel" each other, the levels associated with the electronic ground state shift down in energy, while the levels associated with the electronic excited state shift up by the same amount. The vertical arrows depict the gamma transitions which produce the spectra in part b of Fig. 31. It should be emphasized that the vertical scale has been considerably distorted; in particular the splitting of the electronic levels, which is not shown, is at least an order of magnitude larger than either of the hyperfine interactions.

The spectra which result from situations A and B in Fig. 31 are the usual one and two line patterns. For situation C, with the pseudo-quadrupole interaction, several cases may be distinguished. At high temperatures and slow relaxation times (an unrealistic case) each of the four transition lines will be observed with equal intensity. θ is the splitting of the electronic levels in thermal units. As the temperature decreases, the populations of the two electronic states change, causing the lines associated with the electronic ground state to increase in intensity, the others to decrease. The intensity change causes the center of gravity to shift from zero velocity to a negative velocity. As the relaxation between the electronic states increases (i.e., between

*See also Chap. 1   by B. Bleaney.

the solid and dashed spectrum lines) the pairs of lines corresponding to the same nuclear states begin to merge into single lines.
The positions of the energy levels are not affected by relaxation,
only the spectrum lines. This means that as the relaxation rate
increases, lines a and b merge, first into a broad line, and then
into a single narrow line of approximately natural line width for
fast relaxation. The position of this resultant line is the weighted
average of the positions of lines a and b. The theory of the line
shape is too complicated to present here; it is essentially the same
as for NMR (Anderson, 1954). The spectrum for intermediate relaxation rates is like the spectrum observed in $Tm_2(SO_4)_3 \cdot 8H_2O$
(Fig. 30).

One feature of the last three spectra in Fig. 31 should be
emphasized: The centers of gravity of all three spectra are the
same. The shift of the center of gravity caused by the pseudo-
quadrupole interaction is determined by the relative populations
of the electronic levels. This in turn is a function of temperature,
but not of the relaxation rate. This can be seen in particular for
$T \ll \theta$ in which case only the electronic ground state is occupied.
Then, only the dashed spectrum lines will be seen, regardless of
relaxation rates.

This pseudo-quadrupole shift has been observed in $TmCl_3 \cdot 6H_2O$
at different temperatures (Clauser et al., 1966). The results are
shown in Fig. 32. The data include some results from Tm diluted
in $YCl_3 \cdot 6H_2O$. The dilution has no measurable effect on the positions of the peaks. The solid lines are plots of E_0 Tanh $(\theta/2T)$ for
different θ; for each value of θ, E_0 was chosen to fit the measured
shifts best. Varying both parameters, the best fit is obtained
with $k\theta = 1.11$ cm^{-1}, $E_0 = 2.09 \times 10^{-3}$ cm^{-1}. In the chloride the
lines were sharper than those shown in Fig. 30 for the sulfate, so
that the positions could be determined relatively accurately.

It can be shown generally that the shift must have the temperature dependence:

$$E_c = E_0 \text{ Tanh } (\theta/2T) \qquad (43)$$

where θ is the (undetermined) electronic level splitting. All the
measurements thus far have been done in the "high temperature"
range $T \geq 1°$ where E_c is given approximately by

$$E_c \approx \frac{E_0 \theta}{2T} \qquad (44)$$

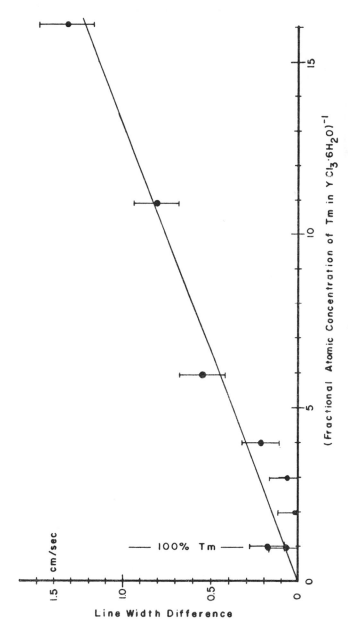

Fig. 33: Line width asymmetry as a function of Tm concentration in $YCl_3 \cdot 6H_2O$. The difference of widths of the two spectrum lines (similar to Fig. 30) is plotted versus the *reciprocal* of the fractional atomic concentration of Tm. All experimental points were measured at 4.2°K (Clauser, 1966).

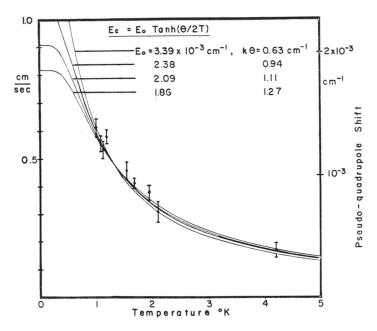

Fig. 32: Pseudo-quadrupole shift for Tm^{169} in $TmCl_3 \cdot 6H_2O$.

in which case E_c is only a function of the product $E_0\theta$, so that neither can be determined individually at present. This situation will be remedied in the near future by making measurements below 1°K.

One might hope to influence the spectrum shape by changing the relaxation time. At low temperatures the predominant mechansim for relaxation is the spin-spin interaction between neighboring paramagnetic ions. By diluting the paramagnetic ions (Tm^{3+}) with a diamagnetic ion (Y^{3+}) the relaxation rate should decrease proportionately. In the transition range from fast to intermediate relaxation rates the widths of the spectral lines are inversely proportional to the relaxation rate, and hence to the concentration. Figure 33 shows just such a dependence for $TmCl_3 \cdot 6H_2O$. Evaluation of these data yields a value of approximately 10^{-11} sec for the relaxation time in undiluted $TmCl_3 \cdot 6H_2O$.

B.   Measurements in Magnetically Ordered States

The total magnetic hyperfine field comes from four contributions:

(i) The "Local" field contribution which consists of the external, demagnetizing, and Lorentz fields. All of these are more or less uniform throughout the sample. They are usually very small, of the order of several kilogauss;

(ii) Electronic orbital contribution which comes from the orbital part of the electronic angular momentum. In iron transition elements it is of the order of 10^4 gauss when the orbital angular momentum is not completely quenched. In rare earths this is the dominant contribution, of the order of $10^6 - 10^7$ gauss. This is due to the fact that the angular momentum is not quenched: J is a good quantum number for the rare earths;

(iii) Electronic spin dipole contribution from surrounding ions. This is relatively small, of the order of 10^4 gauss. In cubic symmetry it drops out entirely;

(iv) Fermi contact contribution which comes from the spin density at the nucleus. This is finite only for s electrons. This contribution is of the order of 10^5 gauss. The Fermi contact contribution can be subdivided into three contributions:

(a) from core s electrons (in closed shells)

(b) from s electrons covalently mixed into "magnetic" electron shells (open shells)

(c) from conduction electrons which have s character.

The magnetic hyperfine portion of the Hamiltonian is then:

$$\mathcal{H} = -g_I \beta_N I \cdot (H_{loc} + H_{el}) \tag{45}$$

with

$$H_{loc} = H_{ext} + \frac{4\pi}{3} M' - DM ,$$

$$H_{el} = -2\beta \left[\frac{\ell}{r^3} + \left(\frac{s}{r^3} - \frac{3r(r \cdot s)}{r^5} \right) + \frac{8\pi}{3} s \delta(r) \right] \tag{46}$$

where g_I is the nuclear g factor, β and β_N are the Bohr and nuclear magnetons, M is the magnetization, M' is the domain magnetization (M' = M in a paramagnet), and D is the demagnetization factor.

Experimentally the contributions to the Fermi contact term cannot be separated out. The theory is very complicated; no derivation from first principles is possible. The experiments have contributed greatly to the understanding of some of the basic mechanisms, particularly in the case of core electron polarization.

The importance of the core electron contribution was realized when the hyperfine field in iron was found to be negative (Hanna, et al., 1960). No other contribution could be found to produce such a large negative contribution. In first order the core s electrons produce no hyperfine field since they are paired. In second order there is an exchange interaction between the s electrons and the unpaired 3d electron spins. This is called a one-electron exchange polarization.* In describing this mechanism, the following sign convention is used: The magnetic hyperfine field is said to be positive when it is parallel to the magnetization, M. In order that positive fields correspond to positive spins, the spins are said to be positive when directed anti-parallel to M, since an electron carries a negative charge.

The exchange interaction between the 3d electrons and the core s electrons causes a repulsion of electrons with anti-parallel spins, which may be understood as follows: The Pauli principle (anti-symmetrization of wave functions) causes the electrons with parallel spins to be farther away from each other on the average than the electrons with antiparallel spin. However, this holds for "non-interacting" electrons. When the Coulomb interaction is switched on, the interaction will be larger for electrons of anti-parallel spin (since they appear to be closer together). This causes a greater repulsion of the anti-parallel spin electrons than of the parallel spin electrons or an effective attraction between parallel spin electrons.* Thus inner shell electrons produce a negative spin density at the nucleus which produces a negative hyperfine field contribution, while the opposite is true of outer shell electrons (see Fig. 34). The net hyperfine field then depends on whether the inner or the outer electrons produce the greater contribution. Table VI shows the hyperfine fields produced by the various s electrons as calculated by Watson and Freeman (1961). As can be seen the 2s electrons are more polarized than the 1s electrons, since the former have a greater overlap with the 3d electrons. On the other hand, the 3s electrons overlap even more, but they are somewhat "confused" since they lie partly inside and partly outside the 3d electrons. The net effect is that the inner electrons predominate, so that a negative hyperfine field results.*

The experiment to determine the sign of the hyperfine field was done by applying an external field to a ferromagnetic iron foil. The external field would then add to or subtract from the electronic

*For a review of these mechanisms and extensive discussions, see Freeman and Watson (1965) and Chap. 2 of this volume.

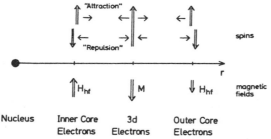

Fig. 34: Spins, magnetic fields, and exchange interactions in an
iron transition ion. The exchange interaction causes an
attraction between the parallel spins.

Table VI: Core electron exchange polarization (Watson and
Freeman, 1961).

Magnetic Field at Nuclei in Kilogauss

	Mn^{++} ($3d^5$)		Fe^{3+} ($3d^5$)	Fe^{2+} ($3d^6$)
1s ↑	2502840			
1s ↓	-2502870	-30	-50	-30
2s ↑	226670			
2s ↓	-228080	-1410	-1790	-1310
3s ↑	31210			
3s ↓	-30470	+740	+1215	+790
Total		-700	-630	-550

hyperfine field, depending on whether the hyperfine field is positive
or negative, respectively. The gamma resonance spectrum was
found to contract upon application of the field, indicating a negative
hyperfine field.

C. Comparison of Methods

In order to obtain good results efficiently in the measurement
of hyperfine interactions, one should be aware of the relative merits
of various experimental methods so that time is not wasted by using an unsuitable method. Of course, one is usually limited to using certain types of equipment in a given laboratory. A brief survey of the relative merits of several experimental techniques will
be given here. The emphasis will be primarily on the gamma

resonance method. It should also be pointed out that many of the methods are complementary rather than competitive.

In contrast to other resonance methods, gamma resonance involves two nuclear states. If the nuclear ground state has zero angular momentum, which is the case for even-even nuclei, conventional resonance methods cannot measure hyperfine interactions. However if there is a low energy excited state, it generally has a finite angular momentum, so that gamma resonance can measure hyperfine interactions in such an isotope. Of course, one can sometimes switch to a different isotope of the same element and use other resonance methods, but there are not always available stable isotopes with a finite nuclear spin. The same remarks apply to nuclear ground states with spin 1/2 with respect to the nuclear quadrupole interaction.

From the measurement of hyperfine magnetic splittings one may obtain the two quantities $\mu_1 H_{eff}$ and $\mu_2 H_{eff}$, where μ_1 and μ_2 are the nuclear ground and excited state magnetic moments respectively, and H_{eff} is the effective magnetic field. From these quantities the ratio of the two nuclear g factors can be obtained. If the ground state nuclear moment is known from other data, the excited state moment and the effective field can then be determined.

One quantity which can be used for a comparison between NMR, EPR and gamma resonance is the linewidth. In gamma resonance, the linewidth is limited by the lifetime of the nuclear excited state. This corresponds to 10^4 - 10^5 gauss, which is quite broad in comparison to NMR linewidths. This has both advantages and disadvantages: it means, of course, that the precision of NMR measurements is much higher; on the other hand, sharp lines are difficult to locate. In this case gamma resonance and NMR may be used in a complementary fashion. Gamma resonance can be used first to locate the lines, then NMR can be used to measure the splittings precisely. When spin-spin interactions between neighboring ions are strong, or the local surroundings are inhomogeneous, the NMR line may be broadened so much that it cannot be observed at all. In contrast, this hardly affects most gamma resonance experiments to the same extent. This is a typical situation in alloys, where it is difficult for NMR to measure hyperfine interactions except in very dilute alloys.

Another problem which both NMR and EPR face in metals is attenuation of the r.f. or microwave signal. This limits the measurements to small particles, whereas gamma resonance can use relatively large single crystals.

To contrast gamma resonance with EPR, it should be mentioned that EPR is generally limited to atoms or ions where the electronic ground state is degenerate. The degeneracy is removed by the application of a magnetic field and transitions are then observed between the resulting levels. It is unusual that electronic levels in the absence of a magnetic field happen to have a splitting which lies within the relatively fixed limits of the microwave frequency range. This is a drawback which does not exist for gamma resonance and NMR.

A few words should be said about one other method, perturbed angular correlation.* As in gamma resonance experiments, the quantities measured are products like μH_{eff}. Angular correlation experiments can be used to help determine nuclear moments, for example by measuring the rotation of the correlation pattern of an ion in a liquid in an external field, where H_{eff} is more readily known. On the other hand, there are corrections to the externally applied field due to polarization of the ion. These corrections must be worked out accurately, as they can be several times larger than the external field. Also, the unperturbed correlation pattern must be known before information can be obtained from the perturbed pattern. This is not always easy to achieve because it is sometimes necessary to work with strongly paramagnetic ions, where the corrections can be large, even in aqueous solution. Furthermore, it is very often difficult to separate the electric quadrupole and the magnetic hyperfine contributions to the perturbations. This is not the case with the gamma resonance method where it is usually very easy to distinguish the two effects. On the other hand, gamma resonance experiments are limited to low energy transitions, which means in most cases that only the first excited nuclear state can be used, providing that it is low enough in energy. There is no such limitation on the angular correlation experiments.

General References

Abragam, A. (1964). "L'Effet Mössbauer, " (Gordon and Breach, New York).

Boyle, A. J. F. and Hall, H. E. (1962). Repts. Progr. Phys. 25, 441.

Frauenfleder, H. (1962). "The Mössbauer Effect, " (Benjamin, New York).

*See S.G. Cohen, Chap. 12.

Muir, A. H. , Jr. , Ando, K. J. , and Coogan, H. M. (1966). "Mössbauer Effect Data Index, " Issue 4, North American Aviation Inc. , Science Center, Thousand Oaks, California.

Wegener, H. (1965). "Der Mössbauer-Effekt und seine Anwendungen in Physik und Chemie, " (Bibliographisches Institut, Mannheim).

Wertheim, G. K. (1964). "Mössbauer Effect: Principles and Applications, " (Academic Press, New York).

References

Anderson, P. W. (1954). J. Phys. Soc. Japan $\underline{9}$, 316.

Barnes, R. G. , Mössbauer, R. L. , Kankeleit, E. , and Poindexter, J. M. (1964). Phys. Rev. $\underline{136}$, A175.

Bersuker, I. B. , Gol'danskii, V. I. , and Makarov, E. F. (1966). Soviet Phys. -JETP $\underline{22}$, 485.

Bloembergen, N. and Sookin, P. P. (1958). Phys. Rev. $\underline{110}$, 865.

Clauser, M. J. (1966). Ph. D. thesis, Physics Dept. , California Institute of Technology, Pasadena, California.

Clauser, M. J. , Kankeleit, E. , and Mössbauer, R. L. (1966). Phys. Rev. Letters $\underline{17}$, 5.

Freeman, A. J. and Watson, R. E. (1965). "Hyperfine Interactions in Magnetic Materials, " in Treatise on Magnetism , edited by G. T. Rado and H. Suhl, Vol. II (Academic Press, New York), p. 167.

Gol'danskii, V. I. (1964). "The Mössbauer Effect and Its Application in Chemistry, " (Consultants Bureau, New York).

Gol'danskii, V. I. , Makarov, E. F. , and Khrapov, V. V. (1963). Phys. Letters $\underline{3}$, 344.

Hafemeister, D. W. , DePasquali, G. , and de Waard, H. (1964). Phys. Rev. $\underline{135}$, B1089.

Hanna, S. S. , Heberle, J. , Perlow, G. J. , Preston, R. S. , and Vincent, D. H. (1960). Phys. Rev. Letters $\underline{4}$, 513.

Kagan, Yu. M. (1961). Doklady Akad. Nauk SSSR $\underline{140}$, 794.

Karyagin, S. V. (1963). Doklady Akad. Nauk SSSR $\underline{148}$, 110.

Kistner, O. C. and Sunyar, A. W. (1960). Phys. Rev. Letters 4, 412.

Kuhn, W. (1929). Phil. Mag. 8, 625.

Lees, J. and Flinn, P. A. (1965). Phys. Letters 19, 186.

Menes, M. and Bolef, D. (1961). Phys. Chem. Solids 19, 79.

Moon, P. B. (1951). Proc. Phys. Soc. (London) 64, 76.

Mössbauer, R. L. (1958). Z. Physik 151, 124.

Pound, R. V. and Rebka, G. A. (1960). Phys. Rev. Letters 4, 274.

Shirley, D. A. (1964). Rev. Mod. Phys. 36, 339.

Snively, F. T. (1965). Ph. D. thesis, Phys. Dept., California Institute of Technology, Pasadena, California (unpublished).

Sternheimer, R. M. (1963). Phys. Rev. 132, 1637.

Watson, R. E. (1959). Solid State and Molecular Theory Group, Technical Rep. No. 12, Massachusetts Institute of Technology.

Watson, R. E. and Freeman, A. J. (1961). Phys. Rev. 123, 2027.

Walker, L. R., Wertheim, G. K., and Jaccarino, V. (1961). Phys. Rev. Letters 6, 98.

12. HYPERFINE INTERACTIONS AND THE ANGULAR DISTRIBUTION AND CORRELATIONS OF NUCLEAR γ-RAYS

S.G. Cohen

Department of Physics
The Hebrew University
Jerusalem, Israel

Table of Contents

I. Introduction

In this chapter we shall mainly discuss the perturbation by
hyperfine fields in solids of angular correlation or angular distribution patterns of γ-rays emitted from excited states of nuclei in
solids, either formed in the process of radioactive decay, or in
nuclear reactions. We shall also, however, give some attention
in passing, to the information on hyperfine interactions which can
be obtained from the investigation into the degree of nuclear orientation obtaining in solids at low temperatures, either by measuring
the angular distribution of nuclear radiations, in the case of radioactive nuclei, or, by measuring the transmission of polarized
neutron beams by the solid containing an appreciable percentage
of orientated nuclei, in the case of stable nuclei.

Until fairly recently, the whole subject of angular distribution or angular correlation of γ-rays was, from the experimental
aspects mainly of interest to the nuclear physicist, in that it provided a valuable tool for the determination of some important
properties of nuclear states, such as spin (angular momentum)
and magnetic moments. And this, despite the fact, that a remarkably thorough and exhaustive theoretical treatment of the subject
of perturbations by internal fields was published in a classic paper
as early as 1953 by Abragam and Pound. In particular, in favourable circumstances, the precession of the angular distribution
pattern in an external magnetic field could often be used for the
determination of nuclear magnetic moments of excited states.
Insofar as the angular distributions were affected or liable to be
affected by the hyperfine or internal magnetic or electric fields,
such perturbations were generally regarded as a nuisance which
had, however, to be understood in order to be able to correctly
interpret experimental results and to obtain correct values for
nuclear magnetic moments from experiments usually carried out
in the presence of external magnetic fields.

However, it is now realised that the study of perturbation of angular correlations is of great interest in its own right and provides a valuable (and in some cases unique) tool for measuring hyperfine interactions in solids and liquids. The nuclear physicist continues to be interested in the subject, because of the importance in measuring moments of short lived states, and the solid state physicist is becoming increasingly aware of its importance for solid state physics. The host of new problems concerning hyperfine fields, particularly in magnetically ordered materials, which have arisen particularly as a consequence of the discovery of the Mössbauer effect, have given a new lease of life to the angular correlation technique. This, together with the recent exciting experimental confirmation (Matthias et al., 1966) of the suggestion that γ angular distribution or correlation measurements might perhaps be used as a detector of nuclear magnetic resonance in relatively short lived states, leads one to predict great activity for the whole field in the future.

An exact description of experiments in which the angular distribution of radiations are measured demands the use of the techniques of angular momentum operators and Racah algebra. We shall limit ourselves, however, to illustrating the basic physical ideas involved and describe in a general way the most important and useful results.

We first describe briefly the basic idea involved in a precession type experiment involving angular distribution of nuclear radiations. We first note that an ensemble of nuclei having no preferred orientation in space will emit radiation isotropically. If, however, we prepare the nuclei, in some way, so that the spins, assumed to be non-zero, are preferentially orientated in space, then the angular distribution of nuclear radiation emitted from such nuclei will, in general, be anisotropic.

Let us concentrate our attention upon the emission of γ-rays from such an orientated or partially orientated ensemble.

We remember that γ-rays are photons emitted from excited states of nuclei, which are characterized by a certain mean-life τ. Mean lifetimes extend over an enormous range of values — as short as 10^{-15} sec and as long as hours or years, for so-called metastable states; however, here, we restrict ourselves for the most part to a more limited range of lifetimes, say 10^{-11} sec to 10^{-6} sec. Now, if during the lifetime of the excited states concerned, appropriate magnetic or electric fields (external magnetic fields, internal hyperfine fields, or both) act on the nuclei, then, we know, on a semiclassical description, that the nuclei will precess in these fields, and this, of course, will give rise to a change in the angular distribution of the emitted radiation. The extent of the change will depend on the strength of the interaction between the nucleus and the fields in question, and also on the lifetime of the excited state, the precession being greater the longer the mean-life. From a measurement of the change in angular distribution and a knowledge of τ, we can derive the strength of the interaction.

A. Properties of the Electromagnetic Radiation Field

Let us summarize some properties of the electromagnetic radiation field appropriate to the emission of gamma-rays from nuclei. A γ-ray photon of energy $h\nu$ is radiated in the de-excitation taking place between an upper and lower nuclear state with spins (angular momentum) I_1 and I_2 respectively and corresponding parities π_1, π_2, which may be odd or even (Fig. 1).

Fig. 1: A γ-ray transition between
two nuclear states.

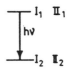

The electromagnetic radiation field can be characterized by a certain multipole character L (equals 1 for dipole, 2 for quadrupole, etc.). The angular momentum carried by the multipole field will be $\hbar L$. The selection rules for L are thus

$$\left| I_1 - I_2 \right| \le L \le \left| I_1 + I_2 \right| \tag{1}$$

and the type of radiation (electric or magnetic) will be determined by the parity selection rule:

No parity change, $\Delta\pi = +1$, M1, E2 etc. (magnetic
dipole, electric qua-
drupole, etc.)

Yes parity change, $\Delta\pi = -1$, E1, M2 etc. (electric
dipole, magnetic qua-
drupole, etc.)

$\tag{2}$

i. e. $\Delta\pi = (-1)^L$ for EL radiation

$\quad = (-1)^{L-1}$ for ML radiation

In any particular transition we are usually limited to the lowest possible multipolarities permitted by the selection rules, since electromagnetic transition probabilities are strongly reduced as we go to higher multipoles (the reduction factor is of the order $(a/\lambda)^{2L}$ where a is the nuclear dimension and λ the wavelength of the radiation). In practice this usually means that only the lowest value of L is present, or at most, some mixture of the lowest multipole with the next $L + 1$ multipole which must have, however, the same parity, since parity is conserved. Thus, for example, in Fig. 2a, showing a transition between two states, each having spin 2 and both having the same parity, one might expect a mixture of the multipole fields, M1 and E2 (magnetic dipole and electric quadrupole respectively); similarly for the transition in Fig. 2b we might expect a mixture of electric dipole (E1) and magnetic quadrupole (M2). But quite often we may expect effectively pure multipole character. In the case of mixed multipoles we introduce the mixing ratio δ, the ratio of amplitudes of the respective multipoles in the transition. Then δ^2 will be the ratio of intensities (integrated over all angles) of the multipole fields. Angular distributions are often sensitive to quite small values of mixed-in amplitudes.

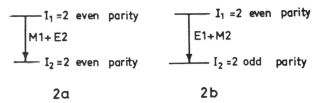

$$\text{2a} \qquad\qquad \text{2b}$$

Fig. 2: γ-ray transitions showing examples of mixed multipoles.

B. γ-γ Angular Correlations and Angular Distribution of γ-Rays

In a typical γ-γ angular correlation experiment we are concerned with nuclei emitting two γ radiations in cascade (Fig. 3). The first radiation is detected selectively by counter 1 and the second radiation by counter 2 (Fig. 4). We record the simultaneous appearance of the two quanta in the two counters (i. e. "coincidences") as a function of the angle θ between them, using appropriate electronics.

A simple example will be given to illustrate the important general rule that we can write the angular correlation function in the form

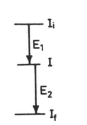

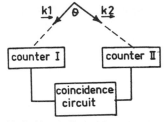

Fig. 3: A γ-ray cascade   Fig. 4: Schematic arrangement of an angular correlation measurement.

$$W(\theta) = \sum_{k(even)} A_k P_k (\cos \theta) \qquad (3)$$

where $k_{max} \lesssim \min (2I, 2L_1, 2L_2)$. $P_k (\cos \theta)$ are the Legendre polynomials. It is customary to normalize the distribution function to $A_0 = 1$. Different, and sometimes convenient, forms of writing $W(\theta)$ are

$$W(\theta) = \sum_k b_k \cos k\theta$$

or $\qquad\qquad\qquad\qquad\qquad\qquad\qquad\qquad\qquad\qquad\qquad$ (4)

$$W(\theta) = \sum_k a_k \cos^k \theta \quad .$$

The algebraic relation between the coefficients A_k, b_k, and a_k can easily be derived. These expressions are valid providing that the correlation is unperturbed, i.e., there are no significant perturbations acting on the nucleus in the intermediate state of the cascade.

As a simple example, let us consider a γ-γ cascade (Fig. 3) where $I_i = I_f = 0$ and I, the spin of the intermediate state, is unity. The selection rules then demand that both gamma transitions have pure dipole character (electric or magnetic according to Eq. (2)).

Let us apply a very weak magnetic field, so weak that we can ignore the perturbation of the correlation in the intermediate state. The I = 1 level is then split into three magnetic substates, m = -1, 0, +1. We choose the axis of quantization along the direction of the fixed counter detecting the γ-radiation of the first transition of the cascade. Then for dipole radiation, the change in the projection of the angular momentum quantum number along the quantization direction will be given by $\Delta m = \pm 1$. Thus the only substates of the intermediate level which will be populated, will be those with m = ± 1.

In this way, we select a certain population of the substates of the intermediate state. From elementary theory of electromagnetic dipole radiation we know that the angular distribution of radiation emitted from each of the m substates to the nuclear ground state with angular momentum zero is given by

$$F_1^{\pm 1}(\theta) = \tfrac{1}{2}(1 + \cos^2\theta), \text{ from the } m = \pm 1 \text{ substates}$$

$$F_1^0(\theta) = \tfrac{1}{2}\sin^2\theta\,, \qquad \text{from the } m = 0 \text{ substates}$$

(5)

If the three m states were equally populated, then, since $W(\theta) = F_1^{+1}(\theta) + F_1^{-1}(\theta) + F_1^0(\theta) = 2$ which is independent of angle, we see that the radiation is isotropic, as indeed it must be. But since, in our example, we have excited only the states with $m = \pm 1$, the angular correlation function in a coincidence experiment will be given by

$$W(\theta) = F_1^{+1}(\theta) + F_1^{-1}(\theta) = 1 + \cos^2\theta$$
$$= 1 + 0.5\, P_2(\cos\theta)\quad.$$

(6)

The principle of spectroscopic stability tells us that the result of our discussion is independent of the application of the weak magnetic field.

By the way, this type of analysis of the angular correlation of a γ-γ cascade applies, essentially, also in the case of nuclear resonance scattering, and particularly, Mössbauer scattering, although no coincidence experiments are performed in this case. One can ask in these latter cases, what is the angular distribution of the scattered radiation with respect to the incident radiation? It is clear that $W(\theta)$ in this case will be the same as in the case of a fictitious cascade in which I_i and I_f both correspond to the nuclear ground state, and I is the excited state (Fig. 5), i.e. we may regard the scattering as a two-step process.

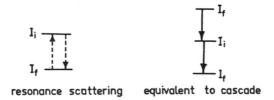

resonance scattering   equivalent to cascade

Fig. 5: Resonant γ-ray scattering and equivalent cascade.

Let us now consider an example of considerable current
interest, namely, the angular distribution of γ-rays emitted from
the excited states of nuclei, produced in the nuclear reaction
known as Coulomb excitation. *

Heavy ions are accelerated in a particle accelerator, and
a well-defined beam of such ions falls on a target. A strong time-
dependent electric field acts between target nuclei and those accelerated ions which make a close approach. This time dependent
Coulomb field may be represented, in the so-called Weiszacker-
Williams description, by a field of virtual photons, and these
virtual photons may have a strong probability of inducing a collective nuclear transition from the ground state to an excited state,
especially in the region of the deformed nuclei. Let us take as an
example, the Coulomb excitation of the first excited state with
spin $I_i = 2$ of an even-even nucleus with ground state spin I_f equal
to zero. Such an excited state de-excites by the emission of pure
electric quadrupole radiation to the ground state.

Consider a special case when the incident particle returns
almost exactly along its path after interaction and excitation of the
nucleus (Fig. 6) i. e. the case of an almost head-on collision.
Suppose we record the γ-rays emitted in the de-excitation of the
excited state of the target nuclei *in coincidence* with the scattered particle. This particle can transfer angular momentum to the
excited nucleus only in a plane perpendicular to its path and therefore, cannot change the projection of the orbital angular momentum
of the target nucleus along the direction of the beam, which we
take to be the axis of quantization. Remembering that the initial
target nuclei have zero angular momentum we see that *this corresponds to a selective excitation of the m = 0 substates of
the spin 2 excited state.*

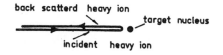

Fig. 6: Head-on collision in Coulomb excitation.

The resulting angular distribution of quadrupole radiation
emitted from the excited state when measured in coincidence with
the back-scattered ions, will have the characteristic distribution

---

*
See discussion by D. Murnick, Chap. S.2.

of an aligned quadrupole antenna, well known in classical electromagnetic theory:

$$W(\theta) = 2 \sin^2 \theta \cos^2 \theta \qquad (7)$$

which may be written in the somewhat more sophisticated form
(more useful for our purpose)

$$W(\theta) = 1 + \frac{5}{7} P_2 (\cos \theta) - \frac{12}{7} P_4 (\cos \theta) \qquad (8)$$

(Note that this distribution function is a very steep function of
angle (Fig. 7) with high anisotropy and therefore very sensitive
to perturbing fields.)

Fig. 7: Angular distribution of quadrupole γ-rays (in coincidence with
back-scattered heavy ions) from 2+
excited states produced in Coulomb
excitation.

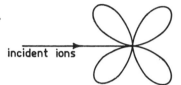

incident ions

In both these examples we have essentially oriented nuclei
in the intermediate state, producing what one may call a state of
alignment, characterized by the preservation of the equality of
population of sub-states with +m to that of -m.

It will be useful to define the following terms:*

(i) A nonequal population of magnetic m-states defines a
state of *nuclear orientation.*

(ii) If states with m plus and m minus are equally populated, then
we say the nuclei are *aligned.*

(iii) If this equality is not conserved, then we have a *polarization.*

We can define moments which measure the degree of orientation of the nuclei. The first order moment f_1 is defined as

$$f_1 = I^{-1} \sum_m a_m \cdot m \qquad (9)$$

where a_m are the relative populations, normalized to $\sum_m a_m = 1$.
The second order moment is defined as

---

* *See N.J. Stone, Chap. S.4.*

$$f_2 = I^{-2} \sum_m \left\{ a_m \cdot m^2 - \tfrac{1}{3} I(I+1) \right\}^2 . \tag{10}$$

Higher moments may be important, but we shall not define them here.

These definitions of the moments f_1, f_2, etc., are useful particularly in the discussion of methods of orientating appreciable fractions of nuclei in bulk matter, at very low temperatures. For example, in the case of magnetic orientation, one employs a strong magnetic field (external or hyperfine field). A significant amount of nuclear polarization will obtain provided the ratio $\mu H/kT$ is sufficiently large, where μ is the nuclear magnetic moment.

Returning now to the general expression for an unperturbed correlation or distribution, Eq. (3), A_k is separable into a product of two coefficients

$$A_k = A_k(1) \cdot A_k(2) \tag{11}$$

where $A_k(1)$ belongs to the first transition only and $A_k(2)$ to the second.

If we are dealing with pure multipoles in a γ-ray cascade, the A_k's are functions of the multipole order and the initial and final spins, of the particular transition:

$$A_k(1) = F_k(L_1 L_1 \; I_i I) \quad ,$$
$$A_k(2) = F_k(L_2 L_2 \; I_f I) \quad . \tag{12}$$

The F_k coefficients have all been calculated and tabulated and can be found, for example, in the appendix to the article on angular correlations by Frauenfelder and Steffen (1965).

When one of the transitions contains a mixture of two multipolarities L, L' (usually, as we have seen, $L' = L + 1$) then, for this transition,

$$A_k(1) = \frac{1}{1+\delta^2} \left\{ F_k(L_1 L_1 \; I_i I) + 2\delta \, F_k(L_1 L_1' I_i I) \right.$$
$$\left. + \delta^2 \, F_k(L_1' \, L_1' \; I_i I) \right\} \tag{13}$$

where δ^2 is the mixing ratio between the two multipoles.

In most cases the angular correlation is suitably described by only two parameters A_2 and A_4, and

$$W(\theta) = 1 + A_2 P_2 (\cos \theta) + A_4 P_4 (\cos \theta) \quad . \tag{14}$$

However, we see that A_2 and A_4, in their turn, are fixed in general by a large number of nuclear parameters (especially in the case of mixed multipoles) including nuclear spins, multipole orders and mixing ratios δ, and in general one will need additional nuclear data to determine the mixing ratios. This may be particularly important in cases where there is some doubt whether a measured angular correlation is truly unperturbed or not. The problem here is to determine the theoretical unperturbed correlation to be compared with experiment. We see this is sensitive to the mixing ratios, which a priori may not be known.

II. The Perturbations of γ-Ray Angular Correlations and Distributions in External and Hyperfine Fields

A. The Detection of Nuclear Magnetic Resonance

This idea is probably, conceptually, the simplest application of angular correlations to the determination of hyperfine interactions, especially to those familiar with NMR techniques. Nevertheless, experimental observations of this type have only been recently reported.* We have seen in the case of a nuclear cascade of γ-rays that an angular correlation exists since essentially we have selected, by the process of measurement, certain magnetic substates from among the total ensemble of nuclei in the intermediate nuclear state. In the presence of a static magnetic field (preferably, as we shall see, in the direction of detection of the first radiation), which may be an external field or the hyperfine field, some kind of magnetic splitting of the intermediate nuclear state will result, and in principle, application of a radio frequency field at a frequency satisfying the usual resonance condition $h\nu =$ level splitting, will induce transitions between the sub-states, thereby changing the relative population of substates and therefore changing the angular distribution of the succeeding radiation. A study of the angular correlation, or simply, the coincidence rate with the two counters in a favourably fixed situation, as a function of the RF frequency in the neighbourhood of the resonance frequency should yield a typical resonance curve.

One of the difficulties in the application of this principle is that large RF amplitudes are needed to induce transitions in nuclear states having only short lifetimes. The elegant experiments of

*See discussion by E. Matthias, Chap. 13.

Matthias et al., have nevertheless detected such resonant transitions in the 74.8 keV excited state of Rh^{100} (mean life 2.3×10^{-7} sec) situated as a dilute impurity in iron, relying on the domain enhancement of RF fields in ferromagnets.[*] Similarly, the resonant change of the angular distribution of γ-rays, emitted from orientated Co^{60} in iron at low temperatures on application of an RF field has also been observed recently (Matthias and Holliday, 1966). The latter experiment is somewhat easier since the Co^{60} ground state is relatively long lived, and also since counter statistics are much better in an angular distribution experiment as compared to a coincidence experiment, for which in general rather low counting rates obtain.

As stated earlier, we anticipate a great development in these types of measurements, which will in favourable circumstances, permit measurement of hyperfine interactions of dilute radioactive nuclei with an accuracy approaching that of normal NMR techniques.

We now turn to the more classical types of situation which have been treated.

B.   Static and Time-Dependent Perturbations Produced by Hyperfine Interactions

The most important part of the hyperfine interactions to be considered are the leading terms in the multipole expansion of the electric and magnetic parts of the interactions. For the magnetic part, this is the magnetic dipole interaction involving the interaction of the nuclear magnetic moment with the magnetic fields at the nucleus produced by the spin and orbital moments of the electrons. For the electric part, there are two terms, the monopole Coulomb interaction (with the small but significant corrections to this arising from the finite size of the nuclear charge distribution), and the electric quadrupole interaction (involving the nuclear quadrupole moment and the electric field gradient set up at the nucleus by the surrounding charge distributions). The monopole part of the interaction can have no effect of the angular distribution of γ-rays, which involves, as we have seen, the creation of at least one unit of angular momentum in the radiation field and so can be ignored in this discussion. (This represents an important difference in comparison with the Mössbauer technique.)[**] Thus, we have to deal with only magnetic dipole and electric quadrupole interactions.

*E. Matthias, Chap. 13.
** See Mössbauer and Clauser, Chap. 11.

In general, it is also of great importance to consider the *time-dependence* of these interactions. We may distinguish between static interactions and those that are time-dependent. Static hyperfine magnetic and quadrupole fields may be found in saturated ferromagnets or in paramagnetic materials at very low temperatures. But at higher temperatures, fluctuation phenomena will occur, in general, thereby complicating the situation. Consider the hyperfine interaction in ferromagnets. Under conditions of ideal magnetic saturation (say, at low enough temperatures), the full hyperfine interaction is operative as a static interaction and the maximum value of H_{eff} is obtained. At higher temperatures, because of the lattice thermal motions, the average value of the magnetization is reduced and correspondingly the average field at the nucleus in the direction of the magnetization will be smaller, but this reduction in the average effective magnetic field will be accompanied by the presence of a randomly fluctuating component of the magnetic field, which gives rise to time dependent perturbations. Relaxation times as short as 10^{-12} - 10^{-13} sec are sufficient for appreciable effects in angular correlations experiments provided the hyperfine fields are sufficiently large. At higher temperatures, H_{eff} may fall to quite low values and the amplitude of the fluctuating part of the field will be correspondingly much higher. In a paramagnetic solid at higher temperatures the hyperfine field, averaged over a long enough period in time, will be zero, in the absence of an external field, but again there may be large fluctuating instantaneous hyperfine fields. In such a solid, the average quadrupole interaction will be the Boltzman average over the various Stark levels excited at a given temperature produced by the crystalline electric field splitting. But over short periods of time there will be fluctuations between the instantaneous interactions corresponding to each level, due to the relaxation processes associated with thermal exchange between these Stark levels. Again, in general, we must expect the nuclear quadrupole interactions in liquids to be essentially time-dependent, since the quadrupole interactions must be strongly influenced by the random molecular collisions.

C. Integral and Time-Differential Angular Correlations

The most complete and valuable information is obtained from time-dependent angular correlation measurements. Such measurements are possible when the resolving time of the electronic coincidence circuits is appreciably shorter than the lifetime of the intermediate state involved. (Today resolving times of the order of 10^{-9} sec or less are often attainable.) One may then measure coincidence counting rates as a function of the time spent by nuclei in the intermediate state before decaying, for a given angular setting between the counters. In practice the coincidence rate is measured as a function of the length of calibrated delay line introduced in one arm of the coincident circuit. The angular correlation will then, in general, change as a function of delay, the perturbation being greater the longer the nuclei remain in the intermediate state before decaying.

An unperturbed angular correlation will not depend on the time elapsed by nuclei in the intermediate state. For unperturbed cases, then $W(\theta, t) = W(\theta, 0)$ (cf. Eq. (3)). In the case of perturbations, however

$$W(\theta, t) = \sum_k G_k(t) A_k P_k(\cos \theta) \tag{15}$$

where $G_k(t)$ are the time dependent functions, describing the attenuation of the correlation coefficients A_k. The G_k's are less than unity. In any actual experiment the counter may detect the second radiation within a finite interval t_1 to t_2 after the first and the measured correlation will be (taking into account the exponential decay of excited states)

$$W(\theta, t_1 t_2) = \frac{\int_{t_1}^{t_2} W(\theta, t) \exp(-t/\tau)\, dt}{\int_{t_1}^{t_2} \exp(-t/\tau)\, dt} . \tag{16}$$

The smallest interval (t_1, t_2) which may be used, is, of course, the resolving time of the experimental set-up.

If the resolving time is much larger than the mean life, as sometime occurs, then we can only measure the integral correlation

$$W(\theta, \infty) = \frac{\int_0^{\infty} W(\theta, t)\exp(-t/\tau)\,dt}{\int_0^{\infty} \exp(-t/\tau)\,dt} = \frac{1}{\tau} \int_0^{\infty} W(\theta, t) \exp(-t/\tau)\,dt . \tag{17}$$

An integral correlation measurement, in general, yields much less information concerning the nature of the hyperfine interactions involved.

III. Theoretical Discussion of Perturbations of Angular Correlations

A. The Density Matrix

A very suitable tool for dealing with the theory of perturbation of angular correlations is the density matrix which is introduced to describe situations where we do not have an ensemble of pure quantum states, but rather "mixed" states. Such situations are common in physics — a good example being the quantum description of an incoherent light source.

For a pure quantum state, $|n\rangle$ we have

$$|n\rangle = \sum_m a_{nm}|m\rangle \tag{18}$$

where there are fixed phase relations between the orthogonal eigenstates $|m\rangle$ of some operator. If we wish to calculate the expectation value of the operator F, for such a pure state, we take

$$\langle n|F|n\rangle = \sum_{mm'} a^*_{nm'}\, a_{nm} \langle m'|F|m\rangle \quad . \tag{19}$$

In the case where we do not have pure states, but, instead, an incoherent mixture of states $|n\rangle$ with relative weight g_n, then the expectation value for such an ensemble will be

$$\langle|F|\rangle = \sum_n g_n \langle n|F|n\rangle$$

$$= \sum_n \sum_{mm'} g^*_n a_{nm'}\, a_{nm} \langle m'|F|m\rangle \quad . \tag{20}$$

We now define the density matrix ρ:

$$\langle m|\rho|m'\rangle = \sum_n g_n a^*_{nm'}\, a_{nm} \quad . \tag{21}$$

This matrix enables us to write the expectation value of F in a compact form:

$$\langle F\rangle = \sum \langle m|\rho|m'\rangle \langle m'|F|m\rangle = \mathrm{Tr}\,(\rho \cdot F) . \tag{22}$$

Now we shall see how the density matrix helps to describe angular correlations.

If, as may often happen, the m substates of the intermediate nuclear level (of spin I) are equally populated, the subsequent radiation will be isotropic. The density matrix is then diagonal and proportional to the unit matrix:

$$\langle m | \rho | m' \rangle = (2I+1)^{-1} \, \delta_{mm'} \quad . \tag{23}$$

As we have seen, the detection of the first radiation of a cascade, with wave vector $\mathbf{k}_1$ in a given direction introduces an unequal population of the m states in the intermediate state, which we may describe by a density matrix. We denote this density matrix by $\rho(\mathbf{k}_1, 0)$ and 0 denotes zero time after the photon emission. If there are no perturbations, the density matrix will be independent of the time t which the nucleus spends in the intermediate state. Explicitly, the form of ρ is given by

$$\langle m | \rho(\mathbf{k}_1, 0) | m' \rangle = (4\pi)^{\frac{1}{2}} \sum_k (-1)^m A_k(1) \begin{pmatrix} I & I & k \\ m' & -m & \mu \end{pmatrix} Y^*_{k\mu}(k_1)$$
$$\tag{24}$$

where the successive factors are: A_k introduced in Eq. (12), a Clebsh-Gordan coefficient; and, the spherical harmonic expressing the angular dependence.

In a similar way we can write down the density matrix corresponding to the second transition associated with wave-vector $\mathbf{k}_2$. We denote this by $\rho(\mathbf{k}_2)$, given explicitly by

$$\langle m' | \rho(\mathbf{k}_2) | m \rangle = (4\pi)^{\frac{1}{2}} \sum_{k'} (-1)^m A_{k'}(2) \begin{pmatrix} I & I & k' \\ m' & -m & \mu \end{pmatrix} Y_{k'\mu'}(k_2) . \tag{25}$$

The unperturbed angular correlation is then given by the trace of the product of the two density matrices:

$$W(\theta, 0) \equiv W(\mathbf{k}_1, \mathbf{k}_2, 0)$$

$$= \mathrm{Tr} \, \{\rho(\mathbf{k}_1, 0), \, \rho(\mathbf{k}_2)\}$$

$$= \sum_{mm'} \langle m | \rho(\mathbf{k}_1, 0) | m' \rangle \langle m' | \rho(\mathbf{k}_2) | m \rangle \quad . \tag{26}$$

If interactions are introduced in the intermediate state, associated with an interaction Hamiltonian $\mathcal{H}$, then the density matrix will change in time

$$\rho(\mathbf{k_1}, 0) \rightarrow \rho(\mathbf{k_1}, t) \tag{27}$$

and

$$W(\theta, t) \equiv W(\mathbf{k_1 k_2}, t) = \sum_{mm'} \langle m | \rho(\mathbf{k_1}, t) | m' \rangle \langle m' | \rho(\mathbf{k_2}) | m \rangle .$$
$$\tag{28}$$

Here t is the delay introduced in the angular correlation coincident experiment. The change of the density matrix with time is given by the Heisenberg equation of motion

$$\frac{\partial \rho}{\partial t} = -\frac{i}{\hbar} [\mathcal{K}, \rho] . \tag{29}$$

Consider now the case of static interactions. Here the formal solution of the equation of motion is

$$\rho(\mathbf{k}, t) = \Lambda(t) \; \rho(\mathbf{k}, 0) \; \Lambda^{-1}(t) . \tag{30}$$

$\Lambda(t)$ is a unitary operator, usually called "the evolution operator" and is given by

$$\Lambda(t) = \exp\left(-\frac{i}{\hbar} \mathcal{K} \cdot t\right) . \tag{31}$$

B. The Time Dependent Attenuation Coefficients

Substituting these expressions for $\rho(\mathbf{k_1}, t)$ into Eq. (28), and comparing with the corresponding expression obtaining without a perturbation, we can derive a general form for the attenuation coefficients $G_k(t)$:

$$G_k(t) = \sum_{\substack{mm' \\ m'' m'''}} \left\{ \left[\begin{array}{l} \text{geometric factors including} \\ \text{"Clebsch-Gordanery"} \end{array} \right] \right.$$

$$\left. \times \; \langle m | \Lambda(t) | m'' \rangle \; \langle m' | \Lambda(t) | m''' \rangle^* \right\} \tag{32}$$

and*

$$W(\mathbf{k_1 k_2}, t) = 4\pi \sum_{\substack{kk' \\ \mu\mu'}} \frac{A_k(1) \; A_k(2)}{(2k+1)(2k'+1)} \; G_{kk'}^{\mu\mu'}(t) \; Y_{k\mu}^*(\mathbf{k_1}) \; \times$$

$$\times \; Y_{k'\mu'}(\mathbf{k_2}) . \tag{33}$$

*This is in fact the most general form for a perturbed angular correlation.

Suppose we now choose a representation $|Im\rangle$ such that the interaction operator $\mathcal{K}$ is diagonal. For example, if $\mathcal{K}$ is produced by a static magnetic field, we shall choose our z axis along its direction. In this representation, ρ is given by

$$\rho(\mathbf{k}, t) = \exp\left(-\frac{i}{\hbar}\,\mathcal{K}t\right)\rho(\mathbf{k}, 0)\exp\left(+\frac{i}{\hbar}\,\mathcal{K}t\right) \tag{34}$$

and the matrix elements by

$$\langle m|\rho(\mathbf{k}, t)|m'\rangle = \langle m|\rho(\mathbf{k}, 0)|m'\rangle\exp\left(\frac{i}{\hbar}\,[E_m' - E_m]t\right) \tag{35}$$

where the E_m's are the energies of the m states and the eigen-values of the interaction Hamiltonian $\mathcal{K}$. The important thing to notice is that the density matrix $\rho(\mathbf{k}, t)$ is thus an oscillating function of time, the frequency of which is determined by the level splitting produced by the interaction. This fact is reflected in the angular correlation pattern, and $G_k(t)$ will also oscillate, har-monically with time, with the same frequency.

If we are not free to choose a diagonal representation for $\mathcal{K}$, for example, if there are magnetic and electric interactions in different directions, then we must first diagonalize the interaction. We must find a unitary matrix U so that

$$V = U\mathcal{K}U^{-1} \qquad \text{is diagonal} \tag{36}$$

The evolution operator $\Lambda(t)$ becomes

$$\Lambda(t) = U^{-1}\exp\left[-\frac{i}{\hbar}\,Vt\right]U \tag{37}$$

and we have to transform the eigenstates $|m\rangle$ and $|m'\rangle$ by the same transformation.

In the particular case where the magnetic field is parallel to the direction of one of the counters, there are no matrix elements connecting different m-states, i.e., the magnetic field cannot induce transitions between m-states in the intermediate state. Thus, a magnetic field parallel to one of the directions of observa-tion will not produce any perturbation. Classically, we can regard this as a static situation of the nuclei precessing about the z axis, a precession that does not change the density matrix. For these reasons, longitudinal static magnetic fields are favourable for the resonance type of experiments mentioned above in Sec. II. A.

One important application of this result is in the use of a magnetic field to remove the perturbations, caused by the presence of hyperfine interactions, in order to measure the unperturbed angular correlation. By applying a sufficiently large magnetic field parallel to one of the counter directions one should be able to decouple the electronic and nuclear moments (a Paschen-Back effect, essentially) and restore the true angular correlation.

For the case of a static magnetic field the exponent in Eq. (37) reduces to $i \omega_L (m' - m)t$, or

$$V = \hbar \omega_L (m' - m) \tag{38}$$

where ω_L is the Larmor frequency $= g \mu_n H / \hbar$.

For a static axially symmetric electric field gradient the exponent becomes

$$V = 3\hbar \ \omega_q (m'^2 - m^2) \tag{39}$$

where

$$\omega_q = \frac{1}{4I(2I - 1)} \cdot \frac{eQ}{\hbar} \frac{\partial^2 V}{\partial z^2} \ ,$$

is the basic quadrupole frequency.

The simplest case to be discussed, and experimentally the most useful one, is that of a static magnetic field perpendicular to the correlation plane. After evaluating the appropriate expression for $G_k(t)$ we indeed get the result expected classically, that is to say, the angular correlation precesses with the Larmor frequency ω_L about the direction of the field. So that after a time t, the angular correlation pattern, has rotated by an angle $\omega_L t$.

The expression of the time dependent angular correlation then becomes simply

$$W(\theta, t) = \sum_k A_k P_k [\cos (\theta - \omega_L t)] \tag{40}$$

which may also be written as

$$W(\theta, t) = \sum_k b_k \cos k(\theta - \omega_L t) \ . \tag{41}$$

If we measure the rate of the delayed coincidences as a function of time, at a fixed angle, we shall then obtain a harmonic function, provided we divide out by the factor $\exp(-t/\tau)$ describing the exponential decay of the intermediate state, as a function of time delay t.

In those cases where the nuclear lifetime is too short for a time dependent measurement, one has to measure the time integral angular correlation. For this, one obtains

$$W(\theta, \infty) = \frac{1}{\tau} \int_0^\infty W(\theta, t) \exp(-t/\tau) \, dt$$

$$= \sum_k b_k \frac{\cos k(\theta - \Delta\theta)}{1 + (k\omega_L \tau)^2} \tag{42}$$

where $k\Delta\theta = \arctan(k\omega_L \tau)$.

As we see from this equation, we obtain an integral rotation $\Delta\theta$, which is, however, accompanied by an attenuation of the angular correlation pattern, given by the factor $1/(1 + [k\omega_L \tau]^2)$. As a check that one has only a magnetic interaction in a particular situation, one can use both the measurements of the average rotation and the attenuation factor, together with the above formulae, to yield independent values of ω_L. If these are not consistent one might suspect in addition the existence of an electric quadrupole interaction.

The preceding formulae, involving, either a differential or integral precession are of great use for measurements of nuclear magnetic moments and, more recently, for measuring hyperfine fields, in those cases where there is a well defined direction of the effective field.

The differential rotation measurement however is clearly capable of yielding much more information concerning hyperfine interactions. In the case of hyperfine magnetic fields which are well-defined in both magnitude and direction, we shall obtain a purely harmonic function of time. For a distribution of fields in solids, corresponding to different sites, one might, in principle, derive this information by a Fourier analysis of the experimental time-differential curve. Little work of this kind has yet been carried out, but it looks promising for a number of problems involving inhomogeneous fields.

A very common situation is one in which a static magnetic field has a well defined value, but is not perpendicular to the correlation plane. For example, in an unorientated ferromagnet there will be an ensemble of static fields pointing in all directions in space. This type of perturbation clearly does not produce any resultant rotation, but nevertheless one still obtains harmonic oscillations in the time delayed curve (with more than a single frequency, however), in addition to an attenuation in the integral correlation.

The pertinent expressions are

$$G_k(t) = \frac{1}{2k+1} \sum_{N=0}^{k} \cos N \omega_L t$$

$$G_k(\infty) = \frac{1}{2k+1} \left(\sum_{N=-k}^{k} \frac{1}{1+(N\omega_L \tau)^2} \right) \qquad (43)$$

but very often, only the term $k = 2$ is important, and we have

$$G_2(\infty) = \frac{1}{5}\left[1 + \frac{2}{1+(\omega_L \tau)^2} + \frac{2}{1+(2\omega_L \tau)^2}\right]. \qquad (44)$$

An important point about this type of interaction is that the angular correlation can never be washed out completely, as we see from the above expressions, even for very large $\omega_L \tau$. We obtain for the limiting value of $G_k(\infty)$, $1/(2k+1)$. This is usually called the "hard core" attenuation.

The perturbed angular correlation technique can similarly be used also to study electric quadrupole interactions. Since this interaction is degenerate with respect to $\pm m$ it clearly cannot produce any rotation of the integral correlation pattern, but we do get attenuation. The time dependent correlation, as in the case previously discussed, is again harmonically modulated, with a set of characteristic frequencies.

In the case of an axially symmetric quadrupole interaction in a polycrystalline material (no preferred direction in the source) the attenuation factors will be

$$G_k(t) = \sum_{n} S_{nk} \cos n \omega_q t$$

$$G_k(\infty) = \sum_{n} S_{nk} \frac{1}{(1+n\omega_q \tau)^2} \qquad (45)$$

where $n = m'^2 - m^2$ and S_{nk} are geometric coefficients, which have been tabulated.

Work on quadrupole interactions has been done also using single crystals. In this case one can change the orientation of the source with respect to the counters. One then expects that the correlation will be a function of the crystal orientation. The general form of the attenuation coefficients remains similar to the above, but is somewhat more complicated.

We shall now discuss time-dependent perturbations. These occur when the fields acting on the nucleus in its intermediate state fluctuate with time in a random manner. The two important cases of time-dependent perturbations are: (i) Electric quadrupole interactions in liquids due to the rapid fluctuations of the electric gradient caused by the Brownian motion. (ii) Magnetic time-dependent interactions in paramagnetic solids and possibly ferro- and ferrimagnetic materials. Assuming that in each individual fluctuation the change is small, or, in other words, adopting a perturbation treatment, one gets for the time-dependent attenuation factor

$$G_k(t) = \exp(-\lambda_k t) \tag{46}$$

and the integral attenuation factor becomes therefore

$$G_k(\infty) = \frac{1}{1 + \lambda_k \tau} \cdot \tag{47}$$

In this case, Eq. (42) may be written

$$W(\theta \, \omega) = 1 + \frac{1}{4} A_2 G_2 \left\{ 1 + \frac{3 \cos 2(\theta - \Delta\theta_{22})}{[1 + (2\omega_L \tau G_2)^2]^{1/2}} \right\}$$
$$+ \frac{1}{64} A_4 G_4 \left\{ 9 + \frac{20 \cos 2(\theta - \Delta\theta_{24})}{[1 + (2\omega_L \tau G_4)^2]^{1/2}} + \frac{35 \cos 4(\theta - \Delta\theta_{44})}{[1 + (4\omega_L \tau G_4)^2]^{1/2}} \right\} \tag{48}$$

where $n(\theta_{nk}) = \arctan(n\omega_L \tau G_k)$, $0 < \Delta\theta_{nk} < \pi/2n$.

For electric quadrupole interaction in liquids, a detailed theory of fluctuations yields for the relaxation parameters λ_k,

$$\lambda_k = (3/80)(\tau_c/\hbar^2)(eQ)^2 V_{zz}^2 \frac{k(k+1)[4I(I+1) - k(k+1) - 1]}{I^2(2I-1)^2} \tag{49}$$

Here τ_c is the correlation time in the liquid.* For the magnetic time dependent interaction

$$\lambda_k = (2/3)\tau_s \omega^2 I(I+1) J(J+1) \cdot [1 - (2I+1)W(I \, |kI| \, II)] ; \tag{50}$$

here τ_s is the spin relaxation time, and ω is the frequency corresponding to the instantaneous hyperfine magnetic field. For sufficiently large λ, the integral angular correlation can be completely wiped out, leaving an isotropic distribution. This is unlike the case of static interactions, where, as we have seen, we are left with a "hard core." When the orbital angular momentum L is quenched (as is usual, for example, in the 3d transition

* See A. Abragam and J. Kirsch, Chap. 8.

ions) one should change J to S in the above relation.

Dillenburg and Maris (1962) have recently challenged the "small change" assumption or perturbation approach, in the treatment of time dependent interactions. Using a more general treatment, independent of the perturbation assumption, they obtain for the attenuation factors, expressions involving the sum of exponentials. For example, the attenuation coefficients may become

$$G_2(t) = \alpha \exp(-\lambda_1 t) + (1-\alpha) \exp(-\lambda_2 t) \ ,$$

$$G_4(t) = \beta \exp(-\lambda_1 t) + (1-\beta) \exp(-\lambda_2 t) \ . \tag{51}$$

In this case we need four parameters to describe the attenuation. To date there is some slight evidence for the necessity for introducing such a more complicated parametrization in one or two cases, but this is not yet convincing.

IV. Special Topics in Perturbed Angular Correlation

A. Measurement of Hyperfine Interactions Using Orientated Nuclei at Low Temperatures

In those cases where the existence of a hyperfine interaction in solids is itself exploited in order to attain a bulk nuclear orientation in solids at low temperatures, the measurement of the degree of orientation at a known temperature permits an estimate of the hyperfine interaction. Statistical mechanics predicts the degree of orientation obtaining in thermodynamic equilibrium as a function of the hyperfine interaction energy and the temperature. In the simplest case, when we have an effective hyperfine magnetic field H_{eff} at the nuclei, which is well defined in value and direction, the degree of orientation will be, in thermodynamic equilibrium, an easily derivable function of the argument $\mu H_{eff}/kT$, and will be appreciable when this argument approaches unity. The degree of orientation may be measured, in the case of radioactive nuclei, by measuring the angular distribution of the emitted radiations. For example, for *aligned* nuclei, (i. e. $f_2 \neq 0$) the directional distribution of γ-radiation will be anisotropic. Thus, for example, for dipole radiation, and nuclear spin change $I \rightarrow I$, we have

$$W(\theta) = 1 - \frac{3I}{2I+1} \ f_2 P_2 (\cos \theta) \ . \tag{52}$$

In considering the angular distribution of γ-radiation, one must take into account that the parent nuclei, supposed aligned, will decay in general by β or α decay, and γ-rays will only be emitted from excited states of the daughter nuclei; however, an appreciable degree of orientation is transmitted to such excited states and proper quantitative account of the situation can usually be made. Of course, the directional distribution of β and α radiation can also be measured, but often this may be inconvenient due to the relatively strong absorption of these latter radiations. Measurements of the degree of polarization of γ-radiation can also provide valuable additional information on the nuclear orientation, particularly if we have only nuclear polarization ($f_1 \neq 0$) and no alignment ($f_2 = 0$).

We list briefly some of the important situations in which hyperfine interactions can be utilized to produce appreciable bulk orientation, as opposed to the "brute force" methods using only external magnetic fields:

(i) Orientation in ferromagnetic and antiferromagnetic materials. In saturated ferromagnetic materials (magnetically orientated perhaps with a small external field) the nuclear magnetic moments in paramagnetic ions experience large directed effective magnetic fields which may be used to orient nuclei at sufficiently low temperatures. These fields are of the order of 10^5 gauss for the 3d group and several million for the 4f rare-earths. Samoilov et al. (1959) and since then, others have successfully oriented diamagnetic ions situated as dilute impurities in ferromagnetic iron and have, from measurements of the degree of alignment, estimated the effective magnetic fields acting on many nuclei, such as In, Sb, Ir, and Au. Alignment in anti-ferromagnetic materials has also been detected.

(ii) In certain paramagnetic single crystals at low temperatures, the effect of the crystalline electronic field is to produce highly aligned orbitals and spins in the paramagnetic ions with respect to the crystalline axis. The resulting magnetic and electric quadrupole fields at the nuclei are correspondingly oriented and will lead to a nuclear orientation at low temperatures, even without an external magnetic field. We note that because of time reversal invariance associated with electric fields, only alignment (symmetry between +z and -z) can be achieved in the absence of an external field. A full discussion of the method would involve the detailed consideration of the full spin Hamiltonian in a crystalline solid, elaborated in Chap. 1 by Prof. Bleaney, who first proposed this approach. The method has been particularly fruitful for orientating many rare-earth nuclei in their paramagnetic salts.

(iii) Similar situations exist in certain crystals, whereby the strongly aligned electric quadrupole interaction alone may produce, at low temperatures, appreciable alignment.

(iv) At very low temperature, paramagnetic ions in solids can be polarized in a relatively small external field (say 1000 Oe at 0.01°K). The internal magnetic fields at the nuclei in these ions may then be large enough to polarize and usually also align the nuclei.

Methods (i) and (ii) have the advantage of not needing such low temperatures. For example, holmium nuclei in ferromagnetic holmium has been polarized at temperatures as high as 1°K. *

A method for detecting the degree of nuclear polarization, which is especially suitable for non-radioactive nuclei, is that of measuring the transmission by a sample of material containing polarized nuclei, of a beam of slow mono-energetic polarized neutrons of energy appropriate to a suitable resonance level in the compound nucleus, formed by neutron capture (kinetic energies of the order of electron volts). The transmission of such a beam of polarized thermal neutrons through a polarized ensemble of nuclei will depend on the relative directions of the neutron and nuclear polarizations.

One may easily see this through the following example. Let us assume a target which contains an ensemble of completely oriented nuclei with spin I. Since very low energy neutrons cannot transmit orbital angular momentum to a capturing resonance state (in other words — we have only "s wave" capture, or scattering) the only levels of the compound nucleus formed by the neutron capture in the target nuclei are those with $I' = I \pm 1/2$, since the intrinsic spin of the neutron is $1/2$. Assume further, that there exists only a resonance level having a spin $I' = I + 1/2$ which can be excited with the mono-energetic neutrons. Then we will obtain appreciably high absorption when the spins of the incident neutrons are parallel to those of the target nuclei, as compared with a rather low absorption when they are antiparallel.

In practice one uses a reactor to prepare a neutron beam of known degree of polarization (produced in general by reflection from a cobalt mirror) having an energy adequate for exciting a known resonance in the compound nucleus. High polarizations approaching 100 percent can be obtained today. By comparing the

*See discussion of its nuclear specific heat in Chap. 10.

transmission of the neutrons when polarized in the two directions, one may calculate the degree of orientation of the target.

The Oak Ridge and Brookhaven groups (see for example, Postma et al., 1962) have done experiments of this type on a variety of nuclei. In recent years experiments have been extended to rare-earth nuclei in a variety of salts, metals, and alloys. Thus the magnitude and sign of the magnetic hyperfine fields in Eu, Gd, and Ho metals have been studied by these methods.

B. "After" and Recoil Effects in γ-Ray Angular Distribution Measurements

One of the frequently debated questions related to perturbed angular distributions is that of the importance, or otherwise, of "after-effects" associated with the preceding radioactive decay or with the "recoil" accompanying a nuclear decay or a nuclear reaction. If our purpose, in experiments, is basically to determine hyperfine interactions obtaining in the normal solid, characteristic of atoms or ions in their normal state and in the normal lattice positions, then clearly, in principle, the question is an important one, since the radioactive decay or nuclear reaction may lead to the production of an ion in some state other than the normal state, and at some peculiar lattice site, interstitial or otherwise, particularly when recoil energies are large. Then one may obtain hyperfine interactions which are not characteristic of the normal state.

In practice, judging from empirical observation, it seems that these "radiation damage" effects are fortunately not at all serious in most cases, at least following *radioactive decay*. We have convincing proof of this in an increasing number of examples, where, for example, good agreement is obtained between the measurement of a nuclear moment of an excited state based on a P. A. C. measurement and the moment of the same state as measured by the Mössbauer splittings in absorbers containing the normal ions. (Note that radiation effects may be important in Mössbauer *sources*, as opposed to absorbers, in which in general, there is no radioactivity.) The Mössbauer effect, by the very nature of the recoil-free process, must leave the ion or atom involved, and in fact the whole lattice in the same initial quantum state obtaining before emission or absorption; there can, therefore, be no doubt that hyperfine interactions measured by the Mössbauer effect must be those characteristic of the normal state. In the case of ferromagnetic and ferrimagnetic materials there are similarly an increasing number of cases where the same hyperfine field is obtained in P. A. C. measurements as in other measurements (Mössbauer,

NMR) not involving possible after-effects. Since hyperfine fields in such materials are sensitive to magnitudes of exchange interactions and exchange intervals, which in their turn, must surely be very sensitive to small changes of position, we conclude that any such changes in position due to recoil must be very small. * The recoil energies (for a medium size nucleus, say $A \sim 100$), in radioactive decay, may be of the order of several eV or less. It seems that these energies are too small to lead to displacement or a serious change in the state of the ions involved. Of crucial importance is the time scale. Although immediately after the decay, there may be quite serious changes produced by the shock of the decay (particularly in the case of K electron-capture, when a hole is produced in the K-shell — this "hole" travels outwards in a succession of Auger transitions, leaving initially, at any rate, a highly ionized state), it seems these changes are "healed" in a time short compared to the lifetime of the excited state concerned ($10^{-10} \sim 10^{-6}$ sec). This is not at all surprising in metal environments, where the conduction electrons must help to heal rapidly. But the healing seems fairly rapid ($< 10^{-9}$ sec) even in insulators, as a rule. This is lucky for the game! However, there is still a lurking suspicion among some workers concerning these radiation effects in P. A. C. measurements. Metals may now be considered to be very safe, however, and even in insulators these effects, if present, are far less serious than once thought.

We leave until the next section remarks concerning these recoil or after effects occurring in Coulomb excitation recoil implantation experiments.

C. Coulomb Excitation and Other Implantation Techniques

We have discussed in the early part of this chapter the exceedingly anisotropic angular distributions occurring in the angular distribution of Coulomb excited γ-rays in coincidence with back-scattered projectile nuclei from the 2+ states of even-even deformed nuclei, when there are no perturbations acting on the

---

*This argument is perhaps a stronger one in the case of insulators than for metals. The theoretical origin of ferromagnetism in metals is still obscure, and perhaps long range effects may tend to reduce the strong dependence of exchange integrals on position suggested here. There is little experimental or theoretical work bearing on this problem, which surely must be of interest from the point of view of ferromagnetic theory.

nuclear excited state. * In the presence of perturbing fields, the anisotropy will be attenuated. In view of the initial high anisotropy, the angular distributions are highly sensitive to the perturbations. In these experiments the excited nuclei are ejected from the target (if thin enough) in the forward direction with considerable energy (several MeV or more in typical experiments), and may be directed into any material situated behind the target. Usually the target material is a thin evaporated layer on the matrix, into which one wishes to embed the recoil nuclei. A number of experiments of this kind (Grodzins et al. , 1966; Boehm et al. , 1966; Gilad et al. , 1966) have been carried out in order to measure the internal fields acting on deformed rare earth nuclei injected into various metals, particularly ferromagnetic iron. Figure 8 shows a graph of results for rare earth ions implanted in this way in iron, as obtained by Boehm et al. (1966). The fields are large and positive in the first half of the shell and negative in the second half. It is not yet clear to what extent quadrupole interactions are important after implantation in cubic metals. Clear evidence for quadrupole interactions in cubic metals would indicate, of course, that a large fraction of recoils end up on asymmetric interstitial sites rather than substitutional sites.

DeWaard and Drentje (1965) and others have used a beam of radioactive ions in a mass-spectrometer to inject radioactive

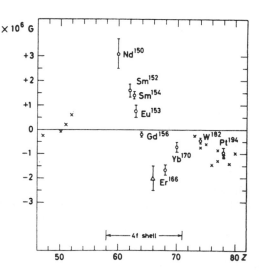

Fig. 8: Internal magnetic fields acting on rare-earth ions (and beyond) in iron, as obtained from Coulomb excitation implantation experiment.

*See also D. Murnick, Chap. S.2.

nuclei into ferromagnetic metals for Mössbauer and P. A. C. experiments, this being another way of avoiding chemical and metallurgical problems in the preparation of sources.

In fact, one of the powerful advantages of these implantation techniques is that they permit one to choose the embedding matrix at will, independent of chemical and metallurgical problems connected with the preparation of dilute alloys or with substitution in insulators. One might hope, therefore, that the technique might be applied to a variety of solid state problems. In the Coulomb excitation implantation method, it should not be difficult to vary and control the temperature of the matrix into which the recoils are shot, to even quite low temperature, provided metals are used for the target. All this will be valuable, of course, provided further experiment confirms the present impression that the recoils end-up in metals for the most part as substitutional ions and not as interstitials. However, it is too early to generalize in this respect and we need further data. To quote from a very recent publication by Borchers et al. (1966), "There are several instances where internal fields have been investigated both with alloys and with implantation technique. For Pt in Fe, fields are the same within 10 to 20 percent. For W in Fe, Mössbauer experiments yield 705 kilogauss which is much higher than 455 kilogauss observed with implantation. For Te in Fe the results are similar." It seems too early to generalize, but it looks as if, in many cases, if not all, the recoil ions end up substitutionally.

One interesting problem which could perhaps be tackled by these methods in a systematic way, might be an investigation into the variation of spin relaxation times of dilute paramagnetic ions in diamagnetic metals at low temperatures. For the case of paramagnetic ions having large hyperfine fields (e. g. rare-earths) one anticipates that the time-dependent perturbations will not average to zero at low enough temperatures if the relaxation times are not very short indeed ($<10^{-13}$ sec). (Such P. A. C. experiments are, of course, possible without resorting to Coulomb excitation implantation. One might incorporate radioactive paramagnetic ions in metals, using chemical or metallurgical techniques, in certain cases.) Figure 9 shows a plot based on the theory of magnetic time-dependent perturbations mentioned earlier, of the integral attenuation factor G_2 (∞) as a function of the ion relaxation time τ_s, for the paramagnetic Dy^{3+} ion, for which the instantaneous value H_{eff} is about 7×10^6 gauss. We indeed see that

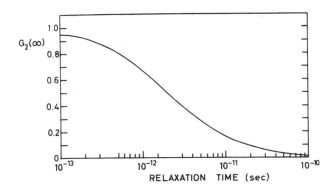

Fig. 9: $G_2(\infty)$ as a function of paramagnetic relaxation time for
instantaneous $H_{eff} \sim 7 \times 10^6$ gauss.

measurable attenuations $[G_2(\infty) \sim 0.9]$ are obtained even for τ_S
as short as 10^{-13} sec. In fact, investigations seem possible in
the range of τ_S between 10^{-13} and 10^{-11}. We know of no other
method capable of measuring such short relaxation times.

D. Possibilities for Research into Hyperfine Fields in Superconductors

We mention a few problems concerning the properties of
superconductors which are of considerable interest and which, it
seems to us, could be usefully studied using the techniques described in these lectures.

(i) The distribution of internal magnetic fields in Type II
superconductors accompanying the Abrikosov-type lattice of flux
vortices postulated to account for the properties of these superconductors in magnetic fields above the first critical field H_{C_1}.
We would then expect a distribution of internal fields f(H) associated with the lattice of quantized fluxoids. Such an inhomogeneous
field distribution could be measured by introducing dilute diamagnetic radioactive nuclei, for which the distribution of Larmor
precession frequencies can be measured using the time dependent
angular correlation technique discussed earlier. The nuclear
cascade in Rh^{100} would seem to be very appropriate for this purpose, because of the high sensitivity to small fields (large nuclear
moment and relatively long lifetime in the intermediate nuclear
state). Such experiments have been proposed by the author and
are now being pursued (Alonso, 1966). In principle, the Mössbauer

nuclei could also be used as a probe for measuring such inhomogeneous fields. However the resolution available with known
Mössbauer isotopes does not seem to be good enough for use in
such experiments.

There may be advantages in using dilute nuclei in paramagnetic ions as probes for measuring the internal field distribution
in such problems, and exploiting the "paramagnetic magnification"
of the external field which will occur, particularly at low temperatures. However, one must then beware of inhomogeneities in
the "magnification" due to crystalline field effects in polycrystalline
samples.

(ii) Measurements of spin relaxation time of paramagnetic
ions in superconductors. Transition rates, in general, change
in going from the normal to superconducting state in BCS theory.
For example, nuclear relaxation times show large and interesting
changes. Provided, as indicated earlier, relaxation times of
paramagnetic ions in metals are not too fast ($> 10^{-13}$ sec) one
might expect to follow such changes by measuring the change of
time-dependent perturbations with temperatures, as we go through
the transition temperature.

(iii) Study of the possible simultaneous co-existence of ferromagnetism and superconductivity. Speculations have been made
concerning such a possibility for certain alloy systems, but the
experimental situation is still most obscure, and no direct proof
of such a "co-existence" has yet been forthcoming.

E. Magnetic Hyperfine Interactions in Ordered Magnetic Solids

Using a variety of techniques, including P. A. C., fairly extensive studies have been made of the internal hyperfine magnetic
fields acting on dilute impurity ions dissolved in the 3d ferromagnetic metals — iron, cobalt, and nickel. This subject has recently
been reviewed by Shirley and Westenbarger (1965). Studies in
ferrimagnetic insulators, particularly the rare earth iron garnets
have been made, using P. A. C. techniques by Caspari et al. (1962)
and by Cohen and Gilat (1962).

The P. A. C. technique has in recent years been used in
Jerusalem to measure the internal fields acting on diamagnetic impurities in the rare-earth metals. The magnetic fields acting on
lutecium and hafnium nuclei have been measured within ferromagnetic gadolinium, terbium, dysprosium, holmium, and erbium.
One measurement has been made using as a host dysprosium metal
in the antiferromagnetic state. For ferromagnetic host metals the

sign of the internal magnetic field was measured in each case. We describe this work in some detail, in order to illustrate some typical problems, and the usefulness of different experimental approaches (Cohen et al. , 1964).

It is generally believed that the ferromagnetic interactions in the pure rare-earth metals, which are known to have a long range character, are essentially indirect interactions between the localized 4f electrons via the conduction electrons. While a number of important theoretical studies have been made on the nature of this indirect interaction and the 4f conduction electron interaction, its precise nature is still to some extent undetermined. In particular, the sign of this spin dependent 4f conduction electron interaction has not yet been unambiguously fixed. However, according to this general picture, one would expect an appreciable extent of spin polarization of the conduction electrons in the ferromagnetic state. The s conduction electrons, if polarized, should then make a serious contribution to the hyperfine field acting on the impurity nuclei, through the Fermi contact interaction. Using a particular model for the s-f interaction — the Kasuya-Yosida theory, which has had a great success in accounting for many detailed properties of the rare-earth metals — one can estimate the local polarization at a particular impurity site in terms of the basic effective exchange integral J_{s-f} acting between the 4f electrons and the s-conduction electrons. * (The Kasuya-Yosida model of course predicts in general a non-homogeneous polarization of the conduction electrons.) It is therefore to be expected that from the sign and magnitude of the observed hyperfine fields one might be able to draw conclusions concerning the sign and magnitude of J_{s-f}, provided, of course, that other contributions to the hyperfine interactions are small.

The 208 - 113 keV γ-γ cascade of Hf^{177} and the 282 - 114 keV cascade of Lu^{175} used in this work were produced in the β-decay of Lu^{177} (half-life 6. 8 days) and Yb^{175} (half-life 101 hours). The mean lives and the nuclear gyromagnetic ratios for the intermediate states are known. For the 113 keV state of Hf^{177}, τ = $(8. 3 \pm 0. 4) \times 10^{-10}$ sec and g = 0. 235 ± 0. 02. For the 114 keV state of Lu^{175}, $\tau = (1. 36 \pm 0. 15) \times 10^{-10}$ sec and g = 0. 49 ± 0. 05. The angular correlation of the 208 - 113 keV cascade of Hf^{177} for a source in the form of an aqueous solution has previously been measured and found to be: $W(\theta) = 1 - (0. 121 \pm 0. 007) \cos 2\theta$. For the 282 - 114 keV cascade of Lu^{175}, the angular correlation

*See discussion by R.E. Watson, Chap. 9.

function obtained in previous measurements was $1 + (0.145 \pm 0.010) \cos 2\theta$.

With a magnetic field directed normal to the correlation plane, the integral angular correlation function has the form (neglecting terms higher than b_2),

$$W(\theta, \pm H) = 1 + \frac{b_2 (\cos 2\theta \mp 2\omega\tau \sin \theta)}{1 + (2\omega\tau)^2} \tag{53}$$

where $\omega = g\mu_n H/\hbar$ (g is the gyromagnetic ratio corresponding to the intermediate level, b_2 is the coefficient of $\cos 2\theta$ for the unperturbed correlation and H is the magnetic field).

For sufficiently soft magnetic materials, in the presence of an external magnetic field, the internal field will be parallel to the external field. For such cases, the above formula is valid and ω is given by $g\mu_n H_{tot}/\hbar$ where H_{tot} is the sum of the external magnetic field, the local dipolar field and the internal magnetic field H_{eff} acting on the nuclei ($H_{tot} = H_{ext} + H_{dip} + H_{eff}$).

The following techniques were used in the present work in order to determine ω:

(i) The coincidence rate $C(H, \theta)$ produced by the relevant cascade at $\theta = 135°$ was measured for the two possible directions of the external magnetic field, up and down (H+ and H-), then

$$R = 2 \frac{C(H^+, 135°) - C(H^-, 135°)}{C(H^+, 135°) + C(H^-, 135°)}$$

$$= (2b_2)(2\omega\tau)/[1 + (2\omega\tau)^2] \tag{54}$$

was determined. Most of the rare-earth metals used in the present work are magnetically hard. With polycrystalline samples the full magnetization corresponding to the temperature of the measurement is not obtained even in the presence of strong external magnetic fields. For these metals the domains are not magnetized in the same direction and there exists an angular distribution of the directions of H_{eff} relative to H_{ext} which depends on the magnitude of H_{ext} and on temperature. It can be shown that ω can still be determined quite accurately if this technique is used for hard ferromagnetic materials, so long as $\omega\tau$ is not large. The relation which is approximately correct in these cases is

$$R = 2 \, \frac{C(H^+, \, 135°) - C(H^-, \, 135°)}{C(H^+, \, 135°) + C(H^-, \, 135°)}$$

$$= 2b_2 \, (M/M_s) \, 2\omega\tau/[(1 + (2\omega\tau)^2] \tag{55}$$

where M is the bulk-magnetization of the sample, which is a function of temperature and H_{ext}, and M_s is the saturation magnetization at the temperature of measurement (i. e. the magnetization obtaining if all the domains were oriented in the direction of H_{ext}).

(ii) For magnetically soft hosts, the anisotropy of the angular correlation was measured in the presence of an external magnetic field directed perpendicular to the correlation plane, then the anisotropy X is given by

$$X = 2 \, \frac{C(H, \, 180°) - C(H, \, 90°)}{C(H, \, 180°) + C(H, \, 90°)}$$

$$= 2b_2/[1 + (2\omega\tau)^2] \quad . \tag{56}$$

ω can be derived from the measured value of the anisotropy.

(iii) Measurement of the anisotropy of the angular correlation without the application of any external magnetic field: the absolute value of H_{eff} is assumed to be the same for all the domains of the ferromagnetic sample which are randomly orientated. No preferred direction exists in the source considered as a whole. The perturbed correlation (assuming that additional perturbations are negligible) was given in Eqs. (15) with G_k defined in Eq. (43). We terminate the series at k = 2 and G_2 is given in Eq. (44) where $\omega = g\mu_n H_{tot}/\hbar$ is the Larmor frequency corresponding to the full magnetic interaction in each domain and is a function of temperature and can be determined from the measurement of the attenuation factor G_2.

The sensitivities of the three methods described depend on the values of $\omega\tau$ and of $M(T)/M_s(T)$. For most cases in the present work, at least two of the techniques described were independently used for the determination of ω. The sign of H_{eff} can be determined only from measurements in which the first technique is used.

Most measurements were carried out with a Lu^{177} source which was prepared by neutron irradiation of pure lutecium metal. The radioactive source was introduced homogeneously into samples of Gd, Tb, Dy, Ho, and Er metals by induction melting the metals in a tantalum crucible; the atomic concentration of lutecium in the samples varied between 0.3 to 0.8 percent. One set of measurements was performed with a Yb^{175} source decaying to Lu^{175}, which was produced by neutron irradiation of ytterbium metal; the radioactive ytterbium was introduced homogeneously into gadolinium metal at an atomic concentration of 7×10^{-4}. The samples used were prepared in the form of thin needles and held perpendicular to the correlation plane. For all the sources that were used, the angular correlations were also measured at temperatures above their Curie and Neel temperatures. The angular correlations for the various sources were identical within the statistical errors.

Figure 10 shows the temperature dependence of H_{eff} acting on Hf^{177} and on Lu^{175} in gadolinium. The values of H_{eff} were obtained from those of H_{tot} after correcting for the small contributions of the external magnetic field (when applied) and the local dipolar field $-4\pi M/3$ (this is a good approximation for an hexagonal lattice). The errors shown in Fig. 10 do not include the possible errors in the values of g and τ, as these errors are not relevant for the comparison of the values of H_{eff} at the same nucleus for various hosts and temperatures. Figure 11 shows the dependence of the saturation effective field, acting on Hf^{177} nuclei, on the spin S of the ions of the host rare-earth metal.

The following general conclusions can be drawn from the experimental results: (a) in all cases for which the sign could be measured H_{eff} is negative, i.e. opposite to the magnetization; (b) in the case of Gd as host metal the magnitude of H_{eff} follows well the magnetization with changing temperature; (c) the magnitude of H_{eff} acting on Hf^{177} nuclei seems to vary linearly with spin S of the ferromagnetic host metal (S for the second half of the rare-earth group also equals the projection of the total angular momentum along the magnetization axis in the fully aligned state), but the curve in Fig. 11 does not pass through the origin, indicating perhaps more than one contribution to the effective fields, of quite different character; (d) at saturation in gadolinium host metal, H_{eff} acting on Hf nuclei seems to be rather greater than on lutecium (380 as compared with 200 kilogauss) although the errors are rather large; (e) in the only case in which a measurement was carried out on an impurity in an antiferromagnetic host (dysprosium at 125°K) a very small value of H_{eff} acting on Hf^{177} was found [$H_{eff} = (0 \pm 50)$ kOe]. We shall not discuss the theoretical implications of these results here, but refer again to the original paper (Cohen et al., 1964).

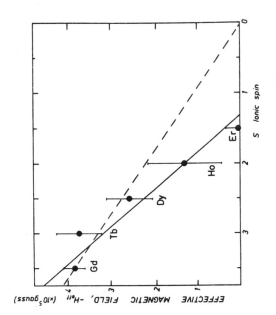

Fig. 11: Dependence of the saturation effective field acting on Hf^{177} nuclei, on the spin S of the ions of the host rare-earth metal.

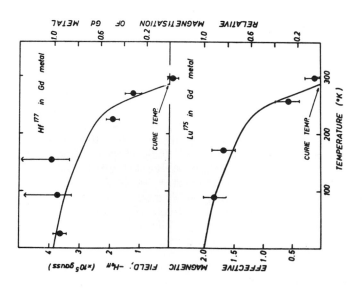

Fig. 10: Temperature dependence of Heff acting on Lu^{175} and Hf^{177} in gadolinium.

V. Conclusion

Finally, we close with some general remarks concerning the advantages and disadvantages of the P. A. C. methods for investigating hyperfine interactions in solids, including a comparison with other techniques, particularly the Mössbauer technique. The two methods both have in common the utilization of nuclear radiations — in particular nuclear γ-rays.

1. We first note that the two methods may be combined. We mentioned earlier in these lectures, that we expect the angular distribution of resonance scattered radiation (including recoil-free scattering as a special case) to be anisotropic — the scattering is formally analogous to a γ-γ coincidence angular correlation. We will then expect an attenuation of the anisotropy of the scattered radiation if hyperfine interactions perturb the excited nuclear state which emits the scattered radiations; we may also expect a simple rotation of the angular distribution for the case of a magnetic field acting at the nuclei, perpendicular to the scattering plane. Knowing the lifetime of the state, hyperfine interactions may be derived from the experimentally observed attenuations or rotations (Chow et al., 1965). A recent theoretical paper (Gorbel and McVoy, 1966) deals with the calculation of Larmor precession frequencies from measurements of the angle of rotation of angular distributions in such experiments. The results are somewhat surprising, at first sight, and show that one must be very careful in interpretation. The authors show that in general the angle of rotation is not simply given by the product of the Larmor angular precession frequency ω and the mean-life τ, but also involves the bandwidth Δ of the incident wave-packet. The rotation varies from $\omega\tau$, for $\Delta << \Gamma$ (Γ is natural width of the excited state) to $2\omega\tau$ for $\Delta >> \Gamma$. When the incident radiation is recoil-free and emitted from an ideal source, $\Delta = \Gamma$ and then the rotation equals $1.5\,\omega\tau$.

2. Hyperfine interactions obtained using the recoil-free technique are usually displayed in the recoil-free spectrum in a very direct and explicit way. We can often infer the nature of the interaction directly from the spectrum, without being biased by previous knowledge or some theory. This is less true in the case of angular correlations. To the extent that the *time-dependent* attenuation can be measured, then indeed the form of the time-dependence of the coefficients $G_k(t)$ does give us some detailed information concerning the hyperfine interaction, but it is not so directly inferred. However, the situation is far worse in the case of an integral attenuation or rotation measurement, and the results can only be interpreted if we have a priori knowledge or

intuition concerning the hyperfine interactions responsible for the attenuation or rotation. *Usually, we need to know what is happening, qualitatively, and then we can infer quantitative information from the measurement.*

3. A few words concerning resolution and sensitivity. Suppose we consider a nuclear excited state which, in principle, could be involved either in a recoil-free experiment, or as an intermediate state in a P. A. C. measurement. Then the limiting energy resolution or bandwidth for *both* experiments is essentially determined by the uncertainty principle and will be the natural width of the level in question, i. e., $\Gamma = \hbar/\tau$, where τ is the mean-life. Of course, in a detailed analysis there may be other factors (geometric or others) affecting the comparative resolution, but these will, in general, be of the order of unity. In a Mössbauer experiment, one could, often, probably without undue difficulty, measure to 10 percent of a linewidth; in a Larmor precession measurement, this would correspond to measuring an angle of rotation equal to 10 percent of one radian i. e. 6°, which again would be rather easy.

But of course, usually we cannot employ the same radio-active species for both types of experiments. In fact, we have a far greater choice of nuclear states available for P. A. C. measurements. In order to get appreciable recoil-free efficiencies in Mössbauer experiments we are limited to low-energy transitions (say less than 150 keV). There is no such energy limitation in angular correlation experiments. It turns out that there are a number of relatively long-lived states, which can be employed as intermediate states in P. A. C. measurements, and which provide rather precise and not inconvenient probes for the measurement of magnetic hyperfine interactions and magnetic fields. (If we wish to measure small magnetic fields, then, of course, a large nuclear magnetic moment helps.) Mössbauer experiments with long-lived states, however, are limited to fewer potential nuclei and are fraught with great difficulties. In general, neither of these methods provides the resolution usually obtainable in NMR; the latter are usually carried out on stable nuclei which have an infinitely long mean-life and hence are infinitely narrow in width. The experimental resolution is then determined by other factors. The energy resolution in the recent NMR experiments on excited or unstable nuclear states, using nuclear radiation detection of the resonance, will be again limited by the width of the states involved. To the extent they are done on long-lived states (e. g. in nuclear polarization experiments) the resolution attainable may be very good.

4. Integral angular correlation measurements break down for very high hyperfine fields, since the rotation angle becomes larger than 2π, and the accompanying attenuation wipes out the anisotropy. In time-dependent correlation experiments, we are again limited at high fields, when the period for one oscillation of the angular correlation — time curve becomes less than the time resolution of the electronic circuits ($\sim 10^{-9}$ sec). There is no such limitation in recoil-free measurements of large hyperfine fields.

5. In view of the great sensitivity of radioactive measurements, P. A. C. measurements and nuclear orientation angular distribution measurements often enable one to introduce the radioactive nuclei into the solid in a state of very high dilution. In cases where we are particularly interested in dilute systems — for example, dilute alloys — these methods present a considerable advantage. Recoil-free hyperfine splittings are usually measured in an *absorber*, and there will be a minimum concentration of the isotope which can be used in order to get measurable effects; this will only rarely be less than a few percent and may often be greater. A dilution two or three orders of magnitude smaller, may often be attainable in P. A. C. measurements.

6. P. A. C. measurements seem to be potentially useful in measuring very short spin relaxation times, especially when the instantaneous hyperfine fields are large.

7. The new Coulomb-excitation experiments permit one to inject recoil radioactive nuclei in any desired solid matrix. This can be useful for both perturbed angular distribution and Mössbauer experiments.

8. Isomer shifts can only be measured in recoil-free spectra.

9. Recoil-free measurements of hyperfine splittings in absorbers are free from radiation damage effects. In principle this is not necessarily true for P. A. C. measurements. Nevertheless, in practice this does not seem to be generally troublesome.

Acknowledgements

My task in preparing these lectures has been considerably lightened by the existence of excellent and comprehensive recent reviews of the whole subject of angular correlations, particularly those by Frauenfelder and Steffen and Alder and Steffen, which I recommend for more details concerning some of the subjects discussed here.

I also wish to thank Ram Avida and Hagai Zmora for their help and assistance in preparing this chapter.

References

Alonso, J. (1966). Private communication.

Boehm, F., Hagemann, G. B., and Winter, A. (1966). Physics Letters 21, 217.

Borchers, R., Bronson, J. D., Murnick, D. E., and Grodzins, L. (1966). Phys. Rev. Letters 17, 1099.

Caspari, M., Frankel, S., and Wood, G. (1962). Phys. Rev. 127, 1514.

Chow, Y. W., Grodzins, L., and Barrett, P. A. (1965). Phys. Rev. Letters 15, 369.

Cohen, S. G., and Gilat, G. (1962). Nucl. Phys. 38, 1.

Cohen, S. G., Ofer, S., and Kaplan, N. (1964). Proceedings of the International Conference on Magnetism (Nottingham, England), p. 233.

De Waard, H. and Drentje, S. A. (1965). Phys. Letters 20, 38.

Dillenburg, D. and Maris, Th. A. J. (1962). Nucl. Phys. 33, 1962.

Gilad, P., Goldring, G., Kalish, R., and Herber, R. (1966). Phys. Rev. 151, 281.

Gorbel, G. T. and McVoy, K. W. (1966). Phys. Rev. 148, 1021.

Grodzins, L., Borchers, R., and Hagemann, G. B., (1966). Phys. Letters 21, 214.

Matthias, E., Shirley, D. A., Klein, M. P., and Edelstein, N. (1966). Phys. Rev. Letters 16, 974.

Postma, H., Marshak, H., Sailov, V. L., Shore, F. J., and Reynolds, C. A. (1962). Phys. Rev. 126, 979.

Samoilov, B. N., Sklyarevskii, V. V., and Stepanov, E. P. (1959). Zh. Eksperim. i Teor. Fiz. 36, 644; [Soviet Phys. -JETP 36, 448]

Shirley, D. A. and Westenbarger, G. A. (1965). Phys. Rev. 138, A170.

General References

Abragam, A. and Pound, R. V. (1953). "Influence of Electric and Magnetic Fields on Angular Correlations," Phys. Rev. 92, 943.

Alder, K. and Steffen, R. M. (1964). "Electromagnetic Moments of Excited Nuclear States," Ann. Rev. Nucl. Sci. 14, 403.

De Groot, S. R. , Tolhoek, H. A. , and Huiskamp, W. J. (1965). "Orientation of Nuclei at Low Temperatures," α-β-λ-Ray Spectroscopy, edited by Kai Siegbahn (North Holland).

Frauenfelder, H. and Steffen, R. M. (1965). "Angular Correlations," α-β-γ-Ray Spectroscopy, edited by Kai Siegbahn (North Holland).

Freeman, A. J. and Watson, R. E. (1965). "Hyperfine Interactions in Magnetic Materials," Magnetism Vol. IIA, edited by T. Rado and H. Suhl (Academic Press).

Heer, E. and Novey, T. B. (1959). "The Interdependence of Solid State Physics and Angular Distribution of Nuclear Radiations," Solid State Physics 9, p. 199, editors F. Seitz and D. Turnbull (Academic Press).

Karlsson, E. , Matthias, E. , and Siegbahn, K. , Editors (1964). Perturbed Angular Correlations (North-Holland Publ. Co. , Amsterdam).

Steffen, R. M. (1955). "Extranuclear Effects on Angular Correlations of Nuclear Radiations," Adv. Phys. 4 293.

13. RECENT APPLICATIONS OF PERTURBED ANGULAR CORRELATIONS

E. Matthias

*University of California
Lawrence Radiation Laboratory* *
Berkeley, California

Table of Contents

Supported by the United States Atomic Energy Commission.

595

I. Introduction

The purpose of this brief review is to sketch the recent experimental development in the field of perturbed angular correlations (PAC).* Considerable progress has been made during the past three years. In particular, three types of experiments have had a great impact on the whole field concerned with measurements of electromagnetic moments and hyperfine interactions of short-lived nuclear levels:

(i) Implantation of recoil atoms into ferromagnetic lattices following Coulomb excitation (Grodzins et al., 1966; Boehm et al., 1966; Gilad et al., 1966). Combined with a systematic knowledge of magnetic hyperfine fields, it will be possible to measure g-factors for the short-lived first vibrational and second rotational states.

(ii) NMR in radioactive states with half lives down to 10^{-8} s using angular correlations or distributions to detect the resonance. For short half lives (10^{-3} s to 10^{-8} s), the experiment has to be performed by making use of some kind of intrinsic enhancement of the external rf field (Matthias et al., 1966a). For half lives longer than 10^{-3} s, the externally applied rf amplitude is sufficient to destroy the angular distribution directly (Sugimoto et al., 1965; 1966). The basic problem in all these experiments, however, is that the polarization of the nuclei has to be preserved for times longer than the lifetime of the state in order to obtain a detectable destruction effect of the rf on the angular distribution.

(iii) Reorientation effects in Coulomb excitation (de Boer et al., 1965) which provides a means to measure quadrupole moments of excited nuclear states without relying on calculated electric field gradients or nuclear models.

We will discuss here some conventional perturbed angular correlation methods, but mainly the development of radioactive NMR detection.** For a detailed and complete description of all conventional methods, the reader is referred to the articles by Steffen and Frauenfelder (1964, 1965).

Perturbed angular correlation measurements with radioactive isotopes and perturbed angular distributions of gamma rays following Coulomb excitation have been widely used to determine magnetic

---

* For an introduction to PAC, see S.G. Cohen, Chap. 12.
** For a discussion of the recoil implantation method, see D. Murnick, Chap. S.2.

moments of short-lived excited, nuclear states. Systematic nuclear information has been gathered for g_R-factors of the first excited rotational states in deformed nuclei and for g-factors of first excited vibrational states in spherical nuclei. Although the PAC technique has been applied to the investigation of hyperfine fields, the information obtained in this way is to date far from systematic. In most of the experiments, the approach was rather to determine the nuclear g-factor by using the known value for the magnetic hyperfine field, obtained from either Mössbauer effect or nuclear magnetic resonance studies.

Apart from a few exceptions, all the work with perturbed angular correlations or distributions has been carried out with short-lived states with half lives in the nanosecond or sub-nanosecond range, where the accuracy is limited by the small rotation angles of the correlation pattern. It is recognized, on the other hand, that for half lives long enough to employ the time-differential method, good accuracy, of the order of one percent, can be obtained. The precision with which interaction frequencies can be measured improves with increasing half life. Surprisingly enough, however, there has not yet been one measurement on a state with a half life longer than 500 nsec. Until the present time, no method for measuring magnetic moments has been proved to work for isomeric states with half lives between 10^{-6} s and 1 s. It seems feasible, however, that the PAC method could be applied at least up to the millisecond range. Although only a limited number of states with lifetimes in this range are known to be populated by cascading radioactive decay, many more isomeric levels can be conveniently produced by nuclear reactions. The generally non-isotropic angular distribution of gamma rays following the reaction process lends itself to either spin rotation or NMR experiments. The basic difficulty of all measurements involving long-lived levels will be to preserve the nuclear orientation for times longer than the half life.

The applicability of the method of perturbed angular correlations and distributions for different half-life ranges is illustrated in Fig. 1. The experiment of Sugimoto et al. (1965, 1966) proved that the polarization of the product nuclei in nuclear reactions can, under special circumstances, be preserved up to about 10 sec, which makes it possible to use the angular distribution as a detector for the NMR in the isomeric states. For the long-lived isomers, it is hoped that the range can be extended up to the half lives where nuclear orientation and atomic beam measurements become possible. Time differential spin rotation measurements will dominate in the region 10^{-6} s to 10^{-9} s, although some experiments with nuclear magnetic resonance in that range might be possible. For half lives

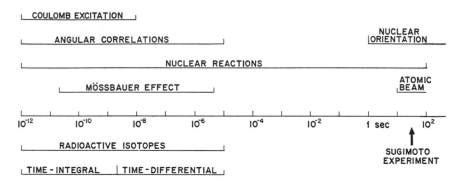

Fig. 1: Comparison of the applicability of different methods to different nuclear lifetime ranges.

shorter than 10^{-9} sec, only time-integral measurements can be performed. For low-lying excited states in which the recoilless resonance absorption is possible, Mössbauer effect measurements are in direct competition with PAC in the range 10^{-10} sec to 10^{-6} sec. In practice, however, both techniques are often complementary in their application.

II. Conventional Perturbed Angular Correlation Techniques

A. Time Integral Method

Time-integral perturbed angular correlations involve mean lives τ between 10^{-12} and 10^{-9} sec. * For very small rotations, the attenuation of the correlation is negligible and the angular shift of the correlation is $\Delta\theta \approx \omega_L \tau$, where ω_L is the Larmor precession frequency, i.e., the effect of the interaction on the angular correlation is linear. It is for these small values of $\omega_L \tau$ that the time-integral angular correlation is a very valuable method, in particular, when used together with the large internal fields in ferromagnetic hosts. The magnitude of the hyperfine fields permits one to measure magnetic moments for nuclear levels with half lives down to 10^{-12} sec. An example demonstrating the accuracy which can be obtained for the quantity $\omega_L \tau$ is shown in Fig. 2. **

---

* See E. Karlsson, Chap. S.1.
** We are grateful to Auerbach et al. (1966) for providing Fig. 2.

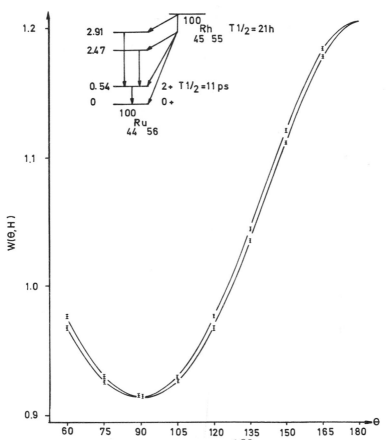

Fig. 2: Integral angular correlation for ^{100}Ru in iron measured by Auerbach et al. (1966). The rotation corresponds to $\omega\tau$ = $-(1.78 \pm 0.12) \times 10^{-2}$ rad, in a polarizing field of ± 10 kG.

This measurement for ^{100}Ru in Fe (Auerbach et al., 1966) gives $\omega_L\tau$ with an uncertainty of $\pm 6.7\%$. In spite of this accuracy for $\omega_L\tau$, the final result for the product $g \cdot H_{eff}$ has a much larger error, as the nuclear mean life τ is not known, in most cases, with a comparable accuracy and the final result for either the nuclear g-factor or the effective field usually carries a rather large error arising from the uncertainty in τ.

B. Time-Differential Method

Experimentally, the time-differential method is of great importance since the time-dependent observation of the interaction matrix elements

$$\langle m_b | \exp\left(-\frac{i}{\hbar}\mathcal{H}t\right) | m_a \rangle \langle m_b' | \exp\left(-\frac{i}{\hbar}\mathcal{H}t\right) | m_a' \rangle^*$$

allows one to obtain good accuracy for the interaction frequency. It is worth noting that the time-spectrum of the perturbed angular correlation is the Fourier transform of the frequency spectrum obtained in NMR. Both techniques are related by the Fourier-transformation

$$f(t) = \frac{1}{2\pi} \int_{-\infty}^{+\infty} g(\omega) \exp(i\omega t)\, d\omega ,$$

$$g(\omega) = \int_{-\infty}^{+\infty} f(t) \exp(-i\omega t)\, dt . \tag{1}$$

In the limit of a large number of rotations of the angular correlation pattern, the accuracy approaches that usually obtained in NMR work. But even with a few observed cycles, the time-differential method is far superior to all time-integral measurements not only because of higher accuracy, but also because it is independent of the mean life τ. Further, it shows directly any additional perturbation present in the source, either in form of amplitude damping or by the occurrence of several superimposed frequencies. A limitation imposed on the time-differential method is that the rotation of the angular correlation pattern should be sufficiently slow that the electronic resolving time, τ_0, permits one to distinguish between successive rotations, which means the condition $\omega_L \tau_0 < \pi$ has to be fulfilled. Very often, this makes it impossible to measure magnetic hyperfine fields in this way.

A typical example of a time-differential PAC measurement is shown in Fig. 3. From such data, the interaction frequency ω_L can be obtained with an accuracy much better than one percent, sufficient in some cases to reveal finer details as, for example, the Knight shift. It should be noticed that up to 1 μsec no attenuation of the angular correlation pattern is visible. This clearly demonstrates that cubic metal lattices are very suitable as perturbation-free host lattices up to the microsecond range. How useful the time-differential technique is for magnetic hyperfine fields becomes obvious from Fig. 4. Measurements can also be performed with randomly oriented magnetic fields as, for example, a completely unmagnetized ferromagnetic sample. In this particular case a superposition of frequencies is observed (Matthias et al., 1965a). An example for this is shown in Fig. 5. Here, the

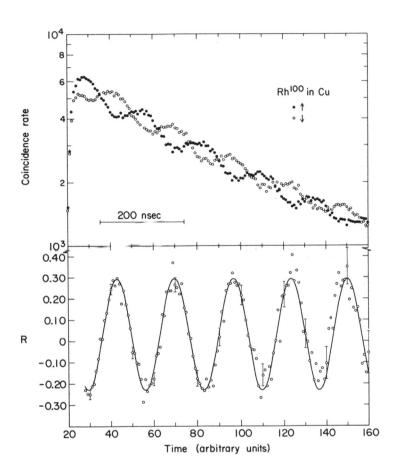

Fig. 3: Time-differential g-factor measurement with a source of
^{100}Rh in copper in an external field of ±2. 22 kG (Matthias
et al. , 1965b). Upper figure: raw data.   Lower figure:
ratios which eliminate exponential dependence.   The
weighted least-squares fit to the data   yields g =
+2. 160 ± 0. 006.

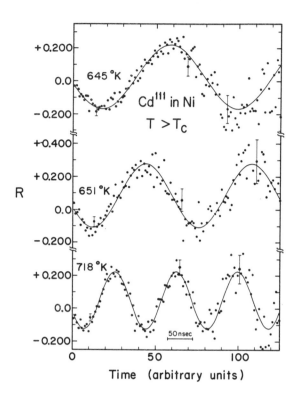

Fig. 4: Time-differential angular correlation for [111]Cd in nickel
above the Curie point in an external magnetic field of
19.6 kG (Rosenblum et al., 1967). The paramagnetic
correction factors for the three temperatures are:
$\beta(645°K) = 0.398 \pm 0.007$; $\beta(651°K) = 0.511 \pm 0.009$,
$\beta(718°K) = 0.879 \pm 0.011$.

frequency could be obtained with good accuracy from the time
spectrum taken at just one angle. For smaller amplitudes, however, one has to measure the anisotropy as a function of time.

C. Digital Analysis of Perturbed Angular Correlations

When trying to use the conventional time-differential method
on half lives longer than 1 μsec, one runs into the following basic
difficulties:(i) the source strength has to be reduced to keep the

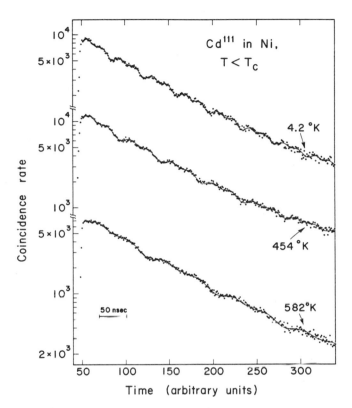

Fig. 5: Time-differential angular correlation for ^{111}Cd in Ni
below the Curie point (Rosenblum et al., 1967) at 180° and
no external polarizing field. The least-squares fit to the
data gives the interaction frequencies: $\omega(4.2°K) = 104.37 \pm$
0.21 MHz, $\omega(454°K) = 82.55 \pm 0.21$ MHz, $\omega(582°K) =$
49.77 ± 0.20 MHz.

ratio of true to accidental coincidences acceptable; (ii) the time
resolution of analog converters is limited and of the order of 1%
of the total time range; (iii) the limited time resolution requires
the use of low magnetic fields. In addition, one has the usual
problems with linearity, stability, and, in most instances, a
memory limitation in the analyzer. One experimental approach to
overcome most of the above weaknesses is a technique called "Digital
Analysis of Perturbed Angular Correlations" (DAPAC) (Matthias
and Shirley, 1966b). The principle is to obtain the data directly in
a digital form and to find the interaction frequency by calculating

the Fourier transform, Eq. (1), of the time spectrum. The use of a digital time-to-height converter automatically offers the advantages that the resolving time is independent of the time range used, there is practically no limitation in channel numbers, and it has perfect linearity and a much greater stability than analog systems. Further, the necessity of an accurate time calibration is completely avoided.

The data analysis is based on the fact that the Fourier transform of the time spectrum $W(t)$ is a function of frequency, $g(\nu)$, with the resonance frequency given by $\nu_L = 2gH(\mu_N/h)$. After normalization for the exponential decay, the time spectrum can be described by the function $W(t) = \Sigma_k A_k P_k [\cos(\theta_0 \pm \omega_L t)]$ for the case of an oriented magnetic dipole interaction. The even and odd parts of the Fourier transform are calculated separately,

$$A(\nu) = \int_{T_{min}}^{T_{max}} W(t) \sin 2\pi \nu t \, dt \;,$$

$$B(\nu) = \int_{T_{min}}^{T_{max}} W(t) \cos 2\pi \nu t \, dt \;. \qquad (2)$$

The phase is defined as

$$\varphi(\nu) = tg^{-1} \left[\frac{-A(\nu)}{B(\nu)} \right] ,$$

in accordance with the normal sign convention of the Fourier transform. This allows the determination of the sign of the magnetic dipole interaction for a certain detector geometry and field direction.

To illustrate this technique, two examples are shown in Figs. 6 and 7. The shift of the resonance in Fig. 7 is the Knight shift for ^{100}Rh in the three different metals. The most striking practical advantage of this method is that it is very time-saving. Since the analysis is based on a frequency search, it does not require such good statistical accuracy as is normally needed when a mathematical function is fitted to the data. Compared to the result of Figs. 6 and 7, it is possible to improve the signal-to-noise ratio more than an order of magnitude by using the autocorrelation function $C(T)/C(0)$ instead of $W(t)$ in Eq. (2). The autocorrelation technique smoothes the discrete data carrying a statistical uncertainty at each point.

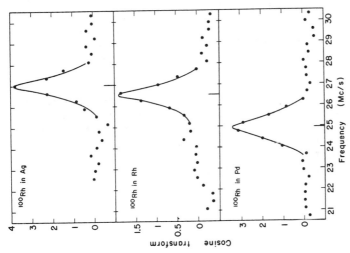

Fig. 7: Cosine transform of the time spectrum obtained with ^{100}Rh in three different host lattices, showing the different Knight shifts. The external field was 8047 ± 15 gauss.

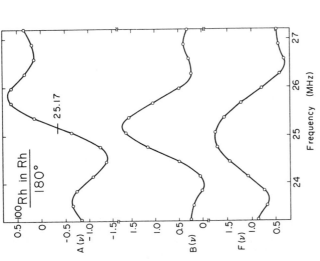

Fig. 6: Digital analysis of perturbed angular correlations with frequency spectrum of: sine transform, $A(\nu)$; cosine transform, $B(\nu)$; absolute function, $F(\nu) = [A(\nu)^2 + B(\nu)^2]^{1/2}$. The measurement was done in an external field of 7636 ± 7 gauss, which gives $g = 2.162 ± 0.005$.

III. Resonance Destruction of Angular Distributions

A. <u>NMR in Angular Correlations</u>

As discussed above one of the limitations of the time-differential method was that it cannot be applied if the time resolution is larger than the precession time for one cycle, $\tau_0 \geq T_L = (\pi/\omega_L)$. This is often the case for magnetic hyperfine fields at impurity atoms in ferromagnetic lattices. We know, on the other hand, that the accuracy of a time-differential measurement is higher, the more spin rotations are observed. This leads necessarily to the question: Is it possible to perform an NMR experiment with the excited state in a case where the rotations of the angular correlation pattern are no longer resolved? The rf-field would then, at resonance, change the non-isotropic population of the substates (see Fig. 8) and thus have a destructive effect on the angular correlation. This effect could then in turn be used for a radiative detection of NMR.

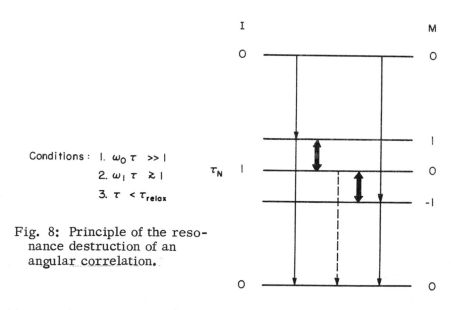

Conditions : 1. $\omega_0 \tau \gg 1$

2. $\omega_1 \tau \gtrsim 1$

3. $\tau < \tau_{relax}$

Fig. 8: Principle of the resonance destruction of an angular correlation.

This question has been discussed by Abragam and Pound (1953), and the following conditions for such an experiment were formulated: (i) The splitting of the substates of the intermediate state (Fig. 8) should be large compared to the natural linewidth, i.e., $\omega_0 \tau \gg 1$. (ii) The rf-field, H_1, must have sufficient amplitude to induce transitions between the substates in times comparable to the nuclear lifetime, i.e., $\omega_1 \tau \gtrsim 1$, where ω_1 is the interaction frequency with a field of amplitude H_1. (iii) Nuclear relaxation times should be longer than the nuclear lifetime, i.e., $\tau < \tau_{rel}$, so as not to broaden or wipe out the resonance line. Conditions (i) and (iii) can easily be met, but (ii) is so stringent that a resonance experiment was considered not to be feasible. For a lifetime of 0.2 μsec and a g-factor of one, for example, one would have to use an rf amplitude of 1 kG which would correspond to a power of 10^6 watts in 1 cm^3 at 40 MHz.

It is possible, however, to fulfill condition (ii) by making use of the enhancement of the effective rf amplitude, H_1^{eff}, in nuclear magnetic resonance in ferromagnets (Portis and Lindquist, 1965). If the resonance is observed in a domain, the externally applied rf field, H_1, is amplified according to the relation

$$2H_1^{eff} = \left(1 + \frac{H_{hf}}{H_O} \right) H_1 \tag{3}$$

where H_{hf} is the magnetic hyperfine field and H_O is the external polarizing field. This means that the nuclear resonance is driven indirectly through the hyperfine coupling between the nucleus and the electrons, rather than directly by the external rf field. With the usual magnitude of magnetic hyperfine fields, it is easy to obtain an enhancement factor, H_{hf}/H_O, of 10^3 or larger which means that it is possible to meet condition (ii) with external rf amplitudes of about 1 gauss.

The geometry for such a resonance experiment is shown in Fig. 9. A thin foil of the ferromagnetic material, into which the activity has been diffused, is mounted with its plane parallel to the axis of either one or both detectors. The polarizing field is applied parallel to this axis which ensures, for a sufficiently large H_O, a completely decoupled (unperturbed) angular correlation. The rf-field, H_1, has to be applied perpendicular to the detector plane and consequently, to H_O. The first resonance destruction effect detected with such an arrangement (Matthias et al., 1966a) is shown in Fig. 10. For this experiment the 84-74.8 keV cascade in ^{100}Rh, which has a large positive anisotropy and a half life of 235 nsec, was used. The resonance was driven by the hyperfine field of Rh in Ni, which is 200 kG. With the detectors arranged at 180°, one observes a decrease in the coincidence counting rate around the point of resonance. The natural linewidth, due to the lifetime, is about 0.5 MHz, i.e., much smaller than the observed one. The interpretation of the large linewidth is difficult, but

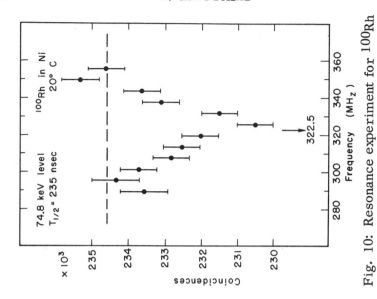

Fig. 10: Resonance experiment for ^{100}Rh in Ni at room temperature. $H_O = 100$ gauss, $2H_1 \simeq 3$ gauss, $H_{hf} = 197 \pm 2$ kG.

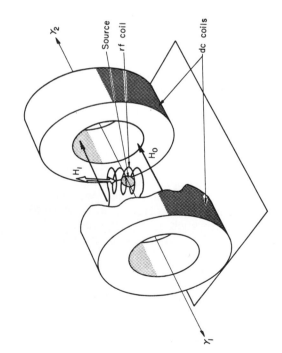

Fig. 9: Sketch of the geometry of a resonance experiment with angular correlations.

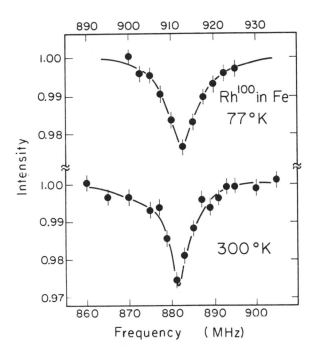

Fig. 11: Resonance experiment for ^{100}Rh in Fe at
two different temperatures. $H_0 = 100$ gauss
and $2H_1 \simeq 1.5$ gauss. The corresponding
internal fields are $H_i(300°K) = 537.0 \pm$
0.6 kG, and $H_i(77°K) = 556.5 \pm 0.6$ kG.

newer results show that the resonance can actually be resolved into
two components, corresponding to two different sites, a main peak
and a satellite about 20 MHz lower. Whether there is an additional
broadening due to relaxation phenomena cannot be determined
until we have a theoretical prediction of the linewidth.

Another example of a resonance with ^{100}Rh in Fe at two different temperatures is given in Fig. 11. The shift between room
temperature and 77°K is obvious. The resonance is much more
symmetrical compared to the Ni case, but the observed linewidth
is still much larger than the natural width. Despite this, it is apparent that the interaction frequency ω_L can be determined from

these data with an accuracy of about 0.1%.

The formalism to describe the resonance destruction has to be developed from the general expression for a PAC (Steffen and Frauenfelder, 1964; 1965)

$$W(\mathbf{k}_1, \mathbf{k}_2, t) = \sum_{\substack{k_1 k_2 \\ N_1 N_2}} A_{k_1}(1) A_{k_2}(2)\, G_{k_1 k_2}^{N_1 N_2}(t)$$

$$\times\, [(2k_1 + 1)(2k_2 + 1)]^{-\frac{1}{2}}\, Y_{k_1}^{N_1 *}(\theta_1, \varphi_1) Y_{k_2}^{N_2}(\theta_2, \varphi_2) \tag{4}$$

where the perturbation factor is defined as

$$G_{k_1 k_2}^{N_1 N_2}(t) = [(2k_1 + 1)(2k_2 + 1)]^{\frac{1}{2}} \sum_{m_a m_b} (-1)^{2I + m_a + m_b}$$

$$\times \begin{pmatrix} I & I & k_1 \\ m_a' & -m_a & N_1 \end{pmatrix} \begin{pmatrix} I & I & k_2 \\ m_b' & -m_b & N_2 \end{pmatrix}$$

$$\times \langle m_b | \exp\left[-\frac{i}{\hbar}\mathcal{H}(t)t\right] | m_a \rangle \langle m_b' | \exp\left[-\frac{i}{\hbar}\mathcal{H}(t)t\right] | m_a' \rangle^*. \tag{5}$$

The interaction Hamiltonian is now time-dependent and has the form well known from NMR theory:

$$\mathcal{H}(t) = -\gamma\hbar[H_0 I_z + H_1 (I_x \cos\omega t + I_y \sin\omega t)]. \tag{6}$$

The time dependence of $\mathcal{H}(t)$ can be eliminated by transforming to a coordinate system which rotates about H_0 (z-axis) with frequency ω. With H_1 along the x-axis we get a transformed (effective) Hamiltonian (Abragam, 1961; Slichter, 1963)

$$\mathcal{H} = -\gamma\hbar\left[\left(\frac{\omega}{\gamma} + H_0\right) I_z + H_1 I_x\right]. \tag{7}$$

For the experimental set-up described in Fig. 9, we have $\theta_1 = 0°$ and $\theta_2 = 180°$, which implies $N_1 = N_2 = 0$ and consequently, $m_a = m_a'$ and $m_b = m_b'$. With these simplifications, we find the time-integrated perturbation factor from Eq. (5)

$$G^{oo}_{k_1 k_2} = [(2k_1 + 1)(2k_2 + 1)]^{\frac{1}{2}} \sum_{m_a m_b} (-1)^{2I + m_a + m_b}$$

$$\times \begin{pmatrix} I & I & k_1 \\ m_a & -m_a & 0 \end{pmatrix} \begin{pmatrix} I & I & k_2 \\ m_b & -m_b & 0 \end{pmatrix} \frac{1}{\tau} \int_0^\infty \exp(-t/\tau)$$

$$\times \left| \langle m_b | \exp\left[-\frac{i}{\hbar} \mathcal{H}t \right] | m_a \rangle \right|^2 dt . \tag{8}$$

The transformation into a rotating coordinate system effects only the interaction Hamiltonian, but not the angular correlation function, since the axis of rotation is chosen parallel to the emission direction of the γ-rays. The square of the matrix element is the probability $P_{m_b m_a}$ of finding the spin I at time t in the state m_b when it was in the state m_a at time t = 0. The matrix elements are non-diagonal which means that the perturbation factor $G^{oo}_{k_1 k_2}$ is best calculated by numerical methods. It is interesting to note that the interference term for $k_1 \neq k_2$ in Eq. (8) is not zero. From Eqs. (4) and (8) it follows that the time-integrated angular correlation function exposed to a destructive rf field with the geometry shown in Fig. 9 is described by

$$W(180^\circ) = \sum_{k_1 k_2} A_{k_1}(1) A_{k_2}(2) G^{oo}_{k_1 k_2} \tag{9}$$

with

$$G^{oo}_{k_1 k_2} = [(2k_1 + 1)(2k_2 + 1)]^{\frac{1}{2}} \sum_{\substack{m_a m_b \\ n \ n'}} (-1)^{2I + m_a + m_b}$$

$$\times \begin{pmatrix} I & I & k_1 \\ m_a & -m_a & 0 \end{pmatrix} \begin{pmatrix} I & I & k_2 \\ m_b & -m_b & 0 \end{pmatrix} \langle n | m_b \rangle^* \langle n | m_a \rangle$$

$$\times \langle n' | m_b \rangle \langle n' | m_a \rangle^* \frac{1}{1 + [(E_n - E_{n'})\tau/\hbar]^2} . \tag{10}$$

In this equation E_n are the eigenvalues and $\langle n | m \rangle$ the corresponding eigenvectors of the interaction Hamiltonian given in Eq. (7).

B. NMR in Statically Polarized Nuclei

The resonance destruction method to detect NMR in a radio-active state can always be employed when the nuclei in this state are oriented. In angular correlations the coincidence between γ_1 and γ_2 selects a certain non-isotropic population of the nuclei in the m-substates. Thus, the γ_2 are emitted from an oriented system with respect to γ_1. Another way of obtaining a polarization of the nuclei is to go to very low temperatures and expose them to a sufficiently large magnetic field, H_{eff}, so that $kT \sim \mu H_{eff}$. This technique is well known* and discussed in detail in the literature (Blin–Stoyle and Grace, 1957).

The angular distribution of γ-rays emitted from polarized nuclei is given by

$$W(\theta) = \sum_{k \text{ even}} B_k \, U_k \, A_k \, P_k (\cos \theta) \tag{11}$$

The coefficients A_k are the angular distribution coefficients. The coefficients U_k account for any disorientation by preceding but unobserved transitions (Blin-Stoyle and Grace, 1957). The orientation parameter, B_k, describes the degree of nuclear orientation and is given by

$$B_k(I) = \sqrt{2I+1} \sum_m (-1)^{I-m} (IIm-m|k0) \frac{\exp[-E_m/kT]}{\sum_m \exp[-E_m/kT]} \tag{12}$$

where $(IIm-m|k0)$ is a Clebsch-Gordon coefficient and E_m are the eigenvalues of the interaction Hamiltonian. Resonance-induced transitions disturb the Boltzmann distribution and, consequently, alter the orientation parameters B_k. The resonance effect should then be observable as a change in radiation intensity at a fixed angle θ.

An experiment of this type was suggested, in principle, by Bloembergen and Temmer (1953) but no successful experiment has been carried out until very recently (Matthias and Holliday, 1966c). The great difficulty is the large heating effect of the rf-field. However, this can be avoided by again taking advantage of the rf-amplitude enhancement in a ferromagnetic sample. According to Eq. (3), the external rf-field can be reduced by a factor of about

---

* See N.J. Stone, Chap. S.4.

10^3, leaving a sufficiently large effective rf-amplitude acting at the nucleus so that an adequate warm-up rate of the sample can be obtained. Note that there are no power requirements here due to a short nuclear lifetime; all radioactive levels suitable for nuclear polarization work have long enough lifetimes to eliminate this problem.

The geometry for such an experiment is sketched in Fig. 12. The radioactive material is diffused into a thin foil of the ferromagnetic host material which is soldered onto copper fins which provide the thermal contact with the demagnetizing salt. A set of superconducting Nb rings produce the polarizing field, H_O, oriented parallel to the plane of the foil. $\mathbf{H_O}$ defines the reference axis for the emission direction θ of the γ-rays. The rf-field is applied perpendicular to the polarizing field, but parallel to the plane of the foil. The effect of the rf on the angular distribution was first observed for ^{60}Co in Fe (Matthias and Holliday, 1966c). Figure 13 shows the warm-up rate for ^{60}Co nuclei as a function of time and frequency (upper part) and with a fixed frequency off resonance (lower part). Summing up the results of repeated demagnetization runs lead to resonance curves like the ones displayed in Fig. 14 which were obtained with two different alloys. Although the resonance frequency is the same, the two measurements give a different linewidth. We attribute the larger linewidth of alloy I to such experimental conditions as, e.g., a larger inhomogeniety of the polarizing field. Alloy I was larger than alloy II and also two frequency scans were made following one demagnetization. The resonance for each second scan was shifted

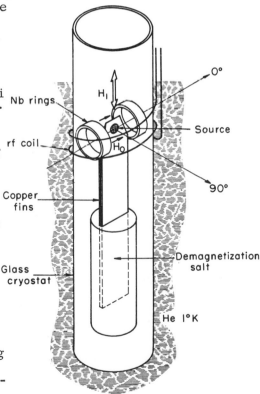

Fig. 12: Experimental arrangement for resonance in statically polarized nuclei

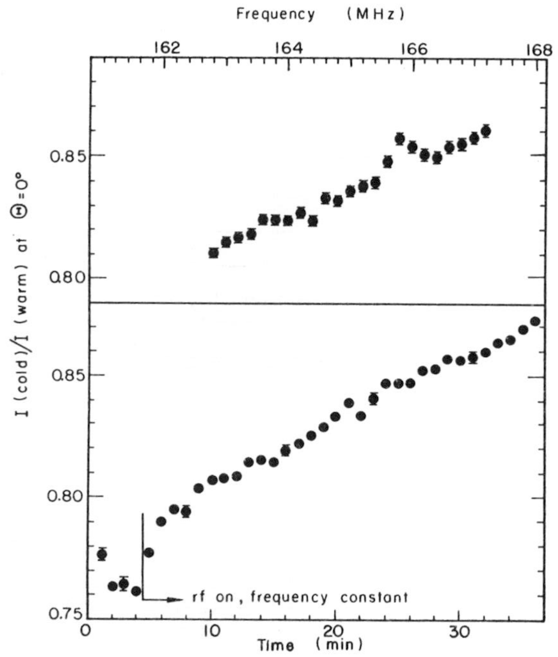

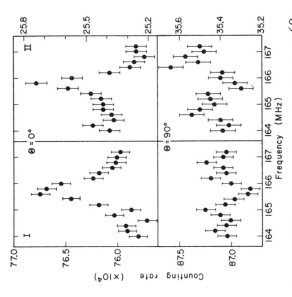

Fig. 14: Resonance effect in polarized ^{60}Co nuclei, observed at 0° and 90° for two different alloys (Matthias and Holliday, 1966c). The internal field obtained from these data is $H_i = 290.6 \pm 0.9$ kG.

Fig. 13: Typical warm-up curves for ^{60}Co in Fe at $\theta = 0°$ (Matthias and Holliday, 1966c). In the upper part: frequency varied with time. Lower part: fixed frequency off resonance, but same rf amplitude.

toward lower frequencies, either because of a change of the trapped magnetic flux in the Nb rings or because of long relaxation times. The measurements with alloy II are more representative for a typical linewidth to be expected in this type of experiment. However, to draw any conclusions from the observed linewidth, one would have to use a more controlled external polarizing field with greater homogeneity.

Independent of these linewidth considerations, it is apparent that the interaction frequency can be obtained from these measurements with an accuracy of about 0.1%. This is at least an order of magnitude better compared to what can be done with conventional nuclear polarization experiments (Shirley, 1966) and characterizes the importance of the method. Further, in contrast to conventional measurements the rf destruction of the polarization gives the interaction frequency independent of any precise knowledge of the temperature scale. It should be noted that the conventional nuclear orientation technique measures an energy $|\mu H_{eff}|$ while the present method gives a frequency $|g H_{eff} \cdot (\mu_N/\hbar)|$. Combining both techniques would determine the spin of the nuclear state. If a sufficiently large polarizing field is applied to completely saturate the ferromagnetic sample, the resonance is observed in domains. In that case, the resonance frequency should shift linearly with the applied field (Portis and Lindquist, 1965) which would make it possible to determine the nuclear g-factor directly. The technique will also prove valuable for studies of the magnetic hyperfine fields of impurities in ferromagnetic lattices. It measures, to a good approximation, the hyperfine field at $T = 0°K$ and allows one to work with extremely small concentrations. A great number of radioactive isotopes and isomeric levels are accessible to this technique, particularly in connection with isotope separators, which provide a way to shoot isotopes into a lattice in cases where chemical procedures fail.

C. NMR in Nuclei Polarized by Nuclear Reactions

Nuclear reactions is another technique in which an appreciable degree of nuclear polarization is achieved. In particular, in (heavy-ion, xn) reactions, the product nucleus is highly aligned and the gamma rays emitted in the decay of the compound state show angular distributions with considerable anisotropies (Diamond et al., 1966). If an isomeric state is populated in this decay, the high degree of alignment could be used to measure electromagnetic hyperfine interactions in that state. One great advantage of this technique would be that very high spin states could be measured, as they are populated with a high yield in reactions with large momentum transfer. Also, systematic measurements of the same spin state in different isotopes could be carried out. A practical advantage is that these measurements involve only singles counting, which eliminates restrictions in the available half-life range caused by accidental coincidences. However, the greatest difficulty which has to be overcome in such an experiment is to preserve the spin orientation in the isomeric level for a period longer than the lifetime τ. Here, the large recoil velocity of the product nucleus is very valuable in getting the nucleus quickly into a suitable environment.

Since the first experiment of Goldring and Scharenberg (1958) angular distributions following Coulomb excitation have been frequently used (Bodenstedt and Rogers, 1964) to measure nuclear g-factors by observing the effect of an external magnetic field on the distribution function. Very recently this technique has been extended to the use of internal magnetic fields (Grodzins et al., 1966; Boehm et al., 1966; Gilad et al., 1966) by using the recoil to implant the Coulomb-excited nuclei into ferromagnetic lattices. However, due to the Coulomb excitation process this technique will be limited to nuclear levels in the nano- and subnano-second range. It will, therefore, hardly be possible to use it for resonance destruction experiments. The first perturbed angular distribution experiment involving a half life longer than 10^{-8} sec was performed by Treacy (1956) on the 198 keV level in ^{19}F, excited in a (p, p') reaction on ^{19}F. This level has a half life of 87 nsec, very convenient for time-differential investigations. Some more work has been done with this level (Freeman, 1961; Sugimoto et al., 1964) but it still remains the only case where an angular distribution following a nuclear reaction was used for time-differential investigations involving a longer half-life.

In a remarkable experiment, Sugimoto et al. (1965, 1966) proved that the polarization of nuclei produced by a nuclear charged particle reaction can be preserved up to 10 sec or longer at room temperature and subsequently used to detect the nuclear magnetic resonance. The principal idea for this experiment was to work with free ions and to decouple the nuclear spin completely from the highly excited electronic states in a strong external field. To achieve this, Sugimoto et al. used the experimental set-up shown in Fig. 15. * The recoil atoms were taken out of the target, separated from the beam and cought by a CaF_2 recoil stopper. This

*We are grateful to Sugimoto et al. (1965; 1966) for permission to publish Fig. 15.

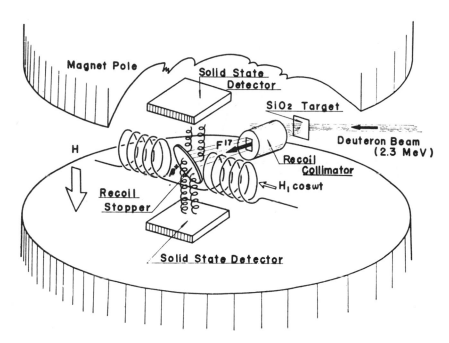

Fig. 15: Sketch of the experimental arrangement used by Sugimoto et al. for measuring the NMR in ^{17}F.

crystal was chosen because it is cubic and known to have long relaxation times for F nuclei. The reaction used was ^{16}O(d, n)^{17}F $(\beta^+)^{17}$O with a half life of 66 sec for the β^+-decay of ^{17}F. The polarization of the ^{17}F nuclei was detected by observing the asymmetry of the β-decay (see Fig. 15). The reconance effect is shown in Fig. 16. *

The experiment sets a standard for what can be done with nuclear alignment following reactions and it demonstrates that, indeed, the whole half-life range from nanoseconds up to seconds is open for investigation. The decoupling technique used by Sugimoto et al. is probably the only way to avoid disorientation of the nuclei by hyperfine interactions with the highly excited ionic state, and would have to be used in the range between 10^{-5} sec and 1 sec. There is also evidence that thick cubic metallic targets are a suitable environment to observe unperturbed angular distributions up to the microsecond range (Matthias et al., 1965b; Yamazaki,

*We are grateful to Sugimoto et al. (1965; 1966) for permission to publish Fig. 16.

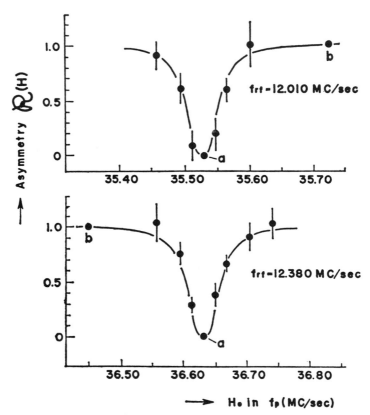

Fig. 16: Experimental result for the NMR in ^{17}F obtained by
Sugimoto et al. (1965; 1966). R(H) is the relative β-
particle asymmetry. The result obtained from these
data is $\mu(F^{17})$ = 4. 7200 ± 0. 0011 nm.

1966). However, no measurements of electromagnetic interactions
involving half lives longer than 10^{-8} sec have been made yet with
metallic targets.

The polarization of the product nuclei following capture of
polarized thermal neutrons should also be mentioned. Connor
(1959) utilized this fact to determine the magnetic moment of ^{8} Li.
The NMR in this system was measured by using the asymmetry of
the β-decay of polarized ^{8} Li nuclei for the detection. In contrast
to charged particle reactions there is no change or disruption in
the electronic shell involved for thermal neutron capture and
hyperfine and relaxation interactions in the target are of the same
nature as encountered in ordinary NMR.

IV. Source Structure Considerations

Any attempt to use time-differential and resonance perturbed angular correlation techniques for half-lives longer than a microsecond faces the major difficulty that the source structure has to be such that time-dependent and static internal perturbations are small enough not to cause an appreciable disorientation during the time interval used for the measurement. Our concern is with time-dependent perturbations which damp the amplitude of the angular correlation pattern with time; static perturbations can never wipe out the correlation completely. The originally non-isotropic population of the substates of the intermediate level becomes randomized as a result of transitions induced by the fluctuating fields. The only, but important, difference between nuclear relaxation effects in NMR and PAC is that in the latter we have the lifetime of the intermediate state which sets a natural time window for the observation. Everything that happens outside this window cannot be observed with angular correlation techniques, i.e., small line broadenings are not measurable as the natural linewidth is comparatively large. Thus, the ratio of the nuclear lifetime, τ, to the relaxation time, τ_{rel}, is the factor which determines the proper choice of the source material. For very long relaxation times, $\tau_{rel} >> \tau$, the observed angular correlation pattern is undamped. If the relaxation time is comparable to the lifetime, $\tau_{rel} \sim \tau$, then the angular correlation is strongly damped and an interaction frequency, ω_L, can only be measured if it is sufficiently large, $\omega_L \tau_{rel} >> 1$. For still shorter relaxation times, $\tau_{rel} << \tau$, the angular correlation is completely wiped out, assuming that the coupling between the fluctuating fields and the nuclear moments is reasonably strong. The angular correlation remains, of course, unperturbed in all cases where the fields fluctuate so fast that the coupling is broken and the fields average to zero within a short time interval. This happens when $\omega_{rel} \tau_c << 1$, where ω_{rel} is the relaxation interaction and τ_c is the time interval during which a local field configuration remains stable.

1. Liquid Sources and Ionic Crystals. Most g-factor measurements on nuclear states in the nanosecond range have been performed with liquid sources. These measurements show that nuclei in paramagnetic ions in liquids are affected by very strong time-dependent perturbations which destroy the angular correlation within a few nanoseconds at room temperature. In diamagnetic liquids, on the other hand, the anisotropy remains unperturbed for very long times; from NMR measurements, the relaxation times are in the range of milliseconds to seconds or sometimes

even longer. In the angular correlation experiments, however, the radioactive decay creates highly excited paramagnetic ions and the time in which the atom reaches its ionic ground state depends greatly on the surroundings. If the ionic ground state is diamagnetic and the atom reaches the ground state in a time short compared to the precession time of the nucleus in the external field (e.g. metals), the correlation will not be further attenuated. If the atom is still excited for times comparable or longer than the nuclear precession time, coherence is lost and the correlation is wiped out by this "after effect" perturbation. The existence of after-effects in non-metallic sources has been established by many experiments, but a quantitative understanding is still missing. The orientation of the nuclei can, however, be preserved by decoupling the nuclear and the electronic spin by a large enough external magnetic field (see for example, Siegbahn and Asaro, 1962; Pettersson et al., 1961).

Similar perturbations are present if the ionic ground state is paramagnetic. The nuclei will then precess in an effective field, H_{eff}, which is the sum of the external magnetic field, H_O, and the field due to the hyperfine interaction, H_{hf}, and which is usually described in terms of the paramagnetic correction factor β,

$$H_{eff} = \beta \cdot H_O . \tag{13}$$

Typical values of β for the trivalent rare-earth ions have been tabulated (Günther and Lindgren, 1964). The calculation of β requires knowledge of the oxidation state and hf constant. The calculation is not possible for those cases where the atom can exist in several oxidation states following conversion processes, electron capture and β^- decay. The hfs constant can be measured by performing a decoupling experiment as was done by Steining and Deutsch (1961) in the case of $^{154}Gd^{3+}$.

Time-dependent electric quadrupole perturbations are also found in liquid sources, because of the fluctuating electric field gradients. Sources which show such an effect should be avoided for g-factor measurements.

2. Non-Magnetic Metallic Sources. Steffen (1953) showed that liquid metal exhibit the unperturbed angular correlation in case of ^{111}Cd. Also, solid cubic metal lattices can be used with advantage for g-factor measurements as a nearly perturbation-free host, as was done in ^{99}Ru (Matthias et al., 1965c), ^{100}Rh (Matthias et al., 1965b), ^{188}Os, ^{190}Os, and ^{192}Os (Goldring et al., 1966).

The reducing action of the conduction electrons brings the daughter atom into chemical equilibrium in a very short time ($< 10^{-13}$ sec) following the decay of the parent. Assuming there is no localized moment and neglecting quadrupole and dipolar interactions, the remaining perturbation arises from the contact interaction of the nuclei with the spin magnetic moments of core s-electrons or s-like conduction electrons (Slichter, 1963). The relaxation times, T_1, determine the upper limit for which PAC measurements are possible; in metals, $T_1 \cdot T \simeq 10^{-2}$ sec °K for heavy elements, increasing to $T_1 \cdot T \simeq 10^{-1}$ sec °K for medium heavy and lighter elements, i. e. , it is possible to measure lifetimes $\sim 10^{-5}$ sec at room temperature. In fact, the time-dependent angular correlation pattern offers an interesting alternative method for determining T_1.

The perturbation-free environment seems to apply not only to radioactive sources, but also to thick metallic targets in nuclear reactions (Yamazaki, 1966) and to recoil implantation following Coulomb excitation (Goldring et al. , 1966). The correction due to the paramagnetism of the conduction electrons does not enter within the accuracy of PAC measurements. Thus, cubic metals seem to be universally good hosts. However, Frauenfelder et al. (1953) found that the angular correlation in ^{204}Pb was attenuated to the hard-core value in the face-centered cubic environment of a Pb_{60}-Tl_{40} alloy, while it was unperturbed in the cubic body-centered phase of Pb between 235°C and 303°C.

3. Ferromagnetic Metallic Sources. For the measurement of magnetic moments of nuclear levels in the sub-nanosecond range large magnetic fields are required to obtain a detectable rotation. The internal fields in cubic ferromagnets have been used successfully. After-effects are not expected because of the metallic state. Thus, if the internal field is known from either NMR or Mössbauer experiments, they can be used to measure magnetic moments by PAC techniques. However, a knowledge of the field is not necessary if a sufficiently large external field H_0 is superimposed onto the internal field. If the ferromagnetic sample is saturated, there should be a linear relationship between $g \cdot H_{eff}$ and H_0. From such a measurement all quantities of interest, i. e. , the g-factor (slope), the internal field (ordinate intercept) and the sign of the internal field (sign of slope) can be determined.

V. Summary

Within the scope of this presentation it was neither possible to treat all problems of perturbed angular correlations in detail nor to touch on all related experiments. The beautiful measurement of the hyperfine splitting of positronium by Deutsch and Brown (1952) was not discussed despite the fact that it was (to the knowledge of the author) the first resonance experiment with gamma-ray detection. Another experiment not mentioned here was the measurement of NMR in ^{19}Ne by means of the β^+-asymmetry from ^{19}Ne polarized in an atomic beam apparatus (Commins and Dobson, 1963). While these experiments certainly fall under the subject of "radioactive detection of NMR" they are less related to perturbed angular correlations and distributions.

Many experiments remain to be done even before the various methods can be understood in detail. (1) For example, there is the question of the form of hyperfine fields for sources prepared by simple melting, diffusion, recoil implantation, and ion implantation with isotope separators. (2) Another problem is the determination of the sign of the interaction frequency in NMR experiments. (3) It has to be proved that NMR experiments in saturated samples show the domain resonance, and that the g-factor can be measured by observing a linear shift of the resonance as a function of the external field. (4) It would be interesting to measure the resonance spectrum of an electric quadrupole interaction, for example, in garnets. (5) The use of the Mössbauer effect to detect the nuclear magnetic resonance is another possibility. It has the interesting aspect that it probably provides a means to detect the Mössbauer effect in long-lived states ($> 10^{-6}$ sec) where the present day velocity spectrometers fail. Instead of measuring a velocity spectrum, the Mössbauer effect would be recorded as a frequency spectrum. (6) The subject of "after effects" needs further investigation to obtain more quantitative results, e.g., by careful decoupling experiments, or the investigation of hyperfine fields in ferromagnetic insulators. (7) Last, but not least, it should not be forgotten that despite the exciting possibilities, no perturbed angular distribution measurement has yet been performed with an isomeric level with a lifetime between 1μ sec and 1 sec.

Acknowledgements

Some of the figures presented in this paper are published or unpublished results of the Berkeley group. It is a pleasure for the author to acknowledge the ideas, the help, the stimulating discussions and the enthusiasm of all collaborators: D.A. Shirley, N. Edelstein, S.S. Rosenblum, H.J. Körner, B.A. Olsen, M.P. Klein, R.J. Holliday, F.S. Stephens, J.O. Newton, and T. Yamazaki.

References

Abragam, A. and Pound, R.V. (1953). Phys. Rev. 92, 943.

Abragam, A. (1961). The Principles of Nuclear Magnetism, (Oxford University Press, Oxford, England).

Auerbach, K., Siepe, K., Wittkemper, J., and Körner, H.J. (1966). (private communication).

Blin-Stoyle, R.J. and Grace, M.A. (1957). "Oriented Nuclei," in Encyclopedia of Physics, edited by S. Flügge, Vol. XLII, (Springer-Verlag, Berlin).

Bloembergen, N. and Temmer, G.M. (1953). Phys. Rev. 89, 883.

Bodenstedt, E. and Rogers, J.D. (1964). Perturbed Angular Correlations, edited by E. Karlsson, E. Matthias, and K. Siegbahn, Chap. II, pg. 92 (North Holland Publ. Co., Amsterdam).

Boehm, F., Hagemann, G.B., and Winther, A. (1966). Phys. Letters 21, 217.

Commins, E.D. and Dobson, D.A. (1963). Phys. Rev. Letters 10, 347.

Connor, D. (1959). Phys. Rev. Letters 3, 429.

de Boer, J., Stokstad, R.G., Symons, G.D., and Winther, A. (1965). Phys. Rev. Letters 14, 564.

Deutsch, M. and Brown, S.C. (1952). Phys. Rev. 85, 1047.

Diamond, R.M., Matthias, E., Newton, J.O., and Stephens, F.S. (1966). Phys. Rev. Letters 16, 1205.

Frauenfelder, H. and Steffen, R.M. (1965). Alpha-, Beta-, and Gamma-Ray Spectroscopy, edited by K. Siegbahn, Chap. 19A, Vol. 2 (North-Holland Publ. Co., Amsterdam).

Frauenfelder, H. , Lawson, J. S. , Jentschke, W. , and De Pasquali, G. (1953). Phys. Rev. 92, 513.

Freeman, R. M. (1961). Nucl. Phys. 26, 446.

Gilad, P. , Goldring, G. , Kalish, R. , and Herber, R. H. (1966). Phys. Rev. 151, 281.

Goldring, G. and Scharenberg, R. P. (1958). Phys. Rev. 110, 701.

Goldring, C. , Kalish, R. , and Spehl, H. (1966). Nucl. Phys. 80, 33.

Grodzins, L. , Borchers, R. , and Hagemann, G. B. (1966). Phys. Letters 21, 214.

Günther, C. and Lindgren, I. (1964). Perturbed Angular Correlations, edited by E. Karlsson, E. Matthias, and K. Siegbahn, (North-Holland Publ. Co. , Amsterdam), pg. 357.

Matthias, E. , Rosenblum, S. S. , and Shirley, D. A. (1965a). Phys. Rev. Letters 14, 46.

Matthias, E. , Shirley, D. A. , Evans, J. S. , and Naumann, R. A. (1965b). Phys. Rev. 140, B264.

Matthias, E. , Rosenblum, S. S. , and Shirley, D. A. (1965c). Phys. Rev. 139, B532.

Matthias, E. , Shirley, D. A. , Klein, M. P. , and Edelstein, N. (1966a). Phys. Rev. Letters 16, 974.

Matthias, E. and Shirley, D. A. (1966b). Nucl. Instr. Methods 45, 309.

Matthias, E. and Holliday, R. J. (1966c). Phys. Rev. Letters 17, 897.

Pettersson, B. G. , Thun, J. E. , and Gerholm, T. R. (1961). Nucl. Phys. 24, 223.

Portis, A. M. and Lindquist, R. H. (1965). Magnetism, edited by G. T. Rado and H. Suhl, Vol. IIA, pg. 35 (Academic Press, Inc. , New York).

Rosenblum, S. S. , Matthias, E. , and Shirley, D. A. (1967). (to be published).

Shirley, D. A. (1966). Ann. Rev. Nucl. Sci. 16, 89.

Siegbahn, K. and Asaro, F. (1962). Phys. Letters 2, 323.

Slichter, C. P. (1963). Principles of Magnetic Resonance, (Harper and Row, New York).

Steffen, R. M. (1953). Phys. Rev. 89, 903.

Steffen, R. M. and Frauenfelder, H. (1964). Perturbed Angular Correlations, edited by E. Karlsson, E. Matthias, and K. Siegbahn, Chap. I (North-Holland Publ. Co., Amsterdam).

Stiening, R. and Deutsch, M. (1961). Phys. Rev. 121, 1484.

Sugimoto, K., Mizobuchi, A., Nakai, K. (1964a). Perturbed Angular Correlations, edited by E. Karlsson, E. Matthias, and K. Siegbahn, pg. 337 (North-Holland Publ. Co., Amsterdam).

Sugimoto, K., Mizobuchi, A., and Nakai, K. (1964b). Phys. Rev. 134, B539.

Sugimoto, K., Mizobuchi, A., Nakai, K., and Matuda, K. (1965). Phys. Letters 18, 38.

Sugimoto, K., Mizobuchi, A., Nakai, K., and Matuda, K. (1966). J. Phys. Soc. Japan 21, 213.

Treacy, P. B. (1956). Nucl. Phys. 2, 239.

Yamazaki, T. (1966). (private communication).

S.1. STUDIES OF HYPERFINE INTERACTIONS IN FERROMAGNETIC ALLOYS BY INTEGRAL ANGULAR CORRELATION TECHNIQUES

Erik Karlsson

Institute of Physics
Uppsala, Sweden

I. Introduction

Since the study of perturbed angular correlations (PAC) by time-differential method is limited to nuclear excited states with lifetimes $\tau > 5 \cdot 10^{-9}$ sec, one has to resort to the less accurate but more widely applicable time-integral method for measurements of interactions with the majority of excited nuclear states. In order to obtain measurable interactions down to the picosecond (10^{-12} sec) region there is at present great interest in the use of the large hyperfine fields present at the nuclei of paramagnetic ions or of atoms introduced as dilute impurities in ferromagnetic Fe, Ni, Co, or Gd. We shall discuss some recent experiments with nuclei in ferromagnetic iron hosts. Although these experiments were performed with the main purpose of obtaining nuclear information, they illustrate how the integral angular correlation is perturbed by the hyperfine field, the orders of magnitude of effects, and the accuracy with which effective hyperfine fields can be derived from the perturbations in typical cases. It will be seen that the integral PAC method is sometimes capable of relatively high accuracy and that it can be applied to many elements, like the magnetically important palladium, for which the Mössbauer effect and differential PAC cannot be used for the study of hyperfine fields. The examples presented below deal with ^{193}Ir, ^{106}Pd, and

^{122}Te in iron matrices and the potential use of ^{127}I as a case for the comparison and combination of PAC and Mössbauer techniques.

II. Experiments

The relevant decay schemes for the isotopes considered here are shown in Fig. 1.

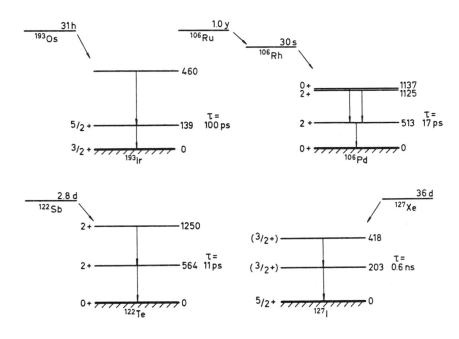

Fig. 1: Relevant parts of decay schemes for ^{193}Os, ^{106}Ru $(^{106}$Rh), ^{122}Sb, and ^{127}Xe leading to excited states in ^{193}Ir, ^{106}Pd, ^{122}Te, and ^{127}I, respectively.

A. ^{193}Ir

Since PAC in connection with hyperfine interactions in magnetic materials is still a method under development, several experiments were carried out to check the consistency of the angular correlation results. Because of the unusually high anisotropy of the correlation in the 321-139 keV γ-γ cascade in ^{193}Ir, it was possible to compare critically three distinct effects on the correlation due to the perturbations in the 139 keV state ($\tau \approx 100$ ps) for ^{193}Ir in Fe: (i) the rotation of the pattern, P; (ii) the attenuation of the pattern, $A_\perp$, with source magnetized perpendicular to the detector plane; (iii) the attenuation, with source demagnetized (isotropic magnetic perturbation), A_0.

Relevant formulas for these cases are given in the chapter by Cohen. * The quantity P is related to the rotation of the pattern and has been defined previously (Karlsson, 1962). As shown in Fig. 2 and presented quantitatively in Table I, all three measured

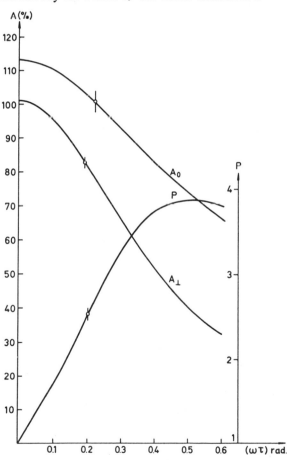

Fig. 2: Effect of hyperfine interactions on the 321-139 angular correlation in ^{193}Ir. Notations P, $A_\perp$, and A_0 are explained in the text. The reason for the different zero-field anisotropies in case $A_\perp$ and A_0 is that different geometries were used in the two measurements.

* See S.G. Cohen, Chap. 12.

Table I: Summary of measurements and quality figures for determinations of hyperfine fields.

	^{193}Ir	^{106}Pd	^{122}Te	^{127}I
$\omega\tau$ in external field (rad)	52.0 kG: 0.0063 ± 0.0007	46.0 kG: 0.00147 ± 0.00016		51.2 kG: 0.088 ± 0.002
$\omega\tau$ in internal field (rad) Fe (300°K)				
From rotation	-0.200 ± 0.014	-0.0167 ± 0.0005	0.0132 ± 0.0013	
From attenuation $A_\perp$	|0.190 ± 0.016|			
From attenuation A_o	|0.220 ± 0.080|			
Range of B_{int} measureable	50 kG - 10 MG	50 kG - 30 MG		10 kG - 1000 kG
Figure of merit: Accuracy obtained in 24 hrs.:				
$\Delta\omega\tau$	± 0.002 rad	± 0.0006 rad		± 0.002 rad
ΔB	± 15 kG	± 15 kG		± 2 kG
	(B < 2 MG)	(B < 2 MG)		(B < 200 kG)

quantities are consistent with the same parameter, $\omega\tau$ (Gustafsson et al., 1966). The direct measurement of $\omega\tau$ in an external field is difficult since the lifetime is short and the g-factor is small. The relative error achieved, $\approx 10\%$, corresponds to several weeks of continuous collection of coincidences. The hyperfine field, which is obtained from the ratio of $\omega\tau$-values in internal and external fields, is therefore given as $B_{int} = 1.65 \pm 0.22$ MGauss. This is to be compared with the value 1.40 MGauss determined by spin-echo NMR (Kontani et al., 1965), bearing in mind that the latter value has a 17 percent error because of un-certainty in the value of the ^{193}Ir ground state moment.

B. ^{106}Pd

The excited state observed in the ^{106}Pd case has a lifetime which is an order of magnitude shorter than in the previous case, but the 0-2-0 γ-γ cascade through the 513 keV level is highly anisotropic. This makes it possible to determine rotations with an error of less than 0.0002 rad (or 0.01 degrees) with the instru-ment used here. Measurements were performed in external fields and in an iron lattice. Preliminary data for the ratio of the inter-action frequencies at room temperature lead however to a hyper-fine field which is 13 percent lower than that observed at 4.2°K by the spin-echo method (Johansson et al., 1966).

We therefore used our cryogenic facility to investigate the temperature dependence of the hyperfine field between helium and room temperatures. The low-temperature equipment used was designed especially for angular correlation work and involved modification of the normal setup (Karlsson, 1962) used for mea-surements of perturbations in an external field. This allowed the tail of a thin-walled helium cryostat to be introduced from above through axial holes in the pole-tips of the electromagnet (Fig. 3). This still allows the application of external fields up to 30 kG which is useful in order to attain large hyperfine fields by "ampli-fication" in paramagnetic salts at low temperatures or polarization of magnetic materials with large magnetic anisotropies. The basic motivation behind this construction is the exploitation of the large hyperfine fields in paramagnetic salts at low temperatures or in those materials which possess a low ferromagnetic transition temperature. Further, it is important to be able to measure the PAC in a magnetic material at the same temperature (usually very low) as that used to measure the hyperfine field by Mössbauer effect, nuclear orientation, nuclear specific heat or spin-echo NMR — before using these fields in calculations to extract nuclear information.

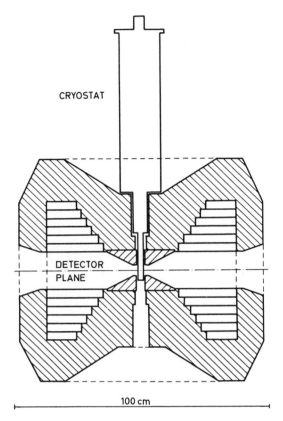

Fig. 3: Low-temperature arrangement for angular correlation
measurements at min. temp. 1.5°K, max. field 30 kG.
Four detectors are placed in the equatorial plane of the
magnet.

The ^{106}Pd in iron results at various temperatures are shown in
Table II with an error of ± 0.04 in all values. Although these
figures are to be considered as preliminary, it is evident that no

Table II: ^{106}Pd hyperfine field measurements at various
temperatures.

Temperature (°K):	1.5	4.2	78	160	300	570	820
Eff. int. field rel. to value at 300°K:	1.05	0.99	1.07	1.00	1.00	0.98	0.70

drastic changes in the hyperfine field occur at low temperatures relative to room temperature. Instead, the hyperfine fields seem to follow the host magnetization at least up to 600°K. The details closer to the Curie point are presently under investigation (Johansson et al., 1966). The reason for the discrepancy with the spin-echo value for the hyperfine field is not yet understood; one possible cause is that the Pd-nuclei in the external field experiment (which was carried out with a liquid source) in fact experience a field different from the applied one; another cause may be differences in environments for nuclei in domain walls and in domains. Furthermore, in the radioactive method one has to introduce small amounts of a third constituent, in this case Ru, to serve as source material and this may change the conditions for magnetism somewhat.

Leaving this problem aside, we observe in anticipation of further experiments which are under way, that the integral PAC-method here yields good accuracy in *relative* measurements of the hyperfine field. When a proper calibration point at low temperatures is agreed upon, the method is capable of giving absolute values to better than 10 kG which corresponds to a relative error of about 2 percent at magnetic saturation. For palladium, this accuracy should make PAC a worthwhile complement to the NMR-method, which is not easily applied at higher temperatures. The former can provide data at any temperature between 1.5°K and the Curie point for any composition in the Pd-Fe system with the above mentioned accuracy. For platinum, e.g., in the analogous Pt-Fe system, the integral PAC-method offers similar possibilities as a complement to Mössbauer studies using ^{195}Pt.

C. ^{122}Te

Here, the hyperfine field acting on the Te-nuclei in ferromagnetic iron had been determined by Frankel et al. (1965) by observation of the splitting of the Mössbauer line from the 35 keV transition in ^{125}Te. These authors used a source of dilute antimony in iron for the resonance experiment. This situation resembled that in the angular correlation measurements, in that the tellurium atoms are also formed in the iron by radioactive decay of antimony, and we were confident that the measured field, +620 kG, could be used in the calculation of the nuclear g-factor. The effect of different temperatures in the two experiments should be insignificant for impurities in iron as seen from experiments with other elements, e.g. the one mentioned above in Pd. The strong hyperfine field at the nucleus made it possible to determine the g-factor of the 2+ state in ^{122}Te as +0.39 ± 0.06. This result is of some importance for the theoretical discussion concerning nuclear vibrational states (Johansson et al., 1966).

D. ^{127}I

This example is mentioned for two reasons: (a) the method of introducing the radioactive nuclei into the host material is by ion bombardment in a mass-separator instead of diffusion or melting, and (b) the element iodine may be of interest in comparing PAC data with Mössbauer data on magnetic fields using the isotope ^{129}I. The radiations used for the study of the interaction with the 203 keV excited state ($\tau \approx 0.6$ ns) are from the 175-203 keV cascade which combines the advantages of a high counting rate with a relatively high angular correlation anisotropy. The lifetime and the g-factor of the 203 keV state are high enough to make possible a rather precise measurement (Svenson et al., 1966) of the parameter $\omega\tau$ in the external magnetic field (Table I). This determination was carried out with the source ions shot into an aluminium backing in order to avoid paramagnetic behaviour as an after-effect of the decay, which otherwise has been observed for this particular case (Leisi, 1966), following K-capture rather than β-decay. The ^{127}Xe ions can easily be introduced into other backings, e.g. iron, nickel, or cobalt foils.

A measurement of iodine in iron by the Mössbauer effect has been reported by DeWaard and Dreutje (1966). Results of similar or better accuracy can be obtained by the PAC-method, especially for hyperfine fields in the region up to 500 kG. Measurements, e.g., in nickel, would provide a good test on the consistency of the two methods for determining hyperfine fields. It is to be noted that such measurements are independent of the lifetime of the nuclear state. Unknown fields are calculated only by taking ratios with values obtained in a known field. In the ^{127}I case, the inherent accuracy in the field determination is of the order of 2 percent although the lifetime is presently uncertain to at least 10 percent.

III. Conclusions

The results discussed above were summarized in Table I. In addition, two more items have been added. The *range of applicability* to magnetic hyperfine determinations is limited for low values by the statistical uncertainty in the measurement of the rotation of the angular correlation pattern and for high values by the gradual smearing out of the angular correlation with increasing perturbation. The practical upper limit for a good determination has somewhat arbitrarily been put at the value where 20 percent of the anisotropy remains. The *figure of merit* of the cascades, which we define here as the accuracy obtainable in a 24 hour run, is valid for the instrument used in the present investigations and depends on the number of detectors used, time resolution of coincidence arrangements, possibilities to eliminate systematic errors, etc. For each isotope it depends on inherent properties of the cascade (number of cascading γ-rays per decay and energies of the γ-rays employed) and the nuclear state (lifetime and g-factor). The attainable accuracy can in many cases be improved by increasing the measuring time, but relative errors lower than 1 percent can hardly be reached because of instrumental instabilities.

In the preceding discussion it was assumed that the perturbations observed are of purely magnetic character. This assumption must in the general case be settled by auxiliary experiments, since integral angular correlations cannot separate magnetic and electric perturbations. So far however, no electric interactions of measurable strengths have been observed for impurities in ferromagnetic iron or nickel in the Mössbauer effect (Wäppling, 1966) or other (Matthias et al., 1965) experiments. The impurities evidently enter in good substitutional sites of cubic symmetry and the recoils from the nuclear decay are not sufficient to destroy this situation (Wäppling, 1966).

As illustrated by the cases described above, it may be stated quite generally that integral angular correlation in combination with other techniques can provide valuable and sometimes unique information about the magnitudes and signs of hyperfine fields.

References

De Waard, H. , Dreutje, S. A. (1966). Phys. Letters 20, 38.

Frankel, R. B. , Huntzicker, J. , Matthias, E. , Rosenblum, S. S. , Shirley, D. A. , and Stone, N. J. (1965). Phys. Letters 15, 163.

Gustafsson, S. , Johansson, K. , Karlsson, E. , Norlin, L. O. , and Svensson, Å. G. (1966). (to be published).

Johansson, K. , Karlsson, E. , Norlin, L. O. , and Tandon, P. (1966). (to be published).

Johansson, K. , Karlsson, E. , and Sommerfeldt, R. W. (1966). Phys. Letters 22, 297.

Karlsson, B. E. (1962). Arkiv Fys. 22, 1.

Kontani, M. , Asayama, K. , and Itoh, J. (1965). J. Phys. Soc. Japan 20, 1737.

Leisi, H. J. (1966). Nucl. Phys. 76, 308.

Matthias, E. , Shirley, D. A. , Evans, J. S. , and Nauman, R. A. (1965). Phys. Rev. 140B, 264.

Svenson, Å. G. , Tandon, P. N. , Sommerfeldt, R. W. , and Norlin, L. O. (1966). (to be published).

Wäppling, R. (1966). (private communication).

S.2. COULOMB EXCITATION ION IMPLANTATION PERTURBED ANGULAR CORRELATION METHOD*

Daniel Murnick

*Department of Physics and
Laboratory for Nuclear Science
Massachusetts Institute of Technology
Cambridge, Massachusetts*

I. Introduction

Utilizing the large anisotropy of gamma radiation emitted from Coulomb excited nuclei, in coincidence with backscattered exciting particles, one can study the hyperfine interactions of nuclear moments with the internal electromagnetic fields of solid state environments. Thus far the Coulomb excitation ion implantation method has been most fruitful in the determination of magnetic moments of short lived nuclear excited states, (Grodzins et al., 1966; Borchers et al, 1966) and for the measurement of hyperfine magnetic fields on dilute impurities in ferromagnetic materials at room temperature (Boehm et al.,1966a; Murnick et al.,1966; Boehm et al.,1966b; Gilad et al.,1966). The versatility, sensitivity, and simplicity of the technique, however, should lead to its use in studying other hyperfine interaction problems such as temperature dependences of internal fields, relaxation phenomena, and electric quadrupole interactions.

Work done in collaboration with L. Grodzins, Dept. of Physics and Laboratory for Nuclear Science, Massachusetts Institute of Technology, Cambridge, Mass. and R. Borchers and J. Bronson, Dept. of Physics, University of Wisconsin, Madison, Wisconsin. Supported by the U.S.A.E.C.

The first hyperfine interaction (hfi) studies using this method were carried out by Grodzins et al. (1966) at the Tandem Accelerator Laboratory, Riso, Denmark, and work has been continued in Denmark by Boehm et al. (1966a, 1966b). Goldring et al. (1966) at the Weizmann Institute in Israel had previously used Coulomb excitation ion implantation techniques with externally applied magnetic fields for determining excited state nuclear magnetic moments; and Gilad et al. (1966) have recently reported hfi studies of tungsten and neodymium implanted into ferromagnetic materials.

In this paper we will describe the experimental arrangement at the Wisconsin Tandem Accelerator, University of Wisconsin, in some detail, comment on the physical processes taking place in the preparation and decay of the nuclear states studied, and illustrate the capabilities of the method with some recent results obtained implanting samarium 150 into various lattices.

II. Experimental

A. Apparatus

A schematic diagram of the experimental apparatus is shown in Fig. 1. A well collimated beam of 33 MeV oxygen ions strikes

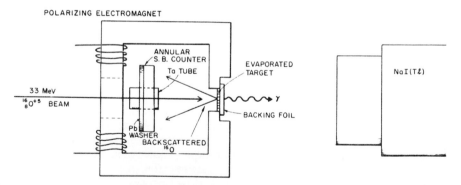

Fig. 1: Schematic drawing of apparatus. Only one of 4 coplanar NaI(Tl) gamma detectors is shown.

the target foil which is held between the pole pieces of a polarizing electromagnet. The target consists of an evaporation 50 to 500 μgm/cm^2 thick of the isotope under study on a thick (5 - 10 mg/cm^2) backing of the chosen host material. Any stable isotope can be implanted into any desired backing matrix, including aligned single crystals. Implantation also insures an impurity concentration of less than 1 part in 10^6 .

Oxygen 16 is chosen as the Coulomb exciting particle, as it is easy to accelerate, yields high Coulomb excitation cross sections and small cross sections for competing nuclear processes, at the energies used. Ions backscattered at center of mass angles of 175. 9° to 161. 7° are detected in an annular surface barrier particle counter. Gamma rays emitted from Coulomb excited nuclei, in coincidence with the selected backscattered O^{16} ions, are detected with four coplanar 3" by 3" sodium iodide (thallium activated) counter assemblies, rotatable from -135° to +135°, and are electronically routed into separate parts of the memory of a multichannel analyzer. Figure 2 is a detailed block diagram of the electronics used in the experiments.

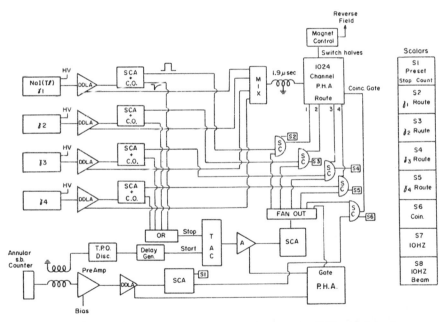

Fig. 2: Electronics block diagram. Legend: HV, high voltage; DDLA, delay line shaping amplifier; SCA + C. O., single channel analyzer and crossover pickoff unit; T. P. O., time pickoff tunnel diode discriminator; TAC, time to amplitude converter (used as a fast coincidence circuit); PHA, pulse height analyzer.

By only recording events initiated by those O^{16} ions which are backscattered close to 180°, one insures that only $m_{\ell} = 0$ photons are included, and that sufficient forward momentum is imparted to the target nuclei to impel them well into the host material. Figure 3 is a typical energy spectrum of O^{16} particles with 33 MeV incident energy backscattered from a samarium 150 on iron target. The sharp peak at about 21 MeV is due to particles backscattered from the thin samarium layer, the lower energy continuum from scattering events in the iron foil.

$$E_{\text{Recoil}} = \left\{ 1 - \left(\frac{M-m}{M+m} \right)^2 \right\} E_0 \qquad (1)$$

is the recoil energy of the heavy atom of mass M, (approximately 12 MeV for Sm^{150}) and is sufficient for implantation into iron to depths greater than 1 mg/cm^2 .

B. Analysis

For hfi studies, it is often most useful to choose for the target an even-even isotope of the element of interest. The first excited nuclear state is then invariably 2^+, and usually has a relatively high Coulomb excitation cross section. The angular distribution function is generally written as a sum of Legendre Polynomials, *

$$W(\theta) = 1 + A_2 P_2 (\cos \theta) + A_4 P_4 (\cos \theta). \qquad (2)$$

For the $(O^{16}_{\theta = 180^{\circ}}, \gamma_{2+ \to 0})$ case, $A_2 = 5/7$ and $A_4 = -12/7$, so that $W(\theta) = 0$ for $\theta = n\pi/2$, and the angular correlation is highly anisotropic.

Geometrical corrections due mainly to finite detector sizes decrease the effective A_2 and A_4, but the coincidence count rate still varies by a factor of about 8 from $\theta = 45^{\circ}$ to $\theta = 90^{\circ}$. Figure 4 shows two angular correlations from samarium 150 implanted into copper and silicon respectively. The solid curves are best fits to Eq. (2), determining A_2 and A_4. The best fit values agree, within experimental and calculational uncertainties, with those calculated assuming no extranuclear perturbations. The dashed curve in the same figure is the normalized theoretical distribution which would be obtained with point (zero solid angle) detectors.

The observed large anisotropy is extremely sensitive to small perturbations induced via hyperfine interactions. General

*See S.G. Cohen, Chap. 12.

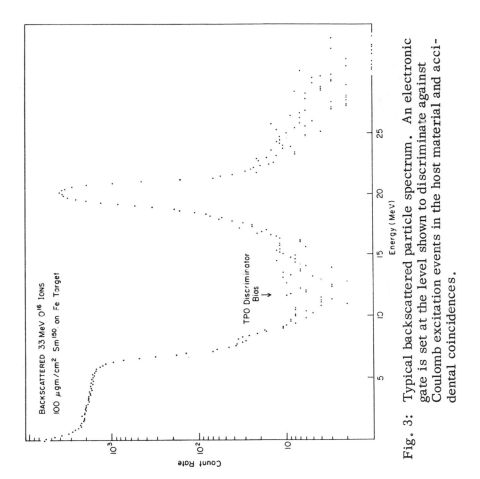

Fig. 3:   Typical backscattered particle spectrum. An electronic gate is set at the level shown to discriminate against Coulomb excitation events in the host material and accidental coincidences.

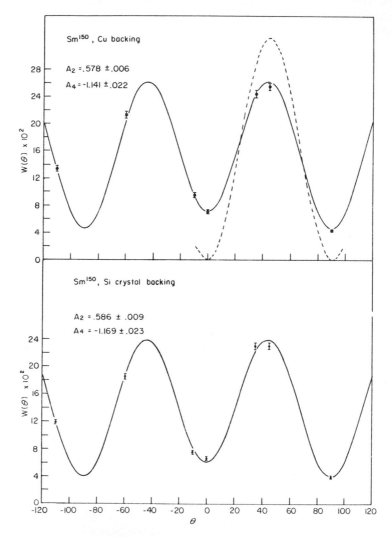

Fig. 4: Angular correlations obtained after Coulomb excitation
         ion implantation into non-magnetic materials. The
         dashed curve is the theoretical correlation for hypothe-
         tical point detectors. The best fit A_2 and A_4 parameters
         agree, within error brackets, with those calculated as-
         suming only geometrical corrections.

expressions for an angular correlation perturbed by electric or magnetic, or electric and magnetic hyperfine interactions are given by Steffen and Frauenfelder (1964). In a magnetic field perpendicular to the counting plane, the time integral perturbed angular correlation

$$W(\theta, H) = b_0 + \frac{b_2}{1 + 4\langle(\omega_H \tau)^2\rangle} (\cos 2\theta - 2\langle\omega_H \tau\rangle \sin 2\theta)$$

$$+ \frac{b_4}{1 + 16\langle(\omega_H \tau)^2\rangle} (\cos 4\theta - 4\langle\omega_H \tau\rangle \sin 4\theta)$$

$$(3)$$

is observed. $\omega_H = -g_R \mu_N H/\hbar$ with g_R the nuclear gyromagnetic ratio and H the effective magnetic field on the excited nucleus; τ is the nuclear meanlife, and b_0, b_2 and b_4 well known linear combinations of A_2 and A_4 (Steffen and Frauenfelder, 1964).

In a typical magnetic hfi experiment, the angular correlation is measured at several angles with a small external polarizing magnetic field alternatively up and down. Each point is normalized to the same number of backscattered particles, eliminating errors due to changes in accelerator beam intensity and variations in target thickness. The measured correlations are then analyzed using Eq. (3) and an $\langle\omega_H \tau\rangle$ value determined. The nuclear meanlife τ is known, or independently measured, so g_R or H_{eff} can be determined, if one or the other is known.

There are several assumptions implicit in the described analysis:

i. The slowing down time of the recoil ion is much less than the nuclear meanlife so that the ion-lattice system rapidly comes to equilibrium and an essentially static interaction is measured. Using the theory of Lindhard et al. (1963) for the energy loss of fast heavy ions in matter, the slowing down times can be roughly calculated and turn out to be about 5 to 8 $\times$ 10^{-13} seconds for the cases of concern here. For states living longer than about 5 picoseconds this first assumption then should be valid.

ii. Perturbations while the ions are slowing down are negligible. The recoiling ion undoubtedly loses and picks up electrons while moving through the host lattice. The time scale for this process is of the order of 10^{-16} seconds (10^{-8} cm, an atomic distance divided by 10^8 cm/sec, an average recoil velocity), however, and the effective magnetic field due to unpaired electrons averages to zero. [It should be emphasized that if the

recoil ion moves in vacuum, significant depolarization effects
are expected and have been found (Goldring et al., 1966)].

iii. Electric quadrupole and time dependent perturbations
are close to zero. The electric quadrupole interaction is characterized by the frequency $\omega_E = -eqQ/4\hbar(2I - 1)$, where Q is the
nuclear quadrupole moment and q the electric field gradient. One
expects q to be small for ions implanted into cubic lattices. The
angular correlation perturbation depends on $(\omega_E \tau)^2$ and for excited
state lifetimes less than 10^{-10} seconds, the calculated quadrupole
attenuation is negligible in all but the most extreme cases (Steffen
and Frauenfelder, 1964). That unperturbed integral correlation
patterns are observed, for most targets studied, on implantation
into copper corroborates these arguments.

III. Recoil Implantation of Sm^{150} into Fe, Co, and Ni

Experiments done at Wisconsin on the angular correlation of
gammas emitted from the first 2^+ level in Sm^{150} at 336 keV confirm the above assumptions and serve as a good example of the
capabilities of the described method.   The nuclear state studied
is an excellent probe for the internal fields on samarium in iron,
cobalt and nickel. The Coulomb excitation probability is high, the
336 keV photopeak is experimentally well resolved from any background radiations, and the lifetime (6.96×10^{-11} sec.) is long
enough to obviate questions of slowing down perturbations, but
short enough to minimize possible quadrupole effects. And, the
resulting $\omega_H \tau$ values are in the range for which the present technique is most sensitive.

Figure 5 displays the experimental results obtained implanting excited Sm^{150} into polarized iron, nickel, and partially
polarized cobalt. In the former two cases, the drawn curves are
best fits to Eq. (3) with $\omega_H \tau$ the only variable parameter. Two fits
are shown for the cobalt data, one varying $\omega_H \tau$ only, and a second
letting $\langle (\omega_H \tau)^2 \rangle$ be different from $\langle \omega_H \tau \rangle^2$.

Unlike iron and nickel, cobalt has a hexagonal crystal structure and it is relatively hard to saturate magnetically using the
small magnet shown in Fig. 1. Nevertheless, in a partially po-
larized sample the angular correlation displacement $\langle \omega_H \tau \rangle$ would
be due to the component of H_{eff} perpendicular to the quantization
axis, while the attenuation of the correlation, related to $\langle (\omega_H \tau)^2 \rangle$,
would depend on the magnitude of H_{eff} only. This point was
checked by repeating the experiment with several external field

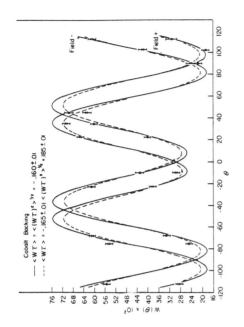

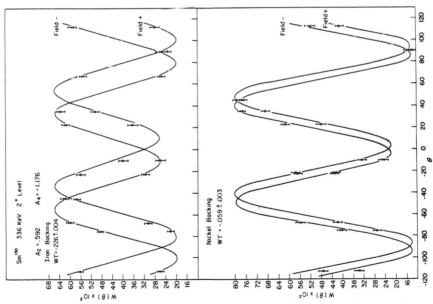

Fig. 5: Angular correlations obtained after ion implantation into magnetized ferromagnetic foils. Data are taken at each angle with the external polarizing field alternatively up and down (+ and −). The two fits shown for the cobalt data are discussed in the text.

values. $\langle \omega_H \tau \rangle$ was found to follow the cobalt magnetization curve for low polarizing fields, while $\langle (\omega_H \tau)^2 \rangle$ did not show significant variation.

In order to extract absolute internal field values on samarium from these results [$(\omega_H \tau)_{Fe}$ = -0.226 ± 0.005, $(\omega_H \tau)_{Co}$ = -0.185 ± 0.01, $(\omega_H \tau)_{Ni}$ = -0.060 ± 0.003] either one value of H_{eff} or g_R must be independently determined. The signs and relative magnitudes of the $(\omega_H \tau)$'s themselves are striking, however. $\omega_H \tau$ and therefore H_{eff} is seen in Fig. 6 to be linearly proportional to the atomic magnetic moment of the host material. This result is somewhat

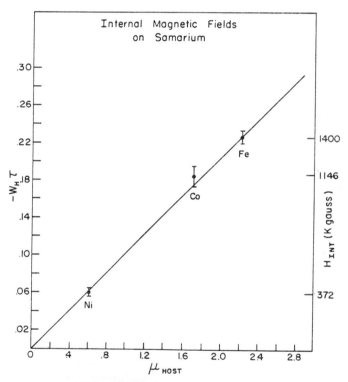

Fig. 6: Experimental $\omega_H \tau$ values for Sm^{150} in ferromagnetic materials plotted against the atomic magnetic moment of the host material. The right hand ordinate scale gives the internal magnetic field in kilogauss.

surprising for samarium where the effective field is due to polarization of the samarium inner 4f electrons, and crystal field effects are thought to be important (Ofer et al., 1965). The internal field is positive, indicating an antiferromagnetic spin exchange coupling between the Sm 4f electrons and the ferromagnetic 3d electrons of the host.

Grodzins et al. (1966) and Boehm et al. (1966a) have determined the effective field on samarium in iron to be 1400 ± 200 kG using the same technique and Sm^{152} as a probe. Adopting the internal field value as 1400 kG, one obtains from our results: g_R (336 keV, Sm^{150}) = 0.482 ± 0.005, $H_{eff}(Co)$ = 1146 ± 65 kG and $H_{eff}(Ni)$ = 372 ± 19 kG. Temperature dependent experiments are now in progress to further elucidate the internal field behavior for these interesting systems.

IV. Discussion

Sm^{150} is such a good experimental probe primarily because its lifetime, 6.96×10^{-11} sec., is in the range for which the discussed assumptions are most secure. For very short lifetimes, less than 5 picoseconds, for example, some modifications should be made in the analysis if only because some nuclei will decay before coming to rest. Surprisingly high g_R factors obtained using this method for the first excited states of Te^{126} and Te^{128} (τ = 5.82 and 4.36 picosec. respectively) (Borchers et al., 1966) have led to an *ad hoc* conjecture that a large transient magnetic field may be present on slow moving tellurium atoms in a polarized iron lattice. Experiments to determine a lower limit on τ for which the method is applicable are in progress.

For long lifetimes, greater than about 1 nanosecond, quadrupole perturbations are likely to be important for some isotope-lattice systems (Grodzins et al., 1966; Boehm and Hagemann, 1966b). In this region, though, time dependent experiments should be capable of separating the magnetic and electric perturbations, providing additional interesting information.

Another interesting and important question relevant to these experiments is the nature of the final site of the recoiling impurity atom in the host lattice. Atomic radii and electron configurations as well as lattice constants must be considered in each case, but the available evidence indicates that the recoil impurity site is unique and often substitutional. The data for impurities implanted into ferromagnetic materials are consistent with a unique effective internal field (Murnick et al., 1966; Gilad et al., 1966) and agrees with internal field data obtained from metallurgically prepared samples in several cases (Borchers et al., 1966; Boehm et al.,

1966a; Agarwal et al., 1966; Buyrn and Grodzins, 1964; Auerbach et al., 1966). At present the only anomaly is tungsten in iron for which implantation perturbed angular correlations yield H_{eff} = 455 ± 30 kG (Boehm et al., 1966a; Gilad et al., 1966) and Mössbauer effect measurements yield 705 ± 25 kG (Kankeleit, 1965; Frankel et al., 1966).

Calculations of Erginsoy et al.(1964, 1965) indicate that the recoil atom should stop substitutionally for projectile and host of the same element. Beginning with a realistic set of interatomic forces in a bcc iron lattice, they have integrated the equations of motion of a large set of atoms for a primary knock-on of energy from 17 to 1500 eV, with many different incident momentum directions with respect to the lattice planes. Their results of primary interest are that, in all cases, the initial knock-on stops in a substitutional position, and that the radiation damage which consists of vacancies and interstitials in the crystal occurs far from the primary site.

Striking confirmation that the recoil ion indeed stops substitutionally in some cases is given by some experiments of Domeij and Bjorquist (1965). Utilizing the string effect in crystals (Lindhard, 1965) they have shown by studying the angular distribution of emitted alpha particles, that at least 72% of 60 keV Rn^{222} atoms implanted into tungsten crystals end up at lattice points.

To summarize briefly, the Coulomb excitation ion implantation technique has many merits for studies of hyperfine interactions in solids. The choice of target and host materials is extremely flexible and adaptation to temperature dependent studies is not difficult. Integral measurements can be used to study interactions with nuclear states having lifetimes in the 10^{-12} to 10^{-10} second range and time dependent measurements can be made using longer lived excited states. The information obtainable is great, and in many cases extends and complements that obtained using NMR, Mössbauer effect, or radioactive source perturbed angular correlation methods.

References

Agarwal, Y., Baba, L., and Bhattacherjee, S. (1966). Nuc. Phys.
    79, 437.

Auerbach, K., Harms, B., Siepe, K., Wittkemper, G., and Körner, H. (1966). Phys. Letters 22, 299.

Boehm, F., Hagemann, G., and Winther, A. (1966a). Phys. Letters 21, 217.

Boehm, F. and Hagemann, G. (1966b). Akad. Nauk USSR (in press).

Borchers, R., Bronson, J., Murnick, D., and Grodzins, L. (1966). Phys. Rev. Letters 17, 1099.

Buyrn, A and Grodzins, L. (1964). Bull. Am. Phys. Soc. 9, 410.

Domeij, B and Björquist, K. (1965). Phys. Letters 14, 127.

Erginsoy, C., Vineyard, G., and Englert, A. (1964). Phys. Rev. 133, A595.

Erginsoy, C., Vineyard, G., and Shimizu, A. (1965). Phys. Rev. 139, A118.

Frankel, R., Chow, Y., and Grodzins, L. (1966).(to be published).

Gilad, P., Goldring, G., Kalish, R., Herber, R. (1966). Phys. Rev. 151, 281.

Goldring, G., Kalish, R., and Spehl, H. (1966). Nucl. Phys. 80, 33.

Grodzins, L., Borchers, R., and Hagemann, G. (1966). Phys. Letters 21, 214.

Kankeleit, E. (1965). Bull. Am. Phys. Soc. 11, 65.

Lindhard, J., Scharff, M., and Schiott, H. (1963). Mat. Fys. Medd. Dan. Vid. Selsk. 33, No. 14.

Lindhard, J. (1965). Mat. Fys. Medd. Dan. Vid. Selsk. 34, No. 14.

Murnick, D., Grodzins, L., Borchers, R., and Bronson, J. (1966).(to be published).

Ofer, S., Segal, E., Nowik, I., Bauminger, E., Grodzins, L., Freeman, A. J., and Schieber, M. (1965). Phys. Rev. 137, A627.

Steffen, R. and Frauenfelder, H. (1964). in Perturbed Angular Correlations (North-Holland Publishing Co., Amsterdam) p. 3.

S.3. A STUDY OF RARE-EARTH HYPERFINE STRUCTURES USING COULOMB EXCITED MÖSSBAUER LEVELS

J.C. Walker

*The Johns Hopkins University
Baltimore, Maryland*

I. Introduction

A considerable amount of work on hyperfine structures has been done using the recoilless emission and recoilless resonant absorption of gamma rays; that is the Mössbauer effect. Among the requirements which must be met if a gamma ray from the decay of a given nuclear level is to be used for Mössbauer effect studies is the requirement that there be a satisfactory means of exciting the level. In most cases the level is excited by the beta-decay of a parent of sufficiently long half-life to permit the experiment to be performed. It is also necessary that the source not produce other non-resonant radiations close in energy to the gamma ray of interest. This requirement, however, is somewhat relieved by the development of high resolution LiGe detectors.

II. Mössbauer Effect in Fe^{57}

It has recently been discovered that the relevant nuclear levels for Mössbauer effect studies can be excited by nuclear reactions (Ruby and Holland, 1965; Hafemeister and Shera, 1965; Seyboth, et al., 1965; Lee et al., 1965; Goldberg, et al., 1965). In one case Mössbauer effect studies of Fe^{57} following Coulomb

excitation were carried out using both metals and oxides for target materials (Ritter et al., 1965). In these experiments the
bombarding particles were 3 MeV protons from a Van de Graaff
accelerator. With the metal target and a single line absorber, a
Mössbauer spectrum showing a hyperfine splitting characteristic
of the metal target was obtained. Examination of the spectrum
indicated that the hyperfine fields in the target foil were identical
to those in an ordinary iron foil. In addition, the fraction of recoilless gamma rays emitted by the Coulomb-excited levels was
equal, within experimental error, to the recoilless fraction for
the level excited by beta decay. Both of these findings are somewhat surprising in that the nuclei of interest receive average recoil energies of hundreds of kilovolts in these Coulomb excitation
processes, which certainly causes them to move from their original lattice sites as typical displacement energies are of the order
of tens of electron volts.

If the recoiling nucleus came to rest in an interstitial position in the lattice before emitting the gamma ray of interest, some
change of either the nuclear hyperfine field or the recoilless
fraction would be anticipated. The fact that this was not seen in
the metal foil indicates that in this case the recoiling nucleus
regains a normal lattice position before emitting a gamma ray.
This is supported by the fact that Coulomb excitation Mössbauer
experiments with oxide targets indicate a significantly diminished
recoilless fraction compared to normal beta decay sources in
oxide form. One might expect that the close packed metal lattice
would behave differently under bombardment than the more open
oxide lattice which has both iron and oxygen sites. While a real
understanding of the behavior of the Coulomb excited nucleus is
lacking, these preliminary investigations indicate that under most
circumstances one can obtain reliable information on hyperfine
structures using the Mössbauer effect following Coulomb excitation.

III. Mössbauer Effect in the Rare Earth Region

The possibility of exciting nuclear levels for Mössbauer
effect studies by Coulomb excitation is particularly interesting in
the rare-earth region ($140 \leq A \leq 180$). In this region there are
many stable isotopes with excited states within 100 keV of the
ground state. The gamma rays emitted by these levels in their
decay to the ground state have sufficiently low energy that at
$4.2°K$ a significant fraction of the decays are recoilless.

Further, cross-sections for Coulomb excitation of these states are in many cases twenty to a hundred times greater than one finds for similar transitions for $A < 140$. Many of these excited levels cannot be reached by means of a suitable beta-decay.

In the present case, we have restricted our attention to the $2+ \rightarrow 0+$ transitions in the even-even rare earth isotopes. These $2+$ levels are interpreted as corresponding to rotational excitations of the nucleus as a whole (Bohr and Mottelson, 1953) rather than intrinsic excitations involving a small number of the nucleons, such as one has in the simple shell model. This collective model relates the energies of these rotational levels to a distortion of the nucleus from a spherical shape and thus relates the large Coulomb excitation cross-sections for these levels to the enhancement of E2 transition probabilities by this nuclear distortion. This also leads to large electric quadrupole moments for the 2+ levels. Using this model and determinations of the E2 transition probabilities by Coulomb excitation, the quadrupole moments Q_0 associated with the deformed nuclear shapes have been determined for the 2+ levels of the even-even rare-earth isotopes. These Q_0's are related to the quadrupole moments Q appearing in the electric quadrupole hyperfine interaction by a projection factor (Bohr and Mottelson, 1953):

$$Q = \left(\frac{3K^2 - I(I+1)}{(I+1)(2I+3)} \right) Q_0 \tag{1}$$

By observing electric quadrupole hyperfine spectra for the 2+ levels of several even-even isotopes of the same element, one can compare the variation of Q with A with that obtained from E2 transition rates and the assumptions of the collective model.

While hyperfine spectra of isotopes of several rare-earth elements in a number of different lattice environments have been obtained using the Mössbauer effect following Coulomb excitation, (Eck et al., 1966) the present discussion will be restricted to several even-even isotopes of ytterbium,* namely Yb^{170}, Yb^{172}, Yb^{174} and Yb^{176}. Electric hyperfine spectra were obtained for the 2+ nuclear levels of these isotopes in Yb_2O_3. The oxide is a complicated lattice for these experiments in that there are two non-equivalent lattice sites. Three-fourths of the Yb^{3+} ions are at sites of C_2 symmetry, while one-fourth are at sites of C_{3i} symmetry. Other Mössbauer experiments involving the oxides

*The work mentioned here was done in collaboration with Y.K. Lee, R. Stevens, and J. Eck.

have demonstrated that the resulting spectra can be satisfactorily explained by considering only the ions at the C_2 sites (Barnes et al., 1964). If we are interested in changes in the spectra as one considers different isotopes, these complications are not particularly serious.

A. Experimental Procedure

The 2+ levels of Yb^{172}, Yb^{174} and Yb^{176} were populated by Coulomb excitation using a beam of 3 MeV protons from the Johns Hopkins University Van de Graaff accelerator. In some cases enriched oxide targets were used. With a beam of 0.2 microamperes the oxide targets produced a counting rate in the gamma ray window of 600 counts per second for a detector solid angle of approximately 5% of 2π steradians. When enriched metallic targets were used, beam currents of 0.1 microamperes produced count rates of 1,000 counts per second in the same detector. A typical excitation gamma spectrum is shown in Fig. 1. The relatively high energies of the gamma rays involved made it necessary to cool both source and absorber to liquid helium temperature to observe appreciable Mössbauer effects. The apparatus used to achieve this cooling, provide the necessary Doppler velocity between target and absorber, and permit the beam to reach the target is shown schematically in Fig. 2 and is described in detail elsewhere (Stevens, 1966). The Doppler velocity drive was of standard form operating in a constant acceleration mode. The gamma rays were detected by a scintillation counter and were recorded in a 256-channel analyzer operating in the time mode.

In all of these experiments, we used ytterbium metal foils and Yb_2O_3 for targets and absorbers. Ytterbium metal is diamagnetic and cubic, and exhibits no hyperfine interaction. It is therefore useful in Mössbauer experiments as it contributes no structure when used in combination with other ytterbium compounds. Yb_2O_3 is paramagnetic, but in this case the Yb^{3+} ion has a very short spin-lattice relaxation time compared to a Larmor period, so that the magnetic hyperfine structure is not seen in a gamma resonance experiment even at $4.2°K$. The quadrupole hyperfine interaction in Yb_2O_3 is complicated by the lack of axial symmetry at the C_2 sites; the electric field gradient at the nucleus therefore cannot be specified by a single component V_{zz}. In our analysis we have assumed that the asymmetry can be described by a single parameter $\eta = (V_{xx} - V_{yy})/V_{zz}$, where V_{zz} is chosen as the largest of the components so that $0 \le |\eta| \le 1$. The quadrupole hyperfine splitting of the 2+ levels as a function of η is shown in Fig. 3. Because of the short half-lives of these

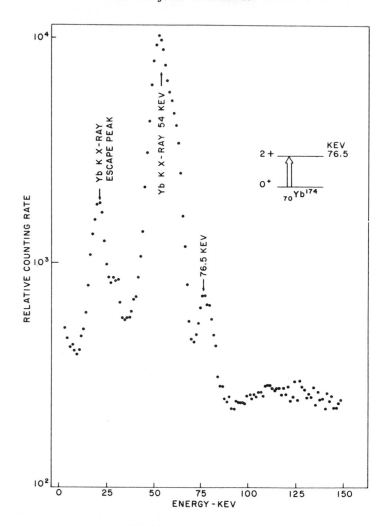

Fig. 1: Coulomb excitation gamma spectrum for Yb^{174} using an enriched Yb$_2$O$_3$ target.

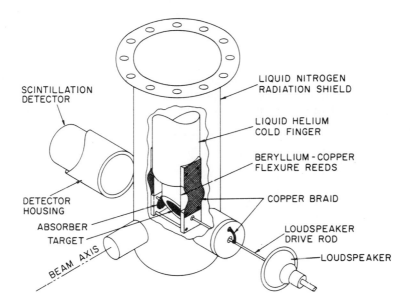

Fig. 2: Schematic drawing of liquid helium system.

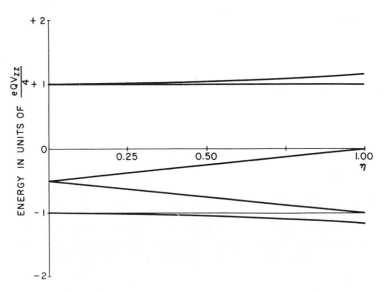

Fig. 3: Energy levels of a 2+ state for a quadrupole interaction
with asymmetry parameter η.

2+ states (about 2 nanoseconds) the natural widths of the lines in the Mössbauer spectra preclude a complete resolution of the five lines which result for $\eta \neq 0$.

The data were fitted by computer to five Lorentzian lines each having the same width and depth parameters and whose positions were determined by adjusting parameters eQV_{ZZ} and η. An example of the data and fit is shown in Fig. 4. To assess possible

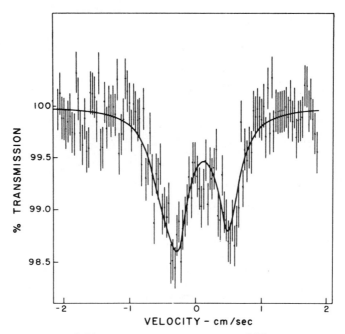

Fig. 4: Yb^{174} metallic target vs. $Yb_2^{174}O_3$ absorber.

radiation damage effects in the spectra, an enriched metallic target was run with a metal absorber. The resulting single line showed a width only 30% greater than that obtained if the natural width were assumed for the emission and absorption process. In addition, experiments were performed with Yb^{174} using first an oxide target versus a metal absorber and then a metal target versus oxide absorber. The values of eQV_{ZZ} determined in each case agree with each other within experimental error.

B. Results

In this fashion values of eQV_{ZZ} for Yb^{172}, Yb^{174} and Yb^{176}

were obtained and compared with the value for Yb^{170} determined by us in a separate experiment using a radioactive source. As one expects V_{ZZ} and η to be the same regardless of the isotope of ytterbium used, the ratio of hyperfine splittings yields the ratio of quadrupole moments. The ratios Q_A/Q_{170} are shown in Fig. 5,

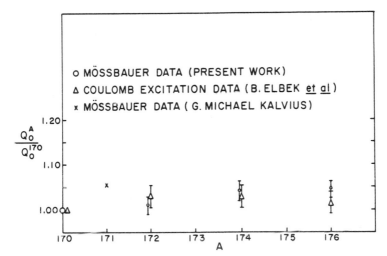

Fig. 5: Relative values of quadrupole moments vs. atomic number.

compared to the ratios of $Q_o(A)/Q_o(^{170})$ obtained from a collective model interpretation of B(E2) from Coulomb excitation measurements (Elbek, et al., 1960). It can be seen that the agreement is excellent. The lack of variation of Q with A for ytterbium isotopes precludes drawing firm conclusions about the validity of the collective model from the ratios. At present, it is not possible to calculate reliable values of V_{zz}, so that absolute values of Q are not available for comparison with the Coulomb excitation values of Q_o. Work has also been done at Johns Hopkins on the even isotopes of gadolinium using a similar method (Stevens et al., 1966). Here there is a pronounced variation of Q with A. In this case agreement is also found between quadrupole moment ratios determined from Mössbauer effect spectra and those obtained from measurements of B(E2).

IV. Conclusion

The use of the Mössbauer effect for a determination of hyperfine structure of excited nuclear levels in the rare earth region has the advantage of providing an explicit spectrum which is often easier to interpret than the hyperfine information obtainable from integral angular correlation techniques. Coulomb excitation can be used to excite the relevant nuclear levels without significant distortion of the hyperfine spectra by the excitation process.

References

Barnes, R. G., Mössbauer, R. L., Kankeleit, E., and Poindexter, J. M. (1964). Phys. Rev. 136, 175.

Bohr, A. and Mottelson, B. R. (1953). Phys. Rev. 89, 316.

Eck, J., Lee, Y. K., Ritter, E. T., Stevens, R. R., Jr., and Walker, J. C. (1966). Phys. Rev. Letters 17, 120.

Elbek, B., Olesen, M. C., and Skilbreid, O. (1960). Nuc. Phys. 19, 523.

Goldberg, D. A., Keaton, P. W., Jr., Lee, Y. K., Madansky, L., and Walker, J. C. (1965). Phys. Rev. Letters 15, 418.

Hafemeister, D. W. and Shera, E. B. (1965). Phys. Rev. Letters 14, 593.

Lee, Y. K., Keaton, P. W., Jr., Ritter, E. T., and Walker, J.C. (1965). Phys. Rev. Letters 14, 957.

Ritter, E. T., Lee, Y. K., Stevens, R. R. Jr., and Walker, J.C. (1965). Bull. Am. Phys. Soc. 10, 1111.

Ruby, S. L. and Holland R. E. (1965). Phys. Rev. Letters 14, 591.

Seyboth, D., Obenshain, F. E., and Czjzek, G. (1965). Phys. Rev. Letters 14, 954.

Stevens, R. R., Jr. (1966). Ph.D. Thesis, Johns Hopkins University.

Stevens, R. R., Jr., Eck, J., Lee, Y. K., and Walker, J. C. (1966). (to be published).

S.4.

SOME LOW TEMPERATURE NUCLEAR ORIENTATION TECHNIQUES AND APPLICATIONS

N.J. Stone

Clarendon Laboratory
Oxford, England

I. Introduction

This chapter aims to fulfill two objectives. The first is to outline the theory and technique of the nuclear orientation method and to give some idea of its scope and its limitations. The second is to give a brief account of nuclear orientation studies at the Clarendon Laboratory, Oxford. Currently, the main object in those studies is the measurement of hyperfine interactions at paramagnetic ions of the iron group present as dilute impurities in metals which, in their pure state, are non-magnetic. In addition, experiments to extend the systematic study of hyperfine fields at diamagnetic impurities in ferromagnets are described.

II. The Experimental Concept

To give the orders of magnitude associated with the low temperature nuclear orientation method we may consider a system of nuclei of spin I, with magnetic moment μ, in a magnetic field H. The hyperfine interaction gives then a system of magnetic sub-levels equally spaced by $\mu H/I$. In thermal equilibrium the population distribution between these levels is a Boltzmann distribution

$$N(M_I) = K \exp[-\mu HM_I/IkT].$$ (1)

To obtain appreciable differences in population, the hyperfine interaction must be of the same order as the thermal energy, i. e., the exponent must be of order unity, or $\mu H \approx kT$. Taking as an example $\mu = 1$ nuclear magneton, the product H/T is then 3×10^7 gauss/$^\circ$K. Thus one needs 10^6 gauss at 0.03°K, and even larger fields at higher temperatures. Such fields cannot be produced in the laboratory but do occur at nuclei in various classes of solids. Hyperfine interactions in solids are of order 10^{-1} $^\circ$K or less, so that the experiments are possible only at temperatures below 0.1°K.

The nuclear ordering may be detected by the spatial anisotropy of emission of radioactive decay products.

III. Outline of the Theory

The angular distribution of emission probability for gamma radiation may be written*

$$W(\theta) = \sum_\nu F_\nu P_\nu (\cos \theta)$$ (2)

where θ is the angle between the direction of emission and the nuclear spin quantization axis, ν is an even integer, and $P_\nu(\cos \theta)$ are the Legendre polynomials.

We will also make the following assumptions:

i. For all other radiation fields connecting states of well-defined angular momentum the distribution has the same form as Eq. (2). In particular, it applies to alpha emission and beta decay. In the latter case, ν can also take on odd integral values as a result of parity non-conservation.

ii. For a sequence of such emissions the multiplication properties of the Legendre polynomials again give the same final form. Thus the difference between nuclear orientation and angular correlation lies in the fact that in the former the nuclear spins are oriented in the initial state. This orientation contains all the information concerning the hyperfine interaction of the parent nuclei and is the concern of this chapter. In angular correlation

*See S. G. Cohen, Chap. 12.

this information can only be obtained by interaction effects in the intermediate, partially ordered, state.

The "moments of orientation," $f_\nu(I)$, for a system of oriented nuclei may also be defined. The first three of these are:

$$f_0 = 1$$

$$f_1 = \frac{1}{I} \sum_{M_I} a_{M_I} M_I \tag{3}$$

$$f_2 = \frac{1}{I^2} \left[\sum_{M_I} a_{M_I} M_I^2 - \frac{1}{3} I(I + 1) \right]$$

where the a_{M_I} are the normalized occupation probabilities for the nuclear spin projections M_I along the axis of orientation. In the low temperature thermal equilibrium methods of nuclear orientation the a_{M_I} are given by a Boltzmann distribution. The f_ν factors were first introduced by Tolhoek and Cox (1953), and the general expression for $f_\nu(I)$ is given by (e.g., de Groot et al., 1965),

$$f_\nu(I) = \binom{2\nu}{\nu}^{-1} I^{-\nu} \sum_{M_I} \sum_{n=0}^{\nu} (-1)^n \frac{(I - M_I)! \, (I + M_I)!}{(I - M_I - n)!(I + M_I - \nu + n)!} \times \binom{\nu}{n}^2 a_{M_I} \tag{4}$$

where the notation $\binom{a}{b} = \frac{a!}{b!(a-b)!}$ has been used. These authors also develop a complete formalism for the description of the angular distribution of radiation from oriented nuclei using the f_ν parameters. A second system of parametrisation for the angular distribution has been developed and is also widely used. Here the parent state order is described by "orientation parameters" $B_\nu(I)$ defined by

$$B_\nu(I) = \sum_{M_I} (2\nu + 1)^{\frac{1}{2}} C(I \, \nu \, I; M_I \, 0) a_{M_I} \tag{5}$$

(Gray and Satchler, 1955). These differ from the $f_\nu(I)$ only in normalisation, and the two are related by

$$B_\nu(I) = \binom{2\nu}{\nu} I^\nu \left[(2\nu + 1)(2I + 1)(2I - \nu)!/2I + \nu + 1)! \right]^{\frac{1}{2}} f_\nu(I). \tag{6}$$

The advantage of this second system is that the final expression for the angular distribution of gamma rays is

$$W(\theta) = \sum_\nu B_\nu U_\nu F_\nu P_\nu (\cos \theta) \tag{7}$$

where the F_ν factors are the same as those used in the theory of angular correlation, tabulated by Ferentz and Rosenzweig (1955). The facility of interchange of information between the two techniques argues strongly for the general adoption of this system. It is described fully in e.g., Blin-Stoyle and Grace (1957), who discuss the orientation parameters with reference to various experimentally important spin Hamiltonians.

In Eq. (7), the U_ν factors are angular momentum coupling constants describing the effect of the unobserved intermediate transition(s) preceding the observed transition, which is described by the appropriate F_ν coefficient. Thus the $U_\nu F_\nu$ products ($=A_\nu$) are functions of the nuclear spins, and transition multipolarities with their various amplitudes. For simplicity, we will assume that for at least one observable gamma transition these parameters are known. If, however, this is not so, the hyperfine interaction may still be obtained, provided the temperature dependence of $W(\theta)$ is measured, as the $B_\nu(I)$ are the only temperature dependent terms in Eq. (7) and the A_ν are simply multiplicative constants.

The general expression (Eq. 7) can be further limited by considering the range of values of ν. We talk of nuclear polarisation if all $B_\nu(I) \neq 0$, and of nuclear alignment if only even terms are non-zero, both cases being known collectively as orientation. The range of the parameter ν depends on three considerations:

i. If the *observed* radiation mechanism conserves parity, only even ν terms can be detected, i.e., even ν for α, γ measurements, but all ν for β measurements.

ii. The series terminates, from angular momentum coupling considerations, at $\nu_{max} \leq \min(2I, 2L)$ where I is the lowest spin in the decay sequence preceding the observed transition and L is the highest multipole component of the observed transition.

iii. In most cases the degree of orientation at attainable temperatures is well below saturation and the $B_\nu(I)$ fall off rapidly for increasing ν. Specifically for gamma radiation often only B_2 and B_4 need be considered, and in many cases only B_2.

In this simplest of all cases we have:

$$W(0^\circ) = 1 + A_2 B_2 ,$$
$$W(90^\circ) = 1 - A_2 B_2/2 . \tag{8}$$

Another widely used parameter is the "anisotropy" ε defined as

$$\varepsilon = 1 - W(0)/W(90) . \tag{9}$$

IV. The Hyperfine Hamiltonian

The general hyperfine Hamiltonian is discussed at length elsewhere in this volume.* The nuclear interaction may be either via the magnetic dipole moment or the electric quadrupole moment of the nucleus. We give here a simple example to show how these may be distinguished by measurement of the temperature dependence of the anisotropy. Table I shows the result of calculating the f_ν parameters for $\nu = 0$, 1, 2 for two Hamiltonians: i) $\mathcal{H}_N = -g\beta_N H \cdot I$, i.e., magnetic hyperfine splitting, levels equally spaced with separation $\Delta = g\beta_N H/I$; ii) $\mathcal{H}_N = P[M_I^2 - \frac{1}{3}I(I+1)]$, where P is the interaction between the nuclear electric quadrupole moment and the electric field gradient at the nucleus. The latter gives a basic splitting $\Delta' = P$. The calculation has been done for the case $I = 1$ and in the high temperature approximation $\Delta/kT \ll 1$, i.e., retaining only the first non-zero term and normalising only to this order.

Table I: Calculation of f_ν parameters for $I = 1$

	Magnetic $\mathcal{H}_N = g\beta_N H \cdot I$	Electric $\mathcal{H}_N = P[M_I^2 - \frac{1}{3}I(I+1)]$
f_0	1	1
f_1	$\frac{2}{3}(\frac{\Delta}{kT})$	0
f_2	$\frac{2}{9}(\frac{\Delta}{kT})^2$	$-\frac{2}{9}(\frac{\Delta'}{kT})$

In the magnetic case polarisation is produced, the leading term in f_2 varies quadratically with $1/T$ and the leading term in f_2 varies quadratically with Δ, so that a simple gamma anisotropy measurement cannot yield the sign of the hyperfine interaction $g\beta_N H$.

*B. Bleaney, Chap. 1.

In the electric case, there is alignment but no polarisation, the leading term in f_2 varies linearly with $1/T$ and the sign of f_2 gives the sign of the hyperfine interaction.

Thus the form of temperature dependence observed allows separation of magnetic and electric interactions but the sign of the interaction is given by a simple gamma ray angular distribution experiment in the electric case only. The sign of magnetic interaction requires a measurement of either β-asymmetry or gamma ray circular polarisation (for details see De Groot et al (1965) or Blin-Stoyle and Grace (1957)).

V. Experimental Methods

The experimental methods of nuclear orientation are described in detail in the reviews already cited. Recent developments are described fully by Shirley (1966), with the exception of the recently developed technique which combines nuclear orientation with NMR (Matthias and Holliday, 1966)*. Here, the basic outline only is given.

i. Low Temperatures. The low temperatures required are attained, presently, by adiabatic demagnetisation of a paramagnetic salt, although the rapidly developing He^3 - He^4 refrigerator technique may soon provide an alternative method with the advantage of continuous operation. One then either a) observes the decay of nuclei in the demagnetised salt itself or b) uses the salt to cool some secondary system via a thermal link. Method b) is more flexible. The choice of salt is determined by its having a large enthalpy in the temperature range required; a review of useful salts is given by Hudson (1961). Currently chrome potassium alum is widely used. When demagnetised from 20 kGauss/°K, it cools to close to $1/T = 100$, where it has a co-operative (antiferromagnetic) specific heat anomaly (Daniels and Kurti, 1954). The thermal contact to the specimen is made by copper foils or wires embedded at one end in the cooled salt with the sample at the other, either soldered (if metallic) or held in pressure contact using oil or varnish (if crystalline). A typical system is shown in Fig. 1.

ii. The Macroscopic Axis. To observe macroscopic orientation an axis must be defined, and since the fields which orient

*See E. Matthias, Chap. 13.

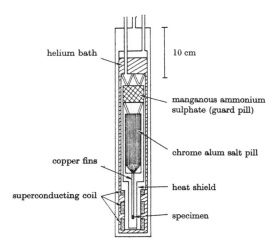

helium bath

10 cm

manganous ammonium
sulphate (guard pill)

chrome alum salt pill

copper fins

heat shield

superconducting coil

specimen

Fig. 1: Contact cooling cryostat arrangement (Campbell et al.,
(1965).

the nuclei are electronic in origin this means that the electron
spins must be ordered. In single crystals this axis may be provided by ionic alignment in the crystalline electric field, but an
external magnetic polarising field is required for ferromagnetic
metallic specimens and for polycrystalline samples.

iii. Thermometry. The most suitable method of thermometry is to observe a second nuclear species, in the same specimen or a second in similar thermal contact with the cooling salt.
If for this second species all the parameters of orientation are
known, the temperature of the specimen may be deduced from the
observed anisotropy. The thermometer nuclei should have a
simple decay scheme and not contribute a large background to the
spectra of the nuclei under study. Common examples are Co^{60} or
Mn^{54} in various hosts as thermometers for contact cooled metallic systems.   Poor thermal conductivity, particularly of
dielectric crystalline materials in this temperature range, makes
it important that the thermometric nuclei have the same distribution in the sample as those under study. Thus a bulk (average)
temperature measurement, as given by magnetic susceptibility,
is generally unsuitable, particularly if the nuclei are in a crystalline surface layer.

iv. The Experiments. The parameters of the system are
obtained by demagnetising to a range of final temperatures, and
observing the count rate as a function of temperature at $0°$ and

$90°$ to the orientation axis, normalising to the count rate at the He bath temperature (where the radiation is isotropic).

VI. Comparison with Other Techniques

1. Nuclear Spectroscopy and Count Rate

Nuclear orientation involves singles counting only (i.e., no coincidences are required). Since no coincidence requirement is made, the counting times can be short, typically a few minutes, and experiments can be done on extremely dilute spin systems. Measurement on activity concentrations as low as 10^{-10} is possible. In practice, one is limited in the lowest concentration range by the purity of available samples. Nevertheless the concentration range is wider than for NMR and the experimental time for a given concentration shorter than for perturbed angular correlation or the Mössbauer effect. The advent of Ge(Li) gamma detectors has widened the applicability of nuclear orientation to complex decay schemes, and the low efficiency of these devices again favours a singles measurement.

2. Range of Applicability

Over 40 elements have been oriented, and suitable isotopes exist for as many others. The requirements are: nuclear spin ≥ 1 ($\geq 1/2$ for parity non-conserving radiations); half life of the isotope, or a parent isotope, ≥ 1 hour; and a sufficiently large magnetic or electric moment. The present limitation lies in finding environments with sufficiently strong hyperfine coupling to give orientation in the accessible temperature range. A recent development in this field is the use of ion implantation techniques (see section VIIb) to study elements in environments not accessible by equilibrium methods of crystal growth or alloy preparation. Although this range is notably wider than that of the Mössbauer effect, nature has provided no suitable iron isotope for orientation!

3. Temperature Range

This is limited to the region $< 0.1°K$ in the vast majority of cases, and the technique thus lacks the flexibility of others in following the variation of hyperfine interactions with temperature.

4. Precision

Hitherto the precision of nuclear orientation results has been comparable with the Mössbauer effect and perturbed angular correlation, i.e., a few percent, where the nuclear Hamiltonian can be assumed to be known. The sensitivity of resolving magnetic and electric hfs is lower in conventional orientation work than in other methods. However the new application of NMR detected by the destruction of the nuclear orientation anisotropy* (Matthias and Holliday, 1966) outdates both these remarks. Accuracy of a few tenths percent is clearly attainable in magnetic metallic systems with good contact with the paramagnetic heat sink. A most useful feature of this combination of techniques is that the conventional orientation experiment, measuring the temperature dependence of the anisotropy, can be done on the same specimen at the same time, greatly reducing the search problem normally present with NMR. Details of the Hamiltonian will also be more easily observed.

5. Magnetic Saturation

In order to interpret the anisotropy from e.g., a simple magnetic hfs, magnetic saturation of the ionic spin system must be achieved. In some cases, notably rare-earth metals, this requirement, which does not apply to other techniques, is difficult to satisfy. Again one can observe that the combined NMR-nuclear orientation technique, as it does not depend upon interpretation of the magnitude of the effect, will not suffer from this limitation.

6. Time Dependent Effects

Nuclear orientation experiments may be used to study time dependent effects, based upon the anisotropy of the electronic Hamiltonian in certain systems (Lubbers, 1966). In addition there is the interesting possibility of measuring both T_1 and T_2 for the oriented nuclear species if the NMR/N.O. technique can be developed to give more complete destruction of the polarisation. By using pulsed NMR to turn the nuclear spins through, say $90°$, one could then observe the restoration of equilibrium orientation by monitoring the count rate along the equilibrium orientation axis and the axis of the NMR inducing field.

VII. Recent Oxford Work

During recent years, the N.O. group at the Clarendon Laboratory has worked exclusively on contact cooled metallic systems. Currently two main lines of research are being followed.

*E. Matthias, Chap. 13.

A. Local Moments

Various dilute alloys of transition metals in noble metal hosts show anomalies in the variation of electrical conductivity, specific heat, and magnetic susceptibility as functions of temperature which would indicate magnetic ordering. Recently, work at Oxford (Cameron et al., 1966) has been devoted to studying these alloys to discover how and when localised magnetic moments occur on the transition metal impurity and to measure associated hyperfine magnetic fields. Interest has developed in possible interactions between these local moments, and the effect of other trace impurities in the alloys is being investigated.

Detection of the localised moment is more easily done by the macroscopic measurements, notably electrical conductivity, mentioned above. However for detailed study of the hyperfine interaction nuclear orientation has several advantages. The concentration range accessible goes lower than that for NMR or nuclear specific heat measurements. Studies with Fe impurities may be done by the Mössbauer effect, whereas nuclear orientation has been observed for isotopes of Sc, V, Mn, Co and Cu. Cr^{51} is being used in attempts to observe an effective field for this element in Ni, Fe, and Au (Williams, 1966).

The simplest approach to these systems is to consider the transition metal impurity, here either Co or Mn at concentrations of order $10^{-8} - 10^{-9}$, as free paramagnetic ions in the host lattice. If the applied field is large enough to fully align the paramagnetic ions, the hyperfine fields will be equal and parallel and the simple magnetic hfs Hamiltonian will apply (as in Table I). From such saturation measurements the magnitude of H_{hf} has been obtained (Table II). The signs of the fields were obtained from measurement of the sense of circular polarisation of the gamma radiation.

In several cases measurements on higher concentration alloys by specific heat methods do not show good agreement with nuclear orientation values, nor do the various specific heat measurements agree (Cameron et al., 1966).

Interactions between the magnetic impurities are evident from hyperfine field measurements for applied external fields lower than that required for saturation. For non-interacting ions at lower fields the magnitude of the average field at the nuclei will be

Table II: Hyperfine fields in dilute alloys

Alloy	$|H_{hf}|$ (kOe)	Sign of H_{hf}
Mn^{54}/Cu	278 ± 10	-
Mn^{54}/Ag	313 ± 15	-
Mn^{54}/Au	400 ± 20	-
Mn^{54}/Pd	370 ± 20	-
Co^{60}/Pd	$140 \pm 20^{(a)}$	+
Co^{60}/Cu	≤ 40	
Co^{60}/Au	≤ 40	

(a) Dependent upon Co concentration. This result is for a few ppm Co. For 500 ppm Co H_{hf} = +205 ± 20 kOe.

$$\overline{H} = H_{hf} \frac{M_Z}{M_{sat}} \pm H_a \qquad (10)$$

where H_a is the applied field and M_Z and M_{sat} are the ionic magnetisations in a field H_a and for complete polarisation respectively. Provided the ionic spin-spin relaxation time is short compared with the nuclear precession time, the nuclear Zeeman level populations will be determined by taking H in Eq. (1) and in the a_{m_I} of Eq. (3) equal to $\overline{H}$. Thus the nuclear hyperfine field will follow the Brillouin function describing the approach to ionic saturation magnetisation.

Experimentally (Fig. 2) this simple behaviour is not found and in all cases the applied fields required to produce the saturation value of H_{hf} were larger than for

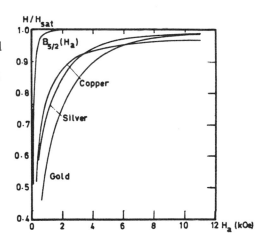

Fig. 2: Saturation behaviour of the hyperfine field at manganese in copper, silver and gold, compared with Brillouin function $B_{5/2}(H_a)$ of the external polarising field at $1/T = 48$.

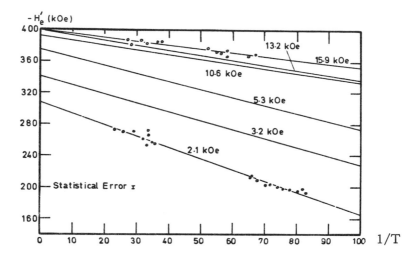

Fig. 3: Variation of the hyperfine field at manganese in Au as a function of $1/T$ for various external polarising fields.

free ions. In addition, the variation with temperature of the degree of saturation for a given H_a differs from free ion behaviour which would predict an increase in ionic polarisation with falling temperature. This is shown in Fig. 3. Present attempts to interpret these departures are based on the presence in these alloys of several parts per million of non-radioactive magnetic impurity, primarily Fe. It is possible to explain the observations if these impurities become magnetically ordered and produce a range of fields at the ions of the radioactive impurity of up to 1 kOe and of either sign. Their random spacing will prevent a sharp transition temperature, but the percentage of ions involved the ordering will increase with reducing temperature.

This work is being extended to alloys with Pt and Pd, and with varying transition element impurity concentration.

B. Hyperfine Fields at Diamagnetic Impurities in Ferromagnets by Ion Implantation

A project still in its infancy is the measurement of nuclear hyperfine fields for dilute diamagnetic impurities in ferromagnets using ion implantation for source preparation. The systematic variation of fields so far measured (Fig. 4) indicates that noble gases, alkali metals, alkaline earths, and the halogens may show large fields in ferromagnets. These fields are of interest for their own sake and as a means of orienting nuclei of these elements to

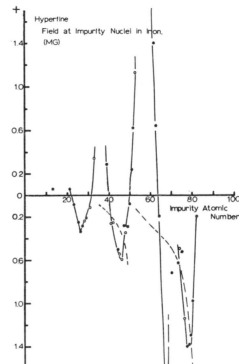

Fig. 4: Hyperfine fields at dilute impurities in iron. Filled circles indicate measured signs, open circles indicate signs based on the systematic trends.

obtain moments and decay scheme parameters. Such systems cannot be prepared by conventional alloying; however, there is considerable evidence to suggest that substitutional implantation results from bombarding an iron foil with ions accelerated in an electromagnetic separator. In conjunction with the separator group at U. K. A. E. A. Harwell, a program of checking the method, by using implantation to make alloy sources which can also be prepared conventionally, has recently started using Mn, Sb, and Au in iron. Preliminary results on Mn^{56} in Fe implantation sources give 75 ± 25% of the conventional source hyperfine interaction.

References

Blin-Stoyle, R. J. and Grace, M. A. , (1957). Handbuch der Physik 42, 555 (Springer, Berlin).

Cameron, J. A. , Campbell, I. A. , Compton, J. P. , Lines, R. A. G. , and Wilson, G. V. H. (1966). Phys. Letters 20, 569.

Campbell, I. A. , Stone, N. J. , and Turrell, B. G. , (1965). Proc. Roy. Soc. A283, 379.

Daniels, J. M. and Kurti, N. , (1954). Proc. Roy. Soc. A221, 243.

DeGroot, S. R. , Tolhoek, H. A. , and Huiskamp, W. J. , (1965). Alpha-, Beta-, and Gamma-Ray Spectroscopy, Vol. II, (North Holland, Amsterdam), p. 1199.

Ferentz, M. and Rosenzweig, N. , (1955). Argonne Natl. Lab. Report 5324.

Gray, T. P. and Satchler, G. R. , (1955). Proc. Phys. Soc. London A68, 349.

Hudson, R. P. , (1961). Prog. in Cryogenics 3, 99.

Lubbers, J. , (1966). Private communication (to be published).

Matthias, E. and Holliday, R. J. , (1966). Phys. Rev. Letters 17, 897.

Shirley, D. A. , (1966). Ann. Rev. Nucl. Sci. 16, (to be published).

Tolhoek, H. A. and Cox, J. A. M. , (1953). Physica 19, 101.

Williams, I. R. , (1966). Private communication.

S.5.   ROTATIONAL COOLING AND NUCLEAR RELAXATION IN A DILUTE PARAMAGNETIC CRYSTAL*

J. Lubbers

University of Leiden
Kamerlingh Onnes Laboratory
The Netherlands

I. Introduction

The use of very low temperatures for orienting nuclei is well known (de Groot et al., 1964; Daniels, 1965).** The temperatures required, generally of the order of 0. 01°K, are reached by means of adiabatic demagnetization of a paramagnetic salt. For some studies, the presence of a rather strong magnetic field is required, in which case it is necessary to cool the sample, which contains the nuclei, by means of a heat conductor to an adiabatically demagnetized salt outside the magnetic field region. Heat transfer problems generally preclude attainment of temperatures below 0. 01°K. A lower temperature in the sample may, however, be attained by the so-called "rotational cooling method" (Wheatley and Estle, 1956). In this method, a single crystal is used, wherein ions are included which have an anisotropic spin-Hamiltonian, e. g., Ce in LaMg-nitrate. By rotating the magnetic field from the direction where the splitting factor g is large to a direction

*This investigation is part of the research program of the "Stichting voor Fundamenteel Onderzoek der Materie," which is financially supported by the "Nederlandse Organisatie voor Zuiver Wetenschappelijk Onderzoek."
**See N.J. Stone, Chap. S.4.

where g is small, the magnetic splitting decreases and if the rotation process is adiabatic (i. e. , the crystal is thermally isolated), a decrease of the temperature is obtained even though the magnetic field remains.

Mn^{54} in (Ce-La) Mg nitrate was studied at low temperatures (Lubbers and Huiskamp, 1967). A two stage cooling process was used consisting of: (i) precooling the sample by a cooling salt outside the field region, while a magnetic field is applied in the direction of the large g-value, and (ii) rotating the field to a low g-value direction, thus demagnetizing the Ce spins. The degree of nuclear orientation of the Mn^{54} spin system was calculated from the observed γ-ray anisotropy, which was measured by observing the intensity of the γ-rays emitted in the direction of the magnetic field. This intensity is denoted as $W(0°)$; $W(0°) = 1$ for unoriented nuclei and $W(0°) = 0$ for completely oriented nuclei.

II. Experimental Results

Measurements of the Mn^{54} nuclear spin-lattice relaxation time were made in the following way. Nuclear orientation of Mn^{54} was produced by rotational cooling. Subsequently the lattice temperature was raised to a certain temperature T and held constant. The degree of nuclear orientation of Mn decreased gradually with time, as could be observed from an increase of $W(0°)$. It was found that the increase had the form of an exponential rise to an equilibrium value and hence could be characterized by a relaxation time τ; the measured values of τ are shown in Fig. 1 for three different magnetic fields as a function of the lattice temperature. It can be seen that the relaxation times are very long for low temperatures and high magnetic fields. This can be understood by assuming that the main relaxation mechanism for Mn^{54} nuclei is a flip of coupled electron and nuclear spins of the same ion (processes II and III of Fig. 2). Electron spin flips, and hence nuclear spin flips, become rare for high values of the Boltzmann-factor $g\mu_B H/kT$. Flips of the nuclear spins alone (process I of Fig. 2) are improbable and do not contribute significantly to the relaxation rate except for low values of H.

The γ-ray intensity $W(0°)$ during rotational cooling of a (0. 1% Ce-La) Mg-nitrate crystal is shown in Fig. 3. The sample was precooled while a magnetic field was applied in a direction which made an appreciable angle θ with the c-axis of the crystal. Under these conditions the spin-lattice relaxation time of Ce is

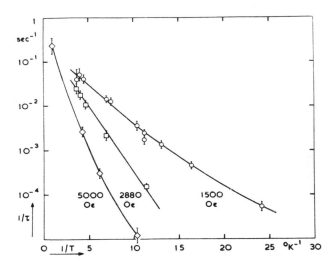

Fig. 1: The inverse of the relaxation time τ for Mn^{54} as a function of the inverse of the lattice temperature $1/T$ for three magnetic fields.

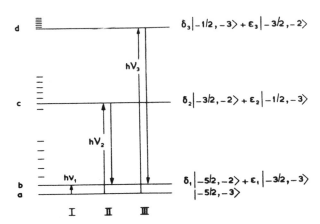

Fig. 2: Energy levels of Mn^{54} and paths for relaxation by phonons between the levels a and b.

short (Ruby et al. , 1962) and thus the Ce could be precooled in a few minutes. When θ was decreased, the energy splitting of Ce and consequently the Ce temperature was decreased; at the same time the spin-lattice relaxation time increased considerably so that the Ce spins were thermally isolated from the lattice. The low Ce-temperature was preserved for many minutes. Because of the long spin-lattice relaxation time of the Mn nuclei, no nuclear orientation was generated during the precooling period (i. e. , $W(0°) = 1.00$). During the rotation, the Mn remained isolated up to a certain angle θ_m, at which point the Mn became polarized, and $W(0°)$ decreased. The value of θ_m depended on the applied magnetic field H. The experimental relation between θ_m and H is depicted by the bars in Fig. 4; the lines represent the theoretically calculated relation between the values of θ_m and H for which the *Zeeman* splitting of Ce equals the *hyperfine* structure splitting of Mn, i. e. ,

$$g_{Ce} \mu_B H = A_{Mn} S I + \text{correction terms} \qquad (1)$$

where $g_{Ce}^2 = g_{\|}^2 \cos^2\theta_m + g_{\perp}^2 \sin^2\theta_m$. The correction terms can be found from a perturbation treatment of the Mn energy levels. Since two different types of Mn ions are present, two lines are drawn in Fig. 4 but it can be seen that the difference is important only in low magnetic fields. Good agreement between experimental points and the theoretical line in found, and thus it can be concluded that nuclear orientation of Mn^{54} is a result of thermal mixing between Ce and Mn which occurs when their energy splittings are equal. The maximum magnetic field for Ce-Mn mixing occurs for the magnetic field oriented along the c axis (i.e., $\theta_m = 0$) where g_{Ce} is a minimum; experimentally, H = 15.4 kOe. With $A/k = -0.0102°K$ (calculated from Kedzie and Jeffries, 1958), it follows from Eq. (1) that for Ce, $g_{\|} = 0.0235 \pm 0.0009$.

After one rotational cooling the orientation of Mn^{54} was not complete, as can be seen in Fig. 3. Repeating the rotational cooling procedure led to $W(0°) = 0.024$, indicating that at least 97.6% of all Mn ions could be completely polarized. Due to the long nuclear spin-lattice relaxation time such a polarization could be maintained for a long time.

III. Discussion

When comparing rotational cooling in dilute paramagnetic crystals to rotational cooling in concentrated paramagnetic crystals,

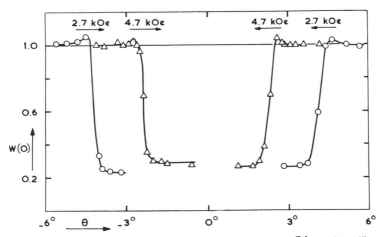

Fig. 3: Four typical series showing $W(0°)$ for Mn^{54} in (0. 1%Ce-
La) Mg-nitrate as the angle θ between magnetic field and
c-axis was decreased in small steps. Steps were taken
every 30 seconds.

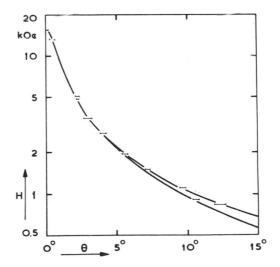

Fig. 4: Relation between field strength H and mixing angle θ_m.
The dashes represent the measurements; the two drawn
lines give the result of the theoretical calculations from
Eq. (1) for the two different Mn sites.

it can be seen that the former method has some attractive features for nuclear orientation:

(i) The oriented nuclei can be isolated from their surroundings, thus giving ample time (several hours) for their study. This isolation occurs because of the mismatch between nuclear splittings and electronic splitting of other ions, which generally relax more rapidly with the lattice. In concentrated crystals the energy levels are generally broadened so that this isolation cannot occur, in which case a long measuring time requires minimization of the heat input to the sample.

(ii) The sharp energy levels give rise to a well defined mixing region, which could be used to deduce some parameters of the spin-Hamiltonian of the two ions (e.g., $g_{||}$ or A).

Finally, we may mention that rotational cooling experiments in dilute paramagnetic crystals have been reported by several authors (Langley and Jeffries, 1964; Robinson, 1963), in which protons were polarized, starting from a temperature of 1°K. The use of a lower initial temperature, as was done here, makes the relaxation processes destroying nuclear polarization slower, but on the other hand, imposes severe limitations on the number of nuclei that can be oriented.

The stimulating interest of Prof. C.J. Gorter and Dr. W.J. Huiskamp, the help of H. F. van der Land, L. Niesen, and H. B. Brom, and the technical assistance of Mr. J. van Weesel is gratefully acknowledged.

References

Daniels, J. M. (1965). Oriented Nuclei (Academic Press, N. Y.).

de Groot, S. R. , Tolhoek, H. A. , and Huiskamp, W. J. (1964). Alpha-, Beta-, and Gamma-Ray Spectroscopy, edited by K. Siegbahn (North-Holland Publ. Co. , Amsterdam).

Kedzie, R.W. and Jeffries, C. D. (1958). Bull. Am. Phys. Soc. 3, 415.

Langley, K. H. and Jeffries, C. D. (1964). Phys. Rev. Letters 13, 808.

Lubbers, J. and Huiskamp, W. J. (1967). Physica (to be published).

Robinson, F. N. H. (1963). Phys. Letters 4, 180.

Ruby, R. H. , Benoit, H. , and Jeffries, C. D. (1962). Phys. Rev. 127, 51.

Wheatley, J. C. and Estle, T. L. (1956). Phys. Rev. 104, 264.

S.6. MAGNETIC RELAXATION EFFECTS IN MÖSSBAUER SPECTRA

A.J. Dekker

Solid State Physics Laboratory
University of Groningen
The Netherlands

I. Introduction

The purpose of this chapter is to introduce the subject of relaxation effects in Mössbauer spectra, particularly with reference to the magnetic hyperfine splitting. Although the arguments given apply to other nuclei as well, Fe^{57} will be used as a specific example. This nucleus has a ground state with $I = 1/2$, $g = 0.18$, and a 14.37 keV excited state with $I^* = 3/2$, $g^* = -0.103$ and a life time $\tau_n = 1.45 \times 10^{-7}$ sec. If the nucleus is subjected to a *constant* magnetic field H, the excited state is split into four levels with Zeeman energies $(-g^* m_I^* \beta_n H)$ and the ground state into two levels with energies $(-g m_I \beta_n H)$ as indicated in Fig. 1 for a positive value of H. For magnetic dipole transitions $(\Delta m_I = 0, \pm 1)$ this leads to the familiar pattern of six absorption lines. Thus, if the field seen by the nuclei is constant, only one condition is required for observable hyperfine splitting of a Mössbauer spectrum, viz. that the separation between successive lines be larger than the natural linewidth $\Gamma = \hbar/\tau_n$,

$$|g| \beta_n H \gtrsim \Gamma \quad \text{or} \quad \omega_{Ln} \tau_n \gtrsim 1 \tag{1}$$

where ω_{Ln} is the nuclear Larmor frequency in the field H. For Fe^{57} this requires $H \gtrsim 10^4$ Oe.

　　　　　　　A.J. DEKKER

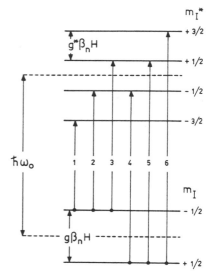

Fig. 1: Zeeman splitting of
the ground state and
first excited state of
Fe^{57}.

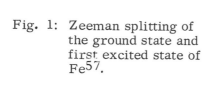

II. The Origin of the Magnetic Hyperfine Field

As discussed previously* the main contribution to the effective magnetic field at an Fe^{57} nucleus in iron compounds arises as a result of the exchange interaction between the 3d-electrons and the s-electrons of the core, which makes the densities at the nucleus of s-electrons of opposite spin orientation, $|\Psi_{s\uparrow}(0)|^2$ and $|\Psi_{s\downarrow}(0)|^2$, unequal; through the Fermi contact interaction this establishes an effective field H_e parallel to S, the net 3d spin, where $H_e \approx 5 \times 10^5$ Oe. The interaction between the nucleus and the ion spin is thus of the form $A\, I \cdot S$ and for the purpose of our discussion all other interactions between the nucleus and its surroundings will be neglected. It must be emphasized that the field seen by a given nucleus is determined by a *single* ionic spin and not, for example, by the magnetization, which is a bulk property. In other words, the origin of H_e at a nucleus in a paramagnetic material is the same as that in a material which exhibits magnetic order. The specific properties of the system of ionic spins enter only indirectly in the hyperfine splitting of Mössbauer spectra, i.e., only insofar as they determine the time dependence or the average value of the single spin S.

*See R.E. Watson and A.J. Freeman, Chap. 2 and R.L. Mössbauer and M.J. Clauser, Chap. 11.

III. A Simple Relaxation Model

From what has just been said about the origin of the magnetic hyperfine field, it is evident that any fluctuations in the ionic spin components will be transmitted directly to the nucleus in the form of fluctuations in the corresponding components of H_e. As a magnetic probe, however, the nucleus will respond to such fluctuations only if they are slow compared to the nuclear Larmor frequency ω_{Ln}. Thus, if τ_S represents the correlation time of the fluctuations of a particular component of S, two extreme cases present themselves immediately: for $\omega_{Ln} \tau_S << 1$, the nuclear spin senses only the *average* value of that component, whereas for $\omega_{Ln} \tau_S >> 1$, the nucleus responds to the instantaneous values of the component. In these extreme situations, the shape of the Mössbauer spectra can usually be predicted without too much difficulty. The most interesting region, however, corresponds to $\omega_{Ln} \tau_S \approx 1$, because relaxation effects should then be observable. In order to illustrate some essential features of relaxation phenomena in Mössbauer spectra, we now sketch briefly the consequences of a simple model employed previously in the interpretation of experimental data (van der Woude and Dekker 1965a; 1965b).

Consider a paramagnetic iron compound subjected to an applied magnetic field H_a at a temperature T. We assume that the precession frequency of the ionic spins around H_a is large compared to ω_{Ln}, so that the nucleus only sees the z-component of S; this will be the case if $H_a \gtrsim 10^2$ - 10^3 Oe. The influence of I on S is neglected, since this corresponds to an effective field ≈ 10 Oe. The effective magnetic field H_e at a nucleus is then at any instant proportional to m_S (t), where m_S represents the magnetic quantum number of the electron spin. In order to obtain an easily calculable case, we first take S = 1/2 and assume that the effect of the surroundings on a given ion leads to fluctuations between the discrete states $m_S = \pm 1/2$. The effective field H_e then also fluctuates between two discrete values of equal magnitude but opposite sign, as indicated in Fig. 2.

Consider now a particular nuclear absorption process, say, from $m_I = -1/2$ to $m_I^* = -3/2$. If H_e is positive, this corresponds to a Mössbauer line of frequency ω_1 in Fig. 1. However, if H_e switches sign, the same nuclear transition produces absorption at ω_6, because a change in sign of H_e is equivalent to changing the signs of all quantum numbers in Fig. 1. The problem of calculating the absorption spectrum corresponding to this particular nuclear transition is very similar to that of motional narrowing in NMR (Abragam, 1961; Anderson, 1954); in the present case the statistical

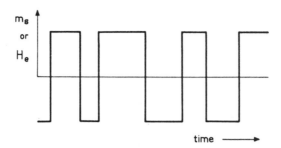

Fig. 2: Schematic representation of the effective field H_e at the nucleus of an ion of spin 1/2.

probabilities for the frequencies ω_1 and ω_2 are unequal as a result of the presence of the magnetic field H_a. In fact, for $S = 1/2$, the ion spin has two Zeeman levels $2\beta m_S H_a$, where β is the Bohr magneton, so that for H_a chosen negative, the probability to find $m_S = +1/2$ is larger than for $m_S = -1/2$. We therefore introduce an order parameter η such that the probabilities for $m_S = \pm 1/2$ are $(1 \pm \eta)/2$, respectively; η is proportional to the magnetization and equal to tanh $[\beta|H_a|/kT]$. We assume that the transitions of the ion spin between the states $m_S = \pm 1/2$ are described by a stationary Markoff process; this implies that if $m_S = +1/2$ at t, the probability for m_S to be $-1/2$ at $t + \Delta t$ is independent of t and is only proportional to Δt,

$$P(+\tfrac{1}{2}, t \mid -\tfrac{1}{2}, t + \Delta t) = \Omega \Delta t . \tag{2a}$$

Similarly,

$$P(-\tfrac{1}{2}, t \mid +\tfrac{1}{2}, t + \Delta t) = \Omega' \Delta t . \tag{2b}$$

Detailed balance requires that the absorption and emission "spin flip frequencies" Ω and Ω' satisfy the relation $\Omega(1+\eta) = \Omega' (1 - \eta)$.

On the basis of this model, the Mössbauer absorption spectrum corresponding to the single nuclear transition from $m_I = -1/2$ to $m_I^* = -3/2$ can be calculated by employing, for example, the procedure outlined by Abragam (1961) for motional narrowing in NMR. If one neglects the natural linewidth, the result first derived explicitly by van der Woude and Dekker (1965a) is

$$I_1(\omega) \propto \frac{2\Omega}{1 - \eta} \frac{\delta^2(1 - \eta^2)}{(\omega^2 - \delta^2)^2 + \dfrac{4\Omega^2}{(1 - \eta)^2}(\omega + \eta \delta)^2} . \tag{3}$$

Here, $\delta = (\omega_6 - \omega_1)/2$ represents half the maximum splitting between lines 1 and 6; the frequency has been scaled such that $\omega = 0$ corresponds to the center of the spectrum $(\omega_1 + \omega_6)/2$. If the spin-flip frequency $\Omega \ll \delta$, this gives rise to two sharp absorption peaks at $\omega = \pm \delta$; note that in this case *the position of the peaks is independent of the magnetization.* For high spin flip frequencies, $\Omega \gg \delta$, only one sharp absorption maximum occurs at $\omega = -\eta \delta$ and in this case the position measures the magnetization. In Fig. 3 we have indicated how the position of absorption peak number 1 shifts from $-\delta$ to $-\eta \delta$ as a function of Ω/δ for the case $\eta = 0.5$.

In general, a complete Mössbauer spectrum for $S = 1/2$ is obtained as a sum of six intensity distributions of the form (3) and three values of δ will occur, viz., $\delta_1 = (\omega_6 - \omega_1)/2$, $\delta_2 = (\omega_5 - \omega_2)/2$, and $\delta_3 = (\omega_4 - \omega_3)/2$. If one chooses an experimental situation for

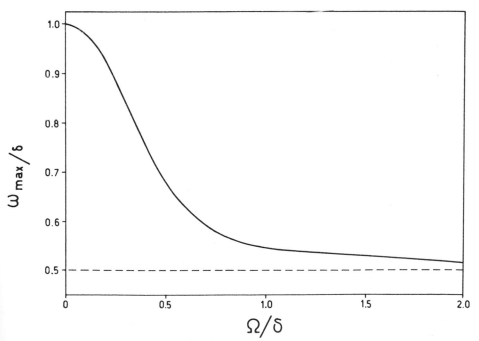

Fig. 3: Position of the absorption maximum according to expression (3) as a function of the spin flip frequency Ω for an order parameter $\eta = 0.5$.

which H_a is parallel to the direction of propagation of the γ-rays, lines 2 and 5 will be absent in the spectrum. Theoretical spectra for this case with $\eta = 0.5$ are given in Fig. 4 for three different values of Ω/δ_1. In these spectra the natural linewidth $\gamma = 1/\tau_n$ has been taken into account to first order, which leads instead of (3) to the more complicated expression,

$$I_1(\omega) \propto \frac{\dfrac{2\Omega}{1-\eta}\,\delta^2\,(1-\eta^2) + \gamma\left(\delta^2 + \omega^2 + \dfrac{4\Omega^2}{(1-\eta)^2} - 2\omega\,\delta\,\eta\right)}{(\delta^2 - \omega^2)^2 + \dfrac{4\Omega^2}{(1-\eta)^2}\,(\omega+\eta\delta)^2 + \dfrac{4\Omega\gamma}{1-\eta}\,(\omega^2 + \delta^2 + 2\omega\,\delta\,\eta)} \cdot (4)$$

In the spectra of Fig. 4 we see clear evidence of the consequences of Fig. 3. In fact, since $\delta_1 = 6.35\,\delta_3$ for Fe^{57}, there exists a range of Ω-values such that the separation between the inner lines is proportional to the magnetization, whereas the maxima of the outer lines still are somewhere between $\pm\delta$ and $\pm\eta\delta$. Also note that in this region the outer lines are still strongly broadened by relaxation effects, whereas the inner ones have nearly the natural linewidth. These striking features explain qualitatively the Mössbauer spectra observed by Obenshain et al. (1965) on the paramagnetic salt $FeNH_4(SO_4)_2 \cdot 12H_2O$ in large external fields at low temperatures, although it should be admitted that a more quantitative comparison requires considerations based on $S = 5/2$ rather than on $S = 1/2$.

IV. Ferro- and Antiferromagnetic Materials

In materials which exhibit magnetic order, the fluctuations in the z-component of the individual spins are due to spin waves, at least for temperatures far below the transition temperature. For a spin wave of thermal energy, the frequency $\omega_s \approx kT/\hbar$, so that for $T = 1°K$, $\omega_s \approx 10^{11}$ rad/sec, which is considerably larger than the nuclear Larmor frequency $\omega_{Ln} \approx 10^8$ rad/sec. In the spin wave region one would therefore expect that the Zeeman splitting of the Mössbauer spectrum is determined by the *average* spin value, i.e. by the magnetization. Nearer to the magnetic transition temperature, one is inclined to replace the collective spin wave model by a Weiss molecular field model, which considers the behavior of a *single* spin in the average field produced by its neighbors. If one accepts this point of view, one has arrived essentially at the model of van der Woude and Dekker (1965a) if one replaces H_a by the Weiss field. In fact, this model was used to

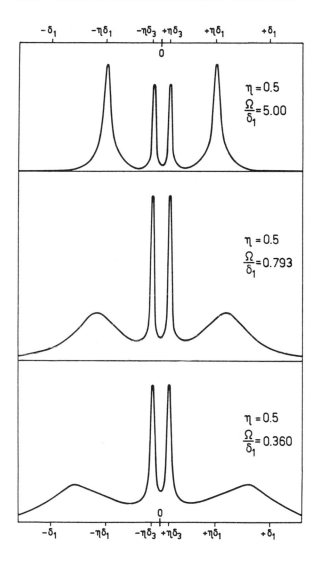

Fig. 4: Mössbauer spectra for three values of Ω/δ_1 calculated from expression (4) for $\eta = 0.5$ and $\gamma = 0.0105$ $\delta_1 = 1.1$ Mc/sec; transitions 2 and 5 in Fig. 1 were assumed to be absent. The vertical scales are different for the three curves shown.

interpret certain anomalies observed in Mössbauer spectra near the transition temperature. For example, a careful study of the shape of Mössbauer spectra as a function of temperature in the antiferromagnetic compound α-FeOOH reveals (van der Woude and Dekker, 1966) that as one approaches the Néel temperature of 393. 3°K, the central portion of the spectrum becomes more and more pronounced until it collapses into a single line at T_N (actually a doublet due to quadrupole splitting); the lines are also broadened. Similar features have been observed, for example, in ferromagnetic alloys (Nakamura et al., 1964). In the latter case one usually has interpreted such results by assuming that the differences in the environment of the individual atoms lead to a distribution of magnetic transition temperatures and thus to a coexistence of "paramagnetic" and "ferromagnetic" regions near the transition temperature. Although such an interpretation may be valid in random alloys, it becomes questionable in the case of a completely ordered arrangement of magnetic atoms, as in perfect α - FeOOH. It should also be emphasized that, in view of these considerations, the effective field measured by a Mössbauer experiment is not necessarily proportional to the magnetization or the sublattice magnetization.

A further application of the arguments given above pertains to Mössbauer spectra of superparamagnetic particles. In fact, if the reversal frequency of the magnetization becomes comparable to the nuclear Larmor frequency, relaxation effects should be observed. Such effects have indeed been detected (Nakamura et al., 1964; Shuele et al, 1965) and lead to line broadening, a decrease in the effective field and finally to a complete destruction of the hyperfine structure *below* the Néel temperature of well-crystallized material.

V. Extension to the Case of $S = 5/2$

Although the model for $S = 1/2$ exhibits some essential features which allow a qualitative comparison with experiment, it is obviously of practical interest to extend the model to $S = 5/2$, corresponding to the Fe^{3+} ion. The procedure will be outlined here briefly (van der Woude, 1966).   For an effective field $H_e(t)$, the absorption frequency for a given nuclear transition from m_I to m_I^* is

$$\omega(t) = \omega_0 - (g^* m_I^* - g m_I) \beta_n H_e(t)/\hbar . \tag{5}$$

Since $H_e(t)$ is proportional to $m_S(t)$, the frequency fluctuates among six discrete values corresponding to $m_S = 5/2, 3/2, \ldots,$ $-5/2$. The quantity that actually determines the spectrum is the relaxation function of the transition considered,

$$G(t) = \left\langle \exp\left\{ i \int_0^t w(t')\,dt' \right\} \right\rangle \tag{6}$$

Referring for details to Abragam's treatment of motional narrowing, the spectrum is given by the Fourier transform of $G(t)$, which for a Markoff process yields

$$I(\omega) = \mathrm{Re} \int_0^\infty G(t) \exp(-i\omega t)\,dt = -\mathrm{Re}\{W \cdot A^{-1} \cdot 1\} \tag{7}$$

In our case, $W = [s^5, s^4, s^3, s^2, s, 1]$ is a row vector which gives the distribution over the electron spin states $m_S = +5/2, \ldots, -5/2$ and $s = \exp(-2\beta H_a/kT)$. The matrix A^{-1} is the inverse of the matrix

$$A = i(\omega - \omega E) + \pi \tag{8}$$

where ω is a diagonal matrix with elements $\omega_{ij} = \omega_i \delta_{ij}$, with $i = 1, 2, \ldots, 6$. E is the unit matrix and the elements π_{ij} play the role of transition probabilities. As an example, we give here the matrix A based on the assumption that the transitions between the electron states satisfy the selection rule $\Delta m_S = \pm 1$.

$$
\begin{bmatrix}
i(5\delta-\omega)-5\Omega_e & 5\Omega_e & 0 & 0 & 0 & 0 \\
5s\Omega_e & i(3\delta-\omega)-(8+5s)\Omega_e & 8\Omega_e & 0 & 0 & 0 \\
0 & 8s\Omega_e & i(\delta-\omega)-(9+8s)\Omega_e & 9\Omega_e & 0 & 0 \\
0 & 0 & 9s\Omega_e & -i(\delta+\omega)-(8+9s)\Omega_e & 8\Omega_e & 0 \\
0 & 0 & 0 & 8s\Omega_e & -i(3\delta+\omega)-(5+8s)\Omega_e & 5\Omega_e \\
0 & 0 & 0 & 0 & 5s\Omega_e & -i(5\delta+\omega)-5s\Omega_e
\end{bmatrix} \tag{9}
$$

In this case, the transition probabilities for $m_s = 5/2 \rightarrow 3/2$, $3/2 \rightarrow 1/2, \ldots, -3/2 \rightarrow -5/2$ are given, respectively, by $5\Omega_e$, $8\Omega_e$, $9\Omega_e$, $8\Omega_e$, $5\Omega_e$ where the numerical factors are Clebsch-Gordon coefficients and where the subscript e refers to emission of an energy quantum $2\beta H_a$ by the electron spin. The reverse transitions involve absorption of energy and the corresponding probabilities are obtained by replacing Ω_e by $\Omega_a = 5\Omega_e$ (compare 2a and 2b, where Ω and Ω' play the same role as Ω_a and Ω_e in the present case). In order to obtain a complete Mössbauer spectrum, it must be realized that there are six possible nuclear transitions and that the spectrum of each of these is given by an expression of the form (7). Consequently, three values of δ will occur which, in accordance with Fig. 1, satisfy the relation

$$\delta_1 : \delta_2 : \delta_3 = (g + 3|g^*|) : (g + |g^*|) : (g - |g^*|) . \tag{10}$$

Some examples of theoretical spectra for Fe^{3+} so obtained will be presented in the lecture by de Waard, * for the region of electonic spin "correlation times" $\tau_s (\equiv 1/14 \ \Omega_e)$ between 0.66×10^{-9} and 330×10^{-9} sec, in the absence of an external field, i.e. for $s = 1$. For the shortest value of τ_s, the spectrum consists of a single line and as τ_s increases, more lines gradually develop until for very large values of τ_s it consists of a superposition of three six-line spectra resulting from $m_s = \pm 5/2$, $\pm 3/2$, and $\pm 1/2$.

An interesting illustration of this extreme situation is provided by the Mössbauer measurements of Wertheim and Remeika (1964) on a paramagnetic solid solution of 0. 08 at. % of Fe_2O_3 in Al_2O_3. These measurements were performed at 78°K, corresponding to a spin-lattice relaxation time of the order of 10^{-6} sec. The crystalline field splits the ^6S state of the Fe^{3+} ion into three Kramers doublets corresponding to $m_s \pm 1/2$, $\pm 3/2$, and $5/2$ in order of increasing energy. The total separation between the lowest and highest doublet is $1 \ cm^{-1}$, so that at 78°K all three are equally populated. The resulting Mössbauer spectrum can be intrepreted as a superposition of two six-line spectra associated with the $\pm 5/2$ and $\pm 3/2$ states. The spectrum corresponding to $\pm 1/2$ is absent, presumably because the relaxation rate of these states is considerably greater than for the others (van der Woude and Dekker, 1965b). More recently, Wickman and Wertheim (1966) have published a detailed experimental and theoretical study on the influence of applied magnetic fields up to 41 kOe on the Mössbauer spectra of single crystals of Fe^{3+} in Al_2O_3.

*See Chap. S.7.

VI. Other Work on Relaxation Effects

Finally we make some brief remarks on work by others. Wegener (1965) has given another interpretation of the measurements by Obenshain et al. (1965), mentioned earlier. Although he assumes a continuous range of values for S_z rather than a discrete set as employed by van der Woude and Dekker (1965a) it can be shown that the two treatments are essentially equivalent. However, Wegener's actual discussion is limited to electron spin correlation times which are short compared to the nuclear Larmor precession time. An interesting treatment has also been given by Boyle and Gabriel (1965).

If the Larmor precession frequency of the electron spin is smaller than the nuclear Larmor frequency, i. e. if $H_a = 0$ or small, the x- and y-components of the $AI \cdot S$ interaction must of course be taken into account. This has been done, for example, in the general treatment for a paramagnetic material in the absence of a magnetic field by Afanas'ev and Kagan (1964) and in the more recent work of Bradford and Marshall (1966); in the latter paper the discussion is limited to electron spin relaxation which is fast, but nevertheless produces observable results.

Blume (1965) has published calculated spectra of asymmetric quadrupole doublets resulting from relaxation effects, based on a model involving motional narrowing; details were not given.

References

Abragam, A. (1961). in The Principles of Nuclear Magnetism (Oxford University Press), pp. 447-451.

Afanas'ev, A. M. and Kagan, Y. (1964). Soviet Phys. -JETP 18, 1139.

Anderson, P. W. (1954). J. Phys. Soc. Japan 9, 316.

Blume, M. (1965). Phys. Rev. Letters 14, 96.

Boyle, A. J. F. and Gabriel, J. R. (1966). Phys. Letters 19, 451.

Bradford, E. and Marshall, W. (1966). Proc. Phys. Soc. 87, 731.

See for example, Nakamura, Y., Shiga, M., and Shikazona, N. (1964). J. Phys. Soc. Japan 19, 1177.

Nakamura, T., Shinjo, T., Endoh, Y., Yamamoto, N., Shiga, M., and Nakamura, Y. (1964). Phys. Letters 12, 178.

Obenshain, F. E. , Roberts, L. D. , Coleman, C. F. , Forester, D. W. , Thomson, J. O. (1965). Phys. Rev. Letters 14, 365.

Shuele, W. J. , Shtrikman, S. , and Treves, D. (1965). J. Appl. Phys. 36, 1010.

van der Woude, F. (1966). "Mössbauer Spectra and Magnetic Properties of Iron Compounds," Thesis, Groningen.

van der Woude, F. and Dekker, A. J. (1965a). Phys. Stat. Sol. 9, 775; (1965b). Solid State Comm. 3, 319; (1966). Phys. Stat. Sol. 13, 181.

Wegener, H. (1965). Zeit. für Phys. 186, 498.

Wertheim, G. K. and Remeika, J. P. (1964). Phys. Letters 10, 14.

Wickman, H. H. and Wertheim, G. K. (1966). Phys. Rev. 148, 211.

S.7. THE MÖSSBAUER EFFECT IN DILUTE FE-ALUM

H. de Waard

Department of Experimental Physics
University of Groningen
The Netherlands

R. M. Housley

North American Aviation Science Center
Thousand Oaks, California

I. Introduction

In the previous chapter, Dekker*has discussed relaxation
phenomena from a theoretical point of view. Here we describe
the use of the Mössbauer effect to study relaxation phenomena
both as a function of temperature and applied magnetic field; as
example we chose $Fe_x^{57}Al_{1-x}(SO_4)_2 \cdot 12H_2O$ (x = 0.01 - 0.03).
Results are reported here for this dilute Fe alum system in zero
field and in a longitudinal field H = 700 Gauss and a tentative explanation is given of the observed temperature and field effects.

In the Fe-alum, the ferric ion is surrounded by a slightly
distorted octahedron of water molecules. The resulting crystal
field splits the $^6S_{5/2}$ state of the ion into three Kramers doublets
whose separation appears to be concentration and temperature
dependent and, though not accurately known, is probably less than
0.1 cm^{-1} in all cases. In the undiluted Fe-alum the Fe^{+++}-ions
are on a face centered cubic lattice with a nearest neighbour separation of 8.7 Å. In this case, the spin-spin interaction strength
is comparable to the crystal field splitting. In the dilute alum, the
average Fe-Fe distance has increased to more than 25 Å; the spin-

---

*See A.J. Dekker, Chap. S.6.

spin interaction is now small compared with the crystal field splitting.

II. Experiments and Theoretical Interpretation

At room temperature and in zero field, the Mössbauer spectrum of the undiluted alum consists of a broad line with half width $\Gamma \approx 2$ mm/sec; on dilution, the width increases to about 3.5 mm/sec (for x = 0.026).

The spectrum of the undiluted alum remains virtually unchanged down to liquid helium temperature, which demonstrates the temperature independence of spin-spin relaxation. The dilute alum spectrum, however, clearly exhibits the strong temperature dependence to be expected if spin lattice relaxation dominates (Fig. 1a). On cooling down from room temperature, the observed broad line first narrows to about 2 mm/sec at 100°K. Below this temperature, the slow relaxation structure developed rapidly, indicating a fast increase of the spin-lattice relaxation time.

The experimental spectra in the region 5° - 100°K may be compared with calculated spectra shown in Fig. 1b. The calculation is based on the relaxation model discussed by Dekker under the following assumptions:

(i) The states can be approximately characterized by Kramers doublets, with $S_z = \pm \frac{1}{2}$, $\pm \frac{3}{2}$, $\pm \frac{5}{2}$ (Bleaney and Trenam (1954)) equally populated. The assumption of equal populations is certainly valid for all temperatures used. (ii) The spin correlation times τ are equal for all transitions between states with $\Delta S_z = \pm 1$ (and zero for all $|\Delta S_z| > 1$). The spectra measured at T = 5°K and T = 20°K of Fig. 1a compare well with the spectra calculated for $\tau = 330$ nsec and $\tau = 166$ nsec in Fig. 1b. The line at zero velocity in the measured spectra arises from Fe in the cryostat windows. We notice that the lines corresponding to the $S_z = \pm \frac{1}{2}$ electronic state (Wertheim and Remeika, 1965) are not visible in the experimental spectra. The hyperfine levels corresponding to this doublet are very sensitive to perturbation. We suggest that superhyperfine interaction with surrounding protons or weak dipole-dipole interactions with other paramagnetic ions may broaden them beyond recognition.

We note that two lines found in the 5°K spectrum at about ± 3 mm/sec have disappeared in the 20° spectrum. This is in

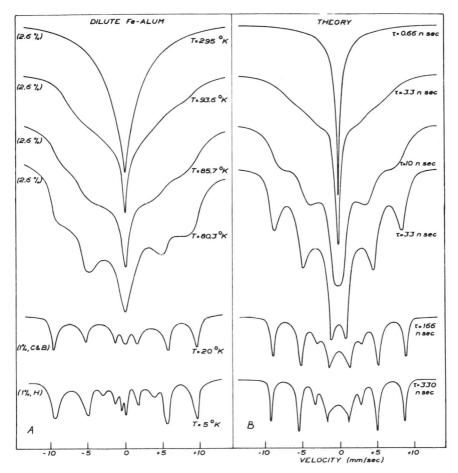

Fig. 1:   a.   Experimental Mössbauer spectra of dilute Fe-alum.
The spectrum at 20°K was taken from the work of
Campbell and DeBenedetti (1966).

b.   Spectra calculated on the basis of the relaxation model
discussed by Dekker in the preceeding paper, for spin
correlation times τ from 0.66 to 330 nsec.

agreement with the behavior of the calculated spectra for decreas-
ing spin correlation time of the $S_z = \pm \frac{3}{2}$ and $S_z = \pm \frac{5}{2}$ components.
The two lines are interpreted as the $m^* = +\frac{1}{2} \rightarrow m = +\frac{1}{2}$ and $m^* =
-\frac{1}{2} \rightarrow m = -\frac{1}{2}$ components of the 14.4 keV line in the $S_z = \pm \frac{3}{2}$ par-
tial spectrum. The $m^* = \frac{3}{2} \rightarrow m = \frac{1}{2}$ and $m^* = -\frac{3}{2} \rightarrow m = -\frac{1}{2}$ compon-

ents, at about ± 5.5 mm/sec, coincide with the $m^* = +\frac{1}{2} \to m = +\frac{1}{2}$ and $m^* = -\frac{1}{2} \to m = -\frac{1}{2}$ components of the partial spectrum with $S_z = \pm\frac{5}{2}$.

The four outer lines of the $S_z = \pm\frac{5}{2}$ partial spectrum remain visible up to about 85°K, corresponding to a spin correlation time $\tau \sim 10$ nsec.

Above 100°K, a serious discrepancy between the measured spectra and the results of the relaxation model appears; whereas the model predicts a narrow line on a broad base if the spin correlation time decreases further, the measured spectra yield very broad lines, incompatible with any value of τ. If, however, a longitudinal magnetic field is applied to the absorber, the expected shape is restored as shown in Fig. 2. We have previously reported similar behavior (Housley and de Waard, 1966).

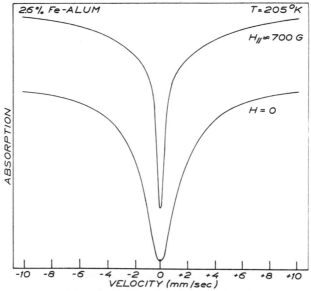

Fig. 2: Line narrowing by a longitudinal field $H_{\parallel} = 700$ Gauss, applied to the dilute Fe-alum absorber.

It seems probable that in order to explain the high temperature, low field data the crystal field splitting must be considered in more detail. There is experimental evidence that the axial term in the spin-Hamiltonian becomes very small at high temperatures (S. Maekawa, 1961). In that case, the crystal field states and the corresponding hyperfine levels will be more complicated than was assumed. When a field of a few hundred Gauss is applied, the Zeeman splitting dominates the crystal field and the simple situation is restored. It is also possible that the off diagonal elements $S_x I_x + S_y I_y$ of the hyperfine interaction must be included to explain the low field data.

References

Bleaney, B. and Trenam, R. S. (1954). Proc. Roy. Soc. A223, 1.

Campbell, L. and DeBenedetti, S. (1966). Phys. Letters 20, 102.

Maekawa, S. (1961). J. Phys. Soc. Japan 16, 2337.

Housley, R. M. and de Waard, H. (1966). Phys. Letters 21, 90.

Wertheim, G. K. and Remeika, J. P. (1965). Proc. of the XIIIth Colloque Ampere, Louvain, Belgium, 1964 (North Holland Publ. Co., 1965), 147.

S.8. POLARIZED RECOIL-FREE GAMMA-RAYS

U. Gonser

North American Aviation Science Center
Thousand Oaks, California

I. Introduction

Soon after the discovery of the Mössbauer effect, it was realized that the use of polarized sources or absorbers and polarized recoil-free γ-rays could advance the understanding of the hyperfine interactions in solids in a fashion similar to magneto- and electro-optical polarization effects in atomic spectra (Boyle, Bunbury, and Edwards, 1960; Dash et al., 1961; Hanna et al., 1960a; Hanna et al., 1960b).

We restrict ourselves here to magnetic dipole radiation and particularly to the 14.4 keV γ-ray of the first excited state of Fe^{57} because most of the important polarization experiments have been performed with this isotope. For higher polarity γ-radiation, see the work of Frauenfelder et al. (1962); for the interpretation of the spectra using the isotope Ni^{61} see Obenshain and Wegener (1961).

The energy levels of the ground state and first excited state of Fe^{57} for a pure magnetic hyperfine interaction and a pure axially symmetric quadrupole interaction are shown in Fig. 1. The multipolarity of the 14.4 keV γ-ray is almost exclusively M1 with the selection rule $\Delta m = 0, \pm 1$; the allowed transitions leading to the six-line Zeeman pattern and the two-line quadrupole pattern are indicated in the figure.

696

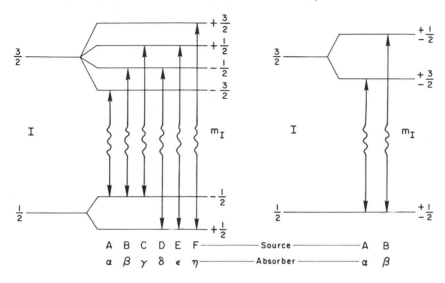

Fig. 1: Magnetic hyperfine splitting (nuclear Zeeman effect) and quadrupole splitting of the ground and first excited state of Fe^{57}. A, B, C, D, E, F, or A, B, and α, β, γ, δ, ε, η, or α, β designate the allowed transitions in ascending order of energy for source and absorber, respectively.

We adopt the following notation, in ascending order of energy: the six Zeeman emission lines are designated by capital letters A, B, C, D, E, F; the two quadrupole split emission lines by the capital letters A, B; the six Zeeman absorption lines by Greek letters α, β, γ, δ, ε, η; and the quadrupole split absorption lines by α, β.

The magnitude of the internal field at the site of the nuclei H_{int} is revealed in the splitting of the Mössbauer lines. Hanna et al. (1960) have shown that the hyperfine field at the iron nuclei is opposite to the electronic magnetic moment direction (indicated in Fig. 2 for the source). Here however, we are mainly concerned with the relative intensities of the Mössbauer lines which depend on the transition probabilities of the allowed transitions and the angle θ between the direction of the emission or absorption of the γ-quantum and the direction of the magnetic field at the Fe^{57} nuclei, H_{int} (see source in Fig. 2) or the principal axis of the axially symmetric electric field gradient (EFG) for the case of the quadrupole splitting. We neglect thickness effects and quote relative intensities in the thin source – thin absorber approximation.

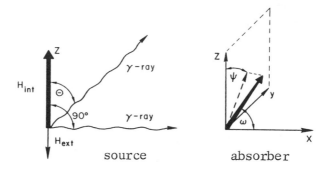

Fig. 2: Schematic for the definition of the angles θ, ω, and Ψ. In the source the angle θ is indicated between the internal magnetic field and the direction of the propagation direction of the γ-radiation. In the absorber the spin direction or the principal axis of the EFG is represented by the bold arrow. ω is the angle between x and the spin direction or the axis of the EFG; Ψ is the angle between the projection of the spin direction or the axis of the EFG on the y-z plane and the z-direction.

Furthermore, we assume that the Debye-Waller factor is directionally invariant, so that the intensities of the quadrupole split lines (Gol'danskii, Makarov, and Khrapov, 1963) or the Zeeman hyperfine lines (Cohen, Gielen, and Kaplow, 1966; Gonser, 1966) do not reflect any lattice anisotropy.

The angular dependence of the γ-radiation for allowed transitions in the hyperfine Zeeman spectrum is shown in Table I. If

Table I: Angular dependence of the allowed transition in the nuclear Zeeman pattern. θ is angle between the magnetic field at the nucleus and the propagation direction of the γ-radiation.

Transition	Δm	Angular Dependence
$\pm 3/2 \rightarrow \pm 1/2$	∓ 1	$3/4\,(1 + \cos^2 \theta)$
$\pm 1/2 \rightarrow \pm 1/2$	0	$\sin^2 \theta$
$\mp 1/2 \rightarrow \pm 1/2$	± 1	$1/4\,(1 + \cos^2 \theta)$

the source *or* the absorber is magnetically ordered, three special arrangements can be distinguished: the relative intensities are 3:0:1:1:0:3 for the case where the propagation direction of the single line γ-rays is parallel or antiparallel to the internal magnetic field, 3:4:1:1:4:3 with the γ-radiation perpendicular to the internal magnetic field, and 3:2:1:1:2:3 for the case of random orientation of the magnetic fields in source or absorber. The angular dependence of the γ-radiation in the case of a pure quadrupole interaction was discussed previously. *

Polarized γ-rays in conjunction with a hyperfine split source *and* a hyperfine split absorber will exhibit a Mössbauer spectrum with relative line intensities which depend on the angular dependence of the γ-rays and on the relative orientation of the magnetic fields or axes of the EFG in source and absorber. We will show how the spin orientation in a magnetic material or the axis of the EFG in a crystal can be determined from these angular dependencies. The analogy of this method to optical polarimetry is apparent.

Polarized 14.4 keV radiation can be produced by magnetizing a Co^{57} in α-iron source. The emitted radiation pattern will consist of six lines, all linearly polarized, if observed perpendicular to H_{int} ($\theta = 90°$). However, only four lines will be emitted along the direction of magnetization ($\theta = 0$); the transitions $\Delta m = 0$ are missing. The γ-radiation of the four lines are circularly polarized and the helicity of the γ-radiation reverses with the reversal of the external field. A γ-ray is called right circularly polarized if its spin lies in the direction of motion (Frauenfelder, 1962). If θ is between 0° and 90°, the observed radiation pattern is elliptically polarized. Polarized 14.4 keV radiation can also be produced by a single crystal with an axially symmetric EFG containing Co^{57}; the lines of the quadrupole split spectrum are linearly polarized if the axis of the EFG is perpendicular to the propagation direction of the γ-rays.

II. Circularly Polarized γ-Rays

First we consider the case where source and absorber are in a colinear longitudinal magnetic field (Blum and Grodzins, 1964). Conservation of angular momentum requires that the helicity of the γ-radiation in the source has to be matched with the one in the absorber. For instance, a γ-ray, due to the transition $+3/2 \rightarrow +1/2$ carrying the angular momentum +1, can only be absorbed in a transition with the corresponding angular momentum change +1.

*See R.L. Mössbauer, Chap. 11.

The relative absorption intensities of parallel and antiparallel internal magnetic fields in source and absorber in the thin source and thin absorber approximation are listed in Table II. The table indicates that eight lines are expected for the parallel and anti-parallel fields and the positions and intensities of the lines as a function of the ratio of the hyperfine fields in source and absorber can be conveniently shown in a nomograph, Fig. 3. The velocity axis is scaled for $H_A = 331$ kOe. The following cases and the occurring degeneracies can easily be distinguished: three lines are expected for $H_S/H_A = 1$ and six lines for $H_S/H_A = -1$. A single line source ($H_S/H_A = 0$) exhibits a four line Zeeman pattern. (The subscript "S" refers always to the source and the subscript "A" to the absorber.)

Table II: Relative absorption intensities (for Fe^{57}) obtained with source and absorber in colinear longitudinal magnetic fields ($\theta = 0$ and $\omega = 0°$ or $180°$, respectively). In this arrangement both source and absorber exhibit four Zeeman lines ($\Delta m = \pm 1$) in conjunction with a single line absorber or source, respectively.

Zeeman$_S \to$ Zeeman$_A$							
H_S parallel to H_A				H_S antiparallel to H_A			
α	γ	δ	η	α	γ	δ	η
A 9	0	3	0	0	3	0	9
C 0	1	0	3	3	0	1	0
D 3	0	1	0	0	1	0	3
F 0	3	0	9	9	0	3	0

III. Linearly Polarized γ-Rays

A. Determination of Spin Directions

The use of linearly polarized recoil free γ-rays is of some special interest because one can determine the spin orientation in a magnetic material by analyzing the line intensities obtained from one single crystal cut in an arbitrary direction. Using a source (e.g., Co^{57} in α-iron) magnetized to saturation (z-direction) normal to the propagation direction of the γ-rays (x-direction) (see Fig. 2), all six Zeeman components of the emission spectrum are linearly polarized either in the x-z plane or x-y plane (y is normal to x and z). A magnetically ordered absorber will show, in general, 36 absorption lines in conjunction with a linearly polarized source. The locations of the lines are derived easily by overlapping the six-line

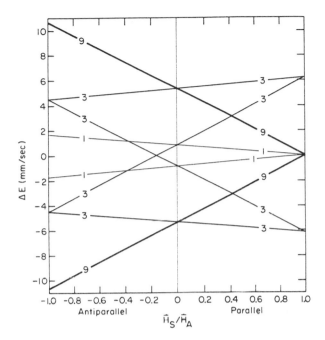

Fig. 3: Nomograph showing the position and intensities of the lines of an absorption spectrum for longitudinal magnetic fields as a function of the ratio of the hyperfine fields in source and absorber. The velocity axis is scaled for **H** = 331 kOe (after Blum and Grodzins, 1964).

patterns of the source and absorber obtained with a single-line absorber or source, respectively. The absorption intensities of the 36 lines are obtained from expressions given by Frauenfelder et al. (1962) and listed in the thin source — thin absorber approximation in Table III. ω is the angle between x and the spin direction in the absorber, Ψ is the angle between the projection of the spin direction on the y-z plane and the z-directions as indicated in Fig. 2. In Table III, (b)-(e) refer to the following limiting cases: Zeeman split source and absorber with spins in the z, y, and x direction (Zeeman$_S$ → Zeeman$_A$, b); Zeeman split source and absorber with axis of the EFG in the z, y, and x direction (Zeeman$_S$ → Q$_A$, c); quadrupole split source and absorber with spins in the z, y, and x direction (Q$_S$ → Zeeman$_A$, d); and quadrupole split source and absorber with axis of the EFG in the z, y, and x direction (Q$_S$ → Q$_A$, e). If the absorber spins lie in the x,

Table III: Relative absorption intensities (for Fe^{57}) obtained with a linearly polarized source and a magnetically ordered absorber or a single crystal with unique axis of the EFG as absorber ($\theta = 90°$).

$Zeeman_S \rightarrow Zeeman_A$

(a)	α, η	β, ϵ	γ, δ
A, F	$9(1-\sin^2 \omega \sin^2 \psi)$	$12 \sin^2 \omega \sin^2 \psi$	$3(1-\sin^2 \omega \sin^2 \psi)$
B, E	$12(1-\sin^2 \omega \cos^2 \psi)$	$16 \sin^2 \omega \cos^2 \psi$	$4(1-\sin^2 \omega \cos^2 \psi)$
C, D	$3(1-\sin^2 \omega \sin^2 \psi)$	$4 \sin^2 \omega \sin^2 \psi$	$(1-\sin^2 \omega \sin^2 \psi)$

$Zeeman_S \rightarrow Zeeman_A$

(b)	$\omega = 90°, \psi = 0$			$\omega = 90°, \psi = 90°$			$\omega = 0, \psi$ indeterminate		
	α, η	β, ϵ	γ, δ	α, η	β, ϵ	γ, δ	α, η	β, ϵ	γ, δ
A, F	9	0	3	0	12	0	9	0	3
B, E	0	16	0	12	0	4	12	0	4
C, D	3	0	1	0	4	0	3	0	1

$Zeeman_S \rightarrow Q_A$

(c)	$\omega = 90°, \psi = 0$		$\omega = 90°, \psi = 90°$		$\omega = 0, \psi$ indeterminate	
	α	β	α	β	α	β
A, F	9	3	0	12	9	3
B, E	0	16	12	4	12	4
C, D	3	1	0	4	3	1

$Q_S \rightarrow Zeeman_A$

(d)	$\omega = 90°, \psi = 0$			$\omega = 90°, \psi = 90°$			$\omega = 0, \psi$ indeterminate		
	α, η	β, ϵ	γ, δ	α, η	β, ϵ	γ, δ	α, η	β, ϵ	γ, δ
A	9	0	3	0	12	0	9	0	3
B	3	16	1	12	4	4	15	0	5

$Q_S \rightarrow Q_A$

(e)	$\omega = 90°, \psi = 0$		$\omega = 90°, \psi = 90°$		$\omega = 0, \psi$ indeterminate	
	α	β	α	β	α	β
A	9	3	0	12	9	3
B	3	17	12	8	15	5

y, or z direction, an appreciable number of the intensities are zero as seen from Table III (see Zeeman$_S$ → Zeeman$_A$ (b)).

When the magnetic vector of the source is parallel or anti-parallel to the spin orientation in the absorber (no quadrupole interaction), the spectrum consists of 20 lines with the following allowed transitions:

$$\Delta m_S = \pm 1 \rightarrow \Delta m_A = \pm 1 , \quad (16)$$

$$\Delta m_S = 0 \quad \rightarrow \Delta m_A = 0 , \qquad (4)$$

$\left. \right\}$ $H_S \parallel H_A$

When the magnetic vector of the source is perpendicular to the spin orientation in the absorber, the spectrum consists of 16 lines with the allowed transitions:

$$\Delta m_S = \pm 1 \rightarrow \Delta m_A = 0 , \qquad (8)$$

$$\Delta m_S = 0 \quad \rightarrow \Delta m_A = \pm 1 , \qquad (8)$$

$\left. \right\}$ $H_S \perp H_A$

The positions of the lines as a function of the ratio of the hyperfine fields in the source and absorber are shown in the nomo-graph of Fig. 4 scaled for the internal field of α-iron, H_S, H_A = 331 kOe. The right-hand side of the figure corresponds to the case where the magnetic fields of source and absorber are paral-lel. The 20 lines with their expected intensities (see Table III(b), $\omega = 90°$, $\Psi = 0$) are indicated. The left-hand side corresponds to the case where the fields are perpendicular to each other and the expected 16 lines (see Table 3(b), $\omega = 90°$, $\Psi = 90°$) are drawn. With the parallel and the perpendicular arrangements of the fields in source and absorber, the resonance condition of the lines of the two spectra on the right and on the left side of Fig. 4 are mutually exclusive. For the individual lines, an absorber may change from opaque to transparent or vice versa by rotating either source or absorber by 90°. Under the condition of $H_S = H_A$, the follow-ing special cases can be distinguished: nine lines are expected for H_S parallel to H_A and six lines for H_S perpendicular to H_A. A single line source or absorber, H_S/H_A; $H_A/H_S = 0$, exhibits the familiar six line Zeeman pattern.

The spin orientation was determined in the antiferromag-netic material $Ca_2[Fe](Fe)O_5$ (Gonser et al., 1966). The Möss-bauer spectrum of a polycrystalline $Ca_2[Fe](Fe)O_5$ absorber at room temperature obtained with a single line source reveals two superimposed Zeeman patterns corresponding to the octahedral ($[\alpha] [\beta] [\gamma] [\delta] [\epsilon] [\eta]$) and tetrahedral ((α) (β) (γ) (δ) (ϵ) (η))

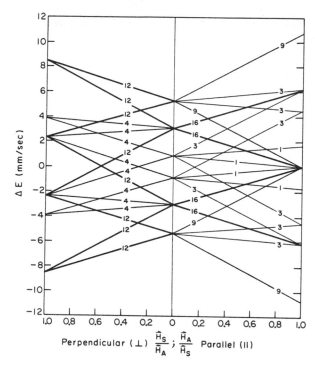

Fig. 4: Nomograph showing the position and intensities of the lines
of an absorption spectrum for parallel and perpendicular
arrangements of the magnetic fields in source and absorber
as a function of the ratio of the hyperfine fields. The magnetic fields in source and absorber are perpendicular to
the propagation direction of the γ-radiation. The velocity
axis is scaled for $H = 331$ kOe.

Fe^{3+} ion sites as shown in Fig. 5. The absorption spectra expected
for the individual sublattices with a Co^{57} in α-iron source polarized in the z-direction and a single crystal absorber are plotted at
the top of Fig. 6a for the cases in which the spins are perpendicular
to z ($\perp$ (Fe), $\perp$[Fe]) and parallel to z ($\parallel$(Fe), $\parallel$[Fe]). Locations
(taking into account the isomer shift) and intensities were obtained
as outlined in the previous paragraph, or in other words, the lines
corresponding to the nomograph in Fig. 4 for the parallel and perpendicular arrangements of the fields for the octahedral and tetrahedral sites were ordered in four subspectra. The capital letters
and Greek letters indicate which lines of the source and absorber

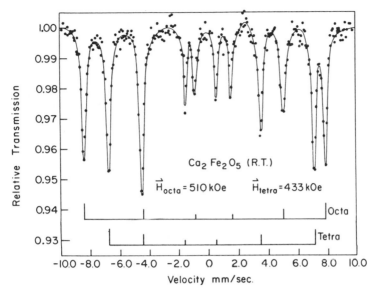

Fig. 5: Mössbauer spectrum obtained with a room temperature
source of Co^{57} diffused into Pt and a polycrystalline absorber of $Ca_2[Fe](Fe)O_5$ at room temperature. Source
approaching absorber is positive velocity.

Fig. 6: Predicted and experimental Mössbauer spectra for a magnetized Co^{57} in α-iron source at room temperature and a
single crystal of $Ca_2[Fe](Fe)O_5$. The crystallographic
b-axis of the $Ca_2[Fe](Fe)O_5$ and the magnetization direction of the source are parallel and perpendicular to the
γ-ray propagation direction, respectively.
(6a) Expected locations and intensities for the octahedral
[Fe] and tetrahedral (Fe) subspectra with the source magnetization direction perpendicular (⊥) and parallel or antiparallel (‖) to the spin orientation in the absorber.
(6b-6c) Observed spectra with crystallographic c-axis
perpendicular (6b) and parallel (6c) to the source magnetization direction.

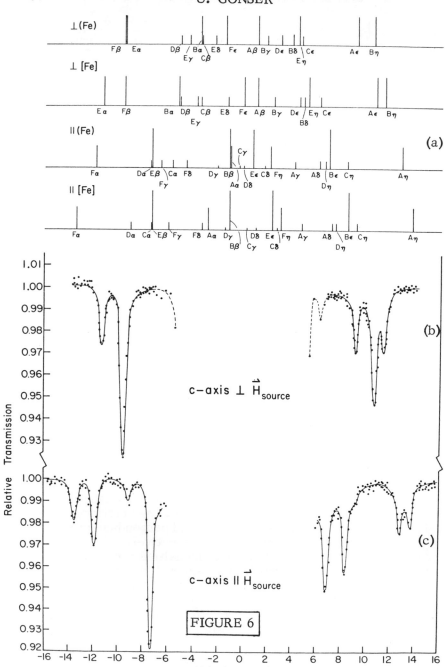

FIGURE 6

are in resonance.   The perturbation of the intensities due to non-zero quadrupole interactions is neglected.

Figure 6a indicates that the differences in the spectra are most easily distinguished in the high velocity range; therefore, data were taken only between ± (6 and 15) mm/sec.   Figures 6b and 6c show spectra with the crystallographic b-axis of the $Ca_2[Fe](Fe)O_5$ absorber in the x-direction, and the c-axis in the y-direction (6b) and in the z-direction (6c).   From comparison with Fig. 6a one can conclude that in $Ca_2[Fe](Fe)O_5$ all spins in the octahedral *and* tetrahedral sites are oriented in the c-direction.

B.   Determination of the Principal Axis of an EFG

As was shown by Johnson et al. (1962), linearly polarized recoil-free γ-rays can also be conveniently used to determine the axis of the EFG of a resonating atom in a crystal.   This method is restricted to resonating atoms with an asymmetry parameter η which is small or zero.*   Under this condition the two lines taken with an unpolarized source correspond to the states $m = \pm 3/2$ and $m = \pm 1/2$.   In the compound $FeSiF_6 \cdot 6H_2O$, the iron atoms are in a unique crystallographic environment and the axially symmetric EFG ($\eta \approx 0$) is parallel to the c-axis.   The Mössbauer spectrum of a single crystal taken with an unpolarized source is shown in Fig. 7a.   The orientation of the c-axis was chosen to be perpendicular to the propagation direction of the γ-rays.   The relative intensities of the two lines (approximately 3:5) indicate that the higher energy line (plus velocity) corresponds to the $m = \pm 1/2$ state and the lower energy line (minus velocity) to the $m = \pm 3/2$ state.   It follows that the quadrupole coupling constant, e^2qQ, has a negative value.

Linearly polarized γ-rays emitted from a magnetized source have the electric vector parallel to the internal magnetic field for the transition $\Delta m = \pm 1$, and the linearly polarized γ-rays corresponding to the transitions $\Delta m = 0$ have the electric vector perpendicular to the internal magnetic field.   Strong absorption in the $m = \pm 3/2$ state takes place if the principal axis of the EFG is parallel to the electric vector of the incident γ-radiation in the $m = \pm 1/2$ state if the axis of the EFG is perpendicular to the electric vector of the γ-radiation.   The expected intensities of the absorption lines are given in Table III, (Zeeman$_S \rightarrow Q_A$ (c)) for a polarized source and a single crystal with a unique axis of the EFG for all iron atoms. For the cases of quadrupole splittings, the bold arrow in the absorber of Fig. 2 represents the axis of the EFG, and ω is then the

*See R.L. Mössbauer, Chap. 11.

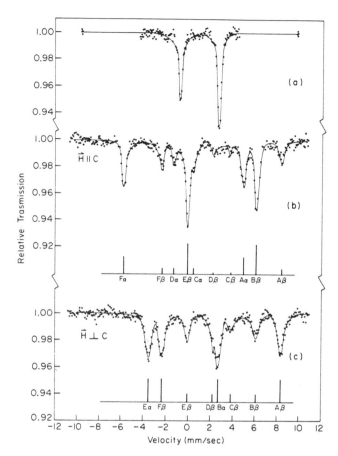

Fig. 7: Absorption spectra of a FeSiF$_6$· 6H$_2$O single crystal taken with a Co^{57}-Pt single line source (a) and with a Co^{57}-α-iron source magnetized parallel to the axis of the EFG (crystallographic c-axis) (b) and perpendicular to the axis of the EFG (c). The stick diagram indicates the expected intensities (according to Table III). The locations for the lines are marked with the appropriate letters for source and absorber.

angle between x and the axis of the EFG, and Ψ is the angle between the projection of the axis of the EFG on the y-z plane and the z-direction. The spectrum of a single crystal of FeSiF$_6$·6H$_2$O absorber with the c-axis parallel to the internal magnetic field in the source, **H** ‖ c, is shown in Fig. 7b. The spectrum in Fig. 7c was taken

after the absorber was rotated by 90°, **H** ⊥ c. The line locations
and expected intensities from Table III (c) are indicated by the
stick diagrams in Figs. 7b and 7c. The spectra show that the axis
of the EFG coincides with the crystallographic c-axis.

In Table III we have also listed the expected intensities for
the cases of a single crystal quadrupole split source with an axis
of the EFG perpendicular to the propagation direction of the γ-rays
and a polarized magnetic absorber, $Q_S \rightarrow Zeeman_A$ (d), and a
single crystal quadrupole absorber, $Q_S \rightarrow Q_A$ (e). The latter
cases indicate that quadrupole split single crystal sources (like
Co^{57} in Be or Zn) should be suited for determining the orientation
of the spins in magnetic materials and the axis of an EFG.

The case of quadrupole split source and absorber scaled to
a line separation of 2 mm/sec both having the axis of the EFG
($e^2qQ > 0$) perpendicular to the propagation direction of the γ-rays
is shown in the nomograph of Fig. 8. The intensities and the
positions of the lines as a function of the ratio of the quadrupole

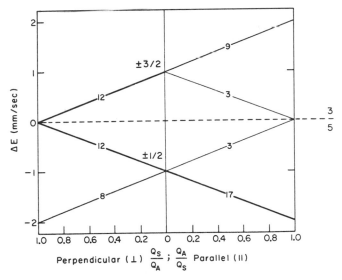

Fig. 8: Nomograph showing the position and intensities of the lines
of an absorption spectrum for parallel and perpendicular
arrangements of the axes of the EFG in source and absorber as a function of the ratio of the quadrupole splittings.
The axes of the EFG's in source and absorber are perpendicular to the propagation direction of the γ-radiation.
The velocity axis is scaled for a quadrupole splitting of
2mm/sec.

splittings are indicated for the situation where the two axes of the EFG are parallel (right-hand side) and for the situation where the two axes are perpendicular (left-hand side). If the axes of the EFG in source and absorber are parallel, four lines are expected. This is reduced to three lines in the case $Q_S = Q_A$. If the axes of the EFG in source and absorber are perpendicular, only three lines are expected with the special case $Q_S = Q_A$ where only two lines result. The ratio of the line intensities of the $\pm 3/2$ and $\pm 1/2$ state (upper half and lower half of figure) remains 3:5 while the individual line components have quite different intensities.

It should be noted that linearly polarized γ-rays with a unique orientation of the electric vector are only observable in transitions to and from the $m = \pm 3/2$ state. The radiation pattern involving the $m = \pm 1/2$ state is more complex.

C. Mössbauer Polarimeter

The technique described here might be regarded as a nuclear or γ-ray polarimeter with extremely high resolution in energy. In the γ-ray polarimeter, the polarized source emits linearly polarized recoil-free γ-rays, and by turning a magnetic material with a unique spin orientation or a single crystal with a principal axis of the EFG perpendicular to the propagation direction of the γ-rays, the absorber becomes transparent or opaque for the individual line components depending on the orientation of the spins and EFG in source and absorber.

A very interesting application of the γ-ray polarimeter was the demonstration by Imbert (1964) of a Faraday effect in linearly polarized recoil-free γ-rays, i.e., a rotation of the polarization passing through a medium in a direction parallel to an applied magnetic field.

Acknowledgement

Discussions with Drs. R. W. Grant, R. M. Housley, A. H. Muir, Jr., and H. Wiedersich are appreciated.

References

Blum, N. and Grodzins, L. (1964). Phys. Rev. 136, A133.

Boyle, A. J. F., Bunbury, D. St. P., and Edwards, C. (1960). Phys. Rev. Letters 5, 553.

Cohen, S. G. , Gielen, P. , Kaplow, R. (1966). Phys. Rev. 141, 423.

Dash, J. G. , Taylor, R. D. , Nagle, D. E. , Craig, P. P. , and Visscher, W. M. (1961). Phys. Rev. 122, 1116.

Frauenfelder, H. (1962). The Mössbauer Effect, (W. A. Benjamin, Inc. , New York).

Frauenfelder, H. , Nagle, D. E. , Taylor, R. D. , Cochran, D. R. F., and Visscher, W. M. (1962). Phys. Rev. 126, 1065.

Gol'danskii, V. I. , Makarov, E. F. , and Khrapov, V. V. (1963). Phys. Letters 3, 344.

Gonser, U. (1966). Z. fur Metallkunde 57, 85.

Gonser, U. , Grant, R. W. , Wiedersich, H. , and Geller, S. (1966). Appl. Phys. Letters 9, 18.

Hanna, S. S. , Heberle, J. , Littlejohn, C. , Perlow, G. J. , Preston, R. S. , and Vincent, D. H. (1960a). Phys. Rev. Letters 4, 177.

Hanna, S. S. , Heberle, J. , Perlow, G. J. , Preston, R. S. , and Vincent, D. H. (1960b). Phys. Rev. Letters 4, 513.

Imbert, P. (1964). Phys. Letters 8, 95; (1966). J. Physique 27, 429.

Johnson, C. E. , Marshall, W. , and Perlow, G. J. (1962). Phys. Rev. 126, 1503.

Obenshain, F. E. and Wegener, H. H. (1961). Proceedings of the Second International Conference on the Mössbauer Effect, Saclay, France, p. 148.

S.9. ELECTRONIC STRUCTURE AND HYPERFINE FIELDS IN METALLIC ALLOYS

E. Daniel

Institut de Physique
Strasbourg, France

I. Introduction

In this lecture, we shall try to show the connection between observed hyperfine fields in metallic alloys and some of the concepts most useful in describing their electronic structure (Friedel 1954, 1958, 1962). These concepts are the screening of positive ionic charge by the conduction electrons and the corresponding phase shifts in partial waves, giving rise to long range oscillations of charge or spin density. We shall also consider the special case of virtual bound states which can give rise to localized magnetic moments and show how it has been recently successfully applied to Heusler alloys. After some comments on binary alloys of transition metals, we shall look at the spin polarization of conduction electrons in iron, as deduced from measurements of the hyperfine field at the nuclei of nonmagnetic impurities.

II. Electronic Structure of Dilute Metallic Alloys

The characteristic feature for the metallic state of a material is the existence of a so-called conduction band, the electronic states of which are but partially occupied, up to some maximum

energy E_F which defines the Fermi level of the metal (at least at
low temperature). Conduction electrons behave in many respects
nearly as free electrons, at least in first approximation.

When an alloy is made by substituting an atom X with valency differing by Z from that of the pure matrix M, the conduction
electrons get perturbed in the vicinity of the solute atom X. The
main effect of the electronic rearrangement which occurs is the
screening of the excess of ionic charge Z by the conduction electrons. In most cases, the screening is nearly complete in the
atomic cell of the impurity, but simultaneously, it produces in
the matrix an oscillation in the electronic charge density, the amplitude of which decreases asymptotically like the inverse cube of
the distance at the impurity for large distances (Fig. 1).

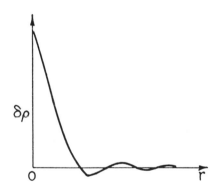

Fig. 1: Screening of an impurity and
oscillations of charge density.

For simple metals with cubic symmetry such as Na, Al, Cu,
Ag, etc...., the conduction electrons can, in first approximation,
be taken as free electrons and the effect of the impurity atom X
on these can be ascribed to a spherically symmetrical potential V
acting as a perturbation on these electrons. It is then convenient
to make a partial wave analysis of the scattering of conduction
electrons by the impurity. Piling up the screening charge of the
impurity produces a phase shift η_l in the lth spherical component of an electron wave function.[*]

*See the description given earlier in Chap. 9 by R.E.Watson.

The phase shifts at the Fermi level are related to the screening charge Z through the Friedel sum-rule,

$$Z = \frac{2}{\pi} \sum_{\ell} (2\ell + 1) \eta_{\ell}(E_F) \ . \tag{1}$$

Usually, these phase shifts become negligibly small for $\ell > 3$ or 4. These phase shifts also give the oscillations δ_{ρ} in charge density in the matrix. Asymptotically, for $r \to \infty$:

$$\delta \to \frac{C}{r^3} \cos (2 k_F r + \varphi), \tag{2}$$

where:

$$k_F^2 = 2 E_F \quad \text{(Hartree atomic units } e = m = \hbar = 1 \\ \text{are used throughout) ,}$$

$$C \sin \varphi = \frac{-1}{2\pi^2} \sum_{\ell} (-1)^{\ell} (2\ell + 1) \sin^2 \eta_{\ell}(k_F) \ ,$$

$$C \cos \varphi = \frac{-1}{2\pi^2} \sum_{\ell} (-)^{\ell} (2\ell + 1) \sin \eta_{\ell}(k_F) \cos \eta_{\ell}(k_F) \ .$$

III. Virtual Bound States and Localized Magnetic Moments

When the potential V is almost strong enough for binding an electron in a state with orbital angular momentum $\ell \neq 0$, the corresponding phase shift η_{ℓ} increases rapidly from zero to almost π in a small energy range Δ around some mean value E_m and then decreases with increasing energy (Fig. 2). The electronic charge almost bound in such a state is strongly localized on the impurity site and usually makes up most of the screening. Such virtual bound states, with d character (that is, corresponding to $\ell = 2$) occur for instance when the solute atom X is a transition element and the matrix is a simple metal such as Mg, Al, Cu, etc. The virtual bound states have their most important effects when their mean energy E_m is close to the Fermi level.

When electrons are localized in a virtual d bound state, as for instance on a Mn atom dissolved in Cu, they experience strong exchange and correlation forces which tend to make their spins

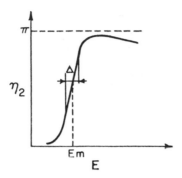

Fig. 2: Virtual d bound state.

parallel, according to Hund's rule for free atoms or ions. If the strength of these forces is large enough to split the energy of virtual bound states with opposite spins, so that they are occupied by unequal numbers of electrons up to the Fermi level, a localized magnetic moment occurs (Fig. 3). In that case, the phase shifts $\eta_{2\uparrow}$ and $\eta_{2\downarrow}$ for opposite spins $\uparrow$ and $\downarrow$ become different; as a result one gets electronic spin density oscillations in the matrix in addition to the oscillations of charge density. This makes magnetic coupling between impurities possible at rather large distances (Fig. 4).

IV. Applications to Heusler Alloys

These are ferromagnetic alloys with cubic structures and the general formula Cu_2MnX where X can be Al, In, Sn, ... (Fig. 5). Nuclear magnetic resonance experiments show that there is a hyperfine field of -212 kOe at Cu in Cu_2MnAl (Sugikuchi and Endo, 1964). Caroli and Blandin (1966) have shown that such a field may result from localized magnetic moments on the Mn atoms only, without any local moment on the Cu atoms, i. e. , without unpaired d electrons on Cu. According to their model, the measured fields arise only from the oscillating spin polarization induced in the conduction band of the alloy by the magnetic moments localized on Mn. They get in this way the right spin and order of magnitude for the hyperfine field on Cu nuclei and predict these quantities for the Al atoms.

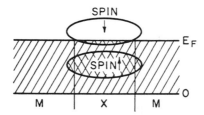

Fig. 3: Localized magnetic moment at impurity X and matrix M.

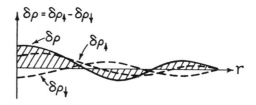

Fig. 4: Oscillations of spin density around a localized
magnetic moment.

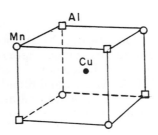

Fig. 5: Crystal structure of Heusler alloys.

Caroli and Blandin make use of the fact that the Mn atoms are rather far apart so that they can be treated as independently inducing their own spin polarization in the conduction band. They assume that this conduction band is built of one electron from each Cu atom, three electrons from each Al and one electron out of the seven 3d and 4s electrons of each Mn atom, the other six being localized in a virtual bound state in such a way as to produce the right screening charge and magnetic moment. This moment is approximately equal to 4 Bohr magnetons per Mn atom.

According to this model, in which most of the screening charge is in the d shell, they assume that in first approximation only the $\ell = 2$ phase shifts $\eta_\uparrow$ for spin up and $\eta_\downarrow$ for spin down are important. The screening condition:

$$Z = \frac{2\ell+1}{\pi} (\eta_\uparrow + \eta_\downarrow) = Z_\uparrow + Z_\downarrow \tag{3}$$

and the size of the magnetic moments in units of Bohr magnetons:

$$\mu = Z_\uparrow - Z_\downarrow = \frac{2\ell+1}{\pi} (\eta_\uparrow - \eta_\downarrow) \tag{4}$$

give, for $Z = 6$, $\mu = 4$, and $\ell = 2$:

$$\eta_\uparrow = \pi \text{ and } \eta_\downarrow = \frac{\pi}{5} .$$

This gives for the asymptotic value of the spin density oscillations arising from each Mn atom:

$$\delta\rho = \delta\rho_\uparrow - \delta\rho_\downarrow = \frac{-5}{4\pi^2 r^3} \sin\frac{\pi}{5} \cos\left(2 k_F r + \frac{\pi}{5}\right) \tag{5}$$

where $k_F \simeq 0.8$ atomic units is the Fermi momentum for the free conduction electrons corresponding to the lattice parameter of the alloy.

The hyperfine field induced by a given Mn atom at a Cu nucleus located at distance r is:

$$H_{hf} = \frac{8\pi}{3} \beta \langle |\psi(0)|^2 \rangle_F \delta\rho(r)$$

where β is the Bohr magneton and $\langle |\psi(0)|^2 \rangle_F$ is the average density of conduction electrons at the Fermi level on the Cu nucleus. Assuming for this last quantity the same value as in pure copper, they find that each of the four Mn neighbours of a given Cu in $Cu_2 MnAl$ contributes approximately -30 kOe, each of the eight second neighbours nearly -10 kOe and each of the third neighbours

between 0. 1 and 0. 2 kOe.   Neglecting small contributions from
more remote shells, this gives $H_{eff} \simeq$ -200 kOe, which is to be
compared to the experimental value -212 kOe.   In fact, such good
agreement is somewhat fortuitous, given the approximations which
have been made; e. g. , there is the use of the asymptotic form of
the spin density oscillations up to the nearest neighbours.   From a
discussion of these various approximations, Caroli and Blandin
reach the conclusion that their estimated hyperfine fields must be
right in the negative sign, and within a factor two of the true value
in order of magnitude.   They predict a negative hyperfine field
equal to -168 kOe on the Al nuclei.   It must be noticed that these
high values of induced hyperfine fields correspond to a spin polarization of conduction electrons not greater than 3 or 4 percent at
the nearest neighbour sites of a Mn atom.   The spin polarization
of the conduction band gives rise to a magnetic coupling between
the Mn atoms, leading to ferromagnetic order below some Curie
temperature.

Caroli and Blandin have computed this Curie temperature and
find theoretical values from the preceding model in good agreement
with experiment.

V. Alloys of Transition Metals

In the simplest scheme, a transition metal is described by an
incompletely filled "d" band in addition to the ordinary "s" conduction band (Fig. 6).   This d band is comparatively narrow with a

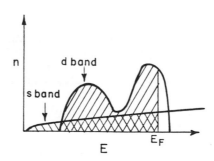

Fig. 6: Density of states per unit energy in a transition metal.

high density of states and is responsible for the magnetic properties of the metal. When both the solute atom X and the matrix M in a dilute alloy MX are transition elements, the screening usually occurs mainly in the d band due to its high density of states. In fact, it is customary to neglect the "s" conduction band and to treat the d band in the tight binding approximation. This allows a treatment of the scattering problem of the type described by Slater and Koster (1954). The perturbation due to the impurity is usually taken as localized in its atomic cell; this means that it has non-zero matrix elements only between d orbitals centered on the impurity. For some cases, such as for instance some Pd based alloys, the perturbation certainly extends farther than the impurity cell. Charge- or spin-density oscillations also result in screening in these metals and virtual bound states can occur also under appropriate conditions. The concept of phase shift can be applied to the d bands in transition metals, using cubic harmonics and irreducible representations of the cubic group for the partial wave analysis (Callaway, 1964; Friedel and Gautier, 1966; Gautier and Lenglart, 1965).

From the theoretical point of view, at least within the approximations made above, the simplest case is probably that of ferromagnetic Ni. Its spin ↑ d band being full, only the spin ↓ d band has states available at the Fermi level, and so takes part in the screening as long as the perturbation is not too strong. This gives a fairly good description of the NiCo alloys for instance. The oscillations in charge density in the matrix from the screening of the impurity give rise to the same amount of oscillations of the magnetization of the atoms of the matrix. The relative change in charge on an atom of the matrix being rather small, let us say a few percent, it is reasonable to assume that in first approximation the relative change in hyperfine field $\delta H_{hf}/H_{hf}$ on such an atom will be equal to the relative change in magnetization $(\delta\rho/\rho)$. As a result, the hyperfine fields in the matrix of a dilute alloy MX will be distributed around the mean value corresponding to the pure matrix and satellite lines may be resolved in nuclear magnetic resonance at least for the first few shells of neighbours of the impurity (Fig. 7) for which the relative shift in resonance frequency may reach 1 to 10 percent. For atoms too far away from an impurity, the satellites cannot be resolved and the distribution of fields results in a broadening of the central line. For finite but small concentrations, the mean frequency of this central line must itself be shifted proportionally to the concentration, as this is the case for the Knight shift in binary alloys of ordinary (i.e., non-transition) metals. These features have been observed for instance by nuclear

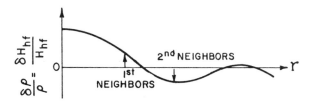

Fig. 7: Hyperfine field distribution in a ferromagnetic alloy.

magnetic resonance on NiCo, CoFe, CoNi alloys (Koi et al., 1961). Theoretical estimates by Gautier (1962, 1965), using a rough approximation to the Fermi surface of Co, show that one gets the right order of magnitude for the satellite line frequencies by ascribing them to the oscillations of spin density in the d band.

Except for the order of magnitude of the shifts in frequency, the quantitative agreement is not very good. In fact, an accurate calculation of the frequency would be very difficult and requires a detailed knowledge of the band structure and shape of the Fermi surface of the metal. Also one should properly take account of the separate contribution of the 4s conduction electrons to the hyperfine fields. The situation is even worse in Fe, where d bands of both spin directions intersect the Fermi surface.

VI. Spin Polarization of Conduction Electrons in Fe

A method for finding the sign of the s conduction electron contribution to the hyperfine field in Fe is to measure the induced field at the nucleus of a nonmagnetic impurity dissolved in Fe. In fact, experimental results, as shown in Fig. 8, give fields of different sign depending upon the atomic number of the impurity (DeWaard and Drentje, 1966; Frankel et al., 1965; Holliday et al., 1966). For a low enough number of external (s,p) electrons, that is up to Sn, the observed field is negative but for a higher number, that is from Sb upwards, the observed field becomes positive. This was predicted in a calculation of the screening of the impurities by the conduction electrons of Fe (Daniel and Friedel, 1963).

According to magnetic measurements, the effect of substituting a nonmagnetic impurity for an Fe atom is simply to diminish by

2.2 Bohr magnetons (just its average value) the magnetization of Fe. This dilution effect suggests that in a tight binding picture of the d bands, the Fe atom which is removed brings out its magnetic d electrons and that the screening of the impurity occurs mainly through the conduction band. Assuming one "4s" conduction electron in pure iron and $Z + 1$ valence electrons for the impurity, the screening charge needed amounts to Z. This will be attracted to the impurity by some perturbative potential well V, the radius of which is taken as the atomic radius of Fe, with the depth adjusted so as to give the right screening charge from the phase-shift and Friedel sum-rule. Now in the ferromagnetic state, because of the s-d ex-

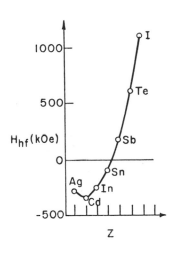

Fig. 8: Hyperfine fields at non-magnetic impurities (DeWaard and Drentje, 1966).

change coupling in the iron matrix, the conduction electrons with spin ↑ (parallel to that of the majority d electrons) will have on the average their energies lowered by some quantity ε while electrons with opposite spin will have their energies raised by the same quantity (a priori, ε can be either positive or negative). This s-d exchange coupling does not exist in the impurity cell. As a result, the electrons with spin ↑ will see an effective potential $V_↑ = V - ε$, while the electrons with spin ↓ will be acted on by $V_↓ = V + ε$ (Fig. 9). If, for instance, one has ε >0, that is, if the spin polarization of conduction electrons is on the average positive, there will be more conduction electrons with spin ↑ than with spin ↓, but they will be attracted by a smaller effective potential $|V_↑| < |V_↓|$. The enhancement of the quantity $|\psi(0)|^2$ on the impurity due to the screening will then be higher for spin ↓ than for spin ↑ electrons. This effect must become less and less important when V becomes very large with respect to ε, that is for high enough values of Z.

The hyperfine field, H_{hf}, at the nucleus of the impurity is given by the proportionality:

$$H_{hf} \propto \int^{E_F} \left[|\psi_↑(0)|^2 \, n_↑(E) - |\psi_↓(0)|^2 \, n_↓(E) \right] dE \, . \qquad (6)$$

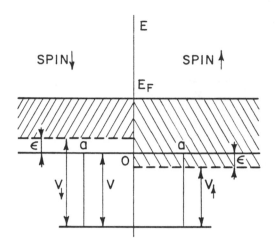

Fig. 9: Effective potentials for conduction
electrons at a nonmagnetic impurity
dissolved in ferromagnetic Fe.

The two following limiting cases are of special interest:

(1) When V is very large with respect to ε, that is when the electrostatic potential is much larger than the exchange potential, one expects $\psi_\uparrow(0)$ and $\psi_\downarrow(0)$ to be very close to each other at each energy, so that the sign at the hyperfine field must be given by

$$\int^{E_F} (n_\uparrow - n_\downarrow)\, dE \ ,$$

which is the overall mean spin polarization of the conduction band;

(2) When V is small compared to ε, that is for vanishingly small value of Z, the difference in $\psi_\uparrow(0)$ and $\psi_\downarrow(0)$ becomes comparatively more important and one gets for the hyperfine field the sign opposite to that given by the mean polarization.

Numerical calculations using this simple model indicate that the sign reversal of the field must occur for Z between 3 and 4, that is between Sn and Sb, in good agreement with experiment. From the positive sign of the field for high values of Z, one deduces that the *average* spin polarization of conduction electrons in Fe must be *positive*. This does not exclude the possibility of finding a local negative spin polarization for instance in the region close to the limits of the atomic cell, outside of the d shells, by means of neutron diffraction or position annihilation measurements.

VII. Conclusion

In conclusion, we note that useful qualitative or semi-quantitative information on their electronic structure have been obtained by using simple schemes which distinguish between "s" and "d" electrons. Even with this simplification, the complicated band structure and Fermi surfaces of these metals prevents getting accurate quantitative results without an enormous amount of numerical calculation. Theoretical estimates of the hyperfine field at the solute atoms in a dilute alloy are especially poor. Finally, in a real transition metal there is no clear cut distinction between "s" and "d" electrons and an accurate theory should take s-d mixing into account.

References

Callaway, J. (1964). J. Math. Phys. 5, 783.

Caroli, B. and Blandin, A. (1966). J. Phys. Chem. Solids 27, 503.

Daniel, E. and Friedel, J. (1963). J. Phys. Chem. Solids 24, 1601.

De Waard, H. and Drentje, S. A. (1966). Phys. Letters 20, 38.

Frankel, R. B., Huntzicker, J., Matthias, E., Rosenblum, S. S., Shirley, D. A., and Stone, N. J. (1965). Phys. Letters 15, 163.

Friedel, J. (1954). Adv. in Phys. 3, 446; (1958). Nuovo Cimento Suppl. No. 2 7, 287; (1962). J. Phys. Rad. 23, 692.

Friedel, J. and Gautier, F. (1966). (in press).

Gautier, F. (1962). J. Phys. Rad. 23, 738; (1965S). Ann. de Phys. 10, 275.

Gautier, F. and Lenglart, P. (1965). Phys. Rev. 139A, 705.

Holliday, R., Shirley, D. A., and Stone, N. J. (1966). Phys. Rev. 143, 130.

Koi, Y., Tsujinura, A., Tadamiki, M., and Kushida, T. (1961). J. Phys. Soc. of Japan 16, 1040.

La Force, R. C., Ravitz, S. F., and Day, G. F. (1961). Phys. Rev. Letters 6, 226.

Slater, J. C. and Koster, G. F. (1954). Phys. Rev. 95, 1167.

Sugikuchi, K. and Endo, K. (1964). J. Phys. Chem. Solids 25, 217.

S.10. NUCLEAR MAGNETIC RESONANCE IN SOME MAGNETICALLY ORDERED SYSTEMS[*]

J.I. Budnick and S. Skalski

Fordham University
Bronx, New York

I. Introduction

Nuclear magnetic resonance spectroscopy has become a useful tool in the study of hyperfine fields in magnetically ordered systems (Portis and Gossard, 1960; Portis and Lindquist, 1965). In a metallic ferromagnetic solid (our principal concern here), a nucleus at $\mathbf{r}$ experiences a hyperfine field which is conveniently taken to be proportional to the local value of the average electronic angular momentum $\langle \mathbf{J}(\mathbf{r}) \rangle$ (Freeman and Watson, 1965). This average most generally includes contributions from several sources, each of which leads to a hyperfine interaction, the strengths of which can be quite different. Because of this complexity, one cannot, from the measured hyperfine field alone, infer the individual contributions to $\langle \mathbf{J}(\mathbf{r}) \rangle$ unless, in a particular system, one source dominates. On the other hand, a determination of the hyperfine field, together with other measurements both local (e. g. neutron scattering) and average (e. g. saturation magnetization, heat capacity) can lead to a fairly complete understanding of the internal fields and their sources.

[*]*Work supported by the National Science Foundation.*

In an NMR experiment done at *low* rf power on a ferromagnet in zero external static field, one observes principally nuclei located in domain walls (Weger, 1962). In most systems (especially alloys) a complete analysis of the NMR spectra requires consideration of the variation of magnetization direction within a domain wall (Murray and Marshall, 1965), as well as the wall configuration and mobility in the actual sample. However, significant information about both the hyperfine field and nuclear spin relaxation is readily obtainable. In systems where a Mössbauer isotope is available, a direct comparison of the two experiments is possible and helpful in interpreting spectra obtained by either method.

The spin-echo technique has been demonstrated to be especially useful in the study of the broad line spectra frequently encountered in ferromagnets (Asayama et al., 1963). In Sec. II we describe briefly our experimental procedure. In the remaining sections we present results on several systems: (i) ferromagnetic solutions of Fe in Pd; (ii) Fe rich solid solutions; (iii) ordered ferromagnetic Fe_3Si; (iv) Laves phase compounds of Gd.

The NMR results discussed herein have been obtained in collaboration with R. E. Gegenwarth, J. Lechaton, T. J. Burch, and J. J. Murphy, all of Fordham University and J. H. Wernick of the Bell Telephone Laboratories.

II. Experimental Method

The large enhancement factors encountered for nuclei in domain walls make it possible to do NMR experiments at low rf power (Portis and Gossard, 1960; Portis and Lindquist, 1965). Although several different excitation conditions for the formation of spin-echoes were used in these studies, our experience favored the use of small ($\lesssim$ 120°) turn angle exciting pulses. The echo-shapes obtained with approximately equal pulses, agreed well with those computed by Mims (1966) in an analysis of the echoes obtained in broad line spectra. The procedure, which gave reproducible results, was to measure the frequency of the *echo* corresponding to each exciting frequency, and to compare the echo amplitude with that of a simulated echo produced by a pulsed signal generator. For long pulses and low turn angles, the echo frequency is essentially the same as the exciting pulse frequency (a result not obtained for short, high turn angle pulses). This effect of the exciting pulse widths, and an indication of the resolution obtainable in our spin-echo experiments, can be seen in the pure Fe spectrum shown in Fig. 1.

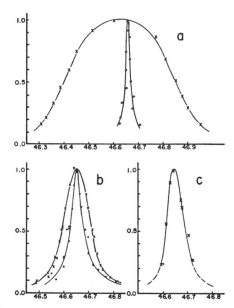

Fig. 1: Uncorrected spin-echo amplitude (arbitrary units) vs. frequency (Mc/sec) for ^{57}Fe in iron sponge (99.999%). The exciting pulse frequencies are shown by crosses and the echo frequencies by open circles. The effect of varying the widths of the two exciting pulses can be seen; (a) pulse widths 2.0 and 1.0 μsec, (b) pulse widths 10 and 10 μsec, and (c) pulse widths 40 and 40 μsec.

The raw data, therefore, is the echo amplitude as a function of *echo* frequency. Because of the broad lines, correction (Kobayashi et al., 1966; Streever and Uriano, 1965) must be made for: (i) the variation of the Boltzmann factor ($\propto \nu$), (ii) the frequency dependence of the detected voltage induced by the pre- cessing magnetization ($\propto \nu$), (iii) the explicit frequency dependence of the enhancement mechanism, and (iv) the variation in relaxation rates. By inductively coupling the calibrating voltage we com- pensate for (ii) above, and because we use a constant turn angle, we expect the frequency dependence of the enhancement, noted in (iii) above, not to be appreciable in analyzing the raw data. Fur- thermore, no significant variation in relaxation rates was ob- served within a given line in these systems. Thus, we take the echo amplitude divided by frequency to be proportional to the number of nuclei with a given hyperfine frequency.

III. Ferromagnetic Solutions of Fe in Pd

Small concentrations of Fe in Pd give rise to a ferromagnetic state in which there is a moment (Crangle, 1960; Crangle and Scott, 1965; Clogston et al., 1962) as high as $12 \mu_B$ associated with each Fe atom (for 0.25 at.% Fe). Neutron scattering (Low and Holden, 1966; Cable et al., 1965) indicates that the Fe moment is essentially constant at a value of about $3 \mu_B$, and for dilute solutions ($\sim$ 1/4 to 1/2 at.% Fe), the Pd matrix is polarized out to a distance of about 10 Å from an Fe site, with a near neighbor Pd moment of about $1/20 \mu_B$. Above 4 at.% Fe in Pd, the neutron scattering cross section is isotropic (Low and Holden, 1966) suggesting a uniform Pd polarization.

A unique Fe hyperfine field, consistent with the long range of the polarization, is observed in Mössbauer experiments (Craig et al., 1965). This field, for concentrations up to 25 at.% Fe, is shown in Fig. 2 which also shows the results of the NMR study (Budnick et al., 1966). The NMR data extrapolates to a low concentration limit in better agreement with a more recent result of -300.8 kOe (Maley et al., 1966) for the saturation field at very dilute Fe in Pd (50 ppm). The concentration dependence of the NMR value for the Fe field is drastically reduced above 4 at.%, the concentration at which the neutron cross section becomes isotropic. An NMR study (Budnick et al., 1966) of an enriched 13.2 at.% foil sample used in the Mössbauer study shows an Fe line asymmetrically broadened to a field value corresponding to the Mössbauer result but having a maximum consistent with the lower concentration NMR data. The difference between the two experimental results above 5 at.% Fe is not yet fully understood.

The smoothed Pd field distribution, for frequencies greater than 10 Mc/sec, is contained in Fig. 3. At low concentrations ($\sim$ 1/4 at.% Fe), the average (over the observed distribution) Pd hyperfine field tends to a value of about 72 kOe. If one analyzes these spectra in terms of the ratio of the average field to average moment (as obtained from other experiments), one finds that this ratio (an average hyperfine coupling constant) approaches a constant value of approximately 525 kOe/μ_B for concentrations above 4 at.% Fe. We believe that the *structure* in the Pd spectra arises from a directly induced moment on the near neighbor Pd atoms of

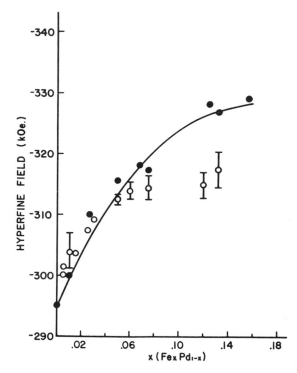

Fig. 2: ^{57}Fe hyperfine field in a series of Pd-Fe alloys. Open circles — NMR data, filled circles — Mössbauer data (uncertainty in Mössbauer field values is about ± 4 kOe). The solid curve gives the concentration dependence expected from the model of Craig and co-workers (1965) using -295 kOe for x =0 and -335 kOe for large x.

an Fe impurity; The *concentration dependence* of the spectra is due to the changing nearest neighbor configuration of a Pd atom, and to the concentration dependence of the average polarization (Lechaton et al., 1966).

IV. Fe Rich Solid Solutions

An investigation of the hyperfine field and magnetic moment at Fe sites in the neighborhood of various substitutional impurities can provide valuable information about the nature and range of the

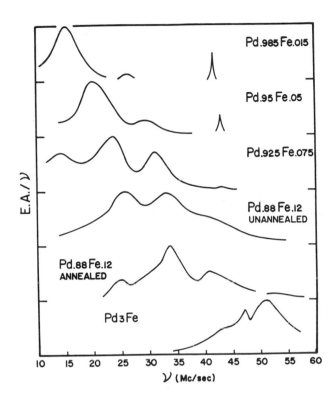

Fig. 3: Smoothed spin-echo spectra for a series of Pd-Fe alloys. The sharp [57]Fe resonance appears near 42 Mc/sec in the 1.5 and 5.0 at.% Fe samples. The remainder of the distribution (Pd) was normalized to the absolute maximum for each spectrum.

exchange polarization mechanisms.* Mössbauer studies (Wertheim et al., 1964; Stearns, 1966) of the Fe field in various solid solutions indicate that discrete values of the field can be assigned to Fe nuclei with a specific configuration of neighbor impurity atoms. One such investigation (Wertheim et al., 1964) considers explicitly only the first and second neighbor effects; more distant neighbors are taken to produce a shift in the overall spectra. One system (Fe-Ru), which has been analyzed in this fashion, has also been studied by us using the NMR spin-echo technique. The Mössbauer result for the field at iron atoms which are first or second

*See Chap. 9 by R.E. Watson.

near neighbors of a Ru impurity are indicated on the NMR spectrum for a 5.0 at.% Ru sample shown in Fig. 4. The high frequency

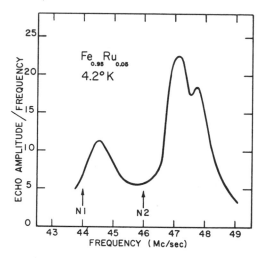

Fig. 4: Spin-echo spectrum for 5.0 at. % Ru in Fe alloy. The arrows labeled N1 and N2 give the location of the first and second neighbor Fe lines as determined from the Mössbauer experiment.

satellite in Fig. 4 is not resolved in the Mössbauer experiment (which has an inherently lower resolution), but appears in the Mössbauer analysis as a shift in the entire spectrum. In this NMR experiment on nuclei in domain walls, the variation of magnetization direction within the wall would cause a broadening (Murray and Marshall, 1965) which would be greatest for the second neighbors to a Ru atom. Thus the N2 line is not clearly resolved in the NMR spectrum, however, it has an appreciable echo amplitude at the corresponding frequencies.

Mössbauer spectra on several other Fe alloy systems have been analyzed to give the shifts in the Fe hyperfine fields out to the 6th neighbors of an impurity (Stearns, 1966). An oscillatory variation in this shift has been interpreted in terms of an oscillating conduction electron spin polarization. J. J. Murphy et al. (1966) have studied* some of these systems by NMR and we will discuss the comparison of these results and the Mössbauer results for Fe-Al. A spectrum for a 4.0 at.% Al sample as shown in Fig. 5 shows a satellite in good agreement with the Mössbauer result for the first near neighbor Fe hyperfine field. At 46 Mc/sec a strong contribution is observed which we associate with the third neighbors of an impurity. The spectra at several

*See also Rubinstein et al. (1966a).

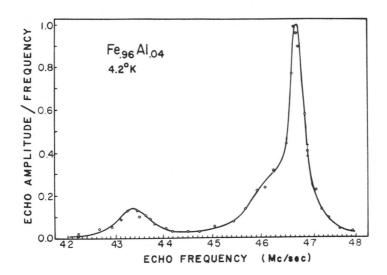

Fig. 5: Spin-echo spectrum for a 4.0 at.% Al in Fe alloy. The
first neighbor contribution is clearly resolved.

concentrations suggest that second neighbor irons are not resolved
probably due to a combination of a small isotropic shift plus dipolar broadening. A Mössbauer study (Cranshaw, 1966) of an
Fe + Si single crystal indicates that the second neighbor irons are
essentially unshifted; our analysis of the NMR spectra from the
similar Fe-Al system is consistent with this result.

        Further information on these systems is available from the
study of the solute resonances (Rubinstein et al., 1966b).*

V. Ordered Fe₃Si

        The Fe-Si system can display Fe₃Si type order for Si con-
centrations above about 10 at.% Fe. It is interesting to study the
effects of this order on the exchange mechanisms by measuring

*These workers have noted a correspondence between the satel-
lite structure of the solute and solvent resonances in Fe-Mn
alloys, but not for Fe-V alloys. We have also observed the
V resonance in Fe-V and the Al resonance in Fe-Al. In the
latter system, the solute spectra are also not in a simple
correspondence to the solvent spectra.

both the Fe and Si hyperfine fields. In ordered Fe_3Si, three sharp lines are observed in the NMR spectra. The earlier Möss-bauer data (Stearns, 1963) on the Fe hyperfine field at the two iron sites* enable us to identify the third line as the ^{29}Si resonance; it occurs at 31.5 Mc/sec at 4.2°K. In a 23.0 at.%Si sample, another line, not previously observed in the Mössbauer experiments appears at about 47 Mc/sec. In samples of 22.3 and 18.4 at.%Si, the 31.5 Mc/sec line is no longer observed but the 47 Mc/sec line persists and grows in intensity. The concentration dependence of the frequencies of these lines is summarized in Fig. 6. One of the two lines labeled X and Y in that figure is for

Fig. 6: The frequencies of the spin-echo maxima in a series of Fe-Si alloys at 4.2°K.
D: Fe sites with 8 Fe n.n.'s;
A_5: Fe sites with 5 Fe n.n.'s;
A_4: Fe sites with 4 Fe n.n.'s.
S is the ^{29}Si line. The curves labeled X and Y are discussed in the text.

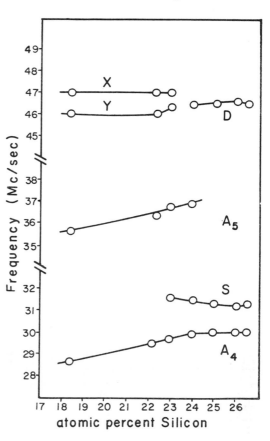

*The A_4 sites have 4 Fe n.n.'s and 4 Si n.n.'s. The D sites have 8 Fe n.n.'s.

the previously identified Fe D site; the other must be the Si line. Intensity arguments preclude the identification of both the X and Y lines with Fe sites. Thus, the Si hyperfine field changes drastically at about 23 at.% Si; at concentrations in this vicinity, there is also a sharp drop in the electrical resistivity.

Even though the Fe fields shift by only about 1% in this concentration range, the Si field could change by a much larger fractional amount since the Si atomic site carries a negligible magnetic moment and should be more sensitive to any change in ordering. If conduction electron polarization is the dominant source of the Si hyperfine field, the abrupt change in the field at 23 at.% may result from an abrupt change in the long range order. The magnitude of the field shift is about 17 kOe which is not very different from the shift (Stearns, 1966) in the Fe field for an Fe which is a first neighbor of a Si impurity in dilute Si in Fe alloys. This result suggests that conduction electron polarization is the dominant mechanism (Rubinstein et al., 1966b).

A similar difference in the Al hyperfine field between ordered and disordered Fe_3Al has also been observed; this difference (30 kOe) is also very close to the magnitude of the first neighbor Fe field shift (Wertheim et al., 1964; Stearns, 1966) in dilute Al in Fe alloys (24 kOe).

VI. Laves Phase Compounds of Gd

Of the magnetic rare-earths, Gd is particularly interesting because it has a small magnetic hyperfine interaction due to the absence of a 4f orbital contribution. Gd does not easily lend itself to a Mössbauer determination of the hyperfine field. In the (hcp) metal, the quadrupole interaction is appreciable and, together with the spatially varying magnetization direction in the ordered state, complicates the analysis of NMR results.

We have made a systematic NMR study of the Gd hyperfine field in magnetically ordered cubic Laves phase compounds of Gd. The results for the Gd field plotted as a function of the rare-earth separation are shown in Fig. 7 along with the Mössbauer results for Dy fields (Nowick, 1966) in similar compounds. The similar variation of these rare-earth hyperfine fields in the presence of the large absolute difference in the fields suggests that (i) the 4f orbital contribution (dominant in the Dy and negligible in the Gd compounds) is essentially unchanged throughout each series and is largely determined by the crystal symmetry, and therefore

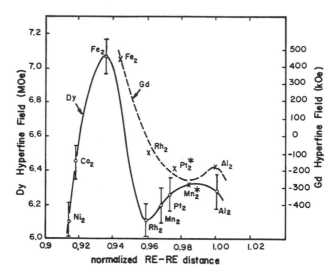

Fig. 7: Gd and Dy hyperfine fields in a series of Laves phase
compounds as a function of rare-earth separation normalized to that in $GdAl_2$. The asterisks on the $GdPt_2$ and
$GdMn_2$ points indicate that the signs of these fields have
not been measured but are believed to be negative.

(ii) the 4f core polarization field is also constant throughout each
series.

The large positive value for the Gd hyperfine field in $GdFe_2$
(see Fig. 7) is about 800 kOe larger than the field value in the
metal and for the Gd^{3+} ion (about -340 kOe) and may be considered
to be the contribution from core polarization (Freeman and Watson,
1965) by the 4f electrons. It is significant that the hyperfine fields
at the Tb, Dy, Tm, and Er nuclei in the analogous Fe_2 compounds
(Nowik, 1966) are also about 800 kOe higher than the fields in the
corresponding pure metals, *independent of the large variation
in the orbital contribution*. The polarization mechanism
responsible for this difference must be attributed to the valence
(5d, 6s) electrons. This polarization could be caused by overlap
of d character electron wave functions localized about the rare-
earth and iron sites respectively; this overlap is probably responsible for the observed high Curie temperatures of the RFe_2 compounds (Wertheim and Wernick, 1962).

References

Asayama, K., Kobayashi, S. and Itoh, J. (1963). J. Phys. Soc. Japan 18, 458.

Budnick, J. I., Lechaton, J. and Skalski, S. (1966). Phys. Letters 22, 405.

Cable, J. W., Wollan, E. O. and Koehler, W. C. (1965). Phys. Rev. 138, A755.

Clogston, A. M., Matthias, B. T., Peter, M., Williams, H. J., Corenzwit, E., and Sherwood, R. C. (1962). Phys. Rev. 125, 541.

Craig, P. P., Mozer, B., and Segnan, R. (1965). Phys. Rev. Letters 14, 895.

Crangle, J. (1960). Phil. Mag. 5, 335.

Crangle, J. and Scott, W. R. (1965). J. Appl. Phys. 36, 921.

Cranshaw, T. (1966). Private communication.

Freeman, A. J. and Watson, R. E. (1965). in Magnetism, edited by G. T. Rado and H. Suhl (Academic Press, New York) Vol. IIA, p. 167.

Kobayashi, S., Asayama, K. and Itoh, J. (1966). J. Phys. Soc. Japan 21, 65.

Lechaton, J., Budnick, J. I. and Skalski (1966). (to be published).

Low, G. G. and Holden, T. M. (1966). Proc. Phys. Soc. (London) 89, 119.

Maley, M. P., Taylor, R. D. and Thompson, J. L. (1966). 12th Annual Conference on Magnetism and Magnetic Materials, Washington, D. C.

Mims, W. B. (1966). Phys. Rev. 141, 499.

Murphy, J. J., Budnick, J. I. and Skalski, S. (1966). (to be published).

Murray, G. A. and Marshall, W. (1965). Proc. Phys. Soc. 86, 315.

Nowik, I. (1966). (to be published).

Portis, A. M. and Gossard, A. C. (1960). J. Appl. Phys. 31, 2058.

Portis, A. M. and Lindquist, R. H. (1965). in Magnetism, edited by G. T. Rado and H. Suhl (Academic Press, New York) Vol. IIA, p. 357.

Rubinstein, M., Stauss, G. H. and Stearns, M. B. (1966a). J. Appl. Phys. 37, 1334.

Rubinstein, M., Stauss, G. H. and Dweck, J. (1966b). Phys. Rev. Letters 17, 1001.

Stearns, M. B. (1963). Phys. Rev. 129, 1136.

Stearns, M. B. (1966). Phys. Rev. 147, 439.

Streever, R. L. and Uriano, G. A. (1965). Phys. Rev. 139, A135.

Weger, M. (1962). Ph. D. Thesis, University of California, Berkeley, unpublished.

Wertheim, G. K. and Wernick, J. H. (1962). Phys. Rev. 125, 1937.

Wertheim, G. K., Jaccarino, V., Wernick, J. H., and Buchanan, D. N. E. (1964). Phys. Rev. Letters 12, 24.

S.11. RELATION BETWEEN g SHIFT OF MAGNETIC IMPURITIES AND KNIGHT SHIFT OF THE HOST NUCLEI IN METALS*

D. Shaltiel

Microwave Division
Department of Physics
The Hebrew University
Jerusalem, Israel

I. Introduction

Experiments done in recent years on the electron paramagnetic resonance (EPR) and g shift of magnetic impurities in metals have shown that a correlation exists between the g shift and the susceptibility of the metal (Peter et al., 1962). This was clearly demonstrated in the intermetallic compound UPd_3, with 1 mole percent Gd in the U site (Shaltiel et al., 1964) where the g shift of Gd was found to be a linear function of the susceptibility (the temperature being the implicit parameter). Experiments on NMR and Knight shift in metals have shown that in many metals the Knight shift is a function (usually linear) of the susceptibility (Clogston and Jaccarino, 1961; Jaccarino, 1964.)

The correlation between the g shift and the Knight shift is due to the fact that both are due to an interaction between a localized magnetic moment and the conduction electrons. Although the nature of the interaction between the conduction electrons and the magnetic impurity or the nuclear magnetic moment is different,

Work done in collaboration with A.C. Gossard and J.H. Wernick, Bell Telephone Labs., Murray Hill, New Jersey.

their effects on various properties have many similarities. Some similarities were already pointed out by Yosida (1956) when he compared his calculations on electron magnetic moments in metals with those of Ruderman and Kittel (1954) on nuclear magnetic moments in metals. It was found that the spatial spin polarization function of conduction electrons around the magnetic moment is the same in both cases.*

II. Theory

The relation between the Knight shift, K, and the g shift, $\Delta g/g$, can be analysed following the method used in NMR (Clogston and Jaccarino 1961). For a d-band metal the susceptibility may be taken, using the rigid band approximation, as the sum of a number of terms,

$$\chi = \chi_s^{spin} + \chi_d^{spin} (T) + \sum_i \chi_i^{orb} + \chi_{dia} . \qquad (1)$$

The first two terms are the Pauli spin susceptibility of the s and d bands. $\sum_i \chi_i^{orb}$ is the sum of the field induced orbital paramagnetism for different elements; χ_{dia} is the diamagnetic susceptibility of the ion cores. Only χ_d^{spin} is appreciably temperature dependent.

The hyperfine field induced by the spin and the orbital currents is proportional to the corresponding susceptibilities.** The resultant Knight shift at the site i is

$$K_i = \alpha H_{(s)i}^{hf} \chi_s^{spin} + \alpha H_{(d)i}^{hf} \chi_d^{spin} + \frac{2}{A} \chi_{(d)i}^{orb} + K_{(dia)i} \qquad (2)$$

where $\alpha = 0.895 \ 10^{-4}$, $H_{(s)i}^{hf}$ and $H_{(d)i}^{hf}$ are the hyperfine fields per unit spin of the s and d bands respectively. A is Avogadro's number and $\langle r_i^{-3} \rangle$ is the average of r^{-3} of the electrons contributing to the orbital paramagnetism. The susceptibilities are per mole.

In the same manner the exchange fields induced by the spin and orbital currents on an electron magnetic impurity are also proportional to the susceptibilities. The resultant g shift is

---

*For a detailed discussion of Ruderman-Kittel theory see R.E. Watson, Chap. 9.
**See A. Narath, Chap. 7.

$$\Delta g/g = \alpha H^{ex}_{(s)i}\chi^{spin}_s + \alpha H^{ex}_{(d)i}\chi^{spin}_d + H^{orb}_i \chi^{orb}_i ,\qquad (3)$$

which is the same expression as in Eq. (2). $H^{ex}_{(s)i}$ and $H^{ex}_{(d)i}$ are the exchange fields per unit spin of the s and d bands respectively. For a scalar exchange interaction of the type $J(S\cdot s)$ between magnetic impurity spin S and the spin s of the conduction electrons, with J the exchange constant, the exchange fields are given by

$$H^{ex}_s = \frac{J^{ex}_s}{g\mu_B} \quad ; \qquad H^{ex}_d = \frac{J^{ex}_d}{g\mu_B} \quad . \qquad (4)$$

The third term in Eq. (3) is due to the magnetic field-induced orbital paramagnetism. Since the magnetic impurity ion has a much wider spatial distribution than the nucleus, the orbital field seen by the impurity ion is smaller than that perceived by the nuclei. We therefore obtain

$$(\Delta g/g)_{orb} < K_{orb} \qquad (5)$$

Equations (2) and (3) show that the Knight shift and the g shift are related via the various susceptibilities of the metal. As each equation has many unknowns, it is possible to evaluate only a few terms through the temperature dependence of the Knight shift or the g shift alone. The combination of both observations enables us to obtain some complementary information and to evaluate additional terms. This combined method is illustrated by the investigation of the system $La_{1-x}Th_xRu_2$ (Shaltiel et al., 1965).

III. Experiment

The properties of the system of intermetallic compounds $La_{1-x}Th_xRu_2$ ($0 < x < 1$) are very interesting. The compounds have the Laves phase structure. Both $LaRu_2$ and $ThRu_2$ are superconductors with superconducting transition temperatures of $4°K$ and $3.5°K$, respectively. The superconducting transition temperature varies strongly with concentration (Shulman et al., 1961). The alloy with equal amounts of La and Th, e.g., $La_{0.5}Th_{0.5}Ru_2$, either has a very low transition temperature or is not a superconductor. Williams and Sherwood (1966) found that the susceptibility, on the other hand, varies only slightly as a function of x at room temperature and has a minimum at x = 0.5. The system is ideal for investigating both K and $\Delta g/g$. The La Knight shift is not affected by quadrupole effects since the La site has cubic symmetry. For EPR measurements, Gd is almost always used as the magnetic impurity since it is readily observed. Gd enters substitutionally into the La site and has a similar electronic environment. The ^{139}La NMR was measured in eleven of these Laves phase compounds as a function of temperature while the ESR of one mole percent of Gd added as impurity in place of La in compounds of the same composition was studied at 20°K.

In LaRu$_2$, χ and K were found to vary with temperature. Figure 1 shows K versus χ with temperature as the implicit parameter. The linear relationship which is evident can be derived from Eqs. (1) and (2) since only χ_d^{spin} and K_d are temperature dependent.

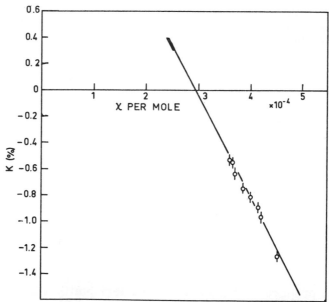

Fig. 1: ^{139}La Knight shift (K) versus magnetic susceptibility χ for LaRu$_2$, temperature being the implicit parameter.

From the experimentally observed slope of K versus χ in Fig. 1, $H^{hf}_{(d)La}$ is determined to be -0.83×10^6 gauss. Neither the various contributions to the total susceptibility nor the 6s and orbital hyperfine fields can be determined unambiguously from the NMR data alone.

The ESR of one percent Gd in place of La in $LaRu_2$ was observed at $20°K$. The line width was 1200 gauss and the g-value of 1.84 may be compared to 2.00 for the unshifted Gd. The g shift is -8%, the largest negative shift observed so far in a non-magnetic host. Measurements were made at temperatures above $20°K$ in order to analyze the g shift in a similar way to that shown in Fig. 1. It was found qualitatively that the absolute value of the g shift decreased with the decrease of the susceptibility as expected from Eq. (3). However, the excessive increase of the line width at higher temperatures prevented quantitative measurements of g versus χ. The g value of Gd at $20°K$ in $La_{1-x}Th_xRu_2$ as a function of x is shown in Fig. 2; there is a strong dependence on

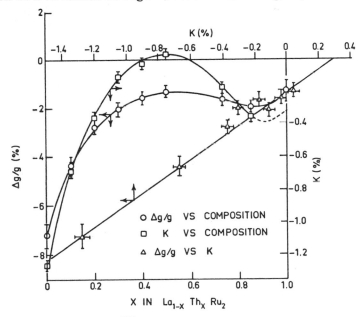

Fig. 2: Upper curves: [139] La Knight shift and g shift of Gd impurities at $20°K$ versus composition.
Lower curve: g shift versus Knight shift.

composition. The [139] La Knight shift measured in similar alloys, without Gd, is also shown in Fig. 2. In the same figure a plot of $\Delta g/g$ against K with x the implicit parameter is also shown. A striking linear relation between $\Delta g/g$ and K is seen.

The large changes of $\Delta g/g$ and K with composition can be shown to be due to the change of the d-band susceptibility by the

following argument. Any shift produced by the field-induced orbital paramagnetism would have to be related by Eq. (5); but Fig. 2
shows that the change in $\Delta g/g$ is nearly five times the change in
K. ESR measurements on various compounds with filled inner
shells indicate that any g shift from 6s electrons would have to be
less than 0.5%, i.e., much smaller than the observed g shifts.
Further, at the extreme point of the K versus x plot in Fig. 2, i.e.
i.e., at $La_{0.5}Th_{0.5}Ru_2$, we find $dK/dT > 0$, indicating a minimum
in the d band density of states for this composition, while for
large negative K, i.e., for small x, $dK/dT < 0$, indicating that the
d band density is high and near a maximum (Shimizu et al., 1963).
Thus the d-band susceptibility and not the s-band or the orbital
induced susceptibility, is the cause of the large shifts observed.
Equations (2) and (3) will therefore lead to a linear relation between the g shift and Knight shift, in agreement with the observed
straight line in Fig. 2. The slope of this line is given by

$$\delta\left(\frac{\Delta g/g}{K}\right) = \frac{J_d^{ex}}{H_{(d)La}^{hf}\, g\mu_B} . \tag{6}$$

With the value of $H_{(d)La}^{hf} = -0.83 \times 10^6$ gauss obtained earlier and
the experimental slope, we obtain $J_{Gd} = -0.05$ eV. It has been
found that the exchange constant is negative in almost-filled d-
band alloys. $LaRu_2$ or $ThRu_2$ also have almost-filled d-bands
and the negative g-shifts are in agreement with the empirical rule.
Further, it is found experimentally that J_{Gd} has a large spread of
values, both in magnitude and sign. For instance, the values of
J_{Gd} in Pd and UPd_3 are -0.01 eV and +0.002 eV, respectively,
compared with -0.05 eV obtained here. The large spread of the
observed values of J_{Gd} results from the various contributions,
both positive and negative, arising from the interaction of Gd
with the conduction band (Koide and Peter, 1964). Implicit in the
linear relationship between $\Delta g/g$ and K is the inference that J_{Gd}
does not change appreciably with composition, indicating that the
d-electron wave function does not change appreciably with composition.

The intercept of the plot of $\Delta g/g$ versus K (Fig. 2) with the
K axis yields the relative distribution of the orbital paramagnetism between the La and the Ru sites. At $\Delta g/g = 0$, K = 0.3%. As
$(\Delta g/g)_s^{spin}$ is not larger than 0.5% and as $(\Delta g/g)_{orb} < K_{orb}$
(Eq. (5)), we obtain $0.3\% < (K_{orb} + K_{spin}) < 0.4\%$. Thus in
Fig. 1, a point in the segment between K = +0.3% and K = +0.4%
corresponds to zero d-band spin susceptibility. From Eq. (1) we

obtain, using calculated values of H_{6s}^{hf} and $\langle r^{-3} \rangle_{\text{La 5d}}$, an upper limit of 0.07×10^{-4} emu/mole for χ_{6s}^{spin} corresponding to 0.4 of a free 6s electron at the La site, and an upper limit of 0.7×10^{-4} emu/mole for $\chi_{\text{La 5d}}^{orb}$. We thus conclude that the orbital paramagnetism in LaRu_2 resides primarily at the Ru sites: 1.8 emu/mole $< \chi_{Ru}^{orb} < 2.4$ emu/mole, which is about 50% of the total susceptibility. The contribution to the orbital susceptibility comes from all the electrons in the d-band and not only from those at the Fermi surface. It is therefore expected that the χ_{Ru}^{orb} will not vary rapidly as a function of band population. In analyzing the total susceptibility as a function of concentration we expect that a large contribution should arise from χ_{Ru}^{orb} and that the χ_d^{spin} contribution should be concentration dependent. The sum of all contributions should produce a susceptibility at room temperature which varies slowly with concentration and has a minimum at $x = 0.5$, in agreement with measurements of Sherwood and Williams (1966).

In conclusion it is seen that the relation between the g shift and the Knight shift can be used to evaluate some properties of the metal with the rigid band model in addition to those properties obtained from independent measurements of the g shift and the Knight shift.

Acknowledgement

The author wishes to thank H. J. Williams and R. C. Sherwood for their private communication.

References

Clogston, A. M. and Jaccarino, V. (1961). Phys. Rev. 121, 1357.

Jaccarino, V. (1964). Proceedings of the International Conference on Magnetism, Nottingham, England, p. 377.

Koide, S. and Peter, M. (1964). Rev. Mod. Phys. 36, 160.

Peter, M., Shaltiel, D., Wernick. J. H., Williams, H. J., Sherwood, R. C. and Mock, J. B. (1962). Phys. Rev. 126, 1395.

Ruderman, M. A. and Kittel, C. (1954). Phys. Rev. 96, 99.

Shaltiel, D., Peter, M., Wernick, J. H. and Williams, H. J. (1964). Phys. Rev. 135, A1346.

Shaltiel, D., Gossard, A. C. and Wernick, H. J. (1965). Phys. Rev. 137, 1027.

Shimizu, M., Takahashi, T., and Katsuki, A. (1963). J. Phys. Soc. Japan 18, 1142.

Shulman, R. G., Wyluda, B. G. and Mathias, B. T. (1961). Bull. Am. Phys. Soc. 6, 103.

Williams, H. J. and Sherwood, R. C. (1966). private communication.

S.12. ELECTRIC FIELD PERTURBATIONS OF HYPERFINE INTERACTIONS

Jonathan F. Reichert

Department of Physics and
Condensed State Center
Western Reserve University
Cleveland, Ohio

I. Introduction

Since we are concerned with understanding all types of hyperfine interactions from both the theoretical and experimental point of view, it would seem appropriate to discuss methods of producing external perturbations of these hyperfine interactions. External electric fields were once thought to produce far too small an effect to measure by either electron spin resonance or nuclear resonance, and indeed early experiments seemed to confirm this conjecture. However, after Bloembergen pointed out the necessary conditions for the existence of a first order or linear Stark shift, many experiments were done which clearly showed the effect. Electric field perturbations of nuclear quadrupole interactions, nuclear magnetic hyperfine interactions in NMR and hyperfine interactions in antiferromagnetic materials, g shifts and crystal field shifts in electron spin resonance all have been observed (Bloembergen, 1962). Electric field effects have been observed in free atom configurations by atomic beam methods as discussed above by Sandars. * This paper will be concerned only with the effects in solids as measured by spin resonance.

---

* See Chap. 4.

II. Conditions for the Occurrence of Linear Electric Field Effects

The question arises as to why such effects were first observed in 1961 when magnetic resonance was discovered in 1945, a span of some 16 years! The answer lies in the peculiar nature of the electric field operator, $\mathcal{H}_E = e\mathbf{E} \cdot \mathbf{r}$ (where e is the electronic charge, $\mathbf{E}$ is the electric field and $\mathbf{r}$ is the electronic radial position vector) which is of odd parity upon inversion of coordinates. Consider the Hamiltonian $\mathcal{H}_0$ of a spin system in a magnetic field with no electric field applied. The energy levels of the system are given by:

$$\mathcal{H}_0 \, \psi_m = \varepsilon_0 \, \psi_m \quad \text{and} \quad \varepsilon_0 = \langle \psi_m | \mathcal{H}_0 | \psi_m \rangle \; . \tag{1}$$

If an external uniform electric field is applied to the system, one can write the new perturbed wave function as:

$$\psi_m^E = \psi_m + \sum_{i \neq m} \frac{\langle \psi_i | \mathcal{H}_E | \psi_m \rangle}{E_m - E_i} \, \psi_i + \text{higher order terms,} \tag{2}$$

considering only the first order corrections. Note here that the electric field admixes the excited state wavefunctions ψ_i into the ground state. Using these new wave functions one can calculate the change in the energy of the system due to this imposed electric field

$$\Delta \varepsilon_E = \langle \psi_m^E | \mathcal{H}_0 | \psi_m^E \rangle - \langle \psi_m | \mathcal{H}_0 | \psi_m \rangle$$

or

$$= \sum_{i \neq m} \frac{\langle \psi_i | \mathcal{H}_E | \psi_m \rangle \langle \psi_i | \mathcal{H}_0 | \psi_m \rangle}{E_m - E_i} + \text{complex conj.}$$

$$+ \sum_{\substack{i \neq m \\ k \neq m}} \frac{\langle \psi_i | \mathcal{H}_E | \psi_m \rangle \langle \psi_i | \mathcal{H}_0 | \psi_k \rangle \langle \psi_k | \mathcal{H}_E | \psi_m \rangle}{(E_m - E_i)^2} \; . \tag{3}$$

The last term in Eq. (3) is quadratic in the electric field perturbation and is in general far too small to observe in condensed materials with their inherent linewidth. In a few cases, where the excited states are low lying (and the energy denominator $(E_m - E_i)$ is small), heroic experiments have observed this effect. The first term (and its complex conjugate) represent a linear electric field perturbation. The question is, under what conditions is this term non-zero?

Consider for a moment the case when $\mathcal{H}_o$ is the Fermi contact hyperfine interaction between nuclear spin $\mathbf{I}$ and electron spin $\mathbf{S}$. This interaction is written*

$$\mathcal{H}_{contact} = \left(\frac{8\pi}{3}\right) g_e g_n \beta_e \beta_n \, \delta(\mathbf{r}_e - \mathbf{r}_n)\mathbf{I} \cdot \mathbf{S} \qquad (4)$$

and is an operator of *even parity* under inversion of the electronic coordinates about the nucleus. However $\mathcal{H}_E$ is of *odd parity* under the same inversion. Thus one might expect expression (3) to vanish, since one of the two matrix elements in this bilinear product will be zero if the ground and excited state have *definite* parity. Indeed it does! The linear electric field effects do not vanish if and *only* if the wave functions of ground state ψ_m or the excited state ψ_i have *mixed* parity. If the nucleus resides in the crystal at a site which *lacks inversion symmetry*, by Neumann's principle (Nye, 1960) the wave function must be of mixed parity. One may generalize this conclusion to include all types of interactions present in the spin Hamiltonian. Any "probe" which allows the measurement of some physical property of a region in a condensed medium (such as a paramagnetic ion or magnetic nucleus) and which is located at a site which lacks inversion symmetry, may have its physical properties depend linearly on an applied uniform electric field. Note carefully that the symmetry upon inversion that is pertinent here, is that of the "probe" site, *not* that of the crystal as a whole. The entire crystal may indeed have a center of inversion and the nucleus (or paramagnetic ion or defect) may have local symmetry which lacks inversion symmetry. It is important not to confuse these electric field effects with piezoelectric induced strains.

III. Electric Field Perturbations of Transferred Hyperfine Interactions

Electric field perturbations of the ligand or transfer hyperfine interactions will be the focus of the remaining part of this discussion. Ligand hyperfine interactions have been measured to a high precision for a number of paramagnetic impurities by the technique of electron nuclear double resonance or ENDOR.** With

*See B. Bleaney, Chap. 1.
**See Geschwind, Chap. 6.

this technique, one can measure not only the various hyperfine interactions of the paramagnetic electrons with their parent nuclei but also the ligand hyperfine interaction (including isotropic and anisotropic magnetic and electric quadrupole interactions) with the first, second, third, etc. nearest neighbors. Such measurements have yielded detailed "road maps" of the electronic ground state wave functions. The motivation for electric field shift measurements of ENDOR spectroscopy is that they might yield the same type of detailed information about the excited-state wave functions as is presently available for the ground state. Reference to Eq. (3) shows that the linear electric field shift involves calculations of the bilinear products of matrix elements of the ground and excited states. Knowing the ground state wave functions, and the energy splitting between the ground and excited states from optical spectroscopy, the hope is to use the electric field shifts to verify the theoretical expressions for the excited states of various electronic configurations. Thus a theoretical analysis of the electric field ENDOR data should give valuable and otherwise inaccessible information about excited states.

IV. Experiment

So far only one electric field ENDOR experiment has been carried out and that in the F-centers in KCl (Reichert and Pershan, 1966). Figure 1 shows the local environment of the F-center (a trapped electron in a chlorine vacancy). Standard ENDOR experiments have been able to measure the electron nuclear hyperfine interaction out to the fourth nearest neighbor (Holton and Blum, 1962). The ENDOR spectrum is accurately represented by the spin Hamiltonian

$$\mathcal{H}_{spin} = g\beta H_o S_z - \beta_n H_o \sum_\alpha g_m^\alpha I_z^\alpha + \mathbf{S} \cdot \sum_\alpha \mathbf{A}^\alpha \cdot \mathbf{I}^\alpha$$

$$+ \sum_\alpha Q'^\alpha \left[(I_z^\alpha)^2 - \frac{I^\alpha (I^\alpha + 1)}{3} \right] \tag{5}$$

where for the α nucleus

$$(A^\alpha)_{ij} = a^\alpha \delta_{ij} + (B^\alpha)_{ij} . \tag{6}$$

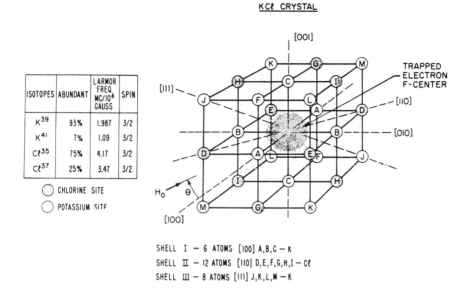

KCl CRYSTAL

ISOTOPES	ABUNDANT	LARMOR FREQ. MC/10⁴ GAUSS	SPIN
K^{39}	93%	1.987	3/2
K^{41}	7%	1.09	3/2
Cl^{35}	75%	4.17	3/2
Cl^{37}	25%	3.47	3/2

◎ CHLORINE SITE
○ POTASSIUM SITE

SHELL I — 6 ATOMS [100] A,B,C — K
SHELL II — 12 ATOMS [110] D,E,F,G,H,I — Cl
SHELL III — 8 ATOMS [111] J,K,L,M — K

Fig. 1: Schematic representation of an F-center in a KCl lattice.

A casual study of the F-center symmetry might lead one to believe that no linear electric field effect could be observed, since the electron resides at a site which clearly has inversion symmetry. Indeed no electric field effects were observed in the electron spin resonance signal, but ENDOR is *not* electron spin resonance. It is *nuclear resonance* using what Prof. Abragam calls "trigger detection." Here the ESR plays the role of the trigger detector for the nuclear resonance of those nuclei which are near the electron. It is quite clear that these nuclei are at sites which lack inversion symmetry, having the trapped electron in the vacancy on one side and the normal ionic configuration on the other. The quadrupole interaction splits the K^{39} ($I = 3/2$) line into three components, two of which are shown in Fig. 2. One notes that the ENDOR transitions, even in the case of zero electric field, have resolved a "super-hyperfine" structure. This structure comes about because of the electron-coupled nuclear-nuclear interaction between equivalent pairs of nuclei on opposite sides of the electron. It is in fact this very interaction, which is destroyed by the applied electric field (removing the symmetry about the F-center), which one observed in these experiments. Physically one can think of the electric field as shifting the electronic cloud

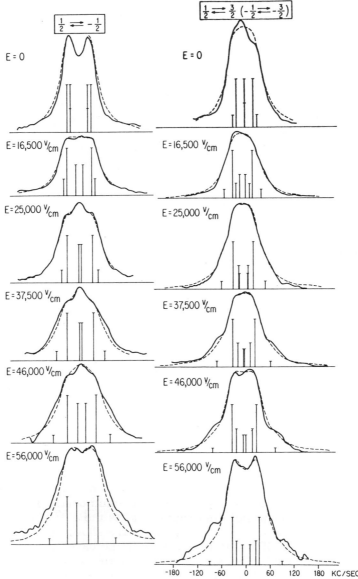

Fig. 2:   The experimental curves of the ENDOR spectrum of F-
centers in KCl with an applied uniform dc electric field.
The bars represent the theoretical line spectrum and the
dashed curves represent a theoretical simulation of the
lines using an assumed linewidth and shape.

in the direction of the electric field. One would then expect a simple splitting of the ENDOR line (one nucleus seeing a larger hyperfine interaction than the other), but the super-hyperfine interaction makes the picture more complicated.

The only electric field shifts observed were for the four nearest neighbor K^{39}, whose hyperfine interaction constants are $A_{zz}/h = 20.6$ kHZ and $Q'/h = 0.2$ kHZ.

Using the approximate wavefunctions derived from LCAO by Gourary and Adrian (1960), the electric field perturbations of the isotropic part of the magnetic hyperfine interaction of the F-center electron with the nearest neighbor potassium nuclei have been calculated. The values of dA_{zz}/dE for several alkali halide F-centers (LiF, NaF, LiCl, NaCl) have been estimated. For KCl, $dA_{zz}/dE = 0.88 + 0.05$ HZ $(V/cm)^{-1}$ was measured and 0.89 HZ $(V/cm)^{-1}$ was theoretically estimated. However this agreement is at present considered accidental, since the theoretical model of four K^{39} ions surrounding a vacancy with a trapped electron completely neglects second neighbor ionic displacement due to the applied electric field. A systematic study is underway at present to measure electric field perturbations in various materials. Hopefully second and possibly even further nearest neighbor interactions will be detected. Such studies may shed some light on the nature of the excited states of F-centers as well as other paramagnetic centers.

References

For a general review article on electric field effects see N. Bloembergen (1962). in Proceedings of the Eleventh Colloque Ampere, edited by J. Smidt, (North-Holland Publishing Co., Amsterdam, 1963), p. 39.

Gourary, B. S. and Adrian, F. J. (1960). Solid State Physics, Vol. 10, edited by Seitz and Turnbull, (Academic Press, New York).

Holton, W. C. and Blum, H. (1962). Phys. Rev. 125, 89.

Reichert, J. F. and Pershan, P. S. (1965). Phys. Rev. Letters 15, 780.

SUBJECT INDEX

Adiabatic demagnetization, 613
  cryostat, 476
Admixture coefficients, 396
Angular correlations (see Perturbations
  of angular correlations)
  density matrix in, 568-570
  theory of, 557ff
Angular distributions of γ-rays
  after Coulomb excitation, 560-561,
    616, 640
  after nuclear reactions, 615
  from oriented nuclei, 561, 660-663
  in angular correlations (see Angular
    correlations)
  in recoilless nuclear resonance,
    513, 698
  in resonance scattering, 559, 589
Atomic beams
  "flop in" apparatus, 116
  isotropic shift measurement, 120
  light source, 175
  standard experiments, 117
  triple resonance, 118
Attenuation coefficients (see Perturbation of angular correlations)

Bethe-Goldstone Equations, 104, 108
Bleaney-Koster Terms
  CO^{2+} in tetrahedral coordination, 252
  HSI^2 term, 257
  independent parameters in I^2S^2,
    255-257
  in spin-Hamiltonian higher order,
    251-257
  IS^3 term, 251-253
  magnetic I^2S^2 term, 253
  quadrupole I^2S^2 term, 255-257
  s-state ions, 253-257
Bloch equations, 295, 374-376, 390

Central field approximation, 134
  deviations, 135
Charge density, 82ff, 513, 414ff, 713
Coherence, 371, 385
  factor δ, 385-386
Comparison of methods, 227, 478,
  547-549, 589, 597-598

Conduction electrons
  interactions, 91, 334ff, 389ff, 421-422,
    445-447, 480
  screening, 713
  spin polarization, 584, 720, 730-733
Configuration interaction, 10-12, 60,
  101-106, 136
Contact interaction, 5, 9-12, 298, 348,
  470-479, 481-484, 545-547
Core polarization, 11-12, 59-60, 169, 348,
  480, 545-547
  in 3d atoms, 64-65
  in 3d ions, 64-68
  in 4d ions, 66-69
  in 4f ions, 69-71, 734
  in atomic phosphorous, 62
  some systematics and $3d^n$ series,
    261, 265-266
Correlation function, 292, 302, 343, 368,
  374, 395
  angular (see Angular correlations)
  time, 292, 369
Coulomb excitation, 579ff, 596-598,
  637-648, 651-658
  and ion implantation, 637-648
Covalency, 65, 81ff, 264
  charge and spin density, 83ff
  electron transfer in EPR, 23-24
Crystal field effects, 22-24, 71ff,
  529-533, 646, 692

Day shift, 389-391, 393
  (see Overhauser shift)
Density matrix, 367, 382, 567-570
  in angular correlations, 568-570
  in nuclear transitions, 567-568
  master equation, 369, 372
Diamagnetic shielding of nucleus, 3-4
Dielectric response theory, 421-422
Diffusion barrier, 398, 402
Doppler effect
  first order, 506, 513
  second order, 513
Dynamic polarization, 376, 378, 380

Effective spin, 24-50

753

MINTZBERG ON MANAGEMENT

MINTZBERG ON MANAGEMENT

*Inside Our Strange
World of Organizations*

Henry Mintzberg

THE FREE PRESS
A Division of Macmillan, Inc.
NEW YORK

Collier Macmillan Publishers
LONDON

104782

The Free Press
A Division of Macmillan, Inc.
866 Third Avenue, New York, N.Y. 10022

Collier Macmillan Canada, Inc.

Printed in the United States of America

printing number

2 3 4 5 6 7 8 9 10

Library of Congress Cataloging-in-Publication Data

Mintzberg, Henry.
   Mintzberg on management: inside our strange world of organizations / Henry Mintzberg.
      p.   cm.
   Bibliography: p.
   Includes index.
   ISBN 0–02–921371–1
   1. Management.   2. Organization.   3. Organizational behavior.
I. Title.
HD31.M4568   1989
658—dc 19   89–1241
                                   CIP

*This book is written for those of us who
spend our public lives dealing with organizations
and our private lives escaping from them.*

*It is dedicated to the memory of Jim Waters,
who spent his career seeking to make those organizations
more humane.*

CONTENTS

Acknowledgment

It is customary here to thank everyone who provided significant help to the book. But since a good part of this book is based on my previous writings, where I already thanked many of those people, I shall not repeat those thank-you's here. They were heartfelt then; they remain so. What I would like to do here, aside from certain special mentions— my colleagues Danny Miller and Frances Westley, who helped my thinking in many ways; Jim Waters, a wonderful friend whose implicit contributions to this book far outweigh the many formally acknowledged in the text and who will be deeply missed; my editor Bob Wallace, who exhibited remarkable tolerance; my support staff Kate Maguire-Devlin and Zinette Khan, who handled my awful scrawl with grace; and my two deans Morty Yalovsky and Wally Crowston, who provided other important kinds of support—is to focus this acknowledgment on one person.

Bill Litwack embodies the word empathy. Not the empathy of the pop psychologist, for he is rude and abrasive, at least to his good friends. But he understands those friends and responds to their needs, not to mention the needs of the books they write.

In 1968, Billy, at the not-so-tender age of twenty, edited my doctoral thesis. It was a harrowing experience. But I learned how to write. In the twenty years since, either I forgot how to write or else his standards went up. I certainly forgot what a harrowing experience it had been. In any event, after our second such experience, I survived, Billy survived, this book survived, and most important, our friendship survived. Billy lived the book for several intense months, getting inside my head and driving me crazy (not so sample comment: "It is hypocrisy to spell 'hypo-cracy' 'hippo-cracy' ") until I turned a portfolio of publications into (what I at least hope is) the book I intended it to be. I thank you for this Bill, but not primarily for this.

The author is supposed to add here, as if anyone doubts it, that despite all the wonderful things everyone else contributed, somehow only he is responsible for what follows. No way. (Billy's not editing this!) I may not have taken his "advice" in some places, may have made some last minute changes he never got to see, but everywhere else Litwack is to blame for any errors or inadequacies that remain in this book. Here's to another twenty years of peace.

Lac Castor
January 1989

OUR WORLD OF ORGANIZATIONS

Ours has become, for better and for worse, a society of organizations. We are born in organizations and are educated in organizations so that we can later work in organizations. At the same time, organizations supply us and entertain us, they govern us and harass us (sometimes concurrently). Finally, we are buried by organizations. Yet aside from a small group of scholars called "organization theorists" who study them, and those managers inclined to look deeply into the subject of their management, few people really understand these strange collective beasts that so influence our daily lives.

If you want to find out about your own psyche, walk into any bookstore and take your pick of dozens of books on how your mind, body, or behavior supposedly works. But if it is your organization you wish to understand, you must instead find a college bookstore and then wade through the dense theory of some academic tome, unless you are willing to settle for a textbook that packages it all very neatly—and probably simplistically.

At least that's what you will find on the management shelves. On those devoted to the older, more traditional disciplines, you will find material that talks around organizations. In economics, the organization takes on the form of a "rational" but otherwise mysterious entity that somehow manages to maximize its profits. I don't know any organizations like that. Psychology teaches us about the behavior of individuals and small groups inside organizations, but not about the behavior of organizations themselves. Political science considers one very important class of organization, government, but more as a legislative or political system than as the network of organizations it significantly is. Sociology and anthropology do consider collective human behavior, but usually in terms of the larger informal society rather than the smaller formal organization.

Organization theory draws on all those disciplines, but it adds something very important, the concept of "organization" itself. Organization to me means collective action in the pursuit of a common mission, a fancy way of saying that a bunch of people have come together under an identifiable label ("General Motors," "Joe's Body Shop") to produce some product or service.

I present this book in the belief that there is a real thirst out there to understand organizations, in society at large no less than among the managers who try to run them (and who often seem as puzzled by their strange behavior as the rest of us). Every time I have discussed organizations with people from diverse backgrounds—including self-employed professionals, homemakers, and others who have *relatively* little contact with them—I have been amazed at the interest in the subject. Someone recounts a bizarre experience in a hospital, another person an incident in an airplane or at an auto dealership. We all need desperately to comprehend these strange beasts that so affect us. The basic conceptual understanding is there; it just has not been readily accessible.

This book presents material on organizations that I have been working on these past twenty years. It contains not just my own ideas, because a certain amount of my work set out to synthesize the work of others, especially that based on systematic research. Over the years, I have considered how managers work; how organizations function, make decisions, develop strategies, and structure themselves; and how power relationships surround and infuse organizations, including how societies try to deal with their organizations.

I present here a series of essays drawing on those parts of my writings that I believe are best suited to a general readership interested in organizations. Some of this material was first published in the more popular business press, while other material received only limited circulation in more obscure academic journals. I have tried to include here, and to render easily readable, that material I believe to be of widest interest. I originally set out to package this material together; I ended up rewriting, or in several cases writing originally, well over half of what appears here. This book is offered, therefore, in the hope of extending the audience for these ideas more deeply inside as well as beyond the management community. Call this "pop org theory" if you like, so long as there is no presumption that I have tried to trivialize the complicated activity of organizations.

I have divided these essays into three sections. The first is on *management,* that process by which the people who are formally in charge of whole organizations or part of them try to direct or at least to guide what they do. The second considers forms of *organizations,* in a way comparable to how biologists consider different species in nature. I believe our greatest mistake in dealing with organizations—one we have made throughout this century and continue to make every day—is in pretending that there is "one best way" to manage every organization. What's good for General Motors is often dead wrong for Joe's Body Shop. We have no more business treating all organizations alike than do doctors in prescribing the same pair of glasses for everyone. The third section looks at *our society of organizations*—how we try to influence them and how they influence us in turn and thereby make our lives happy and miserable.

Read what follows at your leisure; pick and choose, skimming or studying according to your own interests. Whatever you do, think about your own company, your repair shop or supplier of automobiles, the hospital that cured you and the school that made you miserable, the airline you fly, the association that lobbies for the clothing of animals or for the promotion of popcorn. Organizations supply us and exploit us, they nurture us and torment us. We can all escape them occasionally, a few of us can even function relatively free of them. But most of us must resign ourselves to spending a great deal of our public and private lives dealing with them. We all need to understand them better.

Part I
ON MANAGEMENT

In some sense, the twentieth century might be characterized as the age of management. Certainly the more economically developed world has become enamored with the management process over the course of this century. Henri Fayol, the French industrialist, may have done some of the important early thinking on management, but it was really a stream of writers in America, from Frederick Taylor through Peter Drucker and Herbert Simon, among many others, who created and reinforced the love affair America has had with managers and the management process.

That was why the recent Japanese challenge to American industrial supremacy came as such a shock. Here was a people from a very different culture beating America at its own game, the game of management. But it was not the first time. The West Europeans did it first, if not so dramatically. (Volkswagen embarrassed Detroit's Big Three long before Toyota did.) Not so very long ago, in 1968, Jean-Jacques Serven-Schreiber published *The American Challenge*, about how the key to America's economic success lay not in its resources or technologies, but in its attention to the management process itself.[1] Well, America's friends learned that lesson so well that *the European challenge* and later *the Japanese challenge* have been published many times over, if not by those titles.

There has been no such communist challenge. But management has certainly emerged as a critical process in Eastern Europe as well. Indeed, promises of the withering of the state notwithstanding, there is no way to run a communist society without heavy reliance on the management process. In this regard, America and the Soviet Union differ not in their obsession with management but simply in where they tend to locate their most influential managers. Everywhere we look then, where there is economic development there is attention to the management process.

Of course, there is more to organizations than management. Likewise, there is more to economic development than attention to management. Indeed, it can be argued (as I shall in Part III) that the traditional approach to management may now be impeding rather than fostering economic development. But no consideration of organizations is complete without careful attention to the management process. And so we begin our discussion with such attention, at least to management as it really seems to be practiced, not how the traditional literature keeps telling managers how to practice it.

We begin at what I believe should be the beginning: with the nature of managerial work, what those people called "manager" or something equivalent actually do at the office all day long. You may be surprised by what you read—well, not surprised in terms of your own experiences so much as in the light of what decades of literature have made people believe managers are *supposed* to do. This first article will make clear the discrepancy, very common and costly in organizations, between what really does go on and some vague and often misguided ideas of what *should* go on.

Our second article continues in the same vein, but on a different aspect of management. It considers the process of developing strategy. But again, in contrast to the traditional perception of a process of planning, here it is characterized as one of *craft,* which has all kinds of implications for managers and for organizations.

Both articles suggest something else is happening in management, something besides the highly analytical and "rational" processes so long favored. Our third article tries to get at this, drawing on research into the two hemispheres of the human brain to suggest that, in our race to throw the light of analysis on management, we may have lost sight of that darker but no less important process called intuition. The essay that follows, prepared for this book from several sources, probes more deeply into this issue, first considering the fundamental debate between analysis and intuition, then proposing ways in which the two can be coupled to manage complex organizations.

A final essay of this section on management, written especially for this book, takes up a major consequence of this debate, the inclination of our business schools to train MBAs, not managers. I imply here, and argue more fully in the final essay of this book, that this has had serious effects on our organizations, undermining their social as well as their economic effectiveness.

1
THE MANAGER'S JOB
Folklore and Fact

When we think of *organization,* we think of *management.* Of course, there is a great deal more to organizations than managers and the management systems they create. But what distinguishes the formal organization from a random collection of people—a mob, an informal group—is the presence of some system of authority and administration, personified by one manager or several in a hierarchy to knit the whole effort together.

That being the case, and given the love affair the American people in particular have had with the manager for more than a century, from Horatio Alger to Lee Iacocca, it is surprising how little study there has been of what managers actually do. Like thousands of other students at the time, I took an MBA, a degree ostensibly designed to train managers, without questioning the fact that no one ever discussed in a serious way what managers really did. Imagine a program in medicine without ever a comment on the work of the doctor.

There has certainly been no shortage of material on what managers *should* do (for example, follow a whole set of simple prescriptions called "time management" or use computers in the ways recommended by detached technical specialists). Unfortunately, in the absence of any real understanding of managerial work, much of this advice has proved false and wasteful. How can anyone possibly prescribe change in a phenomenon so complex as managerial work without first having a deep comprehension of it?

In the mid-1960s, James Webb, who ran NASA, wanted to be studied. NASA felt the need to justify its existence by spinning off practical applications of its innovations, and Webb counted its management processes among those innovations. Webb raised the idea with a professor of mine at the MIT Sloan School of Management, and since I was the only doctoral student then studying *management* there (as opposed to computer systems or mathematical models or motivating people, etc.), he approached me to study Webb as my doctoral thesis. I declined what seemed to be a crazy idea. This was MIT, after all, the bastion of science. Sitting in a manager's office and writing down what he did all day just didn't seem quite right. (Another professor had told me earlier that what an MIT doctoral thesis had to be above all was "elegant." He was not referring to the results.) In any event, I was going to do a thesis on how to develop a comprehensive strategic planning process for organizations. Luckily, and not for the last time in my life, forces outside of me saved me from myself.

The planning thesis didn't work out, for want of an organization willing to subject itself to such an exercise (or for want of my trying very hard to find one). Then I attended a conference at MIT to which a number of impressive people came to discuss the impact that the computer would have on the manager. They went nowhere; for two days they talked in circles, hardly getting beyond the contention that the managers' use of the computer should have something to do with the fact that their work was "unprogrammed" (whatever that was supposed to mean). It struck me that these people lacked a framework to enable them to understand managerial work. They certainly didn't lack an innate knowledge of the process—they all worked with managers, and a number were managers themselves. What they lacked was a *conceptual* basis to consider the issue.

I learned two things at that conference. The first was that knowing explicitly was different from knowing implicitly, and both had great relevance for running organizations. The second was that there was an urgent need for someone to look carefully at what managers really did, that even at a place like MIT, what mattered in a thesis was not the elegance of the methodology but the relevance of the topic.

And so I did my first research on "the nature of managerial work" (the title of the book that resulted from the thesis). But not with James Webb, who was no longer available. Using a stopwatch (much as Frederick Taylor had done with factory workers years earlier), I observed in the course of one intensive week the activities of five chief executives: of a major consulting firm, a well-known teaching hospital, a school system, a high-technology firm, and a manufacturer of consumer goods. One week was not a long time, but I was more interested in the pace and nature of the work than in the unfolding of issues over the long term. The dissertation was completed in 1968, the book in 1973; two years later, the *Harvard Business Review* published the article that is reprinted here (with minor changes).

In orientation and tone, as well as in some of its central content, this article really set the pattern for my subsequent work. An article that followed in the *New York Times* (on October 29, 1976)[1] labeled this description of managerial work "calculated chaos" and "controlled disorder." It also used a phrase that I have come to prefer for characterizing much of my writing: "celebrating intuition."

If you ask managers what they do, they will most likely tell you that they plan, organize, coordinate, and control. Then watch what they do. Don't be surprised if you can't relate what you see to those four words.

When they are called and told that one of their factories has just burned down, and they advise the caller to see whether temporary arrangements can be made to supply customers through a foreign subsidiary, is that planning, organizing, coordinating, or controlling? How about when they present a gold watch to a retiring employee? Or when they attend a conference to meet people in the trade? Or on returning from that conference, when they tell one of their employees about an interesting product idea they picked up there?

The fact is that those four words, which have dominated management vocabulary since the French industrialist Henri Fayol first introduced them in 1916, tell us little about what managers actually do. At best, they indicate some vague objectives managers have when they work.

My intention here is simple: to break the reader away from Fayol's words and introduce him or her to a more supportable, and what I believe to be a more useful, description of managerial work. This description is based on my own study of the work of five chief executives, supported by a few others on how various managers spent their time.

In some studies, managers were observed intensively ("shadowed" is the term some of them used); in a number of others, they kept detailed diaries of their activities; in a few studies, their records were analyzed. Various kinds of managers were studied—foremen, factory supervisors, staff managers, field sales managers, hospital administrators, presidents of companies and nations, and even street gang leaders. These "managers" worked in the United States, Canada, Sweden, and Great Britain.

A synthesis of these findings paints an interesting picture, one as different from Fayol's classical view as a cubist abstract is from a Renaissance painting. In a sense, this picture will be obvious to anyone who has ever spent a day in a manager's office, either in front of the desk or behind it. Yet at the same time, this picture may turn out to be revolutionary, in that it throws into doubt so much of the folklore that we have accepted about the manager's work.

I first discuss some of this folklore and contrast it with some of the findings of systematic research—the hard facts about how managers spend their time. Then I synthesize those research findings in a description of ten roles that seem to describe the essential content of all managers' jobs. In a concluding section, I discuss a number of implications of this synthesis for those trying to achieve more effective management.

SOME FOLKLORE AND FACTS ABOUT MANAGERIAL WORK

There are four myths about the manager's job that do not bear up under careful scrutiny of the facts.

1. Folklore: The manager is a reflective, systematic planner. The evidence on the issue is overwhelming, but not a shred of it supports this statement.

Fact: Study after study has shown that managers work at an unrelenting pace, that their activities are characterized by brevity, variety, and discontinuity, and that they are strongly oriented to action and dislike reflective activities. Consider this evidence:

• Half the activities engaged in by the five chief executives of my study lasted less than nine minutes, and only 10 percent exceeded one hour.[2] A study of fifty-six U.S. foremen found that they averaged 583 activities per eight-hour shift, one every forty-eight seconds.[3] The work pace for both chief executives and foremen was unrelenting. The chief executives met a steady stream of callers and mail from the moment they arrived in the morning until they left in the evening. Coffee breaks and lunches were inevitably work-related, and ever present subordinates seemed to usurp any free moment.

• A diary study of 160 British middle and top managers found that they worked for a half-hour or more without interruption only about once every two days.[4]

• Of the verbal contacts of the chief executives in my study, 93 percent were arranged on an *ad hoc* basis. Only 1 percent of the executives' time was spent in open-ended observational tours. Only 1 out of 368 verbal contacts was unrelated to a specific issue and could be called general planning.

• No study has found important patterns in the way managers schedule their time. They seem to jump from issue to issue, continually responding to the needs of the moment.

Is this the planner of the classical literature? Hardly. How, then, can we explain this behavior? The manager is simply responding to the pressures of his or her job. I found that my chief executives terminated many of their own activities, often leaving meetings before the end, and interrupted their desk work to call in subordinates. One president not only placed his desk so that he could look down a long hallway but also left his door open when he was alone—an invitation for subordinates to come in and interrupt him.

Clearly, these managers wanted to encourage the flow of current information. But more significantly, they seemed to be conditioned by their own work loads. They appreciated the opportunity cost of their own time, and they were continually aware of their ever present obligations—mail to be answered, callers to attend to, and so on. It seems that no matter what they are doing, managers are plagued by the possibilities of what they might do and what they must do.

When the manager must plan, he or she seems to do so implicitly in the context of daily actions, not in some abstract process reserved for two weeks at the organization's mountain retreat. The plans of the chief executives I studied seemed to exist only in their heads—as flexible, but often specific, intentions. The traditional literature notwithstanding, the job of managing does not breed reflective planners; the manager is a real-time responder to stimuli, an individual who is conditioned by his or her job to prefer live to delayed action.

2. Folklore: The effective manager has no regular duties to perform. Managers are constantly being told to spend more time planning and delegating, and less time seeing customers and engaging in negotiations. Those are not, after all, the true tasks of the manager. To use the popular analogy, the good manager, like the good conductor, carefully orchestrates everything in advance, then sits back to enjoy the fruits of his or her labor, responding occasionally to an unforeseeable exception.

But here again the pleasant abstraction just does not seem to hold up.

Fact: In addition to handling exceptions, managerial work involves performing a number of regular duties, including ritual and ceremony, negotiations, and processing of soft information that links the organization with its environment. Consider some evidence from the research studies:
   • A study of the work of the presidents of small companies found that they engaged in routine activities because their companies could

not afford staff specialists and were so thin on operating personnel that a single absence often required the president to substitute.[5]

• One study of field sales managers and another of chief executives suggest that it is a natural part of both jobs to see important customers, assuming the managers wish to keep those customers.[6]

• Someone, only half in jest, once described the manager as that person who sees the visitors so that everyone else can get on with his or her work. In my study, I found that certain ceremonial duties—meeting visiting dignitaries, giving out gold watches, presiding at special dinners—were an intrinsic part of the chief executive's job.

• Studies of managers' information flow suggest that managers play a key role in securing "soft" external information (much of it available only to them because of their status) and in passing it along to their subordinates.

3. Folklore: The senior manager needs aggregated information, which a formal management information system best provides. In keeping with the classical view of the manager as that individual perched on the apex of a regulated, hierarchical system, the literature's manager is to receive all important information from a giant, comprehensive MIS. But a look at how managers actually process information reveals a very different picture. Managers have five media at their command—documents, telephone calls, scheduled and unscheduled meetings, and observational tours.

Fact: Managers strongly favor the oral media—namely, telephone calls and meetings. The evidence comes from every single study of managerial work. Consider the following:

• In two British studies, managers spent an average of 66 and 80 percent of their time in oral communication.[7] In my study of five American chief executives, the figure was 78 percent.

• These five chief executives treated mail processing as a burden to be dispensed with. One came in Saturday morning to process 142 pieces of mail in just over three hours, to "get rid of all the stuff." This same manager looked at the first piece of "hard" mail he had received all week, a standard cost report, and put it aside with the comment, "I never look at this."

• These same five chief executives responded immediately to just two of the forty routine reports they received during the five weeks of my study and to four items in the 104 periodicals. They skimmed most of these periodicals in seconds, almost ritualistically. In all, these chief executives of good-size organizations initiated on their own—that is, not in response to something else—a grand total of twenty-five pieces of mail during the twenty-five days I observed them.

An analysis of the mail the executives received reveals an interesting picture: Only 13 percent was of specific and immediate use. So now we have another piece in the puzzle. Not much of the mail provides live, current information—the action of a competitor, the mood of a government legislator, the rating of last night's television show. Yet this is the information that drove the managers, interrupting their meetings and rescheduling their workdays.

Consider another interesting finding. Managers seem to cherish "soft" information, especially gossip, hearsay, and speculation. Why? The reason is its timeliness; today's gossip may be tomorrow's fact. The manager who is not accessible for the telephone call informing him that his biggest customer was seen golfing with his main competitor may read about a dramatic drop in sales in the next quarterly report. But then it's too late.

Consider the words of Richard Neustadt who studied the information-collecting habits of three U.S. Presidents:

> It is not information of a general sort that helps a President see personal stakes; not summaries, not surveys, not the *bland amalgams.* Rather . . .
> it is the odds and ends of *tangible detail* that pieced together in his mind illuminate the underside of issues put before him. To help himself, he must reach out as widely as he can for every scrap of fact, opinion, gossip, bearing on his interests and relationships as President. He must become his own director of his own central intelligence.[8]

The manager's emphasis on the oral media raises two important points:

First, oral information is stored in the brains of people. Only when people write this information down can it be stored in the files of the organization—whether in metal cabinets or on magnetic tape—and managers apparently do not write down much of what they hear. Thus the strategic data bank of the organization is not in the memory of its computers so much as in the minds of its managers.

Second, the managers' extensive use of oral media helps to explain why they are reluctant to delegate tasks. When we note that most of the managers' important information comes in oral form and is stored in their heads, we can well appreciate their reluctance. It is not as if they can hand a dossier over to someone; they must take the time to "dump memory"—to tell that someone all they know about the subject. But this could take so long that the managers may find it easier to do the task themselves. Thus the manager is damned by his or her own information system to a "dilemma of delegation"—to do too much him or herself or to delegate to subordinates with inadequate briefing.

4. Folklore: Management is, or at least is quickly becoming, a science and a profession. By almost any definitions of *science* and *profession*, this statement is false. Brief observation of any manager will quickly lay to rest the notion that managers practice a science. A science involves the enaction of systematic, analytically determined procedures or programs. If we do not even know what procedures managers use, how can we prescribe them by scientific analysis? And how can we call management a profession if we cannot specify what managers are to learn?

Fact: The managers' programs—to schedule time, process information, make decisions, and so on—remain locked deep inside their brains. Thus, to describe those programs, we rely on words like *judgment* and *intuition*, seldom stopping to realize that they are merely labels for our ignorance.

I was struck during my study by the fact that the executives I observed—all very competent by any standard—were fundamentally indistinguishable from their counterparts of a hundred years ago. The information they needed differed, but they sought it in the same way—by word of mouth. Their decisions concerned modern technology, but the procedures they used to make them were the same as the procedures of the nineteenth-century manager. Even the computer, so important for the specialized work of the organization, had apparently had no influence on the work procedures of general managers. In fact, the manager is in a kind of loop, with increasingly heavy work pressures but no aid forthcoming from management science.

Considering the facts about managerial work, we can see that the manager's job is enormously complicated and difficult. The manager is overburdened with obligations; yet he or she cannot easily delegate his or her tasks. As a result, he or she is driven to overwork and is forced to do many tasks superficially. Brevity, fragmentation, and oral communication characterize the work. Yet these are the very characteristics of managerial work that have impeded scientific attempts to improve it. As a result, management scientists have concentrated their efforts on the specialized functions of the organization, where they could more easily analyze the procedures and quantify the relevant information. Thus the first step in providing the manager with some help is to find out what his or her job really is.

BACK TO A BASIC DESCRIPTION OF MANAGERIAL WORK

Let us try to put some of the pieces of this puzzle together. The manager can be defined as that person in charge of an organization or one of its subunits. Besides chief executive officers, this definition would include vice presidents, bishops, foremen, hockey coaches, and prime ministers. Can all of these people have anything in common? Indeed they can. For an important starting point, all are vested with formal authority over an organizational unit. From formal authority comes status, which leads to various interpersonal relations, and from these comes access to information. Information, in turn, enables the manager to make decisions and strategies for his or her unit.

The manager's job can be described in terms of various "roles," or organized sets of behaviors identified with a position. My description, shown in Figure 1–1, comprises ten roles.

INTERPERSONAL ROLES

Three of the manager's roles arise directly from formal authority and involve basic interpersonal relationships.

1. First is the *figurehead* role. By virtue of his or her position as head of an organizational unit, every manager must perform some duties of a ceremonial nature. The president greets the touring dignitaries, the foreman attends the wedding of a lathe operator, and the sales manager takes an important customer to lunch.

The chief executives of my study spent 12 percent of their contact time on ceremonial duties; 17 percent of their incoming mail dealt with acknowledgments and requests related to their status. For example, a letter to a company president requested free merchandise for a disabled schoolchild; diplomas were put on the desk of the school superintendent for his signature.

Duties that involve interpersonal roles may sometimes be routine, involving little serious communication and no important decision-making.

FIGURE 1–1
The Manager's Roles

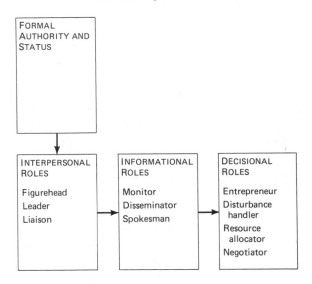

Nevertheless, they are important to the smooth functioning of an organization and cannot be ignored by the manager.

2. Because he or she is in charge of an organizational unit, the manager is responsible for the work of the people of that unit. His or her actions in this regard constitute the *leader* role. Some of those actions involve leadership directly—for example, in most organizations the manager is normally responsible for hiring and training his or her own staff. In addition, there is the indirect exercise of the leader role. Every manager must motivate and encourage his or her employees, somehow reconciling their individual needs with the goals of the organization. In virtually every contact the manager has with those employees, subordinates seeking leadership clues probe his or her actions: "Does he approve?" "How would she like the report to turn out?" "Is he more interested in market share than high profits?"

The influence of the manager is most clearly seen in the leader role. Formal authority vests the manager with great potential power; leadership determines in large part how much of it he or she will in fact use.

3. The literature of management has always recognized the leader role, particularly those aspects of it related to motivation. In comparison,

until recently it has hardly mentioned the *liaison* role, in which the manager makes contacts outside his or her vertical chain of command. This is remarkable in light of the finding of virtually every study of managerial work that managers spend as much time with peers and other people outside their units as they do with their own subordinates, and, surprisingly, very little time with their own superiors (generally on the order of 45, 45, and 10 percent respectively).

The contacts the five CEOs of my study made were with an incredibly wide range of people: subordinates; clients, business associates, and suppliers; managers of similar organizations, government and trade organization officials, fellow directors on outside boards; and so on. Robert Guest's study of foremen shows, likewise, that their contacts were numerous and wideranging, seldom involving fewer than twenty-five individuals, and often more than fifty.

As we shall see shortly, the manager cultivates such contacts largely to find information. In effect, the liaison role is devoted to building up the manager's own external information system—informal, private, oral but nevertheless effective.

INFORMATIONAL ROLES

By virtue of interpersonal contacts, both with subordinates and with the network of contacts, the manager emerges as the nerve center of his or her organizational unit. The manager may not know everything, but he or she typically knows more than any one of his or her subordinates.

Studies have shown this to hold for all managers, from street gang leaders to U.S. Presidents. In *The Human Group,* George C. Homans explains how, because they were at the center of the information flow in their own gangs and were also in close touch with other gang leaders, street gang leaders were better informed than any of their followers.[9] And Richard Neustadt describes the following account from his study of Franklin D. Roosevelt:

> The essence of Roosevelt's technique for information-gathering was competition. "He would call you in," one of his aides once told me, "and he'd ask you to get the story on some complicated business, and you'd come back after a couple of days of hard labor and present the juicy morsel you'd uncovered under a stone somewhere, and *then* you'd find out he knew all about it, along with something else you *didn't* know. Where he got this information from he wouldn't mention, usually, but

after he had done this to you once or twice you got damn careful about *your* information.''[10]

We can see where Roosevelt "got this information" when we consider the relationship between the interpersonal and informational roles. As leader, managers have formal and easy access to each of their subordinates. Hence, as noted earlier, they tend to know more about their own units than anyone else does. In addition, their liaison contacts expose the managers to external information to which their subordinates often lack access. Many of those contacts are with other managers of equal status, who are themselves nerve centers in their own organizations. In this way, managers develops powerful data bases of information.

The processing of information is a key part of the manager's job. In my study, the chief executives spent 40 percent of their contact time on activities devoted exclusively to the transmission of information and 70 percent of their incoming mail was purely informational (as opposed to requests for action). The manager does not leave meetings or hang up the telephone in order to get back to work. In large part, communication *is* his or her work. Three roles describe the informational aspects of managerial work.

4. As *monitor,* the manager perpetually scans his or her environment for information, interrogates liaison contacts and subordinates, and receives unsolicited information, much of it as a result of the network of personal contacts he or she has developed. Remember that a good part of the information the manager collects in the monitor role arrives in oral form, often as gossip, hearsay, and speculation. By virtue of contacts, the manager has a natural advantage in collecting this soft information for his or her organization.

5. Managers must share and distribute much of this information. Information they glean from outside personal contacts may be needed within their organizations. In their *disseminator* role, managers pass some of their privileged information directly to their subordinates, who would otherwise have no access to it. Moreover, when their subordinates lack easy contact with one another, managers will sometimes pass information from one to another.

6. In their *spokesman* role, managers send some of their information to people outside their units—a president makes a speech to lobby for an organizational need, or a foreman suggests a product modification to a supplier. In addition, as part of the role of spokesman, every manager

must inform and satisfy the influential people who control his or her organizational unit. Chief executives especially may spend great amounts of time dealing with hosts of influencers. Directors and shareholders must be advised about financial performance, consumer groups must be assured that the organization is fulfilling its social responsibilities, and so on.

DECISIONAL ROLES

Information is not, of course, an end in itself; it is the basic input to decision-making. One thing is clear in the study of managerial work: The manager plays the major role in his or her unit's decision-making system. As its formal authority, only the manager can commit the unit to important new courses of action; and as its nerve center, only the manager has full and current information to make the set of decisions that determines the unit's strategy. Four roles describe the manager as decision-maker.

7. As *entrepreneur,* the manager seeks to improve his or her unit, to adapt it to changing conditions in the environment. In the monitor role, the president is constantly on the lookout for new ideas; when a good one appears, he or she initiates, in the context of the entrepreneur role, a development project that he or she may supervise or else delegate to an employee (perhaps with the stipulation that the manager must approve the final proposal).

There are two interesting features about development projects at the chief executive level. First, these projects do not involve single decisions or even unified clusters of decisions. Rather, they emerge as a series of small decisions and actions sequenced over time. Apparently, chief executives prolong each project so that they can fit it bit by bit into their busy, disjointed schedule and so that they can gradually come to comprehend the issue, if it is a complex one.

Second, the chief executives I studied supervised as many as fifty of these projects at the same time. Some projects entailed new products or processes; others involved public relations campaigns, resolution of a morale problem in a foreign division, integration of computer operations, various acquisitions, and so on. The chief executives appeared to maintain a kind of inventory of the development projects they themselves supervised—projects at various stages of development, some active and some in limbo. Like a juggler, they seemed to keep a number of projects in the air; periodically, one comes down, is given a new burst of energy and is sent back into orbit. At various intervals, they put new projects onstream and discard old ones.

8. While the entrepreneur role describes the manager as the voluntary initiator of change, the *disturbance handler* role shows the manager involuntarily responding to pressures. Here change is beyond the manager's control: A strike looms, a major customer has gone bankrupt, a supplier reneges on a contract.

It has been fashionable, I noted earlier, to compare the manager to an orchestra conductor, as Peter F. Drucker wrote in *The Practice of Management:*

> The manager has the task of creating a true whole that is larger than the sum of its parts, a productive entity that turns out more than the sum of the resources put into it. One analogy is the conductor of a symphony orchestra, through whose effort, vision and leadership individual instrumental parts that are so much noise by themselves become the living whole of music. But the conductor has the composer's score; he is only interpreter. The manager is both composer and conductor. [11]

Now consider the words of Leonard R. Sayles, who carried out systematic research on the manager's job. The manager

> . . . is like a symphony orchestra conductor, endeavouring to maintain a melodious performance in which the contributions of the various instruments are coordinated and sequenced, patterned and paced, while the orchestra members are having various personal difficulties, stage hands are moving music stands, alternating excessive heat and cold are creating audience and instrument problems, and the sponsor of the concert is insisting on irrational changes in the program. [12]

In effect, every manager must spend a good part of time responding to high-pressure disturbances. No organization can be so well run, so standardized, that it has considered every contingency in advance. Disturbances arise not only because poor managers ignore situations until they reach crisis proportions, but also because good managers cannot possibly anticipate all the consequences of the actions they take.

9. The third decisional role is that of *resource allocator.* To the manager falls the responsibility of deciding who will get what in the organizational unit. Perhaps the most important resource the manager allocates is his or her own time. Access to the manager constitutes exposure to the unit's nerve center and decision-maker. The manager is also charged with designing the unit's structure, that pattern of formal

relationships that determines how work is to be divided and coordinated.

Also, in his or her role as resource allocator the manager authorizes the important decisions of the unit before they are implemented. By retaining this power, the manager can ensure that decisions are interrelated—all must pass through a single brain. To fragment this power is to encourage discontinuous decision-making and a disjointed strategy.

I found that the chief executives of my study faced incredibly complex choices. They had to consider the impact of each decision on other decisions and on the organization's strategy. They had to ensure that the decision would be acceptable to those who influenced the organization, as well as ensure that resources would not be overextended. They had to understand the various costs and benefits as well as the feasibility of the proposal. They also had to consider questions of timing. All this was necessary for the simple approval of someone else's proposal. At the same time, however, delay could lose time, while quick approval could be ill considered and quick rejection could discourage a subordinate who had spent months developing a pet project. One common solution in approving projects seems to have been to pick the person instead of the proposal. That is, managers authorize those projects presented to them by people whose judgment they trust. But they cannot always use this simple dodge.

10. The final decisional role is that of *negotiator*. Studies of managerial work at all levels indicate that managers spend considerable time in negotiations: The president of the football team is called in to work out a contract with the holdout superstar; the corporation president leads his or her company's contingent to negotiate a new strike issue; the foreman argues a grievance problem to its conclusion with the shop steward. As Leonard Sayles puts it, negotiations are a "way of life" for the sophisticated manager.

The negotiations are duties of the manager's job; perhaps routine, they are not to be shirked. They are an integral part of the job, for only the manager has the authority to commit organizational resources in "real time," and only he or she has the nerve center information that important negotiations require.

THE INTEGRATED JOB

It should be clear by now that the ten roles I have been describing are not easily separable. They form a *gestalt,* an integrated whole. No role can be pulled out of the framework and the job be left intact. For example, a manager without liaison contacts lacks external information. As a result, he or she can neither disseminate the information subordinates need nor make decisions that adequately reflect external conditions. (In fact, this is a problem for the new person in a managerial position, since he or she cannot make effective decisions until the network of contacts has been built up.)

Herein lies a clue to the problems of team management. Two or three people cannot share a single managerial position unless they can act as one entity. That means they cannot divide up the ten roles unless they can very carefully reintegrate them. The real difficulty lies with the informational roles. Unless there can be full sharing of managerial information—and, as I pointed out earlier, it is primarily oral—team management breaks down. A single managerial job cannot be arbitrarily split, for example, into internal and external roles, for information from both sources must be brought to bear on the same decisions.

To say that the ten roles form a *gestalt* is not to say that all managers give equal attention to each role. In fact, I found in my review of the various research studies that

- Sales managers seem to spend relatively more of their time in the interpersonal roles, presumably a reflection of the extroverted nature of the marketing activity
- Production managers give relatively more attention to the decisional roles, presumably a reflection of their concern with efficient work flow
- Staff managers spend relatively more time in the informational roles, since they are experts who manage departments that advise other parts of the organization

Nevertheless, in all cases the interpersonal, informational, and decisional roles remain inseparable.

TOWARD MORE EFFECTIVE MANAGEMENT

What are the messages for management in this description? I believe, first and foremost, that this description of managerial work should itself prove more important to managers than any prescription they might derive from it. That is to say, *the managers' effectiveness is significantly influenced by their insight into their own work.* Their performance depends on how well they understand and respond to the pressures and dilemmas of the job.

Let us take a look at three specific areas of concern. For the most part, the managerial logjams—the dilemma of delegation, the data base centralized in one brain, and the problems of working with the management scientist—revolve around the oral nature of the manager's information. There are great dangers in centralizing the organization's data bank in the minds of its managers. When they leave, they take their memory with them. And when subordinates are out of convenient oral reach of the manager, they are at an informational disadvantage.

1. The manager is challenged to find systematic ways to share his or her privileged information. A regular debriefing session with key subordinates, a weekly memory dump on the dictating machine, the maintaining of a diary of important information for limited circulation, or other similar methods may ease the logjam of work considerably. Time spent disseminating this information will be more than regained when decisions must be made. Of course, some will raise the question of confidentiality. But managers would do well to weigh the risks of exposing privileged information against having subordinates who can make effective decisions.

If there is a single theme that runs through this description, it is that the pressures of his job drive the manager to be superficial in his or her actions—to overload him- or herself with work, encourage interruption, respond quickly to every stimulus, seek the tangible and avoid the abstract, make decisions in small increments, and do everything abruptly.

2. Here again, the manager is challenged to deal consciously with the pressures of superficiality by giving serious attention to the issues that require it, by stepping back from tangible bits of information in order to see a broad picture, and by making use of analytical inputs. Although effective managers have to be adept at responding quickly to numerous and varying problems, the danger in managerial work is that they will respond to every issue equally (and that means abruptly) and that they will never work the tangible bits and pieces of informational input into a comprehensive picture of their world.

In dealing with complex issues, the senior manager has much to gain from a close relationship with the management scientists of his or her own organization. They have something important that he lacks—time to probe complex issues. An effective working relationship hinges on the resolution of what a colleague and I have called "the planning dilemma."[13] Managers have the information and the authority; analysts have the time and the technology. A successful working relationship between the two will be effected when the manager learns to share his or her information and the analyst learns to adapt to the manager's needs. For the analyst, adaptation means worrying less about the elegance of the method and more about its speed and flexibility.

3. The manager is challenged to gain control of his or her own time by turning obligations to advantage and by turning those things he or she wishes to do into obligations. The chief executives of my study initiated only 32 percent of their own contacts (and another 5 percent by mutual agreement). And yet to a considerable extent they seemed to control their time. There were two key factors that enabled them to do so.

First, managers have to spend so much time discharging obligations that if they were to view them as just that, they would leave no mark on their organizations. The unsuccessful manager blames failure on the obligations; the effective manager turns obligations to his or her own advantage. A speech is a chance to lobby for a cause; a meeting is a chance to reorganize a weak department; a visit to an important customer is a chance to extract trade information.

Second, managers free some of their time to do those things that they—perhaps no one else—think important by turning them into obligations. Free time is made, not found, in the manager's job; it is forced into the schedule. Hoping to leave some time open for contemplation or general planning is tantamount to hoping that the pressures of the job will go away. The manager who wants to innovate initiates a project and obligates others to report back to him or her; the manager who needs certain external information establishes channels that will automatically keep him or her informed; the manager who has to tour facilities commits him- or herself publicly to doing so.

No job is more vital to our society than that of the manager. It is the manager who determines whether our social institutions serve us well or whether they squander our talents and resources. It is time to strip away the folklore of managerial work so that we can begin the difficult task of making significant improvements in its performance.

2
CRAFTING STRATEGY

One of the more important things managers do is make strategy for their organizations, or at least oversee the process by which they and others make strategies. In a narrow sense, strategy-making deals with the positioning of an organization in market niches, in other words, deciding on what products will be produced and for whom. But in a broader sense strategy-making refers to how the collective system called organization establishes, and when necessary changes, its basic orientation. Strategy-making also takes up the complex issue of collective intention—how an organization composed of many people makes up *its* mind, so to speak.

Strategy-making is a fascinating process, involving more than the simple set of prescriptions called "planning" with which it is usually associated. This subject has been my central interest throughout my career. My first article, in 1967, as a doctoral student and entitled "The Science of Strategy Making," contrasted a Biblical "grand plan" approach with a Darwinian evolutionary approach. My current writing involves a two-volume work entitled "Strategy Formation," whose underlying theme contrasts deliberate and emergent approaches to the subject.

My ideas on this subject developed through a research project initiated in 1971. With the aid of a number of doctoral students and colleagues, especially Jim Waters, the intention was to study how organizations engage in the process by tracking their strategies across decades in their histories. Over the next twelve years or so, we carried out a whole series of studies—on a supermarket chain, a major airline, a government film agency, a small daily newspaper, our own university, and others. As the project neared its end, I began to search for a way to bring the conclusions to a general managerial audience.

All the while, my wife was crafting pottery in the basement. One day she put up a retrospective of her work, and I saw strategy evolving before my own eyes. An idea struck then, or perhaps it had struck when she made a presentation to a combined class of pottery and management students on the source and nature of creativity in craft. I realized I was hearing from her much the same as I had heard from creative strategists in business (for example, the serendipitous role of "mistakes" in pottery and of "opportunities" in business, "a feel for the clay" and "a knowledge of the business"). Thus I decided to use crafting as a metaphor and an analogy to capture the difficulties of creating strategy in a dynamic organization. "Crafting Strategy" appeared in the *Harvard Business Review* in 1987.

My ideas may have developed over the years (though you will see shades of Biblical grand plans and Darwinian evolution here too), but you will find here a tone similar to that of the "manager's job" article. What this article presents is a description of how managers who must work in "calculated chaos" deal with the complex and necessarily collective process of making strategy.

Imagine someone *planning* strategy. What most likely springs to mind is an image of orderly thinking: a senior manager, or a group of them, sitting in an office formulating courses of action that everyone else will implement on schedule. The keynote is reason—rational control, the systematic analysis of competitors and markets, of company strengths and weaknesses, the combination of these analyses producing clear, explicit, full-blown strategies.

Now imagine someone *crafting* strategy. An entirely different image most likely results, as different from planning as craft is from mechanization. Craft evokes traditional skill, dedication, perfection through the mastery of detail. What springs to mind is not so much thinking and reason as involvement, a feeling of intimacy and harmony with the materials at hand, developed through long experience and commitment. Formulation and implementation merge into a fluid process of learning, through which creative strategies evolve.

My thesis is simple: The crafting image better captures the process by which effective strategies come to be. The planning image, long popular in the literature, distorts those processes and thereby misguides organizations that embrace it unreservedly.

In developing this thesis, I shall draw on the experiences of a single craftsman, a potter, and compare them with the results of a research project that tracked the strategies of a number of corporations across several decades. Because the two contexts are so obviously different, my metaphor, like my assertion, may seem far-fetched at first. Yet if we think of a craftsman as an organization of one, we can see that he or she must also resolve one of the great challenges the corporate strategist faces: knowing the organization's capabilities well enough to think deeply about its strategic direction. By considering strategy-making from the perspective of one person, free of all the paraphernalia of what has been called the strategy industry, we can learn something about the formation of strategy in the corporation. For much as our potter has to manage her craft, so too managers have to craft their strategy.

At work, the potter sits before a lump of clay on the wheel. Her mind is on the clay, but she is also aware of sitting between her past experiences and her future prospects. She knows exactly what has and has not worked for her in the past. She has an intimate knowledge of her work, her capabilities, and her markets. As a craftsman, she senses rather than analyzes these things; her knowledge is "tacit." All this is working in her mind as her hands are working the clay. The product that emerges on the wheel is likely to be in the tradition of her past work. But she may break away and embark on a new path. Even so, the past is no less present, projecting itself into the future.

In my metaphor, managers are craftsmen and strategy is their clay. Like the potter, they sit between a past of corporate capabilities and a future of market opportunities. And if they are truly craftsmen, they bring to their work an equally intimate knowledge of the materials at hand. That is the essence of crafting strategy.

We will explore this metaphor by looking at how strategies actually get made as opposed to how they are supposed to get made. Throughout, I will be drawing on the two sets of experiences I have mentioned. One is a research project on patterns in strategy formation that went on at McGill University under my direction beginning in 1971. The second is the stream of work of a successful potter, my wife, who began her craft in 1967.

Strategies are both plans for the future and patterns from the past.

Ask almost anyone what strategy is, and they will define it as a plan of some sort, an explicit guide to future behavior. Then ask them what strategy a competitor or a government or even they themselves have actually pursued. Chances are they will describe consistency in *past* behavior—a pattern in action over time. Strategy, it turns out, is one of those words that people define in one way and often use in another, without realizing the difference.

The reason for this is simple. Strategy's formal definition and its Greek military origins notwithstanding, we need the word as much to explain past actions as to describe intended behavior in the future. After all, if strategies can be planned and intended, they can also be pursued and realized (or not realized, as the case may be). And pattern in past action, or what I call *realized* strategy, reflects that pursuit. Moreover, just as a plan need not produce a pattern (some strategies that are intended are simply not realized), so too a pattern need not result from a plan. An organization can develop a pattern (a realized strategy) without knowing it, let alone making it explicit.

Patterns, like beauty, are of course in the mind of the beholder. But anyone reviewing a chronological lineup of our craftsman's work would have little trouble discerning clear patterns, at least in certain periods. Until 1974, for example, she made small, decorative ceramic animals and objects of various kinds. Then this "knickknack strategy" stopped abruptly, and eventually new patterns formed around waferlike sculptures and ceramic bowls, highly textured and unglazed.

Finding equivalent patterns in action for organizations isn't that much more difficult. Indeed, for such large companies as Volkswagenwerk and Air Canada in our research, it proved simpler! (As well it should. A craftsman, after all, can change what she does in a studio a lot more easily than a Volkswagenwerk can retool its assembly lines.) Mapping the product models at Volkswagenwerk from the late 1940s to the late 1970s, for example, uncovers a clear pattern of concentration on the Beetle, followed in the late 1960s by a frantic search for replacements through acquisitions and internally developed new models, until a strategic reorientation developed around more stylish, water-cooled, front-wheel-drive vehicles in the mid-1970s.

But what about *intended* strategies, those formal plans and pronouncements we think of when we use the term *strategy*? Ironically, here we run into all kinds of problems. Even with a single craftsman, how can we know what her intended strategies really were? If we could go back, would we find expressions of intention? And if we did, would we be able to trust them? We often fool ourselves, as well as others, by denying our subconscious motives. And remember that intentions come cheap, at least when compared with realizations.

READING THE ORGANIZATION'S MIND

If you believe all this has more to do with the Freudian recesses of a craftsman's mind than with the practical realities of producing automobiles, then think again. For who knows what the intended strategies of a Volkswagenwerk really mean, let alone what they are? Can we simply assume in this collective context that the company's intended strategies are represented by its formal plans or by other statements emanating from the executive suite? Might these be just vain hopes, or rationalizations, or ploys to fool the competition? And even if such expressed intentions exist, to what extent do other people in the organization share them? How do we read the collective mind? Who is the strategist anyway?

The traditional view of strategic management resolves these problems quite simply, by what organizational theorists call attribution. You see it all the time in the business press. When General Motors acts, it's because its chief executive has made a strategy. Given realization, there must have been intention, and that is automatically attributed to the chief.

In a short magazine article, this assumption is understandable, even if wrong. Journalists don't have a lot of time to uncover the origins of strategy, and GM is a large, complicated organization. But just consider all the complexity and confusion that get swept under this assumption—all the meetings and debates, the many people involved, the dead ends, the folding and unfolding of ideas. Now consider trying to build a formal strategy-making system around that assumption. Is it any wonder that formal strategic planning is often such a resounding failure?

To unravel some of the confusion—and move away from the artificial complexity we have piled around the strategy-making process—we need to get back to some basic concepts. The most basic of all is the intimate connection between thought and action. That is the key to craft, and so also to the crafting of strategy.

Strategies need not be deliberate—they can also emerge, more or less.

Virtually everything that has been written about strategy-making depicts it as a deliberate process. First we think, then we act. We formulate, then we implement. The progression seems so perfectly sensible. Why would anybody wish to proceed differently?

Our potter is in the studio, rolling the clay to make a waferlike sculpture. The clay sticks to the rolling pin, and a round form appears. Why not make a cylindrical vase? One idea leads to another, until a new pattern forms. Action has driven thinking: A strategy has emerged.

Out in the field, a salesman visits a customer. The product isn't quite right, and together they work out some modifications. The salesman returns to the company and puts the changes through; after two or three more rounds, they finally get it right. A new product emerges, which eventually opens up a new market. The company has changed strategic course.

In fact, most salespeople are less fortunate than this one or than our craftsman. In an organization of one, the implementer is the formulator, so innovations can be incorporated into strategy quickly and easily. In a large organization, the innovator may be ten levels removed from the leader who is supposed to dictate strategy, and may also have to sell the idea to dozens of peers doing the same job.

Some salespeople, of course, can proceed on their own, modifying products to suit their customers and convincing skunkworks in the factory to produce them. In effect, they pursue their own strategies. Maybe no one else notices or cares. Sometimes, however, their innovations do get noticed, perhaps years later, when the company's prevalent strategies have broken down and its leaders are groping for something new. Then the salesperson's own strategy may be allowed to pervade the system, to become organizational.

Is this story far-fetched? Certainly not. We have all heard stories like it. But since we tend to see only what we believe, if we believe that strategies have to be planned, we are unlikely to see the real meaning such stories hold.

Consider how the National Film Board of Canada (NFB) came to adopt a feature-film strategy. The NFB is a federal government agency, famous for its creativity and expertise in the production of short documentaries. Some years back, it funded a filmmaker on a project that unexpectedly ran long. To distribute his film, the NFB turned to theaters and so inadvertently gained experience in marketing feature-length films. Other filmmakers caught on to the idea, and eventually the NFB found itself pursuing a feature-film strategy—a pattern of producing such films.

My point is simple, deceptively simple: Strategies can *form* as well as be *formulated*. A realized strategy can emerge in response to an evolving situation, or it can be brought about deliberately, through a process of formulation followed by implementation. But when these planned intentions do not produce the desired actions, organizations are left with unrealized strategies.

Today we hear a great deal about unrealized strategies, almost always in concert with the claim that implementation has failed. Management has been lax, controls have been loose, the implementers haven't been committed. Excuses abound. At times, they may be valid. But often these explanations prove too easy. So some people look beyond implementation, to formulation. The strategists haven't been smart enough.

While it is certainly true that many intended strategies are ill conceived, I believe that the problem often lies one step beyond that, in the distinction we make in the first place between formulation and implementation, the common assumption that thought must be independent of (and precede) action. Sure, people could be smarter—but not only by conceiving smarter strategies. Sometimes they can be smarter by allowing their strategies to develop gradually, through the organization's actions and experiences. Smart strategists appreciate that they cannot always be smart enough to think through everything in advance.

HANDS AND MINDS

No craftsman thinks some days and works others. The craftsman's mind is going constantly, in tandem with her hands. Yet large organizations try to separate the work of minds and hands. In so doing, they often sever the vital feedback link between the two. The salesperson who finds a customer with an unmet need may possess the most strategic bit of information in the entire organization. But that information is useless if he or she cannot create a strategy in response to it, or else convey the information to someone who can—because the channels are blocked or because the formulators have simply finished formulating. The notion that strategy is something that should happen way up there, far removed from the details of running an organization on a daily basis, is one of the great fallacies of conventional management. And it explains a good many of the most dramatic failures in business and public policy today.

We at McGill call strategies that appear without clear intentions—or in spite of them—*emergent* strategies. Actions simply converge into patterns. They may become deliberate, of course, if the pattern is recognized and then legitimized by senior management. But that is after the fact.

All this may sound rather strange, I know. Strategies that emerge? Managers who acknowledge strategies already formed? Over the years, our research group at McGill has met with a good deal of resistance from people upset by what they perceive to be our passive definition of a word so bound up with proactive behavior and free will. After all, strategy means control—the ancient Greeks used it to describe the art of the army general.

STRATEGIC LEARNING

But we have persisted in this usage for one reason: learning. Purely *deliberate* strategy precludes learning once the strategy is formulated; emergent strategy fosters it. People take actions one by one and respond to them, so that patterns eventually form.

Our craftsman tries to make a freestanding sculptural form. It doesn't work, so she rounds it a bit here, flattens it a bit there. The result looks better but still isn't quite right. She makes another and another and another. Eventually, after days or months or years, she finally has what she wants. She is off on a new strategy.

In practice, of course, all strategy-making walks on two feet, one deliberate, the other emergent. For just as purely deliberate strategy-making precludes learning, so purely emergent strategy-making precludes control. Pushed to the limit, neither approach makes much sense. Learning must be coupled with control. That is why the McGill research group uses the word *strategy* for both emergent and deliberate behavior.

Likewise, there is no such thing as a purely deliberate strategy or a purely emergent one. No organization—not even the ones commanded by those ancient Greek generals—knows enough to work everything out in advance, to ignore learning en route. And no one—not even a solitary potter—can be flexible enough to leave everything to happenstance, to give up all mental control. Craft requires control just as it requires responsiveness to the material at hand. Thus deliberate and emergent strategies form the end points of a continuum along which the strategies that are crafted in the real world may be found. Some strategies may approach either end, but many more fall at intermediate points.

Effective strategies develop in all kinds of strange ways.

Effective strategies can show up in the strangest places and develop through the most unexpected means. There is no "one best way" to make strategy.

The form for a cat collapses on the wheel, and our potter sees in the clay a bull taking shape. Clay sticks to a rolling pin, and a line of cylinders results. Waferlike forms come into being because of a shortage of clay and limited kiln space while the potter is working temporarily in a studio in France. Thus errors become opportunities, and limitations stimulate creativity. The natural propensity to experiment, or sometimes just boredom, likewise encourages strategic change.

Organizations that craft their strategies have similar experiences. Recall the National Film Board with its inadvertently long film that brought about a feature-film strategy. Or consider its experiences with experimental films, which made special use of animation and sound. For twenty years, the NFB produced a thin but steady trickle of such films. In fact, every film but one in that trickle was produced by a single person, Norman McLaren, the NFB's most celebrated filmmaker. McLaren pursued a *personal strategy* of experimentation, deliberate for him perhaps (did he intend the whole stream or simply consider one film at a time?) but not for the organization. Then twenty years later, others followed his lead and the trickle widened, his personal strategy becoming more broadly organizational.

Conversely, in 1952, when television came to Canada, a *consensus strategy* emerged at the NFB. Senior management was not keen on producing films for the new medium. But while the arguments raged, one filmmaker quietly went off and made a single series for TV. That precedent being set, one by one his colleagues leapt in, and within months the NFB—and its management—found themselves committed for several years to a new strategy with an intensity unmatched before or since. That consensus strategy arose spontaneously, as a result of many independent decisions made by the filmmakers about the films they wished to make. Can we call the strategy deliberate? For the filmmakers perhaps; for senior management certainly not. But for the organization? It all depends on your perspective, on how you choose to read the organization's mind.

While the NFB may seem like an extreme case, it highlights behavior that can be found, albeit in muted form, in all organizations. Those who doubt this might read Richard Pascale's account of how Honda stumbled into its enormous success in the American motorcycle market. Brilliant as its strategy may have looked after the fact, Honda's managers made almost every conceivable mistake until the market finally hit them over the head with the right formula. The Honda managers on site in

America, driving their products themselves (and thus inadvertently picking up market reaction), did only one thing right: They learned, firsthand.[1]

GRASSROOTS STRATEGY-MAKING

These strategies all reflect, in whole or part, what we like to call a grassroots approach to strategic management. Strategies grow like weeds in a garden. They take root in all kinds of places, wherever people have the capacity to learn (because they are in touch with the situation) and the resources to support that capacity. These strategies become organizational when they become collective, that is, when they proliferate to influence the behavior of the organization at large.

Of course, this view is overstated. But it is no less extreme than the conventional view of strategic management, which might be labeled the hothouse approach. Neither is right. Reality falls between the two. Some of the most effective strategies we uncovered in our research combined deliberation and control with flexibility and organizational learning.

Consider first what we call the *umbrella strategy*. Here senior management sets out broad guidelines (say, to produce only high-margin products at the cutting edge of technology or to produce products using bonding and coating technologies) and leaves the specifics (such as what those products will be) to others lower down in the organization. This strategy is not only deliberate (in its guidelines) and emergent (in its specifics), but it is also deliberately emergent in that the process is consciously managed to allow strategies to develop en route. IBM used the umbrella strategy in the early 1960s with the impending 360 series, when its senior management approved a set of broad criteria for the design of a family of computers later developed in detail throughout the organization.[2]

Deliberately emergent, too, is what we call the *process strategy*. Here management controls the process of strategy formation—concerning itself with the design of the structure, with staffing, development of procedures, and so on—while leaving the actual content to others.

Both process and umbrella strategies seem to be especially prevalent in businesses that require great expertise and creativity—a 3M, a Hewlett-Packard, a National Film Board. Such organizations can be effective only if their implementers are allowed to be formulators, because it is the people way down in the hierarchy who are in touch with the situation at hand and have the requisite technical expertise. In a sense, these are organizations peopled with craftsmen, all of whom must be strategists.

Strategic reorientations happen in brief, quantum leaps.

The conventional view of strategy in the planning literature claims that change must be continuous: The organization should be adapting all the time. Yet this view proves to be ironic, because the very concept of strategy is rooted in stability, not change. As this same literature makes clear, organizations pursue strategies to set direction, to lay out courses of action, and to elicit cooperation from their members around common, established guidelines. By any definition, and especially from the perspective of planning, strategy imposes stability on an organization. No stability means no strategy (no course to the future, no pattern from the past). Indeed, the very fact of having a strategy, and especially of making it explicit (as the conventional literature implores managers to do), creates resistance to strategic change!

What the conventional view fails to come to grips with, then, is how and when to promote change. A fundamental dilemma of strategy-making is the need to reconcile the forces for stability and for change—to focus efforts and gain operating efficiencies on the one hand, yet adapt and maintain currency with a changing external environment on the other.

QUANTUM LEAPS

Our own research and that of colleagues suggest that organizations resolve those opposing forces by attending first to one and then to the other. Distinct periods of stability and of change can usually be identified in organizations; major shifts in strategic orientation occur only rarely.

In our study of Steinberg Inc., a large supermarket chain headquartered in Montreal, we found only two important reorientations in the sixty years from its founding to the mid-1970s: a shift to self-service in 1933 and the introduction of shopping centers and public financing in 1953. At Volkswagenwerk, we saw only one reorientation between the late 1940s and the 1970s, the major shift from the traditional Beetle to the Audi-type design mentioned earlier. And at Air Canada, we found none over the airline's first four decades, following its initial positioning.

Our colleagues at McGill, Danny Miller and Peter Friesen, found this pattern of change so common in their studies of large numbers of companies (especially the high-performance ones) that they built a theory around it which they labeled the *quantum* theory of strategic change.[3] Their basic point is that organizations adopt two distinctly different modes of behavior at different times.

Most of the time organizations pursue a given strategic orientation. Change may seem continuous, but it occurs in the context of that orientation (perfecting a given retailing formula, for example) and usually amounts to doing more of the same, perhaps better as well. Most organizations favor these periods of stability because they achieve success not by changing strategies but by exploiting the ones they have. They, like craftsmen, seek continuous improvement by using their distinctive competencies on established courses.

While this goes on, however, the world continues to change, sometimes slowly, occasionally in dramatic shifts. As a result, whether gradually or suddenly, the organization's strategic orientation moves out of sync with its environment. Then what Miller and Friesen call a strategic revolution must take place. That long period of evolutionary change is suddenly punctuated by a brief bout of revolutionary turmoil in which the organization quickly alters many of its established patterns. In effect, it tries to leap to a new stability quickly to reestablish an integrated posture among a new set of strategies, structure, and culture.

But what about all those emergent strategies, growing like weeds around the organization? What the quantum theory suggests is that the really novel ones are generally held in check in some corner of the organization until a strategic revolution becomes necessary. Then as an alternative to having to develop new strategies from scratch or having to import generic strategies from competitors, the organization can turn to its own emerging patterns to find its new orientation. As the old, established strategy disintegrates, the seeds of the new one begin to spread.

This quantum theory of change seems to apply particularly well to large, established, mass-production organizations. Because they are especially reliant on standardized procedures, their resistance to strategic reorientation tends to be especially fierce. So we find long periods of stability broken by short disruptive periods of revolutionary change.

Volkswagenwerk is a case in point. Long enamored of the Beetle and armed with a tightly integrated set of strategies, the company ignored fundamental changes in its markets throughout the late 1950s and 1960s. The bureaucratic inertia of its mass-production organization combined with the psychological inertia of its leader, the person most responsible for the strategies it had been realizing. When change finally did come, it was tumultuous: The company groped its way through a hodgepodge of models before it settled on a new set of vehicles championed by a new leader. Strategic reorientations really are cultural revolutions.

CYCLES OF CHANGE

In more creative organizations like the National Film Board, we see a somewhat different pattern of change and stability, one that is more balanced. Organizations in the business of producing novel outputs apparently need to fly off in all directions from time to time to sustain their creativity. Yet they also need to settle down after such periods to find some order in the resulting chaos.

The NFB showed a marked tendency to move in and out of focus through remarkably balanced periods of convergence and divergence. Concentrated production of films to aid the war effort in the 1940s gave way to great divergence after the war as the organization sought a new raison d'être. Then the advent of television brought back a very sharp focus in the early 1950s, as noted earlier. But in the late 1950s, this dissipated almost as quickly as it began, giving rise to another period of exploration. Then the social changes in the early 1960s evoked a new period of convergence around experimental films and films on social issues.

We use the label "adhocracy" for organizations, like the National Film Board, that produce individual, or custom-made, products (or designs) in an innovative way, on a project basis.[4] Our craftsman is an adhocracy of sorts too, since each of her ceramic sculptures is unique. And her pattern of strategic change was much like the NFB's, with evident cycles of convergence and divergence: a focus on knickknacks from 1967 to 1972; then a period of exploration to about 1976, which resulted in a refocus on ceramic sculptures; that continued to about 1981, followed by a period of searching for new directions.

Whether through quantum revolutions or cycles of convergence and divergence, however, organizations seem to need to separate in time the basic forces for change and stability, reconciling them by attending to each in turn. Many strategic failures can be attributed either to mixing the two or to an obsession with one of these forces at the expense of the other.

The problems are evident in the work of many craftsmen. On the one hand, there are those who seize on the perfection of a single theme and never change. Eventually the creativity disappears from their work and the world passes them by—much as it did Volkswagenwerk until the company was shocked into its strategic revolution. And then there are those who are always changing, who flit from one idea to another and never settle down. Because no theme or strategy ever emerges in their work, they cannot exploit or even develop any distinctive competence. And because their work lacks definition, identity crises are likely to develop, with neither the craftsmen nor those interested in the craft knowing what to make of it. Miller and Friesen found this behavior in conventional business too; they labeled it "the impulsive firm running blind."[5] How often have we seen it in companies that go on acquisition sprees?

To manage strategy, then, is to craft thought and action, control and learning, stability and change.

The popular view sees the strategist as a planner or as a visionary, someone sitting on a pedestal dictating brilliant strategies for everyone else to implement. While recognizing the importance of thinking ahead and especially of the need for creative vision in a prosaic world, I wish to propose an additional view of the strategist—as a pattern recognizer, a learner if you will, who manages a process in which strategies (and visions) can emerge as well as be deliberately conceived. I also wish to redefine that strategist, to replace that individual with a collective entity, made up of many actors whose interplay expresses an organization's mind. This strategist *finds* strategies no less than creates them, often in patterns that form inadvertently in its own behavior.

What, then, does it mean to craft strategy? Let us return to the words associated with craft: dedication, experience, involvement with the material, the personal touch, mastery of detail, a sense of harmony and integration. Managers who craft strategy do not spend much time in executive suites reading MIS reports or studying industry analyses. They are involved, responsive to their materials, learning about their organizations and industries through personal touch. They are also sensitive to experience, recognizing that while individual vision may be important, other factors must help determine strategy as well.

TO MANAGE STABILITY. To manage strategy is in the first place mostly to manage stability, not change. Indeed, most of the time senior managers should not be formulating strategy at all; they should be getting on with making their organizations as effective as possible in pursuing the strategies they already have. Like distinguished craftsmen, organizations become distinguished because they master the details.

To manage strategy, then, at least in the first instance, is not so much to promote change as to know *when* to do so. Advocates of strategic planning often urge managers to plan for perpetual instability in the environment (for example, by rolling over five-year plans annually). But this obsession with change is dysfunctional. Organizations that reassess their strategies continuously are like individuals who reassess their jobs or their marriages continuously—in both cases, they can drive themselves crazy, or else reduce themselves to inaction. The formal planning process repeats itself so often and so mechanically that it can desensitize organizations to real change, programming them more and more deeply into set patterns, and thereby encouraging them to make only minor adaptations.

So-called strategic planning must be recognized for what it is: a means, not to create strategy, but to program a strategy already created—to work out its implications formally. It is essentially analytic in nature, based on decomposition, while strategy creation is essentially a process of synthesis. That is why trying to create strategies through formal planning most often leads to the extrapolation of existing strategies or to the copying of the strategies of competitors.

This is not to say that planners have no role to play in strategy formation. In addition to programming strategies created by other means, they can feed ad hoc analyses into the strategy-making process at the front end to be sure that the hard data are taken into consideration. They can also stimulate others to think strategically. And of course people called planners can be strategists too, so long as they are creative thinkers who are in touch with what is relevant. But that has nothing to do with the technology of formal planning.

TO DETECT DISCONTINUITY. Environments do not change on any regular or orderly basis. And they seldom undergo continuous dramatic change, claims about our "age of discontinuity" and environmental "turbulence" notwithstanding. (Go tell those claims to people who lived through the Great Depression or survivors of the siege of Leningrad during World War II.) Much of the time, change is minor and even temporary and requires no strategic response. Once in a while there is a truly significant discontinuity or even less often, a *gestalt* shift in the environment, where everything important seems to change at once. But these events, while critical, are also easy to recognize.

The real challenge in crafting strategy lies in detecting the subtle discontinuities that may undermine an organization in the future. And for that, there is no technique, no program, just a sharp mind in touch with the situation. Such discontinuities are unexpected and irregular, essentially unprecedented. They can be dealt with only by minds that are attuned to existing patterns yet able to perceive important breaks in them. Unfortunately, this form of strategic thinking tends to atrophy during the long periods of stability that most organizations experience (just as it did at Volkswagenwerk during the 1950s and 1960s). So the trick is to manage within a given strategic orientation most of the time yet be able to pick out the occasional discontinuity that really matters.

The Steinberg chain was built and run for more than half a century by a man named Sam Steinberg. For twenty years, the company concentrated on perfecting a self-service retailing formula introduced in 1933. Installing fluorescent lighting and figuring out how to package meat in cellophane wrapping were the "strategic" issues of the day. Then in 1952, with the arrival of the first shopping center in Montreal, Steinberg realized he had to redefine his business almost overnight. He knew he needed to control those shopping centers and that control would require public financing and other major changes. So he reoriented his business. The ability to make that kind of switch in thinking is the essence of strategic management. And it has more to do with vision and involvement than it does with analytic technique.

TO KNOW THE BUSINESS. Sam Steinberg was the epitome of the entrepreneur, a man intimately involved with all the details of his business, who spent Saturday mornings visiting his stores. As he told us in discussing his company's competitive advantage:

> Nobody knew the grocery business like we did. Everything has to do with your knowledge. I knew merchandise, I knew cost, I knew selling, I knew customers. I knew everything, and I passed on all my knowledge; I kept teaching my people. That's the advantage we had. Our competitors couldn't touch us.

Note the kind of knowledge involved: not intellectual knowledge, not analytical reports or abstracted facts and figures (though these can certainly help), but personal knowledge, intimate understanding, equivalent to the craftsman's feel for the clay. Facts are available to anyone; this kind of knowledge is not. Wisdom is the word that captures it best. But wisdom is a word that has been lost in the bureaucracies we have built for ourselves, systems designed to distance leaders from operating details. Show me managers who think they can rely on formal planning to create their strategies, and I'll show you managers who lack intimate knowledge of their businesses or the creativity to do something with it.

Craftsmen have to train themselves to see, to pick up things other people miss. The same holds true for managers of strategy. It is those with a kind of peripheral vision who are best able to detect and take advantage of events as they unfold.

TO MANAGE PATTERNS. Whether in an executive suite in Manhattan or a pottery studio in Montreal, a key to managing strategy is the ability to detect emerging patterns and help them take shape. The job of the manager is not just to preconceive specific strategies but also to recognize their emergence elsewhere in the organization and intervene when appropriate.

Like weeds that appear unexpectedly in a garden, some emergent strategies may need to be uprooted immediately. But management cannot be too quick to cut off the unexpected, for tomorrow's vision may grow out of today's aberration. (Europeans, after all, enjoy salads made from the leaves of the dandelion, America's most notorious weed!) Thus some patterns are worth watching until their effects have more clearly manifested themselves. Then those that prove useful can be made deliberate and incorporated into the formal strategy, even if that means shifting the strategic umbrella to cover them.

To manage in this context, then, is to create the climate within which a wide variety of strategies can grow. In more complex organizations, this may mean building flexible structures, hiring creative people, defining broad umbrella strategies, and watching for the patterns that emerge.

TO RECONCILE CHANGE AND CONTINUITY. Finally, managers considering radical departures need to keep the quantum theory of change in mind. As Ecclesiastes reminds us, there is a time to sow and a time to reap. Some new patterns must be held in check until the organization is ready for a strategic revolution, or at least a period of divergence.

Managers who are obsessed with either change or stability are bound eventually to harm their organizations. As pattern recognizer, the manager has to be able to sense when to exploit an established crop of strategies and when to encourage new strains to displace the old.

While strategy is a word that is usually associated with the future, its link to the past is no less central. As Kierkegaard once observed, life is lived forward but understood backward. Managers may have to live strategy in the future, but they must understand it through the past.

Like a potter at the wheel, organizations must make sense of the past if they hope to manage the future. Only by coming to understand the patterns that form in their own behavior do they get to know their capabilities and their potential. Thus crafting strategy, like managing craft, requires a natural synthesis of the future, present, and past.

3
PLANNING ON THE LEFT SIDE, MANAGING ON THE RIGHT

The article reprinted here preceded the last by more than a decade and took me into a somewhat different although perhaps more fundamental issue: the relationship between analysis and intuition, as manifested in the long and sometimes strained relationship between "staff" and "line," with special reference to planners and managers. The first two articles of this book grew out of years of research and contemplation; this third one developed rather spontaneously. In the summer of 1975, on a small farm in the Perigord region of France, I read Robert Ornstein's *The Psychology of Consciousness,* a popular account of the findings on the two hemispheres of the human brain. Although attention to these findings had become faddish at the time, to me they provided a basis for much of what I had been finding in my own research.

There is a lovely irony in the fact that intuition was in some sense brought back to life by the biologists. You see, intuition should really be a psychological concept. But most psychologists, in order to be perceived as good scientists, have long slighted it, when not ignoring it altogether. After all, if intuition is a thought process inaccessible to the *conscious* mind, how could they use *scientific* methods to describe it? Then along came people like Roger Sperry—real scientists, who cut tissue with knives and the like—and they were the ones to rediscover intuition, in a sense hiding all along in the mute right hemisphere of the human brain!

In reading Ornstein's book, I came to realize that I had really been celebrating intuition in my own research, uncovering it in all kinds of odd and clandestine places. This was at odds with the mainline management literature—applied no less than academic—that emphasized, almost to the point of obsession, the role of analysis in organizations, especially under so-called professional management. The title hit me first, then I wrote the article. (Usually it has been the other way around.) My writing almost always goes through many drafts before the editors get their hands on it and propose further changes. "Planning on the Left Side and Managing on the Right" appeared in the *Harvard Business Review* in 1976 almost as I first put it down on that small farm in the Perigord.

In the folklore of the Middle East, the story is told about a man named Nasrudin, who was searching for something on the ground. A friend came by and asked: "What have you lost, Nasrudin?"

"My key," said Nasrudin.

So the friend went down on his knees too, and they both looked for it. After a time, the friend asked: "Where exactly did you drop it?"

"In my house," answered Nasrudin.

"Then why are you looking here, Nasrudin?"

"There is more light here than inside my own house."

This little story has some timeless, mysterious appeal which has much to do with what follows. But let me leave that aside for a moment while I pose some questions—also simple yet mysterious—that have long puzzled me.

• First: Why are some people so smart and so dull at the same time, so capable of mastering certain mental activities yet so incapable of mastering others? Why is it that some of the most creative thinkers cannot comprehend a balance sheet, and that some accountants have no sense of product design? Why do some brilliant management scientists have no ability to handle organizational politics, while some of the most politically adept individuals seem unable to understand the simplest elements of management science?

• Second: Why do people sometimes express such surprise when they read or learn the obvious, something they already must have known? Why is a manager so delighted, for example, when he or she reads a new article on decision-making, every part of which must be patently obvious to him or her even though never before seen in print?

• Third: Why is there such a discrepancy in organizations, at least at the top levels, between formal planning on the one hand and informal managing on the other? Why have none of the techniques of planning and analysis really had much effect on how top managers function?

I intend below to weave answers to those three questions around the theme of the specialization of the hemispheres of the human brain. Later

I shall use my own research to draw out some implications of this for management, returning to our story of Nasrudin.

THE TWO HEMISPHERES OF THE HUMAN BRAIN

Let us first try to answer the three questions by looking at what is known about the hemispheres of the human brain.

QUESTION ONE

Scientists—in particular, neurologists, biologists, and psychologists—have known for a long time that the brain has two distinct hemispheres. They have known, further, that the left hemisphere controls movements on the body's right side while the right hemisphere controls movements on the left. What some have discovered more recently, however, is that the two hemispheres are specialized in more fundamental ways.

In the left hemisphere of most people's brains (lefthanders largely excepted), the mode of operation appears to be largely linear, information being processed sequentially, one bit after another, in an ordered way. Perhaps the most obvious linear faculty is language. In sharp contrast, the right hemisphere appears to be specialized for simultaneous processing; that is, it seems to operate in a more holistic, relational way. Perhaps its most obvious faculty is comprehension of visual images.

Although relatively few specific mental activities have yet been associated with one hemisphere or the other, research has provided some important clues. For example, an article in *The New York Times* cited research which suggests that emotion may be a right-hemispheric function.[1] This notion is based on the finding that victims of right-hemispheric strokes are often comparatively untroubled about their incapacity, while those with strokes of the left hemisphere often suffer profound mental anguish.

What does this specialization of the brain mean for the way people function? Speech, being linear, is a left-hemispheric activity, but other forms of human communication, such as gesturing, are relational and visual rather than sequential and verbal so tend to be associated with the right hemisphere. Imagine what would happen if the two sides of a human brain were detached so that, for example, in reading stimuli, words would be separate from gestures. In other words, in the same person, two separate brains—one specialized for verbal communication, and the other for gestures—would react to the same stimulus.

This, in fact, describes how the main breakthrough in the research on the human brain took place. In trying to treat certain cases of epilepsy, neurosurgeons found that by severing the corpus callosum, which joins the two hemispheres of the brain, they could "split the brain," isolating the epilepsy. A number of experiments run on these "split-brain" patients produced some fascinating results.

In one experiment, doctors showed a woman epileptic's right hemisphere a photograph of a nude woman. (This is done by showing it to the left half of each eye.) The patient said she saw nothing, but almost simultaneously blushed and seemed confused and uncomfortable. Her "conscious" left hemisphere, including her verbal apparatus, was aware only that something had happened to her body, but not what had caused the emotional response. Only her "unconscious" right hemisphere knew. Here neurosurgeons observed a clear split between the two independent consciousnesses that are normally in communication and collaboration.[2]

Scientists have found further that some common human tasks activate one side of the brain while leaving the other largely at rest. For example, learning a mathematical proof might evoke activity in the left hemisphere of the brain, while viewing a piece of sculpture or assessing a political opponent might evoke activity in the right.

So now we seem to have the answer to the first question. An individual may be smart and dull at the same time simply because one side of his or her brain is more developed than the other. Some people—perhaps most lawyers, accountants, planners—may have better developed left-hemispheric thinking processes, while others—perhaps, artists, athletes, politicians—may have better developed right-hemispheric processes. Thus an artist may be incapable of expressing certain feelings in words, while a lawyer may have no facility for painting. Or a politician may not be able to learn mathematics, while a management scientist may be constantly manipulated in political situations.

QUESTION TWO

A number of word opposites have been proposed to distinguish the two hemispheric modes of "consciousness," for example: explicit versus implicit; verbal versus spatial; argument versus experience; intellectual versus intuitive; and analytic versus gestalt.

I should interject at this point that these words, as well as much of the evidence for these conclusions, can be found in the remarkable book entitled *The Psychology of Consciousness* by Robert Ornstein, a research psychologist in California. Ornstein uses the story of Nasrudin to further the points he is making. Specifically, he refers to the linear left hemisphere as synonymous with lightness, with thought processes that we know in an explicit sense. We can *articulate* them. He associates the right hemisphere with darkness, with thought processes that are mysterious to us, at least "us" in the Western world.

Ornstein also points out how the "esoteric psychologies" of the East (Zen, Yoga, Sufism, and so on) have focused on right-hemispheric consciousness (for example, altering pulse rate through meditation). In sharp contrast, Western psychology has been concerned almost exclusively with left-hemispheric consciousness, with logical thought. Ornstein suggests that we might find an important key to human consciousness in the right hemisphere, in what to us in the West has been the darkness.

Now, reflect on this for a moment. (Should I say meditate?) There is a set of thought processes—linear, sequential, analytical—that scientists as well as the rest of us know a good deal about. And there is another set—simultaneous, relational, holistic—that we know little about. More importantly, here we do not "know" what we "know" or more exactly, our left hemispheres do not seem able to articulate explicitly what our right hemispheres know implicitly.

So here, seemingly, is the answer to the second question as well. The feeling of revelation about learning the obvious can be explained with the suggestion that the "obvious" knowledge was implicit, apparently restricted to the right hemisphere. The left hemisphere never "knew." Thus it seems to be a revelation to the left hemisphere when it learns explicitly what the right hemisphere knew all along implicitly.

Now the third question—the discrepancy between planning and managing—remains.

QUESTION THREE

By now, it should be obvious where my discussion is leading (at least, to the reader's right hemisphere and, now that I write it, perhaps to the reader's left hemisphere as well). It may be that management researchers have been looking for the key to management in the lightness of logical analysis whereas perhaps it has always been lost in the darkness of intuition.

Specifically, I propose that there may be a fundamental difference between formal planning and informal managing, a difference akin to that between the two hemispheres of the human brain. The techniques of planning and analysis are sequential and systematic; above all, articulated. Planners and management scientists are expected to proceed in their work through a series of logical, ordered steps, each one involving explicit analysis. (The argument that the successful application of these techniques requires considerable intuition does not really change my point. The occurrence of intuition simply means that the analyst is departing from his or her science.)

Formal planning, then, seems to use processes akin to those identified with the brain's left hemisphere. Furthermore, planners and management scientists seem to revel in a systematic, well-ordered world, and many show little appreciation for the more relational, holistic processes.

What about managing? More exactly, what about the processes used by top managers? (Let me emphasize here that I am focusing this discussion at the senior levels of organizations, where I believe the dichotomy between planning and managing is most pronounced.) Managers plan in some ways, too (that is, they think ahead), and they engage in their share of logical analysis. But I believe there is more than that to the effective managing of an organization. I hypothesize, therefore, that *the important processes of managing an organization rely to a considerable extent on the faculties identified with the brain's right hemisphere.* Effective managers seem to revel in ambiguity, in complex, mysterious systems with relatively little order.

If true, this hypothesis would answer the third question about the discrepancy between planning and managing. It would help to explain why each of the new analytic techniques of planning and analysis has, one after the other, had so little success at the senior levels. PPBS, strategic planning, "management" information systems, and models of the firm—all have been greeted with great enthusiasm, then, in many instances, a few years later quietly ushered out the back door.

MANAGING FROM THE RIGHT HEMISPHERE

Because research has so far told us little about the right hemisphere, I cannot support with evidence my claim that a key to managing lies there. I can only present to the reader a "feel" for the situation, not a reading of concrete data. A number of findings from my own research on senior management processes do, however, suggest that they possess characteristics of right-hemispheric thinking.

One fact recurs repeatedly in all of this research. The key managerial processes are enormously complex and mysterious (to me as a researcher, as well as to the managers who carry them out), drawing on the vaguest of information and using the least articulated of mental processes. These processes seem to be more relational and holistic than ordered and sequential, more intuitive than intellectual; they seem, in other words, to be most characteristic of right-hemispheric activity.

Here are some general findings:

1. The five chief executives I observed strongly favored the oral media of communication, especially meetings, over the written forms, namely reading and writing. Of course oral communication is linear, too, but it is more than that. Managers seem to favor it for two fundamental reasons that suggest a relational mode of operation.

First, oral communication enables the manager to "read" facial expressions, tones of voice, and gestures. As I mentioned earlier, these stimuli seem to be associated with the right hemisphere of the brain. Second, and perhaps more important, oral communication enables the manager to engage in the "real-time" exchange of information. Managers' concentration on the oral media, therefore, suggests that they desire relational, simultaneous methods of acquiring information, rather than the ordered and sequential ones.

2. In addition to noting the media managers use, it is interesting to look at the content of managers' information, and at what they do with it. The evidence here is that a great deal of the managers' inputs are soft and speculative—impressions and feelings about other people, hearsay, gossip, and so on. Furthermore, the very analytical inputs—reports, documents, and hard data in general—seem to be of relatively little interest to many managers.

What can managers do with this soft, speculative information? They "synthesize" rather than "analyze" it, I should think. (How do you analyze the mood of a friend or the grimace someone makes in response to a suggestion?) A great deal of this information helps the manager understand implicitly his or her organization and its environment, to "see the big picture." This very expression, so common in management, implies a relational, holistic use of information.

A number of words managers commonly use suggest this kind of mental process. For example, the word "hunch" seems to refer to the results of using the implicit models that managers develop subconsciously in their brains. "I don't know why, but I have a hunch that if we do x, then they will respond with y.'' Managers also use the word ''intuition'' to refer to thought processes that work but are unknown to them. This seems to be a word that the verbal intellect has given to the mysterious thought processes. Maybe ''a person has good intuition'' simply means that person has good implicit models in his or her right hemisphere.

3. Another consequence of the oral nature of the managers' information is of interest here. Managers tend to be the best-informed members of their organization, but they have difficulty disseminating their information to their subordinates. Therefore, when managers overloaded with work find a new task that needs doing, they face a dilemma: They must either delegate the task without the background information or simply do the task themselves, neither of which is satisfactory.

When I first encountered this ''dilemma of delegation,'' I described it in terms of time and of the nature of the manager's information: Because so much of a manager's information is oral (and stored in his or her head), the dissemination of it consumes much time. But now the split-brain research suggests a second, perhaps more significant, reason for the dilemma of delegation. The manager may simply be incapable of disseminating some relevant information because it is inaccessible to his or her consciousness.

4. Earlier in this article I wrote that managers revel in ambiguity, in complex, mysterious systems without much order. Let us look at evidence of this. What I have discussed so far about the managers' use of information suggests that their work is geared to action, not reflection. We see further evidence for this in the pace of their work (''Breaks are rare. It's one damn thing after another.''); the brevity of their activities (half of the chief executives' activities I observed were completed in less than nine minutes); the variety of their activities (these chief executives had no evident patterns in their workdays); the active preference for interruption in their work (stopping meetings, leaving their doors open); and the lack of routine in their work (few regularly scheduled contacts, and hardly any issues related to general planning).

Clearly, the manager does not operate in a systematic, orderly, and intellectual way, puffing on a pipe in a mountain retreat, as problems are analyzed. Rather, the manager deals with issues in the context of daily activities—one hand on the telephone, the other shaking hands with a departing guest. The manager is involved, plugged in; the mode of operating is relational, simultaneous, experiential, that is, encompassing all the characteristics associated with the right hemisphere.

5. If the most important managerial roles of the ten described in my research were to be isolated, leader, liaison, and disturbance handler would certainly be among them. Yet these are the roles least understood. *Leader* describes how the manager deals with his or her own subordinates. It is ironic that despite an immense amount of research, managers and researchers still know virtually nothing about the essence of leadership, about why some people follow and others lead. Leadership remains a mysterious chemistry; catchall words such as *charisma* proclaim our ignorance.

In the *liaison* role, the manager builds up a network of outside contacts, which serve as his or her personal information system. Again, the activities of this role remain almost completely outside the realm of articulated knowledge. And as a *disturbance handler* the manager handles problems and crises in his or her organization. Here again, despite an extensive literature on analytical decision-making, virtually nothing is written about decision-making under pressure. These activities remain outside the realm of management science, inside only the realm of intuition and experience.

6. Let us turn now to our research on strategic decision-making processes.[3] Two aspects of this—the *diagnosis* of decision situations and the *design* of custom-made solutions—stand out in that almost nothing is known about them. Yet these two stand out for another reason as well: They seem to be the most important aspects. In particular, diagnosis seems to be *the* crucial step in strategic decision-making, for it is here that the whole course of decision-making is set. It is a surprising fact, therefore, that diagnosis goes virtually without mention in the literature of planning or management science, most of which deals with the formal evaluation of given alternatives. The question becomes, *where* and *how* does diagnosis take place? Apparently in the darkness of judgment and intuition.

7. Another point that emerges from studying strategic decision-making processes is the existence and profound influence of a set of dynamic factors. Strategic decision-making processes are stopped by interruptions, delayed and speeded up by timing responses, and forced repeatedly to branch and cycle. Yet it is these dynamic factors that the ordered, sequential techniques of analysis are least able to handle. Thus, despite their importance, the dynamic factors go virtually without mention in the literature of management science.

Let us look at timing, for example. It is evident that timing is crucial in virtually everything the manager does. No manager takes action without considering the effects of moving more or less quickly, of seizing initiatives or of delaying to avoid complications. Yet in one review of the literature of management, the authors found fewer than ten books in 183 that refer directly to the subject of timing.[4] Essentially, managers are left on their own to deal with dynamic factors, which involve simultaneous, relational modes of thinking.

8. When managers do have to make serious choices from among options, how do they in fact make them? Three fundamental modes of selection can be distinguished—analysis, judgment, and bargaining. The first involves the systematic evaluation of options in terms of their consequences on stated organizational goals; the second is a process in the mind of a single decision-maker; and the third involves negotiations between different people.

One of the most surprising facts about how managers made the strategic decisions we studied is that so few reported using explicit analysis. There was considerable bargaining, but in general the selection mode most commonly used was judgment. Typically, the options and all kinds of data associated with them entered the mind of a manager, and somehow a choice later came out. *How* was never explained. *How* is never explained in any of the literature either.

9. Finally, we turn to our research on strategy-making in organizations. This process does not turn out to be the regular, continuous, systematic process depicted in so much of the planning literature. It is most often an irregular, discontinuous process, proceeding in fits and starts. There are periods of stability in strategy development, but also there are periods of flux, of groping, and of global change. To my mind, "strategy" represents the mediating force between a dynamic environment and a stable operating system. Strategy is the organization's "conception" of how to deal with its environment for a time.

Now, the environment does not change in any set pattern. And even if it did, the human brain would be unlikely to perceive it that way. People tend to underreact to mild stimuli and overreact to strong ones. It stands to reason, therefore, that strategies that mediate between environments and organizations cannot change in regular patterns.

How does strategic planning account for these fits and starts? The fact is that it does not. So again, the burden to cope falls on the manager, specifically on his or her mental processes—intuitional and experiential—that can deal with the irregular inputs from the environment.

10. Where do new strategies come from? This is not the place to probe into that complex question. But research does make one thing

clear. Formal, analytical processes that generally go under the label of planning are not likely to produce innovative strategies so much as "mainline" ones common to organizations in a given industry.[5] Innovative strategies seem to result from informal processes—vague, interactive, and above all oriented to the synthesis of disparate elements. No management process is more demanding of holistic, relational thinking than the creation of an integrated strategy to deal with a complex, intertwined environment. How can analysis, under the label strategic planning, possibly produce such a strategy?

Another famous old story has relevance here. It is the one about the blind men trying to identify an elephant by touch. One grabs the trunk and says the elephant is long and soft; another holds the leg and says it is massive and cylindrical; a third touches the skin and says it is rough and scaly. As Ornstein points out:

> Each person standing at one part of the elephant can make his own limited, analytic assessment of the situation, but we do not obtain an elephant by adding "scaly," "long and soft," "massive and cylindrical" together in any conceivable proportion. Without the development of an overall perspective, we remain lost in our individual investigations. Such a perspective is a province of another mode of knowledge, and cannot be achieved in the same way that individual parts are explored. It does not arise out of a linear sum of independent observations.[6]

What can we conclude from these findings? I must first reemphasize that everything I write about the two hemispheres of the brain falls into the realm of speculation. Researchers have yet to formally relate any management process to the functioning of the human brain.* Nevertheless, these findings do seem to support the hypothesis stated earlier: *The important policy-level processes required to manage an organization rely to a considerable extent on the faculties identified with the brain's right hemisphere.*

This conclusion does not imply that the left hemisphere is unimportant for policy-makers. Every manager engages in considerable explicit calculation when he or she acts, and much intuitive thinking must be translated into the linear order of the left hemisphere if it is to be articulated and

---

* Almost concurrently with the publication of this article, Robert Doktor was, in fact, reporting on research with senior line managers and staff analysts which uncovered physiological evidence (through EEG measurement of brainwaves) for the lateral specialization implied here. See R. Doktor, "Problem Solving Styles of Executives and Management Scientists," *TIMS Studies in the Management Sciences,* no. 8 (1978), pp. 123–34.

eventually put to use. The great powers that appear to be associated with the right hemisphere are obviously useless without the faculties of the left. The artist can create without verbalizing; the manager cannot.

Truly outstanding managers are no doubt the ones who can couple effective processes of the right (hunch, intuition, synthesis) with effective processes of the left (articulateness, logic, analysis). But there will be little headway in the field of management if managers and researchers continue, like Nasrudin, to search for the key to management in the "lightness" of ordered analysis. Too much will stay unexplained in the "darkness" of intuition.

IMPLICATIONS FOR THE LEFT HEMISPHERE

What does all this mean for those associated with management?

First, I would not like to suggest that planners and management scientists pack up their bags of techniques and leave organizations, or that they take up basket-weaving or meditation in their spare time. (I haven't—at least not yet!) It seems to me that the left hemisphere is alive and well; the analytic community is firmly established, and indispensable, at the operating and middle levels of most organizations. Its real problems occur at the senior levels. Here analysis must coexist with—perhaps even take its lead from—intuition, a fact that many analysts and planners have been slow to accept. To my mind, organizational effectiveness does not lie in that narrow-minded concept called "rationality"; it lies in a blend of clear-headed logic *and* powerful intuition.

For one thing, only under certain circumstances should planners try to plan. When an organization is in a stable environment and has no use for an innovative strategy, then the development of formal, systematic strategic plans (and main-line strategies) may be in order. But when the environment is unstable or the organization needs an innovative strategy, then strategic planning may not be the best approach to strategy making, and planners have no business pushing their organizations to use it. Further, effective decision-making at the senior level requires good analytical input; it is the job of the planner and management scientist to ensure that top management gets it. Managers are very effective at securing soft information. But they tend to underemphasize analytical input that is often important as well. The planners and management scientists can serve their organizations effectively by carrying out ad hoc analyses and feeding the results to top management (need I say orally?), ensuring that the very best of analysis is brought to bear on policy-making.

For teachers of management, if the suggestions in this article turn out to be valid, then educators had better revise drastically some of their notions about management education. Unfortunately, the revolution in that sphere over the last fifteen years—while it has brought so much of value—has virtually consecrated the modern management school to the worship of the left hemisphere.

Should educators be surprised that so many of their graduates end up in staff positions, with no intention of ever managing anything? Some of the best-known management schools have become virtual closed systems in which professors with little interest in the reality of organizational life teach inexperienced students the theories of mathematics, economics, and psychology as ends in themselves. In these management schools, management is accorded little place. There is a need for a new balance in our schools, the balance that the best of human brains can achieve, between the analytic and the intuitive.

As for managers, the first conclusion should be a call for caution. The findings of the human brain should not be taken as license to shroud activities in darkness. Artificially mystifying behavior is a favorite ploy of those seeking to protect a power base; this helps no organization and neither does trying to impose intuition on activities that can be handled effectively by analysis. But a misplaced obsession with analysis is no better, and to my mind represents a far more prevalent problem today.

A major thrust of development in our organizations, ever since Frederick Taylor began experimenting in factories late in the last century, has been to shift activities out of the realm of intuition, toward conscious analysis. That trend will continue. But managers, and those who work with them, need to be careful to distinguish that which is best handled analytically from that which must remain in the realm of intuition. That is where we shall have to continue looking for the lost keys to management.

4

COUPLING ANALYSIS AND INTUITION IN MANAGEMENT

"Planning on the Left Side, Managing on the Right" did not resolve any issue so much as open up a number of difficult and, I believe, fundamental ones. First among these is the question of how our organizations should make use of the processes of analysis and intuition. Excessive use of intuition, perhaps common a century ago, can drive organizations toward idiosyncratic and arbitrary behaviors. But excessive reliance on analysis, which I believe to be the common case now, can make their behavior indifferent and unresponsive. How we couple these two processes has major implications, not only for the effectiveness of our organizations but for the society we are to live in.

I began on the analytic side of management. I was trained in engineering and accepted my first full-time job in the Operational Research Branch of Canadian National Railways. Operational research (called operations research, or OR, in the United States, also known as management science), seeks to apply systematic analysis to the problems of management. Later, when I did my masters degree at the MIT Sloan School of Management, I shifted my attention to the softer side of the field—the policy processes of senior management. But my interest in the role of analysis remained, and one stream of my articles has been directed to that group with which I first identified, the staff analysts of organizations—OR people, planners, information systems designers. Nothing in management has frustrated me more than what has been called the "rule of the tool," the use of technique for its own sake ("Give a little boy a hammer and it just so happens that everything needs pounding!").* These articles sought to help correct that.

---

* One of the founders of operational research during World War II in Britain, P. M. S. Blackett, defined it as "merely the scientific method applied to the complex data of human society."[1] By the 1970s, a prominent American practitioner would define it as "a comprehensive array of tested and proven tools."[2]

I have always considered Herbert Simon the most distinguished organization theorist of our time. Simon was trained in political science but early on joined the Graduate School of Industrial Administration at Carnegie-Mellon University, where he served as a major intellectual force in the development of the contemporary management school.

In the 1950s GSIA, as it is called, literally invented contemporary management education—the notions of basing it in the fundamental disciplines of economics, psychology, and mathematics, and of teaching theory derived from research, which was viewed at GSIA as the main task of the business school academic. Carnegie-Mellon in these respects was at least ten years ahead of other business schools, almost all of which now do (I shall soon argue overdo) these things as their natural way of functioning.

Simon's impact on our understanding of organizations, as well as on our attitudes toward research, has been profound, reflected in a publication list that numbers over five hundred items, including several major books in the field.[3] His contribution was recognized in 1978, when he was awarded the Nobel Prize. This was the prize in Economics, but Simon won it for his work in organization theory. In fact, since the early 1970s Simon has made his home in Carnegie-Mellon's psychology department, where he pursues his interests in decision-making through studies of human cognition.

I sent Simon a copy of "Planning on the Left Side and Managing on the Right" shortly after it was accepted for publication. He responded soon after, suggesting my argument was false. Just then receiving a telegram from the publisher requesting the article immediately, I spent a miserable forty-eight hours. I finally decided to proceed with the publication, which I feel represents a turning point in my career.

To that time, I was a fairly conventional scholar. I toyed with notions of intuition etc., but it was only after I decided to publish the article that I really opened up to them. Herbert Simon knew a great deal more than I about human cognition in decision-making; my problem during those forty-eight hours was to conclude whether he knew enough, in essence whether anyone really understood the full meaning of intuition. By concluding that no one did (I mean formally, not intuitively!), I was also concluding that society has paid a terrible price by rejecting it over the course of almost a century—in organizations, the study of organizations, and, behind that, the field of psychology itself.

I believe it is worth taking the space here to repeat some of the correspondence I had with Herbert Simon about the article, partly because it may be of interest in itself, but primarily because I believe it helps to introduce a critical issue that is addressed in the text that follows.

In earlier correspondence, Simon had mentioned he was revising *The New Science of Management Decision,* a small but important book about the impact of computers on organizations and especially about the need to bring the "modern techniques" of systematic analysis to bear on the "traditional," "nonprogrammed" decision processes of senior management. On March 17, 1976, I wrote him, in part:

> I have one question about that revision, which is implied in the enclosed paper. All of my work to date has proceeded on the assumption that we must specify as precisely as possible—"program," if you like—the organizational decision processes. I continue to work in this direction . . . but some reading I have recently done on the brain's two hemispheres (notably the book by Robert Ornstein entitled *The Psychology of Consciousness*) has upset this assumption somewhat. Perhaps the processes we call intuition are fundamentally different from those we can specify or program. Do we really yet understand the meaning of synthesis? This reading as well as gnawing questions which have remained in all of my own research stimulated me to write "Planning on the Left Side, and Managing on the Right," more to raise questions than to answer them. In any event, I am curious whether you will address this issue in the revision, and if so, how. I am beginning to believe that this may be a fundamental issue for us.

His letter of March 24, 1976, read as follows:

> I do not discuss the left–right brain evidence in the new revision, but I do discuss ill-structured problem solving. I believe that the left–right distinction is important, but not (a) that Ornstein has described it correctly, or (b) that it has anything to do with the distinction between planning and managing or conscious-unconscious.
>
> What I think it *does* have to do with is the role of perceptual recognition in problem solving. On this, we have done a good deal of work, in the environment of chess. I enclose a couple of reprints, which will give you a general idea of our local views on the matter, and I have incorporated some of these views in the revision. If you want to substitute "right hemisphere" for visual pattern recognition, you will have a first approximation of what I believe to be the case.
>
> The temptations are so great to romanticize about human performance

(and even to credit it with ESP for which there is no real evidence)! I will paraphrase one of the French philosophers: ''I have no need for that hypothesis.'' Was that Diderot? Perhaps one of your colleagues at Aix-en-Provence can identify the quotation.

We are now starting some research on managers' versus students' analysis of policy cases, using our perceptual hypothesis as a guide for what kinds of differences to look for. Perhaps in some months, we will have some results. Meanwhile, I would be inclined to go slow with left–right brain explanations of intuition. It is just the latest of a long series of fads—not the phenomenon, but this particular romantic explanation of it.

Simon's comment about ESP was in reference to two sentences in my original paper that both I and the *Harvard Business Review* editor, independently, deleted as too provocative. (In reference to the roles of oral communication and gestures in managerial work, they read in the original version: "I am tempted to raise the issue of extra-sensory perception here. There is clearly too much evidence to dismiss this as a medium of communication, at least for some people, and as Ornstein suggests, it is presumably a right hemisphere activity.") In fact, my decision to publish ultimately turned on that comment of Simon: While the presence of ESP may not have been *proved* in any scientific sense, to dismiss it for "no real evidence" suggested to me more about Simon's thinking than about ESP. The text of my letter to Simon of May 4, 1976, follows:

Your letter about my paper on managing and the two hemispheres of the human brain stimulated me to review it very carefully. When your letter arrived, the paper was already accepted for publication, but I was able to make changes. On balance, while I chose to tone down some of the specific comments linking management process to one hemisphere or the other, and to make clearer what is fact and what is speculation, I feel that it is important to proceed with the general theme. I believe that a number of the points in the paper need to be made, especially to management schools that I find have moved increasingly away from real management process.

As for your disagreement with Ornstein, the issue seems to come down to a question of whether or not there are two fundamentally different thought processes. I am concerned about a number of unexplained phenomena, for example the sudden discovery of a creative insight after a period of intellectual incubation. I'm tempted to side with Ornstein for the moment (that there are fundamentally different thought processes; that they do or not fall into distinct hemispheres interests me less; that is an issue for the physiologists, although the evidence seems tempting), while keeping a watchful eye on how far researchers like yourself can push the frontiers of linear simulation into real-world decision-making. It seems to me that you are uncomfortable with Ornstein's extrapolations from the tangible evidence of the research to date. I am not so uncomfortable, partly because they suggest so much to me and partly, I am sure, because I know so much less than you do about human cognition. But when we get right down to it, how much does anyone really know about creativity, concept formation, and the like? Ornstein's work does have all the trappings of a fad. I am generally opposed to fads; this one is the exception because it seems to explain so much behavior that I have observed informally. (May I say that my right hemisphere "feels" that Ornstein is on to something?) In any event, all of my other papers in one way or another have roots in your work; this one provides a counterpoint. My intention is primarily to provoke, to open some new channels of debate, not to make any definitive claims.

Incidentally, concerning "no real evidence" for ESP, have you by chance seen a book entitled "Psychic Discoveries Behind the Iron Curtain"? No one can invent that many lies. If only one of the hundreds of research studies reported there is valid, then the phenomenon cannot be dismissed as a "residual." The signal may not be identified, but the presence of communication is. Did you know that Turing,* in his paper reprinted in the Feigenbaum and Feldman book, while refuting in an elegant way a number of the arguments about why computers cannot think, hesitates on only one, commenting as follows:

> "I assume that the reader is familiar with the idea of extrasensory perception, and the meaning of the four items of it, viz., telepathy, clairvoyance, precognition and psychokinesis. These disturbing phenomena seem to deny all our usual scientific ideas. How we should like to descredit them! Unfortunately the statistical evidence, at least for telepathy, is overwhelming. It is very difficult to rearrange one's ideas so as to fit these new facts in. . . . This argument is to my mind quite a strong one. One can say in reply that many scientific theories seem to remain workable in practice, in spite of clashing with ESP; that in fact one can get along very nicely if

* An eminent British mathematician of the 1930s and 1940s.

one forgets about it. This is rather cold comfort, and one fears that thinking is just the kind of phenomenon where ESP may be especially relevant.'' (p. 29)

A year later, I published a review of Simon's revised *The New Science of Management Decision.* In later publications, in reference to the left and right hemisphere discussion, Simon has made clear his use of the word intuition in management. In the text that follows, I begin with excerpts from my book review, concentrating on my critique of Simon's view of intuition in management. I conclude with the juxtaposition of two single sentence quotations that diametrically oppose each other—one by Herbert Simon, the other by Roger Sperry, who also won a Nobel Prize, in his case in physiology, in 1981 for the split brain research. I then present Simon's more recent views on intuition, quoting from an article in a management journal of 1987. (In my request to him to reprint this correspondence, which also stated my wish to quote his more recent ideas, he suggested this particular article.)

While I continue to disagree with Simon's view of intuition, I agree fully with his final conclusion, that effectiveness in management depends ultimately on the coupling of analytic and intuitive processes. Accordingly, the rest of this chapter presents excerpts from three of my publications that sought to do that, with regard to the practice of strategic decision-making, of management information systems design, and of planning.

REVIEW OF THE NEW SCIENCE
OF MANAGEMENT DECISION

A brief word on history: *The New Science of Management Decision* was first published in 1960 as a fifty-page book, based on a series of lectures Herbert Simon gave at New York University on the nature of the executive decision process and the impact of new techniques on organizational decision-making and structure. A second version appeared in 1965 . . . under the title, *The Shape of Automation.* . . . "What we have in 1977 is a 175-page revised edition of the 1965 book with the 1960 title. . . . But the changes are not fundamental: ". . . revising this volume, although the revision is extensive, has been more a matter of updating the evidence and treating a number of topics more fully, than it has been a matter of altering the main findings and conclusions.''[4]

The New Science of Management Decision seeks to understand the effects that the computer has had, and by extrapolation will have, on organizations, the people who work in them, and the society in which they are embedded. . . .

If the essence of *The New Science of Management Decision* were to be captured in a single phrase, it would be that the book celebrates the results of technology, particularly of the information processing variety, on decision-making and structure in organizations, on the work of the executives at the top and the workers at the bottom, even on society and its capacity to solve the problems of pollution and overpopulation. . . .

> The processes of nonprogrammed decision making are beginning to undergo as fundamental a revolution as the one that is currently transforming programmed decision making in business organizations. Basic discoveries have been made about the nature of human problem solving, and their first potentialities for business application have already emerged. (p. 63)

My own research as well as my review of others' on the work of senior managers—those people most involved with nonprogrammed decision making—led to a very different conclusion, namely that "there is as yet no science in managerial work" . . . [and] that "even the computer . . . has apparently done little to alter the working methods of the general manager."[5]

[The review then considers the evidence Simon presents for his assumption, including his own research in the psychology laboratory, and ends with:] The sparseness of evidence cited notwithstanding, Simon draws a rather strong conclusion:

> The first thing we have learned—and the evidence for this is by now substantial—is that these human processes (problem solving, thinking, and learning) can be explained *without* postulating mechanisms at subconscious levels that are different from those that are partly conscious and partly verbalized. Much of the iceberg is, indeed, below the surface and inaccessible to verbalization, but its concealed bulk is made of the same kind of ice as the part we can see. The secret of problem solving is that there is no secret. It is accomplished through complex structures of familiar simple elements.[6]

I read [Simon's argument] with a good deal of incredulity. But my biggest surprise came when I discovered that Simon had written essentially the same thing in the 1960 edition of the book.* I had read that version in the mid-60s without surprise; indeed, I positively shared Simon's vision of the coming managerial revolution. What has changed since then? My own research on the work and decision processes of senior managers has certainly opened my eyes to a very different perspective, but that is beside the point in this review. Two fundamental events have taken place in those intervening years which have changed my views. . . . One exposed a fundamental problem with technology and analysis; the other suggests a possible explanation for the problem. . . .

Vietnam represented a critical turning point in the perceptions of many of us toward analysis. It would be trite to say that a reading of Halberstam's *The Best and the Brightest*[7] signaled that the honeymoon with analysis was over. Its relationship with management, which began in the factory with Frederick Taylor, flourished in the office with the introduction of Operations Research, and culminated in Robert McNamara's application of the Hitch and McKean[8] proposals for PPBS and cost-benefit analysis at the policy level, started to come apart in the rice paddies of Vietnam. Halberstam's carefully documented story makes it quite clear that this was no ordinary failure of analysis, not yet another one to be explained away in "implementation." Something was fundamentally wrong with the "formulation," that is, with analysis itself. Here the best and the brightest—not politicians or bureaucrats, but America's finest analytic talent, drawn from the centers of liberal intelligentsia—applied the modern techniques to the White House's nonprogrammed decisions, and the result was a war effort both ill-conceived and fundamentally immoral.

What went wrong? Could it have been the inability of analysis to handle the soft data—the expression on a peasant's face as opposed to a body count, the will of the enemy as opposed to the number of bombs needed to defoliate a jungle? "When [civilian advisers] said the Diem government was losing popularity with the peasants because of the Buddhist crisis, McNamara asked, well, what percentage was dropping off,

---

* The [above] quotation appears almost word-for-word. The only substantive change is the addition in 1977 of the phrase "and inaccessible to verbalization." Most curious is the statement seventeen years after the first edition: "It is only in the past twenty years that we have begun to have a good scientific understanding of the information processes that humans use in problem solving and nonprogrammed decision making." [Much of the research Simon cites is, in fact, discussed in the 1960 edition of the book as well.]

what percentage did the government have and what percentage was it losing? He asked for facts, some statistics, something he could run through the data bank, not just this poetry they were spouting.''[9] Could the facts have represented values?* In other words, can values inadvertently creep into the analysis when the number of dead bodies or the acres of defoliated jungle are measurable while the worth of a single human life is not?

Facts become impregnated with value when they consistently line up behind a single set of goals. In Vietnam they supported the military goals; the humanitarian goals, supported only by soft data, were driven out of the analysis. We see the same thing in corporations when the hard data line up behind the economic goals—cost reduction, profit increase, growth in market share—leaving the social goals—product quality, employee satisfaction, protection of the environment—to fend for themselves.[10] And in society itself, when pollution endures pending calculation of its costs, and chemicals continue to be pumped into our bodies until some scientist can "prove" that they are killing us (presumably by more body counts). When these things happen, analysis can no longer be called amoral: It drives even well-intentioned decision makers to make decidedly immoral choices. Shortly after the Bay of Pigs incident, Chester Bowles wrote of the Kennedy administration:

> The question which concerns me most about this new Administration is whether it lacks a genuine sense of conviction about what is right and what is wrong. . . .
>
> Anyone in public life who has strong convictions about the rights and wrongs of public morality, both domestic and international, has a very great advantage in times of strain, since his instincts on what to do are clear and immediate. Lacking such a framework of moral conviction or sense of what is right and what is wrong, he is forced to lean almost entirely upon his mental processes; he adds up the pluses and minuses of any question and comes up with a conclusion. Under normal conditions, when he is not tired or frustrated, this pragmatic approach should successfully bring him out on the right side of the question.
>
> What worries me are the conclusions that such an individual may reach when he is tired, angry, frustrated or emotionally affected. The Cuban fiasco demonstrates how far astray a man as brilliant and well intentioned as Kennedy can go who lacks a basic moral reference point.[11]

---

* In *Administrative Behavior,* Herbert Simon makes what has become a well-known distinction between facts and values in decision-making. See also Chapter 16 of this book.

If Vietnam exposed the problem, then a psychobiologist at the California Institute of Technology may have found the explanation. [The review then presents Roger Sperry's notions of the two hemispheres of the brain, much as discussed in "Planning on the Left Side, Managing on the Right," concluding that the right hemisphere] appears to be the seat of what we call judgment or intuition, the "instincts" Bowles found missing in the Kennedy administration, a likely place to deal with the soft data analysis cannot handle.

[Sperry's] speculation, of course, diametrically opposes that of Simon. To Sperry, the ice is not the same on both sides of the human brain; Simon's [research accesses] only one kind of ice; and sequential programming cannot simulate gestalt thinking.* In fact, Sperry has spoken out on this last point. In sharp contrast to Simon's statement that "We now know a great deal about what goes on in the human head when a person is exercising judgment or having an intuition, to the point where many of these processes can be simulated on a computer," Sperry has written . . . "The right [hemisphere], by contrast [with the left] is spatial, mute and performs with a synthetic spatio-perceptual and mechanical kind of information processing *not yet simulateable in computers*"[13]. . . .

On page 7 of his book, Simon asks: "How does one choose among experts? The easiest and commonest way is to accept an expert who confirms one's present beliefs and prior prejudices." As reviewer, I have not hidden my beliefs or prior prejudices. But then Simon adds, "We choose among experts by forcing the experts to disclose how they reached their conclusions, what reasoning they employed, *what evidence they relied upon*. . . . We do not have to be championship boxers to referee a fight."[14] I suppose that being the reviewer puts me in the ring as referee; I am certainly not here as a championship psychologist. Given the evidence Simon and Sperry rely upon in this match of speculations, I declare Sperry's two modes of thinking, only one that can be simulated in computers, the winner by a technical knockout!

---

* In discussing the simulation of human thought, Simon writes: "In solving problems, human thinking is governed by programs that organize myriads of simple information processes—or symbol manipulating processes if you like—into orderly, complex *sequences* that are responsive to and adaptive to the task environment and the clues that are extracted from that environment as the sequences unfold. Since programs of the same kind can be written for computers, these programs can be used to describe and simulate human thinking."[12]

To conclude, Simon's *The New Science of Management Decision* celebrates the effects of technology, analysis as well as automation. It does so to the point of concluding that all modes of thinking can be represented in sequential form, that what we call judgment or intuition can be simulated in the computer, and that the modern techniques of analysis must be applied to that judgment if society is to solve its problems. But we have also seen that other important [scientists] disagree. And of equal importance, we have seen that the issue has to do with much more than just the physiology of the brain; it may be the key to the management of our organizations and even to the ultimate survival of mankind itself. Many of us are coming to question increasingly the extent to which we can trust analysis untempered by intuition, to question whether truly humanitarian decisions will always have to be made in places inaccessible to Herbert Simon's computer.

SIMON'S CURRENT VIEW OF INTUITION

In an article published in the *Academy of Management Executive* of February 1987, entitled "Making Management Decisions: The Role of Intuition and Emotion," Herbert Simon reviews some evidence from physiological research and then notes that "the more romantic issues of the split-brain doctrine extrapolate this evidence into the two polar forms of thought labelled . . . as analytical and creative." But

> The evidence for this romantic extrapolation does not derive from the physiological research. As I indicated above, that research has provided evidence only for some measure of specialization between the hemispheres. It does not in any way imply that either hemisphere (especially the right hemisphere) is capable of problem solving, decision making, or discovery independent of the other. The real evidence for two different forms of thought is essentially the observation that, in everyday affairs, men and women often make competent judgments or reach reasonable decisions rapidly—without evidence indicating that they have engaged in systematic reasoning, and without their being able to report the thought processes that took them to their conclusion.
>
> There is also some evidence for the very plausible hypothesis that some people, confronted with a particular problem, make more use of intuitive processes in solving it, while other people make relatively more use of analytical processes.[15]

Simon then discusses some research on the "expert's intuition," particularly the ability of chess grandmasters to glance at a chessboard and quickly size up the situation. He argues that the expert recognizes familiar patterns, that "the secret of the grandmaster's intuition or judgment" is "previous learning that has stored the patterns and the information associated with them." Simon's own extrapolation is that "the experienced manager, too, has in his or her memory a large amount of knowledge, gained from training and experience and arranged in terms of recognizable chunks and associated information,"[16] and that the essence of intuition lies in the *organization* of knowledge for quick identification, and not in its rendering for inspired design. He cites, for example, one study in which business people could identify the key features of a case far faster than MBA students.

Simon concludes that "intuition is not a process that operates independently of analysis; rather the two processes are essential complementary components of effective decision-making systems." Therefore:

> It is a fallacy to contrast "analytic" and "intuitive" styles of management. Intuition and judgment—at least good judgment—are simply *analyses frozen into habit* and into the capacity for rapid response through recognition. Every manager needs to be able to analyze problems systematically (and with the aid of the modern arsenal of analytical tools provided by management science and operations research). Every manager needs also to be able to respond to situations rapidly, a skill that requires cultivation of intuition and judgment over many years of experience and training. The effective manager does not have the luxury of choosing between "analytic" and "intuitive" approaches to problems. Behaving like a manager means having command of the whole range of management skills and applying them as they become appropriate.[17]

Simon's view of intuition as "analyses frozen into habit" appears to me to be overly narrow, slighting especially the important phenomenon of creative insight (where did those famous new chess moves come from, anyway?). In none of the evidence he cites do I get a sense of how decision-makers see deeply into a complex problem, how they size up novel situations, how they leap to creative solutions.

Simon is well known for his concept of "bounded rationality," that people are limited in the amount of information they can process at any one time. In one rendition of this by psychologist George Miller, this amounts to about seven "bits" or "chunks" of information in our short and intermediate term memories.[18] The question remains, however, whether other things are going on deeper inside our brains—whether we are in fact restricted to processing discreet units of information (as are computers), as opposed, say, to vague "impressions" or "images," whatever form they may take, and, concomitantly, whether there are complex processes of synthesis taking place there that cannot be studied by the research methods of the cognitive psychologist.

Remember that much of Simon's work has been based on verbal protocols—voice articulations of the person's thoughts as he or she makes a decision. Words are bits; they express the results of thought processes that are available to the conscious mind, and they must be emitted in linear order. Thus, research that accesses the *conscious,* that does so via people's *input/output* devices (notably speech), and that assumes a posture that is essentially reductionist in nature, and therefore basically *analytic* (reflecting conventional "rationality," however "bounded"), has been used to draw inferences about *processes* that appear to be *subconscious* and based in a good part on *synthesis.* Is it any wonder then that intuition gets reduced to "analyses frozen into habit"?

Can attention to the bounded rationality of bits and chunks of information really capture feats of synthesis that take place in human minds—for example, Edwin Land's conception of the instant camera one day in Santa Fe? Can it explain the writing of Simon's own books, full of insights and representing tremendous integration of all kinds of ideas and information? Land himself has commented that during his intense periods of creative insight "atavistic competencies seem to come welling up. You are handling *so many variables* at a barely conscious level that you can't afford to be interrupted"[19] (presumably, even by the researcher's request for protocols!).

As human beings, we may have to articulate the results of our insightful syntheses in the linear order of words. But the processes by which we arrive at them seem to remain mysterious, not irrational so much, perhaps, as *a*rational, locked deep inside our subconscious minds.

But then again, will anyone ever be able to resolve this type of disagreement? If intuition is, by definition, a thought process in the subconscious, then how can we ever know we have probed deeply enough inside anyone's head to be sure we have captured what is going on there? (For example, what if Turing was right about ESP? That would leave not even "cold comfort" for anyone intent on understanding intuitive thought processes through research.) The researcher's tool is essentially analytical, as is the scholar's in debating this issue—words in linear order. How can rational analysis be used to prove or disprove the existence of an arational, nonanalytical thought process?

There is, however, cold comfort in the implication of Herbert Simon's final conclusion: that no matter what intuition really is—anything from the rapid recognition of the expert to the extrasensory perception of the psychic—clearly it must be combined with analysis in managerial decision-making. No organization can afford the luxury of being purely analytic or purely intuitive.

STRENGTHS AND WEAKNESSES OF ANALYSIS AND INTUITION

An expert has been defined as someone who avoids all the many pitfalls on his or her way to the grand fallacy. What makes this quotation of relevance here is that analytical and planning people in the field of management have long been inclined to blame their failures on a set of pitfalls, mostly of "implementation." They have claimed that managers don't understand analysis, that they don't support planning sufficiently, that the politicized climates of organizations impede the use of planning and analysis, and so on. But pitfalls are to organizations what sins are to religions—blemishes to be removed, so that people can get on with the more noble task of serving the almighty. These pitfalls ignore the more deeply rooted causes of the resistance to planning and analysis, which I believe should be labeled the fallacies of formulation—essentially misperceptions of how planning and analysis, as well as managers and organizations, need to work.

Implicit in a good deal of management science, information systems design, and formal planning have long been the assumptions that strategy making is a relatively static, orderly process (it is anything but); that discontinuities can be forecast through systematic procedures (there is no support for this whatsoever); that strategic management can be detached from operating management, with the senior managers informed by "hard" (namely computer-generated) data (managers who believe this are ignorant in two ways); and ultimately that the processes of making decisions and developing strategies can be formalized, or programmed, by systems that rely above all on decomposition. All these fallacies, to my mind, reduce to one grand fallacy: that to decompose is to recombine, in other words, that analysis includes synthesis. In the final analysis (so to speak), synthesis is not analysis, but rather is rooted in the mysteries of intuition.

Analysis and intuition differ not only in how they work but also in their respective strengths and weaknesses. Let us consider several of these.

COST. Ask almost anyone which process is more costly and the quick response will be "analysis." After all, it takes time to study an issue systematically, whereas intuition is right there with an answer. Well, this might be an example of intuition itself leaping to the wrong conclusion, because the question turns out to be more involved than it first seems. The fact is that analysis has a high *operating* cost, but its *investment* cost is relatively low (just hire a few freshly minted MBAs). Intuition, on the other hand (again, so to speak), has almost no operating cost ("Hey, Fred, should we expand into Guadeloupe?"). But its investment cost is high: A person has to know a subject deeply, has to have long and intimate experience with it, to be able to deal with it effectively through intuition. (Simon comments in his article about the need for at least ten years before a chess grandmaster or other "expert" can recognize those chunks quickly.)

ERROR. Also, again on first thought, analysis appears to be systematic, intuition haphazard. But several studies have shown that although analysis, when correct, tends to be precisely correct, when it errs it can produce strange answers. "Analytic thinking involves measurement and calculation and 'resembles the switching of trains at a multiple junction, with each of the possible courses being well organized and of machine-like precision yet leading to drastically different destinations.' "[20] Switch one track incorrectly and you might head in exactly the opposite direction to the one desired; misplace one decimal point, and you might be off by a factor of ten. Intuition, in contrast, while not usually precise, is generally close enough on certain kinds of issues. Figure 4–1 demonstrates this in one experiment, where the intuitive approach had a narrower range of errors while the analytic approach was more often precisely correct.[21] Thus, just as organizations need to confirm the speculations of intuition with systematic analysis, so too do they need to "eyeball" the results of formal analysis with "commonsense" intuition. When they need precision, they must rely on analysis, but when they don't, it is sometimes easier, even safer, to rely on intuition.

EASE. While intuition is subject to the biases of emotion and experience, analysis can sometimes prove terribly cumbersome at tasks that prove simple for intuition. As Polanyi has noted for what here may be an analogy if not an example, any five-year-old can ride a bicycle without conscious thought. But for analysis, "to ride a bicycle . . . it is necessary at any given angle of unbalance for the rider to give a turn to the front

FIGURE 4–1

Distribution of Errors in an Experiment of Intuitive and Analytical Thinking
(in Peters et al., 1974:128)

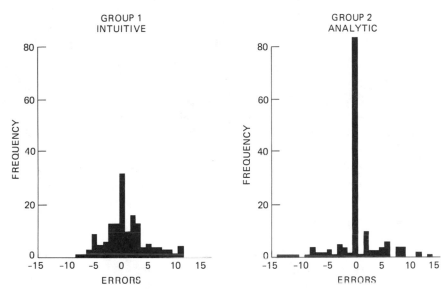

wheel that is by some measure inversely proportional to the square of the speed at which he is proceeding.''[22] Curtis put it well when he claimed: ''The [intuitive] people tend to act before they think, if they ever think; and the [analytic] people think before they act, if they ever act.''[23] Or more succinctly, being forced to choose only one may amount to either ''extinction by instinct'' or ''paralysis by analysis.''[24]

COMPLEXITY. Jay Forrester has argued in a paper entitled ''The Counter-Intuititve Behavior of Social Systems'' that intuitive interventions in complex social systems (such as urban decay) have often worked to aggravate rather than correct the problem, because our brains cannot comprehend complex feedback loops without the aid of formal models.[25] But someone could also write ''the counter-*analytic* behavior of social systems,'' because an understanding of some such systems is also dependent on the use of soft data inaccessible to computers, indeed sometimes even to analysis in any form.

CREATIVITY. Then there is the achievement of creativity. That too requires a form of synthesis beyond just analysis. That is why analytic techniques—planning included—have tended to produce incremental adaptations more than innovative breakthroughs. "Premature closure" is a major problem in analysis. It tends to impose structure on problems too early, by seizing upon convenient alternatives so that the analysts can get on with the process of evaluating them, which is where most of their techniques apply. As McKinney and Keen have stated, "The systematics preferred program-type problems while the intuitives liked open-ended ones, especially those that required ingenuity or opinion."[26] On the other hand, while intuition may be the source of creativity, it can also be constrained by experience and tradition. "That's not thirty years of experience; that's one year of experience thirty times," the analyst tells the experienced manager. Thus, while analysis may provide moderate change and limited creativity, intuition would seem to provide either dramatic creativity or none at all, indeed sometimes resistance to change.

Given these strengths and weaknesses, it becomes clear why organizations need to couple analysis with intuition. Let us now consider the roles of analysis alongside intuition in decision-making, in the design of information systems, and in strategy formation.

THE ROLE OF ANALYSIS IN STRATEGIC DECISION-MAKING

The first generally recognized operations research study, "a quite elementary analysis of fighter losses over France in May 1940, which helped in the momentous decision not to send any more British fighters over France,"[27] was, according to the group leader, "an impromptu two-hour study."[28]

Operations research seems to have worked best when it involved clever people, comfortable with numbers, who could bring common sense alongside analytical thinking (as opposed to analytical technique) to bear on complex organizational problems. Managers, many of whom are inclined to overlook the hard data, can be helped by analysts who have the time and the inclination to feed such analysis into decision-making. What this amounts to is "soft analysis," in which teams of interdisciplinary analysts couple a certain amount of intuitive sense with their more systematic thinking.

> The good systems analyst is a "chochem," a Yiddish word meaning "wise man," with overtones of "wise guy." His forte is creativity. Although he sometimes relates means to ends and fits ends to match means,

he ordinarily eschews such pat processes, preferring instead to relate elements imaginatively into new systems that create their own means and ends.[29]

Soft analysis can provide managers not with solutions so much as perspectives they may be inclined to overlook because of the time pressures of their jobs and their orientation toward oral forms of communication. It can suggest new means to consider market or economic forces, or new conceptions of the functioning of their own organizations. Soft analysis can expose errors in intuitive thinking and question long held assumptions. It can be "quick and dirty analysis" on complex, pressing problems, so that a manager who must make a decision in a busy week can benefit from the equivalent of several weeks of the work of a team of analysts.

THE ROLE OF *MIS* IN INFORMATION PROCESSING

Many *management* information systems (MIS) seem not to be for management at all. They are *computer* information systems and proceed on the assumption that managers care that the information has been processed by a machine. In fact, as discussed earlier, what managers seem to care about is that their information is timely and relevant, and much information that comes from the computer is not. As a result, managers have to build their own MIS. The "rule of the tool" strikes again.

What MIS people tend to overlook are the limitations of formal information. In a monograph for the Canadian and American management accounting associations, entitled "Impediments to the Use of Management Information," I reviewed some reasons why managers seem to fail to use information as they apparently should. A number of the reasons lay in the inadequacies of formal information, while others pertained to problems in the functioning of organizations and ones rooted in the human brain.

INADEQUACIES OF FORMAL INFORMATION

1. Formal information is often too limited. Much formal management information is simply not sufficiently rich for the manager (e.g., ignoring information on lost sales or on risk); it precludes much that is nonquantitative (politics, personality, quality, etc.) and noncommunicable (tone of voice, gesture, facial expression, etc.); moreover, it tends to be weak on the external situation.

2. Formal information, by aggregating data, is often too general for the manager. It is not the cumulative data on the sales drop that may count so much as the specific reason why a particular Mrs. Consumer didn't buy your toothpaste last month. In other words, one informal discussion can sometimes be far more revealing than reams of statistics.

3. Much formal information is too late. It takes time for events to become facts, more time for those facts to be recorded and aggregated, to appear in a periodic report. Thus, while the American leaders in Washington were reading about the dead body counts of Vietnam, live Vietcong were marching down the jungle paths. It is often the necessarily quick response in the short run that dictates performance in the long run, even for the most senior managers of the largest organizations.

4. Some formal information is unreliable. Which statistics can anyone be sure of? In those body counts, who was a Vietcong and who an innocent bystander? What about scores on IQ-type tests? In business, what do quality figures really measure; can anyone be sure of market data; does increased profit reflect better performance or forgone investment mistakenly recorded as cut costs?

FUNCTIONING PROBLEMS IN ORGANIZATIONS

Formal information systems do not, of course, contain the only inadequacies. Organizations too have their limitations with regard to the processing of information.

5. Rigid, dysfunctional objectives can encourage the use of inappropriate information. Maintenance can, for example, be cut or research forgone as managers react to the pressures of short-term profit measures.

6. Politics can cause the distortion of information. People are inclined to send up the hierarchy information that makes them look good. In fact, Robert McNamara, who as U.S. Secretary of Defense probably did more than any other manager to promote analysis in government, is reported to have deliberately distorted the cost estimates sent to Congress on the Vietnam war.[30]

7. The nature of managerial work introduces a bias in favor of oral channels of information at the expense of documented sources. This point has already been discussed at length; suffice it here to note that oral channels have their obvious limitations too, in terms of inconsistencies and superficialities.

LIMITATIONS OF THE HUMAN BRAIN

Finally, beyond the inadequacies of information itself and of the arrangements of the organization lie our inadequacies as human beings to process correctly all the information we receive.

8. Cognitive limitations restrict the amount of information that people consider in a complex decision process. Herbert Simon has argued this point in much of his work. People can focus on only a few elements at a time; they lose detail in what can be retained in short-term memory and stored in long-term memory. Simon quotes an all too common newspaper story about how the State Department, "drowning in a river" of 15 million words a month, "has turned to the computer for help." Officials claimed that would "eliminate bottlenecks in the system" by "absorbing cable messages electronically at a rate of 1,200 lines a minute." Simon remarks: "A touching faith in more water as an antidote to drowning! Let us hope that Foreign Ministers will not feel themselves obliged to process those 1,200 lines of messages per minute just because they are there."[31]

9. The brain systematically filters information in line with its established patterns of experience. In other words, to reverse the old adage, believing is seeing. Marketing people see problems as marketing related, finance people as having to do with the numbers.

10. Psychological failures and threats further impede the brain's openness to information. All of our psychological problems get reflected in the information we end up processing and retaining. There is a good deal of evidence on these last two points from psychology.

To summarize, of all the available information, the formal systems capture only a subset; of what is captured, the managers receive only a subset; of what is received, the brain absorbs only a subset; and of what the brain absorbs, only a subset is relevant and accurate in the first place. With all of these impediments, it is a wonder that organizations get anything right!

Of course, they usually do. But there are clear messages for the designer of a true MIS. Above all, it must exist in good part independent of the computer. Systems should feed managers the information they need when and how they need it, based on what they actually use, whether or not that happens to be convenient to the tool called a computer. That tool is a means for handling large quantities of quantitative information, nothing more. Oral channels should be used alongside documentary ones, and information should be stored in convenient places, in paper files and assistants' heads no less than on magnetic disks. The MIS should also filter information for managers on an *intelligent* basis, for example, reducing it not just by aggregating it but also by isolating its key messages. Despite the excitement about so-called expert systems, that will probably continue to require human brains, not electronic ones, in my opinion.

THE ROLE OF PLANNING (AND PLANNERS) IN STRATEGY-MAKING

"Strategic planning" was very popular in the 1960s; by the 1980s, a series of setbacks, not least the energy crisis of the 1970s, to which planning had great difficulty responding, had seriously reduced its role in organizations. But there was no need to throw out the baby with the bathwater—planning as well as planners have important roles to play in organizations.

The grand fallacy expressed itself here in the belief that strategy could be formulated formally, that the analytic procedures of planning could generate the synthesis required in strategy. It was the old machine assumption: Assemble all the parts (steps, checklists, techniques) and you have an operating whole. But machines are first designed somewhere else, whereas the planning machine itself was supposed to produce the blueprint—the strategy. That is why the phrase "strategic planning"—like Progressive Conservative or fresh frozen (or civil engineer?)—has proved to be an oxymoron.

In a forthcoming book on strategic planning, I consider the evidence on this process and its pitfalls and fallacies before considering the roles that planning, plans, and planners might play in various types of organizations.

Part of the problem has been with the definition used for planning itself. To associate planning with future thinking in general, as has often been done, is to render the term so broad as to lose all practical meaning. ("If Planning Is Everything, Maybe It's Nothing," is the title Aaron Wildavsky used for an article.[32]) So too is to associate planning with decision-making, as has also been done. If planning means, as I think it most logically does, formalized procedure to produce articulated results about coordinated systems of decisions, then one thing I think becomes clear: Planning is not a means to create strategy but one to operationalize strategies already created by other means.

Strategic programming would thus seem to be a more appropriate label, entailing the working out of the consequences of strategies in terms of budgets, programs, action plans, and the like. Thus, organizations would logically engage in planning when they already have viable intended strategies and need to formalize them into a future that appears to be stable or at least predictable.

That is not, of course, to deny roles for people called planners, aside from operating the systems of strategic programming. Planners are, in some sense, the analysts of the strategy-making system. They can carry out ad hoc studies to feed managers information they might otherwise overlook: that a market is being undermined by a new technology, that competitor postures seem to be changing, that organizational strengths may be faltering in a certain area. Planners can also scrutinize the viability of strategies managers intend to pursue, and even undertake the search for potentially viable strategies that may be emerging in strange places around the organization itself. These things would, of course, involve a good deal of soft analysis.

Planners can be catalysts too, but not to promote strategic planning as some kind of religion so much as to encourage strategic *thinking* to keep the organization viable. In some sense, the planners are the ones most inclined to think conceptually about the strategy-making process in organizations. They must try to understand its complexities and nuances (including when it is best to avoid formal planning), and feed that understanding to the managers charged with running that process.

Of course, planners can be strategists too—anyone can who happens to be bright, creative, well informed, and adept at synthesis. But that has nothing to do with the fact that they are planners; their techniques give them no advantage in this regard, indeed perhaps a disadvantage.

In a sense, we end up with a planner for each side of the brain. On one hand, we have the highly analytic planner, the strategic programmer who brings order to the managers' strategies for purposes of implementation, and also carries out analyses to feed hard data into the front end of the strategy-making process. On the other hand, we have the soft planner, a more creative, divergent thinker, rather intuitive in addition to being analytical, who seeks to open up the strategy-making process by conducting quick and dirty studies, finding emergent strategies in strange places, and stimulating others to think strategically, perhaps sometimes doing so himself or herself. As we shall see, some organizations need to rely more on the traditional "righthanded planners," others on the less traditional "lefthanded planners." But in the spirit of coupling analysis with intuition, most need some degree of both.

5

TRAINING MANAGERS,
NOT MBAs

There remains one last consequence of the analysis–intuition issue, alluded to earlier. In "Planning on the Left Side, Managing on the Right," I commented on how business school education has been virtually consecrated to the worship of the brain's left hemisphere. To my mind, the balance that Simon seeks has been totally lost in most of our business schools.*

In 1980, two Harvard Business School professors, Hayes and Abernathy, published an award-winning article entitled "Managing Our Way to Economic Decline."[1] They argued, among other things, that overly analytical business schools were partly responsible for a misguided obsession with technique and analysis in practice. Few disagreed. Well, since then I have watched business school education become more analytic, not less. I have seen professors of finance continue to search for the respect of economists by teaching increasingly irrelevant mathematical models. I have watched many of the behavioral scientists who have infiltrated business schools strut around like high priests seeking to ensure a degree of "scientific" rigor in research sufficient to detach researchers from the very organizations they are supposed to understand. The field of management information systems, ostensibly concerned with application, continues to try to define itself by what a machine is claimed able to do (but never quite does, although no one dares to find out). Even my own field of strategy, which maintained a balance before 1980, has since tilted in favor of the "number crunchers" more inter-

* Though this can be traced to the indiscriminate embracing of the very changes in business school education—an emphasis on rigorous research and theory development rooted in the basic disciplines of economics, psychology, and mathematics—that Simon and his colleagues at Carnegie-Mellon so vigorously promoted in the 1950s. In his book *The Sciences of the Artificial*,[2] Simon does, however, deplore the reluctance of business schools to teach ''design'' (to train ''in the core professional skills'') alongside the fundamental disciplines.

ested in the techniques of "competitive analysis" than the nuances of crafting strategies. I do not exaggerate one bit by claiming that if those people in business and government who support today's business schools really knew what was going on inside many of them, including some of the best known, really took the trouble, for example, to interview the professors at random, they would be demanding revolutionary changes in faculty and curriculum instead of passively writing checks.

I don't write such checks, but I do receive them. A few years ago I decided to put my money where my mind was and do the kind of management training I believed in. I proposed a reduction in my teaching and my salary at McGill in order to restrict my academic work to research and doctoral training while focusing my managerial training on experienced practitioners in the field.

My research and writing have always come first in my professional life. Some years ago, in a *Fortune* article entitled "The MBA—the Man, the Myth, and the Method," Zalaznick made the interesting point that the real contribution of the American business school lay not in its graduates from teaching so much as in its insights from research.[3] I still believe this to be true, at least for that portion of research that remains creative and applied to organizations.

I have long had concerns about undergraduate education in management and have not done it for many years (although I do believe in accounting training at that level, since accounting really is a profession). More recently I developed similar concerns about the conventional MBA. Increasingly I have come to believe that it is wrong—socially as well as economically—to train relatively inexperienced people in management. A few years of prior experience does help, but that does not resolve the fundamental problem. We cannot afford to have a society of elitist managers, preselected at a young age on the basis of academic criteria and then promoted on a "fast track" outside of the difficult work of making products and serving customers. Thus, I have come to believe that management training should be directed at people who have substantial organizational experience coupled with proven leadership ability as well as the requisite intelligence.

As a result, three years ago, with the understanding cooperation of the McGill administration, I taught my last MBA class. About a year later I addressed a meeting of the directors of MBA programs in Canada about these issues. What follows is the material of that talk, prepared for publication in this book. It may sound like a diatribe; I stand behind every word of it. Its implications will be pursued further in the final chapter of this book.

I propose to address my concerns about conventional MBA training in terms of how students get into the program in the first place, how they then go through it, and finally how they come out of it—in systems terms, input, throughput, and output.

APPLICANT INPUT

People come into MBA programs largely on the basis of two sets of criteria. First, they select themselves, by virtue of applying to the program in the first place. In other words, the pool of applicants from which the students are chosen is not defined by any leadership ability, real or potential, but simply by their desire for an MBA. This may reflect an interest in management, but all too often it simply reflects an interest in income. Business schools can certainly screen candidates for leadership or managerial potential, but at the age of, say, twenty-four, usually with no more than two or three years of full-time work experience, this is a chancy means of selection at best.

The other set of criteria is the hard numbers of performance. There are no hard numbers of work performance (beyond years of simply doing it), but there certainly are ones of test performance: grades on examinations (the grade point average, or GPA) and the notorious GMAT (Graduate Management Aptitude Test). Don't underestimate business schools' use of these. After all, they provide objective criteria for selection, and anything to do with management (or at least the teaching of management) has to be above all else objective. No matter what the object.

I know of no evidence that relates high GMAT score to success in the practice of management. Certainly a low score (by a native English speaker at least) may signal a problem of intelligence, and good managers must be intelligent. But how intelligent? It has long been known that there is no correlation between intelligence (as measured on IQ tests) and creativity above a certain moderate level. In other words, intelligent people range widely in their creativity. So too, I believe, do they in their managerial ability. In fact, when I see a score of 796 on a GMAT or a GPA of 4.9, I wonder if I am not as likely to be facing an "idiot-savant" as someone who is worldly, a person who can ace tests but can't talk to a customer.

I am a graduate of the MIT Sloan School masters program (yes, a young MBA). In their magazine recently,[4] they published statistics on their 1986 class. "Over 1,500 men and women vied for 185 places." Applicants were put into twelve levels, "based roughly on their numerical addition," which is made up of a variety of factors, including GMAT scores and GPA. "Admission is granted primarily to applicants falling in the top three levels." In fact, no one was rejected or waitlisted in the first two levels (some were deferred), while every single candidate in levels eight to twelve was rejected. The average GMAT scores for Levels I and II were both 680, and the GPAs, 4.6 and 4.5. For Levels VIII to XII, those averages ranged from 590 to 615 and 4.1 to 4.3.* Associate Dean Barks takes issue with my suggestion that MIT makes its decisions on the basis of these two scores. But surely the results suggest considerable attention to them,† unless of course there is a remarkable correlation between these scores and other, softer factors in assessing managerial potential.

A famous article of years ago, entitled "The Myth of the Well-Educated Manager,"[5] by Harvard's Professor Stirling Livingston, in fact suggested contrary evidence for that correlation—the lack of relationship between grades at the Harvard Business School and subsequent success in management jobs. Livingston's implication was that there was a need to assess intuitive skills and street sense, not just academic prowess.

There is a problem with assessing the intuition of MBA applicants, however: Intuition hardly gets a chance to manifest itself at a young age. A person simply cannot be effectively intuitive about things of which he or she has only superficial understanding. So it becomes difficult to know if even the potential for good intuition is present in most MBA applicants.

Moreover, even if the potential for intuition were there, its absence in *developed* form means that it cannot be used in the training process. Thus much of the conventional MBA program reduces to the formally analytical. The students can only appreciate formal knowledge, generally in the form of technique. And that, of course, is what they promote

---

* Which group of applicants would my 1963 GMAT of 602 and GPA of well under 4 have put me in 1986?

† Early in his article, Barks writes: "The aspects of quality that can be measured [for those applying] are indeed impressive, with a median GMAT of 630 and a mean GPA of 4.3 for all applicants" (p. 3). But can management *quality* in fact be measured? In the Zalaznick article in *Fortune,* it can be seen how far back this inclination to rely on numbers goes: He reports that the incoming Stanford class in 1958 was close to the median GMAT of 500; by 1968, it had attained the 96th percentile at 650 (p. 171).

immediately after they graduate—at least if their two years of training in business school is to have had any purpose. No wonder young MBA graduates run around putting down intuition whenever it rears its mysterious head. (In a subsequent talk I gave on these ideas to a class of MBA students, one young student came up with the marvelous comment that "How can you select for intuition when you can't even measure it!")

My criterion for entry to management education is very simple: proven success in managerial work. This would mean two things. First, applicants would need extensive practical experience; most would be in their thirties before even being considered for such education. My preference would be for intensive experience, well within at least one industry, preferably one organization, so that the knowledge base is deep, or "thick," as anthropologists might put it. I would not favor accepting "professional managers," those "birds of passage" who flit from one situation to another. Second, the candidates' leadership and management ability would have to be proven. They would, in other words, be selected not by themselves but by the subordinates who follow them, the peers who respect them, the supervisors who appreciate them. In this way, management training would not be wasted on people who are unlikely to be effective managers—a sizable number of today's MBA students, I should think.

I am, of course, making the assumption here that the MBA means to combine the B with the A. In other words, we are seeking to train for administration as well as for business. It could also be argued that we should decouple the two, train people for certain positions in business—namely the more analytical, such as marketing research or accounting—without pretending that we are training them to be managers. But that would require changing a great many established expectations, including those of the applicants who believe they will attain positions of power quickly because they sat in a classroom for a couple of years, the many recruiting firms that believe they are hiring their future leaders, and the business schools whose budgets are predicated on continuation of the production of about 60,000 MBAs annually (in the United States at least).

I do not mean to suggest that education for management is ineffective, only that it makes little sense when the student lacks the knack for leadership. Some years ago, Herbert Simon suggested in reference to the nature–nurture debate that if you wish to develop a star athlete, you must begin with someone who has the "natural endowment" (not me for instance) and then "by dint of practice, learning and experience develops that . . . into a mature skill."[6] We have good things to teach in management; let's teach them to people who can use them.

Management theory, like any other, is conceptual and abstract. People without experience cannot appreciate it. They are bound to run around like loose cannons believing that linear programming or portfolio models are the answer to all the world's problems. Seasoned managers, in contrast, have the experience on which to hang the concepts. Some of these run around half-cocked too, looking for the quick fix. But at least experience enables one to question the validity of a theory. And philosophers of science like Karl Popper notwithstanding (a secretary of mine once typed his name as Propper), the best test of an applied theory is still whether intelligent practioners find it more helpful than any other to deal with their problems.

CONTENT THROUGHPUT

What to teach those who get into management training? Given a class of the relatively inexperienced, you certainly don't stress the subtleties of intuition. You inundate them with methods and techniques, the more quantitative the better. After all, the teachers are researchers who may well have even less experience and higher GMAT scores than the students. Teach them statistics (for its own sake), mathematics (labeled "finance"), and behaviorial psychology (under "marketing"). Never, absolutely never, utter the word "judgment," let alone "intuition." Under "strategy," teach them to process reams of hard data on markets and competitors, like good economists. I recently had a vigorous exchange with a psychologist teaching in a business school who did not appreciate my assertion that psychologists, mathematicians, and economists who have no interest in adopting an organizational perspective should not be taking up places in the business schools. Business schools may have to *draw* on these disciplines, within limits (which in my opinion have long been surpassed). But that hardly justifies them in trying to *replicate* these disciplines.

My ideal management education would change the priorities. It would contain less analysis and prescription, more soft material and insights into how the world of organizations really does work, as opposed to how it should work. Incidentally, it need not be an MBA program, or even a form of the so-called executive MBA (although that is a fine idea). It might just be a series of ad hoc short courses for busy practioners. (And I have no concern about the B in the MBA. We need to teach *management,* and it really makes little difference whether that be for hospital directors, government administrators, or business people. I believe management schools should call their degree master in administration and then let the students add the B in the middle if they wish to emphasize business.)

First, in my ideal management program I would emphasize *skill training,* "experiential" education if you like, devoting perhaps a third of the effort to it. This would involve much more than the usual interpersonal skills, however. Equally important are skills at collecting information, at conducting negotiations, at making decisions under conditions of ambiguity, and so on. Of course, I refer not only, not even primarily, to skills exercised through systematic technique, but to those that rely on the softer processes of intuition as well.

In fact, a good deal is known about inculcating such skills, but not in the business schools. A few years ago, we started using a simulation called the "Looking Glass" at McGill, developed at the Center for Creative Leadership in Greensboro, North Carolina. It is a kind of elaborate in-basket exercise in which teams of managers compete with each other in a simulated (but not computer) setting. Watching our MBA students run around the building playing manager, it struck me that this was the first time I ever saw anybody practicing management in the management school (unless you put that label on what the dean does!). Finally we were teaching management, even if only for two days a year.*

The fact is that our management schools do not generally hire people capable of teaching true managerial skills. The PhD is the license to teach in a business school. But that degree neither preselects nor trains for skill in pedagogy, certainly not of the experiential kind. The PhD is a research degree, and in good part it attracts introverts, people who want to bury themselves in a library or under a stack of data. (That is why the questionnaire is such a popular research device—not so much because it has any intrinsic advantage as because it allows academics to do research without ever leaving their offices.) There are certainly

---

* I was also struck by the superficiality of the exercise—the "managers" were "managing" something they learned about only a few days earlier. But then it struck me that I had sometimes seen exercises not much less superficial in real-life executive suites! Perhaps it was an all-too-realistic simulation after all!

academics who are great teachers, even some who are great at skill teaching. But that is purely coincidental, and in any event, these are few in my opinion.

Without the innate ability to teach, teacher training (like management training) is of little help. But we don't even try. Some years ago, in the development of our own PhD program in management, we proposed a course in pedagogy. One course. Just 3 percent of the total program devoted to pedagogy, with 97 percent left for research, for a degree, it should be noted, that licenses people to spend about as much time teaching as doing research. Some of my colleagues disagreed—excessive attention to pedagogy, I guess they believed—but we managed to get it accepted. I'll bet there are not many other such courses around.

The ability to train for managerial skills resides largely in the field, with people who teach "in-house" for the big organizations or who work on a consulting basis. These people devote their efforts exclusively to pedagogy, with no need to be skilled at research. Thus, we do have some natural division of labor between scholarship and management training, but we have not pursued it to its logical conclusion. Perhaps the universities have no business trying to train managers, at least not in the sphere of skill development.

Second—and here I believe the universities *do* have the natural advantage—I would devote perhaps another third of my management education to *descriptive insight,* informing managers about how their world works. I refer here to understanding in a formal or conceptual sense, theory based on systematic research—the domain of the scholar.

The trouble with prescription is that it cannot be applied in general. No one approach can solve the problems of managers from many different organizations, all sitting in one classroom. Prescription belongs in context: It has to be done in a specific situation, tailored to the needs of that place at that particular time.

Critical to effective prescription is effective diagnosis, and that depends on the best possible understanding of the situation in question. In management, we simply lack generic categories of problems and their symptoms—quick ways to diagnose issues and prescribe solutions, as perhaps exist in medicine. Each management problem, at least at senior levels, has usually to be studied on its own terms. That is why I believe *de*scription is the most powerful *pre*scriptive tool we have, in the right hands—those of the *informed* practitioner. (And that is why I see my role as researcher not to create technique but to develop insight, and my role as educator not to prescribe change but to disseminate that insight. Only when I serve as a consultant, in a specific context, do I have any business being prescriptive. Which I guess is what I am doing now—as self-proclaimed consultant to management educators!)

The actual content of this descriptive material could cover two areas. First is the basic functioning of organizations—how they make decisions and form strategies, how they process information, how their managers work, and so on. Second is the basic knowledge about the environments of organizations—the economic, political, social, financial, etc., contexts. But this material must be presented not to preclude intuition, as is so often done now, but to make the very best use of it alongside more formal knowledge.

Theory is a dirty word in some quarters. But we all function on the basis of theories, whether they are formal and explicit or informal and subconscious. Keynes has been paraphrased frequently on this point: The "practical" person is often the prisoner of some defunct theorist. Our job as trainers is to get managers to hold their implicit theories up to scrutiny by challenging them with alternate theories, ones developed more systematically. Managers have to consider when it is beneficial to watch the world through a different lens, for example to think of strategy formation as an informal craft instead of a process of formal planning.

Clearly, there is no shortage of bad theory in our field. You can usually tell it by the ugliness of its labels—the "vertical dyad linkage model" (believe it or not, about leadership) is my favorite example. Abraham Kaplan, in *The Conduct of Inquiry,* talks about the "esthetic qualities of a theory,"[7] and I suspect he is correct that a harmonious theory, one that is nicely constructed and labeled, is more likely to be valid and useful than an ugly one. In any event, intelligent managers with deep-rooted knowledge of their practice can usually sort out the more and less useful theories.

From the outset of my teaching career, I emphasized descriptive theory in the classroom. But soon the questions came: "Hey, listen, Prof, it's fine to hear about how managers do work and how organizations do make strategies, but when·are you going to tell us how these things should be done, something we can use the day we graduate." "Wait," I would answer, "it's coming at the end of the course." I stopped saying that a few years later (since I had little to say about it at the end of the course). Instead I began to shoot back: "If you didn't know how the doorknob worked, you would never have been able to get inside this classroom. What makes you think you understand how organizations work? These are immensely complicated systems. What would you do with prescription even if I gave it to you?'' I now say much the same thing to the executives I teach: "Don't expect prescription from me; the best thing I can do for you—in fact, anyone standing up here in front of all your different organizations can do for you—is to provide you with rich description, alternate ways to view your world. If it's good, you'll know what to do with it.''

Why do we in the field of management persist in this premature, all-embracing prescription? It has taken us off course time and time again throughout this century, whether it was participative management (change your leadership style the way you change your clothing), strategic planning (creativity by checklist), or the current obsession with the bottom line (making profits by managing, not products, markets, or customers, but profits themselves). God spare us yet another finance professor arguing that the reason managers are so bored with his teaching is that he is so far ahead of them.

Imagine a student in an engineering class saying, "Hey, listen, Prof, it's fine to hear about how atoms *do* work, but when are you going to tell us how they *should* work?'' Engineering students learn physics, and medical students physiology, because everyone knows that you cannot practice those jobs without a deep understanding of the phenomena in question. Why do we persist in thinking management is any different in this regard?

Third, I would give some attention to *technique* in my management program. Managers do need to be exposed to certain methods that have proved broadly useful, if only to have a sense of how to deal with the people who promote them. Clearly they need to understand accounting, computers, and certain statistical techniques, among others. But since anyone (with one of those fancy GMAT scores, anyway) can quickly and easily learn many of these things, my ideal management program would give far less time to them than MBA programs now do.

Before we leave throughput, I wish to add a word of caution on the case study method of teaching—not so much on the use of cases as on how cases are used. Cases are a powerful device to bring varieties of reality into the classroom for descriptive purposes. But used in a prescriptive way, I believe they are part of the problem, not the solution.

The game is quite simple. As an eager young MBA student at Harvard, you are handed a neat twenty-page package on General Motors or the Mitsubishi Group, which you read the night before, along with the other cases for the next day. Then you arrive in class all prepared to discuss what it is that the denizens of Detroit or the chiefs of some distant Japanese corporation must do to resolve their problems. Don't claim ignorance, lack of sufficient knowledge: Good managers are decisive, therefore good management students must take a stand. The environment of General Motors must be assessed, its distinctive competencies identified, alternate strategies proposed, these strategies evaluated, and one selected, all before class is dismissed in eighty minutes. All based on that neat twenty-page package. All repeated hundreds of times over the course of the MBA program. Imagine the result.

Of course, the students do not implement the strategy they choose. How can they? But that's okay, because the professor makes a convenient distinction between formulation and implementation. For perhaps no more than "the sake of orderly presentation," as the Harvard authors of a well-known textbook put it,[8] tomorrow's captains of industry are left with the impression that good managers pronounce from on high based on a quick reading of a pithy report, without ever leaving their offices, while everyone else scurries around down below doing the implementing. And we believe the secret to the Japanese success lies in the things *they* do *right*!

When the students are seasoned practitioners, the trainer in fact has an opportunity to use something far better than the case study—the students' own experiences. They need only raise current examples or, better still, work up small "caselettes" of problems they have dealt with in the past, to which the conceptual insights and techniques of the classroom can be applied. This can make for especially powerful pedagogy when all the students come from a single organization, or from just a few whose experiences can be compared.

Let me provide one example from my own experience. When organizations ask me to do in-house programs, I now ask that we do workshops on actual issues that they face. That way they learn better, maybe even help in solving a problem in the process, while I learn too. I lose some work this way, but what I get keeps me stimulated. When I requested this of David Frances, who was working with the Thorn-EMI group in the United Kingdom, the result was a wonderful experience.

The participants were a group of practitioners in organizational development from various divisions of the company. They had been using my book on organizational structuring, so there was a common base of conceptual material. Three division managers from very different contexts—the Computer Software division, the Lighting division, and the Music and Distribution Services division—each drew up a kind of live case, essentially a collection of materials on structural issues they currently faced. The class read this material in advance and then, to begin each of three half-day sessions, the division manager outlined the problem, finishing with a series of questions. The class then split into groups to discuss the questions, after which they presented their conclusions to the division manager and me. The two of us then engaged in a discussion of the issues and the recommendations, the division manager drawing mainly on his understanding of the problem, and I on the concepts that might help to deal with it. What emerged was an intriguing combination of teaching and fishbowl consulting, which helped to drive home the conceptual materials (showing how they might be applied) and perhaps to make a bit of progress on the issues themselves.

MBA OUTPUT

We may accept the wrong people for management training and we may train them in the wrong way, but what *really* bothers me about all this is what happens after they leave. An MBA is a license to bypass the very things that organizations do, to leapfrog over the realities of organizational life into its abstractions, where innate intuition, even if it does exist, hardly gets a chance to develop. This encourages an approach to the practice of management that is "thin" and superficial, to my mind close to the root of certain problems facing American business today.

Organizations generally do only two things of consequence: They make things and they sell things. Not market things, not plan things, not control things, not communicate in retreats or feed masses of data into computers. Just physically make something, or provide some service, and then get someone to buy or use it. It can be said, then, without great overstatement, that our MBA programs take people who have hardly ever made anything or sold anything and then make damn sure they never will. How many MBA graduates go into sales or production? How many even manage these things, let alone do them? I recently polled two MBA classes. One student expressed an interest in production, none in sales.

Just consider the most popular jobs of the graduates: finance, where the abstractions of money, so compatible with the whole thrust of quantitative MBA training, shield them from the messiness of people and products; consulting, where the case study lives on in the quick fix of the detached expert; planning, where specialists dream about the abstract futures of organizations they seldom get a chance to know; and marketing, where manipulating concepts and numbers in the aggregate replaces selling one-on-one.

In his article, Livingston condemns the second-handedness of management education; here we have it perpetuated in the world of work. By the time these whiz kids reach the executive suite, having won the race down the "fast track," they may never have had their hands on anything more than sheets of numbers and abstractions, may never have dirtied themselves with anything beyond a malfunctioning photocopying machine, may never have met a customer who was not a statistic in a computer. And then they pretend to practice what they like to call "hands-on" management, while ceding their markets to those clever Japanese.

My ideal management education would take proven leaders well steeped in the making and the buying of one industry and then superimpose on their tacit knowledge and innate intuition the best of skill development, conceptual knowledge, and practical technique, so that they can take a fresh perspective on the very things they know well. Sure any intelligent person can learn good things in the classroom. But let's not promote widespread superficiality in the name of so-called professional management. Our organizations are simply too important for that.

Part II
ON
ORGANIZATIONS

As noted earlier, we can no more talk of *the* organization than we can talk of *the* mammal, no more prescribe one best way to run all organizations than prescribe one pair of glasses for all people. There are species in the world of organizations much as there are species in the world of biology. Too much effort has been wasted in trying to treat all organizations alike—governments that require the same procedures of all their ministries, conglomerates that do the same with their many divisions, consulting firms that seek to impose the latest technique on all their clients, whether they be post offices or hospitals, stable mass producers or fast-moving firms in high technology.

Much of my work has focused on trying to classify organizations, first from the perspective of structure and later from the perspective of power. We like to think of categorizing schemes as fixed by some law of nature. After all, dogs are different from elephants. But any classification scheme is also somewhat arbitrary, especially in the number of categories presented. In other words, every such scheme is to some degree the invention of the classifier and exists as much for convenience of understanding as to represent some scientific truth. Biologists define species by their mating capacity, but we have no such simple rule to classify organizations. (Besides, horses can mate with donkeys, even though the offspring mules are sterile.)

In a famous article entitled "The Magic Number Seven Plus or Minus Two: Some Limits on Our Capacity for Processing Information," the psychologist George Miller suggested that our inclination as human beings to classify things into sevens (the seven wonders of the world, the seven days of the week, and so on) reflects the number of "chunks" of information we are able to retain in our short-term memories.[1] Three wonders of the world would fall a little flat, so to speak, while eighteen would be daunting.

In my book *The Structuring of Organizations,* I proposed five types of organizations. I added two more—more or less—in my book *Power In and Around Organizations.* So I too happened to end up with seven, another of one of those "pernicious Pythagorean coincidences" Miller referred to. In this section, I present these seven—labeled entrepreneurial, machine, diversified, professional, innovative, missionary, and political—as a way to help identify and sort out the variety of things that happen in organizations.

I begin with a derivation of the seven in terms of a number of basic attributes, or building blocks, of organizations that can be used to understand how they function. These attributes include the component parts of organizations, the mechanisms they use to coordinate their work, and elements of their structures, power systems, and contexts. My basic point is that these attributes tend to *configure* in various ways, hence I refer to the different types of organizations as *configurations.* The seven chapters that follow discuss each of the configurations identified, adding other attributes (strategy-making processes, the nature of their managerial work, strengths and weaknesses, social issues, and so forth), while a final chapter of this section looks "beyond configuration" at the broader issues of forces and forms in organizations—really presenting a theory of organizational effectiveness.

6

DERIVING CONFIGURATIONS
Combining the Basic Attributes of Organizations

A few years ago, Danny Miller (my first doctoral student) and I published a paper entitled "The Case for Configuration." To introduce this chapter, which derives the seven basic configurations discussed in this section of the book, I would like to present the argument we developed in that paper.

That argument in fact originated in the earlier work of another colleague at McGill, Pradip Khandwalla, who found in his doctoral thesis at Carnegie-Mellon that the success of different businesses could be explained not by their use of any single organizational attribute (such as a particular type of planning system or form of decentralization), but by how they interrelated various attributes.[1] In other words, there were alternate paths to success, based on an organization's ability to configure the attributes it used. "Getting it all together" proved more important than any "one best way." Configuration subsequently became an important theme in my work.

In making the case for configuration, Danny and I argued that academic research on organizations has tended to limit its insight by favoring analysis over synthesis. In particular, it has tended to focus on how individual variables arrange themselves along linear scales rather than on how sets of attributes configure into types, referred to as configurations, archetypes, or gestalts. On one hand, an organization might be described as more or less decentralized, with the research seeking to correlate that variable with a second (say, the amount of planning). On the other hand, a type of decentralization (say, to grant autonomy to division managers) might be combined with other attributes (say, the use of performance controls and giving each manager responsibility over a distinct set of products) to suggest a type of organization (the divisionalized form).

Configurations are, in essence, systems, in which it makes more sense to talk of networks of interrelationships than of any one variable driving another.

Danny and I presented a number of reasons for the existence of configurations, some to do with the needs of organizations themselves, others with the needs of people trying to understand organizations. Of the former, one is that Darwinian-type forces may encourage only a few basic forms of organizations to survive in a given setting. In other words, like species, perhaps organizations survive only if they evolve in ways suitable to particular niches in the environment. Given that the types of environments are limited, then so too must be the types of organizations.

Our second argument was that organizations may be drawn toward configuration in order to achieve consistency in their internal characteristics, to create synergy in their working processes, and to establish a fit with their external contexts. Configuration in essence means harmony. Instead of trying to do everything well, the effective organization may be able to adapt *itself* (unlike the member of a Darwinian species, it should be noted) by concentrating on a specific theme around which it can configure its attributes.

Third, based on some of the findings of Danny's own research, we argued that it makes more sense for organizations to change, not by adapting continuously and gradually, in piecemeal fashion, but rather by engaging in quantum leaps from one integrated configuration to another. (This is akin to the current notions in ecology of "punctuated equilibrium," except that in our case, individual organizations rather than generations of them can adapt). In effect, it may be more efficient to hold on to a form that is going out of synchronization with its environment until a major transition can be made to a new, more suitable one. That way, internal configuration can be maintained, even if at the expense of external fit, and the costliness and disruption of organizational change can be concentrated into brief periods of "strategic revolution."

But configuration exists also in the mind of the beholder. As we argued in the paper, visitors to an art museum first consider a painting holistically, roaming over the entire canvas with their eyes to take in the gestalt of the work, its image, mood, and theme. Only afterward might attention be focused on a particular attribute—say, the coarseness of brushstrokes, the intensity of hues, the flow of lines. In other words, we appreciate a complex system first through synthesis, perhaps only later through analysis (even though it might have been created in the opposite order). Only a world controlled by a malevolent deity would force us to perceive systems in the reverse order, for example, having to study a painting a square inch at a time before putting it all together ourselves. In such a world, either paintings would be very small or museums would be very empty.

In our opinion, the main reason the museums of organizational theory have been so empty (even though its archives are rather busy) is that most of the writings ask the reader to do just that—survey the attributes of organizations one at a time without ever exposing the whole. The readers need organizational theory for the same reason some viewers need paintings: to gain insight into their world. And the observer of organizations perceives much as does the appreciator of art. Thus we need configuration also to help us understand our world—to allow us to observe whole canvases, if you like. Unlike the famous blind men, each of whom touched a different part of the elephant and then argued about its nature, describing organizations as configurations can open the eyes of the beholder to the nature of whole beasts. Each can be seen as a logical combination of its own particular attributes, similar to other members of its own species (configurations) but fundamentally different from other ones.

Hence, we proceed from the perspective of configuration. But first we must understand the attributes that make them up. This chapter presents those attributes and shows how they were combined into seven distinct forms of configuration. We begin with the people and parts of organizations, then consider the basic mechanisms by which they coordinate their work, look next at various elements of structure and how they are influenced by context (the latter in the spirit of the traditional, analytical research), and conclude by deriving the configurations.

I shall introduce a diagram here that, since first developed for my book on structuring, has become my personal "logo" in a sense, the symbol of my work. Organizations are not linear, but words to describe them in a book must be. So it helps to rely on diagrams as much as possible. I shall use this one in various ways in the discussion that follows.

I have had great fun with this diagram. The young woman artist I first engaged to draw it properly immediately saw but one thing there and claimed everyone else would. Well, I hadn't, and in China recently, someone saw an upside-down mushroom; others have seen lungs, the female uterus, a fly's head, a kidney bean; one person even told me he believed AT&T was using my book in executive programs because it looked like a telephone! In any event, while this may be a kind of Rorschach, I see only an organization. Feel free to experiment with this diagram; just let me know if you find anything interesting!

THE PARTS AND PEOPLE OF AN ORGANIZATION

At the base of any organization can be found its operators, those people who perform the basic work of producing the products and rendering the services. They form the *operating core*. All but the simplest organizations also require at least one full-time manager who occupies what we shall call the *strategic apex,* where the whole system is overseen. And as the organization grows, more managers are needed—not only managers of operators but also managers of managers. A *middle line* is created, a hierarchy of authority between the operating core and the strategic apex.

As the organization becomes still more complex, it generally requires another group of people, whom we shall call the analysts. They, too, perform administrative duties—to plan and control formally the work of others—but of a different nature, often labeled "staff." These analysts form what we shall call the *technostructure,* outside the hierarchy of line authority. Most organizations also add staff units of a different kind, to provide various internal services, from a cafeteria or mailroom to a legal counsel or public relations office. We call these units and the part of the organization they form the *support staff.*

Finally, every active organization has a sixth part, which we call its *ideology* (an alternate popular term recently has been "culture"). Ideology encompasses the traditions and beliefs of an organization that distinguish it from other organizations and infuse a certain life into the skeleton of its structure.

This gives us six basic parts of an organization. As shown in Figure 6–1, our logo, we have a small strategic apex connected by a flaring middle line to a large, flat operating core at the base. These three parts of the organization are drawn in one uninterrupted sequence to indicate that they are typically connected through a single chain of formal authority. The technostructure and the support staff are shown off to either side to indicate that they are separate from this main line of authority, influencing the operating core only indirectly. The ideology is shown as a kind of halo that surrounds the entire system.

These people, all of whom work inside the organization to make its decisions and take its actions—full-time employees or, in some cases, committed volunteers—may be thought of as *influencers* who form a kind of *internal coalition*. By this term, we mean a system within which people vie among themselves to determine the distribution of power.

FIGURE 6-1
Six Basic Parts of the Organization

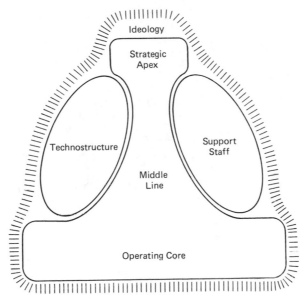

In addition, as shown in Figure 6-2, various outside people also try to exert influence on the organization, seeking to affect the decisions and actions taken inside. These external influencers, shown in Figure 6-2 as creating a field of forces around the organization, can include owners, unions and other employee associations, suppliers, clients, partners, competitors, and all kinds of publics, in the form of governments, special interest groups, and so forth. Together they can all be thought to form an *external coalition.*

Sometimes the external coalition is relatively *passive* (as in the typical behavior of the shareholders of a widely held corporation or the members of a large union). Other times it is *dominated* by one active influencer or some group of them acting in concert (such as an outside owner of a business firm or a community intent on imposing a certain philosophy on its school system). And in still other cases, the external coalition may be *divided,* as different groups seek to impose contradictory pressures on the organization (as in a prison buffeted between two community groups, one favoring custody, the other rehabilitation).

FIGURE 6–2
Internal and External Influencers of an Organization

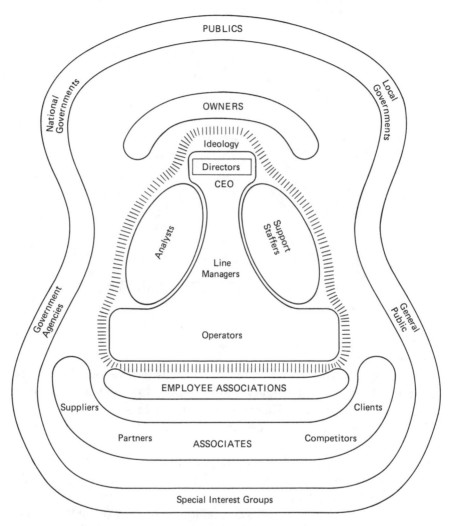

THE ESSENCE OF ORGANIZATIONAL STRUCTURE

Every organized human activity—from the making of pottery to the placing of a man on the moon—gives rise to two fundamental and opposing requirements: the *division of labor* into various tasks to be performed and the *coordination* of those tasks to accomplish the activity. The structure of an organization can be defined simply as the total of the ways in which its labor is divided into distinct tasks and then its coordination achieved among those tasks.

COORDINATING MECHANISMS

A number of coordinating mechanisms seem to describe the fundamental ways in which organizations can coordinate their work, shown in Figure 6–3 and listed below.

1. *Mutual adjustment,* which achieves coordination by the simple process of informal communication (as between two operating employees)
2. *Direct supervision,* in which coordination is achieved by having one person issue orders or instructions to several others whose work interrelates (as when a boss tells others what is to be done, one step at a time)
3. *Standardization of work processes,* which achieves coordination by specifying the work processes of people carrying out interrelated tasks (those standards usually being developed in the technostructure to be carried out in the operating core, as in the case of the work instructions that come out of time-and-motion studies)
4. *Standardization of outputs,* which achieves coordination by specifying the results of different work (again usually developed in the technostructure, as in a financial plan that specifies subunit performance targets or specifications that outline the dimensions of a product to be produced)
5. *Standardization of skills* (as well as *knowledge),* in which different work is coordinated by virtue of the related training the workers have received (as in medical specialists—say a surgeon and an anesthetist in an operating room—responding almost automatically to each other's standardized procedures)
6. *Standardization of norms,* in which it is the norms infusing the work that are controlled, usually for the entire organization, so that everyone functions according to the same set of beliefs (as in a religious order)

These coordinating mechanisms can be considered the most basic elements of structure, the glue that holds organizations together. They seem to fall into a rough order: As organizational work becomes more complicated, the favored means of coordination seems to shift from mutual adjustment (the simplest mechanism) to direct supervision, then

FIGURE 6–3
The Coordinating Mechanisms

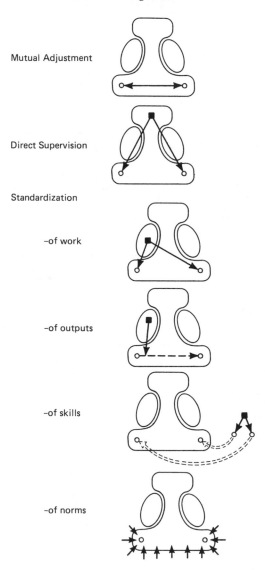

Mutual Adjustment

Direct Supervision

Standardization

   –of work

   –of outputs

   –of skills

   –of norms

to standardization, preferably of work processes or norms, otherwise of outputs or of skills, finally reverting back to mutual adjustment (paradoxically also the mechanism best able to deal with the most complex forms of work).

No organization, of course, can rely on a single one of those mechanisms. The mechanisms may be somewhat substitutable for each other, but all will typically be found in every reasonably developed organization. In particular, mutual adjustment and direct supervision are almost always important, no matter what use is made of the various forms of standardization. Contemporary organizations simply cannot exist without leadership and informal communication, even if only to override the rigidities of standardization.

But the important point for us here is that many organizations do favor one mechanism over the others, at least at certain stages of their lives. In fact, organizations that favor none seem most prone to becoming politicized, simply because of the conflicts that naturally arise when people have to vie for influence in a relative vacuum of power (bearing in mind, for example, that little use of direct supervision means a weak system of authority, little use of standardization of norms means a weak ideology, and so on).

DESIGN PARAMETERS

The essence of organizational design is the manipulation of a series of parameters that determine the division of labor and the achievement of coordination. Some of these concern the design of individual positions, others the design of the superstructure (the overall network of subunits, reflected in the organizational chart), some the design of lateral linkages to flesh out that superstructure, and a final group concerns the design of the decision-making system of the organization. Listed below are the main parameters of structural design, with links to the coordinating mechanisms.

- *Job specialization* refers to the number of tasks in a given job and the worker's control over these tasks. A job is *horizontally* specialized to the extent that it encompasses a few narrowly defined tasks, *vertically* specialized to the extent that the worker lacks control of the tasks performed. *Unskilled* jobs are typically highly specialized in both dimensions; skilled or *professional* jobs are typically specialized horizontally but not vertically. "Job enrichment" refers to the enlargement of jobs in both the vertical and horizontal dimensions.
- *Behavior formalization* refers to the standardization of work processes by the imposition of operating instructions, job descriptions,

rules, regulations, and the like. Structures that rely on any form of standardization for coordination may be defined as *bureaucratic*, those that do not as *organic*.

- *Training* refers to the use of formal instructional programs to establish and standardize in people the requisite skills and knowledge to do particular jobs in organizations. Training is a key design parameter in all work we call professional. Training and formalization are basically substitutes for achieving the standardization (in effect, the bureaucratization) of behavior. In one, the standards are learned as skills, in the other they are imposed on the job as rules.

- *Indoctrination* refers to programs and techniques by which the norms of the members of an organization are standardized, so that they become responsive to its ideological needs and can thereby be trusted to make its decisions and take its actions. Indoctrination too is a substitute for formalization, as well as for skill training, in this case the standards being internalized as deeply rooted beliefs.

- *Unit grouping* refers to the choice of the bases by which positions are grouped together into units, and those units into higher-order units. Grouping encourages coordination by putting different jobs under common supervision, by requiring them to share common resources and achieve common measures of performance, and by facilitating mutual adjustment among them. The various bases for grouping—by work process, product, client, area, and so on—can be reduced to two fundamental ones—the *function* performed and the *market* served. The former refers to a single link in the chain of processes by which products or services are produced, the latter to the whole chain for specific end products.

- *Unit size* refers to the number of positions (or units) contained in a single unit. The equivalent term, *span of control*, is not used here, because sometimes units are kept small despite an absence of close supervisory control. For example, when experts coordinate extensively by mutual adjustment, as in an engineering team in a space agency, they will form into small teams. In this case, unit size is small and span of control is low despite a relative absence of direct supervision. In contrast, when work is highly standardized (because of either formalization or training), unit size can be very large, because there is little need for direct supervision. One foreman can supervise dozens of assemblers, because they work according to very tight instructions.

- *Planning and control systems* are used to standardize outputs. They may be divided into two types: *action planning* systems, which specify the results of specific actions before they are taken (for example, that holes should be drilled with diameters of 3 centimeters); and *performance control* systems, which specify the desired results of whole ranges of actions after the fact (for example, that sales of a division should grow by 10 percent in a given year).
- *Liaison devices* refer to a whole series of mechanisms used to encourage mutual adjustment within and between units. They range from *liaison positions* (such as the purchasing engineer who stands between purchasing and engineering), through *task forces* and *integrating managers* (such as brand managers), finally to fully developed *matrix structures*.
- *Decentralization* refers to the diffusion of decision-making power. When all the power rests at a single point in an organization, we call its structure centralized; to the extent that the power is dispersed among many individuals, we call it relatively decentralized. We can distinguish *vertical decentralization*—the delegation of formal power down the hierarchy to line managers—from *horizontal decentralization*—the extent to which formal or informal power is dispersed out of the line hierarchy to nonmanagers (operators, analysts, and support staffers). We can also distinguish *selective* decentralization—the dispersal of power over different decisions to different places in the organization—from *parallel* decentralization—where the power over various kinds of decisions is delegated to the same place. Six forms of decentralization may thus be described: (1) vertical and horizontal centralization, where all the power rests at the strategic apex; (2) limited horizontal decentralization (selective), where the strategic apex shares some power with the technostructure that standardized everybody else's work; (3) limited vertical decentralization (parallel), where managers of market-based units are delegated the power to control most of the decisions concerning their line units; (4) vertical and horizontal decentralization, where most of the power rests in the operating core, at the bottom of the structure; (5) selective vertical and horizontal decentralization, where the power over different decisions is dispersed to various places in the organization, among managers, staff experts, and operators who work in teams at various levels in the hierarchy; and (6) pure decentralization, where power is shared more or less equally by all members of the organization.

STRUCTURE IN CONTEXT

A number of "contingency" or "situational" factors influence the choice of these design parameters, and vice versa. They include the age and size of the organization; its technical system of production; various characteristics of its environment, such as stability and complexity; and its power system, for example, whether or not it is tightly controlled by outside influencers. Some of the effects of these factors, as found in an extensive body of research literature, are summarized below as hypotheses.

AGE AND SIZE

• *The older an organization, the more formalized its behavior.* What we have here is the "we've-seen-it-all-before" syndrome. As organizations age, they tend to repeat their behaviors: as a result, these become more predictable and so more amenable to formalization.

• *The larger an organization, the more formalized its behavior.* Just as the older organization formalizes what it has seen before, so the larger organization formalizes what it sees often. ("Listen mister, I've heard that story at least five times today. Just fill in the form like it says.")

• *The larger an organization, the more elaborate its structure; that is, the more specialized its jobs and units and the more developed its administrative components.* As organizations grow in size, they are able to specialize their jobs more finely. (The big barbershop can afford a specialist to cut children's hair; the small one cannot.) As a result, they can also specialize—or "differentiate"—the work of their units more extensively. This requires more effort at coordination. And so the larger organization tends also to enlarge its hierarchy to effect direct supervision and to make greater use of its technostructure to achieve coordination by standardization, or else to encourage more coordination by mutual adjustment.

• *Structure reflects the age of the industry from its founding.* This is a curious finding, but one that we shall see holds up remarkably well. An organization's structure seems to reflect the age of the industry in which it operates, no matter what its own age. Industries that predate the industrial revolution seem to favor one kind of structure, those of the age of the early railroads another, and so on. We should obviously expect different structures in different periods; the surprising thing is that these structures seem to carry through to new periods, old industries remaining relatively true to earlier structures.

TECHNICAL SYSTEM

Technical system refers to the instruments used in the operating core to produce the outputs. (This should be distinguished from "technology," which refers to the knowledge base of an organization.)

- *The more regulating the technical system—that is, the more it controls the work of the operators—the more formalized the operating work and the more bureaucratic the structure of the operating core.* Technical systems that regulate the work of the operators—for example, mass production assembly lines—render that work highly routine and predictable, and so encourage its specialization and formalization, which in turn create the conditions for bureaucracy in the operating core.

- *The more complex the technical system, the more elaborate and professional the support staff.* Essentially, if an organization is to use complex machinery, it must hire staff experts who can understand that machinery—who have the capability to design, select, and modify it. And then it must give them considerable power to make decisions concerning that machinery, and encourage them to use the liaison devices to ensure mutual adjustment among them.

- *The automation of the operating core transforms a bureaucratic administrative structure into an organic one.* When unskilled work is coordinated by the standardization of work processes, we tend to get bureaucratic structure throughout the organization, because a control mentality pervades the whole system. But when the work of the operating core becomes automated, social relationships tend to change. Now it is machines, not people, that are regulated. So the obsession with control tends to disappear—machines do not need to be watched over—and with it go many of the managers and analysts who were needed to control the operators. In their place come the support specialists to look after the machinery, coordinating their own work by mutual adjustment. Thus, automation reduces line authority in favor of staff expertise and reduces the tendency to rely on standardization for coordination.

ENVIRONMENT

Environment refers to various characteristics of the organization's outside context, related to markets, political climate, economic conditions, and so on.

• *The more dynamic an organization's environment, the more organic its structure.* It stands to reason that in a stable environment—when nothing changes—an organization can predict its future conditions and so, all other things being equal, can easily rely on standardization for coordination. But when conditions become dynamic—when the need for product change is frequent, labor turnover is high, and political conditions are unstable—the organization cannot standardize but must instead remain flexible through the use of direct supervision or mutual adjustment for coordination, and so it must use a more organic structure. Thus, for example, armies, which tend to be highly bureaucratic institutions in peacetime, can become rather organic when engaged in highly dynamic, guerilla-type warfare.

• *The more complex an organization's environment, the more decentralized its structure.* The prime reason to decentralize a structure is that all the information needed to make decisions cannot be comprehended in one head. Thus, when the operations of an organization are based on a complex body of knowledge, there is usually a need to decentralize decision-making power. Note that a simple environment can be stable or dynamic (the manufacturer of dresses faces a simple environment yet cannot predict style from one season to another), as can a complex one (the specialist in perfected open heart surgery faces a complex task, yet knows what to expect).

• *The more diversified an organization's markets, the greater the propensity to split it into market-based units, or divisions, given favorable economies of scale.* When an organization can identify distinct markets—geographical regions, clients, but especially products and services—it will be predisposed to split itself into high-level units on that basis, and to give each a good deal of control over its own operations (that is, to use what we called "limited vertical decentralization"). In simple terms, diversification breeds divisionalization. Each unit can be given all the functions associated with its own markets. But this assumes favorable economies of scale: If the operating core cannot be divided, as in the case of an aluminum smelter, also if some critical function must be centrally coordinated, as in purchasing in a retail chain, then full divisionalization may not be possible.

• *Extreme hostility in its environment drives any organization to centralize its structure temporarily*. When threatened by extreme hostility in its environment, the tendency for an organization is to centralize power, in other words, to fall back on its tightest coordinating mechanism, direct supervision. Here a single leader can ensure fast and tightly coordinated response to the threat (at least temporarily).

POWER

• *The greater the external control of an organization, the more centralized and formalized its structure*. This important hypothesis claims that to the extent that an organization is controlled externally, for example by a parent firm or a government that dominates its external coalition—it tends to centralize power at the strategic apex and to formalize its behavior. The reason is that the two most effective ways to control an organization from the outside are to hold its chief executive officer responsible for its actions and to impose clearly defined standards on it. Moreover, external control forces the organization to be especially careful about its actions.

• *A divided external coalition will tend to give rise to a politicized internal coalition, and vice versa*. In effect, conflict in one of the coalitions tends to spill over to the other, as one set of influencers seeks to enlist the support of the others.

• *Fashion favors the structure of the day* (*and of the culture*), *sometimes even when inappropriate*. Ideally, the design parameters are chosen according to the dictates of age, size, technical system, and environment. In fact, however, fashion seems to play a role too, encouraging many organizations to adopt currently popular design parameters that are inappropriate for themselves. Paris has its salons of haute couture; likewise New York has its offices of "haute structure," the consulting firms that sometimes tend to oversell the latest in structural fashion.

BASIC TYPES OF ORGANIZATIONS

We have now introduced various attributes of organizations—parts, coordinating mechanisms, design parameters, situational factors. How do they all combine?

For years, the literature of management promoted the "one best way"; it largely still does. A good structure was one with a rigid hierarchy of authority, spans of control no greater than six, heavy use of strategic planning, and so on. In the 1960s, organizational theory developed the contingency approach—"it all depends"—characterized by the situational hypotheses we have just presented. Organizations were to pick their attributes independently, but according to context, much as diners pick their food at a buffet table. As discussed earlier, we have come to favor a third approach, which we characterize as "getting it all together"—the configuration approach. The elements of structure, even those of situation, should be selected to achieve consistency.

Our basic premise here is that a limited number of configurations can help explain much of what can be observed in organizations. We have introduced in our discussion six basic parts of the organization, six basic mechanisms of coordination, as well as six basic types of decentralization. In fact, there seems to be a fundamental correspondence between all of these sixes, which can be explained by a set of pulls exerted on the organization by each of its six parts, as shown in Figure 6–4. When conditions favor one of these pulls, the organization is drawn to design itself as a particular configuration. We list below and then introduce briefly the six resulting configurations, together with a seventh that tends to appear when no one pull or part dominates.

Configuration	Prime Coordinating Mechanism	Key Part of Organization	Type of Decentralization
Entrepreneurial organization	Direct supervision	Strategic apex	Vertical and horizontal centralization
Machine organization	Standardization of work processes	Technostructure	Limited horizontal decentralization
Professional organization	Standardization of skills	Operating core	Horizontal decentralization
Diversified organization	Standardization of outputs	Middle line	Limited vertical decentralization
Innovative organization	Mutual adjustment	Support staff	Selected decentralization
Missionary organization	Standardization of norms	Ideology	Decentralization
Political organization	None	None	Varies

FIGURE 6–4
Basic Pulls on the Organization

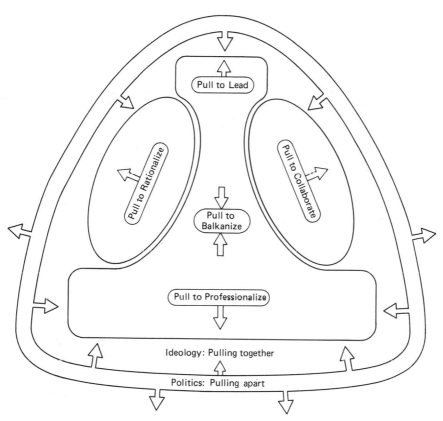

• The strategic apex exerts a pull to *lead,* by which it retains control over decision-making, with coordination achieved by direct supervision. When the organization cedes to this pull, often due to an overriding need for strategic vision, the centralized configuration called *entrepreneurial* results. As shown in Figure 6–5, the strategic apex sits over the operating core directly, with little else in the way of line managers or staff specialists.

• The technostructure exerts its pull to *rationalize,* ideally through the standardization of work processes, encouraging only limited horizontal decentralization (which empowers itself). Organizations that cede to this pull, usually due to an overriding need for routine efficiency, take on the *machine* configuration, shown in Figure 6–6 with a fully elaborated line and staff structure concentrated on controlling and

FIGURE 6–5
The Entrepreneurial Organization

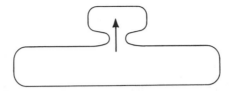

FIGURE 6–6
The Machine Organization

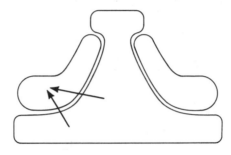

protecting the operating core. (Machine organizations that rationalize on behalf of a dominant external constituency may be called *instruments;* those on behalf of their own administrators, *closed systems.*)

• In their search for autonomy, the managers of the middle line exert a pull to *balkanize* the structure, to concentrate power in their own units through only limited (and parallel) vertical decentralization to themselves. When the organization cedes to this pull, generally by dividing itself into distinct units in order to serve different markets effectively, restricting itself to controlling the performance of those units largely through the standardization of outputs, the *diversified* configuration results. As indicated in Figure 6–7, a small strategic apex at "headquarters" supported by small staff units oversees a set of divisions usually structured as machine configurations (for reasons to be explained later).

• The members of the operating core exert a pull to *professionalize,* in order to minimize the influence that others, colleagues as well as line and technocratic administrators, have over their work. When the organization cedes to this pull, generally due to an overriding need to perfect expert programs, the *professional* configuration results, with full horizontal and vertical decentralization of power to the operating

FIGURE 6–7
The Diversified Organization

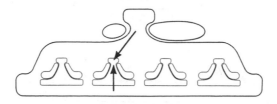

core, with coordinating achieved largely through the standardization of knowledge and skills. As shown in Figure 6–8, the organization has only a small technostructure and middle line, since there is little need for administrative control. But it has a large support staff to back up its high-priced professionals.

• The support staff exerts a pull to *collaborate* in order to involve itself in the central activity of the organization. The organization that has need for sophisticated innovation must usually cede to this pull, welding staff and line, and sometimes operating personnel as well, into multidisciplinary teams of experts that achieve coordination within and between themselves through mutual adjustment. The organization takes on the *innovative* configuration, shown in Figure 6–9, with many of the distinctions of conventional organizations falling away, as its various parts meld into a single system of vertical and horizontal decentralization on a selective basis.

• Ideology exists primarily as a force in organizations of other types, encouraging their members to *pull together,* as shown in Figure 6–10. But sometimes it too can dominate, as the standardization of norms becomes the prime coordinating mechanism. Then the organization takes on the *missionary* configuration, achieving the purest form of decentralization, as each member is trusted to decide and act for the overall good of the organization.

FIGURE 6–8
The Professional Organization

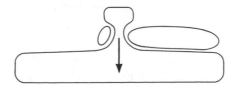

FIGURE 6–9

The Innovative Organization

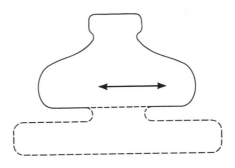

FIGURE 6–10

The Missionary Organization

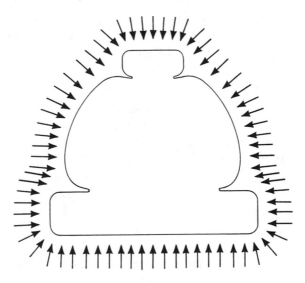

• Finally, politics also exists in organizations of other types, the force of conflict that causes people to *pull apart,* as shown in Figure 6–11. But it too can sometimes dominate, especially when no one part of the organization and no one mechanism of coordination is dominant. Then the organization takes on the *political* configuration, with no stable form of centralization or decentralization.

Together these configurations, as well as the pulls and needs represented by each, seem to encompass and integrate a good deal of what we

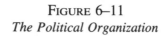

FIGURE 6–11
The Political Organization

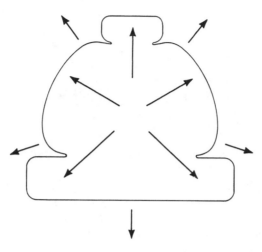

know about organizations. It should be emphasized that, as presented, each configuration is idealized—a simplification, really a caricature of reality. No real organization is ever exactly like any one of them. But some do come remarkably close, while others seem to reflect combinations of them, sometimes in transition from one to another.

Individually then, these configurations reflect leading tendencies in organizations, while collectively they seem to define the boundaries of a space within which real organizations may be considered to lie. In order to map a space, however, the boundaries must first be identified. Thus we begin by describing, in the seven chapters that follow, each of the configurations. Then, in a final chapter we can consider the whole space, by using the framework of the seven to describe the many and varied forms that real-world organizations seem to take.

7

THE ENTREPRENEURIAL ORGANIZATION

Simple organizations that are run firmly and personally by their leaders (even if not strictly entrepreneurs, in the sense of being owner-managers), are fun to consider: They make for wonderful stories of the building of great empires and of dramatic turnarounds. They are also the place where strategic vision most clearly manifests itself, a hot topic these days, though largely remaining in the darkness of human intuition. But, like every other configuration, the entrepreneurial one has its problems too. Indeed, it is not coincidental that this form of organization declined in popularity during much of this century, although it has experienced a resurgence recently as the big bureaucracies have faltered.

Here I set out to describe the entrepreneurial organization: how it organizes itself (or at least resists doing so); how it functions, and especially makes its strategy; the conditions that are likely to foster its development; the problems it encounters; and finally, what can be said about its strategic vision, based on studies we have done at McGill of visionary leaders.

The Entrepreneurial Organization

Structure: • simple, informal, flexible, with little staff or middle-line hierarchy
   • activities revolving around the chief executive, who controls personally, through direct supervision
Context: • simple and dynamic environment
   • strong leadership, sometimes charismatic, autocratic
   • startup, crisis, and turnaround
   • small organizations, "local producers"
Strategy: • often visionary process, broadly deliberate but emergent and flexible in details
   • leader positions malleable organization in protected niches
Issues: • responsive, sense of mission
      but
   • vulnerable, restrictive
   • danger of imbalance toward strategy or operations

Consider an automobile dealership with a flamboyant owner, a brand-new government department, a corporation or even a nation run by an autocratic leader, or a school system in a state of crisis. In many respects, those are vastly different organizations. But the evidence suggests that they share a number of basic characteristics. They form a configuration we shall call the *entrepreneurial organization*.

THE BASIC STRUCTURE

The structure of the entrepreneurial organization is simple, characterized above all by what it is not: elaborated. As shown in the opening figure, typically it has little or no staff, a loose division of labor, and a small managerial hierarchy. Little of its activity is formalized, and it makes minimal use of planning procedures or training routines. In a sense, it is nonstructure; in my "structuring" book, I called it *simple structure*.

Power focuses on the chief executive, who exercises it personally. Formal controls are discouraged as a threat to that person's authority, as are strong pockets of expertise and even aspects of ideology that are not in accord with his or her vision. Under the leader's watchful eye, politics cannot arise. Should outsiders, such as particular customers or suppliers, seek to exert influence, the leader is as likely as not to take the organization to a less exposed niche in the marketplace.

Thus, it is not uncommon in small entrepreneurial organizations for everyone to report to the chief. Even in ones not so small, communication flows informally, much of it between the chief executive and others. As one group of McGill MBA students commented in their study of a small manufacturer of pumps: "It is not unusual to see the president of the company engaged in casual conversation with a machine shop mechanic. [That way he is] informed of a machine breakdown even before the shop superintendent is advised."

Decision-making is likewise flexible, with a highly centralized power system allowing for rapid response. The creation of strategy is, of course, the responsibility of the chief executive, the process tending to be highly intuitive, often oriented to the aggressive search for opportunities. It is not surprising, therefore, that the resulting strategy tends to reflect the chief executive's implicit vision of the world, often an extrapolation of his or her own personality.

Handling disturbances and innovating in an entrepreneurial way are perhaps the most important aspects of the chief executive's work. In contrast, the more formal aspects of managerial work—figurehead duties, for example—receive less attention, as does the need to disseminate information and allocate resources internally, since knowledge and power remain at the top.

CONDITIONS OF THE ENTREPRENEURIAL ORGANIZATION

The entrepreneurial configuration is fostered by an external context that is both simple and dynamic. It must be relatively simple (say retailing food as opposed to designing jet aircraft) in order for one person at the top to retain so much influence, and it is the dynamic context that requires the flexible structure, which in turn enables this organization to outmaneuver the bureaucracies. Entrepreneurial leaders are naturally attracted to such conditions.

The classic case of this is, of course, the entrepreneurial firm, where the leader is the owner. Entrepreneurs often found their own firms to escape the procedures and control of the bureaucracies where they previously worked. At the helm of their own enterprises, they continue to loathe the ways of bureaucracy, and the staff analysts that accompany them, and so they keep their organizations lean and flexible. Figure 7–1 shows the organigram for Steinberg's, a supermarket chain we shall be discussing shortly, during its most classically entrepreneurial years. Notice the identification of people above positions, the simplicity of the structure (the firm's sales by this time were on the order of $27 million), and the focus on the chief executive (not to mention the obvious family connections).

Entrepreneurial firms are often young and aggressive, continually searching for the risky markets that scare off the bigger bureaucracies. But they are also careful to avoid the complex markets, preferring to remain in niches that their leaders can comprehend. Their small size and focused strategies allow their structures to remain simple, so that the leaders can retain tight control and maneuver flexibly. Moreover, business entrepreneurs are often visionary, sometimes charismatic or autocratic as well (sometimes both, in sequence!). Of course, not all "entrepreneurs" are so aggressive or visionary; many settle down to pursue common strategies in small geographic niches. Labeled the *local producers,* these can include the corner restaurant, the town bakery, the regional supermarket chain.

But an organization need not be owned by an entrepreneur, indeed need not even operate in the profit sector, to adopt the configuration

FIGURE 7–1

Organization of Steinberg's, an Entrepreneurial Firm (circa 1948)

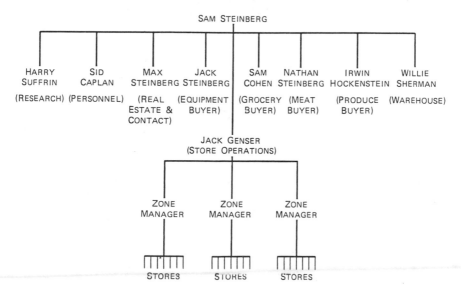

we call entrepreneurial. In fact, most new organizations seem to adopt this configuration, whatever their sector, because they generally have to rely on personalized leadership to get themselves going—to establish their basic direction, or *strategic vision,* to hire their first people and set up their initial procedures. Of course, strong leaders are likewise attracted to new organizations, where they can put their own stamp on things. Thus, we can conclude that most organizations in business, government, and not-for-profit areas pass through the entrepreneurial configuration in their formative years, during *startup.*

Moreover, while new organizations that quickly grow large or that require specialized forms of expertise may make a relatively quick transition to another configuration, many others seem to remain in the entrepreneurial form, more or less, as long as their founding leaders remain in office. This reflects the fact that the structure has often been built around the personal needs and orientation of the leader and has been staffed with people loyal to him or her.

This last comment suggests that the personal power needs of a leader can also, by themselves, give rise to this configuration in an existing organization. When a chief executive hoards power and avoids or destroys the formalization of activity as an infringement on his or her right to rule by fiat, than an autocratic form of the entrepreneurial organization will tend to appear. This can been seen in the cult of personality of the leader, in business (the last days of Henry Ford) no less than in government (the leadership of Stalin in the Soviet Union). Charisma can have a similar effect, though different consequences, when the leader gains personal power not because he or she hoards it but because the followers lavish it on the leader.

The entrepreneurial configuration also tends to arise in any other type of organization that faces severe crisis. Backed up against a wall, with its survival at stake, an organization will typically turn to a strong leader for salvation. The structure thus becomes effectively (if not formally) simple, as the normal powers of existing groups—whether staff analysts, line managers, or professional operators, etc., with their perhaps more standardized forms of control—are suspended to allow the chief to impose a new integrated vision through his or her personalized control. The leader may cut costs and expenses in an attempt to effect what is known in the strategic management literature as an *operating turnaround,* or else reconceive the basic product and service orientation, to achieve *strategic turnaround.* Of course, once the turnaround is realized, the organization may revert to its traditional operations and, in the bargain, spew out its entrepreneurial leader, now viewed as an impediment to its smooth functioning.

STRATEGY FORMATION IN THE ENTREPRENEURIAL ORGANIZATION

How does strategy develop in the entrepreneurial organization? And what role does that mysterious concept known as "strategic vision" play? We know something of the entrepreneurial mode of strategy-making, but less of strategic vision itself, since it is locked in the head of the individual. But some studies we have done at McGill do shed some light on both these questions. Let us consider strategic vision first.

VISIONARY LEADERSHIP

In a paper she co-authored with me, my McGill colleague Frances Westley contrasted two views of visionary leadership. One she likened to a hypodermic needle, in which the active ingredient (vision) is loaded into a syringe (words) which is injected into the employees to stimulate all kinds of energy. There is surely some truth to this, but Frances prefers another image, that of drama. Drawing from a book on theater by Peter Brook,[1] the legendary director of the Royal Shakespeare Company, she conceives strategic vision, like drama, as becoming magical in that moment when fiction and life blend together. In drama, this moment is the result of endless "rehearsal," the "performance" itself, and the "attendance" of the audience. But Brook prefers the more dynamic equivalent words in French, all of which have English meanings—"repetition," "representation," and "assistance." Frances likewise applies these words to strategic vision.

"Repetition" suggests that success comes from deep knowledge of the subject at hand. Just as Sir Laurence Olivier would repeat his lines again and again until he had trained his tongue muscles to say them effortlessly,[2] so too Lee Iacocca "grew up" in the automobile business, going to Chrysler after Ford because cars were "in his blood."[3] The visionary's inspiration stems not from luck, although chance encounters can play a role, but from endless experience in a particular context.

"Representation" means not just to perform but to make the past live again, giving it immediacy, vitality. To the strategist, that is vision articulated, in words and actions. What distinguishes visionary leaders is their profound ability with language, often in symbolic form, as metaphor. It is not just that they "see" things from a new perspective but that they get others to so see them.

Edwin Land, who built a great company around the Polaroid camera he invented, has written of the duty of "the inventor to build a new gestalt for the old one in the framework of society."[4] He himself described photography as helping "to focus some aspect of [your] life"; as you look through the viewfinder, "it's not merely the camera you are focusing: you are focusing yourself . . . when you touch the button, what is inside of you comes out. It's the most basic form of creativity. Part of you is now permanent."[5] Lofty words for fifty tourists filing out of a bus to record some pat scene, but powerful imagery for someone trying to build an organization to promote a novel camera. Steve Jobs, visionary (for a time) in his promotion, if not invention, of the personal computer, placed a grand piano and a BMW in Apple's central foyer, with the claim that "I believe people get great ideas from seeing great products."[6]

"Assistance" means that the audience for drama, whether in the theater or in the organization, empowers the actor no less than the actor empowers the audience. Leaders become visionary because they appeal powerfully to specific constituencies at specific periods of time. That is why leaders once perceived as visionary can fall so dramatically from grace—a Steve Jobs, a Winston Churchill. Or to take a more dramatic example, here is how Albert Speer, arriving skeptical, reacted to the first lecture he heard by his future leader: "Hitler no longer seemed to be speaking to convince; rather, he seemed to feel that he was experiencing what the audience, by now transformed into a single mass, expected of him."[7]

Of course, management is not theater; the leader who becomes a stage actor, playing a part he or she does not live, is destined to fall from grace. It is integrity—a genuine feeling behind what the leader says and does—that makes leadership truly visionary, and that is what makes impossible the transition of such leadership into any formula.

This visionary leadership is style and strategy, coupled together. It is drama, but not play-acting. The strategic visionary is born and made, the product of a historical moment. Brook closes his book with the following quotation:

> In everyday life, "if" is a fiction, in the theatre "if" is an experiment.
> In everyday life, "if" is an evasion, in the theatre "if" is the truth.
> When we are persuaded to believe in this truth, then the theatre and life are one.

This is a high aim. It sounds like hard work.
To play needs much work. But when we experience the work as play,
then it is not work any more.
A play is play.[8]

In the entrepreneurial organization, at best "theater," namely strategic vision, becomes one with "life," namely organization. That way leadership creates drama; it turns work into play.

Let us now consider the entrepreneurial approach to strategy formation in terms of two specific studies we have done, one of a supermarket chain, the other of a manufacturer of women's undergarments.

THE ENTREPRENEURIAL MODE OF STRATEGY FORMATION IN A SUPERMARKET CHAIN

Steinberg's is a Canadian retail chain that began with a tiny food store in Montreal in 1917 and grew to sales in the billion-dollar range during the almost sixty-year reign of its leader. Most of that growth came from supermarket operations. In many ways, Steinberg's fits the entrepreneurial model rather well. Sam Steinberg, who joined his mother in the first store at the age of eleven and personally made a quick decision to expand it two years later, maintained complete formal control of the firm (including every single voting share) to the day of his death in 1978. He also exercised close managerial control over all its major decisions, at least until the firm began to diversify after 1960, primarily into other forms of retailing.

It has been popular to describe the "bold stroke" of the entrepreneur.[9] In Steinberg's we saw only two major reorientations of strategy in the sixty years, moves into self-service in the 1930s and into the shopping center business in the 1950s. But the stroke was not bold so much as tested. The story of the move into self-service is indicative. In 1933 one of the company's eight stores "struck it bad," in the chief executive's words, incurring "unacceptable" losses ($125 a week). Sam Steinberg closed the store one Friday evening, converted it to self-service, changed its name from "Steinberg's Service Stores" to "Wholesale Groceteria," slashed its prices by 15–20 percent, printed handbills, stuffed them into neighborhood mailboxes, and reopened on Monday morning. That's strategic change! But only once these changes proved successful did he convert the other stores. Then, in his words, "We grew like Topsy."

This anecdote tells us something about the bold stroke of the entrepreneur—"controlled boldness" is a better expression. The ideas were bold, the execution careful. Sam Steinberg could have simply closed the one unprofitable store. Instead he used it to create a new vision, but he tested that vision, however ambitiously, before leaping into it. Notice the interplay here of problems and opportunities. Steinberg took what most businessmen would probably have perceived as a *problem* (how to cut the losses in one store) and by treating it as a *crisis* (what is wrong with our *general* operation that produces these losses) turned it into an *opportunity* (we can grow more effectively with a new concept of retailing). That was how he got energy behind actions and kept ahead of his competitors. He "oversolved" his problem and thereby remade his company, a characteristic of some of the most effective forms of entrepreneurship.

But absolutely central to this form of entrepreneurship is intimate, detailed knowledge of the business or of analogous business situations, the "repetition" discussed earlier. The leader as conventional strategic "planner"—the so-called architect of strategy—sits on a pedestal and is fed aggregate data that he or she uses to "formulate" strategies that are "implemented" by others. But the history of Steinberg's belies that image. It suggests that clear, imaginative, integrated strategic vision depends on an involvement with detail, an intimate knowledge of specifics. And by closely controlling "implementation" personally, the leader is able to reformulate en route, to adapt the evolving vision through his or her own process of learning. That is why Steinberg tried his new ideas in one store first. And that is why, in discussing his firm's competitive advantage, he told us: "Nobody knew the grocery business like we did. Everything has to do with your knowledge." He added: "I knew merchandise, I knew cost, I knew selling, I knew customers, I knew everything . . . and I passed on all my knowledge; I kept teaching my people. That's the advantage we had. They couldn't touch us."

Such knowledge can be incredibly effective when concentrated in one individual who is fully in charge (having no need to convince others, not subordinates below, not superiors at some distant headquarters, nor market analysts looking for superficial pronouncements) and who retains a strong, long-term commitment to the organization. So long as the business is simple and focused enough to be comprehended in one brain, the entrepreneurial approach is powerful, indeed unexcelled. Nothing else can provide so clear and complete a vision, yet also allow the flexibility to elaborate and rework that vision when necessary. The conception of a new strategy is an exercise in synthesis, which is typically best carried out in a single, informed brain. That is why the entrepreneurial approach is at the center of the most glorious corporate successes.

But in its strength lies entrepreneurship's weakness. Bear in mind that strategy for the entrepreneurial leader is not a formal, detailed plan on paper. It is a personal vision, a concept of the business, locked in a single brain. It may need to get "represented," in words and metaphors, but that must remain general if the leader is to maintain the richness and flexibility of his or her concept. But success breeds a large organization, public financing, and the need for formal planning. The vision must be articulated to drive others and gain their support, and that threatens the personal nature of the vision. At the limit, as we shall see in the case of Steinberg's in the next chapter, the leader can get captured by his or her very success.

In Steinberg's, moreover, when success in the traditional business encouraged diversification into new ones (new regions, new forms of retailing, new industries), the organization moved beyond the realm of its leader's personal comprehension, and the entrepreneurial mode of strategy formation lost its viability. Strategy-making became more decentralized, more analytic, in some ways more careful, but at the same time less visionary, less integrated, less flexible, and ironically, less deliberate.

CONCEIVING A NEW VISION IN A GARMENT FIRM

The genius of an entrepreneur like Sam Steinberg was his ability to pursue one vision (self-service and everything that entailed) faithfully for decades and then, based on a weak signal in the environment (the building of the first small shopping center in Montreal), to realize the need to shift that vision. The planning literature makes a big issue of forecasting such discontinuities, but as far as I know there are no formal techniques to do so effectively (claims about "scenario analysis" notwithstanding). The ability to perceive a sudden shift in an established pattern and then to conceive a new vision to deal with it appears to remain largely in the realm of informed intuition, generally the purview of the wise, experienced, and energetic leader. Again, the literature is largely silent on this. But another of our studies, also concerning entrepreneurship, did reveal some aspects of this process.

Canadelle produces women's undergarments, primarily brassieres. It too was a highly successful organization, although not on the same scale as Steinberg's. Things were going well for the company in the late 1960s, under the personal leadership of Larry Nadler, the son of its founder, when suddenly everything changed. A sexual revolution of sorts was accompanying broader social manifestations, with bra-burning a symbol of its resistance. For a manufacturer of brassieres the threat was obvious. For many other women the miniskirt had come to dominate the fashion scene, obsoleting the girdle and giving rise to pantyhose. As the executives of Canadelle put it, "the bottom fell out of the girdle business." The whole environment—long so receptive to the company's strategies—seemed to turn on it all at once.

At the time, a French company had entered the Quebec market with a light, sexy, molded garment called "Huit," using the theme, "just like not wearing a bra." Their target market was 15–20-year-olds. Though the product was expensive when it landed in Quebec and did not fit well in Nadler's opinion, it sold well. Nadler flew to France in an attempt to license the product for manufacture in Canada. The French firm refused, but, in Nadler's words, what he learned in "that one hour in their offices made the trip worthwhile." He realized that what women wanted was a more natural look, not no bra but less bra. Another trip shortly afterward, to a sister American firm, convinced him of the importance of market segmentation by age and life-style. That led him to the realization that the firm had two markets, one for the more mature customer, for whom the brassiere was a cosmetic to look and feel more attractive, and another for the younger customer who wanted to look and feel more natural.

Those two events led to a major shift in strategic vision. The CEO described it as sudden, the confluence of different ideas to create a new mental set. In his words, "all of a sudden the idea forms." Canadelle reconfirmed its commitment to the brassiere business, seeking greater market share while its competitors were cutting back. It introduced a new line of more natural brassieres for the younger customers, for which the firm had to work out the molding technology as well as a new approach to promotion.

We can draw on Kurt Lewin's three-stage model of unfreezing, changing, and refreezing to explain such a gestalt shift in vision.[10] The process of *unfreezing* is essentially one of overcoming the natural defense mechanisms, the established "mental set" of how an industry is supposed to operate, to realize that things have changed fundamentally. The old assumptions no longer hold. Effective managers, especially effective strategic managers, are supposed to scan their environments continually, looking for such changes. But doing so continuously, or worse, trying to use technique to do so, may have exactly the opposite effect. So much attention may be given to strategic monitoring when nothing important is happening that when something really does, it may not even be noticed. The trick, of course, is to pick out the discontinuities that matter, and as noted earlier that seems to have more to do with informed intuition than anything else.

A second step in unfreezing is the willingness to step into the void, so to speak, for the leader to shed his or her conventional notions of how a business is supposed to function. The leader must above all avoid premature closure—seizing on a new thrust before it has become clear what its signals really mean. That takes a special kind of management, one able to live with a good deal of uncertainty and discomfort. "There is a period of confusion," Nadler told us, "you sleep on it . . . start looking for patterns . . . become an information hound, searching for [explanations] everywhere."

Strategic *change* of this magnitude seems to require a shift in mind-set before a new strategy can be conceived. And the thinking is fundamentally conceptual and inductive, probably stimulated (as in this case) by just one or two key insights. Continuous bombardment of facts, opinions, problems, and so on may prepare the mind for the shift, but it is the sudden *insight* that is likely to drive the synthesis—to bring all the disparate elements together in one "eureka"-type flash.

Once the strategist's mind is set, assuming he or she has read the new situation correctly and has not closed prematurely, then the *refreezing* process begins. Here the object is not to read the situation, at least not in a global sense, but in effect to block it out. It is a time to work out the consequences of the new strategic vision.

It has been claimed that obsession is an ingredient in effective organizations.[11] Only for the period of refreezing would we agree, when the organization must focus on the pursuit of the new orientation—the new mindset—with full vigor. A management that was open and divergent in its thinking must now become closed and convergent. But that means that the uncomfortable period of uncertainty has passed, and people can now get down to the exciting task of accomplishing something new. Now the organization knows where it is going; the object of the exercise is to get there using all the skills at its command, many of them formal and analytic. Of course, not everyone accepts the new vision. For those steeped in old strategies, *this* is the period of discomfort, and they can put up considerable resistance, forcing the leader to make greater use of his or her formal powers and political skills. Thus, refreezing of the leader's mindset often involves the unfreezing, changing, and refreezing of the organization itself! But when the structure is simple, as it is in the entrepreneurial organization, that problem is relatively minor.

LEADERSHIP TAKING PRECEDENCE IN THE ENTREPRENEURIAL CONFIGURATION

To conclude, entrepreneurship is very much tied up with the creation of strategic vision, often with the attainment of a new concept. Strategies can be characterized as largely deliberate, since they reside in the intentions of a single leader. But being largely personal as well, the details of those strategies can emerge as they develop. In fact, the vision can change too. The leader can adapt en route, can learn, which means new visions can emerge too, sometimes, as we have seen, rather quickly.

In the entrepreneurial organization, as shown in Figure 7–2, the focus of attention is on the leader. The organization is malleable and responsive to that person's initiatives, while the environment remains benign for the most part, the result of the leader's selecting (or "enacting") the correct niche for his or her organization. The environment can, of course, flare up occasionally to challenge the organization, and then the leader must adapt, perhaps seeking out a new and more appropriate niche in which to operate.

FIGURE 7–2
Leadership Taking Precedence in
the Entrepreneurial Organization

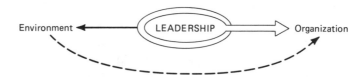

SOME ISSUES ASSOCIATED WITH THE ENTREPRENEURIAL ORGANIZATION

We conclude briefly with some broad issues associated with the entrepreneurial organization. In this configuration, decisions concerning both strategy and operations tend to be centralized in the office of the chief executive. This centralization has the important advantage of rooting strategic response in deep knowledge of the operations. It also allows for flexibility and adaptability: Only one person need act. But this same executive can get so enmeshed in operating problems that he or she loses sight of strategy; alternatively, he or she may become so enthusiastic about strategic opportunities that the more routine operations can wither for lack of attention and eventually pull down the whole organization. Both are frequent occurrences in entrepreneurial organizations.

This is also the riskiest of organizations, hinging on the activities of one individual. One heart attack can literally wipe out the organization's prime means of coordination. Even a leader in place can be risky. When change becomes necessary, everything hinges on the chief's response to it. If he or she resists, as is not uncommon where that person developed the existing strategy in the first place, then the organization may have no means to adapt. Then the great strength of the entrepreneurial organization—the vision of its leader plus its capacity to respond quickly—becomes its chief liability.

Another great advantage of the entrepreneurial organization is its sense of mission. Many people enjoy working in a small, intimate organization where the leader—often charismatic—knows where he or she is taking it. As a result, the organization tends to grow rapidly, with great enthusiasm. Employees can develop a solid identification with such an organization.

But other people perceive this configuration as highly restrictive. Because one person calls all the shots, they feel not like the participants on an exciting journey, but like cattle being led to market for someone else's benefit. In fact, the broadening of democratic norms into the sphere of organizations has rendered the entrepreneurial organization unfashionable in some quarters of contemporary society. It has been described as paternalistic and sometimes autocratic, and accused of concentrating too much power at the top. Certainly, without countervailing powers in the organization the chief executive can easily abuse his or her authority.

Perhaps the entrepreneurial organization is an anachronism in societies that call themselves democratic. Yet there have always been such organizations, and there always will be. This was probably the only structure known to those who first discovered the benefits of coordinating their activities in some formal way. And it probably reached its heyday in the era of the great American trusts of the late nineteenth century, when powerful entrepreneurs personally controlled huge empires. Since then, at least in Western society, the entrepreneurial organization has been on the decline. Nonetheless, it remains a prevalent and important configuration, and will continue to be so as long as society faces the conditions that require it: the prizing of entrepreneurial initiative and the resultant encouragement of new organizations, the need for small and informal organizations in some spheres and of strong personalized leadership despite larger size in others, and the need periodically to turn around ailing organizations of all types.

8

THE MACHINE
ORGANIZATION

These are supposedly the big bad guys of the organization world, the homes of red tape and the sources of curious tales. Yet if we think of McDonald's or the Swiss railroad, a different impression develops, of organizations—when they get it right—that can be enormously efficient and can provide an unmatchable reliability of service (can you think any other way to deliver millions of pieces of mail every day?). Thus, like every other configuration, the machine one cuts both ways too: It can serve us or drive us crazy (or the two concurrently). I am not terribly partial to these personally—you won't find me working in one, except to flit in and out on a consulting basis—but I do not hesitate to fly them to conferences, have them print my books or deliver my mail, even provide me and the kids with the occasional hamburger. Like many other people, I can't live without them even though I choose not to live within them.

In my structuring book, I called these *machine bureaucracies.* To most people, bureaucracy is a pejorative term—the locus of excessive controls, of managers lording authority over workers and workers lording control over the clients. Just as it is always the other guy who causes pollution, so too do we never think of ourselves as the bureaucrats. Well, I hope in this chapter I can dispel these two myths: first, as noted above, by showing that there is a constructive side to machine bureaucracy (though no lack of that destructive side too, as we shall see), and second, by showing that we can all be bureaucrats. Like the tango, it can take only two to make a bureaucracy—two who set up procedures, two obsessed with control to avoid the unexpected, two intent on sticking to the plans. The spirit of bureaucracy is to set course and to stay on it, to ensure that everything comes out as intended. Bureaucracy means no surprises. It is epitomized by the comment of a General Motors chairman some years ago that "In the automotive business, uncertainty is the biggest enemy."[1]

I begin with a description of the machine bureaucracy structure, then consider the well-defined conditions of machine organizations, raising a distinction between this configuration as an externally controlled "instrument" and as an internally controlled "closed system." I then consider some social issues associated with the machine organization—critical ones in a society inundated with these types. Finally, I close by drawing again on our McGill research to describe how these configurations make strategy or, more commonly in this case, use formal planning to resist making strategy, so that they can get on with being the bureaucratic machines that they are designed to be.

The Machine Organization

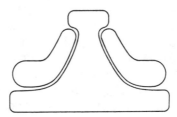

Structure:
- centralized bureaucracy
- formal procedures, specialized work, sharp divisions of labor, usually functional groupings, extensive hierarchy
- key is technostructure, charged with standardizing the work, but clearly separated from middle line (itself highly developed)
- also extensive support staff to reduce uncertainty

Context:
- simple and stable environment
- usually larger, more mature organization
- rationalized work, rationalizing (but not automated) technical system
- external control→*instrument* form
- otherwise can be *closed system* form
- common in mass production mass service, government, organizations in business of control and safety

Strategy:
- ostensibly planning process, but that is really strategic programming
- resistance to strategic change, necessary to overlay innovative configuration for revitalization or else revert to entrepreneurial configuration for turnaround
- hence quantum pattern of change: long periods of stability interrupted by occasional bursts of strategic revolution

Issues:
- efficient, reliable, precise, consistent
    but
- obsession with control leads to
- human problems in operating core, leads to
- coordination problems in administrative center, leads to
- adaptation problems at strategic apex

A national post office, a custodial prison, an airline, a giant automobile company, even a small security agency—all these organizations appear to have a number of characteristics in common. Above all, their operating work is routine, the greatest part of it rather simple and repetitive; as a result, their work processes are highly standardized. These characteristics give rise to the machine organizations of our society, structures fine-tuned to run as integrated, regulated, highly bureaucratic machines.

THE BASIC STRUCTURE

A clear configuration of the attributes has appeared consistently in the research: highly specialized, routine operating tasks; very formalized communication throughout the organization; large-size operating units; reliance on the functional basis for grouping tasks; relatively centralized power for decision making; and an elaborate administrative structure with a sharp distinction between line and staff.

THE OPERATING CORE AND ADMINISTRATION

The obvious starting point is the operating core, with its highly rationalized work flow. This means that the operating tasks are made simple and repetitive, generally requiring a minimum of skill and training, the latter often taking only hours, seldom more than a few weeks, and usually in-house. This in turn results in narrowly defined jobs and an emphasis on the standardization of work processes for coordination, with activities highly formalized. The workers are left with little discretion, as are their supervisors, who can therefore handle very large spans of control.

To achieve such high regulation of the operating work, the organization has need for an elaborate administrative structure—a fully developed middle-line hierarchy and technostructure—but the two clearly distinguished.

The managers of the middle line have three prime tasks. One is to handle the disturbances that arise in the operating core. The work is so standardized that when things fall through the cracks, conflict flares, because the problems cannot be worked out informally. So it falls to managers to resolve them by direct supervision. Indeed, many problems get bumped up successive steps in the hierarchy until they reach a level of common supervision where they can be resolved by authority (as with a dispute in a company between manufacturing and marketing that may have to be resolved by the chief executive). A second task of the middle-line managers is to work with the staff analysts to incorporate their standards down into the operating units. And a third task is to support the vertical flows in the organization—the elaboration of action plans flowing down the hierarchy and the communication of feedback information back up.

The technostructure must also be highly elaborated. In fact this structure was first identified with the rise of technocratic personnel in early-nineteenth-century industries such as textiles and banking.[1a] Because the machine organization depends primarily on the standardization of its operating work for coordination, the technostructure—which houses the staff analysts who do the standardizing—emerges as the key part of the structure. To the line managers may be delegated the formal authority for the operating units, but without the standardizers—the cadre of work-study analysts, schedulers, quality control engineers, planners, budgeters, accountants, operations researchers, and many more—these structures simply could not function. Hence, despite their lack of formal authority, considerable informal power rests with these staff analysts, who standardize everyone else's work. Rules and regulations permeate the entire system: The emphasis on standardization extends well beyond the operating core of the machine organization, and with it follows the analysts' influence.

A further reflection of this formalization of behavior are the sharp divisions of labor all over the machine organization. Job specialization in the operating core and the pronounced formal distinction between line and staff have already been mentioned. In addition, the administrative structure is clearly distinguished from the operating core; unlike the entrepreneurial organization, here managers seldom work alongside operators. And they themselves tend to be organized along functional lines, meaning that each runs a unit that performs a single function in the chain that produces the final outputs. Figure 8–1 shows this, for example, in the organigram of a large steel company, traditionally machinelike in structure.

All this suggests that the machine organization is a structure with an obsession—namely, control. A control mentality pervades it from top to bottom. At the bottom, consider how a Ford Assembly Division general foreman described his work:

> I refer to my watch all the time. I check different items. About every hour I tour my line. About six thirty, I'll tour labor relations to find out

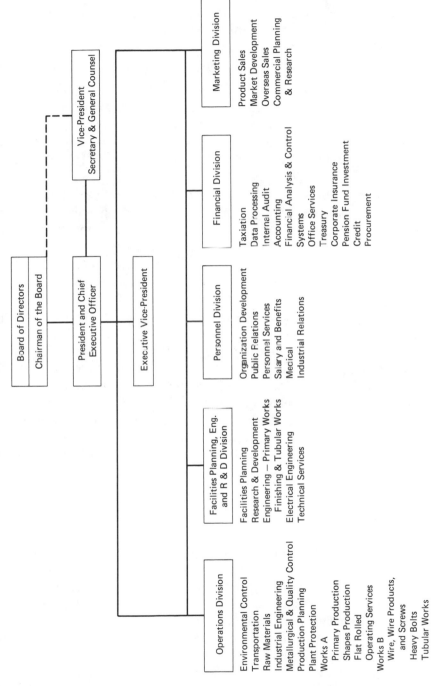

FIGURE 8–1
Organigram of a Large Steel Company

Board of Directors
Chairman of the Board

President and Chief Executive Officer

Executive Vice-President

Vice-President
Secretary & General Counsel

Operations Division

Environmental Control
Transportation
Raw Materials
Industrial Engineering
Metallurgical & Quality Control
Production Planning
Plant Protection
Works A
    Primary Production
    Shapes Production
    Flat Rolled
    Operating Services
Works B
    Wire, Wire Products,
        and Screws
    Heavy Bolts
    Tubular Works

Facilities Planning, Eng. and R & D Division

Facilities Planning
Research & Development
Engineering – Primary Works
    Finishing & Tubular Works
Electrical Engineering
Technical Services

Personnel Division

Organization Development
Public Relations
Personnel Services
Salary and Benefits
Medical
Industrial Relations

Financial Division

Taxation
Data Processing
Internal Audit
Accounting
Financial Analysis & Control
Systems
Office Services
Treasury
Corporate Insurance
Pension Fund Investment
Credit
Procurement

Marketing Division

Product Sales
Market Development
Overseas Sales
Commercial Planning
    & Research

who is absent. At seven, I hit the end of the line. I'll check paint, check my scratches and damage. Around ten I'll start talking to all the foremen. I make sure they're all awake. We can't have no holes, no nothing.

And at the top, consider the words of a chief executive:

When I was president of this big corporation, we lived in a small Ohio town, where the main plant was located. The corporation specified who you could socialize with, and on what level. (His wife interjects: "Who were the wives you could play bridge with."). In a small town they didn't have to keep check on you. Everybody knew. There are certain sets of rules.[2]

The obsession with control reflects two central facts about these organizations. First, attempts are made to eliminate all possible uncertainty, so that the bureaucratic machine can run smoothly, without interruption, the operating core perfectly sealed off from external influence. Second, these are structures ridden with conflict; the control systems are required to contain it. The problem in the machine organization is not to develop an open atmosphere where people can talk the conflicts out, but to enforce a closed, tightly controlled one where the work can get done despite them.

The obsession with control also helps to explain the frequent proliferation of support staff in these organizations. Many of the staff services could be purchased from outside suppliers. But that would expose the machine organization to the uncertainties of the open market. So it "makes" rather than "buys," that is, it envelops as many of the support services as it can within its own structure in order to control them, everything from the cafeteria in the factory to the law office at headquarters.

THE STRATEGIC APEX

The managers at the strategic apex of these organizations are concerned in large part with the fine-tuning of their bureaucratic machines. Theirs is a perpetual search for more efficient ways to produce the given outputs.

But not all is strictly improvement of performance. Just keeping the structure together in the face of its conflicts also consumes a good deal of the energy of top management. As noted, conflict is not resolved in the machine organization; rather it is bottled up so that the work can get done. And as in the case of a bottle, the cork is applied at the top: Ultimately, it is the top managers who must keep the lid on the conflicts through their role of handling disturbances. Moreover, the managers of the strategic apex must intervene frequently in the activities of the middle line to ensure that coordination is achieved there. The top managers are the only generalists in the structure, the only managers with a perspective broad enough to see all the functions.

All this leads us to the conclusion that considerable power in the machine organization rests with the managers of the strategic apex. These are, in other words, rather centralized structures: The formal power clearly rests at the top; hierarchy and chain of authority are paramount concepts. But so also does much of the informal power, since that resides in knowledge, and only at the top of the hierarchy does the formally segmented knowledge of the organization come together.

Thus, our introductory figure shows the machine organization with a fully elaborated administrative and support structure—both parts of the staff component being focused on the operating core—together with large units in the operating core but narrower ones in the middle line to reflect the tall hierarchy of authority.

CONDITIONS OF THE MACHINE ORGANIZATION

Work of a machine bureaucratic nature is found, above all, in environments that are simple and stable. The work associated with complex environments cannot be rationalized into simple tasks, and that associated with dynamic environments cannot be predicted, made repetitive, and so standardized.

In addition, the machine configuration is typically found in mature organizations, large enough to have the volume of operating work needed for repetition and standardization, and old enough to have been able to settle on the standards they wish to use. These are the organizations that have seen it all before and have established standard procedures to deal with it. Likewise, machine organizations tend to be identified with technical systems that regulate the operating work, so that it can easily be programmed. Such technical systems cannot be very sophisticated or automated (for reasons that will be discussed later).

Mass production firms are perhaps the best-known machine organizations. Their operating work flows through an integrated chain, open at one end to accept raw materials, and after that functioning as a sealed system that processes them through sequences of standardized operations. Thus, the environment may be stable because the organization has acted aggressively to stabilize it. Giant firms in such industries as transportation, tobacco, and metals are well known for their attempts to influence the forces of supply and demand by the use of advertising, the development of long-term supply contacts, sometimes the establishment of cartels. They also tend to adopt strategies of "vertical integration," that is, extend their production chains at both ends, becoming both their own suppliers and their own customers. In that way they can bring some of the forces of supply and demand within their own planning processes.

Of course, the machine organization is not restricted to large, or manufacturing, or even private enterprise organizations. Small manufacturers—for example producers of discount furniture or paper products—may sometimes prefer this structure because their operating work is simple and repetitive. Many service firms use it for the same reason, such as banks or insurance companies in their retailing activities. Another condition often found with machine organizations is external control. Many government departments, such as post offices and tax collection agencies, are machine bureaucratic not only because their operating work is routine but also because they must be accountable to the public for their actions. Everything they do—treating clients, hiring employees, etc.—must be seen to be fair, and so they proliferate regulations.

Since control is the forte of the machine bureaucracy, it stands to reason that organizations in the business of control—regulatory agencies, custodial prisons, police forces—are drawn to this configuration, sometimes in spite of contradictory conditions. The same is true for the special need for safety. Organizations that fly airplanes or put out fires must minimize the risks they take. Hence they formalize their procedures extensively to ensure that they are carried out to the letter: A fire crew cannot arrive at a burning house and then turn to the chief for orders or discuss informally who will connect the hose and who will go up the ladder.

MACHINE ORGANIZATIONS AS INSTRUMENTS AND CLOSED SYSTEMS

Control raises another issue about machine organizations. Being so pervasively regulated, they themselves can easily be controlled externally, as the *instruments* of outside influencers. In contrast, however, their obsession with control runs not only up the hierarchy but beyond, to control of their own environments, so that they can become *closed systems* immune to external influence. From the perspective of power, the instrument and the closed system constitute two main types of machine organizations.

In our terms, the instrument form of machine organization is dominated by one external influencer or by a group of them acting in concert. In the "closely held" corporation, the dominant influencer is the outside owner; in some prisons, it is a community concerned with the custody rather than the rehabilitation of prisoners.

Outside influencers render an organization their instrument by appointing the chief executive, charging that person with the pursuit of clear goals (ideally quantifiable, such as return-on-investment or prisoner escape measures), and then holding the chief responsible for performance. That way outsiders can control an organization without actually having to manage it. And such control, by virtue of the power put in the hands of the chief executive and the numerical nature of the goals, acts to centralize and bureaucratize the internal structure, in other words, to drive it to the machine form. (Recall the proposition in Chapter 6 about the centralizing and formalizing effects of the external control of an organization.)

In contrast to this, Charles Perrow, the colorful and outspoken organizational sociologist, does not quite see the machine organization as anyone's instrument:

> Society is adaptive to organizations, to the large, powerful organizations controlled by a few, often overlapping, leaders. To see these organizations as adaptive to a "turbulent," dynamic, very changing environment is to indulge in fantasy. The environment of most powerful organizations is well controlled by them, quite stable, and made up of other organizations with similar interests, or ones they control.[3]

Perrow is, of course, describing the closed system form of machine organization, the one that uses its bureaucratic procedures to seal itself off from external control and control others instead. It controls not only its own people but its environment as well: perhaps its suppliers, customers, competitors, even government and owners too.

Of course, autonomy can be achieved not only by controlling others (for example, buying up customers and suppliers in so-called vertical integration) but simply by avoiding the control of others. Thus, for example, closed system organizations sometimes form cartels with ostensible competitors or, less blatantly, diversify markets to avoid dependence on particular customers, finance internally to avoid dependence on particular financial groups, and even buy back their own shares to weaken the influence of their own owners. Key to being a closed system is to ensure wide dispersal, and therefore pacification, of all groups of potential external influence.

What goals does the closed system organization pursue? Remember that to sustain centralized bureaucracy the goals should be operational, ideally quantifiable. What operational goals enable an organization to serve itself, as a system closed to external influence? The most obvious answer is growth. Survival may be an indispensable goal and efficiency a necessary one, but beyond those what really matters here is making the system larger. Growth serves the system by providing greater rewards for its insiders—bigger empires for managers to run or fancier private jets to fly, greater programs for analysts to design, even more power for unions to wield by virtue of having more members. (The unions may be external influencers, but the management can keep them passive by allowing them more of the spoils of the closed system.) Thus the classic closed system machine organization, the large, widely held industrial corporation, has long been described as oriented far more to growth than to the maximization of profit per se.[4]

Of course, the closed system form of machine organization can exist outside the private sector too, for example in the fundraising agency that, relatively free to external control, becomes increasingly charitable to itself (as indicated by the plushness of its managers' offices), the agricultural or retail cooperative that ignores those who collectively own it, even government that becomes more intent on serving itself than the citizens for which it supposedly exists.

The communist state seems to fit all the characteristics of the closed system bureaucracy. It has no dominant external influencer (at least in the case of the Soviet Union, if not the other East European states, its "instruments"). And the population to which it is ostensibly responsible must respond to its own plethora of rules and regulations. Its election procedures, traditionally offering a choice of one, are similar to those for the directors of the "widely held" Western corporation. The government's own structure is heavily bureaucratic, with a single hierarchy of authority and a very elaborate technostructure, ranging from state planners to KGB agents. (As James Worthy noted, Frederick Taylor's "Scientific Management had its fullest flowering not in America but in Soviet Russia."[5]) All significant resources are the property of the state—the collective system—not the individual. And, as in other closed systems, the administrators tend to take the lion's share of the benefits, as one writer noted some time ago:

> . . . far from increased productivity benefiting the majority, increases in productive capacity primarily benefit the bureaucracy itself. In the case of the Soviet Union, the standard of living of the bureaucracy has risen far more than that of any other group, and its tendency is to go higher still.[6]*

SOME ISSUES ASSOCIATED WITH THE MACHINE ORGANIZATION

No structure has evoked more heated debate than the machine organization. As Michel Crozier, one of its most eminent students, has noted:

> On the one hand, most authors consider the bureaucratic organization to be the embodiment of rationality in the modern world, and, as such, to be intrinsically superior to all other possible forms of organizations. On the other hand, many authors—often the same ones—consider it a sort of Leviathan, preparing the enslavement of the human race.[7]

Max Weber, who first wrote about this form of organization, emphasized its rationality; in fact, the word *machine* comes directly from his writings.[8] A machine is certainly precise; it is also reliable and easy to control; and it is efficient—at least when restricted to the job it has been designed to do. Those are the reasons many organizations are structured as machine bureaucracies. When an integrated set of simple, repetitive tasks must be performed precisely and consistently by human beings, this is the most efficient structure—indeed, the only conceivable one.

But in these same advantages of machinelike efficiency lie all the disadvantages of this configuration. Machines consist of mechanical parts; organizational structures also include human beings—and that is where the analogy breaks down.

---

*On the day that Alexei Kosygin, Chairmain of the USSR Council of Ministers, died, a Canadian diplomat who knew him was interviewed on the CBC radio network. Kosygin reminded him of an American businessman more than the head of a totalitarian state, he said, seemingly surprised at the point. He should not have been. The Soviet Union is organized much like a large Western business, with its divisions, planning procedures, and performance control measures, and, conversely, in many fundamental respects the large Western business is managed internally much like a centralized state.

HUMAN PROBLEMS IN THE OPERATING CORE

James Worthy, when he was an executive of Sears, wrote a penetrating and scathing criticism of the machine organization in his book *Big Business and Free Men*. Worthy traces the root of the human problems in these structures to the "scientific management" movement led by Frederick Taylor that swept America early in this century. Worthy acknowledges Taylor's contribution to efficiency, narrowly defined. Worker initiative did not, however, enter into his efficiency equation. Taylor's pleas to remove "all possible brain work" from the shop floor also removed all possible initiative from the people who worked there: The "machine has no will of its own. Its parts have no urge to independent action. Thinking, direction—even purpose—must be provided from outside or above." This had the "consequence of destroying the meaning of work itself," which has been "fantastically wasteful for industry and society," resulting in excessive absenteeism, high worker turnover, sloppy workmanship, costly strikes, even outright sabotage.[9] Of course, there are people who like to work in highly structured situations. But increasing numbers do not, at least not *that* highly structured.

Taylor was fond of saying, "In the past the man has been first; in the future the system must be first."[10] Prophetic words, indeed. Modern man seems to exist for his systems; many of the organizations he created to serve him have come to enslave him. The result is that several of what Victor Thompson has called "bureaupathologies"—dysfunctional behaviors of these structures—reinforce each other to form a vicious circle in the machine organization.[11] The concentration on means at the expense of ends, the mistreatment of clients, the various manifestations of worker alienation—all lead to the tightening of controls on behavior. The implicit motto of the machine organization seems to be, "When in doubt, control." All problems have to be solved by the turning of the technocratic screws. But since that is what caused the bureaupathologies in the first place, increasing the controls serves only to magnify the problems, leading to the imposition of further controls, and so on.

COORDINATION PROBLEMS IN THE ADMINISTRATIVE CENTER

Since the operating core of the machine organization is not designed to handle conflict, many of the human problems that arise there spill up and over, into the administrative structure.

It is one of the ironies of the machine configuration that to achieve the control it requires, it must mirror the narrow specialization of its operating core in its administrative structure (for example, differentiating marketing managers from manufacturing managers, much as salesmen are differentiated from factory workers). This, in turn, means problems of communication and coordination. The fact is that the administrative structure of the machine organization is also ill suited to the resolution of problems through mutual adjustment. All the communication barriers in these structures—horizontal, vertical, status, line/staff—impede informal communication among managers and with staff people. "Each unit becomes jealous of its own prerogatives and finds ways to protect itself against the pressure or encroachments of others."[12] Thus narrow functionalism not only impedes coordination; it also encourages the building of private empires, which tends to produce topheavy organizations that can be more concerned with the political games to be won than with the clients to be served.

ADAPTATION PROBLEMS IN THE STRATEGIC APEX

But if mutual adjustment does not work in the administrative center—generating more political heat than cooperative light—how does the machine organization resolve its coordination problems? Instinctively, it tries standardization, for example, by tightening job descriptions or proliferating rules. But standardization is not suited to handling the nonroutine problems of the administrative center. Indeed, it only aggravates them, undermining the influence of the line managers and increasing the conflict. So to reconcile these coordination problems, the machine organization is left with only one coordinating mechanism, direct supervision from above. Specifically, nonroutine coordination problems between units are "bumped" up the line hierarchy until they reach a common level of supervision, often at the top of the structure. The result can be excessive centralization of power, which in turn produces a host of other problems. In effect, just as the human problems in the operating core become coordination problems in the administrative center, so too do the coordination problems in the administrative center become adaptation problems at the strategic apex. Let us take a closer look at these by concluding with a discussion of strategic change in the machine configuration.

STRATEGY FORMATION IN THE MACHINE ORGANIZATION

Strategy in the machine organization is supposed to emanate from the top of the hierarchy, where the perspective is broadest and the power most focused. All the relevant information is to be sent up the hierarchy, in aggregated, MIS-type form, there to be formulated into integrated strategy (with the aid of the technostructure). Implementation then follows, with the intended strategies sent down the hierarchy to be turned into successively more elaborated programs and action plans. Notice the clear division of labor assumed between the formulators at the top and the implementors down below, based on the assumption of perfectly deliberate strategy produced through a process of planning.

That is the theory. The practice has been shown to be another matter. Drawing on our strategy research at McGill, we shall consider first what planning really proved to be in one machinelike organization, how it may in fact have impeded strategic thinking in a second, and how a third really did change its strategy. From there we shall consider the problems of strategic change in machine organizations and their possible resolution.

PLANNING AS PROGRAMMING IN A SUPERMARKET CHAIN

What really is the role of formal planning? Does it produce original strategies? Let us return to the case of Steinberg's in the later years of its founder, as large size drove the organization toward the machine form, and as is common in that form, toward a planning mode of management at the expense of entrepreneurship.

One event in particular encouraged the start of planning at Steinberg's: the company's entry into capital markets in 1953. Months before it floated its first bond issue (stock, always nonvoting, came later), Sam Steinberg boasted to a newspaper reporter that "not a cent of any money outside the family is invested in the company." And asked about future plans, he replied: "Who knows? We will try to go everywhere there seems to be a need for us." A few months later he announced a $5 million debt issue and with it a $15 million five-year expansion program, one new store every two months for a total of thirty, the doubling of sales, new stores to average double the size of existing ones.

What happened in those ensuing months was Sam Steinberg's realization, after the opening of Montreal's first shopping center, that he needed to enter the shopping center business himself to protect his supermarket chain and that he could not do so with the company's traditional methods of short-term and internal financing. And, of course, no company is allowed to go to capital markets without a plan. You can't just say: "I'm Sam Steinberg and I'm good," though that was really the issue. In a "rational" society, you have to plan (or at least appear to do so).

But what exactly was that planning? One thing for certain: It did not formulate a strategy. Sam Steinberg already had that. What planning did was justify, elaborate, and articulate the strategy that already existed in Sam Steinberg's mind. Planning operationalized his strategic vision, programmed it. It gave order to that vision, imposing form on it to comply with the needs of the organization and its environment. Thus, planning followed the strategy-making process, which had been essentially entrepreneurial.

But its effect on that process was not incidental. By specifying and articulating the vision, planning constrained it and rendered it less flexible. Sam Steinberg retained formal control of the company to the day of his death. But his control over strategy did not remain so absolute. The entrepreneur, by keeping his vision personal, is able to adapt it at will to a changing environment. But by being forced to program it, the leader loses that flexibility. The danger, ultimately, is that the planning mode forces out the entrepreneurial one; procedure replaces vision. As its structure became more machinelike, Steinberg's required planning in the form of strategic programming. But that planning also accelerated the firm's transition toward the machine form of organization.

Is there, then, such a thing as "strategic planning"? I suspect not. To be more explicit, I do not find that major new strategies are formulated through any formal procedure. Organizations that rely on planning procedures to formulate strategies seem to extrapolate existing strategies, perhaps with marginal changes in them, or else copy the strategies of other organizations. This came out most clearly in another of our McGill studies.

PLANNING AS AN IMPEDIMENT TO STRATEGIC THINKING IN AN AIRLINE

From about the mid-1950s, Air Canada engaged heavily in planning. Once the airline was established, particularly once it developed its basic route structure, a number of factors drove it strongly to the planning mode. Above all was the need for coordination, both of flight schedules with aircraft, crews, and maintenance, and of the purchase of expensive aircraft with the structure of the route system. (Imagine someone calling out in the hangar: "Hey, Fred, this guy says he has two 747s for us; do you know who ordered them?") Safety was another factor: The intense need for safety in the air breeds a mentality of being very careful about what the organization does on the ground, too. That is the airlines' obsession with control. Other factors included the lead times inherent in key decisions, such as ordering new airplanes or introducing new routes, the sheer cost of the capital equipment, and the size of the organization. You don't run an intricate system like an airline, necessarily very machinelike, without a great deal of formal planning.

But what we found to be the consequence of planning at Air Canada was the absence of a major reorientation of strategy during our study period (up to the mid-1970s). Aircraft certainly changed—they became larger and faster—but the basic route system did not, nor did markets. Air Canada gave only marginal attention, for example, to cargo, charter, and shuttle operations. Formal planning, in our view, impeded strategic thinking.

The problem is that planning, too, proceeds from the machine perspective, much as an assembly line or a conventional machine produces a product. It all depends on the decomposition of analysis: You split the process into a series of steps or component parts, specify each, and then by following the specifications in sequence you get the desired product. There is a fallacy in this, however, noted back in Chapter 4. Assembly lines and conventional machines produce standardized products, while planning is supposed to produce a novel strategy. It is as if the machine is supposed to design the machine; the planning machine is expected to create the original blueprint—the strategy. To repeat another point made there, planning is analysis oriented to decomposition, while strategy-making depends on synthesis oriented to integration. That is why the term "strategic planning" has proved to be an oxymoron.

STRATEGIC CHANGE IN AN AUTOMOBILE FIRM

How then does the planning-oriented machine bureaucracy change its strategy when it has to? Volkswagenwerk was an organization that had to. We interpreted its history from 1934 to 1974 as one long life cycle of a single strategic perspective. The original "people's car," the famous "Beetle," was conceived by Ferdinand Porsche; the factory to produce it was built just before the war but did not go into civilian automobile production until after. In 1948, a man named Heinrich Nordhoff was given control of the devastated plant and began the rebuilding of it, as well as of the organization and the strategy itself, rounding out Porsche's original conception. The firm's success was dramatic.

By the late 1950s, however, problems began to appear. Demand in Germany was moving away from the Beetle. The typically machine-bureaucratic response was not to rethink the basic strategy—"it's okay" was the reaction—but rather to graft another piece onto it. A new automobile model was added, larger than the Beetle but with a similar no-nonsense approach to motoring, again air-cooled with the engine in the back. Volkswagenwerk added position but did not change perspective.

But that did not solve the basic problem, and by the mid-1960s the company was in crisis. Nordhoff, who had resisted strategic change, died in office and was replaced by a lawyer from outside the business. The company then underwent a frantic search for new models, designing, developing, or acquiring a whole host of them with engines in the front, middle, and rear; air- and water-cooled; front- and rear-wheel drive. To paraphrase the humorist Stephen Leacock, Volkswagenwerk leaped onto its strategic horse and rode off in all directions. Only when another leader came in, a man steeped in the company and the automobile business, did the firm consolidate itself around a new strategic perspective, based on the stylish front-wheel-drive, water-cooled designs of one of its acquired firms, and thereby turn its fortunes around.

What this story suggests, first of all, is the great force of bureaucratic momentum in the machine organization. Even leaving planning aside, the immense effort of producing and marketing a new line of automobiles locks a company into a certain posture. But here the momentum was psychological, too. Nordhoff, who had been the driving force behind the great success of the organization, became a major liability when the environment demanded change. Over the years, he too had been captured by bureaucratic momentum. Moreover, the uniqueness and tight integration of Volkswagenwerk's strategy—we labeled it *gestalt*—impeded strategic change. Change an element of a tightly integrated gestalt and it *dis*integrates. Thus does success eventually breed failure.

BOTTLENECK AT THE TOP

Why the great difficulty in changing strategy in the machine organization? Here we take up that question and show how changes generally have to be achieved in a different configuration, if at all.

As discussed earlier, unanticipated problems in the machine organization tend to get bumped up the hierarchy. When these are few, which means conditions are relatively stable, things work smoothly enough. But in times of rapid change, just when new strategies are called for, the number of such problems magnifies, resulting in a bottleneck at the top, where senior managers get overloaded. And that tends either to impede strategic change or else to render it ill-considered.

A major part of the problem is information. Senior managers face an organization decomposed into parts, like a machine itself. Marketing information comes up one channel, manufacturing information up another, and so on. Somehow it is the senior managers themselves who must integrate all that information. But the very machine bureaucratic premise of separating the administration of work from the doing of it means that the top managers often lack the intimate, detailed knowledge of issues necessary to effect such an integration. In essence, the necessary power is at the top of the structure, but the necessary knowledge is often at the bottom.

Of course, there is a machinelike solution to that problem too—not surprisingly in the form of a system. It is called a management information system, or MIS, and what it does is combine all the necessary information and package it neatly so that top managers can be informed about what is going on—the perfect solution for the overloaded executive. At least in theory.

Unfortunately, a number of real-world problems arise in the MIS. For one thing, in the tall administrative hierarchy of the machine organization, information must pass through many levels before it reaches the top. Losses take place at each one. Good news gets highlighted while bad news gets blocked on the way up. And "soft" information, so necessary for strategy formation, cannot easily pass through, while much of the hard MIS-type information arrives only slowly. In a stable environment, the manager may be able to wait; in a rapidly changing one, he or she cannot. The president wants to be told right away that the firm's most important customer was seen playing golf yesterday with a main competitor, not to find out six months later in the form of a drop in a sales report. Gossip, hearsay, speculation—the softest kinds of information—warn the manager of impending problems; the MIS all too often records for posterity ones that have already been felt. The manager who depends on an MIS in a changing environment generally finds himself or herself out of touch.

The obvious solution for top managers is to bypass the MIS and set up their own informal information systems, networks of contacts that bring them the rich, tangible, instant information they need. But that violates the machine organization's presuppositions of formality and respect for the chain of authority. Also, that takes the managers' time, the lack of which caused the bottleneck in the first place. So a fundamental dilemma faces the top managers of the machine organization as a result of its very own design: In times of change, when they most need the time to inform themselves, the system overburdens them with other pressures. They are thus reduced to acting superficially, with inadequate, abstract information.

THE FORMULATION / IMPLEMENTATION DICHOTOMY

The essential problem lies in one of the chief tenets of the machine organization, that strategy formation must be sharply separated from strategy implementation. One is thought out at the top, the other then acted out lower down. For this to work assume two conditions: first, that the formulator has full and sufficient information, and second, that the world will hold still, or at least change in predictable ways, during the implementation, so that there is no need for *re*formulation.

Now consider why the organization needs a new strategy in the first place. It is because its world has changed in an unpredictable way, indeed may continue to do so. We have just seen how the machine bureaucratic structure tends to violate the first condition—it misinforms the senior manager during such times of change. And when change continues in an unpredictable way (or at least the world unfolds in a way not yet predicted by an ill-informed management), then the second condition is violated too—it hardly makes sense to lock in by implementation a strategy that does not reflect changes in the world around it.

What all this amounts to is a need to collapse the formulation/implementation dichotomy precisely when the strategy of machine bureaucracy must be changed. This can be done in one of two ways.

In one case, the formulator implements. In other words, power is concentrated at the top, not only for creating the strategy but also for implementing it, step by step, in a personalized way. The strategist is put in close personal touch with the situation at hand (more commonly a strategist is appointed who has or can develop that touch) so that he or she can, on one hand, be properly informed and, on the other, control the implementation en route in order to reformulate when necessary. This, of course, describes the entrepreneurial configuration, at least at the strategic apex.

In the other case, the implementers formulate. In other words, power is concentrated lower down, where the necessary information resides. As people who are naturally in touch with the specific situations at hand take individual actions—approach new customers, develop new products, etc.—patterns form, in other words, strategies emerge. And this, as we shall see, describes the innovative configuration, where strategic initiatives often originate in the grass roots of the organization, and then are championed by managers at middle levels who integrate them with one another or with existing strategies in order to gain their acceptance by senior management.

We conclude, therefore, that the machine configuration is ill-suited to change its fundamental strategy, that the organization must in effect change configuration temporarily in order to change strategy. Either it reverts to the entrepreneurial form, to allow a single leader to develop vision (or proceed with one developed earlier), or else it overlays an innovative form on its conventional structure (for example, creates an informed network of lateral teams and task forces) so that the necessary strategies can emerge. The former can obviously function faster than the latter; that is why it tends to be used for drastic *turnaround*, while the latter tends to proceed by the slower process of *revitalization*. (Of course, quick turnaround may be necessary because there has been no slow revitalization.) In any event, both are characterized by a capacity to *learn*—that is the essence of the entrepreneurial and innovative configurations, in one case learning centralized for the simpler context, in the other, decentralized for the more complex one. The machine configuration is not so characterized.

This, however, should come as no surprise. After all, machines are specialized instruments, designed for productivity, not for adaptation. In Hunt's words, machine bureaucracies are performance systems, not problem-solving ones.[13] Efficiency is their forte, not innovation. An organization cannot put blinders on its personnel and then expect peripheral vision. Managers here are rewarded for cutting costs and improving standards, not for taking risks and ignoring procedures. Change makes a mess of the operating systems: Change one link in a carefully coupled system, and the whole chain must be reconceived. Why, then, should we be surprised when our bureaucratic machines fail to adapt?

Of course, it is fair to ask why we spend so much time trying to make them adapt. After all, when an ordinary machine becomes redundant, we simply scrap it, happy that it served us for as long and as well as it did. Converting it to another use generally proves more expensive than simply starting over. I suspect the same is often true for bureaucratic machines. But here, of course, the context is social and political. Mechanical parts don't protest, nor do displaced raw materials. Workers, suppliers, and customers do, however, protest the scrapping of organizations, for obvious reasons. But that the cost of this is awfully high in a society of giant machine organizations will be the subject of the final chapter of this book.

STRATEGIC REVOLUTIONS IN MACHINE ORGANIZATIONS

Machine organizations do sometimes change, however, at times effectively but more often it would seem at great cost and pain. The lucky ones are able to overlay an innovative structure for periodic revitalization (in ways I shall suggest in the closing chapter of this section), while many of the other survivors somehow manage to get turned around in entrepreneurial fashion.

Overall, the machine organizations seem to follow what my colleagues Danny Miller and Peter Friesen call a "quantum theory" of organization change.[14] They pursue their set strategies through long periods of stability (naturally occurring or created by themselves as closed systems), using planning and other procedures to do so efficiently. Periodically these are interrupted by short bursts of change, which Miller and Friesen characterize as "strategic revolutions" (although another colleague, Mihaela Firsirotu, perhaps better labels it "strategic turnaround as cultural revolution"[15]).

ORGANIZATION TAKING PRECEDENCE IN THE MACHINE ORGANIZATION

To conclude, as shown in Figure 8–2, it is organization—with its systems and procedures, its planning and its bureaucratic momentum—that takes

FIGURE 8–2
Organization Takes Precedence

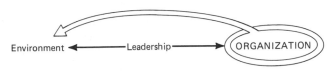

precedence over leadership and environment in the machine configuration. Environment fits organization, either because the organization has slotted itself into a context that matches its procedures, or else because it has forced the environment to do so. And leadership generally falls into place too, supporting the organization, indeed often becoming part of its bureaucratic momentum.

This generally works effectively, though hardly nonproblematically, at least in times of stability. But in times of change, efficiency becomes ineffective and the organization will falter unless it can find a different way to organize for adaptation.

All of this is another way of saying that the machine organization is a configuration, a species, like the others, suited to its own context but ill-suited to others. But unlike the others, it is the dominant configuration in our specialized societies. As long as we demand inexpensive and so necessarily standardized goods and services, and as long as people continue to be more efficient than real machines at providing them, and remain willing to do so, then the machine organization will remain with us—and so will all its problems.

9
THE DIVERSIFIED ORGANIZATION

The waves of mergers that have taken place in American business over the last century, first to combine businesses into larger entities, sometimes enormous trusts, then to add activities at either end of the production chain under the label "vertical integration" (though always, for some curious reason, displayed horizontally), and finally, especially, to move the firms into new businesses, have led to the formation of giant corporations and to the so-called divisionalized forms of structure. The "conglomerate" is, of course, the ultimate example of this, where a corporation doesn't much care about any relationship among its different businesses other than financial.

American business probably reached its peak of conglomerate diversification sometime in the 1970s, after the great merger movement of the 1960s, when so-called professional management—the assumption that a good manager could manage anything—was itself at its peak. But then conglomeration waned. Perhaps there was a realization that it sometimes helps to know a business deeply, more deeply than can executives at a distant headquarters who have to deal with chinaware in the morning and steam shovels in the afternoon. Or maybe it was simply the market forces taking over, the failure of conglomeration allowing outside financial types, even more removed from products and services than the professional managers inside, to strip and restructure excessively diversified corporations.

In any event, the strategy of diversification and the associated structure of divisionalization have hardly disappeared. A chief concern of almost all large corporations remains how to expand while exercising some control over the range of business they are in, and then how to knit these various businesses together to exploit what is now popularly called "synergy" (the 2 + 2 = 5 effect).

In fact, enormous amounts of energy have gone into trying to figure out what to do with overgrown and overextended businesses. It's been great for the consulting professional and the financial houses, but I'm not sure anyone else has benefited very much. The large corporation may have achieved its initial success by being smarter in its core business, but I am not sure that many have been very smart in their programs of conglomerate diversification. A few have persevered and achieved new and viable definition (that is, strategy), but many have been forced into expensive bouts of divestment.

"Put him down as undecided," a friend of mine would say. Well, my biases stem from a belief that power has been allowed to take precedence over performance, rooted in a most superficial view of what it means to manage a business. The relevant distinction for me is between what I prefer to call "thick" and "thin" management. Thin management involves moving pieces around a chessboard, throwing money at people to motivate them and money at facilities to improve them; in the diversified corporation it has meant "portfolio management" and "restructuring" and "shareholder value." Thick management means getting deeply inside a business, coming to know its needs and its processes and its people well enough to weld them all together into a smoothly functioning entity that serves its markets with care and understanding. Conglomerate diversification has given us more than enough of the former, in my opinion.

Severe as those problems have been on the economic side, I believe the greatest ones have been social. Organizations that become too large, too diversified, and too superficial have deadening effects on the people who work for them, and they pose grave threats to the social order, including democracy itself. This applies not only to business but to other spheres as well, governments run as giant conglomerates, multiversities likewise managed, massive divisionalized school systems, and so on through almost every social service. All have caused a great deal of misery.

After discussing the divisionalized form of structure, the conditions that foster it, and the stages that lead up to its fully developed (conglomerate) form, this chapter will delve at some length into what I believe are the threatening social issues that accompany it. I hope you will bear with me as I display my biases rather openly in this latter discussion.

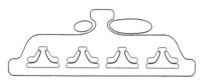

The Diversified Organization

Structure: • market based "divisions" loosely coupled together under central administrative headquarters

• divisions run businesses autonomously (implying no more than limited decentralization to division managers), subjected to performance control system that standardizes their outputs

• tendency to drive structures of divisions toward machine configuration, as instruments of headquarters (though tendency of overall organization to be closed system type)

Context: • market diversity, especially of products and services (as opposed to clients or regions); by-product and related-product diversification encourages intermediate forms, conglomerate diversification being purest form

• typically found in largest and most mature organizations, especially business corporations but also, increasingly, government and other public spheres (e.g. multiversities)

Strategy: • headquarters manages "corporate" strategy as portfolio of businesses, divisions manage individual business strategies

Issues: • resolves some problems of integrated functional (machine) structures (spreading risk, moving capital, adding and deleting businesses, etc.)

      but

• conglomerate diversification sometimes costly and discouraging of innovation; improvements in functioning of capital markets and boards may make independent businesses more effective than divisions

• performance control system risks driving organization toward socially unresponsive or irresponsible behavior

• despite tendency to use in public sphere, dangers there even greater due to nonmeasurable nature of many goals

THE BASIC DIVISIONALIZED STRUCTURE

The diversified organization is not so much an integrated entity as a set of semi-autonomous units coupled together by a central administrative structure. The units are generally called *divisions,* and the central administration, the *headquarters.* This is a widely used configuration in the private sector of the industrialized economy; the vast majority of the Fortune 500, America's largest corporations, use this structure or a variant of it. But, as we shall see, it is also found in other sectors as well.

In what is commonly called the "divisionalized" form of structure, units, called "divisions," are created to serve distinct markets and are given control over the operating functions necessary to do so, as shown

FIGURE 9–1

Typical Organigram for a Divisionalized Manufacturing Firm

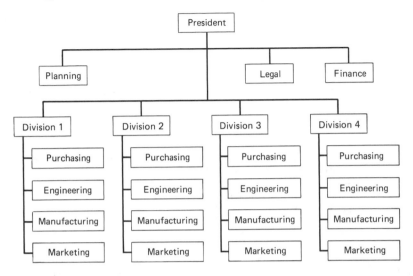

in Figure 9–1. Each is therefore relatively free of direct control by head-quarters or even of the need to coordinate activities with other divisions. Each, in other words, appears to be a self-standing business. Of course, none is. There *is* a headquarters, and it has a series of roles that distinguish this overall configuration from a collection of independent businesses providing the same set of products and services.

ROLES OF THE HEADQUARTERS

Above all, the headquarters exercises performance control. It sets standards of achievement, generally in quantitative terms (such as return on investment or growth in sales), and then monitors the results. Coordination between headquarters and the divisions thus reduces largely to the standardization of outputs. Of course, there is some direct supervision—headquarters' managers have to have personal contact with and knowledge of the divisions. But that is largely circumscribed by the key assumption in this configuration that if the division managers are to be responsible for the performance of their divisions, they must have considerable autonomy to manage them as they see fit. Hence there is extensive delegation of authority from headquarters to the level of division manager.

Certain important tasks do, however, remain for the headquarters. One is to develop the overall *corporate* strategy, meaning to establish the portfolio of businesses in which the organization will operate. The headquarters establishes, acquires, divests, and closes down divisions in order to change its portfolio. Popular in the 1970s in this regard was the Boston Consulting Group's "growth share matrix," where corporate managers were supposed to allocate funds to divisions on the basis of their falling into the categories of dogs, cash cows, wildcats, and stars. But enthusiasm for that technique waned, perhaps mindful of Pope's warning that a little learning can be a dangerous thing.

Second, the headquarters manages the movement of funds between the divisions, taking the excess profits of some to support the greater growth potential of others. Third, of course, the headquarters, through its own technostructure, designs and operates the performance control system. Fourth, it appoints and therefore retains the right to replace the division managers. For a headquarters that does not directly manage any division, its most tangible power when the performance of a division lags—short of riding out an industry downturn or divesting the division—is to replace its leader. Finally, the headquarters provides certain support services that are common to all the divisions—a corporate public relations office or legal counsel, for example.

STRUCTURE OF THE DIVISIONS

It has been common to label divisionalized organizations "decentralized." That is a reflection of how *certain* of them came to be, most notably DuPont early in this century. When organizations that were structured functionally (for example, in departments of marketing, manufacturing, and engineering, etc.) diversified, they found that coordination of their different product lines across the functions became increasingly complicated. The central managers had to spend great amounts of time intervening to resolve disputes. But once these corporations switched to a divisionalized form of structure, where all the functions for a given business could be contained in a single unit dedicated to that business, management became much simpler. In effect, their structures became *more* decentralized, power over distinct businesses being delegated to the division managers.

But more decentralized does not mean *decentralized*. That word, as was noted in Chapter 6, refers to the dispersal of decision-making power in an organization, and in many of the diversified corporations much of the power tended to remain with the few managers who ran the businesses. Indeed, the most famous case of divisionalization was one of relative *centralization:* Alfred P. Sloan introduced the divisionalized structure to General Motors in the 1920s to *reduce* the power of its autonomous business units, to impose systems of financial controls on what had been a largely unmanaged agglomeration of different automobile businesses.

In fact, I would argue that it is the *centralization* of power within the divisions that is most compatible with the divisionalized form of structure. In other words, the effect of having a headquarters over the divisions is to drive them toward the machine configuration, namely a structure of centralized bureaucracy. That is the structure most compatible with headquarters control, in my opinion. If true, this would seem to be an important point, because it means that the proliferation of the diversified configuration in many spheres—business, government, and the rest—has the effect of driving many suborganizations toward machine bureaucracy, even where that configuration may be inappropriate (school systems, for example, or government departments charged with innovative project work).

The explanation for this lies in the standardization of outputs, the key to the functioning of the divisionalized structure. Bear in mind the headquarters' dilemma: to respect divisional autonomy while exercising control over performance. This it seeks to resolve by after-the-fact monitoring of divisional results, based on clearly defined performance standards. But two main assumptions underlie such standards.

First, each division must be treated as a single integrated system with a single, consistent set of goals. In other words, although the divisions may be loosely coupled with each other, the assumption is that each is tightly coupled internally.*

Second, these goals must be operational ones, in other words, lend themselves to quantitative measurement. But in the less formal configurations—entrepreneurial and innovative—which are less stable, such performance standards are difficult to establish, while in the professional configuration, the complexity of the work makes it difficult to establish such standards. Moreover, while the entrepreneurial configuration may

---

* Unless, of course, there is a second layer of divisionalization, which simply takes this conclusion down another level in the hierarchy.

lend itself to being integrated around a single set of goals, the innovative and professional configurations do not. Thus, only the machine configuration of the major types fits comfortably into the conventional divisionalized structure, by virture of its integration and its operational goals.

In fact, when organizations with another configuration are drawn under the umbrella of a divisionalized structure, they tend to be forced toward the machine bureaucratic form, to make them conform with *its* needs. How often have we heard stories of entrepreneurial firms recently acquired by conglomerates being descended upon by hordes of headquarters technocrats bemoaning the loose controls, the absence of organigrams, the informality of the systems? In many cases, of course, the very purpose of the acquisition was to do just this, tighten up the organization so that its strategies can be pursued more pervasively and systematically. But other times, the effect is to destroy the organization's basic strengths, sometimes including its flexibility and responsiveness. Similarly, how many times have we heard tell of government administrators complaining about being unable to control public hospitals or universities through conventional (meaning machine bureaucratic) planning systems?

This conclusion is, in fact, a prime manifestation of one of the hypotheses presented in Chapter 6: that concentrated external control of an organization (through what was called a dominated external coalition) has the effect of formalizing and centralizing its structure, in other words, of driving it toward the machine configuration. Headquarters' control of divisions is, of course, concentrated; indeed, when the diversified organization is itself a *closed system,* as I shall argue later many tend to be, then it is a most concentrated form of control. And, the effect of that control is to render the divisions its *instruments.*

There is, in fact, an interesting irony in this, in that the less society controls the overall diversified organization, the more the organization itself controls its individual units. The result is increased autonomy for the largest organizations coupled with decreased autonomy for their many activities. In other words, the systems are free, the people are not!

To conclude this discussion of the basic structure, the diversified configuration is represented in the opening figure, symbolically in terms of our logo, as follows. Headquarters has three parts: a small strategic apex of top managers, a small technostructure to the left concerned with the design and operation of the performance control system, and a slightly larger staff support group to the right to provide support services common to all the divisions. Each of the divisions is shown below the headquarters as a machine configuration.

CONDITIONS OF THE DIVERSIFIED ORGANIZATION

While the diversified configuration may arise from the federation of different organizations, which come together under a common headquarters umbrella, more often it appears to be the structural response to a machine organization that has diversified its range of product or service offerings. In either case, it is the diversity of markets above all that drives an organization to use this configuration. An organization faced with a single integrated market simply cannot split itself into autonomous divisions; the one with distinct markets, however, has an incentive to create a unit to deal with each.

There are three main kinds of market diversity—product and service, client, and region. In theory, all three can lead to divisionalization. But when diversification is based on variations in clients or regions as opposed to products or services, divisionalization often turns out to be incomplete. With identical products or services in each region or for each group of clients, the headquarters is encouraged to maintain central control of certain critical functions, to ensure common operationg standards for all the divisions. And that seriously reduces divisional autonomy, and so leads to a less than complete form of divisionalization.

Thus, one study found that insurance companies concentrate at headquarters the critical function of investment, and retailers concentrate that of purchasing, also controlling product range, pricing, and volume.[1] One need only look at the individual outlets of a typical retail chain to recognize the absence of divisional autonomy: Usually they all look alike. The same conclusion tends to hold for other businesses organized by regions, such as bakeries, breweries, cement producers, and soft drink bottlers: Their "divisions," distinguished only by geographical location, lack the autonomy normally associated with ones that produce distinct products or services.

What about the conditions of size? Although large size itself does not bring on divisionalization, surely it is not coincidental that most of America's largest corporations use some variant of this configuration. The fact is that as organizations grow large, they become inclined to diversify and then to divisionalize. One reason is protection: Large organizations tend to be risk-averse—they have too much to lose—and diversification spreads the risk. Another is that as firms grow large, they come to dominate their traditional market, and so must often find growth opportunities elsewhere, through diversification. Moreoever, diversification feeds on itself. It creates a cadre of aggressive general managers, each running his or her own division, who push for further diversification and further growth. Thus, most of the giant corporations—with the exception of the "heavies," those with enormously high fixed-cost operating systems, such as the oil or aluminum producers—not only were able to reach their status by diversifying but also feel great pressures to continue to do so.

Age is another factor associated with this configuration, much like size. In larger organizations, the management runs out of places to expand in its traditional markets; in older ones, the managers sometimes get bored with the traditional markets and find diversion through diversification. Also, time brings new competitors into old markets, forcing the management to look elsewhere for growth opportunities.

As governments grow large, they too tend to adopt a kind of divisionalized structure. The central administrators, unable to control all the agencies and departments directly, settle for granting their managers considerable autonomy and then trying to control their results through planning and performance controls. Indeed, the "accountability" buzzword so often heard in governments these days reflects just this trend—to move closer to a divisionalized structure.

One can, in fact, view the entire government as a giant diversified configuration (admittedly an oversimplification, since all kinds of links exist among the departments), with its three main coordinating agencies corresponding to the three main forms of control used by the headquarters of the large corporation. The budgetary agency, technocratic in nature, concerns itself with performance control of the departments; the public service commission, also partly technocratic, concerns itself with the recruiting and training of government managers; and the executive office, top management in nature, reviews the principal proposals and initiatives of the departments.

In the preceding chapter, the communist state was described as a closed system machine bureaucracy. But it may also be characterized as the ultimate closed system diversified configuration, with the various state enterprises and agencies its instruments, machine bureaucracies tightly regulated by the planning and control systems of the central government.

STAGES IN THE TRANSITION TO THE DIVERSIFIED ORGANIZATION

There has been a good deal of research on the transition of the corporation from the functional to the diversified form. Figure 9–2 and the discussion that follows borrow from this research to describe four stages in that transition.

At the top of Figure 9–2 is the pure *functional* structure, used by the corporation whose operating activities form one integrated, unbroken chain from purchasing through production to marketing and sales. Only

FIGURE 9–2

Stages in the Transition to the Pure Diversified Form

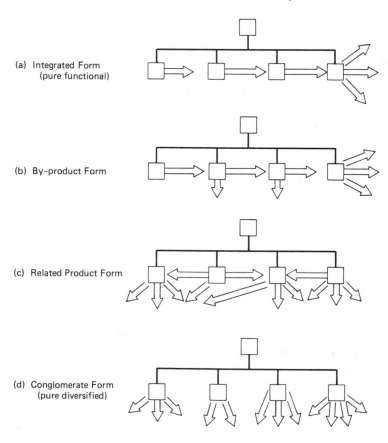

(a) Integrated Form
    (pure functional)

(b) By-product Form

(c) Related Product Form

(d) Conglomerate Form
    (pure diversified)

the final output is sold to the customers.* Autonomy cannot, therefore, be granted to the units, so the organization tends to take on the form of one overall machine configuration.

As an integrated firm seeks wider markets, it may introduce a variety of new end products and so shift all the way to the pure diversified form. A less risky alternative, however, is to start by marketing its intermediate products on the open market. This introduces small breaks in its processing chain, which in turn calls for a measure of divisionalization in its structure, giving rise to the *by-product* form. But because the processing chain remains more or less intact, central coordination must largely remain. Organizations that fall into this category tend to be vertically integrated, basing their operations on a single raw material, such as wood, oil, or aluminum, which they process to a variety of consumable end products. The example of Alcoa is shown in Figure 9–3.

Some corporations further diversify their by-product markets, breaking down their processing chain until what the divisions sell on the open market becomes more important than what they supply to each other. The organization then moves to the *related-product* form. For example, a firm manufacturing washing machines may set up a division to produce the motors. When the motor division sells more motors to outside customers than to its own sister division, a more serious form of divisionalization is called for. What typically holds the divisions of these firms together is some common thread among their products, perhaps a core skill or technology, perhaps a central market theme, as in a corporation such as 3M that likes to describe itself as being in the coating and bonding business. A good deal of the control over the specific product-market strategies can now revert to the divisions, but the central strategic theme means that headquarters may retain certain functions common to the divisions, such as research and development.

As a related-product firm expands into new markets or acquires other firms with less regard to a central strategic theme, the organization moves

---

* It should be noted that this is in fact the definition of a functional structure: Each activity contributes just one step in a chain toward the creation of the final product. Thus, for example, engineering is a functionally organized unit in the firm that produces and markets its own designs, while it would be a market organized unit in a consulting firm that sells its design services, among others, directly to clients.

FIGURE 9–3
By-Product and End-Product Sales of Alcoa[2]

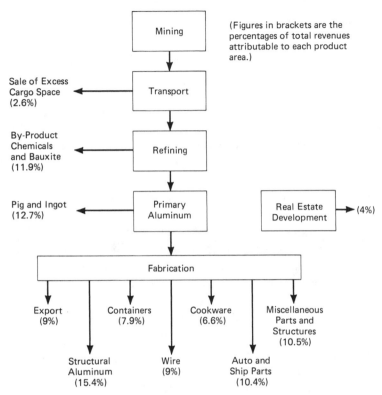

Note: Percentages for 1969 prepared by Richard Rumelt from data in company's annual reports.

See Notes section, page 379, for source.

to the *conglomerate* form and so adopts a pure diversified configuration, the one described at the beginning of this chapter. Each division serves its own markets, producing products unrelated to those of the other divisions—chinaware in one, steam shovels in a second, and so on.* The result is that the headquarters planning and control system becomes simply a vehicle for regulating performance, and the headquarters staff can diminish to almost nothing—a few general and group managers supported by a few financial analysts with a minimum of support services.

* I wrote this example here and in the introduction to this chapter somewhat whimsically before I encountered a firm in Finland with divisions that actually produce, among other things, the world's largest icebreaker ships and fine pottery!

SOME ISSUES ASSOCIATED WITH THE DIVERSIFIED ORGANIZATION

THE ECONOMIC ADVANTAGES OF DIVERSIFICATION?

It has been argued that the diversified configuration offers four basic advantages over the functional structure with integrated operations, namely an overall machine configuration. First, it encourages the efficient allocation of capital. Headquarters can choose where to put its money and so can concentrate on its strongest markets, milking the surpluses of some divisions to help others grow. Second, by opening up opportunities to run individual businesses, the diversified configuration helps to train general managers. Third, this configuration spreads its risk across different markets, whereas the focused machine bureaucracy has all its strategic eggs in one market basket, so to speak. Fourth, and perhaps most important, the diversified configuration is strategically responsive. The divisions can fine-tune their bureaucratic machines while the headquarters can concentrate on the strategic portfolio. It can acquire new businesses and divest itself of old, unproductive ones.

But is the single machine organization the correct basis of comparison? Is not the real alternative, at least from society's perspective, the taking of a further step along the same path, to the point of eliminating the headquarters altogether and allowing the divisions to function as independent organizations? Beatrice Foods, described in a 1976 *Fortune* magazine article, had 397 different divisions.[3] The issue is whether this arrangement was more efficient than 397 separate corporations.* In this regard, let us reconsider the four advantages discussed above.

In the diversified corporation, headquarters allocates the capital resources among the divisions. In the case of 397 independent corporations, the capital markets do that job instead. Which does it better? Studies suggest that the answer is not simple.

Some people, such as the economist Oliver Williamson, have argued that the diversified organization may do a better job of allocating money

---

* The example of Beatrice was first written as presented here in the 1970s, when the company was the subject of a good deal of attention and praise in the business press. At the time of this writing, in 1988, the company is being disassembled. It seemed appropriate to leave the example as first presented, among other reasons to question the tendency to favor fashion over investigation in the business press.

because the capital markets are inefficient.[4] Managers at headquarters who know their divisions can move the money around faster and more effectively. But others find that arrangement more costly and, in some ways, less flexible. Moyer, for example, argued early on that conglomerates pay a premium above stock market prices to acquire businesses, whereas the independent investor need pay only small brokerage fees to diversify his or her own portfolio, and can do so easier and more flexibly.[5] Moreover, that provides the investor with full information on all the businesses owned, whereas the diversified corporation provides only limited information to stockholders on the details inside its portfolio.

On the issue of management development, the question becomes whether the division managers receive better training and experience than they would as company presidents. The diversified organization is able to put on training courses and to rotate its managers to vary their experience; the independent firm is limited in those respects. But if, as the proponents of diversification claim, autonomy is the key to management development, then presumably the more autonomy the better. The division managers have a headquarters to lean on—and to be leaned on by. Company presidents, in contrast, are on their own to make their own mistakes and to learn from them.

On the third issue, risk, the argument from the diversified perspective is that the independent organization is vulnerable during periods of internal crisis or economic slump; conglomeration offers support to see individual businesses through such periods. The counter-argument, however, is that diversification may conceal bankruptcies, that ailing divisions are sometimes supported longer than necessary, whereas the market bankrupts the independent firm and is done with it. Moreover, just as diversification spreads the risk, so too does it spread the consequences of that risk. A single division cannot go bankrupt; the whole organization is legally responsible for its debts. So a massive enough problem in one division can pull down the whole organization. Loose coupling may turn out to be riskier than no coupling!

Finally, there is the issue of strategic responsiveness. Loosely coupled divisions may be more responsive than tightly coupled functions. But how responsive do they really prove to be? The answer appears to be negative: This configuration appears to inhibit, not encourage, the taking of strategic initiatives. The problem seems to lie, again, in its control system. It is designed to keep the carrot just the right distance in front of the divisional managers, encouraging them to strive for better and better financial performance. At the same time, however, it seems to dampen their inclination to innovate. It is that famous "bottom line" that creates the problem, encouraging short-term thinking and shortsightedness; attention is focused on the carrot just in front instead of the fields of vegetables beyond. As Bower has noted:

> [T]he risk to the division manager of a major innovation can be considerable if he is measured on short-run, year-to-year, earnings performance. The result is a tendency to avoid big risk bets, and the concomitant phenomenon that major new developments are, with few exceptions, made outside the major firms in the industry. Those exceptions tend to be single-product companies whose top managements are committed to true product leadership. . . . Instead, the diversified companies give us a steady diet of small incremental change.[6]

Innovation requires entrepreneurship, or intrapreneurship, and these, as we have already argued, do not thrive under the diversified configuration. The entrepreneur takes his or her own risks to earn his or her own rewards; the intrapreneur (as we shall see) functions best in the loose structure of the innovative adhocracy. Indeed, many diversified corporations depend on those configurations for their strategic responsiveness, since they diversify not by innovating themselves but by acquiring the innovative results of independent firms. Of course, that may be their role—to exploit rather than create those innovations—but we should not, as a result, justify diversification on the basis of its innovative capacity.

THE CONTRIBUTION OF HEADQUARTERS

To assess the effectiveness of conglomeration, it is necessary to assess what actual contribution the headquarters makes to the divisions. Since what the headquarters does in a diversified organization is otherwise performed by the various boards of directors of a set of independent firms, the question then becomes, what does a headquarters offer to the divisions that the independent board of directors of the autonomous organization does not?

One thing that neither can offer is the management of the individual business. Both are involved with it only on a part-time basis. The management is, therefore, logically left to the full-time managers, who have the required time and information. Among the functions a headquarters *does* perform, as noted earlier, are the establishment of objectives for the divisions, the monitoring of their performance in terms of these objectives, and the maintenance of limited personal contacts with division managers, for example to approve large capital expenditures. Interestingly, those are also the responsibilities of the directors of the individual firm, at least in theory.

In practice, however, many boards of directors—notably those of widely held corporations—do those things rather ineffectively, leaving business managements carte blanche to do what they like. Here, then, we seem to have a major advantage of the diversified configuration. It exists as an administrative mechanism to overcome another prominent weakness of the free-market system, the ineffective board.

There is a catch in this argument, however, for diversification by enhancing an organization's size and expanding its number of markets, renders the corporation more difficult to understand and so to control by its board of part-time directors. Moreover, as Moyer has noted, one common effect of conglomerate acquisition is to increase the number of shareholders, and so to make the corporation more widely held, and therefore less amenable to director control. Thus, the diversified configuration in some sense resolves a problem of its own making—it offers the control that its own existence has rendered difficult. Had the corporation remained in one business, it might have been more narrowly held and easier to understand, and so its directors might have been able to perform their functions more effectively. Diversification thus helped to create the problem that divisionalization is said to solve. Indeed, it is ironic that many a diversified corporation that does such a vigorous job of monitoring the performance of its own divisions is itself so poorly monitored by its own board of directors!

All of this suggests that large diversified organizations tend to be classic closed systems, powerful enough to seal themselves off from much external influence while able to exercise a good deal of control over not only their own divisions, as instruments, but also their external environments. For example, one study of all 5,995 directors of the Fortune 500 found that only 1.6 percent of them represented major shareholder interests,[7] while another survey of 855 corporations found that 84 percent of them did not even formally require their directors to hold any stock at all![8]

What does happen when problems arise in a division? What can a headquarters do that various boards of directors cannot? The chairman of one major conglomerate told a meeting of the New York Society of Security Analysts, in reference to the headquarters vice presidents who oversee the divisions, that "it is not too difficult to coordinate five companies that are well run."[9] True enough. But what about five that are badly run? What could the small staff of administrators at a corporation's headquarters really do to correct problems in that firm's thirty operating divisions or in Beatrice's 397? The natural tendency to tighten the control screws does not usually help once the problem has manifested itself, nor does exercising close surveillance. As noted earlier, the headquarters managers cannot manage the divisions. Essentially, that leaves them with two choices. They can either replace the division manager, or they can divest the corporation of the division. Of course, a board of directors can also replace the management. Indeed, that seems to be its only real prerogative; the management does everything else.

On balance, then, the economic case for one headquarters versus a set of separate boards of directors appears to be mixed. It should, therefore, come as no surprise that one important study found that corporations with "controlled diversity" had better profits than those with conglomerate diversity.[10] Overall, the pure diversified configuration (the conglomerate) may offer some advantages over a weak system of separate boards of directors and inefficient capital markets, but most of those advantages would probably disappear if certain problems in capital markets and boards of directors were rectified. And there is reason to argue, from a social no less than an economic standpoint, that society would be better off trying to correct fundamental inefficiencies in its economic system rather than encourage private administrative arrangements to circumvent them, as we shall now see.

THE SOCIAL PERFORMANCE OF THE PERFORMANCE CONTROL SYSTEM

This configuration requires that headquarters control the divisions primarily by quantitative performance criteria, and that typically means financial ones—profit, sales growth, return on investment, and the like. The problem is that these performance measures often become virtual obsessions in the diversified organization, driving out goals that cannot be measured—product quality, pride in work, customers well served. In effect, the economic goals drive out the social ones. As the chief of a famous conglomerate once remarked, "We, in Textron, worship the god of New Worth."[11]

That would pose no problem if the social and economic consequences of decisions could easily be separated. Governments would look after the former, corporations the latter. But the fact is that the two are intertwined; every strategic decision of every large corporation involves both, largely inseparable. As a result, its control systems, by focusing on economic measures, drive the diversified organization to act in ways that are, at best, socially unresponsive, at worst, socially irresponsible. Forced to concentrate on the economic consequences of decisions, the division manager is driven to ignore their social consequences.* Thus, Bower found that "the best records in the race relations area are those of single-product companies whose strong top managements are deeply involved in the business."[12]

Robert Ackerman, in a study carried out at the Harvard Business School, investigated this point. He found that social benefits such as "a rosier public image . . . pride among managers . . . an attractive posture for recruiting on campus" could not easily be measured and so could not be plugged into the performance control system. The result was that

> . . . the financial reporting system may actually inhibit social responsiveness. By focusing on economic performance, even with appropriate safeguards to protect against sacrificing long-term benefits, such a system directs energy and resources to achieving results measured in financial terms. It is the only game in town, so to speak, at least the only one with an official scoreboard.[13]

Headquarters managers who are concerned about legal liabilities or the public relations effects of decisions, or even ones personally interested in broader social issues, may be tempted to intervene directly in the divisions' decision-making process to ensure proper attention to social matters. But they are discouraged from doing so by this configuration's strict division of labor: Divisional autonomy requires no meddling by the headquarters in specific business decisions.

As long as the screws of the performance control system are not turned too tight, the division managers may retain enough discretion to consider the social consequences of their actions, if they so choose. But when those screws are turned tight, as they often are in the diversified corporation with a bottom-line orientation, then the division managers wishing to keep their jobs may have no choice but to act socially unresponsively, if not actually irresponsibly. As Bower has noted of the General Electric price-fixing scandal of the 1960s, "a very severely managed system of reward and punishment that demanded yearly improvements

* Indeed, that manager is also driven to ignore the intangible economic consequences too, such as product quality or research effort, another manifestation of the problem of the short-term, bottom-line thinking mentioned earlier.

in earnings, return and market share, applied indiscriminately to all divisions, yielded a situation which was—at the very least—conducive to collusion in the oligopolistic and mature electric equipment markets.''[14]

THE DIVERSIFIED ORGANIZATION IN THE PUBLIC SPHERE

Ironically, for a government intent on dealing with these social problems, solutions are indicated in the very arguments used to support the diversified configuration. Or so it would appear.

For example, if the administrative arrangements are efficient while the capital markets are not, then why should a government hesitate to interfere with the capital markets? And why shouldn't it use those same administrative arrangements to deal with the problems? If Beatrice Foods really can control those 397 divisions, then what is to stop Washington from believing it can control 397 Beatrices? After all, the capital markets don't much matter. In his book on "countervailing power," John Kenneth Galbraith argued that bigness in one sector, such as business, promotes bigness in other sectors, such as unions and government.[15] That has already happened. How long before government pursues the logical next step and exercises direct controls?

While such steps may prove irresistible to some governments, the fact is that they will not resolve the problems of power concentration and social irresponsibility but rather will aggravate them, but not just in the ways usually assumed in Western economics. All the existing problems would simply be bumped up to another level, and there increase. By making use of the diversified configuration, government would magnify the problems of size. Moreover, government, like the corporation, would be driven to favor measurable economic goals over intangible social ones, and that would add to the problems of social irresponsibility— a phenomenon of which we have already seen a good deal in the public sector.

In fact, these problems would be worse in government, because its sphere is social, and so its goals are largely ill-suited to performance control systems. In other words, many of the goals most important for the public sector—and this applies to not-for-profit organizations in spheres such as health and education as well—simply do not lend themselves to measurement, no matter how long and how hard public officials continue to try. And without measurement, the conventional diversified

There are, of course, other problems with the application of this form of organization in the public sphere. For example, government cannot divest itself of subunits quite so easily as can corporations. And public service regulations on appointments and the like, as well as a host of other rules, preclude the degree of division manager autonomy available in the private sector. (It is, in fact, these central rules and regulations that make governments resemble integrated machine configurations as much as loosely coupled diversified ones, and that undermine their efforts at "accountability.")

Thus, we conclude that, appearances and even trends notwithstanding, the diversified configuration is generally not suited to the public and not-for-profit sectors of society. Governments and other public-type institutions that wish to divisionalize to avoid centralized machine bureaucracy may often find the imposition of performance standards an artificial exercise. They may thus be better off trying to exercise control of their units in a different way. For example, they can select unit managers who reflect their desired values, or indoctrinate them in those values, and then let them manage freely, the control in effect being normative rather than quantative (and their structure therefore a hybrid between the diversified and the missionary configurations). But as we shall see in Chapter 12, managing ideology, even creating it in the first place, is no simple matter, especially in a highly diversified organization.

IN CONCLUSION: A STRUCTURE ON THE EDGE OF A CLIFF

Our discussion has led to a "damned if you do, damned if you don't" conclusion. The pure (conglomerate) diversified configuration emerges as an organization perched symbolically on the edge of the cliff, at the end of a long path. Ahead, it is one step away from disintegration— breaking up into separate organizations on the rocks below. Behind it is the way back to a more stable integration, in the form of the machine configuration at the start of that path. And ever hovering above is the eagle, representing the broader social control of the state, attracted by the organization's position on the edge of the cliff and waiting for the chance to pull it up to a higher cliff, perhaps more dangerous still. The edge of the cliff is an uncomfortable place to be, perhaps even a temporary one that must inevitably lead to disintegration on the rocks below, a trip to that cliff above, or a return to a safer resting place somewhere on that path behind.

10
THE PROFESSIONAL ORGANIZATION

I work in a professional organization, and probably chose to do so initially because it is the one place in the world where you can act as if you were self-employed yet regularly receive a paycheck. These seemingly upside-down organizations, where the workers sometimes appear to manage the bosses, are fascinating in the way they work. As the nursery rhyme goes, when they're good, they're very, very good, but when they're bad, they're horrid. It all hinges on that fine line between collegiality (working for the common good) and politics (working for self-interest). We need professional organizations to carry out highly skilled yet highly stable tasks in society, such as replacing someone's heart or auditing a company's books. But as a society we have yet to learn how to control their excesses: professionals who mistreat their clients, professional organizations that mistreat their supporters.

The place to start, as always for me, is in understanding how they work. MIT just doesn't function like McDonald's; everyone knows that, but I suspect few people fully appreciate the differences. I begin, once again, by describing the unique structure, internal processes, and context of this configuration. Then, drawing from an article I co-authored with Cynthia Hardy, Ann Langley, and Janet Rose, I explain the very unusual ways in which the professional organization makes and changes its strategy, probing into the issue of collegiality versus politics. The chapter closes with a discussion of some of the social issues surrounding the professional organization, including a comment on the threat that I believe unionization poses for the practice of professional work.

The Professional Organization

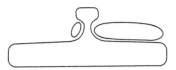

Structure: • bureaucratic yet decentralized, dependent on training to standardize the skills of its many operating professionals

• key to functioning is creation of system of pigeonholes within which individual professionals work autonomously, subject to controls of the profession

• minimal technostructure and middle-line hierarchy, meaning wide spans of control over professional work, and large support staff, more machinelike, to support the professionals

Context: • complex yet stable

• simple technical system

• often, but not necessarily, service sector

Strategy: • many strategies, largely fragmented, but forces for cohesion too

• most made by professional judgment and collective choice (collegially and politically), some by administrative fiat

• overall strategy very stable but in detail continually changing

Issues: • advantages of democracy and autonomy

     but

• problems of coordination between the pigeonholes, of misuse of professional discretion, of reluctance to innovate

• public responses to these problems often dysfunctional (machinelike)

• unionization exacerbates these problems

THE BASIC STRUCTURE

An organization can be bureaucratic without being centralized. This happens when its work is complex, requiring that it be carried out and controlled by professionals, yet at the same time remains stable, so that the skills of those professionals can be perfected through standardized operating programs. The structure takes on the form of *professional* bureaucracy, which is common in universities, general hospitals, public accounting firms, social work agencies, and firms doing fairly routine engineering or craft work. All rely on the skills and knowledge of their operating professionals to function; all produce standardized products or services.

THE WORK OF THE PROFESSIONAL OPERATORS

Here again we have a tightly knit configuration of the attributes of structure. Most important, the professional organization relies for coordination on the standardization of skills, which is achieved primarily through formal training. It hires duly trained specialists—professionals—for the operating core, then gives them considerable control over their own work.

Control over their work means that professionals work relatively independently of their colleagues but closely with the clients they serve—doctors treating their own patients and accountants who maintain personal contact with the companies whose books they audit. Most of the necessary coordination among the operating professionals is then handled automatically by their set skills and knowledge—in effect, by what they have learned to expect from each other. During an operation as long and as complex as open-heart surgery, "very little needs to be said [between the anesthesiologist and the surgeon] preceding chest opening and during the procedure on the heart itself . . . [most of the operation is] performed in absolute silence."[1] The point is perhaps best made in reverse by the cartoon that shows six surgeons standing around a patient on an operating table with one saying, "Who opens?"

Just how standardized the complex work of professionals can be is illustrated in a paper read by Spencer before a meeting of the International Cardiovascular Society. Spencer notes that an important feature of surgical training is "repetitive practice" to evoke "an automatic reflex." So automatic, in fact, that this doctor keeps a series of surgical "cookbooks" in which he lists, even for "complex" operations, the essential steps as chains of thirty to forty symbols on a single sheet, to "be reviewed mentally in sixty to 120 seconds at some time during the day preceding the operation."[2]

But no matter how standardized the knowledge and skills, their complexity ensures that considerable discretion remains in their application. No two professionals—no two surgeons or engineers or social workers—ever apply them in exactly the same way. Many judgments are required.

Training, reinforced by indoctrination, is a complicated affair in the professional organization. The initial training typically takes place over a period of years in a university or special institution, during which the skills and knowledge of the profession are formally programmed into the students. There typically follows a long period of on-the-job training, such as internship in medicine or articling in accounting, where the formal knowledge is applied and the practice of skills perfected. On-the-job training also completes the process of indoctrination, which began during the formal education. As new knowledge is generated and new skills develop, of course (so it is hoped) the professional upgrades his or her expertise.

All that training is geared to one goal, the internalization of the set procedures, which is what makes the structure technically bureaucratic (structure defined earlier as relying on standardization for coordination). But the professional bureaucracy differs markedly from the machine bureaucracy. Whereas the latter generates its own standards—through its technostructure, enforced by its line managers—many of the standards of the professional bureaucracy originate outside its own structure, in the self-governing associations its professionals belong to with their colleagues from other institutions. These associations set universal standards, which they ensure are taught by the universities and are used by all the organizations practicing the profession. So whereas the machine bureaucracy relies on authority of a hierarchical nature—the power of office—the professional bureaucracy emphasizes authority of a professional nature—the power of expertise.

Other forms of standardization are, in fact, difficult to rely on in the professional organization. The work processes themselves are too complex to be standardized directly by analysts. One need only try to imagine a work-study analyst following a cardiologist on rounds or timing the activities of a teacher in a classroom. Similarly, the outputs of professional work cannot easily be measured and so do not lend themselves to standardization. Imagine a planner trying to define a cure in psychiatry, the amount of learning that takes place in a classroom, or the quality of an accountant's audit. Likewise, direct supervision and mutual adjustment cannot be relied upon for coordination, for both impede professional autonomy.

THE PIGEONHOLING PROCESS

To understand how the professional organization functions at the operating level, it is helpful to think of it as a set of standard programs—in effect, the repertoire of skills the professionals stand ready to use—that are applied to known situations, called contingencies, also standardized. As Weick notes of one case in point, "schools are in the business of building and maintaining categories."[3] The process is sometimes known as *pigeonholing.* In this regard, the professional has two basic tasks: (1) to categorize, or "diagnose," the client's need in terms of one of the contingencies, which indicates which standard program to apply, and (2) to apply, or execute, that program. For example, the management consultant carries a bag of standard acronymic tricks: MBO, MIS, LRP, OD. The client with information needs gets MIS; the one with managerial conflicts, OD. Such pigeonholing, of course, simplifies matters enormously; it is also what enables each professional to work in a relatively autonomous manner.

It is in the pigeonholing process that the fundamental differences among the machine organization, the professional organization, and the innovative organization (to be discussed next) can best be seen. The machine organization is a single-purpose structure. Presented with a stimulus, it executes its one standard sequence of programs, just as we kick when tapped on the knee. No diagnosis is involved. In the professional organization, diagnosis is a fundamental task, but one highly circumscribed. The organization seeks to match a predetermined contingency to a standardized program. Fully open-ended diagnosis—that which seeks a creative solution to a unique problem—requires the innovative form of organization. No standard contingencies or programs can be relied upon there.

THE ADMINISTRATIVE STRUCTURE

Everything we have discussed so far suggests that the operating core is the key part of the professional organization. The only other part that is fully elaborated is the support staff, but that is focused very much on serving the activities of the operating core. Given the high cost of the professionals, it makes sense to back them up with as much support as possible. Thus, universities have printing facilities, faculty clubs, alma mater funds, publishing houses, archives, libraries, computer facilities, and many, many other support units.

The technostructure and middle-line management are not highly elaborated in the professional organization. They can do little to coordinate the professional work. Moreover, with so little need for direct supervision of, or mutual adjustment among, the professionals, the operating units can be very large. For example, the McGill Faculty of Management functions effectively with fifty professors under a single manager, its dean, and the rest of the university's academic hierarchy is likewise thin.

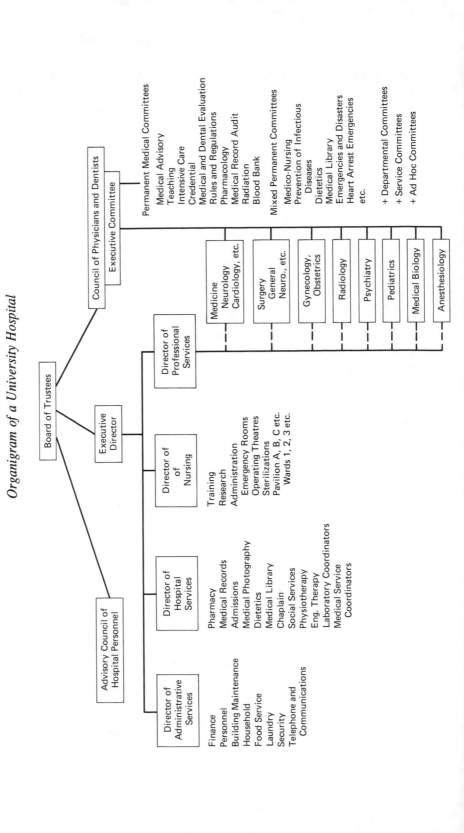

FIGURE 10–1
Organigram of a University Hospital

Thus, the diagram at the beginning of this chapter shows the professional organization, in terms of our logo, as a flat structure with a thin middle line, a tiny technostructure, but a fully elaborated support staff. All these characteristics are reflected in the organigram of a university hospital, shown in Figure 10–1.

Coordination within the administrative structure is another matter, however. Because these configurations are so decentralized, the professionals not only control their own work but they also gain much collective control over the administrative decisions that affect them—decisions, for example, to hire colleagues, to promote them, and to distribute resources. This they do partly by doing some of the administrative work themselves (most university professors, for example, sit on various administrative committees) and partly by ensuring that important administrative posts are staffed by professionals or at least sympathetic people appointed with the professionals' blessing. What emerges, therefore, is a rather democratic administrative structure. But because the administrative work requires mutual adjustment for coordination among the various people involved, task forces and especially standing committees abound at this level, as is in fact suggested in Figure 10–1.

Because of the power of their professional operators, these organizations are sometimes described as inverse pyramids, with the professional operators on top and the administrators down below to serve them—to ensure that the surgical facilities are kept clean and the classrooms well supplied with chalk. Such a description slights the power of the administrators of professional work, however, although it may be an accurate description of those who manage the support units. For the support staff—often more numerous than the professional staff, but generally less skilled—there is no democracy in the professional organization, only the oligarchy of the professionals. Such support units as housekeeping in the hospital or printing in the university are likely to be managed tightly from the top, in effect as machinelike enclaves within the professional configuration. Thus, what frequently emerges in the professional organization are parallel and separate administrative hierarchies, one democratic and bottom-up for the professionals, a second machinelike and top-down for the support staff.

THE ROLES OF THE ADMINISTRATORS OF PROFESSIONAL WORK

Where does all this leave the administrators of the professional hierarchy, the executive directors and chiefs of the hospitals and the presidents and deans of the universities? Are they powerless? Compared with their counterparts in the entrepreneurial and machine organizations, they certainly lack a good deal of power. But that is far from the whole story. The administrator of professional work may not be able to control the professionals directly, but he or she does perform a series of roles that can provide considerable indirect power.

First, this administrator spends much time handling disturbances in the structure. The pigeonholing process is an imperfect one at best, leading to all kinds of jurisdictional disputes between the professionals. Who should perform mastectomies in the hospitals, surgeons who look after cutting or gynecologists who look after women? Seldom, however, can one administrator impose a solution on the professionals involved in a dispute. Rather, various administrators must often sit down together and negotiate a solution on behalf of their constituencies.

Second, the administrators of professional work—especially those at higher levels—serve in key roles at the boundary of the organization, between the professionals inside and the influencers outside: governments, client associations, benefactors, and so on. On the one hand, the administrators are expected to protect the professionals' autonomy, to "buffer" them from external pressures. On the other hand, they are expected to woo those outsiders to support the organization, both morally and financially. And that often leads the outsiders to expect these administrators, in turn, to control the professionals, in machine bureaucratic ways. Thus, the external roles of the manager—maintaining liaison contacts, acting as figurehead and spokesman in a public relations capacity, negotiating with outside agencies—emerge as primary ones in the administration of professional work.

Some view the roles these administrators are called upon to perform as signs of weakness. They see these people as the errand boys of the professionals, or else as pawns caught in various tugs of war—between one professional and another, between support staffer and professional, between outsider and professional. In fact, however, these roles are the very sources of administrators' power. Power is, after all, gained at the locus of uncertainty, and that is exactly where the administrators of professionals sit. The administrator who succeeds in raising extra funds for his or her organization gains a say in how they are distributed; the one who can reconcile conflicts in favor of his or her unit or who can effectively buffer the professionals from external influence becomes a valued, and therefore powerful, member of the organization.

We can conclude that power in these structures does flow to those professionals who care to devote effort to doing administrative instead of professional work, so long as they do it well. But that, it should be stressed, is not laissez-faire power; the professional administrator maintains power only as long as the professionals perceive him or her to be serving their interests effectively.

CONDITIONS OF THE PROFESSIONAL ORGANIZATION

The professional form of organization appears wherever the operating work of an organization is dominated by skilled workers who use procedures that are difficult to learn yet are well defined. This means a situation that is both complex and stable—complex enough to require procedures that can be learned only through extensive training yet stable enough so that their use can become standardized.

Note that an elaborate technical system can work against this configuration. If highly regulating or automated, the professionals' skills might be amenable to rationalization, in other words, to be divided into simple, highly programmed steps that would destroy the basis for professional autonomy and thereby drive the structure to the machine form. And if highly complicated, the technical system would reduce the professionals' autonomy by forcing them to work in multidisciplinary teams, thereby driving the organization toward the innovative form. Thus the surgeon uses a scalpel, and the accountant a pencil. Both must be sharp, but both are otherwise simple and commonplace instruments. Yet both allow their users to perform independently what can be exceedingly complex functions.

The prime example of the professional configuration is the personal-service organization, at least the one with complex, stable work not reliant on a fancy technical system. Schools and universities, consulting firms, law and accounting offices, and social work agencies all rely on this form of organization, more or less, so long as they concentrate not on innovating in the solution of new problems but on applying standard programs to well-defined ones. The same seems to be true of hospitals, at least to the extent that their technical systems are simple. (In those areas that call for more sophisticated equipment—apparently a growing number, especially in teaching institutions—the hospital is driven toward a hybrid structure, with characteristics of the innovative form. But this tendency is mitigated by the hospital's overriding concern with safety.

Only the tried and true can be relied upon, which produces a natural aversion to the looser innovative configuration.)

So far, our examples have come from the service sector. But the professional form can be found in manufacturing too, where the above conditions hold up. Such is the case of the craft enterprise, for example the factory using skilled workers to produce ceramic products. The very term *craftsman* implies a kind of professional who learns traditional skills through long apprentice training and then is allowed to practice them free of direct supervision. Craft enterprises seem typically to have few administrators, who tend to work, in any event, alongside the operating personnel. The same would seem to be true for engineering work oriented not to creative design so much as to modification of existing dominant designs.

STRATEGY FORMATION IN THE PROFESSIONAL ORGANIZATION

It is commonly assumed that strategies are formulated before they are implemented, that planning is the central process of formulation, and that structures must be designed to implement these strategies. At least this is what one reads in the conventional literature of strategic management. In the professional organization, these imperatives stand almost totally at odds with what really happens, leading to the conclusion either that such organizations are confused about how to make strategy, or else that the strategy writers are confused about how professional organizations must function. I subscribe to the latter explanation.

Using the definition of strategy as pattern in action, strategy formation in the professional organization takes on a new meaning. Rather than simply throwing up our hands at its resistance to formal strategic planning or, at the other extreme, dismissing professional organizations as "organized anarchies" with strategy-making processes as mere "garbage cans,"[4] we can focus on how decisions and actions in such organizations order themselves into patterns over time.

Taking strategy as pattern in action, the obvious question becomes, which actions? The key area of strategy-making in most organizations concerns the elaboration of the basic mission (the products or services offered to the public); in professional organizations, we shall argue, this is significantly controlled by individual professionals. Other important areas of strategy here include the inputs to the system (notably the choice of professional staff, the determination of clients, and the raising of external funds), the means to perform the mission (the construction of buildings and facilities, the purchase of research equipment, and so on), the structure and forms of governance (design of the committee system, the hierarchies, and so on), and the various means to support the mission.

Were professional organizations to formulate strategies in the conventional ways, central administrators would develop detailed and integrated plans about these issues. This sometimes happens, but in a very limited number of cases. Many strategic issues come under the direct control of individual professionals, while others can be decided neither by individual professionals nor by central administrators, but instead require the participation of a variety of people in a complex collective process. As illustrated in Figure 10–2, we examine in turn the decisions controlled

FIGURE 10–2
Three Levels of Decision-Making in the Professional Organization

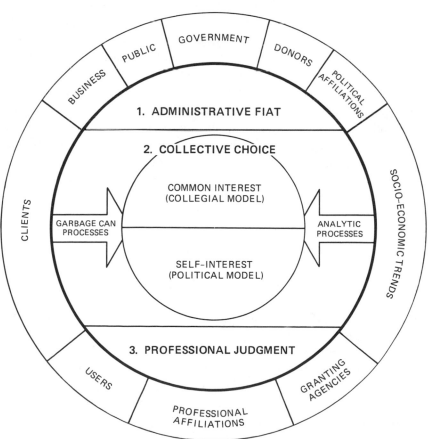

by individual professionals, by central administrators, and by the collectivity.

DECISIONS MADE BY PROFESSIONAL JUDGMENT

Professional organizations are distinguished by the fact that the determination of the basic mission—the specific services to be offered and to whom—is in good part left to the judgment of professionals as individuals. In the university, for example, each professor has a good deal of control over what is taught and how, as well as what is researched and how. Thus the overall product-market strategy of McGill University must be seen as the composite of the individual teaching and research postures of its 1,200 professors.

That, however, does not quite constitute full autonomy, because there is a subtle but not insignificant constraint on that power. Professionals are left to decide on their own only because years of training have ensured that they will decide in ways generally accepted in their professions. Thus professors choose course contents and adopt teaching methods highly regarded by their colleagues, sometimes even formally sanctioned by their disciplines; they research subjects that will be funded by the granting agencies (which usually come under professional controls); and they publish articles acceptable to the journals refereed by their peers. Pushed to the limit, then, individual freedom becomes professional control. It may be explicit freedom from administrators, even from peers in other disciplines, but it is not implicit freedom from colleagues in their own discipline. Thus we use the label ''professional judgment'' to imply that while judgment may be the mode of choice, it is informed judgment, mightily influenced by professional training and affiliation.

DECISIONS MADE BY ADMINISTRATIVE FIAT

Professional expertise and autonomy, reinforced by the pigeonholing process, sharply circumscribe the capacity of central administrators to manage the professionals in the ways of conventional bureaucracy— through direct supervision and the designation of internal standards (rules, job descriptions, policies). Even the designation of standards of output or performance is discouraged by the intractable problem of operationalizing the goals of professional work.

Certain types of decisions, less related to the professional work per se, do however fall into the realm of what can be called administrative fiat, in other words, become the exclusive prerogative of the administrators. They include some financial decisions, for example, to buy and sell property and embark on fundraising campaigns. Because many of the support services are organized in a conventional top-down hierarchy, they too tend to fall under the control of the central administration. Support services more critical to professional matters, however, such as libraries or computers in the universities, tend to fall into the realm of collective decision-making, where the central administrators join the professionals in the making of choices.

Central administrators may also play a prominent role in determining the procedures by which the collective process functions: what committees exist, who gets nominated to them, and so on. It is the administrators, after all, who have the time to devote to administration. This role can give skillful administrators considerable influence, however indirect, over the decisions made by others. In addition, in times of crisis administrators may acquire more extensive powers, as the professionals become more inclined to defer to leadership to resolve the issues.

DECISIONS MADE BY COLLECTIVE CHOICE

Many decisions are, however, determined neither by administrators nor by individual professionals. Instead they are handled in interactive processes that combine professionals with administrators from a variety of levels and units. Among the most important of these decisions seem to be ones related to the definition, creation, design, and discontinuation of the pigeonholes, that is, the programs and departments of various kinds. Other important decisions here include the hiring and promotion of professionals and, in some cases, budgeting and the establishment and design of the interactive procedures themselves (if they do not fall under administrative fiat).

Decision-making may be considered to involve the three phases of *identification* of the need for a decision, *development* of solutions, and *selection* of one of them. Identification seems to depend largely on individual initiative. Given the complexities of professional work and the rigidities of pigeonholing, change in this configuration is difficult to imagine without an initiating ''sponsor'' or ''champion.'' Development may involve the same individual but often requires the efforts of collective task forces as well. And selection tends to be a fully interactive process, involving several layers of standing committees composed of professionals and administrators, and sometimes outsiders as well (such as government representatives). It is in this last phase that we find the full impact and complexity of mutual adjustment in the administration of professional organizations.

MODELS OF COLLECTIVE CHOICE

How do these interactive processes in fact work? Some writers have traditionally associated professional organizations with a *collegial* model, where decisions are made by a "community of individuals and groups, all of whom may have different roles and specialties, but who share common goals and objectives for the organization."[5] *Common interest* is the guiding force, and decision-making is therefore by consensus. Other writers instead propose a *political* model, in which the differences of interest groups are irreconcilable. Participants thus seek to serve their *self-interest,* and political factors become instrumental in determining outcomes.

Clearly, neither common interest nor self-interest will dominate decision processes all the time; some combination is naturally to be expected. Professionals may agree on goals yet conflict over how they should be achieved; alternatively, consensus can sometimes be achieved even where goals differ—Democrats do, after all, sometimes vote with Republicans in the U.S. Congress. In fact, we need to consider motivation, not just behavior, in order to distinguish collegiality from politics. Political success sometimes requires a collegial posture—one must cloak self-interest in the mantle of the common good. Likewise, collegial ends sometimes require political means. Thus, we should take as collegial any behavior that is *motivated* by a genuine concern for the good of the institution, and politics as any behavior driven fundamentally by self-interest (of the individual or his or her unit).

A third model that has been used to explain decision-making in universities is the *garbage can.* Here decision-making is characterized by "collections of choices looking for problems, issues and feelings looking for decision situations in which they may be aired, solutions looking for issues to which they might be an answer, and decision makers looking for work."[6] Behavior is, in other words, nonpurposeful and often random, because goals are unclear and the means to achieve them problematic.

Furthermore, participation is fluid because of the cost of time and energy. Thus, in place of the common interest of the collegial model and the self-interest of the political model, the garbage can model suggests a kind of *disinterest*.

The important question is not whether garbage can processes exist—we have all experienced them—but whether they matter. Do they apply to key issues or only to incidental ones? Of course, decisions that are not significant to anyone may well end up in the garbage can, so to speak. There is always someone with free time willing to challenge a proposal for the sake of so doing. But I have difficulty accepting that individuals to whom decisions are important do not invest the effort necessary to influence them. Thus, like common interest and self-interest, I conclude that disinterest neither dominates decision processes nor is absent from them.

Finally, *analysis* may be considered a fourth model of decision-making. Here calculation is used, if not to select the best alternative, then at least to assess the acceptability of different ones. Such an approach seems consistent with the machine configuration, where a technostructure stands ready to calculate the costs and benefits of every proposal. But, in fact, analysis figures prominently in the professional configuration too, but here carried out mostly by professional operators themselves. Rational analysis structures arguments for communication and debate and enables champions and their opponents to support their respective positions. In fact, as each side seeks to pick holes in the position of the other, the real issues are more likely to emerge.

Thus, as indicated in Figure 10–2, the important collective decisions of the professional organization seem to be most influenced by collegial and political processes, with garbage can pressures encouraging a kind of haphazardness on one side (especially for less important decisions) and analytical interventions on the other side encouraging a certain rationality (serving as an invisible hand to keep the lid on the garbage can, so to speak!).

STRATEGIES IN THE PROFESSIONAL ORGANIZATION

Thus, we find here a very different process of strategy-making, and very different resulting strategies, compared with conventional (especially machine) organizations. While it may seem difficult to create strategies in these organizations, due to the fragmentation of activity, the politics, and the garbage can phenomenon, in fact the professional organization is inundated with strategies (meaning patterning in its actions). The standardization of skills encourages patterning, as do the pigeonholing process and the professional affiliations. Collegiality promotes consistency of behavior; even politics works to resist changing existing patterns. As for the garbage can model, perhaps it just represents the unexplained variance in the system; that is, whatever is not understood looks to the outside observer like organized anarchy.

Many different people get involved in the strategy-making process here, including administrators and the various professionals, individually and collectively, so that the resulting strategies can be very fragmented (at the limit, each professional pursues his or her own product-market strategy). There are, of course, forces that encourage some overall cohesion in strategy too: the common forces of administrative fiat, the broad negotiations that take place in the collective process (for example, on new tenure regulations in a university), even the forces of habit and tradition, at the limit ideology, that can pervade a professional organization (such as hiring certain kinds of people or favoring certain styles of teaching or of surgery).

Overall, the strategies of the professional organization tend to exhibit a remarkable degree of stability. Major reorientations in strategy—"strategic revolutions"—are discouraged by the fragmentation of activity and the influence of the individual professionals and their outside associations. But at a narrower level, change is ubiquitous. Inside tiny pigeonholes, services are continually being altered, procedure redesigned, and clientele shifted, while in the collective process, pigeonholes are constantly being added and rearranged. Thus, the professional organization is, paradoxically, extremely stable at the broadest level and in a state of perpetual change at the narrowest one.

SOME ISSUES ASSOCIATED WITH THE PROFESSIONAL ORGANIZATION

The professional organization is unique among the different configurations in answering two of the paramount needs of contemporary men and women. It is democratic, disseminating its power directly to its workers (at least those lucky enough to be professional). And it provides them with extensive autonomy, freeing them even from the need to coordinate closely with their colleagues. Thus, the professional has the best of both worlds. He or she is attached to an organization yet is free to serve clients in his or her own way, constrained only by the established standards of the profession.

The result is that professionals tend to emerge as highly motivated individuals, dedicated to their work and to the clients they serve. Unlike the machine organization, which places barriers between the operator and the client, this configuration removes them, allowing a personal relationship to develop. Moreover, autonomy enables the professionals to perfect their skills free of interference, as they repeat the same complex programs time after time.

But in these same characteristics, democracy and autonomy, lie the chief problems of the professional organization. For there is no evident way to control the work, outside of that exercised by the profession itself, no way to correct deficiencies that the professionals choose to overlook. What they tend to overlook are the problems of coordination, of discretion, and of innovation that arise in these configurations.

PROBLEMS OF COORDINATION

The professional organization can coordinate effectively in its operating core only by relying on the standardization of skills. But that is a loose coordinating mechanism at best; it fails to cope with many of the needs that arise in these organizations. One need is to coordinate the work of professionals with that of support staffers. The professionals want to give the orders. But that can catch the support staffers between the vertical power of line authority and the horizontal power of professional expertise. Another need is to achieve overriding coordination among the professionals themselves. Professional organizations, at the limit, may be viewed as collections of independent individuals who come together only to draw on common resources and support services. Though the pigeonholing process facilitates this, some things inevitably fall through the cracks between the pigeonholes. But because the professional organization lacks any obvious coordinating mechanism to deal with these, they inevitably provoke a great deal of conflict. Much political blood is spilled in the continual reassessment of contingencies and programs that are either imperfectly conceived or artificially distinguished.

PROBLEMS OF DISCRETION

Pigeonholing raises another serious problem. It focuses most of the discretion in the hands of single professionals, whose complex skills, no matter how standardized, require the exercise of considerable judgment. Such discretion works fine when professionals are competent and conscientious. But it plays havoc when they are not. Inevitably, some professionals are simply lazy or incompetent. Others confuse the needs of their clients with the skills of their trade. They thus concentrate on a favored program to the exclusion of all others (like the psychiatrist who thinks that all patients, indeed all people, need psychoanalysis). Clients incorrectly sent their way get mistreated (in both senses of that word).

Various factors confound efforts to deal with this inversion of means and ends. One is that professionals are notoriously reluctant to act against their own, for example, to censure irresponsible behavior through their professional associations. Another (which perhaps helps to explain the first) is the intrinsic difficulty of measuring the outputs of professional work. When psychiatrists cannot even define the words *cure* or *healthy,* how are they to prove that psychoanalysis is better for schizophrenics than chemical therapy?

Discretion allows professionals to ignore not only the needs of their clients but also those of the organization itself. Many professionals focus their loyalty on their profession, not on the place where they happen to practice it. But professional organizations have needs for loyalty too— to support their overall strategies, to staff their administrative committees, to see them through conflicts with the professional associations. Cooperation is crucial to the functioning of the administrative structure, yet many professionals resist it furiously.

PROBLEMS OF INNOVATION

In the professional organizaton, major innovation also depends on cooperation. Existing programs may be perfected by the single professional, but new ones usually cut across the established specialties—in essence, they require a rearrangement of the pigeonholes—and so call for collective action. As a result, the reluctance of the professionals to cooperate with each other and the complexity of the collective processes can produce resistance to innovation. These are, after all, professional *bureaucracies,* in essence, performance structures designed to perfect given programs in stable environments, not problem-solving structures to create new programs for unanticipated needs.

The problems of innovation in the professional organization find their roots in convergent thinking, in the deductive reasoning of the professional who sees the specific situation in terms of the general concept. That means new problems are forced into old pigeonholes, as is excellently illustrated in Spencer's comments: "All patients developing significant complications or death among our three hospitals . . . are reported to a central office with a narrative description of the sequence of events, with reports varying in length from a third to an entire page." And six to eight of these cases are discussed in the one-hour weekly "mortality-morbidity" conferences, including presentation of it by the surgeon and "questions and comments" by the audience.[7] An "entire" page and ten minutes of discussion for a case with "significant complications"! Maybe that is enough to list the symptoms and slot them into pigeonholes. But it is hardly enough even to begin to think about creative solutions. As Lucy once told Charlie Brown, great art cannot be done in half an hour; it takes at least forty-five minutes!

The fact is that great art and innovative problem-solving require *inductive* reasoning—that is, the inference of the new general solution from the particular experience. And that kind of thinking is *divergent;* it breaks away from old routines or standards rather than perfecting existing ones. And that flies in the face of everything the professional organization is designed to do.

PUBLIC RESPONSES TO THESE PROBLEMS

What responses do the problems of coordination, discretion, and innovation evoke? Most commonly, those outside the profession see the problems as resulting from a lack of external control of the professional and the profession. So they do the obvious: try to control the work through other, more traditional means. One is direct supervision, which typically means imposing an intermediate level of supervision to watch over the professionals. But we already discussed why this cannot work for jobs that are complex. Another is to try to standardize the work or its outputs. But we also discussed why complex work cannot be formalized by rules, regulations, or measures of performance. All these types of controls really do, by transferring the responsibility for the service from the professional to the administrative structure, is destroy the effectiveness of the work. It is not the government that educates the student, not even the school system or the school itself; it is not the hospital that delivers the baby. These things are done by the individual professional. If that professional is incompetent, no plan or rule fashioned in the technostructure, no order from any administrator or government official, can ever make him or her competent. But such plans, rules, and orders can impede the competent professional from providing his or her service effectively.

Are there then no solutions for a society concerned about the performance of its professional organizations? Financial control of them and legislation against irresponsible professional behavior are obviously in order. But beyond that, solutions must grow from a recognition of professional work for what it is. Change in the professional organization does not *sweep* in from new administrators taking office to announce wide reforms, or from government officials intent on bringing the professionals under technocratic control. Rather, change *seeps* in through the slow process of changing the professionals—changing who enters the profession in the first place, what they learn in its professional schools (norms as well as skills and knowledge), and thereafter how they upgrade their skills. Where desired changes are resisted, society may be best off to call on its professionals' sense of public responsibility or, failing that, to bring pressure on the professional associations rather than on the professional bureaucracies.

A NOTE ON THE UNIONIZATION OF PROFESSIONALS

Professionals subjected to dysfunctional administrative pressures have sometimes been driven to unionization. But that, in my opinion, aggravates the problem, diminishing the quality of the professional service even further.

Much like unskilled workers, it is when professionals feel powerless that they are most inclined to unionize. Governments are often at the root of such pressures, with efforts to impose machine bureaucratic controls. That is presumably why the vast majority of faculty unions in the United States are found in the public universities. Of course, internal university administrators with the same intentions can have the same effect. Also, weak professionals may favor unionization to protect themselves from their clients and even from their more capable colleagues. In effect, they may try to use collective power to conceal the illegitimacy of their individual power. Thus, even in states with laws supporting the unionization of university faculty, the few institutions that have not been organized "include most of the largest and most prestigious schools."[8]

Probably no group of specialists has been more subjected to technocratic controls, nor has any been more prone to unionize, than that of public school systems. The controls reflect a number of factors—the high cost of education, the absence of a technical mystique in this field, the zeal of certain politicians, the callousness of certain teachers, the sensitivity of certain parents, and so on. So rules are piled on rules. Yet true education remains, as someone so aptly put it, a teacher and a pupil on a log. In other words, the process, when it works well, simply brings a competent educator face to face with a receptive student.* The role of the institution is to facilitate the exchange between these two, not to interfere with it. All manners of standards cannot make an incompetent teacher competent or a callous one responsible. They can, however, discourage the competent, responsible teacher and turn him or her to unionization.

Thus, we have a vicious circle of dysfunction. Bottom-up professional organizations are progressively transformed through increasing technocratic controls and administrative centralization into top-down machine ones; the response of the professionals is to seek unionization, which, instead of arresting the process, only accelerates it.

The key to the effective functioning of the professional organization is *individual* responsibility: the dedication of the professional to his or her client. Individual responsibility is often based on a personal working relationship between the professional and the client—the professor with the students, the physician with the patient. A subtle but crucial point must be stressed here. Professional bureaucracy may be a highly decentralized structure in which the professionals hold a good deal of the power. But they do so, first individually and then in small specialist units, but

---

* I say competent educator rather than *professional* because this example is unfortunate in one respect. In general, the professional is someone who "knows better" than his or her client. The client must therefore remain rather passive in the exchange, as does a patient operated on by a surgeon. But education is not like that, and teachers who take their professional status to mean that they must largely control the learning process— for example, through detailed curriculum design and the like—in my opinion diminish the commitment of the learner and so damage the learning process. It is for this reason that I have mixed feelings about the "professionalization" of education as well (although not about teacher autonomy).

not in one homogeneous collectivity. Professional organizations typically house all kinds of professionals, each with his or her own needs and interests.

Unionization, by blurring professional and subunit differences and by undermining *individual* control of the operating work, can seriously damage professional responsibility. It provides collective action instead, but that can never replace individual responsibility in the professional organization. Unionization can also damage another characteristic critical to the effective functioning of these organizations, a close coordination of operating and administrative efforts through the involvement of the same professionals in both. Unionization assumes a conflict of interest between these two levels. It takes a we–they attitude, which views administrators as authority figures or "bosses" instead of colleagues. The result is that unionization either drives a wedge between the operating core and the administrative structure or else drives an existing wedge in deeper.

More significantly, unionization diminishes the influence of professionals in the administrative structure. Unionized professionals act collectively through their representatives, who bargain with senior administrators directly, as if they were outside suppliers. The effect, ironically, is to cede control of the organization's administrative apparatus to the senior administrators, thereby centralizing power in the organization. Middle-level administrators and professionals on administrative committees are bypassed in the play of power between union representative and senior administrator. And once these wedges are driven in and held fast by collective bargaining, the likelihood of removing them becomes remote. "Thus far, [academic] institutions once unionized have maintained their status."[9]

Through collective bargaining, the union seeks to impose specific demands on the organization on behalf of its membership at large. But what needs do the various groups of professionals of one organization have in common? On many issues, they in fact disagree. But having to present a united front in its negotiations with the administration, the union must deny these differences and focus instead on the uniformities. And so it tends to be left with the one need the professionals have in common: remuneration in its various forms. Unionization may thus benefit the professionals on this one parochial dimension, but at a great price on some others of great importance to most of them as well, including the quality of their work and their control over it. Thus, clients may have suffered as a result of unionization, but no less than the professionals themselves, especially the most competent and responsible of these.

Note that many union demands amount to standards, in the form of rules and regulations, imposed on the entire organization—not professional standards, but machinelike ones. In other words, though ostensibly imposed on behalf of the professionals, these demands serve to formalize the structure and strengthen the senior administration, which, ironically, implements the standards negotiated by the union. Thus, the direct effect of unionization is to drive whatever is left of professional bureaucracy toward machine bureaucracy, which may be precisely opposite of the reasons professionals unionized in the first place. Everyone loses in the bargain, save a few union officials and some weak members who should never have been allowed into the profession in the first place. The other professionals would have been better off to fight through the administrative system for the reinstatement of collegiality instead.

11
THE INNOVATIVE ORGANIZATION

There is this wonderful passage in A. A. Milne's Introduction to *Winnie-the-Pooh:*

> There are some people who begin the Zoo at the beginning, called WAYIN, and walk as quickly as they can past every cage until they get to the one called WAYOUT, but the nicest people go straight to the animal they love the most, and stay there.

Well, without claiming to be a nice person, I will admit that this is the organizational beast I love the most. Not to live there, mind you, but at least to observe it from a safe distance (the professional organization being just that, since it is the more subdued alternative for expert-type work).*

The label I use here for this configuration is the *innovative organization,* although I shall also make use of the one in my structuring book, *adhocracy.* Some people refer to this type as "high technology," and to its basic orientation as "intrapreneurship," an indication that whereas the entrepreneurial configuration innovates from a central individual at the top, this one depends on a variety of people for its strategic initiatives.

These initiatives tend to be many, because what adhocracy provides is sophisticated innovation. That comes at the price of a good deal of disruption, if not chaos, and wasted resources. As I note in the text, this type achieves its effectiveness by being *in*efficient. Perhaps that explains why it confuses many people: The innovative organization may be necessary, but it is not conventional, at least not by the standards of the traditional literature of management.

A personal anecdote might explain this best. Some time ago, I submitted an article on the different configurations to the *Harvard Business Review.* They accepted it, but the question came back,

---

* Incidentally, you might get an interesting surprise if you go back to the quotation and trace back the reference to the word "one."

"What's adhocracy?" I didn't quite understand; the description seemed clear enough. But I fixed it up a bit and sent the article back. A call came a little while later: "We're ready to go, just one last question: What's adhocracy?" "Wait a minute," I pleaded, "we've been through this already." The editor with whom I was working, Liza Collins, read through her colleagues' comments. When she came to "Is this the lack of structure?" I suddenly understood. The problem lay not with adhocracy, but with the machine organization.

To many people—especially conventional consultants and government people, as well as at least one *Harvard Business Review* editor—machine bureaucracy is not just one possible form of structure, it *is* structure. It is not the "one best way," it is the *only* way. Structure to those people means hierarchy of authority, top-down control, unity of command, detailed planning, formalization of procedure, and all the rest. Like water to the fish, these are the concepts they have swum around in for the better part of a century. Adhocracy, which violates every one of those notions, therefore looks to them like chaos, like the absence of structure.

But it is nothing of the kind. Make no mistake about it, adhocracy is structure too, in its proper context as logical and as reasonable as any other. That context is, above all, one of complexity and unpredictability. "It's all so simple, Anjin-san," was a comment in the novel *Shogun,* "just change your concept of the world." And many conventional management thinkers will have to, because a fascinating thing I found in my book on structure is that almost every major industry established since World War II relies on the innovative configuration. (One of the few important exceptions is the airline industry, which seems to be a classic machine type.) Adhocracy is the structure of *our* age.

The first part of our discussion considers structure, process, context, and then issues. The second part considers the strange ways in which these organizations form their strategies (strange, at least, to those who think the chief executive has to be the architect of strategy, and all the others "implementors"). So on to my favorite beast. But beware!

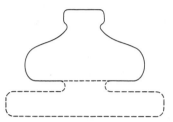

The Innovative Organization

Structure: • fluid, organic, selectively decentralized, "adhocracy"

• functional experts deployed in multidisciplinary teams of staff, operators, and managers to carry out innovative projects

• coordination by mutual adjustment, encouraged by liaison personnel, integrating managers, and matrix structure

Context: • complex and dynamic environment, including high technology, frequent product change (due to severe competition), temporary and mammoth projects

• typically young due to bureaucratic pressure with aging

• common in young industries

• two basic types: operating adhocracy for contract project work, administrative adhocracy for own project work, the latter often when operating core truncated or automated

Strategy: • primarily learning, or "grassroots" process

• largely emergent, evolving through a variety of bottom-up processes, shaped rather than directed by management

• characteristic cycles of convergence and divergence in strategic focus

Issues: • combines more democracy with less bureaucracy, and so fashionable structure

• effective at innovation (an *extra*ordinary configuration)

but

• effectiveness achieved at the price of inefficiency

• also human problems of ambiguity and dangers of inappropriate transition to another configuration

None of the configurations so far discussed is capable of sophisticated innovation, the kind required of a high-technology research organization, an avant-garde film company, or a factory manufacturing complex prototypes. The entrepreneurial organization can certainly innovate, but only in relatively simple ways. The machine and professional organizations are performance, not problem-solving types, designed to perfect standardized programs, not to invent new ones. And although the diversified organization resolves some problem of strategic inflexibility found in the machine organization, as noted earlier it too is not a true innovator. A focus on control by standardizing outputs does not encourage innovation.

Sophisticated innovation requires a very different configuration, one that is able to fuse experts drawn from different disciplines into smoothly functioning ad hoc project teams. To borrow the word coined by Bennis and Slater in 1964 and later popularized in Alvin Toffler's *Future Shock,* these are the *adhocracies* of our society.[1]

THE BASIC STRUCTURE

Here again we have a distinct configuration of the attributes of design: highly organic structure, with little formalization of behavior; specialized jobs based on expert training; a tendency to group the specialists in functional units for housekeeping purposes but to deploy them in small project teams to do their work; a reliance on teams, on task forces, and on integrating managers of various sorts in order to encourage mutual adjustment, the key mechanism of coordination, within and between these teams; and considerable decentralization to and within these teams, which are located at various places in the organization and involve various mixtures of line managers and staff and operating experts.

To innovate means to break away from established patterns. Thus the innovative organization cannot rely on any form of standardization for coordination. In other words, it must avoid all the trappings of bureaucratic structure, notably sharp divisions of labor, extensive unit differentiation, highly formalized behaviors, and an emphasis on planning and control systems. Above all, it must remain flexible. A search for organigrams to illustrate this description elicited the following response from one corporation thought to have an adhocracy structure: ''[W]e would prefer not to supply an organization chart, since it would change too quickly to serve any useful purpose.'' Of all the configurations, this one shows the least reverence for the classical principles of management, especially unity of command. Information and decision processes flow flexibly and informally, wherever they must, to promote innovation. And that means overriding the chain of authority if need be.

The entrepreneurial configuration also retains a flexible, organic structure, and so is likewise able to innovate. But that innovation is restricted to simple situations, ones easily comprehended by a single leader. Innovation of the sophisticated variety requires another kind of flexible structure, one that can draw together different forms of expertise. Thus the adhocracy must hire and give power to experts, people whose knowledge and skills have been highly developed in training programs. But unlike the professional organization, the adhocracy cannot rely on the standardized skills of its experts to achieve coordination, because that would discourage innovation. Rather, it must treat existing knowledge and skills as bases on which to combine and build new ones. Thus the adhocracy must break through the boundaries of conventional specialization and differentiation, which it does by assigning problems not to individual experts in preestablished pigeonholes but to multidisciplinary teams that merge their efforts. Each team forms around one specific project.

Despite organizing around market-based projects, the organization must still support and encourage particular types of specialized expertise. And so the adhocracy tends to use a matrix structure: Its experts are grouped in functional units for specialized housekeeping purposes—hiring, training, professional communication, and the like—but are then deployed in the project teams to carry out the basic work of innovation.

As for coordination in and between these project teams, as noted earlier standardization is precluded as a significant coordinating mechanism. The efforts must be innovative, not routine. So, too, is direct supervision precluded because of the complexity of the work: Coordination must be accomplished by those with the knowledge, namely the experts themselves, not those with just authority. That leaves just one of our coordinating mechanisms, mutual adjustment, which we consider foremost in adhocracy. And, to encourage this, the organization makes use of a whole set of liaison devices, liaison personnel and integrating managers of all kinds, in addition to the various teams and task forces.

The result is that managers abound in the adhocracy: functional managers, integrating managers, project managers. The last-named are particularly numerous, since the project teams must be small to encourage mutual adjustment among their members, and each, of course, needs a designated manager. The consequence is that "spans of control" found in adhocracy tend to be small. But the implication of this is misleading, because the term is suited to the machine, not the innovative configuration: The managers of adhocracy seldom "manage" in the usual sense of giving orders; instead, they spend a good deal of time acting in a liaison capacity, to coordinate the work laterally among the various teams and units.

With its reliance on highly trained experts, the adhocracy emerges as highly decentralized, in the "selective" sense. That means power over its decisions and actions is distributed to various places and at various levels according to the needs of the particular issue. In effect, power flows to wherever the relevent expertise happens to reside—among managers or specialists (or teams of those) in the line structure, the staff units, and the operating core.

To proceed with our discussion and to elaborate on how the innovative organization makes decisions and forms strategies, we need to distinguish two basic forms that it takes.

THE OPERATING ADHOCRACY

The *operating adhocracy* innovates and solves problems directly on behalf of its clients. Its multidisciplinary teams of experts often work under contract, as in the think-tank consulting firm, creative advertising agency, or manufacturer of engineering prototypes.

In fact, for every operating adhocracy, there is a corresponding professional bureaucracy, one that does similar work but with a narrower orientation. Faced with a client problem, the operating adhocracy engages in creative efforts to find a novel solution; the professional bureaucracy pigeonholes it into a known contingency to which it can apply a standard program. One engages in divergent thinking aimed at innovation, the other in convergent thinking aimed at perfection. Thus, one theater company might seek out new avant-garde plays to perform, while another might perfect its performance of Shakespeare year after year.

A key feature of the operating adhocracy is that its administrative and operating work tend to blend into a single effort. That is, in ad hoc project work it is difficult to separate the planning and design of the work from its execution. Both require the same specialized skills, on a project-by-project basis. Thus it can be difficult to distinguish the middle levels of the organization from its operating core, since line managers and staff specialists may take their place alongside operating specialists on the project teams.

Figure 11–1 shows the organigram of the National Film Board of Canada, a classic operating adhocracy (even though it does produce a chart—one that changes frequently, it might be added). The Board is an agency of the Canadian federal government and produces mostly short films, many of them documentaries. At the time of this organigram, the characteristics of adhocracy were particularly in evidence: It shows a large number of support units as well as liaison positions (for example,

FIGURE 11–1

The National Film Board of Canada: An Operating Adhocracy
(circa 1975; used with permission)

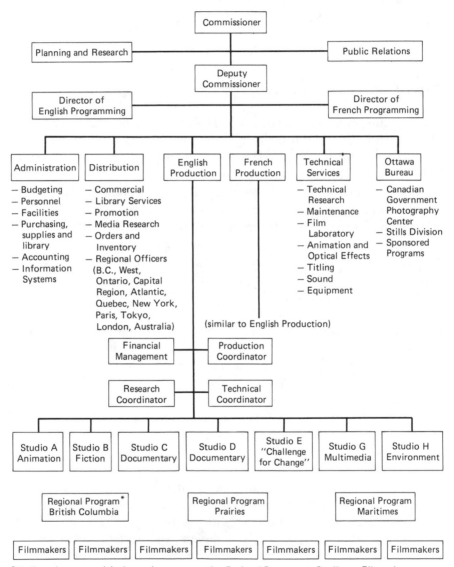

*No lines shown on original organigram connecting Regional Programs to Studios or Filmmakers.

research, technical, and production coordinators), with the operating core containing loose concurrent functional and market groupings, the latter by region as well as by type of film produced and, as can be seen, some not even connected to the line hierarchy!

THE ADMINISTRATIVE ADHOCRACY

The second type of adhocracy also functions with project teams, but toward a different end. Whereas the operating adhocracy undertakes projects to serve its clients, the *administrative adhocracy* undertakes projects to serve itself, to bring new facilities or activities on line, as in the administrative structure of a highly automated company. And in sharp contrast to the operating adhocracy, the administrative adhocracy makes a clear distinction between its administrative component and its operating core. That core is *truncated*—cut right off from the rest of the organization—so that the administrative component that remains can be structured as an adhocracy.

This truncation may take place in a number of ways. First, when the operations have to be machinelike and so could impede innovation in the administration (because of the associated need for control), it may be established as an independent organization. Second, the operating core may be done away with altogether—in effect, contracted out to other organizations. That leaves the organization free to concentrate on the development work, as did NASA during the Apollo project. A third form of truncation arises when the operating core becomes automated. This enables it to run itself, largely independent of the need for direct controls from the administrative component, leaving the latter free to structure itself as an adhocracy to bring new facilities on line or to modify old ones.

Oil companies, because of the high degree of automation of their production process, are in part at least drawn toward administrative adhocracy. Figure 11–2 shows the organigram for one oil company, reproduced exactly as presented by the company (except for modifications to mask its identity, done at the company's request). Note the domination of "Administration and Services," shown at the bottom of the chart; the operating functions, particularly "Production," are lost by comparison. Note also the description of the strategic apex in terms of standing committees instead of individual executives.

FIGURE 11–2

Organigram of an Oil Company: An Administrative Adhocracy

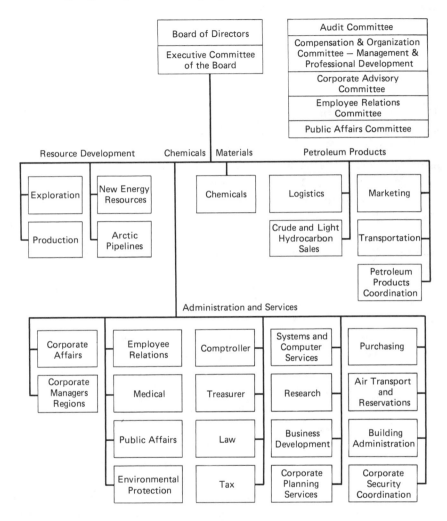

THE ADMINISTRATIVE COMPONENT OF THE ADHOCRACIES

The important conclusion to be drawn from this discussion is that in both types of adhocracy the relation between the operating core and the administrative component is unlike that in any other configuration. In the administrative adhocracy, the operating core is truncated and becomes a relatively unimportant part of the organization; in the operating adhocracy, the two merge into a single entity. Either way, the need for traditional direct supervision is diminished, so managers derive their influence more from their expertise and interpersonal skills than from formal position. And that means the distinction between line and staff blurs. It no longer makes sense to distinguish those who have the formal power to decide from those who have only the informal right to advise. Power over decision-making in the adhocracy flows to anyone with the required expertise, regardless of position.

In fact, the support staff plays a key role in adhocracy, because that is where many of the experts reside (especially in administrative adhocracy). As suggested above, however, that staff is not sharply differentiated from the other parts of the organization, not off to one side, to speak only when spoken to, as in the bureaucratic configurations. The other type of staff, however, the technostructure, is less important here, because the adhocracy does not rely for coordination on standards that it develops. Technostructure analysts may, of course, be used for some action planning and other forms of analysis—marketing research and economic forecasting, for example—but these analysts are as likely to take their place alongside the other specialists on the project teams as to stand back and design systems to control them.

To summarize, the administrative component of the adhocracy emerges as an organic mass of line managers and staff experts, combined with operators in the operating adhocracy, working together in ever shifting relationships on ad hoc projects. Our logo figure at the start of this chapter shows adhocracy with its parts mingled together in one amorphous mass in the middle. In the operating adhocracy, that mass includes the middle line, support staff, technostructure, and operating core. Of these, the administrative adhocracy excludes just the operating core, which is truncated, as shown by the dotted section below the central mass. The reader will also note that the strategic apex of the figure is shown partly merged into the central mass as well, for reasons we shall present in our discussion of strategy formation.

THE ROLES OF THE STRATEGIC APEX

The top managers of the strategic apex of this configuration do not spend much time formulating explicit strategies (as we shall see). But they must spend a good deal of their time in the battles that ensue over strategic choices and in handling the many other disturbances that arise all over these fluid structures. The innovative configuration combines fluid working arrangements with power based on expertise, not authority. Together those breed aggressiveness and conflict. But the job of the managers here, at all levels, is not to bottle up that aggression and conflict so much as to channel them to productive ends. Thus, the managers of adhocracy must be masters of human relations, able to use persuasion, negotiation, coalition, reputation, and rapport to fuse the individualistic experts into smoothly functioning teams.

Top managers must also devote a good deal of time to monitoring the projects. Innovative project work is notoriously difficult to control. No MIS can be relied upon to provide complete, unambiguous results. So there must be careful personal monitoring of projects to ensure that they are completed according to specifications, on schedule and within budget (or, more likely, not excessively late and not too far in excess of cost estimates).

Perhaps the most important single role of the top management of this configuration (especially the operating adhocracy form) is liaison with the external environment. The other configurations tend to focus their attention on clearly defined markets and so are more or less assured of a steady flow of work. No so the operating adhocracy, which lives from project to project and disappears when it can find no more. Since each project is different, the organization can never be sure where the next one will come from. So the top managers must devote a great deal of their time to ensuring a steady and balanced stream of incoming projects. That means developing liaison contacts with potential customers and negotiating contracts with them. Nowhere is this more clearly illustrated than in the consulting business, particularly where the approach is innovative. When a consultant becomes a partner in one of these firms, he or she normally hangs up the calculator and becomes virtually a full-time salesperson. It is a distinguishing characteristic of many an operating adhocracy that the selling function literally takes place at the strategic apex.

Project work poses related problems in the administrative adhocracy. Reeser asked a group of managers in three aerospace companies, "What are some of the human problems of project management?" Among the common answers: "[M]embers of the organization who are displaced because of the phasing out of [their] work . . . may have to wait a long time before they get another assignment at as high a level of responsibility" and "the temporary nature of the organization often necessitates 'make work' assignments for [these] displaced members."[2] Thus senior managers must again concern themselves with a steady flow of projects, although in this case, internally generated.

CONDITIONS OF THE INNOVATIVE ORGANIZATION

This configuration is found in environments that are both dynamic and complex. A dynamic environment, being unpredictable, calls for organic structure; a complex one calls for decentralized structure. This configuration is the only type that provides both. Thus we tend to find the innovative organization wherever these conditions prevail, ranging from guerrilla warfare to space agencies. There appears to be no other way to fight a war in the jungle or to put the first man on the moon.

As we have noted for all the configurations, organizations that prefer particular structures also try to "choose" environments appropriate to them. This is especially clear in the case of the operating adhocracy. Advertising agencies and consulting firms that prefer to structure themselves as professional bureaucracies seek out stable environments; those that prefer the innovative form find environments that are dynamic, where the client needs are difficult and unpredictable.*

A number of organizations are drawn toward this configuration because of the dynamic conditions that result from very frequent product change. The extreme case is the unit producer, the manufacturing firm that custom-makes each of its products to order, as in the engineering company that produces prototypes or the fabricator of extremely expensive machinery. Because each customer order constitutes a new project, the organization is encouraged to structure itself as an operating adhocracy.

Some manufacturers of consumer goods operate in markets so competitive that they must be constantly changing their product offerings, even though each product may itself be mass-produced. A company that records rock music would be a prime example, as would some cosmetic and

---

* I like to tell a story of the hospital patient with an appendix about to burst who presents himself to a hospital organized as an adhocracy: "Who wants to do another appendectomy? We're into livers now," as they go about exploring new procedures. But the patient returning from a trip to the jungle with a rare tropical disease had better beware of the hospital organized as a professional bureaucracy. A student came up to me after I once said this and explained how hospital doctors puzzled by her bloated stomach and not knowing what to do took out her appendix. Luckily, her problem resolved itself, some time later.

pharmaceutical companies. Here again, dynamic conditions, when coupled with some complexity, drive the organization toward the innovative configuration, with the mass production operations truncated to allow for adhocracy in product development.

Youth is another condition often associated with this type of organization. That is because it is difficult to sustain any structure in a state of adhocracy for a long period—to keep behaviors from formalizing and thereby discouraging innovation. All kinds of forces drive the innovative configuration to bureaucratize itself as it ages. On the other hand, young organizations prefer naturally organic structures, since they must find their own ways and tend to be eager to innovate. Unless they are entrepreneurial, they tend to become intrapreneurial.

The operating adhocracy is particularly prone to a short life, since it faces a risky market which can quickly destroy it. The loss of one major contract can literally close it down overnight. But if some operating adhocracies have short lives because they fail, others have short lives because they succeed. Success over time encourages metamorphosis, driving the organization toward a more stable environment and a more bureaucratic structure. As it ages, the successful organization develops a reputation for what it does best. That encourages it to repeat certain activities, which may suit the employees who, themselves aging, may welcome more stability in their work. So operating adhocracy is driven over time toward professional bureaucracy to perfect the activities it does best, perhaps even toward the machine bureaucracy to exploit a single invention. The organization survives, but the configuration dies.

Administrative adhocracies typically live longer. They, too, feel the pressures to bureaucratize as they age, which can lead them to stop innovating or else to innovate in stereotyped ways and thereby to adopt bureaucratic structure. But this will not work if the organization functions in an industry that requires sophisticated innovation from all its participants. Since many of the industries where administrative adhocracies are found do, organizations that survive in them tend to retain this configuration for long periods.

In recognition of the tendency for organizations to bureaucratize as they age, a variant of the innovative configuration has emerged—"the organizational equivalent of paper dresses or throw-away tissues"[3]— which might be called the "temporary adhocracy." It draws together specialists from various organizations to carry out a project, and then it disbands. Temporary adhocracies are becoming increasingly common in modern society: the production group that performs a single play, the election campaign committee that promotes a single candidate, the guerrilla group that overthrows a single government, the Olympic committee that plans a single games. Related is what can be called the "mammoth project adhocracy," a giant temporary adhocracy that draws on thousands of experts for a number of years to carry out a single major task, the Manhattan Project of World War II being one famous example.

Sophisticated and automated technical systems also tend to drive organizations toward the administrative adhocracy. When an organization's technical system is sophisticated, it requires an elaborate, highly trained support staff, working in teams, to design or purchase, modify, and maintain the equipment. In other words, complex machinery requires specialists who have the knowledge, power, and flexible working arrangements to cope with it, which generally requires the organization to structure itself as an adhocracy.

Automation of a technical system can evoke even stronger forces in the same direction. That is why a machine organization that succeeds in automating its operating core tends to undergo a dramatic metamorphosis. The problem of motivating bored workers disappears, and with it goes the control mentality that permeates the structure; the distinction between line and staff blurs (machines being indifferent to who turns their knobs), which leads to another important reduction in conflict; the technostructure loses its influence, since control is built into the machinery by its own designers rather than having to be imposed on workers by the standards of the analysts. Overall, then, the administrative structure becomes more decentralized and organic, emerging as an adhocracy. Of course, for automated organizations with simple technical systems (as in the production of hand creams), the entrepreneurial configuration may suffice instead of the innovative one.

Fashion is most decidedly another condition of the innovative configuration. Every one of its characteristics is very much in vogue today: emphasis on expertise, organic structure, project teams, task forces, decentralization of power, matrix structure, sophisticated technical systems, automation, and young organizations. Thus, if the entrepreneurial and machine forms were earlier configurations, and the professional and the diversified forms yesterday's, then the innovative is clearly today's.

This is the configuration for a population growing ever better educated and more specialized, yet under constant encouragement to adopt the "systems" approach—to view the world as an integrated whole instead of a collection of loosely coupled parts. It is the configuration for environments that are becoming more complex and more insistent on innovation, and for technical systems that are growing more sophisticated and more highly automated. It is the only configuration among our types appropriate for those who believe organizations must become at the same time more democratic and less bureaucratic.

Yet despite our current infatuation with it, adhocracy is not the structure for all organizations. Like all the others, it too has its place. And that place, as our examples make clear, seems to be in the new industries of our age—aerospace, electronics, think-tank consulting, research, advertising, filmmaking, petrochemicals—virtually all of which experienced their greatest development since World War II. The innovative adhocracy appears to be the configuration for the industries of the last half of the twentieth century.

STRATEGY FORMATION IN THE INNOVATIVE ORGANIZATION

The structure of the innovative organization may seem unconventional, but its strategy-making is even more so, upsetting virtually everything we have been taught to believe about that process.

Because the innovative organization must respond continuously to a complex, unpredictable environment, it cannot rely on deliberate strategy. In other words, it cannot predetermine precise patterns in its activities and then impose them on its work through some kind of formal planning process. Rather, many of its actions must be decided upon individually, according to the needs of the moment. It proceeds incrementally; to use Charles Lindblom's words, it prefers "continual nibbling" to a "good bite."[4]

Here, then, the process is best thought of as strategy *formation,* because strategy is not formulated consciously in one place so much as formed implicitly by the specific actions taken in many places. That is why action planning cannot be extensively relied upon in these organizations: Any process that separates thinking from action—planning from execution, formalization from implementation—would impede the flexibility of the organization to respond creatively to its dynamic environment.

STRATEGY FORMATION IN THE OPERATING ADHOCRACY

In the operating adhocracy, a project organization never quite sure what it will do next, the strategy never really stabilizes totally but is responsive to new projects, which themselves involve the activities of a whole host of people. Take the example of the National Film Board. Among its most important strategies are those related to the content of the hundred or so mostly short, documentary-type films that it makes each year. Were the Board structured as a machine bureaucracy, the word on what films to make would come down from on high. Instead, when we studied it some years ago, proposals for new films were submitted to a standing committee, which included elected filmmakers, marketing people, and the heads of production and programming—in other words, operators, line managers, and staff specialists. The chief executive had to approve the committee's choices, and usually did, but the vast majority of the proposals were initiated by the filmmakers and the executive producers lower down. Strategies formed as themes developed among these individual proposals. The operating adhocracy's strategy thus evolves continuously as all kinds of such decisions are made, each leaving its imprint on the strategy by creating a precedent or reinforcing an existing one.

STRATEGY FORMATION IN THE ADMINISTRATIVE ADHOCRACY

Similar things can be said about the administrative adhocracy, although the strategy-making process is slightly neater there. That is because the organization tends to concentrate its attention on fewer projects, which involve more people. NASA's Apollo project, for example, involved most of its personnel for almost ten years.

Administrative adhocracies also need to give more attention to action planning, but of a loose kind—to specify perhaps the ends to be reached while leaving flexibility to work out the means en route. Again, therefore, it is only through the making of specific decisions—namely, those that determine which projects are undertaken and how these projects unfold—that strategies can evolve.

STRATEGIES NONETHELESS

With their activities so disjointed, one might wonder whether adhocracies (of either type) can form strategies (that is, patterns) at all. In fact, they do, at least at certain times.

At the Film Board, despite the little direction from the management, the content of films did converge on certain clear themes periodically and then diverge, in remarkably regular cycles. In the early 1940s, there was a focus on films related to the war effort. After the war, having lost that raison d'être as well as its founding leader, the Board's films went off in all directions. They converged again in the mid-1950s around series of films for television, but by the late 1950s were again diverging widely. And in the mid-1960s and again in the early 1970s (with a brief period of divergence in between), the Board again showed a certain degree of convergence, this time on the themes of social commentary and experimentation.

This habit of cycling in and out of focus is quite unlike what takes place in the other configurations. In the machine organization especially, and somewhat in the entrepreneurial one, convergence proves much stronger and much longer (recall Volkswagenwerk's concentration on the Beetle for twenty years), while divergence tends to be very brief. The machine organization, in particular, cannot tolerate the ambiguity of change and so tries to leap from one strategic orientation to another. The innovative organization, in contrast, seems not only able to function at times without strategic focus, but positively to thrive on it. Perhaps that is the way it keeps itself innovative—by periodically cleansing itself of some of its existing strategic baggage.

THE VARIED STRATEGIES OF ADHOCRACY

Where do the strategies of adhocracy come from? While some may be imposed deliberately by the central management (as in staff cuts at the Film Board), most seem to emerge in a variety of other ways (mentioned back in Chapter 2).

In some cases, a single ad hoc decision sets a precedent which evokes a pattern. That is how the National Film Board got into making series of films for television. While a debate raged over the issue, with management hesitant, one filmmaker slipped out and made one such series, and when many of his colleagues quickly followed suit, the organization suddenly found itself deeply, if unintentionally, committed to a major new strategy. It was, in effect, a strategy of spontaneous but implicit consensus on the part of its operating employees. In another case, even the initial precedent-setting decision wasn't deliberate. One film inadvertently ran longer than expected, it had to be distributed as a feature, the first for the organization, and as some other filmmakers took advantage of the precedent, a feature film strategy emerged.

Sometimes a strategy will be pursued in a pocket of an organization (perhaps in a clandestine manner, in a so-called "skunkworks"), which then later becomes more broadly organizational when the organization, in need of change and casting about for new strategies, siezes upon it. Some salesman has been pursuing a new market, or some engineer has developed a new product, and is ignored until the organization has need for some fresh strategic thinking. Then it finds it, not in the vision of its leaders or the procedures of its planners, not elsewhere in its industry, but hidden in the bowels of its own operations, developed through the learning of its workers.

What then becomes the role of the leadership of the innovative configuration in making strategy? If it cannot impose deliberate strategies, what does it do? The answer is that it manages patterns, seeking partial control over strategies but otherwise attempting to influence what happens to those strategies that do emerge lower down.

These are the organizations in which, as noted earlier in this book, trying to manage strategy is a little like trying to drive an automobile without having your hands on the steering wheel. You can accelerate and brake but cannot determine direction. But there do remain important forms of control. First the leaders can manage the *process* of strategy-making if not the content of strategy. In other words, they can set up the structures to encourage certain kinds of activities and hire the people who themselves will carry out these activities. Second, they can provide general guidelines for strategy—what we have called *umbrella* strategies—seeking to define certain boundaries outside of which the specific patterns developed below should not stray. Then they can watch the patterns that do emerge and use the umbrella to decide which to encourage and which to discourage, remembering, however, that the umbrella can be shifted too.

A GRASSROOTS MODEL OF STRATEGY FORMATION

We can summarize this discussion in terms of a "grassroots" model of strategy formation, comprising six points.

1. Strategies grow initially like weeds in a garden, they are not cultivated like tomatoes in a hothouse. In other words, the process of strategy formation can be overmanaged; sometimes it is more important to let patterns emerge than to force an artificial consistency upon an organization prematurely. The hothouse, if needed, can come later.

2. These strategies can take root in all kinds of places, virtually anywhere people have the capacity to learn and the resources to support that capacity. Sometimes an individual or unit in touch with a particular opportunity creates his, her, or its own pattern. This may happen inadvertently, when an initial action sets a precedent. Even senior managers can fall into strategies by experimenting with ideas until they converge on something that works (though the final result may appear to the observer to have been deliberately designed). At other times, a variety of actions converge on a strategic theme through the mutual adjustment of various people, whether gradually or spontaneously. And then the external environment can impose a pattern on an unsuspecting organization. The point is that organizations cannot always plan where their strategies will emerge, let alone plan the strategies themselves.

3. Such strategies become organizational when they become collective, that is, when the patterns proliferate to pervade the behavior of the organization at large. Weeds can proliferate and encompass a whole garden; then the conventional plants may look out of place. Likewise, emergent strategies can sometimes displace the existing deliberate ones. But, of course, what is a weed but a plant that wasn't expected? With a change of perspective, the emergent strategy, like the weed, can become what is valued (just as Europeans enjoy salads of the leaves of America's most notorious weed, the dandelion!).

4. The processes of proliferation may be conscious but need not be; likewise they may be managed but need not be. The processes by which the initial patterns work their way through the organization need not be consciously intended, by formal leaders or even informal ones. Patterns may simply spread by collective action, much as plants proliferate themselves. Of course, once strategies are recognized as valuable, the processes by which they proliferate can be managed, just as plants can be selectively propagated.

5. New strategies, which may be emerging continuously, tend to pervade the organization during periods of change, which punctuate periods of more integrated continuity. Put more simply, organizations, like gardens, may accept the biblical maxim of a time to sow and a time to reap (even though they can sometimes reap what they did not mean to sow). Periods of convergence, during which the organization exploits its prevalent, established strategies, tend to be interrupted periodically by periods of divergence, during which the organization experiments with and subsequently accepts new strategic themes. The blurring of the separation between these two types of periods may have the same effect on an organization that the blurring of the separation between sowing and reaping has on a garden—the destruction of the system's productive capacity.

6. To manage this process is not to preconceive strategies but to recognize their emergence and intervene when appropriate. A destructive weed, once noticed, is best uprooted immediately. But one that seems capable of bearing fruit is worth watching, indeed sometimes even worth building a hothouse around. To manage in this context is to create the climate within which a wide variety of strategies can grow (to establish flexible structures, develop appropriate processes, encourage supporting ideologies, and define guiding "umbrella" strategies) and then to watch what does in fact come up. The strategic initiatives that do come "up" may in fact originate anywhere, although often low down in the organization, where the detailed knowledge of products and markets resides. (In fact, to be successful in some organizations, these initiatives must be recognized by middle-level managers and "championed" by combining them with each other or with existing strategies before promoting them to the senior management.) In effect, the management encourages those initiatives that appear to have potential, otherwise it discourages them. But it must not be too quick to cut off the unexpected: Sometimes it is better to pretend not to notice an emerging pattern to allow it more time to unfold. Likewise, there are times when it makes sense to shift or enlarge an umbrella to encompass a new pattern—in other words, to let the organization adapt to the initiative rather than vice versa. Moreover, a management must know when to resist change for the sake of internal efficiency and when to promote it for the sake of external adaptation. In other words, it must sense when to exploit an established crop of strategies and when to encourage new strains to displace them. It is the excesses of either—failure to focus (running blind) or failure to change (bureaucratic momentum)—that most harms organizations.

I call this a "grassroots" model because the strategies grow up from the base of the organization, rooted in the solid earth of its operations rather than the ethereal abstractions of its administration. (Even the strategic initiatives of the senior management itself are in this model rooted in its tangible involvement with the operations.)

Of course, the model is overstated. But no more so than the more widely accepted deliberate one, which we might call the "hothouse" model of strategy formulation. Management theory must encompass both, perhaps more broadly labeled the *learning* model and the *planning* model, as well as a third, the *visionary* model.

I have discussed the learning model under the innovative configuration, the planning model under the machine configuration, and the visionary model under the entrepreneurial configuration. But in truth, all organizations need to mix these approaches in various ways at different times in their development. For example, our discussion of strategic change in the machine organization concluded, in effect, that they had to revert to the learning model for revitalization and the visionary model for turnaround. Of course, the visionary leader must learn, as must the learning organization evolve a kind of strategic vision, and both sometimes need planning to program the strategies they develop. And overall, no organization can function with strategies that are always and purely emergent; that would amount to a complete abdication of will and leadership, not to mention conscious thought. But none can function either with strategies that are always and purely deliberate; that would amount to an unwillingness to learn, a blindness to whatever is unexpected.

ENVIRONMENT TAKING PRECEDENCE IN THE INNOVATIVE ORGANIZATION

To conclude our discussion of strategy formation, as shown in Figure 11–3, in the innovative configuration it is the environment that takes precedence. It drives the organization, which responds continuously and eclectically, but does nevertheless achieve convergence during certain periods.* The formal leadership seeks somehow to influence both sides

---

* We might take this convergence as the expression of an "organization's mind"—the focusing on a strategic theme as a result of the mutual adjustments among its many actors.

FIGURE 11–3
Environment Taking the Lead in Adhocracy

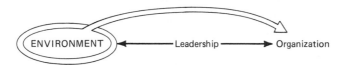

in this relationship, negotiating with the environment for support and attempting to impose some broad general (umbrella) guidelines on the organization.

If the strategist of the entrepreneurial organization is largely a concept attainer and that of the machine organization largely a planner, then the strategist of the innovative organization is largely a *pattern recognizer,* seeking to detect emerging patterns within and outside the strategic umbrella. Then strategies deemed unsuitable can be discouraged while those that seem appropriate can be encouraged, even if that means moving the umbrella. Here, then, we may find the curious situation of leadership changing its intentions to fit the realized behavior of its organization. But that is curious only in the perspective of traditional management theory.

SOME ISSUES ASSOCIATED WITH THE INNOVATIVE ORGANIZATION

Three issues associated with the innovative configuration merit attention here: its ambituities and the reactions of people who must live with them, its inefficiencies, and its propensity to make inappropriate transitions to other configurations.

HUMAN REACTIONS TO AMBIGUITY

Many people, especially creative ones, dislike both structural rigidity and the concentration of power. That leaves them only one configuration, the innovative, which is both organic and decentralized. Thus they find it a great place to work. In essence, adhocracy is the only structure for people who believe in more democracy with less bureaucracy.

But not everyone shares those values (not even everyone who professes to). Many people need order, and so prefer the machine or professional type of organization. They see adhocracy as a nice place to visit but no place to spend a career. Even dedicated members of adhocracies periodically get frustrated with this structure's fluidity, confusion, and ambiguity. "In these situations, all managers some of the time and many managers all the time, yearn for more definition and structure."[5] The managers of innovative organizations report anxiety related to the eventual phase-out of projects; confusion as to who their boss is, whom to impress to get promoted; a lack of clarity in job definitions, authority relationships, and lines of communication; and intense competition for resources, recognition, and rewards.[6] This last point suggests another serious problem of ambiguity here, the politicization of these configurations. Combining its ambiguities with its interdependencies, the innovative form can emerge as a rather politicized and ruthless organization—supportive of the fit, as long as they remain fit, but destructive of the weak.

PROBLEMS OF EFFICIENCY

No configuration is better suited to solving complex, ill-structured problems than this one. None can match it for sophisticated innovation. Or, unfortunately, for the costs of that innovation. This is simply not an efficient way to function. Although it is ideally suited for the one-of-a-kind project, the innovative configuration is not competent at doing *ordinary* things. It is designed for the *extra*ordinary. The bureaucracies are all mass producers; they gain efficiency through standardization. The adhocracy is a custom producer, unable to standardize and so be efficient. It gains its effectiveness (innovation) at the price of efficiency.

One source of inefficiency lies in the unbalanced workload, mentioned earlier. It is almost impossible to keep the personnel of a project structure—high-priced specialists, it should be noted—busy on a steady basis. In January they may be working overtime with no hope of completing the new project on time; by May they may be playing cards for want of work.

But the real root of inefficiency is the high cost of communication. People talk a lot in these organizations; that is how they combine their knowledge to develop new ideas. But that takes time, a great deal of time. Faced with the need to make a decision in the machine organization, someone up above gives an order and that is that. Not so in the innovative one, where everyone must get into the act—managers of all kinds (functional, project, liaison), as well as all the specialists who believe their point of view should be represented. A meeting is called, probably to schedule another meeting, eventually to decide who should participate in the decision. The problem then gets defined and redefined, ideas for its solution get generated and debated, alliances build and fall around different solutions, until eventually everyone settles down to the hard bargaining over which one to adopt. Finally a decision emerges—that in itself is an accomplishment—although it is typically late and will probably be modified later.

THE DANGERS OF INAPPROPRIATE TRANSITION

Of course, one solution to the problems of ambiguity and inefficiency is to change the configuration. Employees no longer able to tolerate the ambiguity and customers fed up with the inefficiency may try to drive the organization to a more stable, bureaucratic form.

That is relatively easily done in the operating adhocracy, as noted earlier. The organization simply selects the set of standard programs it does best, reverting to the professional configuration, or else innovates one last time to find a lucrative market niche in which to mass produce, and then becomes a machine configuration. But those transitions, however easily effected, are not always appropriate. The organization came into being to solve problems imaginatively, not to apply standards indiscriminately. In many spheres, society has more mass producers than it needs; what it lacks are true problem-solvers—the consulting firm that can handle a unique problem instead of applying a pat solution, the advertising agency that can come up with a novel campaign instead of the common imitation, the research laboratory that can make the really serious break-through instead of just modifying an existing design. The television networks seem to be classic examples of bureaucracies that provide largely standardized fare when the creativity of adhocracy is called for (except, perhaps, for the newsrooms and the specials, where an ad hoc orientation encourages more creativity).

The administrative adhocracy can run into more serious difficulties when it succumbs to the pressures to bureaucratize. It exists to innovate for itself, in its own industry. Unlike the operating adhocracy, it often cannot change orientation while remaining in the same industry. And so its conversion to the machine configuration (the natural transition for an administrative adhocracy tired of perpetual change), by destroying the organization's ability to innovate, can eventually destroy the organization itself.

To reiterate a central theme of our discussion throughout this section: In general, there is no one best structure; in particular, there may be at a cost of something forgone, so long as the different attributes combine to form a coherent configuration that is consistent with the situation.

12
IDEOLOGY AND THE MISSIONARY ORGANIZATION

In my book on structure, I discussed five configurations. There were no more than hints of a sixth in that literature at the time (the mid-1970s), and since the book was designed to be "a synthesis of the literature" (its subtitle), I mentioned it only as a brief afterthought in the book's final pages, mostly to suggest that we needn't limit our perspective to five types.

Well, our Japanese friends have changed all that. I subsequently found a sixth configuration in the literature of organizational sociology while doing my book on power. But ever since the Japanese showed us how to manage organizations through the use of ideology—norms and beliefs in place of standards and procedures—these concepts came out of the classrooms of sociology and moved into the boardrooms of management. Now you can hardly avoid them, or at least the homilies that accompany them—the four easy steps to the building of a better culture promoted by some management consultants.

Well, homilies are to culture what rules are to wisdom—superficial distillations that distort the phenomenon. You can't change an organization's culture the way those consultants change their clients. So we had better understand the roots of this important concept.

I shall use the word *ideology* in this chapter, rather than *culture.* Every organization has a culture, which describes its own way of doing things. Our concern here is a very special culture—a richly developed and deeply rooted system of values and beliefs that distinguishes a particular organization from all others. I prefer to call this an ideology, which I mean in the organizational, not the political sense. (An organization that reflects a common political ideology—say, bottom-line economic or participative liberal—cannot be described as having its own unique set of beliefs, in other words, its own particular ideology.)

Sometimes an organization's ideology becomes so strong that its whole structure is built around it. Then a sixth configuration appears, which I labeled the *missionary* in my power book. But more commonly, it seems to me, organizational ideologies "overlay" on more conventional structures—a McDonald's, classic machine structure that uses its own vigorous culture to fire up its employees, a Hewlett-Packard that seems to blend its own particular ideology with, perhaps, an innovative, adhocracy-type structure. Accordingly, in this chapter (like the next on politics), I shall depart from the format of the previous five and focus on *force* as much as *form.* In other words, the discussion will be concerned with ideology as a force in organization as much as with the missionary as a distinct form of organization.

Organizations with established ideologies of their own are fascinating ones, once again for better and for worse. They represent some of the most exciting moments in organizational history as well as some of the worst violations of human rights. (Try the Chinese Cultural Revolution for both.) While we adore the way a Toyota motivates its workers for production, we abhor the way a Jonestown drives its members to destruction, perhaps without stopping to realize the similarities in their methods of control. Ideologies can serve us and can enslave us, sometimes indistinguishably.

This chapter begins with a brief discussion of the development of organizational ideology through three stages. It then considers the structure of the missionary configuration, where ideology predominates, and finally concludes with a brief discussion of ideology as an overlay on more conventional types of organizations.

Ideology

- rich system of values and beliefs that distinguishes an organization
- rooted in sense of mission associated with charismatic leadership, developed through traditions and sagas and then reinforced through identifications
- can be overlaid on conventional configuration, most commonly entrepreneurial, followed by innovative, professional, and then machine
- sometimes so strong that evokes own configuration:

The Missionary Organization

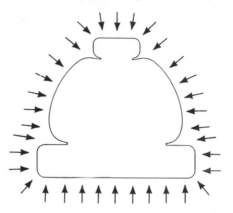

- clear, focused, inspiring, distinctive mission
- coordination through the standardization of norms ("pulling together"), reinforced by selection, socialization, and indoctrination of members
- small units ("enclaves"), loosely organized and highly decentralized but with powerful normative controls
- reformer, converter, and cloister forms
- threats of isolation on one side, assimilation on the other

---

We all know that 2 + 2 = 4. But general systems theory, through the concept of synergy, suggests that it can also equal 5, that the parts of a system may produce more working together than they can apart. A flashlight and a battery add up to just so many pieces of hardware; together they form a working system. Likewise an organization is a working system that can entice from its members more than they would produce apart—more effort, more creativity, more output (or, of course, less). This may be "strategic"—deriving from the way components have been combined in the organization. Or it may be motivational: The group is said to develop a "mood," an "atmosphere," to have some kind of "chemistry." In organizations, we talk of a "style," a "culture," a "character." One senses something unique when one walks into the offices of IBM; the chemistry of Hewlett-Packard just doesn't feel the same as that of Texas Instruments, even though the two have operated in some similar businesses.

All these words are used to describe something—intangible yet very real, over and above the concrete components of an organization—that we refer to as its *ideology*. Specifically, an ideology is taken here to mean a rich system of values and beliefs about an organization, shared by its members, that distinguishes it from other organizations. For our purposes, the key feature of such an ideology is its unifying power: It ties the individual to the organization, generating an "esprit de corps," a "sense of mission," in effect, an integration of individual and organizational goals that can produce synergy.

THE DEVELOPMENT OF AN ORGANIZATIONAL IDEOLOGY

The development of an ideology in an organization will be discussed here in three stages. The roots of the ideology are planted when a group of individuals band together around a leader and, through a sense of mission, found a vigorous organization, or invigorate an existing one. The ideology then develops over time through the establishment of traditions. Finally, the existing ideology is reinforced when new members enter the organization and identify with its system of beliefs.

STAGE 1: THE ROOTING OF IDEOLOGY IN A SENSE OF MISSION

Typically, an organization is founded when a single prime mover identifies a mission—some product to be produced, service to be rendered—and collects a group around him or her to accomplish it. Some organizations are, of course, founded by other means, as when a new agency is created by a government or a subsidiary by a corporation. But a prime mover often can still be identified behind the founding of the organization.

The individuals who come together don't do so at random, but coalesce because they share some values associated with the fledgling organization. At the very least they see something in it for themselves. But in some cases, in addition to the mission per se there is a "sense of mission," that is, a feeling that the group has banded together to create something unusual and exciting. This is common in new organizations for a number of reasons.

First, unconstrained by procedure and tradition, new organizations offer wide latitude for maneuver. Second, they tend to be small, enabling the members to establish personal relationships. Third, the founding members frequently share a set of strong basic beliefs, sometimes including a sense that they wish to work together. Fourth, the founders of new organizations are often "charismatic" individuals, and so energize the followers and knit them together. Charisma, as Weber used the term, means a sense of "personal devotion" to the leader for the sake of his or her personal qualities rather than formal position.[1] People join and remain with the organization because of dedication to the leader and his or her mission. Thus the roots of strong ideologies tend to be planted in the founding of organizations.

Of course, such ideologies can also develop in existing organizations. But a review of our above points suggests why this should be much more difficult to accomplish. Existing organizations *are* constrained by procedures and traditions, many are *already* large and impersonal, and their *existing* beliefs tend to impede the establishment of new ones. Nonetheless, with the introduction of strong charismatic leadership reinforced by a strong new sense of mission, an existing organization can sometimes be invigorated by the creation of a new ideology.

To my mind, key to the development of an organizational ideology, in a new or existing organization, is a leadership with a genuine belief in mission and an honest dedication to the people who must carry it out. Mouthing the right words might create the veneer of an organizational ideology, but it is only an authentic feeling on the part of the leadership—which followers somehow sense—that sets the roots of the ideology deep enough to sustain it when other forces, such as impersonal administration (bureaucracy) or politics, challenge it.

STAGE 2: THE DEVELOPMENT OF IDEOLOGY THROUGH TRADITIONS AND SAGAS

As a new organization establishes itself or an existing one establishes a new set of beliefs, it makes decisions and takes actions that serve as commitments and establish precedents. Behaviors reinforce themselves over time, and actions become infused with value. When those forces are strong, ideology begins to emerge in its own right. That ideology is strengthened by stories—sometimes called "myths"—that develop around important events in the organization's past. Gradually the organization establishes its own unique sense of history. All of this—the precedents, habits, myths, history—form a common base of tradition, which the members of the organization share, thus solidifying the ideology. Gradually, in Selznick's terms, the organization is converted from an expendable "instrument" for the accomplishment of externally imposed goals into an "institution," a system with a life of its own. It "acquires a self, a distinctive identity."[2]

Thus Clark described the "distinctive college," with reference particularly to Reed, Antioch, and Swarthmore. Such institutions develop, in his words, an "organizational saga," "a collective understanding of a unique accomplishment based on historical exploits," which links the organization's present with its past and "turns a formal place into a beloved institution."[3] The saga captures allegience, committing people to the institution.[4]

STAGE 3: THE REINFORCEMENT OF IDEOLOGY THROUGH IDENTIFICATIONS

Our description to this point makes it clear that an individual entering an organization does not join a random collection of individuals, but rather a living system with its own culture. He or she may come with a certain set of values and beliefs, but there is little doubt that the culture of the organization can weigh heavily on the behavior he or she will exhibit once inside it. This is especially true when the culture is rich—when the organization has an emerging or fully developed ideology. Then the individual's *identification* with and *loyalty* to the organization can be especially strong. Such identification can develop in a number of ways:

- Most simply, identification occurs *naturally* because the new member is attracted to the organization's system of beliefs.
- Identification may also be *selected*. New members are chosen to "fit in" with the existing beliefs, and positions of authority are likewise filled from among the members exhibiting the strongest loyalty to those beliefs.
- Identification may also be *evoked*. When the need for loyalty is especially great, the organization may use informal processes of

socialization and formal programs of *indoctrination* to reinforce natural or selected commitment to its system of beliefs.

- Finally, and most weakly, identification can be *calculated.* In effect, individuals conform to the beliefs not because they identify naturally with them nor because they even necessarily fit in with them, not because they have been socialized or indoctrinated into them, but simply because it pays them to identify with the beliefs. They may enjoy the work or the social group, may like the remuneration, may work to get ahead through promotion and the like. Of course, such identification is fragile. It disappears as soon as an opportunity calculated to be better appears.

Clearly, the higher up this list an organization's member identifications tend to be, the more likely it is to sustain a strong ideology, or even to have such an ideology in the first place. Thus, strong organizational belief systems can be recognized above all by the presence of much natural identification. Attention to selected identification indicates the presence of an ideology, since it reflects an organization's efforts to sustain its ideology, as do efforts at socialization and indoctrination. Some organizations require a good deal of the latter two, because of the need to instill in their new members a complex system of beliefs. When the informal processes of socialization tend to function naturally, perhaps reinforced by more formal programs of indoctrination, then the ideology would seem to be strong. But when an organization is forced to rely almost exclusively on indoctrination, or worse to fall back on forms of calculated identification, then its ideology would appear to be weakening, if not absent to begin with.

THE MISSIONARY ORGANIZATION

Organizations whose identifications are so strong and natural (whether at the outset or after selection, socialization, and indoctrination) that they can be used to effect much of the necessary coordination—in place of the more conventional mechanisms such as direct supervision or the standardization of work, output, or skills—tend to adopt a configuration we label the *missionary*. Here rich traditions and a unique history combine to form an especially strong ideology. What counts above all in such organizations is the mission, some endeavor that is typically (1) clear and focused, so that its members are easily able to identify with it, (2) inspiring, so that the members do, in fact, develop such identifications, and (3) distinctive, so that the organization and its members are deposited into a unique niche where the ideology can flourish.

That is not, however, to conclude that all organizations with such missions end up taking the missionary form. When private interests and needs—for example, those of the administrators or of the members at large—are allowed to take precedent, then even the most noble of missions can be overwhelmed. After all, bingo sometimes ends up being more important in some churches than service to the Almighty. Likewise, there is the story in the literature of sociology of certain rehabilitation agencies that kept their "desirable blind" clients in a state of dependence in order to use them to help raise funds, while ignoring the greater needs of older, less attractive blind people.[5] In these organizations, the mission serves the administrators rather than vice versa, and so the configuration, in our terms, ends up being a closed system machine.

The missionary form is another distinct configuration of the attributes of structure, internally highly integrated yet different from the other configurations we have discussed. What holds this organization together—that is, provides for its coordination—is the standardization of its norms, in other words, the sharing of values and beliefs among its members. As was noted, that can happen informally, either through natural selection or else the informal process of socialization. But from the perspective of structural design—meaning systematic intervention to determine behavior—the key attribute is indoctrination, meaning formalized programs to develop or reinforce identification with the ideology. And once the new member has been selected, socialized, and indoctrinated, he or she is accepted into the system as an equal partner, able to participate in decision-making alongside everyone else. Thus, at the limit, the missionary organization can achieve the purest form of decentralization: All who are accepted into the system share its power.

But that does not mean an absence of control. Quite the contrary. No matter how subtle, control tends to be very powerful in this configuration. For here, the organization controls not just people's behavior but their very souls. The machine organization buys the "workers'" attention through imposed rules; the missionary organization captures the "members'" hearts through shared values. As Jay noted in his book *Management and Machiavelli,* teaching new Jesuit recruits to "love God and do what you like" is not to do what they like at all but to act in strict conformance with the order's beliefs.[6] In this way, of course, the missionary organization minimizes political conflict. The only acceptable debates concern interpretation of the established ideology.

But in another important respect, the missionary organization is not unlike the machine one: Because it too relies on a form of standardization for coordination, it is also fundamentally a bureaucracy. Its form of bureaucracy may seem loose, for, after all, standardized norms allow for more fluid structure than do standardized work processes. But don't be misled by this. The standards of the missionary can be so deeply internalized (not just accepted from nine to five in return for a paycheck) that this can turn out to be the most bureaucratic structure of all, at least in the sense of being the most rigid. Bear in mind that ideological standards tend to be immutable: The missionary organization is more inclined to change the world than to change itself. In other words, it is usually too busy interpreting "the word" to call that word into question.

Because the standardization of norms is so powerful in these organizations, other forms of coordination need hardly be relied upon, neither standards of work or output nor direct supervision, nor even much mutual adjustment. Everyone simply acts in accordance with the pervasive beliefs and so can do the operating work relatively independently. This means there tends to be few *formal* rules and regulations in the missionary organization, not much planning or formal control, not even much managerial control, and so hardly any technostructure or hierarchy of authority. (In the Chinese Cultural Revolution, for example, the managers had to work in the factories for a certain number of days each year.) Leadership then becomes not the imposition of direction so much as the protection and enhancement of the common ideology; the leader is expected to inspire others to pursue the mission, perhaps also to interpret the mission, but never to change the mission.

Even professional skills may be discouraged in the missionary organization as incompatible with the ideology. A dependence on particular bodies of expertise might force the organization to surrender some "normative" control to the professional institutions that train and license its members and also introduce status differences between members that true missionary organizations try to minimize. For example, the Foundation for Infantile Paralysis, a missionary organization that ran the famous March of Dimes campaign, forbade medical doctors to hold office in its local chapters to avoid the establishment of a specialized elite.[7]

Thus, as shown in the logo, the missionary organization tends to end up as an amorphous mass of members all pulling together within the common ideology, with minimum specialization as to job, differentiation as to part, division as to status. At the limit, managers, staffers, and operators, once selected, socialized, and indoctrinated, all seem rather alike and may, in fact, rotate into each other's positions.

Important for the missionary organization, however, is that its units remain small, because strong ideology depends on personal contact. Thus, when the missionary organization grows past a certain size, beyond which its members can no longer interact with one another on a personal basis, it tends to divide itself, like an amoeba, forming what may best be thought of as enclaves, self-contained replicas of the initial unit, based on the same ideology.

The traditional Israeli kibbutz is a classic example of the missionary configuration. In certain seasons, everyone pitches in and picks fruit in the fields by day and then attends the meetings to decide administrative issues by night. Managerial positions exist but are generally filled on a rotating basis so that no one emerges with the status of office for long. Likewise, staff support positions exist, but they too tend to be filled on a rotating basis from the same pool of members, as are the operating positions in the fields. (Kitchen duty is, for example, considered drudgery that everyone must do periodically.)

As mentioned, this describes the traditional kibbutz. Internal growth was found to threaten the kibbutz's traditional ideology, with the result that efforts were made to keep them small (six hundred adults being considered the upper limit), or to encourage the spinning off of new ones—the creation of what amount to new "enclaves"—from those that became large. A more serious threat to the traditional ideology was the conversion from agriculture to industry, which became necessary as the kibbutzim sought to enhance their influence and wealth. As suggested, it was relatively easy to sustain the egalitarian ideology when the work was agricultural. Industry, in contrast, generally called for greater levels of technology, specialization, and expertise, with a resulting increase in the need for administrative hierarchy and functional differentiation, all of these, as already noted, threatening to the missionary orientation. The kibbutzim continue to struggle with this problem.

A number of our points about the traditional kibbutz are summarized in a table developed by Rosner, which contrasts the "principles of kibbutz organization"—classic missionary—with those of "bureaucratic organization," in our terms, the classic machine.

Principles of Bureaucratic Organization	*Principles of Kibbutz Organization*
1. Permanency of office	Impermanency of office
2. The office carries with it impersonal, fixed privileges and duties.	The definition of office is flexible—privileges and duties are not formally fixed and often depend on the personality of the official.
3. A hierarchy of functional authorities expressed in the authority of the officials	A basic assumption of the equal value of all functions without a formal hierarchy of authority
4. Nomination of officials is based on formal objective qualifications.	Officials are elected, not nominated. Objective qualifications are not decisive, personal qualities are more important in election.
5. The office is a full-time occupation.	The office is usually supplementary to the full-time occupation of the official.[8]

FORMS OF THE MISSIONARY ORGANIZATION

We can distinguish three different forms of the pure missionary configuration. Some missionary organizations are *reformers*. They set out to change the world directly—anything from overthrowing a government to ensuring that all domestic animals are "decently" clothed. Of course, the label "missionary" comes from the religious orders that are basically reformers. A secular example is the Foundation for Infantile Paralysis, already mentioned, whose mission was to help eradicate that dreaded disease.

Other missionaries can be called *converters*. Their mission is to change the world indirectly, by attracting members and changing them. The difference between the first two types of missionaries is the difference between the Women's Christian Temperance Union and Alcoholics Anonymous. Their ends were similar, but their means differed, seeking to reduce alcoholism in one case by promoting a general ban on liquor sales, in the other by discouraging certain individuals, namely joined members, from drinking. Converters often take the form of what Erving Goffman labeled "total institutions," meaning organizations that house all aspects of their members' private and working lives so that they can control them totally.[9]

Finally there are the *cloister* missionaries, total institutions too, but ones that seek not to change things so much as to allow their members to pursue a unique style of life. The monasteries that close themselves off from the outside world are good examples, as are groups that go off to found new isolated colonies. These are "closed system," but not in the sense that term was used earlier, of an organization that deflects external influence in order to control its environment. The cloisters are not interested in controlling anything but their members' own behavior: They try to close themselves off in every respect.

Of course, no organization can completely seal itself off from the world. All missionary organizations, in fact, face the twin opposing pressures of isolation and assimilation. Together these make them vulnerable, as configurations if not as organizations. On one side is the threat of *isolation,* of growing ever inward in order to protect the unique ideology from the pressures of the ordinary world until the organization eventually dies for lack of renewal. The cloister missionary especially faces the problem of not replenishing its membership (how can it find new people when it is so detached). On the other side is the threat of *assimilation,* of reaching out so far to promote the ideology that it eventually gets compromised. The reformer missionary especially runs this risk, since it must develop intimate contacts with the very world of "contaminated" reality that it wishes to change. When this happens, the organization may survive but the ideology dies, and so the configuration changes (typically to the machine form).

IDEOLOGY AS AN OVERLAY ON CONVENTIONAL ORGANIZATIONS

So far we have discussed what amounts to the extreme form of ideological organization, the missionary. But more organizations have strong ideologies that can afford to structure themselves in this way. In Max Weber's terms, the missionary is an "ideal type," something to be approached but perhaps seldom attained. It may work for an Israeli kibbutz in a remote corner of the Negev desert, but this is hardly a way to run a Hewlett-Packard or a McDonald's, let alone a dynamic university or perhaps even a kibbutz closer to the worldly pressures of Tel Aviv.

What such organizations, with strong ideologies but also important needs for centralized authority or sophisticated expertise, tend to do is overlay ideological characteristics on a more conventional structure— perhaps machinelike in the case of McDonald's and that second kibbutz, professional in the case of Clark's distinctive colleges, innovative in the case of Hewlett-Packard. The mission may sometimes seem ordinary— serving hamburgers, teaching students, developing instruments—but it is carried out with a good dose of ideological fervor by employees firmly committed to it.

Best known for this are, of course, certain of the Japanese corporations, Toyota being a prime example. Ouchi and Jaeger contrast in the table reproduced below the typical large American corporation (Type A) with its Japanese counterpart (Type J):

Type A (for American)	*Type J (for Japanese)*
Short-term employment	Lifetime employment
Individual decision-making	Consensual decision-making
Individual responsibility	Collective responsibility
Rapid evaluation and promotion	Slow evaluation and promotion
Explicit, formalized control	Implicit, informal control
Specialized career path	Nonspecialized career path
Segmented concern	Holistic concern[10]

Every characteristic of what these authors call the Type J firm is consistent with our description of the effects of an ideology on an organization: the personal relationship between the individual and the organization, the collective nature of responsibility and choice, the holistic concern in place of specialization, the discouragement of formal controls in favor of implicit (normative) ones. All point to loyalty and ideology as the central elements in the system. Ouchi and Jaeger in fact make their point best with an example in which a classic Japanese ideological orientation confronts a conventional American bureaucratic one:

> [D]uring one of the author's visits to a Japanese bank in California, both the Japanese president and the American vice-presidents of the bank accused the other of being unable to formulate objectives. The Americans meant that the Japanese president could not or would not give them explicit, quantified targets to attain over the next three or six months, while the Japanese meant that the Americans could not see that once they understood the company's philosophy, they would be able to deduce for themselves the proper objective for any conceivable situation.[11]

In another study, however, Ouchi together with Johnson discusses a native American corporation that does resemble the Type J firm (labeled

"Type Z"; Ouchi later published a best-seller about such organizations[12]). In it, they found greater loyalty, a strong collective orientation, less specialization, and a greater reliance on informal controls. For example, "a new manager will be useless for at least four or five years. It takes that long for most people to decide whether the new person really fits in, whether they can really trust him." That was in sharp contrast to the "auction market" atmosphere of a typical American firm: It "is almost as if you could open up the doors each day with 100 executives and engineers who had been randomly selected from the country, and the organization would work just as well as it does now."[13]

We have suggested above that ideology can overlay on any of the conventional configurations and have provided several different examples of this. But it is perhaps better to conclude that ideology is more likely to be found overlaid on some configurations than others. Some tentative conclusions in this regard are summarized below:

• Ideologies are perhaps to be most commonly expected overlaid on the *entrepreneurial* configuration. That is because it is the one that can most easily develop a sense of mission, and is most likely to be led by a charismatic individual. Indeed, it is here that we are most likely to find the first stage in the development of an ideology, as described at the beginning of this chapter. But it should be noted that the missionary configuration is fundamentally different from the entrepreneurial one, in that power is centralized in one, widely shared in the other. Thus, we might expect to find the beginnings of ideology in this configuration more commonly than a fully developed one (although the latter may follow after the leader departs and his or her beliefs get institutionalized).

• Ideologies can be overlaid on a *machine* configuration too, as suggested in the examples of McDonald's and Toyota. But because formalization is anathema to ideology—turning informal beliefs into formal rules imposed down a centralized hierarchy of authority—we would also expect to find strong forces for the destruction of fledgling ideologies in this configuration. Thus, while this overlay may not be a rarity, it is not likely to be common.

• A similar conclusion might be reached for the *diversified* configuration, only more so. The debilitating effects of formality and of detached calculation, especially as manifested in "bottom line" thinking, are there, and so too is a diversity of missions that makes it difficult to engender enthusiasm for any one. Thus, while we may be able to find diversified configurations overlaid with ideological energy, we should expect these to be relatively rare.

• Expertise acts, as noted, to introduce status differences that work against the egalitarian nature of organizational ideologies. This discourages ideological overlays on the *professional* and *innovative* configurations, where expertise is pervasive. Moreover, the professional configuration promotes fragmentation of effort, while the innovative one gives rise to considerable political activity, both of which are incompatible with the cooperative needs of ideology. On the other hand, these organizations often have missions that are either intrinsically noble or exciting (such as curing the ill or developing high-technology products). Therefore, ideological overlays may in fact occur with some frequency, as in the earlier examples of Clark's distinctive colleges or Hewlett-Packard. This may be especially true for the operating adhocracy, which tends to combine youth, energy, and informality with the excitement of an ever changing stream of products and services.

The trends in American businesses over several decades—"professional" management, emphasis on technique and rationalization, "bottom-line" mentality—have certainly worked against the development of organizational ideologies. Certainly the missionary configuration has hardly been fashionable in the West, especially the United States. But ideology may have an important role to play there, given the enormous success many Japanese firms have had in head-on competition with American corporations organized in machine and diversified ways, with barren cultures. At the very least, we might expect more ideological overlays on the conventional forms of organizations in the West. But this, as we hope our discussion has made clear, may be both for better and for worse.

13
POLITICS AND THE POLITICAL ORGANIZATION

So far this discussion of the different configurations has revolved around the various mechanisms by which organizations achieve coordination. Politics is obviously something very different. In fact, if coordination is the means by which organizations find order and integration, then politics acts to the detriment of coordination, by *dis*ordering and *dis*integrating what currently exists. Politics has to do with power, not structure, and so it was in my book on that subject that I developed my ideas on politics and on the political organization, which I there called the "political arena." I was also reminded there how much politics can influence all of the processes normally considered alongside structure—managerial work, decision-making, strategy formation, and so on. Thus, no description of the basic forces and forms of organizations can be complete without the consideration of politics.

I am no fan of politics in organizations. But neither am I a fan of illness. Yet I know we have to understand one like the other. In fact, politics can be viewed as a form of organizational illness, working both against and for the system. On one hand, politics can undermine healthy processes, infiltrating them to destroy them. But on the other, it can also work to strengthen a system, acting like fever to alert a system to a graver danger, even evoking the system's own protective and adaptive mechanisms.

Political activity can be found in every organization, indeed every human system, more or less. So it is necessary to discuss politics as a general force in organizations, much as we so discussed ideology in the preceding chapter. Accordingly, we begin this chapter with a discussion of the role of politics in organizations and then consider a variety of political games that tend to be played there. Thirteen are discussed in all, a rough but fascinating little group that most of us have encountered in one form or another.

But again, like ideology, politics can also capture an organization, dominating its processes. Thus, we turn next to a discussion of the political organization, how it arises and evolves, based on the different forms it can take. We have "confrontation," the "shaky alliance," the "politicized organization," and the "complete political arena," each a nasty little viper in its own way, but all capable of doing constructive good in certain circumstances (as, of course, do real vipers). Thus, the chapter concludes with a discussion of how politics can serve a functional role in organizations.

Politics

- means of power technically illegitimate, often in self-interest, resulting in conflict that pulls individuals or units apart
- expresses itself in political games, some coexistent with, some antagonistic to, some that substitute for legitimate systems of power
- usually overlaid on conventional organization, but sometimes strong enough to create own configuration:

The Political Organization

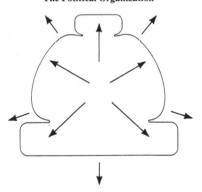

- conventional notions of concentrated coordination and influence absent, replaced by the play of informal power
- dimensions of conflict—moderate/intense, confined/pervasive, as well as enduring/brief—combine into four forms: confrontation, shaky alliance, politicized organization, complete political arena
- can trace development of forms through life cycle of impetus, development, resolution of the conflict
- politics and political organizations serve a series of functional roles in organizations, especially to help bring about necessary change blocked by legitimate systems of influence

---

How does conflict arise in an organization, why, and with what consequences? Years ago, the literature of organization theory avoided such questions. But in the last decade or so, conflict and the politics that go along with it have become not just acceptable topics but fashionable ones. Yet these topics, like most others in the field, have generally been discussed in fragments. Here we seek to consider them somewhat more comprehensively, first by themselves and then in the context of what will be called the political organization—the organization that comes to be dominated by politics and conflict.

POLITICS IN ORGANIZATIONS

What do we mean by "politics" in organizations? An organization may be described as functioning on the basis of a number of systems of influence: authority, ideology, expertise, politics. The first three can be considered legitimate in some sense: Authority is based on legally sanctioned power, ideology on widely accepted beliefs, expertise on power that is officially certified. The system of politics, in contrast, reflects power that is technically illegitimate (or, perhaps more accurately, *a*legitimate), in the means it uses, and sometimes also in the ends it promotes. In other words, political power in the organization (unlike government) is not formally authorized, widely accepted, or officially certified. The result is that political activity is usually divisive and conflictive, pitting individuals or groups against the more legitimate systems of influence and, when those systems are weak, against each other.

POLITICAL GAMES IN ORGANIZATIONS

Political activity in organizations is sometimes described in terms of various "games." The political scientist Graham Allison, for example, has described political games in organizations and government as "intricate and subtle, simultaneous, overlapping," but nevertheless guided by rules: "some rules are explicit, others implicit, some rules are quite clear, others fuzzy. Some are very stable; others are ever changing. But the collection of rules, in effect, defines the game."[1] I have identified thirteen political games in particular, listed here together with their main players, the main reasons they seem to be played, and how they relate to the other systems of influence.

- *Insurgency game:* usually played to resist authority, although can be played to resist expertise or established ideology or even to effect change in the organization; ranges "from protest to rebellion,''[2] and is usually played by "lower participants,"[3] those who feel the greatest weight of formal authority

- *Counterinsurgency game:* played by those with legitimate power who fight back with political means, perhaps with legitimate means as well (e.g., excommunication in the church)
- *Sponsorship game:* played to build power base, in this case by using superiors; individual attaches self to someone with more status, professing loyalty in return for power
- *Alliance-building game:* played among peers—often line managers, sometimes experts—who negotiate implicit contracts of support for each other in order to build power base to advance selves in the organization
- *Empire-building game:* played by line managers, in particular, to build power bases, not cooperatively with peers but individually with subordinates
- *Budgeting game:* played overtly and with rather clearly defined rules to build power base;[4] similar to last game, but less divisive, since prize is resources, not positions or units per se, at least not those of rivals
- *Expertise game:* nonsanctioned use of expertise to build power base, either by flaunting it or by feigning it; true experts play by exploiting technical skills and knowledge, emphasizing the uniqueness, criticality, and irreplaceability of the expertise,[5] also by seeking to keep skills from being programmed, by keeping knowledge to selves; nonexperts play by attempting to have their work viewed as expert, ideally to have it declared professional so they alone can control it
- *Lording game:* played to build power base by "lording" legitimate power over those without it or with less of it (i.e., using legitimate power in illegitimate ways); manager can lord formal authority over subordinate or civil servant over a citizen; members of missionary configuration can lord its ideology over outsiders; experts can lord technical skills over the unskilled
- *Line versus staff game:* a game of sibling-type rivalry, played not just to enhance personal power but to defeat a rival; pits line managers with formal decision-making authority against staff advisers with specialized expertise; each side tends to exploit legitimate power in illegitimate ways
- *Rival camps game:* again played to defeat a rival; typically occurs when alliance or empire-building games result in two major power

blocs, giving rise to two-person, zero-sum game in place of n-person game; can be most divisive game of all; conflict can be between units (e.g., between marketing and production in manufacturing firm), between rival personalities, or between two competing missions (as in prisons split between custody and rehabilitation orientations)

• *Strategic candidates game:* played to effect change in an organization; individuals or groups seek to promote through political means their own favored changes of a strategic nature; many play—analysts, operating personnel, lower-level managers, even senior managers and chief executives (especially in the professional configurations), who must promote own candidates politically before they can do so formally; often combines elements of other games—empire-building (as purpose of game), alliance-building (to win game), rival camps, line versus staff, expertise, and lording (evoked during game), insurgency (following game), and so on

• *Whistle-blowing game:* a typically brief and simple game, also played to effect organizational change; privileged information is used by an insider, usually a lower participant, to "blow the whistle" to an influential outsider on questionable or illegal behavior by the organization

• *Young Turks game:* played for highest stakes of all, not to effect simple change or to resist legitimate power per se, but to throw the latter into question, perhaps even to overthrow it, and institute major shift; small group of "young Turks," close to but not at center of power, seeks to reorient organization's basic strategy, displace a major body of its expertise, replace its ideology, or rid it of its leadership; Zald and Berger discuss a form of this game they call "organizational coup d'état," where the object is "to effect an unexpected succession"—to replace *holders* of authority while maintaining *system* of authority intact[6]

Some of these games, such as sponsorship and lording, while themselves technically illegitimate, can nevertheless *coexist with* strong legitimate systems of influence, as found for example in the machine and missionary configurations; indeed, they could not exist without these systems of influence. Other political games, such as insurgency and young Turks—usually highly divisive games—arise in the presence of legitimate power but are *antagonistic to it,* designed to destroy or at least weaken it. They work against configurations such as the machine.

And still others, such as rival camps, often arise when legitimate power is weak and *substitute for* it, for example in the professional and innovative configurations.

The implication of this is that politics and conflict may exist at two levels in an organization. They may be present but not dominant, existing as an overlay on a more conventional organization, perhaps a kind of fifth column acting on behalf of some challenging power. Or else politics may be the dominant system of influence, and conflict strong, having weakened the legitimate systems of influence or having arisen in their weakness. It is this second level that gives rise to the configuration we shall call the *political organization*.

FORMS OF POLITICAL ORGANIZATIONS

What characterizes the organization dominated by politics is a lack of any of the forms of order found in conventional organizations. In other words, the organization is best described in terms of power, not structure, and that power is exercised in ways not legitimate in conventional organizations. Thus, there is no preferred method of coordination, no single dominant part of the organization, no clear type of decentralization. Everything depends on the fluidity of informal power, marshaled to win individual issues.

How does such an organization come to be? There is little published research on the question. But some ideas can be advanced tentatively. First, conflict would seem to arise in a circumscribed way in an organization, say between two units (such as marketing and production) or between an influential outside group and a powerful insider (such as between a part owner and the CEO). That conflict may develop gradually or it may flare up suddenly. It may eventually be resolved, but when it becomes intense, it may tend to spread, as other influencers get drawn in on one side or the other. But since few organizations can sustain intense political activity for long, that kind of conflict must eventually moderate itself (unless it kills off the organization first). In moderated form, however, the conflict may endure, even when it pervades the whole system, so long as the organization can make up for its losses, perhaps by being in a privileged position (as in the case of a conflict-ridden regulatory agency that is sustained by a government budget, or a politicized corporation that operates in a secure cartel).

What we end up with are two dimensions of conflict, first moderate or intense and second confined or pervasive. A third dimension—enduring or brief—really combines with the first (intense conflict having to be typically brief, moderate conflict possibly enduring). Combining these dimensions, we end up with four forms of the political organization:

- *Confrontation,* characterized by conflict that is *intense, confined,* and *brief* (unstable)
- *Shaky alliance,* characterized by conflict that is *moderate, confined,* and possibly *enduring* (relatively stable)
- *Politicized organization,* characterized by conflict that is *moderate, pervasive,* and possibly *enduring* (relatively stable, so long as it is sustained by privileged position)
- *Complete political arena,* characterized by conflict that is *intense, pervasive,* and *brief* (unstable)*

One of these forms is called *complete* because its conflict is both intense and pervasive. In this form, the external influencers disagree among themselves; they try to form alliances with some insiders, while clashing with others. The internal activities are likewise conflictive, permeated by divisive political games. Authority, ideology, and expertise are all subordinated to the play of political power. An organization so politicized can pursue no goal with any consistency. At best, it attends to a number of goals inconsistently over time, at worst it consumes all its energy in disputes and never accomplishes anything. In essense, the complete political arena is less a coherent organization than a free-for-all of individuals. As such, it is probably the form of political organization least commonly found in practice, or, at least, the most unstable when it does appear.

In contrast, the other three forms of political organization manage to remain partial, one by moderating its conflict, a second by containing it, and the third by doing both. As a result, these forms are more stable than the complete form and so are probably more common, with two of them in particular appearing to be far more viable.

In the *confrontational* form, conflict may be intense, but it is also contained, focusing on two parties. Typical of this is the takeover situation, where, for example, an outside stockholder tries to seize control of a closed system corporation from its management. Another example is the situation, mentioned earlier, of two rival camps in and around a

---

*I do not consider conflict that is moderate, confined, and brief to merit inclusion under the label of political organization.

prison, one promoting the mission of custody, the other that of rehabilitation.

The *shaky alliance* commonly emerges when two or more major systems of influence or centers of power must coexist in roughly equal balance. The symphony orchestra, for example, must typically combine the strong personal authority of the conductor (entrepreneurial orientation) with the extensive expertise of the musicians (professional orientation). As Fellini demonstrated so well in his film *Orchestra Rehearsal,* this alliance, however uncomfortable (experts never being happy in the face of strong authority), is nevertheless a necessary one. Common today is the professional organization operating in the public sector, which must somehow sustain an alliance of experts and government officials, one group pushing upward for professional autonomy, the other downward for technocratic control.

Our final form, the *politicized organization,* is characterized by moderate conflict that pervades the entire system of power. This would appear to describe a number of today's largest organizations, especially ones in the public sector whose mandates are visible and controversial—many regulatory agencies, for example, and some public utilities. Here it is government protection, or monopoly power, that sustains organizations captured by conflict. This form seems to be increasingly common in the private sector too, among some of the largest corporations that are able to sustain the inefficiencies of conflict through their market power and sometimes by their ability to gain government support as well.

LIFE CYCLES OF POLITICAL ORGANIZATIONS

How do these forms of political organizations develop over time and relate with one another? To describe this, we can postulate a life cycle model of political organizations, presented in three stages—impetus, development, and resolution.

IMPETUS

A necessary, and sometimes also a sufficient, condition for the appearance of a political organization is substantial pressure on the part of some influencer, or influencing group, to realign the basic system of power. For example, an outside owner group may seek to consolidate power over an entrepreneurial firm it has just bought, or a group of inside experts, hitherto not influential, may seek to exploit a new and necessary technology to enhance its own power, for example by demanding seats on key administrative committees.

Such pressures may arise by themselves—certain influencers simply demand a new deal—or else they may be provoked by other changes. As in the examples presented—change of ownership, advent of a new technology—some fundamental condition of the organization may have shifted, leading to new demands for influence. Or else the established order of power may have weakened of its own accord, creating a power vacuum that other influencers seek to fill, as when the autocratic chief of an entrepreneurial configuration falls gravely ill.

DEVELOPMENT

Such pressures challenge the existing order of power, if there is one; if not, they produce challenges among different groups vying for new influence in a power vacuum. Of course, since it is the challenge that leads to the conflict, quick resolution of it can avoid politicization, as when a shift of power at the top of a hierarchy is so long overdue and therefore so widely supported that it takes place as a kind of instant coup d'état.

But many important power challenges are not resolved quite so easily. They instead incite resistance, and so it falls to politics to lubricate their movement. As noted earlier, such conflicts tend to be confined at first, for example between "young Turks" promoting change and an "old guard" resisting it. But they can spread.

When the conflict erupts with suddenness and intensity—taking the confrontation form of political organization—unless soon checked it can spread to become a complete political arena. But that form, being intense and pervasive, must be resolved before it kills the entire organization. When the conflict develops gradually, however, it may lead to the more stable form we called the politicized organization, and so can endure (hence we shall discuss it under "resolution"). Of course, the moderate conflict of the politicized form can itself flare up at any time, leading to the confrontation form and then perhaps the complete form of political arena.

RESOLUTION

Three results of such political conflicts are likely. In the simplest case, someone wins—challenger or those challenged—and the organization settles down again to a quiet, relatively nonconflictive existence. That is what we would usually expect from a confrontation. If, however, the side that wins reflects sheer power as opposed to organizational need, then subsequent confrontations may be expected, at least if the organization is to remain effective.

The second possible result is that the conflict kills the organization. When this happens, it is likely to take place via the form of complete political arena. On one hand, this form may arise of its own accord (for example, through a major confrontation that endures and so pervades the organization) and thereby kill the organization. On the other hand, the complete political arena may arise in the death throes of an organization already doomed for other reasons (say, because its technology is hopelessly outmoded or its markets have disappeared). Here, the intense and pervasive conflict of the complete political arena represents a kind of free-for-all in which individuals try to extract whatever resources are left for their own benefit, and so quickly destroy the organization.

The third possible result is that the conflict continues, but in moderated form so that the organization can survive. The shaky alliance and politicized organization are the two moderate forms of political configuration.

When the result of a confrontation is a standoff, we might expect to see the rise of a shaky alliance. Neither side can win, neither wishes to give up, yet both know they must moderate their conflict if the organization is to survive. So they reach some kind of implicit accord, agreeing to tolerate each other. Of course, there are also organizations that must exist in perpetuity as shaky alliances, as in our example of the symphony orchestra or of the professionals who must coexist with government technocrats. In these cases, confrontation does not lead to the shaky alliance so much as the opposite: The alliance, being shaky, flares up into confrontation periodically.

The politicized organization form tends to arise when conflict builds up slowly and spreads throughout an organization, also perhaps when the pervasive conflict of the complete political arena abates, as influencers back off to allow the organization to survive. But as noted earlier, an organization cannot generally survive even with the politicized organizational form unless it is able to exploit a privileged position, such as an established hold on a market or artificial support from a granting agency.

Of course, there is really no such thing as true and final resolution of conflict. Any organization, even the most stable, can flare up into conflict at any time. Even the most formalized bureaucracy, the most secure entrepreneur, the most established ideology can be challenged, either arbitrarily by some group in search of power or because changed conditions have undermined its basis of power. Likewise, the shaky alliance is just that: shaky. The potential for intense conflict—hot war in place of cold—is never far from the surface. Any small perturbation can upset the delicate balance, driving it to outright confrontation. Thus, its power system may best be described as one of homeostasis—a dynamic balance. In the same way, the politicized organization can easily flare up into the intense conflict of the complete political arena. Most of the time, however, most organizations seem to be relatively free of major conflict, which allows them to get on with performing their missions. But politics is never far away. Thus, the only true and permanent stability, for organizations as for all other living systems, is death!

POLITICS IN THE CONVENTIONAL CONFIGURATIONS

Clearly the level of politics will vary in the conventional configurations, some being more prone to this kind of activity (or even to easy transition to a political configuration) than others. Let us consider each in turn.

• The *entrepreneurial* configuration should experience a minimum of politics, since one powerful individual closely supervises all activity. Political games are clearly not encouraged, especially those that cannot coexist with the personalized rule of the chief executive. Sponsorship may take place, but given that the chief does most of the sponsoring, that is hardly political. Likewise, strategic candidates may sometimes be promoted by the chief, but that too is hardly political. Confrontations or shaky alliances may arise between the chief executive and important outside influencers, or a group of young Turks may challenge a faltering chief, but these games are so incompatible with the entrepreneurial organization that they will generally drive it to a new configuration, the political one, for the duration of the conflict in order, perhaps, to make a transition to another stable type.

• The *machine* configuration and the *diversified* one have strong systems of formal authority, which should discourage political activity. But the rigidities of those systems in fact give rise to the milder forms of conflict, as things fall through the bureaucratic cracks. Thus, the political games that can coexist with legitimate authority tend to be prevalent here—empire building, budgeting, sponsorship, strategic candidates, line versus staff, and lording. In effect, machinelike and diversified structures, by introducing sharp divisions of labor, focus attention on the individual unit and so encourage parochialism and efforts to enhance narrow bases of power. That is what all these games do, each in its own way (through accumulating subordinates, enlarging budgets, adding programs, and so on). Games that challenge formal authority—insurgency (responded to by counter-insurgency), young Turks, and whistle-blowing—may also arise periodically to correct deficiencies in the system of formal authority, especially in the closed system form of these configurations where the authority is not constrained by external influence. Given the number of games played here, and the relatively moderate nature of most of them, these configurations can easily tilt over to the politicized organization form. While this tendency tends to be muted in the instrument form, where the presence of external control can discourage excessive political activity, it tends to be exaggerated in the closed system form, where insiders are drawn to share in the distribution of surpluses, and the administrators, on shaky grounds of external legitimacy to begin with, may simply defer to them (e.g., give in to strong union demands so as to avoid the embarrassment of a strike). Moreover, in the closed system form, external influencers may eventually be drawn to challenge the legitimacy of the administration's authority and so further politicize the organization.

• The *professional* and *innovative* configurations have relatively weak systems of authority, though strong ones of expertise. This means that their power tends to be rather diffused, distributed in a fluid way among many individuals. As a result, there is considerable room for political games in these configurations, especially ones that pit groups of insiders against each other—rival camps, alliance building, and young Turks. There is, in addition, a propensity to play the games that build narrow power bases, such as sponsorship, empire building, budgeting, and strategic candidates. Also, of course, the games associated with highly skilled operating work, namely expertise games and those of lording, are commonly played. The professional configuration may have a relatively stable operating core, where activities are highly standardized, but its administrative structure, where all kinds of professionals and managers interact to make choices, is hardly stable and, in fact, very supportive of games such as strategic candidates, empire building, and rival camps. The innovative configuration is far less stable, generally having a highly fluid structure throughout that literally promotes games such as alliance building, rival camps, and strategic candidates. Given the number of games played and the intensity of some of them in these two configurations, transition to a form of the political organization, at least temporarily, would seem to be a natural occurrence, particularly that of confrontation (say, between conflicting groups of experts, each professing to represent pure truth) or the politicized organization, where political activity spreads across the entire system. Transition can also occur to the shaky alliance form, for example when the experts are confronted by an influential group of outside influencers (such as government technocrats), or even to the complete form of political arena for a time, when the experts engage in outright wars with each other.

• The *missionary* is probably the configuration least tolerant of political activity, since the belief system and the encouragement to cooperate are so strong. People in these organizations are not supposed to build private alliances or empires, not hoard budgets, not blow the whistle on their colleagues, not challenge the existing ideology. In fact, the occurrence of these games would suggest the demise of the ideology as well as the configuration, if not the organization itself. Of course, strategic candidates may sometimes be promoted, and lording is one game that might be commonly found, as members flaunt their ideology over outsiders. Conflicts can arise over the interpretation of the ''word''—indeed, these can sometimes become quite heated, as each side professes to be the purer. But these must be decidedly internal, the missionary organization always being very careful to present a united front to the outside world. It might be added in closing that ideology as an overlay on another configuration should have a similar, although muted, effect in reducing political activity, for example by discouraging some of the more divisive political games in a machine configuration or encouraging cooperation over conflict in a professional one.

THE FUNCTIONAL ROLE OF POLITICS IN ORGANIZATIONS

Little space need be devoted to the dysfunctional influence of politics in organizations. Politics is divisive and costly; it burns up energies that could instead go into the operations. It can also lead to all kinds of aberrations. Politics is often used to sustain outmoded systems of power, and sometimes to introduce new ones that are not justified. Politics can also paralyze an organization to the point where its effective functioning comes to a halt and nobody benefits. The purpose of an organization, after all, is to produce goods and services, not to provide an arena in which people can fight with one another.

What does deserve space, however, because they are less widely appreciated, are those conditions in which politics and the political organization serve a functional role. Let us first consider in this regard the force of politics, and then the form of political organization.

In general, the system of politics is necessary in an organization to correct certain deficiencies in its other, legitimate systems of influence—above all to provide for certain forms of flexibility discouraged by those other systems. The other systems of influence were labeled legitimate because their *means*—authority, ideology, or expertise—have some basis of legitimacy. But sometimes those means are used to pursue *ends* that are illegitimate (as in the example of the lording game, where legitimate power is flaunted unreasonably). In contrast, the system of politics, whose *means* are (by definition) illegitimate, can sometimes be used to pursue *ends* that are in fact legitimate (as in certain of the whistle-blowing and young Turks games, where political pressures are used against formal authority to correct irresponsible or ineffective behaviors). We can elaborate on this in terms of four specific points.

First, politics as a system of influence can act in a Darwinian way to ensure that the strongest members of an organization are brought into positions of leadership. Authority favors a single chain of command; weak leaders can suppress strong subordinates. Politics, on the other hand, can provide alternate channels of information and promotion, as when the sponsorship game enables someone to leap over a weak superior. Moreover, since effective leaders have been shown to exhibit a need for power,[7] the political games can serve as tests to demonstrate the potential for leadership. The second-string players may suffice for the scrimmages, but only the stars can be allowed to meet the competition. Political games not only suggest who those players are but also help to remove their weak rivals from contention.

Second, politics can also ensure that all sides of an issue are fully debated, whereas the other systems of influence may promote only one. The system of authority, by aggregating information up a central hierarchy, tends to advance only a single point of view, often the one already known to be favored above. So, too, does the system of ideology, since every issue is interpreted in terms of "the word," the prevailing set of beliefs. As for the system of expertise, people tend to defer to the expert on any particular issue. But experts are often closed to new ideas, ones that developed after they received their training. Politics, however, by obliging "responsible men . . . to fight for what they are convinced is right,"[8] encourages a variety of voices to be heard on any issue. And, because of attacks by its opponents, each voice is forced to justify its conclusions in terms of the broader good. That means it must marshal arguments and support proposals that can at least be justified in terms of the interests of the organization at large rather than the parochial needs of a particular group. As Burns has noted in an amusing footnote:

> It is impossible to avoid some reference from the observations made here to F. M. Cornford's well known "Guide for the Young Academic Politician." Jobs "fall into two classes, My Jobs and Your Jobs. My Jobs are public-spirited proposals, which happen (much to my regret) to involve the advancement of a personal friend, or (still more to my regret) of myself. Your Jobs are insidious intrigues for the advancement of yourself and your friends, spuriously disguised as public-spirited proposals."[9]

Third, the system of politics is often required to stimulate necessary change that is blocked by the legitimate systems of influence. Internal change is generally threatening to the "vested interest" of an organization. Even when the change must be from one form of legitimate power to another, say from the personalized leadership of an entrepreneur to the more formalized leadership of administrators, it is often illegitimate power—namely political power—that must bring it about. The system of authority concentrates power up the hierarchy, often in the hands of those who were responsible for initiating the existing strategies in the first place. It also contains the established controls, which are designed to sustain the status quo. Similarly, the system of expertise concentrates power in the hands of senior and established experts, not junior ones who may possess newer, more necessary skills. Likewise, the system of ideology, because it is rooted in the past, in tradition, acts as a deterrent to change. In the face of these resistances, it is politics that is able to work as a kind of "invisible hand"—"invisible underhand"' would be a better term—to promote necessary change, through such games as strategic candidates, whistle-blowing, and young Turks.

Fourth and finally, the system of politics can ease the path for the execution of decisions. Senior managers, for example, often use politics to gain acceptance for their decisions, playing the strategic candidates game early in promoting proposals to avoid having to play the more divisive and risky counterinsurgency game later in the face of resistance to them. They persuade, negotiate, and build alliances to smooth the path for the decisions they wish to make.

If the system of politics can sometimes be functional, then so too, presumably, can the organization in which it dominates, the one captured by conflict. Specifically, the political configuration would appear to be functional when:

1. It encourages a realignment in the organization's power necessitated by change in one of its fundamental conditions or breakdown in its established focus of power
2. It corrects an earlier change in power that was itself dysfunctional
3. It exists as a shaky alliance that reflects natural, balanced, and irreconcilable forces in the organization
4. It speeds up the death of a spent organization

The first point argues that when the established order of power has outlived its usefulness, then a confrontation form of political organization that flares up to change it can itself be useful. In effect, extensive politics can sometimes be the only way to displace legitimate power that itself has become counterproductive—outmoded expertise, inappropriate controls, a spent ideology, detached leadership. Then the political organization must be viewed as productive. No matter how illegitimate and disruptive its own power may be, it serves as the functional bridge from one legitimate system of power to another. In effect, the organization reverts to the political configuration for a time to achieve a necessary change. For example, a detached leadership is confronted and the organization becomes politicized until a new, more in-touch leadership is installed. We can conclude that the political configuration serves as a prime means by which society corrects deficiencies in its organizations.

Obviously, political confrontation does not always correct a bad situation. Sometimes it aggravates it; the solution proves worse than the problem. Likewise, politics can be used by those at the center of power to block change that the organization requires. But, as argued earlier, such situations are unlikely to remain stable for long. Our second point argues that renewed confrontation is to be expected, with political pressures building up until they burst their confines to effect the necessary change. Just as anarchists, who lurk in all societies, are able to foment revolution only when large segments of the population feel the need for change, so too does politics, which lurks in all organizations, tend to become dominant only when change widely regarded as necessary has been repeatedly thwarted.

Some political challenges are, of course, arbitrary or neutral. An influencer simply wants a new deal. In those cases, we cannot label the resolution of the conflict functional or dysfunctional. We can, however, call the period during which the conflict endures dysfunctional, since it wastes resources that could have been doing other things. Thus a shaky alliance—an enduring political organization—that reflects no natural set of forces on the organization may be considered dysfunctional because of the resources it uses up. But a third point argues that a shaky alliance that does reflect opposing forces that are natural, roughly equal in importance, and irreconcilable—say, between research people promoting innovation and manufacturing people promoting efficiency in a firm that needs the two in balance—must be considered functional. This is because the organization could not function if it did not accommodate each of these forces. It has no choice but to take the form of a shaky alliance. Some conflict is the inevitable consequence of getting its work done.*

Our final point considers the organization that is about to succumb anyway, perhaps because it can no longer perform its mission effectively or because that mission is no longer required. Little hope exists for improving the organization's effectiveness or for converting to another mission (or, more to the point, it may be more efficient to allow new organizations to arise in its place). In any event, when demise is inevitable, from society's perspective the sooner it comes the better. That way a minimum of resources is wasted during the organization's death throes. Thus, the complete political arena that tends to arise as an organization dies, by speeding up its demise, can be considered functional. Much as the scavengers that swarm over a carcass serve a positive function in nature, so too can the political conflicts that engulf a dying organization serve a positive function in society. Both help to speed up the recycling of useful resources.

To be sure, this assumes that the final conflict is allowed to take its natural course. When, however, artificial forces sustain an organization in a state of pervasive conflict—as governments will sometimes do with giant, essentially bankrupt corporations for fear of the political ramifications of their demise—then the political organization must be considered significantly dysfunctional.

To conclude our discussion, while I am not personally enthusiastic about organizational politics and have no desire to live in a political organization, even the forms I have described as functional, I do accept, and hope I have persuaded the reader to accept, that this configuration, like the others, does have useful roles to play in a society of organizations. Organizational politics may irritate us, but it can also serve us.

---

* I do not draw the same conclusion for the politicized organization, because the pervasiveness of its conflict usually means that too much energy is wasted in political activity.

14

BEYOND
CONFIGURATION
Forces and Forms in
Effective Organizations

I originally saw this chapter as a kind of mopping-up operation, to tie together some loose ends and encourage the reader to look beyond the configurations per se. But in an intense period of two or three weeks just before this book went into production (and, to the chagrin of some very tolerant people at The Free Press, again after) things began to develop. As discussed in the text, a student some years earlier had upset my thinking with his question about playing "jigsaw puzzle" or LEGO. That and a number of comments on an earlier draft of this chapter, as well as some consulting experiences just when I was revising it, all suddenly converged to lead me to what has emerged as a statement on organizational effectiveness—the first time I have written directly on this issue. I found myself going not just beyond the actual configurations of my earlier work but beyond the whole notion of configuration that has driven my thinking for almost fifteen years. I am personally excited about the result.

The discussion that follows goes beyond configuration in two ways: It goes back to one and goes past seven. It goes back to one by treating the *forms* as *forces,* in other words by viewing the configurations as a single integrative framework of fundamental forces that act on every organization. And it goes past seven by suggesting that truly creative organizations design forms uniquely suited to their own needs.

Were I asked to state the single most important prescription for developing effective theory, I would answer without hesitation "cherish anomalies." Weak theorists, in my view, dismiss anomalies; they ignore what they cannot readily explain. Breakthroughs, in contrast, come from anomalies that have been identified and held onto, sometimes in the conscious mind, probably more often somewhere below it, until they are explained. The same seems to be true of organizations: The real advances in practice seem to come from difficulties that are put aside and periodically mulled over until they are resolved creatively.

Our discussion of the last seven chapters has all been very pat, a game of jigsaw puzzle with seven ways to combine the pieces. Here, to conclude and integrate that discussion, I set out to play "organizational LEGO" with some of the anomalies I have encountered over the years.

I read somewhere of a professor who told his doctoral students: "Keep your theories simple; reality is complex enough." Well, the discussion of our seven configurations has been simple enough; it is time to face some of the complexities of reality.

LUMPING AND SPLITTING

Charles Darwin once made the distinction between "lumpers" and "splitters." Lumpers categorize; they are the synthesizers, prone to consistency. Once they have pigeonholed something into one box or another, they are done with it. To a lumper in management, strategies are generic, structures are types, managers have a style (X, Y, Z, 9–9, etc.). Splitters nuance; they are the analyzers, prone to distinction. Since nothing can ever be categorized, things are never done with. To a splitter in management, strategies, structures, and styles all vary infinitely.

I believe a key to the effective organization lies in this distinction, specifically in its simultaneous acceptance and rejection (which themselves amount to lumping and splitting). Both are right and both are wrong. Without categories, it would be impossible to practice management. With only categories, it could not be practiced effectively.

For several years I worked as a lumper, seeking to identify types of organizations. Much as in the field of biology, I felt we in management needed some categorization of the "species" with which we dealt. We long had too much of "one best way" thinking, that every organization needed every new technique or idea that came along (like MBO or formal planning or participative management). Thus, in my books on structure and power, I developed various "configurations" of organizations. My premise was that an effective organization "got it all together" as the saying goes—achieved consistency in its internal characteristics, harmony in its processes, fit with its context.

JIGSAW PUZZLE AND LEGO

Every once in a while someone asks you a question that stops you dead in your tracks. Some years back, a doctoral student of mine, Alain Noël, after reading this material on structure and power, asked whether I was intending to play "jigsaw puzzle" or LEGO with it. In other words, did I mean all these elements of organizations to fit together in set ways—to create known images—or were they to be used creatively to build new ones? I had to answer that I had been promoting jigsaw puzzle even if I was suggesting that the pieces could be combined into several images instead of the usual one. But I immediately began to think about playing "organizational LEGO." All of the anomalies I had encountered—all those nasty, well-functioning organizations that refused to fit into one or another of my neat categories—suddenly became opportunities to think beyond configuration. I could become a splitter too.

This chapter is presented in the spirit of playing "organizational LEGO." It tries to show how we can use splitting as well as lumping to understand what makes organizations effective as well as what causes many of their fundamental problems.

FORMS AND FORCES

I shall refer to the configurations of organizations as *forms*. The original five of my structure book—here labeled entrepreneurial, machine, diversified, professional, and innovative—are laid out at the nodes of a pentagon, shown in Figure 14–1. (I shall return to the other two configurations of my power book—the missionary and the political—shortly.)

Many organizations seem to fit naturally into one or another of these categories, *more or less*. We all know the small aggressive entrepreneurial firm, the perfectly machinelike Swiss hotel, the diversified conglomerate, the professional collegial university, the free-wheeling intrapreneurial Silicon Valley innovator. But some organizations do not fit, much to the chagrin of the lumpers. And even many that may seem to, on closer examination reveal curious anomalies. It is difficult to imagine a more machinelike organization than McDonald's; why then does it seem to be rather innovative, at least in its own context? And why is it that whenever I mention to an executive group about a 3M or a Hewlett-Packard as innovative in form, someone from the audience leaps up to tell me about their tight control systems. Innovative adhocracies are not supposed to rely on tight controls.

FIGURE 14–1
An Integrating Pentagon of Forces and Forms

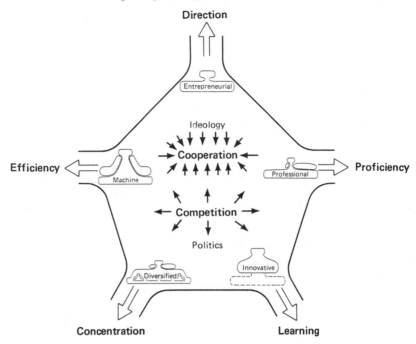

All this of course pleases the splitters. "Come on, Henry," a colleague chided me recently, "in my consulting practice I never see any one of these forms. I can find all of them in all serious organizations." To him, organizations float around the inside of my pentagon; they never make it to any one node. In response, therefore, to the valid claims of the splitters, I recently added *forces* to the pentagon, shown as arrows emanating out from each of the forms. In other words, every form can be thought to represent a force too:

- The entrepreneurial form represents the force for *direction*, for people looking up to the apex of authority, or the leader looking down, and saying, "What we need around here is some *direction*, someone to tell everybody where we all should go."
- The machine form represents the force for *efficiency*, for the staff analysts of the technostructure to look across at everyone else and say, "What they all need there is some order, some work rules and standards to make sure everything comes out as planned."*

---

* Recalling that this, and the diversified configuration, can take the form of instrument or closed system, it should be added that this force for efficiency can be thought to

- The professional form represents the force for *proficiency*, for those in the operating core of the organization to look up and say, "Leave us alone, we're professionals; let us hone our skills and apply them autonomously and all will be well."
- The diversified form represents the forces for *concentration*, for managers in the middle line looking up and down, and saying, "No, we're the ones who should be left alone, to receive clear product–market mandates and then be free to manage them as we see fit, subject only to the performance controls."
- And the innovative form represents the force for *learning*, for experts throughout the organization to look around and say, "What this place really needs is change, adaptation; let's all work together to innovate."

I have so far left out the two forms from my book on power. We can certainly find examples of the missionary configuration, as in the traditional Israeli kibbutz or some radical political movements. Likewise, such organizations as regulatory agencies, sometimes even business corporations, can become so captured by conflict for a time that they come to look like political organizations. But these forms are relatively rare, at least compared with the other five, and so I prefer to show them only as forces (placed in the middle of the pentagon for reasons to be discussed later).

- Ideology represents the force for *cooperation*, for "pulling together" (hence the arrows focus in toward the middle).
- And politics represents the force for *competition*, for "pulling apart" (hence the arrows flare out).

To recap to this point, we have two views of organizational effectiveness. One, for the lumpers, concentrates on a *portfolio of forms*, from which organizations are encouraged to choose if they wish to become effective. The other, for the splitters, focuses on a *system of forces*, with which organizations are encouraged to play in order to become effective. If the lumpers are right, form works; if the splitters are right, we must turn to the forces.

The basis of my argument here is that both views are critical to the practice of management. One represents the most fundamental forces that act on organizations: All serious organizations experience all seven of them, at one time or another if not all the time. And the other represents

---

represent service to a dominant external constituency or else to the organization (and its administrators) as a system unto itself.

the most fundamental forms that organizations can take, which some of them do some of the time. Together, as conceived on the pentagon, these forces and forms appear to constitute a powerful diagnostic framework by which to understand what goes on in organizations and to prescribe effective change in them.

Sometimes one force dominates the behavior of an organization; then we get *configuration*—the appearance of a form. The problem with configuration, however, is that the dominant force can get too powerful, and so have a *contaminating* effect on the other forces. Then the organization risks going *out of control*. Thus the other forces, however secondary, are needed to counterbalance, or *contain*, the dominant one. The lumpers need the splitters.

Some other times, no one force logically dominates, but rather two or more have to exist in a rough balance, as a *combination*. But that creates another problem, which can be called *cleavage*—conflict between the opposing forces. And then there are organizations that experience *conversion*, having to make the transition from one form or combination to another. This also produces opposing forces and cleavage. Splitting has its disadvantages too.

Now containment and cleavage give rise to the need to manage *contradiction*, to reconcile opposing forces. And here the forces of the center of the pentagon come into play, those of cooperation and competition. Lumping for splitters, splitting for lumpers.

We now proceed to lump and to split, to begin by playing jigsaw puzzle and then move quickly to play LEGO. We consider first the configuration of forms, then the combination and conversion of forces (also discussed in a postscript), and finally the management of contradiction, before concluding with a discussion of what makes an organization competent.

CONFIGURATION

When one force dominates the others, based on an organization's particular needs or perhaps just the arbitrary exercise of power, then we should look for the organization to fall close to one of the nodes, to take the form of one of our configurations, more or less. In other words, a force becomes a form when the organization yields to it. Much of what takes place within the configuration then reflects that dominant force. The sociologist Max Weber used the label "ideal type" for the caricatures of reality that our configurations represent. He meant the word "ideal" as pure, not perfect, and we shall refer to our configurations as pure forms. While no real organization matches any one of our pure forms perfectly, as in the examples presented earlier some do come remarkably close.

In the earlier summary chapter of my book on structure, I posed a question: "Do any of these configurations really exist?" I believe my answer to that question bears repeating here.

In one sense, these configurations do not exist at all. After all, they are mere words and pictures on pieces of paper, not reality itself. Real organizations are enormously complex, far more so than any of these caricatures. What these constitute is a kind of theory, or at least the components of a theory, and every theory necessarily simplifies and therefore distorts the reality. The problem, of course, is that in some areas at least, we cannot get by without theory (implicit if not explicit), much as a library cannot get by without a cataloging system.

Thus, our choice is often not between theory and reality but between alternate theories. No one carries reality around in his or her head, no head is that big. Instead we carry around impressions of reality, which amount to implicit theories. Sometimes these are supplemented with explicit frameworks for identifying concepts and interrelating them—in other words, with formal theories, built on systematic investigation known as research, or at least on systematic consideration of experience. In fact, some phenomena cannot be comprehended without such formal aid—how is one to develop an implicit theory of nuclear fission, for example?*

Therefore, I prefer to conclude that the configurations do exist. If I have done my job correctly, they exist where all knowledge ultimately has to exist—in people's minds. With *this* in mind, let us consider some evidence on the occurrence of configurations.

For several years, we have sent out our MBA students at McGill to study organizations in the Montreal area, exposing them, among other things, to my book on structure. At year end, I have circulated a question-naire asking them if they would categorize their organization as one of the forms, a hybrid of two or more, or none of the above. While the results are only the impressions of a group of students after an exercise of a few months, they do give a rough indication of how the world of organizations appears to a group of intelligent observers. In just over

---

* Sometimes, of course, what we think of as personal implicit theories are just formal ones we have internalized long ago. As John Maynard Keynes put it, "Practical men who believe themselves to be quite exempt from any intellectual influences, are usually the slaves of some defunct economist."

half the cases—66 out of 123—the students felt that a single form fitted best. There were 25 entrepreneurial, 13 machine, 11 diversified, 9 innovative, and 8 professional.* All the rest were labeled combinations, in most cases of two of the forms.

Lumping is, of course, convenient; it appeals to our sense of order. Organizations can be quickly and easily understood. Sometimes we find specific forms favored in particular sectors, for example, the machine configuration in such mass industries as automobile production and airline and postal services, the professional configuration in such highly skilled areas as education and health care, the innovative configuration in the dynamic industries of high technology. Of course, there are also sectors where organizations can choose their form according to how they choose their niche. In restauranting, for example, there is the small "greasy spoon" personally controlled by its entrepreneurial owner, the fast-food machine obsessed with standardizing everything, and, of course, that epitome of professional craft, the gourmet French restaurant. Likewise, consulting firms can be divided into the innovators, which look upon every new client as an opportunity to solve a novel problem in a creative way, and the professionals, which seek to slot all new contracts into some existing category or other and so get on with applying to it a well-established program.

For the lumpers who like cultural stereotypes, we can even extend the idea of forms to national preferences. Perhaps that might reveal some comparative advantages. For example, the Swiss, with their love of order, seem eminently well suited to the machine form. Perhaps that is why their hotels, banks, and railroads function so effectively. And studies of the overseas Chinese suggest that they have a strong propensity to favor the entrepreneurial form, sometimes building up huge empires on a base of personal initiative.[1] And to return to our last two configurations momentarily, the Japanese preference for the ideology of the missionary form is well known, as perhaps is the Italian predisposition toward the political organization.

My own suspicion is that the innovative form works best in Sweden, where the work force is highly educated, there is a long history of creative design, and the preferences for collaboration and consensus

---

* The high incidence of entrepreneurial forms may be thought to reflect the students' bias toward studying small organizations, but I think not. There are many more small organizations (in business and otherwise) than large ones, in many cases entrepreneurial in form. Of the larger ones, I would expect the machine form to predominate in any Western society.

are quite strong in contrast to the tendency to denigrate leadership. In casting about for the nation that seems most suitable to the professional form, where the experts work alone and less creatively, I discovered it right around me. Canadians too have a highly educated work force and a tendency to denigrate leadership, but we lack the Swedish inclinations to innovate and to collaborate—we prefer to let people work on their own. That, I believe, makes us quite good at managing professional organizations: We have the most collegial universities I have found anywhere in the world and a health care system that seems to strike the right balance between private initiative and public control.

Big American business, and for that matter big organizations in many spheres of American life, tend to favor the diversified form. Ironically, the same can be said for Eastern bloc nations, where communism can be seen to drive all organizations into one giant divisionalized structure. Indeed, there is a second irony here, because one would expect Americans, with their emphasis on individual initiative and their preference for innovation, to favor the entrepreneurial or at least the intrapreneurial (innovative) configuration. That they may do in principle; there is certainly no shortage of either in the United States. But American industry and other sectors today seem to me to be inundated with machine organizations, as divisions of large diversified ones. I believe this derives from the enormous growth of American organizations over the past several decades, a reflection of the exercise of power as much as the consequence of economic forces. As American organizations grew, as they embraced the concepts of "professional" management, and as they increasingly diversified and tried to manage their divisions as instruments subjected to bottom-line controls, they greatly bureaucratized their activities. Earlier I argued that the advantages of configuration come with internal harmony coupled with external fit. But here external fit seems to be lacking—markets seem increasingly to want more quality and innovation than many American organizations offer—while internal harmony is disrupted by workers (even managers) who don't particularly relish their roles as cogs in the bureaucratic machinery. Remove harmony and fit, and configuration becomes dysfunctional.

When it does fit, however, configuration helps not only to understand organizations but also to manage them. It facilitates diagnosis—everything new that comes along can be assessed in terms of a clear model of the organization—and that in turn facilitates prescription. We know a good deal about each of the common forms—their structures and strategies, their managerial work and management styles, many of their expected problems and opportunities, their people and their systems. We also have a sense of the concepts and techniques that seem to work best in each of them: work-study procedures in the machine form, financial control systems in the diversified, leadership vision in the entrepreneurial, collegiality in the professional, project management and matrix structure in the innovative.

Configuration can also help people who try to make sense of an organization from the outside. A few simple questions can sometimes suggest what form might be expected:

- What are the main groups of operators?
- For each, is their work unskilled or does it require considerable training?
- Do they work alone or must they interact in groups?
- Are their outputs standardized or customized?

Unskilled, standardized work carried out alone suggests the machine configuration. Extensively trained and standardized work done alone suggests the professional one. And the presence of extensively trained workers who require group collaboration and produce customized outputs suggests the innovative form.

Other obvious factors that might be considered in categorizing an organization are the size of its support staff compared with its operators (ratios of three or four to one suggest the professional configuration, sometimes the innovative), the clarity of definition between line and staff (which implies machine or diversified, its absence implying the innovative), the lack of staff altogether (implying the entrepreneurial), and so on. One must, of course, also look for evidence of a preferred mechanism of coordination and clear indications of a center of power. As we shall see, the answers to such questions need not always be unambiguous. But it sure makes things simple when they are.

It can also make them fun. For example, each configuration can be associated with a metaphor (the machine itself, the portfolio for the diversified, the halo for the missionary, the crystalline structure for the innovative, etc.), or with a corresponding animal (the circle of musk-oxen, or perhaps lemmings, for the missionary, the bucket of crabs for the political, the team of beavers for the innovative, etc.). Some configurations also seem to fit naturally with certain sports, American football being the perfect machine (formal leadership, sharp division of labor, preprogrammed work, all highly specialized), perhaps Canadian hockey for the innovative (or is it the political?!).

Thus, for classification, for comprehension, for diagnosis, and for prescription, configuration is most convenient. But it is not without its problems.

CONTAMINATION

Configuration, as noted, represents harmony, consistency, fit. The organization knows what it must do and how; the structure, the distribution of power, and even the culture are clear—you can quickly tell the difference, for example, between a machine and an innovative organization (by who greets you at the door, how he or she is dressed, what the offices—or space in the absence of them—look like). Herein lies its great strength. And its debilitating weakness.

The fact is that configuration contaminates. Just try to be the innovative pocket in an otherwise machine organization, say the research lab in a mass production firm of mature products. Your facility was built in the country, in the belief that distance would shield you from the forces of technocracy. Well, lead may block radiation, but there is no known medium to block the influence of an organizational culture. A director drops in to have a look—''What, no shoes?'' Or the controller schedules a visit: ''It's 9:15. Where is everybody?'' (They quit at 2 A.M.) Of course, contamination is not a problem restricted to the machine configuration. Every time I have done a session with an innovative organization, the question ''Who's the most miserable person in adhocracy?'' evokes the same response: brief silence, then a few smiles, finally growing laughter as everyone turns to some poor person cowering in the corner. Of course, it is the controller, the person who is supposed to keep the lid on all the madness, the victim of adhocracy's contamination.

Contamination is really just another way of saying that the configurations are not just structures, not even just power systems: They are cultures. Being machinelike or innovative is not just a way of organizing; it's a way of life!

CONTAINMENT

Of course, the argument could be made that this is the price an organization must pay for achieving configuration. No organization can be all things to all people. It is better to select and then concentrate than try to be comprehensive and so end up diffusing efforts. Contamination of innovation is the price paid by the machine organization in order to be efficient, just as contamination of efficiency is the price paid by the innovative organization in order to concentrate on learning. Small prices both. Maybe. And for a time. Until things go out of control.

The fact seems to be that truly successful configurations exist not in pure form. The other forces of our pentagon may be secondary, but their presence is necessary to contain the dominant one. Otherwise the organization risks running out of control. Remove all the arrows but one in our pentagon, and the balance is lost. Without the other forces to anchor it, the organization will fly off in the direction of that remaining arrow. For example, people inclined to break rules may feel hard pressed in the machine organization. But without some of them, the organization may be unable to deal with unexpected problems. Similarly, administration may not be the strongest in the professional organization, but when really weak, anarchy arises as the absolute power of the professionals corrupts them absolutely.

Each configuration thus contains the seeds of its own destruction, residing in its own dominant force. Too much technocratic control destroys the machine organization, unimpeded leadership destroys the entrepreneurial one, and so on. But held in check by the other forces, each configuration can be very effective (in its own favored context). Without what we call *containment,* however, each must eventually become dysfunctional.

My colleagues Danny Miller and Manfred Kets de Vries have published a book that considers neuroses in organizations.[2] They present a cheerful set of five—the dramatic organization, the paranoid organization, the schizoid organization, the compulsive organization, and the depressive organization—each a system having run out of control. Very roughly, if I can be pardoned this lumping, I believe these capture the directions in which each of our five forms tend to run out of control.

Entrepreneurial organizations tend to become dramatic as their leaders, unconstrained by, say, the efficiency forces of the analysts or the proficiency forces of the workers, take their systems off on personal ego trips. Machine organizations, for their part, seem predisposed to compulsion once those analysts, with their obsession for efficiency controls through the intricacy of procedures, take over completely. As for the professional organization, anyone who works in a university or the like well understands their paranoid tendencies. Professionals feel set upon at the best of times; a whole organization of them free to pursue their obsessions with proficiency, independent of the forces of administration or innovation, cannot help but become collectively paranoid. I need not dwell on the depressing effects of the obsession with that mercenary bottom line in the diversified organization; the effect of turning the financial screws on morale, on innovation, and on commitment and culture are now widely appreciated. Finally, the problem in innovative organizations is that while they must continually innovate, which requires divergence, they must also exploit the benefits of their innovation, which requires more of a convergent orientation. The presence of forces other than learning can help balance that pressure; without them the organization can easily become schizoid, as it fails to make up its collective mind what to do.

In discussing the containing effects of the other forces, I do not wish to destroy my case for configuration. The point is not that every organization must do everything, rather that the dominant force must somehow be tempered by the secondary ones.

COMBINATION

The world of management would be awfully convenient (for us lumpers at least) if organizations simply pigeonholed themselves neatly into one category or another. Fortunately, many organizations refuse to cooperate, forcing us to play LEGO. IBM makes my life miserable by appearing to be so efficient in its operations (''the big blue machine'') and then turning around periodically and innovating in a most adhocratic way. Equally unnerving is the symphony orchestra that blends the personal leadership of its conductor with the trained skills of its musicians. Is it top-down entrepreneurial or bottom-up professional? There are diversified organizations that work wonderfully well with loose formal controls and innovative organizations that thrive with unexpectedly tight ones.

We can understand these organizations as *combinations* of the forces, sometimes as *hybrids* of the forms. They attend to different forces without letting only one dominate, doing so either in a steady-state balance or else at least in a dynamic equilibrium over time.

The symphony orchestra is an example of a stable and uniform combination. The organization cannot exist without great levels of proficiency coupled with strong central direction. (The Russians apparently tried a leaderless symphony orchestra shortly after their revolution but soon gave it up as unworkable.*) Here combination pervades the entire system as a balance among forces rather than forms.

In other cases, however, the organization combines different forms that dominate different parts. For example, newspapers must couple machine structures in their printing function with what are probably best described as professional structures in their editorial function.† Banks sometimes combine a machinelike retailing service for the mass market with a more innovative wholesaling service for merchant banking. And mass production firms that experience frequent or at least important changes in market demand must somehow achieve a balance between innovation in their development work and machinelike efficiency in their production—apparently the case of an IBM. In fact, an employee of Apple of Canada, upon hearing these ideas, suggested to me that in his firm I would have to add the entrepreneurial form in sales due to a dynamic chief, the professional form in marketing as well as in the training unit, and the innovative form also in the new venture unit.

As I noted earlier, in the McGill MBA student reports combinations appeared almost as frequently as configurations. They so labeled 57 of the 123 organizations, 51 as hybrids of two forms, 5 of three, and 1 of four. These combinations ranged widely—there were seventeen different types in all, with diversified machines being the most common (9), followed by innovative professionals (8), entrepreneurial professionals (6), and entrepreneurial machines (5).††

---

* The state administrative apparatus did not wither away either, as predicted. Machine bureaucracy hardly has less of a need for administration than the symphony orchestra!

† Earlier in the book, I described the editorial function as adhocracy. But a study by a group of students at Laval University suggested that reporters work on relatively standardized assignments from rather well-defined pigeonholes ("beats"), as in professional bureaucracy. (Indeed, for one story that fell between the pigeonholes, reporters from three different beats showed up!) Some of my own work with engineering groups likewise suggests that when engineering is oriented toward modifying standard designs rather than creating new ones, the structure of this function is better described as professional than as innovative.

†† I personally believe that the diversified and innovative forms are the most difficult to sustain in pure configuration (the former a conglomerate with no links between the divisions, the latter a very loose and free-wheeling structure). Thus they should be common in hybrid combinations. Also, some of these hybrids reflect common transitions in organization life cycles (as in the entrepreneurial firm that eventually settles down as a mature mass production machine), which suggests that hybrids occur commonly during transitions between the forms as well (as I shall discuss below).

Of course, since most people see it when they believe it, students exposed to my structure book are apt to see organizations at least as hybrids of the configurations if not as pure types. But real "organizational LEGO" involves playing with the forces and forms in broader ways. I encountered one successful Dutch company in computer software whose founder prided himself on having diversified his firm into regional divisions all over Holland yet not having the machinelike divisions I would have predicted. In front of an audience of six hundred of his compatriots, he said he could not find his organization in my pentagon. He was looking for it at the nodes. I suggested I could find it in the middle. Since he wanted entrepreneurial or intrapreneurial divisions, he relied for control not on the performance systems of the traditional diversified configuration, but on the norms of ideology. Division managers shared ideas and so developed their own approaches, to which they all conformed. That allowed him to eliminate most of the staff groups normally found at corporate headquarters, which tend to impose machinelike structure on the divisions. The regional divisions were thus free to be more innovative. But as a modest Dutchman, he left out one other important element, in my opinion, at the top of the pentagon: Without his central direction, it was doubtful the whole thing would have held together as it did. His organization thus seemed to combine very effectively the force of concentration with those of cooperation and direction, in order to promote that of innovation. Of course, he may not have needed my pentagon to do this, but I could still use it to help explain what was going on in his firm and, more importantly perhaps, to help predict and deal with what might go wrong later.

Even for an organization that has achieved configuration, we must sometimes play LEGO too. The Brookhaven National Laboratory used my book on structure to classify nuclear power plants for purposes of assessing supervisory influences on plant safety. They concluded that with their plethora of controls and standards, these plants looked primarily like machine organizations. I concurred. But on examination of the plants, we found more going on. For one thing, the design of the facility in the first place, and its construction, required another form of organization, professional or innovative, depending on how established was the technology at the time of construction. And the design of the standards—the system "software" in a sense—an ongoing activity that involved great numbers of engineers in the technostructures, looked rather professional in nature. (Indeed, there was so much of this going on that the plants could almost be characterized as professional organizations in the business of writing standards!) It was the execution of the design, the day-to-day operations and maintenance of the facility, that looked machinelike, because compliance to the standards was so critical. But further consideration suggested that these systems had a need for learning too, that the operators occasionally had to cope with unexpected problems in the short term and to ensure their correction in the long term by communicating their occurrence back to the engineers (in their plants and others). This seemed to require an innovative overlay on the machine structure. And finally, the managers of all this had to deal with the contradiction between machinelike compliance on the one hand and innovative learning on the other. To do that effectively, as I shall discuss later, they probably had to turn to the forces in the center of our pentagon.

My point is that there is always the splitting of gray between the black-and-white of lumping. Theories are used in management not to mirror reality but to help explain it. They may do so deductively by helping us to slot the behavior of organizations into categories, but they must also do so inductively by providing the concepts through which we can see new things, and so make better diagnoses. In our pentagon, we identify the nodes so that we can map the space.

CLEAVAGE

Combinations may not experience contamination—since one strong force can hold another in check—but they instead experience *cleavage*. That is, they tend to conflict along their natural fault lines, where their strong forces meet. Thus, the musicians dispute with the conductor, for they are, after all, professionals who do not need anyone to tell them what to do. Of course, that is not true, as Fellini illustrated so graphically in his film *Orchestra Rehearsal*. The revolting musicians, after experiencing complete anarchy, finally defer to the leader they realize is so necessary to their performance. (Fellini was supposed to have meant the film as an allegory on Italian politics, which suggests that our pentagon may have relevance for governments too.)

Likewise the researchers promoting innovation in a manufacturing firm will often conflict with the manufacturing people who want to get the system stabilized for operating efficiency. Newspapers may be fortunate in this regard, since cleavage is alleviated by the formal decoupling of its different functions (referred to as "truncation" in Chapter 11): Editorial produces camera-ready copy, which it hands over to the printing department. The two functions are thus independent in a way that the *inter*dependent industry people in research and manufacturing, who must not only interact closely but often even reach joint decisions, can only envy.

Cleavage is a necessary evil, an expected cost of organizing in combination. My own belief is that, newspapers and the like aside, it must usually be managed by alleviation more than elimination, or, perhaps better, by its redirection to constructive ends. Thus I conclude that configuration is the preferred way of organizing, that combination is effective only so long as the organization has no choice. Configuration promotes definition and discipline rather than conflict and contradiction. The organization knows what its dominant orientation must be and so can get on with pursuing it. For example, it can act like a bureaucratic machine and be proud of its efficiency even if that means a reduced capacity to innovate.

Most of the examples of hybrid combinations given above appeared in organizations that seemed to have no choice. For example, a management in need of significant degrees of productive efficiency as well as research innovation has to combine these different forces. But there is no shortage of examples of hybrid combinations that are dysfunctional because they are arbitrary, or because they reflect a management that cannot make up its mind. In wanting the best of more than one world, it often ends up with the worst of several. There are, for example, firms whose human resource people promote the professionalism of worker participation while their work-study analysts continue to impose stifling efficiency controls on those same workers. And there are those diversified corporations that no sooner give operating autonomy to their division managers to manage as they see fit than they usurp it by centralizing some function critical to that management at headquarters. Sometimes this may be necessary—retail chains with regional divisions, for example, often need to centralize certain merchandising functions. But at other times such behavior is arbitrary, as management wavers between the forces for central efficiency and divisional concentration.

Unfortunately, there are times when the arbitrary forces are imposed on the organizations from without. A common instance is the public school system subject to the controls of government people who believe that all organizations, no matter how professionally trained their people, should be managed like bureaucratic machines. To these technocrats, the machine configuration is not just *a* structure, it *is* structure; it is not *one* way to organize, it is *the only* sensible way to organize. Common too, for the same reason, is the diversified corporation or even government department that tries to force all its units, no matter what their own needs for learning or proficiency, to organize like bureaucratic machines. (In a seminar I gave recently for people in the Australian government, one frustrated manager who had seen enough of such things offered me a label for it to go along with my "bureaucracies" and "adhocracies"—"hypo-cracy," he called it. It amounts to saying one thing while doing another, such as the common practice of centralizing in the name of decentralization. Alongside our configurations, conversions, etc., we might call this just plain "con"!)

Organizations certainly need to give attention to conflicting forces, but not in ways that confuse and frustrate their people. Closely controlled workers may not be happier than more autonomous ones, but they are certainly better off than confused ones. Innovative or professional divisions may not be as *efficient* as machinelike ones, but they can sometimes be more *effective*. Diversified corporations unable to respect the intrinsic needs of certain of their divisions are better off divesting them. And governments have no business trying to force all professional institutions to act like bureaucratic machines.

CONVERSION

Sometimes organizations have to convert from one configuration, or combination, to another, usually because of a change in the forces acting upon them.

That change may be external to the organization or intrinsic. To consider the former, the appearance of a new operating technology may require much higher levels of worker training and so force a machine form to become more professional. Of course, such transitions can also be temporary, the result of forces that arise for a limited time. Thus, for example, when faced with dramatic external change, a machinelike organization may have to turn temporarily to a strong entrepreneurial leader for new direction. Some organizations even oscillate between two forms, making periodic transitions back and forth, for example favoring the efficiency of the machine form during recessions when customers are price conscious and the learning of the innovative form as economic growth favors product differentiation.[3]

But change does not always come arbitrarily from the outside. Sometimes it is intrinsic to the organization's very nature, often a reflection of its own internal development and so necessitating a permanent conversion. In these cases, forces within a configuration sow the seeds of its destruction and drive it to another form. For example, the intrinsic vulnerability of the entrepreneurial form stems from its centralization of power in the hands of a single individual. So long as the organization remains small and simple, this may not pose a problem—assuming containment of the dramatic neurosis. But growth and increasing complexity can undermine such personalized power, and stabilization of markets can require more efficiency than is usually provided by this configuration. A transition to the machine form may then become necessary. In a consulting firm, the tendency to be innovative at the outset may wane over time as the consultants tire of constant change; in their efforts to settle on more standardized applications of their skills, they naturally drive the organization toward the professional form.

While the externally driven conversions may be inflicted on the organization unexpectedly, the internally driven ones are somewhat predictable: They tend to sequence themselves in particular ways over time, known as "life cycles." Common, for example, is the sequence along the left side of our pentagon, from entrepreneurial to machine to diversified forms as a business first establishes itself, settles down eventually to exploit a secure market, and later enters new businesses once its traditional one has been saturated. The postscript to this chapter presents a fairly elaborate model of organization life cycles, based on transitions of power.

Either way, conversion can occur quickly or slowly. When it is intrinsically natural and long overdue, it may take place very rapidly, much as a super-saturated liquid freezes as soon as it is disturbed. But more commonly, it would seem, whether internally or externally driven, transitions tend to be prolonged and agonizing, as the organization sits suspended between its old and new forms, with one group promoting change and another resisting it. The period during the transition amounts, of course, to a hybrid combination, and given the inevitable confrontation between the two forces, generally leads to cleavage. Thus a John Sculley trying to settle Apple down confronts its founder, Steve Jobs, who wishes to sustain its free-wheeling entrepreneurial spirit. Or those consultants who wish to keep innovating challenge their colleagues who wish to converge on more standardized activities. Of course, conversion becomes combination when the organization gets stalled in such a transition and so remains suspended between the opposing forces.

CONTRADICTION

One important conclusion that comes out of our discussion so far is that the achievement of effectiveness in an organization generally requires the management of *contradiction*. This was especially evident in the point about cleavage in the combinations and conversions, but it is also true of contamination and the need for containment in the configurations. Here, I believe, is especially where the two forces in the center of our pentagon came into play. Each has much to do with contradiction, acting to exacerbate it or working to alleviate it. Indeed, I believe that these two forces themselves represent a contradiction that must be managed if an organization is not to run out of control.

I have placed the cooperative pulling together of ideology and the competitive pulling apart of politics in the center of the pentagon for two reasons. First, as noted earlier, while examples of their corresponding forms (the missionary and political organization) can be found, I believe that compared to the others, it is the forces that are common here, not the forms. Certainly one is hard pressed to find any reasonably large organization that is free of politics. And ideologies, while hard pressed themselves in these days of restructuring, etc., are nonetheless somewhat common.

But instead of considering these forces as merely two more alongside the other five, I prefer to see them differently, as *catalytic* forces that *infuse* organizations in which the other five interplay. This is my second reason for placing them in the center of the pentagon.

COOPERATION

Ideology represents the force for cooperation in an organization, for collegiality and consensus. People ''pull together'' for the common good—''we'' are in this together.

I use the word ideology here to describe an organizational culture that is rich and unique and so binds the members tightly to the organization. They commit themselves personally to it and identify with its needs. Such ideologies usually arise with a charismatic leader who has a vision for his or her organization; hence they are commonly associated with the entrepreneurial form, at least initially. But ideologies often outlive their developers and so can infuse other forms of organization as well. Thus we have the ideological machine called McDonald's that Ray Kroc created and the ideological innovator that Messrs. Hewlett and Packard built up. And in Chapter 12 we discussed Clark's "distinctive" colleges, small liberal arts colleges such as Swarthmore and Antioch whose professional forms were infused with powerful ideologies.[4]

Ideology encourages people to look inward—to take their lead from the imperatives of the organization's own vision instead of looking outward to what comparative organizations are doing. (Of course, when ideology is strong, there are no comparable organizations!) Is that not one meaning of Hewlett-Packard's famous "next bench syndrome"— that product designers get their stimulus for innovation not from the aggregations of marketing research reports but from the needs of particular colleagues working alongside them. This notion is indicated by the direction of the arrows in the pentagon—a circle facing inward, as if to shield the organization from outside forces. Such ideology above all draws people to cooperate with each other, to work together to take the organization where they, all of them, duly indoctrinated into its norms, believe it must go. In this sense, ideology should be thought of as the spirit of the organization, the life force that infuses the skeleton of its formal structure.

The important effect of this is to reduce cleavage and contamination, which in turn facilitates the management of contradiction. People in the organization can more easily reconcile opposing forces when it is the organization itself they believe in rather than any one of its particular parts. This is what helps me to understand how big blue machines like IBM are able to innovate—"snappy bureaucracies" is what I like to call such organizations. The presence of strong internal ideologies— related in IBM as well as McDonald's to owner or family control in the recent past—allows them to overlay adhocracy as a kind of shadow structure on their machine form to promote necessary change. If you believe in IBM instead of productive efficiency or marketing finesse per se, then when things really matter you will suspend your departmental rivalries to enable IBM to adapt. Great organizations simply pull together when they have to, because they are rooted in great systems of beliefs.

In his popular book *Competitive Strategy,* Michael Porter warns against getting "stuck in the middle" between a strategy of "cost leadership" (corresponding to the machine force for routine efficiency) and one of "differentiation" (including an emphasis on quality or innovation).[5] How, then, has Toyota been able to produce such high-quality automobiles at such reasonable cost? Why didn't it get stuck in the middle?

I believe Porter's admonition stems from the view, prevalent in American management circles throughout this century, and reflected equally in my own case for configuration, that if an organization favors one particular orientation, others must suffer. If the efficiency experts have the upper hand, quality must get slighted; if it is the elite designers who get their way, productive efficiency lags; and so on. This may be true so long as an organization is treated as just a collection of different activities—a portfolio of products and functions, etc. But when the spirit of ideology is infused into the bones of its structure, the organization takes on an integrated life of its own and this ceases to be true.

Workers on the American automobile assembly lines have long had good reason to consider themselves only cogs in their bureaucratic machines. Indeed, even within the administrative structure of a General Motors, critics continue to bemoan the effects on engineering design of having had all those financial people in the chief executive's chair. But at Toyota, one has the impression that even if you sweep the floor you do not regard yourself as doing a menial job of little consequence; rather you are doing your part to make Toyota great. Is that not why the assembly workers are allowed to shut down the line? Each and every one can be treated as an individual capable of making decisions for the good of Toyota. The only thing that gets stuck in the middle at Toyota, then, is conventional Western management theory!

The infusion of ideology into a configuration can alleviate the effects of contamination; in a combination it can alleviate the effects of cleavage. Contradictory forces are not just tolerated but respected, however, grudgingly: "Old Joe, over there, that nut in the engineering office—we accountants sometimes wonder about him. But we know this place could never function without him." Or in the symphony orchestra, the musicians respect their conductor because together they produce great music.

Even better than reconciling the contradictory forces expressed by different parts of the organization, ideology can cause these forces to be expressed within individuals themselves. Instead of building a laboratory out in the country and hoping it will be able to impose innovation on the rest of the system, everyone in the organization is charged with innovation alongside his or her regular job, as in those quality circles in Japan. Or, to take the opposite case, control in the ideological innovative organization is not reserved for that poor controller cowering in the corner; even the most creative scientist is expected to worry about costs and efficiency too. That presumably explains the tolerance for rather tight control systems in companies like 3M or H-P. In metaphorical terms, it is not so difficult to change hats in an organization when they are all emblazoned with the same insignia!

All in all it sounds like a great thing, this ideology. Unfortunately, consulting promises notwithstanding, it is not there for the taking, to be plucked off the tree of management systems like just another piece of technological fruit. As Karl Weick has argued, "A corporation doesn't *have* a culture. A corporation *is* a culture. That's why they're so horribly difficult to change."[6] The fact is that there are no techniques for building ideologies, no five easy steps to a better culture. These are built slowly and patiently by committed leaders who have found interesting missions for their organizations and care deeply about the people who perform them. To my mind, the critical ingredient is authenticity. In fact, I believe in a kind of psychic law of management here: that workers, customers, every one involved with a management, no matter how physically distant, can tell when it is genuine in its beliefs and when it is just mouthing the right words.

At best, those five easy steps overlay a thin veneer of culture that washes off in the first political storm. Usually, however, these steps don't even do that; instead they often destroy whatever is left of the ideology that existed before. Indeed, any one of a number of the easy steps of "modern" management can do that with great effectiveness: "Focus on the bottom line, as if you make money by managing money." Or "move managers around so they can never get to know anything but 'management' well." Or "hire and fire workers the way you buy and sell machines (for everything is, after all, just a portfolio)."

But is ideology always such a great thing? An answer to this question lies in the arrows of the pentagon. While those of ideology form what looks like a protective halo around the organization, the fact that they all face inward means that in the absence of other forces to anchor them, they too can go out to control: Their inward thrust leads eventually to *implosion*. Earlier I claimed that ideologies cause people to look within the organization for direction. Too much of this and the organization loses touch with its context, closes in on itself. Even its capacity to innovate can become a liability as it continues to improve outmoded strategies, themselves rooted in ideology and so immutable. We have no need for the extreme example of a Jonestown to appreciate the negative consequences of ideology; we all know firms with strong cultures that, like the proverbial bird, flew in ever diminishing circles until they disappeared up their own rear ends!*

COMPETITION

Politics represents the force for competition in an organization, for conflict and confrontation. People pull apart for their own benefit. "They" get in our way.

Politics can infuse any of the configurations or combinations, exacerbating contamination or cleavage. Indeed, both problems were characterized as intrinsically conflictive in the first place; politics only worsens them. The people behind the dominant force in a configuration—the technocrats in the machine organization, the creative types in the innovative one—lord their power over everyone else, while those behind each of the main forces in a combination relish any opportunity to do battle with the other to gain advantage. Thus, in contrast to a machinelike Toyota pulling together is the Chrysler Iaccoca found when he arrived pulling apart; the culture of an innovative Hewlett-Packard stands in contrast to the politics of a NASA during the Challenger tragedy; for every "distinctive" college there are other "destructive" ones.

Of course, it is clear from the outward facing arrows of the pentagon what politics can do to an organization when unconstrained by other forces: cause *explosion,* as everything pulls apart.

Politics seems to be a more natural force in organizations than ideology. That is to say, organizations left alone seem to pull apart rather more easily. Getting systems of human beings to pull together, in contrast, appears to require continual deliberate effort on the part of dedicated managers. In fact, those easy steps listed above that inadvertently kill ideology generally do so by encouraging politics in its place. The quick fix in place of careful consideration, superficial pronouncements instead of genuine commitments, worrying about the numbers while people are treated as objects—all these are breeding grounds for political conflict.

---

* This may seem to contradict the point just made about how an infusion of ideology can make a machine organization capable of change. But it must be borne in mind what kind of change that is: *within* the perspective of the ideology. To reiterate an earlier example, McDonald's introduction of Egg McMuffin constituted the addition of a position within its existing perspective—in other words, the product brought the firm into the breakfast market, but it remained purely McDonald's. In fact, the company would probably have great difficulty changing perspective. (How about McDuckling à l'Orange served at your candle-lit table?)

Thus in contrast to ideology as ostensibly all things good, we have politics as the force for evil. Or do we? The fact is that politics can also act as a catalytic force for the benefit of an organization.

In my own work with organizations, the single most commonly asked question—the virtual obsession of today's managers—is how can we get bureaucracies to change. I have already tried to show how ideology, alongside entrepreneurial direction and intrapreneurial innovation, can be a force for revitalization, and also a force for the opposite, for resistance to fundamental change. Likewise some of the other forces in organizations—especially those for efficiency, for proficiency, and for concentration—often act to resist fundamental change. When these all team up and overwhelm an organization's entrepreneurial and intrapreneurial capabilities, then, ironically, politics may be the only force available to stimulate the necessary change. The organization must, in other words, pull apart before it can adapt: "Young Turks" must confront the "old guard." Even when the protagonists act out of pure self-interest, the effect of their actions can be to shock the organization into adapting despite itself. It appears to be an inevitable fact of organizational life today that a great deal of the most significant change is driven, not by managerial insight or specialized expertise or ideological commitment, let alone the technology of planning, but by political challenge.

To recap, both ideology and politics can promote organizational effectiveness or undermine it. Ideology infused into another configuration can be a force for revitalization, energizing the organization and making its people more responsive. But that same ideology can also hinder fundamental change, since everything must be interpreted in terms of "the word." Likewise, politics can impede change and waste resources. But it can also promote change that may be available in no other way, by allowing those who recognize the need for the change to challenge those who do not. Thus ideology, that harmonizing force for cooperation, can make an organization insular; politics, that mercenary force for competition, can enable an organization to adapt.

COOPERATION COMBINED WITH COMPETITION

How do organizations counter the imploding effects of ideology and the exploding effects of politics? My belief is that these two catalytic forces in the center of the pentagon must naturally counter each other. In fact, I suspect that another clue to the effective organization lies in

FIGURE 14–2
Combining the Catalytic Forces

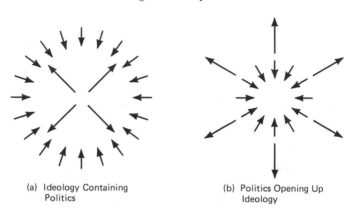

(a) Ideology Containing
   Politics

(b) Politics Opening Up
   Ideology

maintaining a balance between these forces of cooperation and competition: They must form their own combination, must exist in a kind of dynamic tension. Politics challenges the insularity of ideology, ideology constrains the destructiveness of politics.

Again the arrows can tell the story. As shown in Figure 14–2, enveloping the exploding circle of politics within the imploding circle of ideology creates one kind of balance. Consider, for example, those Talmudic scholars who fight furiously with each other over the interpretation of every word in their ancient books yet close ranks to present a united front to the outside world. Is this not exactly the behavior we find in some of the most effective business corporations, IBM among others? Likewise, is not surrounding the converging force of ideology by the diverging force of politics, in order to challenge the organization's most basic assumptions, not the most effective way to counter its inclination to implode?*

Of course, these two catalytic forces need not interact continuously. My own belief is that the pulling together of ideology is probably the preferred state most of the time, so that the organization can pursue its given mission with full vigor. But periodically it must pull apart through

---

* A doctoral student at McGill, Joe Lampel, came up with the ingenious idea, in the spirit of LEGO, that we think of the children's game of paper, scissors, and stone, extending the rules a bit to consider the interplay of these forces—for example, paper (ideology) covers scissors (politics), but scissors cut paper; stone (machine form) crumples paper (ideology), but paper also covers stone, and so on.

the force of politics to ensure necessary change that has been discouraged by the prevailing ideology.

COMPETENCE

One final issue in this summary chapter on organizations: competence. What makes an organization effective? The question has been an elusive one in organizational theory, and I have no intention of dwelling on it here. In fact, I believe this whole section, indeed this whole book, addresses that question, in a variety of ways. What I do wish to do in closing is summarize briefly the various views of organizational effectiveness that have infiltrated our discussion, presented below as a series of hypotheses. Some have been mentioned previously, but this discussion draws them all together.

CONVERGENCE. First is the *convergence* hypothesis. "One best way" is its motto, the single lens its image. There is a proper way to view, and so to design, an organization. As we saw, this is usually associated with the machine form. A good structure is one with a rigid hierarchy of authority, with spans of control no greater than six, with heavy use of strategic planning, MIS, and whatever else happens to be in the current fashion of the rationalizers.

Of course, "one best way" thinking need not always promote the machine configuration. In *In Search of Excellence,* Peters and Waterman argued that ideology was the key to an organization's success.[7] We concurred for a time here too, but later pointed out the negative effect ideology can have on organizations. (In fact, Peters and Waterman give little attention to the need for strategic renewal in their book, concentrating instead on how ideology can promote operating excellence.)

Thus, while we cannot dismiss this hypothesis—sometimes there *are* proper things to do in most if not all organizations—we must take issue with its general thrust. Society has paid an enormous price for "one best way" thinking over the course of this century, on the part of all its organizations that have been drawn into using what is fashionable rather than functional. We need to look beyond the obvious, beyond the convergence hypothesis.

CONGRUENCE. Beyond convergence is the *congruence* hypothesis, "it all depends" being its motto, the buffet table its image. Introduced in organization theory in the 1960s, it suggests that running an organization is like choosing dinner from such a table—a little bit of this, a little bit of that, all selected according to specific needs. Organizational effectiveness thus becomes a question of matching a given set of internal attributes, treated as a kind of portfolio, with various situational factors. The hypotheses presented in Chapter 6—what attributes of structure best suit large size, a stable environment, an automated technical system, etc.—were presented in the spirit of this view of organizational effectiveness. The congruence hypothesis has certainly been an improvement, but like a dinner plate stacked with an odd assortment of foods, it has not been good enough.

CONFIGURATION. And so the *configuration* hypothesis was introduced and became the basis for the seven previous chapters of this section. "Getting it all together" is its motto, the jigsaw puzzle its image, the lumpers its champions. Design your organization as you would do a jigsaw puzzle, fitting all the pieces together to create a coherent, harmonious picture. There is certainly reason to believe that organizations succeed in good part because they are consistent in what they do; they are certainly easier to manage that way. Configuration entered our discussion as structure, then became also situation and later power, and finally emerged as all of them woven together into culture. But, as we have seen, configuration has its limitations too.

CONTRADICTION. While the lumpers may like the configuration hypothesis, the splitters prefer the *contradiction* hypothesis. Manage the dialectic, the dynamic tension, is their call, perhaps "to each his own" their motto, the tug of war their image. They point to the common occurrence of combinations and conversions, where organizations are forced to manage contradictory forces. And while those in favor of the convergence approach might applaud the role of ideology, even that of politics (cooperation, or competition, as the one best way), the splitters would respond with justification that these two are themselves contradictory, and so must be managed as a dialectic. This is an important hypothesis, together with that of configuration (in their own dynamic tension) certainly an important clue to organizational effectiveness. But still it is not sufficient.

CREATION. The truly great organization transcends convergence, congruence, configuration, and contradiction, while building on them to achieve something more. It respects the *creation* hypothesis. Creativity is its forte, "understand your inner nature" is its motto, LEGO its image. The most interesting organizations live at the edges, far from the logic of conventional organizations, where as Raphael has pointed out in biology (for example, between the sea and the land, or at the forest's edge),[8] the richest, most varied, and most interesting forms of life can be found. These organizations invent novel approaches that solve festering problems and so provide all of us with new ways to deal with our world of organizations. Their effectiveness depends on the two things we have sought to promote throughout this book: a rich understanding of the world of organizations and a propensity to play with that knowledge in creative ways.*

POSTSCRIPT: A LIFE CYCLE MODEL OF ORGANIZATIONS

Earlier, the notion of life cycles of organizations was mentioned. Here we return to it, presenting an elaborate model of how organizations undergo sequences of conversions as they develop over time. In presenting this, I put my natural colors back on: This is lumping with a vengeance (even the sixth and seventh forms return to our discussion). I believe this model has important consequences for a society of organizations; this point will be discussed briefly in conclusion here but pursued vigorously in the final chapter of this book.

Given our seven configurations, it is not difficult to think of examples of all the possible transitions between pairs of them, forty-two in all counting both directions, or really forty-nine adding in the transition that each configuration can make to another form of itself (for example, replacing the leader in the entrepreneurial form). But certain transitions do seem to be far more common, for example from the entrepreneurial configuration to the machine configuration as an organization grows and matures.

It is the transitions that reflect the *intrinsic* forces on organizations that appear to be most common—the naturally occurring forces that sow the seeds of the destruction of one configuration and drive it toward another (or drive the organization itself to demise). The less common

---

* In this spirit, I would like to invite anyone who has been able to play organizational LEGO constructively with these forces and forms to write to me at McGill University (Montreal H3A 1G5, Canada) about their experiences. I hope to collect this for a subsequent book.

transitions, in contrast, appear to reflect the external changes that occur independently of the organization—for example, a shift in technology, new government legislation, the arrival of a new competitor. The variety of these is far wider, as are their causes, and so they cannot be predicted (at least not by studying the organization itself). Moreover, there are configurations that appear most often in young organizations, notably the entrepreneurial, or in more established organizations, notably the machine, or during decline, notably the politicized. This suggests a life cycle model of organizations.

Two key assumptions underlie life cycle models of organizations. The first is that organizations spend most of their lives in steady states, in other words as forms that are stable and enduring, but that these states change periodically as an organization undergoes brief periods of transition. Earlier we referred to this as a "quantum theory" of organizational change. The ecologists call it "punctuated equilibrium," while in organization theory, William Starbuck has referred to "metamorphosis models," in which organizations grow not in "a smooth continuous process" so much as in one "marked by abrupt and discrete changes" in conditions and structures.[9] The second assumption is that the actual steady-state forms organizations adopt over time tend to arrange themselves in sequences according to their stage of life. In other words, there are forms associated with birth, growth, maturity, and decline, perhaps even with the death of organizations.

Life cycle models have long been popular in the literature of organization theory. They have also long been criticized, since particular organizations exhibit all kinds of idiosyncratic changes over time, caused by the changes I called external. Moreover, some organizations settle into particular forms for long periods of time, while others break common sequences by reverting back to what seem to be earlier stages. Nonetheless, life cycle models do capture something important about organizations, namely *leading tendencies* in many of them if not compulsory changes in all of them—in other words, sequences that are common rather than imperative.

Most of the well-known life cycle models track changes in structure. The model I shall present here is oriented more to changes in power (though particular structures do, of course, correspond to particular systems of power). Thus, it reintroduces to our discussion forms that I earlier associated with power, namely the missionary and political configurations, as well as the instrument and closed system forms of the machine configuration.

Figure 14–3 presents our life cycle model in four stages, labeled

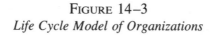

FIGURE 14-3
Life Cycle Model of Organizations

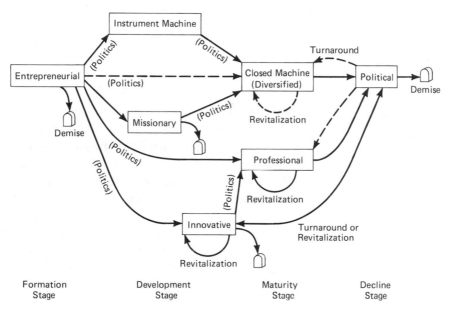

formation (as an entrepreneurial configuration), *development* (as a missionary, instrument-machine, or perhaps innovative configuration), *maturity* (as a closed-machine, professional, or perhaps innovative configuration), and *decline* (as a political configuration, which is also shown accompanying some of the earlier transitions). The demise of the organization is shown (by a tombstone) as common at certain points of the formation and development stages as well as after decline. The model is described below as a series of propositions, each with a label. Note that these propositions are presented in declarative form to highlight them as hypotheses to be considered, not as definitive conclusions. They appear to me to represent leading tendencies in many organizations, but while there is evidence for some, others are in the realm of speculation. All remain to be verified by systematic research.

FORMATION

1. Organizations are typically established in the entrepreneurial form ("personal creation"). A new organization generally finds itself with a mission, some resources, and a leader. The rest must be created. That usually gives the founding leader great personal power: Others defer to him or her to get on with the building of the organization. Moreover, new organizations (even in nonprofit areas, including government) tend to attract forceful leaders, people who prefer to "do their own thing" free of the bureaucratic pressures of established organizations. Hence the entrepreneurial form tends to appear at the outset in all kinds of situations.

2. Many young organizations remain in the entrepreneurial form as long as their founding leaders remain in office ("perpetuation of entrepreneurship"). Forces may soon appear in the new organization (such as the need for expertise or for technocratic controls) to drive it toward another configuration. But many organizations delay making an obvious transition so long as their founders remain in office. For one thing, the organization was built around its leader's personal style, as well as his or her strategic vision. For another, people tend to remain loyal to the leader who hired them and with whom they have been able to develop a personal relationship. Furthermore, founding leaders, because they tend to be strong-willed individuals to begin with, are often able to sustain personal power.

DEVELOPMENT

3. Entrepreneurial organizations tend to be vulnerable; many die, while others tend sooner or later to make a transition to another configuration ("precariousness"). There are some entrepreneurial organizations that remain under the personal control of their founders for long periods. But the entrepreneurial configuration is fundamentally precarious, relying as it does on a single individual. As mentioned earlier, one heart attack can literally wipe out its prime mechanism of coordination. Moreover, entrepreneurial leaders, because they have so much personal power, can easily lose touch. Some get so involved with the operating detail that they loose touch with the need to change strategy. Others become so opportunistic, constantly flitting from one strategic change to another, that they lose touch with the operations.

No matter what its manifestation, the fundamental problem for the entrepreneurial configuration is that there is usually no rational mechanism for self-correction. So much power focuses on the leader that there is often no one able or willing to make things right, at least not in the context of the entrepreneurial configuration. Hence, the demise of the organization or, failing that, of the configuration would seem likely to follow leadership problems in the entrepreneurial organization.

4. The most natural, if not common, transition for the entrepreneurial organization is to the missionary configuration, at least after the departure of a charismatic, visionary leader ("institutionalization of charisma"). Left on their own, with a strong sense of mission after the departure of a revered leader, the followers who remain have a tendency (in the vocabulary of sociology) to *institutionalize* his or her charisma, in other words to form a missionary configuration in which selection, socialization, and indoctrination are used to reinforce the established system of beliefs. But relatively few such organizations seem to be left on their own.

5. New organizations dependent on expertise tend to make a relatively quick transition to the innovative or the professional configuration ("meritocratization"). A new organization that is highly dependent on expert skills and knowledge will be likely to make a relatively rapid transition to one of the expert configurations, the innovative form if its mission focuses on creative design, or the professional form if it applies standardized skills. This transition tends to happen quickly, because experts are generally hired with their skills already in place; hence they generally insist on power early, rather than defer to the personalized power of a leader. For example, a new hospital can adopt the professional configuration in a surprisingly short period of time simply because its staff, imported from other hospitals, brings long-established medical procedures along with them.

6. Given a choice between the professional and the innovative configuration, many young organizations will opt for the innovative one, although some will later be inclined to make a transition to the professional one ("early experimentation"; *later* "institutionalization of innovation"). New expert organizations, given the choice (as in theater companies or consulting firms, less so in hospitals!), are often experimental. The system is new, the people are enthusiastic, there are unexploited opportunities to be pursued and the organization itself may have to be differentiated from its competitors to survive. The innovative configuration may be preferred to the professional in the developmental stage. But later, as things settle down—procedures get established, the experts develop preferences, client needs recur, and so on—there may be a tendency, again given the choice, to make a transition to the professional configuration. In other words, the ad hoc development of novel solutions is replaced by the routine delivery of standardized ones.

7. Entrepreneurial organizations not susceptible to ideological pressures and not dependent on expertise tend to be driven eventually to the machine configuration, usually first in its instrument form ("takeover"). Being vulnerable after the departure of their founding leaders, or even during the leaders' reign, developing organizations largely free of expertise and ideology become prime candidates for takeover and so tend to fall prey to external influencers (or sometimes yield to them voluntarily, for protection). And as noted in Chapter 8, the way in which an external influencer consolidates power over an organization is by encouraging the establishment of technocratic controls through a subservient management. In other words, the natural tendency for the organization taken over in this way is to convert to the machine configuration, in its instrument form.

The classic example of this is, of course, the entrepreneurial firm that comes under the control of a large diversified corporation, whether it sells out or gets seized by it. But a similar process occurs when a government finally consolidates its control over a new agency hitherto personally controlled by its strong-willed founder.

It will be recalled that the difference between the instrument and closed system forms of the machine configuration is that in one power resides with an external influencer (or a group of them acting in concert), while in the other power rests with the internal administrators. The former tends to appear first simply because there is usually no firmly established administrative apparatus to seize the power when the founder departs. A small organization may simply not have had a chance to develop; moreover, entrepreneurial leaders often expressly discourage formalized administration because they consider it a threat to their personalized control. The instrument form of the machine configuration that follows therefore becomes the means to establish the administrative apparatus.

But some organizations do manage to grow quite large under entrepreneurial leadership, including the development of an extensive administrative apparatus to cope with their size. In effect, they develop a hybrid of the entrepreneurial and machine configurations. And these can, of course, make a transition directly to the closed system form of machine, as the administrators take over directly from the founder after he or she departs. Government dictatorships, for example, are sometimes succeeded by closed system bureaucratic regimes, as in the Soviet Union after Stalin. The same thing tends to happen in a large labor union after the departure of the leader who built it (unless that leader has established a strong ideology, in which case we might look for a transition to the missionary configuration instead). Despite these examples, however, I show this transition as a dotted line in Figure 14–3 because I believe it to be less natural—personalized leadership and formalized administration being somewhat incompatible—and therefore less likely to occur.

MATURITY

8. *Missionary configurations, barring the commonly occurring demise of the organization, as well as instrument machine configurations, tend eventually to make a transition to the closed system machine configuration* (the "imperatives of administration"). This is an important proposition, suggesting (as can be seen in Figure 14–3) that organizations not dependent on expertise tend to end up as machine bureaucracies largely impervious to the exercise of external influence. In effect, the administrators come to think of the organization as serving not some external constituency or noble mission, but rather themselves. Yet at the same time, ironically, it may be only through this transition that organizations in certain sectors are able to achieve a scale large enough for the full and efficient exploitation of their products or services.

Many organizations with missionary configurations simply die. As discussed in Chapter 12, those organizations exist on a knife edge between isolation and assimilation. Isolation may protect the ideology, but it can kill the organization. Thus, many religious communities, political movements, even missionary-type business firms die for want of members or resources, or else simply burn themselves out in their ideological fervor.

Those that do survive are instead subjected to the pressures of assimilation. And in a society of large bureaucratic organizations, it is clear what those pressures are. Over time, the organization may have to build an administrative apparatus, especially if it is intent on carrying its mission far and wide; that acts to bureaucratize the structure. Eventually, then, the organization may yield to what I prefer to call the "imperatives of administration," what sociologists might label (paraphrasing Max Weber) the routinization of ideology. Indeed, the Italian political scientist Robert Michels, writing early in this century, was so convinced of the inevitability of this transition (in our terms, from missionary to closed machine) that he labeled it the "iron law of oligarchy."[10] In effect, time blunts the ideology, converting enthusiasm into obligation, traditions into dogmas, norms into rules. Administration thereby replaces ideology at the center of power.

Organizations as instrument machines tend not to die because they are protected by external influencers. But these commonly undergo a similar kind of conversion, to the closed system machine, which seems an almost imperatively iron law in its occurrence. The instrument machine serves an external constituency directly; that is its purpose and its major strength. But this arrangement contains the seeds of its own destruction, namely the difficulty of maintaining external surveillance of internal behavior. The external influencers may have the formal power, but they can exercise it only through the internal administrators, and it is they who develop the information base necessary to manage the organization. And in information, of course, lies power. Furthermore, it is the administrators who have the time and energy to devote full time to the organization. Thus, as an instrument machine organization grows larger and more complex, its internal administrators are able to enhance their power at the expense of the external influencers. A transition to the closed form of machine may become inevitable.

This process is evident in many business corporations, whose growth to large size has been shown to be accompanied by a dispersal of their shareholding until the internal managers rather than the external "owners" exercise effective control.[11] The same result has been shown for large government corporations, in which the internal managers tend gradually to wrest effective control from the government officials until they are able to run the organizations as systems unto themselves.[12]

9. *The closed system nature of the machine configuration encourages, and is in turn encouraged by, a transition to the diversified configuration* ("diversification"). Closed system organizations prefer to retain their earnings (in whatever form), and use them to enhance their own size and influence. A prime way to do this is through diversification, in other words, extending the mission across different sectors of activity, which also helps to spread their risk and to reduce external influence. (As was noted in Chapter 9, for example, diversification may help to diffuse shareholding in a business corporation.) Thus, the closed machine configuration has an incentive to diversify, in order to strengthen its closed system nature.

But conversion to the diversified form does not really induce a major transition, because the diversified configuration is really just an elaborated form of the machine one (typically comprising a set of machine configurations as divisions grouped together under a headquarters umbrella). Thus, this transition tends to amount to an enhancement of the status of the organization as a bureaucratic structure controlled by its administrators and closed to external influencers.

Let me review our discussion to this point, particularly with respect to the identification of different configurations with the various stages of an organization's development. The entrepreneurial configuration has been clearly and solely associated with the formation stage. The missionary and instrument machine configurations, because they are susceptible to transition to the closed machine configuration, have been discussed, and are shown in Figure 14–3, in the development stage. In other words, they are considered to be means by which an organization develops beyond formation toward maturity. The closed machine form, however, is shown in the maturity stage, because the organization by this time tends to be large and firmly established in one or several sectors, to have a well-developed administrative apparatus with highly standardized procedures, and to be relatively free of external influence.

So too is the professional configuration shown at the stage of maturity, for similar reasons. It also tends to be firmly established, with well-defined (if highly skilled) standardized procedures. It is likewise able to seal itself from much external influence and concentrate its power in the hands of insiders (in its case, operating professionals), who are similarly able to use much of it to serve themselves.

Both of these configurations, for all of these reasons, are considered to be highly stable and therefore enduring, it being difficult to displace entrenched administrators or experts. Hence, both are associated with maturity. We can therefore conclude that, barring unpredictable external changes, organizations that survive and grow tend to end up as closed machine configurations (whether or not diversified) when they are fully developed, unless their need for expertise drives them toward the professional configuration in their maturity instead.

The innovative configuration is shown between development and maturity, because on one hand that form of organization is sometimes inclined to make a transition to the more stable professional form (as described earlier), and on the other hand the innovative form can also constitute a basic state (if never fully stable) in its own right. (Recall our discussion in Chapter 11 of the two types of innovative organizations, the operating adhocracy, as found in consulting firms, which tends to be drawn to the professional form as it ages, and the administrative adhocracy, as found in automated or high-technology sectors, which must often remain in the innovative form.)

10. Most of the transitions so far discussed tend to be driven and impeded by forms of the political configuration, typically brief confrontations, although sometimes prolonged by shaky alliances ("transitional politicization"). The transition from the entrepreneurial to the missionary configuration, as the beliefs of a charismatic leader get institutionalized, tends to be smooth, without conflict. All the other transitions so far discussed can be divisive, as an old guard representing the established system of power resists those promoting the change. Outright confrontation may occur and recur, or else, to avoid damaging an organization that is slow to make the transition, the two sides may form a shaky alliance for a time, a transitional hybrid, with considerable cleavage.

Considering the various transitions that have been introduced above, the founder of an entrepreneurial organization, or his or her successors, may resist takeover by a group of external influencers intent on rendering the organization their instrument. Confrontations will thus result unless the transition either is realized through a sudden seizure of power or takes place gradually and the two sides settle down to forming a shaky alliance. Much of the same should happen in the transition from the entrepreneurial directly to the closed machine configuration, except that the conflict here will be between the leader who favors personalized control and the administrators inclined toward the formalized systems that enhance their own influence.

As for organizations dependent on expertise, the transition from the entrepreneurial founding configuration to one of the expert configurations should be similar. The experts would normally be expected to try to gain considerable influence quickly while the leader might try to hang on to his or her personal control, in which case the two will do battle, or else form a shaky alliance until the transition is completed. In the case of the transition between the two expert configurations, from an innovative to a professional one, the experts will be likely to do battle with each other or to settle into a temporary shaky alliance, one side representing creative adhocracy, the other stable professionalism.

Considering the transition from instrument to closed machine, the external influencers probably will not cherish relinquishing power to the administrators they hired to run the organization as their instrument. But the odds are not in their favor, simply because it is the internal administrators who control decision-making directly. At best, the external influencers can form an implicit shaky alliance with the administrators in the hope of stemming their gradual loss of power. Of course, they can also confront the administrators on visible issues, though not too often. (In the case of the publicly owned Air Canada, for example, over the years the government has challenged it on the selection of new aircraft, the location of a new maintenance base, even on a change in the airline's name.) The external influencers may even win these occasional confrontations—social legitimacy is, after all, on the side of the external constituency the organization is supposed to serve. But the external influencers are likely to lose out eventually, at least if the organization grows rather large, simply because they cannot control the great many internal decisions made on a daily basis. In effect, though they may win the wars, they are likely to lose the peace.

Our remaining transition is from the missionary configuration to the closed system machine. Here we should expect both forms of political configuration, as a combination of what was described above. Members of an organization who remain true to the norms of its traditional ideology will not take kindly to administrative types trying to routinize it, to enhance their own formalized power at the expense of the established system of beliefs. Furious confrontations are to be expected. But like the transition previously described, the power of the administrators can be more subtle and pervasive, allowing them to gain influence gradually through the many small decisions they make regularly. Those people true to the ideology may be drawn into a shaky alliance to try to hold their ground, but like the external influencers of the instrument configuration, this may just prolong the inevitable transition to administrative control.

DECLINE

11. The absence of external control tends to have a corrupting influence on the mature configurations, closed machine and professional, driving them eventually toward the political configuration ("eventual politicization"). The seeds of the destruction of the two mature configurations are sown by the very power of their own dominant insiders. To quote Lord Acton, while "power tends to corrupt, absolute power corrupts absolutely." The power of the administrators of the closed system machine or of the experts of the professional configuration can sometimes get so close to absolute that corruption becomes inevitable, first of all in the form of arrogant exercise of that power.

In universities, for example, students can become incidental pawns, there to support what the professors really want to do, namely research.

But that research itself may get done for no constituency other than the professors themselves. To serve is considered cross; the real object of the research becomes methodological elegance, as small communities of "scholars" publish for each other in progressively narrower and more irrelevant journals. In business, it is the customers who get that treatment from the closed system bureaucracies (the students, of course, never being acknowledged as customers in the university). Thus, there was that General Motors chief executive who claimed there was "something wrong" with people who bought small cars, while another commented that "what's good for General Motors is good for the country." And so-called social responsibility can become the closed system executives' smokescreen for ensuring that external influencers cannot penetrate their power base—if they are "responsible," their behavior need not be monitored.

If power produces corruption, then corruption produces conflict. Without the constraint of service beyond themselves, these insiders must be drawn into conflicts with one another. The professionals strut around trying to be superior to each other, while the administrators battle over the building of private empires. The internal coalition then becomes increasingly politicized.

Meanwhile, external influencers, long pacified by the myth of expertise or by the power of the administrative system, begin to take notice of these conflicts. What these indicate is the fundamental illegitimacy of the organization's power system. The organization may have to rely on professionalism or on the formal authority of its administrators to function, but the arrogance and conflicts make it increasingly evident to outsiders that these legitimate means are being used to further illegitimate ends. And so they begin to challenge the insiders, as well as the legitimacy of their power, and thereby politicize the external coalition as well. Students and government administrators question the goals of the university and the actions of its professors. Ralph Nader, listening to the utterances of General Motors executives, begins a series of attacks on the corporation—the safety of its products, its record on pollution, the criteria by which people are named to its board of directors.

With conflict infusing the organization from both inside and outside, the organization begins to take on the form earlier labeled the politicized organization, in which conflict is pervasive but, because it is moderate, also tends to be enduring.

Of course, this need not happen quickly. Organizations can remain in the stage of maturity for long periods, held in check perhaps by a certain degree of market competition or by professional standards. (Or the advent of new competition or renewed professional standards may drive ones on the way to conflictive decline back to more viable maturity.) The vestiges of an earlier ideology can have the same effect. Indeed, the longevity of a healthy state of maturity in certain closed machine or professional organizations is probably best explained by strong ideology in their earlier lives. (It is my suspicion that this last factor is what explains the "excellence" of the companies Peters and Waterman wrote about. In effect, *In Search of Excellence* seems largely to be about the exceptions, those few companies that managed to remain responsive despite growing to a very large size. Thus it should have come as no surprise that many soon slipped out of the ranks of excellence.[13])

Figure 14-3 also shows a line from the innovative to the political configuration, but this conclusion must be qualified. This configuration is certainly predisposed to internal conflict, indeed, far more than the closed machine if not the professional configuration. But this is conflict of a different kind. The structure is so organic, the work so variable, that friction inevitably arises in the normal functioning of the organization. It is true that the experts of the innovative organization tend to have a good deal of power. But external legitimacy is less of a question here because these organizations are characterized by responsiveness to their markets. If anything, adhocracies are too quick to react to external changes. Thus, transition to a political status here may reflect more a temporary difficulty than a permanent shift to a state of decline. (That probably happens to the innovative organization via transition first to a more bureaucratic configuration.)

12. *Barring renewal or some form of artificial support, an enduring political configuration eventually leads to the demise of the organization* ("artificial support," "political demise"). The politicized organization is hardly effective in the long run. As noted in the last chapter, organizations are in the business of producing products and services, not providing a forum for people to fight with one another. So sustained pervasive politicization should lead to the demise of the organization. That is, of course, a common enough occurrence (or, perhaps more accurately, as demise becomes imminent, conflict increases as those who remain fight over the leftovers, giving rise to a complete political arena that finally destroy the organization). But two things can impede it.

One is organizational renewal, to be described below. The other is the presence of artificial support. An organization that can find an artificial means to sustain itself may be able to maintain a state of pervasive politics for a long time. In the last chapter, examples given of this included the controversial regulatory agency whose funding keeps coming from the government and the politicized business corporation that sustains itself by means of a privileged position already established in a market place. But even artificial support cannot last forever, especially since politics feeds on itself and when left unchecked tears an organization apart. Thus, demise must come eventually unless there is renewal.

RENEWAL

13. Organizational renewal may take place in the form of gradual revitalization or, in the absence of that, dramatic turnaround, the former likely during maturity, the latter during demise ("revitalization," "turn-around"). Every organization must adapt eventually if it is to survive. Some do seem capable of renewing themselves; others do not and simply die. Ironically, the latter occurrence seems to be more common in the earlier stages of the life cycle, as shown by the tombstones in Figure 14–3. As already noted, the missionary configuration often kills organizations that use it simply because it isolates them from the rest of the world. Likewise, entrepreneurial configurations tend to kill organizations when their leaders lose their ability to adapt (or adapt too freely, the main reason why innovative configurations are also often implicated in the death of organizations).

Faced with crisis, therefore, an organization in an early stage of its life seems more likely to survive by moving on to a subsequent stage, making the transition to another configuration, than by renewing itself with the configuration it has. Threatened entrepreneurial configurations tend to become instrument machines or expert organizations, as the leaders are replaced not by other entrepreneurs but by different centers of power; threatened missionary organizations tend to become closed system machines, since their ideologies must be destroyed if the organizations are to adapt beyond them; and so on.

Thus, renewal seems to be a phenomenon of the later stages of the organizational life cycle. This would seem to make sense, because by then the organization may have no choice. The mature configuration can only move on to decline, the declining one to demise. Moreover, while the demise of an entrepreneurial or missionary organization may not concern many people, because it tends to be small and insular and often to operate in an inconsequential market niche, the threatened organization that has reached maturity usually attracts a great deal of attention: It is typically large and entrenched in a central market with all kinds of trading relationships established around it, not to mention the institutional status that comes from a long history. Thus, there tends to be a great incentive to save the organization, often even when the organization is not worth saving.

Renewal can take two forms, as was suggested in Chapter 8. Some organizations are capable of revitalizing themselves periodically. Others, which are not, must be subjected to turnaround under crisis if they are to survive.

Revitalization is a gradual process that operates within, reflecting the capacity of an organization to renew itself, in other words to change while maintaining its basic configuration. As implied by points made earlier in this chapter, revitalization would seem to be encouraged by a healthy mixture of politics and ideology in an organization, the former stimulating all kinds of people to promote changes that challenge the status quo, the latter creating the culture that facilitates their acceptance. Thus, we should not expect to find revitalization so much in the decline stage, where politicization has already undermined the healthy functioning of an organization, as in the mature stage, where remaining vestiges of ideology can function alongside the inevitable political games. Of course, we should expect the capacity for revitalization to be greatest in organizations whose ideologies are sufficiently strong to allow them to sustain the various forces of our pentagon concurrently.

The configurations of maturity are the closed system machine, the professional, and, in part, the innovative. Each is shown in Figure 14–3 with a loop underneath to represent this capacity for revitalization. In other words, these alone are considered able to make a natural transition to a renewed form of themselves. (Of course, it is this capacity for self-renewal that helps to define maturity, since this allows an organization to sustain itself in its state for a long time.)

The innovative configuration is the one most naturally amenable to revitalization. After all, it exists to change, to revitalize itself continually in direct response to changes in its environment through its grassroots process of strategy-making. Indeed, its main problem is not to change but to direct that change, find convergence periodically in its many strategic initiatives. Ideology can help in this regard, by focusing perspective.

As its strategy-making process was presented in Chapter 10, the professional organization tends to be in a state of incessant revitalization. But that is at its narrowest level, in the creation of particular pigeonholes and in activities inside of each. It is at the broadest level that the professional organization has difficulty revitalizing itself because its power tends to be so diffuse. Professional organizations are spinning all the time, even when they are headed in the wrong direction. The problem is to get them to change overall direction periodically. Again ideology may help: Politics can promote individual changes, but ideology may be necessary to weave them together into systematic revitalization. Thus, it is the professional organization devoid of ideology that seems most susceptible to decline through transition to the political configuration.

In both of these expert configurations, revitalization, of one kind or another, is driven by forces intrinsic to the configuration itself. In our third mature configuration, the closed system machine, such natural forces for change do not exist. So to revitalize itself, the configuration needs a push from something beyond itself (hence, the loop underneath is shown as dotted). That push appears to come from the two forces in the center of a pentagon, working in concert. Politics helps to generate and to promote strategic initiatives, for example, through games such as strategic candidates and young Turks, while ideology helps to engender a climate of receptivity to such initiatives, at least for the ones that fit the strategic perspective. Thus, the revitalizing machine configuration, what we earlier labeled the "snappy bureaucracy," really has need for both ideology and politics to adapt.

Mature organizations unable to revitalize themselves may coast until their advantages run out, and then become politicized and decline. In decline, they may try to protect themselves politically by exploiting some artificial means of support. But when that fails, and their survival becomes threatened, efforts may be made to renew them economically, through *turnaround.*

Operating turnaround is the popular label for acting on the cost side of an organization's benefit-cost ratio, by economizing; *strategic turnaround,* for acting on the benefit side, by changing direction. (*Political turnaround* should be added as the label for acting externally, through artificial means to protect themselves.) One involves surgery, the removal or reduction of diseased parts; the other involves reconstruction through the improvement or addition of parts. (And the third involves projecting the problem, and the cost of solving it, onto others.) Generally, as noted in Chapter 8, turnaround appears to involve reversion to the entrepreneurial configuration temporarily, as the exercise of established power is suspended to allow a forceful leader with vision (or determination to cut costs) to resolve the crisis in a personal way.

Of the mature configurations, the closed machine seems most amenable to turnaround. For one thing, its centralization of authority facilitates takeover by a single leader. (Zald and Berger write of the "organizational coup d'etat" in such organizations, where the leader is replaced while the structure remains intact.[14]) For another, these organizations tend to be so large and influential that there is bound to be tremendous pressure for renewal when they decline. (Illustrative of both these points is the Chrysler turnaround effected by Lee Iacocca.) For a third, lacking ideology, as many machine configurations do, revitalization does not occur, and so when the crisis eventually arises, turnaround is the only hope.

On the other hand, true turnaround is not easy to effect here. These are machines; they do not take kindly to dramatic change. That is why political and operating turnarounds, which keep the strategies and systems intact, tend to be favored over strategic turnarounds. (Again, consider the Chrysler turnaround, with its heavy dose of the political, in the form of loan guarantees from the government, and the operating, including cost cuts and layoffs of all kinds.) But these forms of turnaround are often just palliatives, cosmetic or temporary relief that only delays recurrence of the real problem.

Thus the line on Figure 14–3 labeled "turnaround," from the political configuration of decline back to the closed machine configuration of maturity, is dotted, to suggest that true turnaround, permanent resolution of the fundamental problem, may not be all that natural here, or all that common. Indeed, it may not be all that necessary: The costs of such turnarounds can be large yet the effort fruitless. Sometimes it simply does not pay to try to save a sick institution, no matter how important it once was and how strong are the social pressures for doing so. (Witness the steady decline of British Leyland.)

In the professional configuration, power is so diffused that it is almost impossible for an entrepreneurial leader to effect a serious turnaround. Even in the best of times, with the aid of a strong ideology, it is no simple matter to change these organizations in an integrated way. Politics having taken over hardly makes this easier. Sometimes it seems that an organization of professionals is more inclined to destroy itself through conflict than to cede its power to a single leader for turnaround. (Of course, why not? Most of the professionals can simply join another professional organization and pick up right where they left off. If the organization is for them just a shell that provides support, then why should they care if it dies?)

On the other hand, the professionals themselves will sometimes reduce their own political activities to allow the organization to survive, if for nothing more than the convenience of being able to get back to what they most want to do, namely practice their professions. Thus, a dotted line is shown from the political organization back to the professional, though it is not labeled turnaround.

The line from the political organization back to the innovative one is solid, because that transition is considered to be more natural, and common. As noted earlier, innovative organizations slip easily into a political state, not because of decline but simply because their fluid structures easily go out of control. Likewise they are easily brought back, as indicated by the use of one solid line in Figure 14–3, with arrows going both ways. This may be done by an entrepreneurial leader who effects a turnaround, probably strategic through the imposition of a new strategic umbrella, but possibly also operating, simply by bringing order to all the chaos. Or it may take place through the organization's own internal processes of revitalization that, ironically, can use politics to focus direction and so to convert a politicized structure back into an innovative one.

One final issue concerning renewal: Can the mature or declining organization begin the overall life cycle anew, emerging as a fresh entrepreneurial configuration, much as the mythical phoenix arises from its own ashes every five hundred years? Despite intimations of this in the popular management press, I think not. Some organizations captured by politics in an enduring way may be turned around, to revert to a machine or expert configuration, though our conclusions were not very optimistic even on this. But to be turned around by entrepreneurship does not mean to become entrepreneurial, in the sense of becoming a simple, supple, and flexible structure ready to go on adapting.

Turnaround tends to be a one-time event, a temporary, sometimes even superficial change during which normal practices are suspended to allow for change. In the machine organization, the procedures do not go away, nor do the analysts who design them or the managers who supervise them. They merely wait for the organization to be secured so that they can continue to get on with their own tasks. Likewise, turnaround of the innovative or professional configuration does not dispense with the power of its experts. The mythical phoenix may arise in the freshness of youth; the real organization does not. Legacies remain, which influence behavior. The organization may be the wiser for its experiences, but it must also be the wearier.

If reversion to the entrepreneurial form on a sustained basis is unlikely, what about reversion to some earlier configuration of the development stage? Again, I find this equally unlikely. There are certainly examples of old, lethargic organizations having developed bright new systems of beliefs. But for every one that truly internalizes a rich new ideology, let alone becomes a missionary configuration, there appear to be a great many others whose beliefs amount to a thin veneer that washes off in the first storm. At best, with a dedicated, patient, and charismatic leadership, the mature organization gets an infusion of ideology, which may be able to exist alongside its conventional structure for a time.

Likewise, reversion to the instrument form does happen, but it is also difficult to sustain in a machine organization that has already become large and established. Corporate raiders may be able to capture large, sick organizations, turning closed systems into their instruments for a time to restructure them. But restructuring these monoliths is different from controlling them externally on a regular basis, much as turning them around is different from sustaining entrepreneurial management of them.

The one reversion that seems possible in our model is from the political back to innovative configuration, as noted above, because the former state tends to be a frequent, natural, and, most important, temporary one for these organizations. But another reversion is less likely: While I have come across many examples of the less stable innovative form (sitting between the stages of development and maturity) making a transition to the more stable professional one (in maturity), I cannot recall a single example of the opposite transition.

Once having commenced this life cycle, therefore, many organizations seem more or less destined to complete it, unless, of course, they stall or die along the way, or get diverted by external changes that have nothing to do with the forces within themselves. Our model suggests that as organizations survive and develop, they become more diffuse in their power relationships, more complex in their functioning, more ambiguous in their intentions, and eventually less functional in their performance, though, ironically, more stable in their makeup. The forces of direction, belief, and service to an external constituency give way to protection of themselves as systems and of their influential members, and later to pervasive conflict.

At some point, as a result, organizations tend to peak in their service to society and then they decline. But there seems to be no going back, at least not in any sustained way. Applying the model to our world of organizations, we would therefore expect a healthy society to maintain a steady level of the replacement of old, spent organizations by fresh new ones. In other words, *it is not the renewal of single organizations that should concern us so much as the renewal of our system of organizations.* But the two would seem to call for very different approaches.

Organizations cannot be renewed very easily, at least not in terms of invigorating long-established ones with the energy of youth. What we have called a life *cycle* model then, is really a life *sequence;* it is the society of organizations that experiences the cycle.

Or at least it should. The problem is that in contemporary society we seem to discourage this cycle of organizational life by allowing spent organizations to survive, indeed even by protecting them artificially. This is done at the expense of new organizations that ought to be able to grow up in their place, using their freed-up resources more judiciously and more productively. That doing this has grave consequences for our society of organizations will be the subject of the closing chapter of this book.

Part III
ON OUR SOCIETY OF ORGANIZATIONS

As I noted in the first sentence of this book, ours is a society of organizations for better *and* for worse. We create organizations to serve us, but somehow they also force us to serve them. Sometimes it feels as if our institutions have run out of control, like the machinery of Charlie Chaplin's film *Modern Times.* Why we should become slaves to our servants is the theme taken up in this section of the book. With an understanding of management developed in the first section and an understanding of organizations developed in the second, we can begin to suggest some answers.

A society of organizations is one in which organizations enter our lives as influential forces in a great many ways—in how we work, what we eat, how we get educated and cured of our illnesses, how we get entertained, and how our ideas get shaped. The ways in which we try to control our organizations and our organizations in turn try to control us become major issues in the lives of all of us.

Foremost among the organizations that influence us may be the large business corporation. Yet the debate over the control of it has advanced hardly at all over the course of more than half a century. This section therefore opens with the question, "Who should control the corporation?," suggesting a series of answers around a "conceptual horseshoe," which represents the political spectrum.

Then we consider "A note on that dirty word efficiency," because an important message lies in the fact that efficiency, that paragon of all good things organizational, should have developed such a reputation. While that message is considered in the second chapter, its full implication is really addressed in the third one of this section, and the final essay of this book. Based on an unpublished speech I gave a few years ago, it seems to bring together virtually every major point made in this book. Its conclusion is not an encouraging one, but is presented in the belief that we must understand our problems before we can deal with them. This closing essay is entitled "Society Has Become Unmanageable as a Result of Management."

15
WHO SHOULD CONTROL THE CORPORATION?

The life cycle model has suggested that as organizations grow large, they tend to seal themselves off from external influence and instead exert their own influence as powerful closed systems, under the control of their own insiders. But clearly, society cannot sit by and be dictated to by systems that were created to serve it. And so a debate arose and has raged for more than half a century,* particularly over the large, widely held business corporation: Who should control it, how, and for whose benefit? As the shareholding of these powerful institutions spread, so that none of their official owners held enough stock to exercise direct control, effective power over many of them passed to their full-time managers. But this was unacceptable to many people, and a host of proposals arose to temper that control, even, in some cases, to eliminate it altogether.

These proposals have run the whole gamut of political persuasions. Yet the issue remains as muddied and unresolved today as it ever was. Indeed, the issue is as important for the "communist" East, which is right now struggling over how to control its large enterprises, as for the "capitalist" West and, in that West, as important for other large public and parapublic institutions as it is for business. How is society to bring its large organizations under adequate social control without endangering their capacity to produce goods and services efficiently?

In discussing the various answers that have been proposed and suggesting a way to reconcile them, I here take less a political stand than an organizational one, arguing in essence that the resolution of the issue may have less to do with debates over "radical left" or "reactionary right" than with the teachings of organization theory:

---

* The publication in 1932 of the Berle and Means book *The Modern Corporation and Private Property* (Macmillan Publishing Company), while not the start of this debate, certainly brought it into sharp focus by presenting evidence that the large business corporation was more likely to be controlled by its managers than its shareholders.

what works in an administrative or organizational sense. "A plague on both your houses" is my response to extremist positions on both sides, simply because they seldom work, not even from the perspective of the proponents themselves. As we shall see, nationalization of industry does not engender social responsibility, often not even service to the state, while absolute shareholder control can lead to concentrations of power that threaten the free market itself. Again, we must understand how organizations work and how and why they get broken before we run off half-cocked trying to fix them.

In a sense, I guess that does position me politically: as a pragmatist. I believe capitalism is no less a failure than communism when pushed to the extreme end of the political spectrum. Extremism is the problem, and ironically, from the perspective of organization theory, the two extremes look remarkably alike. Both, I argue, assume the organization to be the instrument of some dominant group of external influencers, and so a machine configuration. The influencers may differ, even in the goals they ostensibly pursue, but the nature of the resultant organizations does not, nor do the consequences on how they function. My own inclination, therefore, is to favor the combination of proposals that range from the moderate left to the moderate right.

This paper was first published, in a somewhat longer version, in the *California Management Review,* Fall 1984, that version itself based on a fairly long final section of my book *Power In and Around Organizations.* In addressing the issue in question, the paper also shows how organization theory can be used to consider such issues. "Who should control the corporation?" has been considered from the perspective of economics, political science, law, industrial relations, sociology, and a range of other disciplines. I believe organization theory is able to bring special insight to it. In my opinion, nowhere in this book are the benefits of using organization theory better demonstrated than right here.

Who should control the corporation? How? And for the pursuit of what goals?

Historically, the corporation was controlled by its owners—through direct control of its managers if not through direct management—for the pursuit of economic goals. But as shareholding became dispersed, owner control weakened; and as the corporation grew to very large size, its economic actions came to have increasing social consequences. The giant, widely held corporation came increasingly under the implicit control of its managers, and the concept of social responsibility—the voluntary

consideration of public social goals alongside the private economic ones—
arose to provide them with a basis legitimacy for their actions.

To some, including those closest to the managers themselves, this
was accepted as a satisfactory arrangement for the large corporation.
"Trust it" to the goodwill of the managers was their credo; these people
will be able to achieve an appropriate balance between social and economic
goals.

But others viewed this basis of control as unacceptable. The corporation
was too large, too influential, its actions too pervasive to be left free
of the direct and concerted influence of outsiders. At the extreme were
those who believed that managerial control alone was fundamentally
illegitimate and had to be subjected to formal and direct external control.
"Nationalize it," said those at one end of the political spectrum, to
put ultimate control in the hands of the government so that the corporation
would pursue public social goals. No, said those at the other end, "restore
it" to direct shareholder control, so that it will not waver from the
pursuit of private economic goals.

Other people took less extreme positions. "Democratize it" became
the rallying cry for some, to open up the governance of the large, widely
held corporation to a variety of affected groups—if not the workers,
then the customers, or conservation interests, or minorities. "Regulate
it" was also a popular position, with its implicit premise that only by
being subjected to certain government controls would the corporation's
managers attend to particular social goals. Then there were those who
accepted direct management control so long as it was tempered by other,
less formal types of influence. "Pressure it," said a generation of social
activists, to ensure that social goals are taken into consideration. But
others argued that because the corporation is an economic instrument,
you must "induce it" by providing economic incentives to encourage
the resolution of social problems.

Finally, there were those who argued that this whole debate was
unnecessary, that a kind of invisible hand ensures that the economic
corporation acts in a socially responsible manner. "Ignore it" was their
implicit conclusion.

What this implies is that the various positions concerning who should
control the corporation, and how, can be laid out along a political continuum, from nationalization at one end to the restoration of shareholder
power at the other. From the organization theory perspective, however,
those two extremes are not so far apart. Both call for direct control of
the corporation's managers by specific outsiders, in one case the govern-

FIGURE 15–1
The Conceptual Horseshoe

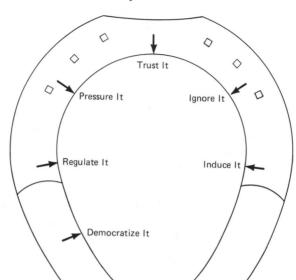

ment to ensure the pursuit of social goals, in the other case the shareholders to ensure the pursuit of economic ones. It is the moderate positions—notably, trusting the corporation to the social responsibility of its managers—that are farthest from the extremes. Hence, we can fold our spectrum around so that it takes the shape of a horseshoe.

Figure 15–1 shows our "conceptual horseshoe," with "nationalize it" and "restore it" at the two ends. "Trust it" is at the center, because this position postulates a natural balance of social and economic goals. "Democratize it," "regulate it," and "pressure it" are shown on the left side of the horseshoe, because all seek to temper economic goals with social ones. "Induce it" and "ignore it," both of which favor the pursuit of economic goals, are shown on the right side.

This conceptual horseshoe provides a basic framework to help clarify the issues in this important debate. We begin by discussing each of these positions in turn, circling the horseshoe from left to right. Finding that each (with one exception) has a logical context, we conclude—in keeping with our organization theory perspective—that they should be thought of as forming a portfolio from which society can draw to deal with the issue of who should control the corporation and how.

"NATIONALIZE IT"

Nationalization of the business corporation is a taboo subject in the United States . . . in general, but not in particular. Whenever a major corporation runs into serious difficulty (i.e., faces bankruptcy with possible loss of many jobs), massive government intervention, often including direct nationalization, inevitably comes up as an option. And this option has been exercised: U.S. travelers now ride on Amtrak; Tennessee residents have for years been getting their power from a government utility; indeed, the Post Office was once a private enterprise. Other nations have, of course, been much more ambitious in this regard.

From an organizational theory perspective, the question is not whether nationalization is legitimate, but whether it works—at least in particular, limited circumstances. As a response to concerns about the social responsibility of large corporations, the answer seems to be no. The evidence suggests that social difficulties arise more from the size of an organization and its degree of bureaucratization than from its form of ownership. On the other hand, contrary to popular belief in the United States, nationalization does not necessarily harm economic efficiency. Renault was long one of the most successful automobile companies outside Japan; it was nationalized by the French government shortly after World War II. Likewise, the state-owned Canadian National has long been an innovative and effective railroad. The prophecy may be a self-fulfilling one: When people believe that government ownership leads to interference, politicization, and inefficiency, that may be exactly what happens. However, when they believe that nationalization *has* to work, then state-owned enterprises may be able to attract the very best talent in the country and thereby work well.

But economic efficiency provides no more reason to favor nationalization than does concern about social responsibility. Nationalization does, however, seem to make sense in at least two particular circumstances. The first is when a mission deemed necessary in a society will not be provided adequately by the private sector. That is presumably why America has its Amtrak and why third world nations often create state enterprises. The second is when the activities of an organization must be so intimately tied to government policy that it is best managed as a direct arm of the state. The Canadian government created Petrocan to act as a "window," a source of knowledge, on the sensitive oil industry.

Thus, it is not rhetoric but requirement that should determine the use of this position as a solution to who should control the corporation. "Nationalize it" should certainly not be embraced as a panacea. But neither should it be rejected as always irrelevant.

"DEMOCRATIZE IT"

A less extreme position—at least in the context of the American debate—is one that calls for formal devices to broaden the governance of the corporation. The proponents of this position either accept the legal fiction of shareholder control and argue that the corporation's power base is too narrow, or else respond to the reality that has evolved and question the legitimacy of managerial control. Why, they ask, do stockholders or self-selected managers have any greater right to control the profound decisions of these major institutions than do workers or customers or the neighbors downstream?

This stand is not to be confused with what is known as "participative management." The call to "democratize it" is a legal rather than an ethical one and is based on power, not generosity. Management is not asked to share its power voluntarily; rather, that power is to be reallocated constitutionally. That makes this position a fundamental and important one, *especially* in the United States, with its strong tradition of pluralist control of its institutions.

The debate over democratization of the corporation has been confusing in part because many of the proposals have been so vague. We can bring some order to it by considering, in organization theory terms, two basic means of democratization and two basic constituencies that can be involved. As shown in Figure 15–2, they suggest four possible forms of corporate democracy. One means is through the election of representatives to the board of directors, which we call *representative democracy*. The other is through formal but direct involvement in internal decision-making processes, which we call *participatory democracy*. Either can focus on the *workers* or else on a host of outside interest groups, the latter giving rise to a *pluralistic* form of democracy. These are basic forms of corporate democracy in theory. With one exception, however, they have hardly been approached—let alone achieved—in practice. But they suggest where the "democratize it" debate may be headed.

FIGURE 15–2

Four Basic Forms of Corporate Democracy

GROUPS INVOLVED

		Internal Employees	External Interest Groups
FOCUS OF ATTENTION	Board of Directors	Worker Representative Democracy (European style, e.g., "co-determination" or worker ownership)	Pluralistic Representative Democracy (American style, e.g., "public interest" directors)
	Internal Decision-Making Process	Worker Participatory Democracy (e.g., works councils)	Pluralistic Participatory Democracy (e.g., outsiders on new product committees)

WORKER REPRESENTATIVE DEMOCRACY. The European debate has focused on worker representative democracy. This has, in some sense, been achieved in Yugoslavia, where the workers of all but the smallest firms elect the members of what is the equivalent of the American board of directors. In Germany, under the so-called *Mitbestimmung* (''co-determination''), the workers and the shareholders each elect half of the directors.

The evidence on this form of corporate democracy has been consistent, and it supports neither its proponents nor its detractors. Workers' representation on the board seems to make relatively little difference one way or the other. The worker representatives concern themselves with wage and welfare issues but leave most other questions to management. Worker-controlled firms (not unlike the state-owned ones) appear to be no more socially responsible than private ones.

On the other hand, worker representative democracy may have certain positive benefits. Helmut Schmidt, when Chancellor of West Germany, is reported to have said that ''the key to [this] country's postwar economic miracle was its sophisticated system of workers' participation.''[1] While no one can prove this statement, co-determination certainly does not seem to have done the German economy much harm. By providing an aura of legitimacy to the German corporation and by involving the workers (at least officially) in its governance and opening up some lines of communication, co-determination may perhaps have enhanced the spirit of enterprise in Germany (while having little real effect on how decisions are actually made). More significantly, co-determination may have fostered greater understanding and cooperation between the managers and the union members who fill most of the worker seats on the boards.

PLURALISTIC REPRESENTATIVE DEMOCRACY. The embryonic debate over representative democracy in the United States has shown signs of moving in a different direction. Consistent with the tradition of pluralism in America's democratic institutions—the town council and the school board, if not the corporation itself—there has been increasing pressure to elect outside directors who represent a wide variety of special interest groups, consumers, minorities, environmentalists, and so on.

Critics have pointed out the problems of defining constituencies and finding the means to hold elections. "One-person, one-vote" may be easily applied to electing representatives of the workers, but no such simple rule can be found in the case of the consumer or environmental representatives, let alone ones of the "public interest." Yet it is amazing how quickly things become workable in the United States when Americans decide to put their collective mind to it. Indeed, the one case of public directors that I came across is telling in this regard. According to a Conference Board report, the selection by the Chief Justice of the Supreme Court of New Jersey of six of the twenty-four members of the board of Prudential Insurance as public directors has been found by the company to be "quite workable."[2]

THE POWER OF THE BOARD. Proposals for representative democracy, indeed those for nationalization and the restoration of shareholder control as well, rest on assumptions about the power of the board of directors. It may, therefore, be worth considering at this point the roles that boards of directors play in organizations and the board's resulting powers.

In law, traditionally, the business of a corporation was to be "managed" by its board. But of course, the board does no such thing. Managers manage, although some may happen to sit on the board. What then are the roles of the board, particularly of its "outside" directors?

The most tangible role of the board, and clearly provided for in law, is to name, and of course to dismiss as well, the chief executive officer, that person who in turn names the rest of the management. A second role may be to exercise direct control during periods of crisis, for example when the management has failed to provide leadership. And a third is to review the major decisions of the management as well as its overall performance.

These three constitute the board's roles of control, in principal at least because there is no shortage of evidence that boards have difficulty doing even these effectively, especially outside directors. Their job is, after all, part-time, and in a brief meeting once in a while they face a complex organization led by a highly organized management that deals with it every day. The result is that board control tends to reduce to naming and replacing the chief executive, and that person's knowledge of that fact, nothing more. Indeed, even that power is circumscribed, because a management cannot be replaced very often. In a sense, the board is like a bee hovering near a person picking flowers. The person must proceed carefully, so as not to provoke the bee, but can proceed with the task. But if the bee does happen to be provoked, it only gets to sting once. Thus many boards try to know only enough to know when the management is not doing its job properly, so that they can replace it.

But if boards tend to be weak in exercising *control over* the organization, they also tend to be strong in providing *service to* the organization. Here board membership plays at least four other roles. First, it "co-opts" influential outsiders: The organization uses the status of a seat on its board to gain the support of people important to it (as in the case of the big donors who sit on university boards). Second, board membership may be used to establish contacts for the organization (as when retired military officers sit on the boards of weapons manufacturing firms). This may be done to help in such things as the securing of contracts and the raising of funds. Third, seats on the board can be used to enhance an organization's reputation (as when an astronaut or some other type of celebrity is given a seat). And fourth, the board can be used to provide advice for the organization (as in the case of many of the bankers and lawyers who sit on the boards of corporations).

How much do boards serve organizations, and how much do they control them? Some boards do, of course, exercise control, particularly when their members represent a well-defined constituency, such as the substantial owner of a corporation. But, as noted, this tends to be a loose control at best. And other boards hardly do even that, especially when their constituencies are widely dispersed.

To represent everyone is ultimately to represent no one, especially when faced with a highly organized management that knows exactly what it wants. (Or from the elector's point of view, having some distant representative sitting on a board somewhere hardly brings him or her closer to control over the things that impinge on daily life—the work performed, the products consumed, the rivers polluted.) In corporations, this has been shown to be true of the directors who represent many small shareholders no less than those who represent many workers or many customers, perhaps even those who represent government, since that can be just a confusing array of pressure groups. These boards become, at best, tools of the organization, providing it with the variety of the services discussed above, at worst mere façades of formal authority. That is why we cannot expect a great deal from the representative forms of corporate democracy.

WORKER PARTICIPATORY DEMOCRACY. Despite its problems, representative democracy is crystal clear compared with participatory democracy. This describes a kind of bottom-up, grassroots democracy in which the workers participate directly in decision-making (instead of overseeing management's decisions from the board of directors) and also elect their own managers (who then become more administrators than bosses). Yet proposals to this effect are inevitably vague, and I have heard of no large mass production or mass service firm—not even one owned by workers themselves or by a union—that comes close to this.

What has impeded worker participatory democracy? In my opinion, something rather obvious has stood in its way, namely the structure required by the very organizations in which the attempts have been made to apply it. Worker participatory democracy—and worker representative democracy too, for that matter—have been attempted primarily in organizations containing large numbers of workers who do highly routine, rather unskilled jobs that are typical of most mass production and service, in other words, ones structured as machine bureaucracies. The overriding requirement in machine bureaucracy is for tight coordination, the kind that can be achieved only by central administrators. For example, the myriad of decisions associated with producing an automobile at Volvo's Kalmar works in Sweden cannot be made by autonomous groups, each doing as it pleases. The whole car must fit together in a particular way at the end of the assembly process. These decisions require a highly sophisticated system of bureaucratic coordination. That is why automobile companies are structured into rigid hierarchies of authority.

Participatory democracy *is* approached in other kinds of organizations, for example in autonomous professional ones such as universities and hospitals or the innovative ones in such fields as high technology, which have very different needs for central coordination. But the proponents of organizational democracy are not lobbying for changes in hospitals or high technology. It is the giant mass producers they are after, and unless the operating work in those corporations becomes largely skilled and professional in nature, nothing approaching participative democracy can be expected.

PLURALISTIC PARTICIPATORY DEMOCRACY. In principal, the pluralistic form of participatory democracy means that a variety of groups external to the corporation can somehow control its decision-making processes directly. In practice, of course, this concept is even more elusive than the worker form of participatory democracy. To fully open up the internal decision-making processes of the corporation to outsiders would mean chaos. Yet certain very limited forms of outside participation would seem to be not only feasible but perhaps even desirable. Imagine telephone company executives resolving rate conflicts with consumer groups in quiet offices instead of having to face them in noisy public hearings.

To conclude, corporate democracy—whether representative or participatory in form—may be an elusive and difficult concept, but it cannot be dismissed. It is not just another social issue, like river pollution or forced retirement, but one that strikes at the most fundamental of values. In a more detailed article on this subject, I argued "why America needs but cannot have corporate democracy." It cannot have it, at least not in organizations that depend on the efforts of many relatively unskilled workers, because effective coordination precludes it. The important decisions must be made at one center, and no part-time representatives of the many workers who produce the outputs or the many customers who buy them, etc., can change that fact. (One Yugoslav has written, regarding industrial democracy in his country, that "decisions are no longer made at the top; they are only integrated and coordinated there."[3] Only!)

But America, alongside other developed nations, must pursue corporate democracy, because in a society of organizations democracy can have meaning only if it applies to the organizational activities that most impinge upon citizens in their daily lives—as workers, consumers, and neighbors. Organizations that prove unresponsive to other forces will have to be opened up to external control, one way or another. Indeed, as the legitimacy of large closed system organizations becomes increasingly questioned by workers inside as well as pressure groups outside, generating greater levels of politicization, the issue will become no less one of economic efficiency than of social democracy.

"REGULATE IT"

In theory, regulating the corporation is about as simple as democratizing it is complex. Practice is, of course, another matter. To the proponents of "regulate it," the corporation can be made responsive to social needs by having its actions subjected to the controls of a higher authority, typically government, in the form of a regulatory agency or legislation backed up by the courts. Under regulation, constraints are imposed externally on the corporation while its internal governance is left to its managers.

Regulation of business is at least as old as the Code of Hammurabi, and has increased steadily through this century, although in recent years it has experienced waves of reduction. To some, regulation is a clumsy instrument that should never be relied upon; to others, it is the only means of ensuring social responsibility. The truth lies in between. At best, regulation sets minimum and usually crude standards of acceptable behavior; when it works, it does not make any organization socially responsible so much as stop some from being grossly irresponsible. Because it is inflexible, regulation tends to be applied slowly and conservatively, usually lagging behind public sentiment. Also, regulation often does not work because of difficulties in enforcement. The problems of the regulatory agencies are legendary—limited resources and information compared with the industries they are supposed to regulate, the co-optation of the regulators by those industries, and so on. When applied indiscriminately, regulation either fails dramatically or else succeeds and creates havoc.

Yet there are obvious places for regulation. A prime one is to control tangible "externalities"—costs incurred by corporations that are passed on to the public at large. When, for example, costly pollution or worker health problems can be attributed directly to a corporation, then there seems to be every reason to force it (or its customers) to bear those costs directly, or else to terminate the actions that generate them. Likewise, regulation may have a place where severe competition pulls all firms down to some base level of behavior, forcing even the well-intentioned manager to ignore the social consequences of his or her actions. Indeed, in such cases, the socially responsible behavior is to encourage sensible regulation. "Help us to help ourselves," businesspeople who want to be socially responsible should be telling the government.

Most discouraging, however, is Theodore Levitt's revelation some years ago that business has fought every piece of proposed regulatory or social legislation throughout this century, from the Child Labor Laws on up. In Levitt's opinion, much of that legislation has been good for business—dissolving the giant trusts, creating a more honest and effective stock market, and so on. Yet, "the computer is programmed to cry wolf."[4]

In summary, regulation is a clumsy instrument but not a useless one. Were the business community to take a more enlightened view of it, regulation could be applied more appropriately, and we would not need those periodic waves of deregulation to eliminate the excesses.

"PRESSURE IT"

"Pressure it" is designed to provoke corporations to act beyond some base level of behavior, usually in areas that regulation misses entirely. Here, activists bring ad hoc campaigns of pressure to bear on one or a group of corporations to keep them responsive to the activists' interpretation of social needs.

"Pressure it" is a distinctively American position. While Europeans debate the theories of nationalization and corporate democracy in their cafés, Americans read about the exploits of Ralph Nader et al. in their morning newspapers. Note that "pressure it," unlike "regulate it," implicitly accepts management's right to make the final decisions. Perhaps that is one reason why it is favored in America.

While less radical than the other positions so far discussed, "pressure it" has nevertheless proved far more effective in eliciting behavior sensitive to social needs. Activist groups have pressured for everything from the dismemberment of diversified corporations to the development of day care centers. Of special note is the class action suit, which has opened up a whole new realm of corporate social issues. But the effective use of the pressure campaign has not been restricted to the traditional activist. President Kennedy used it to roll back U.S. Steel price increases in the early 1960s, and business leaders in Pittsburgh used it in the late 1940s by threatening to take their freight-haulage business elsewhere if the Pennsylvania Railroad did not replace its coal burning locomotives to help clean up their city's air.

"Pressure it" has been highly successful because it is an informal, flexible, and focused way to change corporate behavior. Yet it is irregular and ad hoc, with different pressure campaigns sometimes making contradictory demands on management. Compared to the positions to its right on the horseshoe, "pressure it," like the other positions to its left, is based on confrontation rather than cooperation.

"TRUST IT"

To a large and vocal contingent which parades under the banner of corporate "social responsibility," the corporation has no need to act irresponsibly, and there is thus no reason for it to be nationalized by the state, democratized by its different constituencies, regulated by the government, or pressured by activists. This contingent believes that the corporation's leaders can be trusted to attend to social goals for their own sake, simply because it is the noble thing to do. This is the twentieth-century version of *noblesse oblige,* literally "nobility obliges."

We call this position "trust it," or, more exactly, "trust the corporation to the goodwill of its managers," although looking at it from outside the corporation, it might just as well be called "socialize it." We place it in the center of our conceptual horseshoe because it alone postulates a natural balance between social and economic goals—a balance that is to be attained in the heads (or perhaps the hearts) of responsible business-people. And, as a not necessarily incidental consequence, power can be left in the hands of the managers: The corporation can be trusted to those who reconcile social and economic goals.

ATTACKS ON SOCIAL RESPONSIBILITY. The attacks on social responsibility have been many and varied, from the right as well as the left. They boil down to whether corporate managers should be trusted when they claim to pursue social goals; if so, whether they are capable of pursuing such goals; and finally, whether they have any right to pursue such goals.

The simplest attack is that managerial discussion of social responsibility is all rhetoric, no action. E. F. Cheit refers to the "Gospel of Social Responsibility" as "designed to justify the power of managers over an ownerless system."[5]

Others argue that businessmen lack the personal capabilities required to pursue social goals. Levitt claims that professional managers reach the top of the hierarchy by dedication to their firms and their industries; as a result, their knowledge of social issues is highly restricted.[6] Others argue that an orientation to efficiency renders business leaders inept at handling complex social problems (which require flexibility and political finesse, often involving solutions that are uneconomic).

The most far-reaching criticism, however, is that businesspeople have no right to pursue social goals. "Who authorized them to do that?" asks Braybrooke,[7] attacking from the left. What business have they—self-selected or at best appointed by shareholders—to impose *their* interpretation of the public good on society? Let the elected politicians, directly responsible to the population, look after the social goals.

But that attack comes from the right, too. Milton Friedman writes that social responsibility amounts to spending other people's money—if not that of shareholders, then of customers or employees. Drawing on the pejorative vocabulary of right-wing ideology, Friedman concludes that social responsibility is a "fundamentally subversive doctrine," representing "pure and unadulterated socialism," supported by businessmen who are "unwitting puppets of the intellectual forces that have been undermining the basis of a free society these past decades." To Friedman, "there is one and only one social responsibility of business—to use its resources and engage in activities designed to increase its profits so long as it stays within the rules of the game."[8] Let businessmen, in other words, stick to their own business, which is business itself.

EVIDENCE ON SOCIAL RESPONSIBILITY. The empirical evidence on social responsibility is hardly more encouraging. Brenner and Molander, comparing their 1977 survey of *Harvard Business Review* readers with one conducted fifteen years earlier, concluded that the "respondents are somewhat more cynical about the ethical conduct of their peers" than they were previously. Close to half the respondents agreed with the statement that "the American business executive tends not to apply the great ethical laws immediately to work. He is preoccupied chiefly with gain."[9] Only 5 percent listed social responsibility as a factor "influencing ethical standards" whereas 31 and 20 percent listed different factors related to pressure campaigns and 10 percent listed regulation.

The modern corporation has been described as a rational, amoral institution—its "professional" managers "hired guns" who pursue any goals asked of them in an "efficient" manner. The problem (for reasons that will be discussed in the next chapter) is that efficiency really means measurable efficiency, so that the guns load only with goals that can be quantified. Social goals, unlike economic ones, just don't lend themselves to quantification. As a result, the performance control systems—on which modern corporations so heavily depend—tend to drive out social goals in favor of economic ones.[10]

In the contemporary large corporation, then, professional amorality turns into economic morality. And when the screws of these performance control systems are turned really tight, economic morality can turn into social immorality. And it happens often: A *Fortune* writer found that "a surprising number of [big companies] have been involved in blatant illegalities" in the 1970s, at least 117 of 1,043 firms studied.[11]

How, then, is anyone to "trust it"?

THE NEED FOR SOCIAL RESPONSIBILITY. The fact is that we have to trust it. Social responsibility may be a naive concept, but it is also a necessary one, for two reasons. First, the strategic decisions of large organizations inevitably involve social as well as economic consequences that are inextricably intertwined. The neat distinction between economic goals in the private sector and social goals in the public sector just doesn't hold up in practice. Every important decision of the large corporation—to introduce a new product line, to close an old plant, whatever—generates all kinds of social consequences. There is no such thing as a purely economic decision in big business. Only a conceptual ostrich, with his head deeply buried in the abstractions of economic theory, could possibly use the distinction between economic and social goals to dismiss social responsibility.

The second reason we have to "trust it" is that there is always some degree of discretion involved in corporate decision-making, discretion to thwart social needs or to attend to them. Things could be a lot better in today's corporation, but they could also be worse. It is primarily our ethics that keep us responsible. If the performance control systems favored by large, diversified corporations cut too deeply into our ethical standards, then we shall have to rethink how these corporations are organized—rethink their size, their bureaucratization, their diversification.

To dismiss corporate social responsibility is to allow corporate behavior to drop to the lowest level, propped up only by external controls such as regulation and pressure campaigns. Solzhenitsyn, who has experienced "a society without any objective legal scale," warns us (in sharp contrast to Friedman) that "a society with no other scale but the legal one is not quite worthy of man either. A society which is based on the letter of the law and never reaches any higher is scarcely taking advantage of the high level of human possibilities."[12]

This is not to suggest that we must "trust it" categorically. We certainly cannot trust it unconditionally by accepting the claim popular in some quarters that only business can solve the social ills of society. Business has no business using its resources without constraint in the social sphere—whether to support political candidates or to dictate through its donations how nonprofit institutions should allocate their efforts.

But in situations where business is necessarily involved, where its decisions have inherent social consequences of importance, that is where social responsibility has a role to play: where business creates externalities that cannot be measured and attributed to it (in other words, where regulation is ineffective); where regulation would work if only business would cooperate with it; where the corporation can fool its customers or suppliers or government through superior knowledge; where useful products can be marketed instead of wasteful or destructive ones. In other words, we have to realize that in many spheres we must "trust it," or at least we must socialize it (and perhaps change it) so that we can trust it. None of us will want to live in a society without responsible, ethical, and committed people in important posts.

"IGNORE IT"

"Ignore it" differs from the other positions on the horseshoe in that explicitly or implicitly it calls for no change in corporate behavior. It assumes that social needs are met in the course of pursuing economic goals. We include this position in our horseshoe because it is held by many influential people and also because its validity would make the other positions irrelevant. We must therefore investigate it alongside the others.

It should be noted at the outset that "ignore it" is not the same position as "trust it." In the latter, to be good is the right thing to do; in the present position, "it pays to be good." The distinction is subtle but important, for now it is economics, not ethics, that elicits the desired behavior. One need not strive to be ethical; economic forces will ensure that social needs fall conveniently into place. Thus by moving one notch to the right on our horseshoe, we enter the realm where the economic goals dominate.

"Ignore it" is sometimes referred to as "enlightened self-interest," although some of its proponents are more enlightened than others. Many a true believer in social responsibility has used the "it pays to be good" argument to ward off attacks from the right that corporations have no business pursuing social goals. After all, even Milton Friedman must admit that they have every right to do so if it pays them economically.

The danger of such arguments, however—and a prime reason "ignore it" differs from "trust it"—is that they tend to support the status quo: Corporations need not change their behavior because it already pays to be good.

Sometimes the case for "ignore it" is made in terms of corporations at large, that the whole business community will benefit from socially responsible behavior. Other times the case is made in terms of the individual corporation, that it will benefit directly from its own socially responsible actions. Others make the case for "ignore it" in "social investment" terms, claiming that socially responsible behavior pays off in a better image for the firm, a more positive relationship with customers, and ultimately a healthier and more stable society in which to do business.

Then, there is what can be called the "them" argument: "If we're not good, *they* will move in"—"they" being Ralph Nader, the government, whoever. In other words, "Be good or else." The trouble with this argument is that reducing social responsibility to simply a political tool for sustaining managerial control of the corporation in the face of outside threats tends to encourage general pronouncements instead of concrete actions, unless, of course, "they" actually deliver with pressure campaigns.

I conclude that the "ignore it" position rests on some shaky ground. It promotes average behavior at best—the status quo of corporate social responsiveness—and we have already seen that for many people that average is not good enough. In fact, the "ignore it" position cannot stand alone; its argument collapses without the "pressure it" position. For without the pressure campaign of the activist, corporations need not worry about their behavior. And if this position cannot stand alone, then by its very nature it cannot stand at all.

"INDUCE IT"

Continuing around to the right, our next position drops all concern with social responsibility per se and argues simply: "Pay it to be good," or, from the corporation's point of view, "be good only where it pays." Here, the corporation does not actively pursue social goals at all, whether as ends in themselves or as means to economic ends. Rather, it undertakes socially desirable *programs* when it is induced economically to do so— usually through government incentives. If society wishes to clean up urban blight, then let its government provide subsidies for corporations that renovate buildings. If pollution is the problem, then let corporations be rewarded for reducing it.

"Induce it" faces "regulate it" on the opposite side of the horseshoe for good reason. While one can penalize the corporation for what it does do, the other rewards it for doing what it would not otherwise do. Hence the two positions can be direct substitutes: Pollution can be alleviated by introducing penalties for the damage done or by offering incentives for the improvements rendered.

Logic does, however, dictate an appropriate role for each of these positions. Where a corporation is doing society a specific, attributable harm—as in the case of pollution—then paying it to stop hardly seems to make sense. If society does not wish to outlaw the harmful behavior altogether, then surely it must charge those responsible for it. Offering financial incentives to stop causing harm would be to invite a kind of blackmail—for example, encouraging corporations to pollute so as to get paid to stop. And every citizen would be charged for the harm done by only a few.

On the other hand, where social problems exist that cannot be attributed to specific corporations yet require the skills of business for solution, then financial incentives clearly make sense (so long, of course, as solutions can be clearly defined and tied to tangible economic rewards). Here, then, and not under "trust it," is where the "only business can do it" argument belongs. When it is true that only business can do it (and business has not done it to us in the first place), then business should be encouraged to do it.

"RESTORE IT"

Our last position on the horseshoe tends to be highly ideological, the first since "democratize it" to seek a fundamental change in the governance and the goals of the corporation. Like the proponents of "nationalize it," those of this position believe that managerial control is illegitimate and must be replaced by a more acceptable form of external control. The corporation should be restored to its former status as a "closely held" instrument, in other words, returned to the direct control of its "rightful" owners, the shareholders. The only way to ensure the relentless pursuit of economic goals—and that means the maximization of profit, free of the "subversive doctrine" of social responsibility—is to put control directly into the hands of those to whom profit means the most.

THE FRIEDMAN DOCTRINE. Some years ago this may have seemed to be an obsolete position. But thanks to its patron saint Milton Friedman, it has come back into prominence. Friedman has written:

> In a free-enterprise, private-property system, a corporate executive is an employee of the owners of the business. He has direct responsibility to his employers. That responsibility is to conduct the business in accordance with their desires, which generally will be to make as much money as possible while conforming to the basic rules of the society, both those embodied in law and those embodied in ethical custom.[13]

Interestingly, what seems to drive Friedman is a belief that the shift over the course of this century from owner to manager control, with its concerns about social responsibility, represents an unstoppable skid around our horseshoe. In the opening chapter of his book *Capitalism and Freedom,* Friedman seems to accept only two possibilities—traditional capitalism and state socialism as practiced in Eastern Europe. The absence of the former must inevitably lead to the latter, with social responsibility acting as the catalyst.

> The preservation and expansion of freedom are today threatened from two directions. The one threat is obvious and clear. It is the external threat coming from the evil men in the Kremlin who promise to bury us. The other threat is far more subtle. It is the internal threat coming from men of good intentions and good will who wish to reform us.[14]

The problem of who should control the corporation thus reduces to a war between two ideologies—in Friedman's terms, "subversive" socialism and "free" enterprise. In this world of black and white, there can be no middle ground, no moderate position between the black of "nationalize it" and the white of "restore it," none of the gray of "trust it." Either the owners will control the corporation or else the government will. Hence, " 'restore it' or else." Anchor the corporation on the right side of the horseshoe, Friedman seems to be telling us, the only place where "free" enterprise and "freedom" are safe.

All of this rests on a series of assumptions—some technical, some economic, some political—that I believe are faulty. The issues are important enough in my opinion to merit their consideration at some length.

ASSUMPTION OF SHAREHOLDER CONTROL. First is the technical assumption of shareholder control. Most large corporations are simply beyond the reach of individual shareholders. Those people's vehicle of control, formally at least, is the board of directors. But the boards of widely held corporations are typically controlled by the managers, not the shareholders. Traditions have grown up whereby it is the full-time chairmen who propose new board members, and there is a good deal of evidence that the selection is based not on shareholding per se, certainly not on any inclination by the managers to chose people who will control their behavior, but at best on the ability of the directors to serve the organization, at worst on their propensity to sit quietly and leave the management alone.

It is true that occasionally someone amasses enough stock to wrest control of a board from the management. But more often the volume of the publicly traded stock is so huge that even the largest private shareholders cannot hope to own more than an insignificant portion of it, far too little to challenge the management. (Of course, one corporation, or financial institution, can amass considerable stock ownership of another, but that just bumps our argument up one level, to the question of who can control the controller.)

Every trend in stock ownership throughout this century refutes the assumption that small shareholders are either able or willing to exercise control over the large corporation. As was pointed out in our earlier discussion of the board of directors, wherever power is widely dispersed among a constituency—shareholders no less than workers or customers— those who share it tend to remain passive. It simply does not pay any one of them to invest the effort to exercise it. If shareholders are unhappy with the behavior of a corporation, it is so much easier for them simply to sell their stock.

Interestingly, then, the one place where the free market still clearly exists is in stock ownership, and that has served to detach property from control. Shareholding has become more and more dispersed, and the ease of the market transaction discourages the exercise of control. To use the terms of a fascinating little book by Albert Hirschman, "exit" is preferred to "voice," let alone "loyalty."[15] Thus, while there may occasionally be shareholder *autocracy*—control of the corporation by a single important shareholder—there is never likely to be shareholder *democracy*—true control of the management by many small shareholders.

ASSUMPTION OF COMPETITIVE MARKETS. The economic assumptions of free markets have been discussed at length in the literature. Whether there exists vibrant competition, unlimited entry, open information, consumer sovereignty, and labor mobility is certainly subject to debate. Less subject to debate, though, is the assertion that the larger the corporation, the greater is its ability to interfere with those things. The issues we are discussing center on the giant corporation. It is not Joe's Body Shop that Ralph Nader is after, but General Motors, a corporation that employs more than half a million people and earns greater revenues than many national governments.

Those who laid the foundation for conventional economic theory—such as Adam Smith and Alfred Marshall—never dreamed of chemical complexes that cost more than a billion dollars; of the massive amounts now spent for advertising campaigns, designed for affect more than for effect; of the waves of conglomeration that have combined all kinds of diverse businesses into single corporate entities; and of the intimate relationships that now exist among giant corporations and between them and governments, as customers and partners as well as supporters. The concept of the arms-length relationship in such conditions is, at best, nostalgic.

How does government contract objectively for a major weapons system when only a few firms are capable of supplying it, ones that are likely to have been involved in the previous development of the technologies to be used, not to mention staffed with ex-military personnel with ties deep in its defense department? And the coffers of the politicians who must make the decision have been filled with funds from the corporate managers, if not the corporations themselves (however indirectly)? What happens to consumer sovereignty when Ford knows more about its gas tanks than do its customers? And what does labor mobility mean in the presence of an inflexible pension plan, or commitment to a special skill, or to a one-factory town? Indeed, it is an ironic twist of conventional economic theory that the worker is the one who typically stays put, rendering false the assumption of labor mobility, while the shareholder is the mobile one, thus spoiling the case for owner control.

ASSUMPTION OF FREEDOM THROUGH "FREE" ENTERPRISE. The political assumptions are more ideological in nature, although usually implicit, namely that the corporation is essentially amoral, society's instrument for producing goods and services, and, more broadly, that a society is "free" and "democratic" so long as its governmental leaders are elected by universal suffrage and do not interfere with the legal activities of its businesspeople. Freedom becomes associated with "free" enterprise. But many people—a large majority of the general public, if the polls are to be believed—seem to subscribe to one or more contrary assumptions.

One is that the large corporation is a social and political institution as much as an economic instrument. Economic activities, as noted previously, produce all kinds of social consequences. Jobs get created and rivers get polluted, cities get built and workers get injured. These social consequences cannot be factored out of corporate strategic decisions and assigned to government.

Another contrary assumption is that society cannot achieve the necessary balance between social and economic needs so long as the private sector attends only to economic goals. Given the influence of business in society, it is argued that the acceptance of Friedman's prescriptions would lead to a one-dimensional society—excessively materialistic and mercenary. Economic morality, as noted earlier, can amount to a social immorality.

Finally, the question is asked: Why the owners? In a democratic society, what justifies owner control of the corporation any more than worker control, or consumer control, or pluralistic control? This is not Adam Smith's society of small proprietors and shopkeepers. His butcher, brewer, and baker have become Swift, Anheuser-Busch, and Ralston Purina. What was once a case for individual democracy now becomes a case for oligarchy.

Free enterprise comes to mean, not the freedom of individual entrepreneurs to maneuver in a market place, but the autonomy of large established organizations to sustain their power in good part free of external influence. And there is, as already noted, no democracy within those organizations. They are technically oligarchies, structures of hierarchical authority in which the few at the top direct the activities of the many down below. There is nothing wrong with this, at least not so long as it is viewed for what it is: not freedom itself but rather the suspension of freedom for the sake of productive efficiency. Indeed, it must be considered a curious fact that, as argued back in Chapters 8 and 9, "free" enterprise is structured on the business level in America in much the same way that "subversive" socialism is structured on the state level in the Soviet Union.

Thus, I personally see Friedman's form of "restore it" as a rather quaint position in a society of giant corporations, managed economies, and dispersed shareholders—a society in which the collective power of corporations is coming under increasing scrutiny and in which the tradeoff between economic and social goals is being reconsidered.

OTHER WAYS TO RESTORE IT. Of course, there are ways other than those of Milton Friedman to "restore it." In some cases, divestment can return the corporation to the business or central theme it knows best, restoring the role of allocating funds between different businesses to capital markets. Likewise, it may sometimes be advantageous to do away with certain forms of vertical integration, so that the large corporation trades with its suppliers and customers instead of ingesting them indiscriminately. Boards could be restored to positions of influence by increasing the directors' legal responsibility for their actions and by making them more independent of the management (for example, by giving them the right to personal staffs and by excluding full-time managers from their ranks, especially the position of chairman). And the size of large enterprises can be reduced where that reflects not current economic competitiveness but rather the legacies of historical successes or other political powers.*

Some of these proposals may not be much more easily attainable in today's society than those of Friedman, even though they may be desirable to large segments of the population. "Restore it" is the nostalgic position on our horseshoe, a return to our fantasies of a glorious past. In this society of giant organizations, it flies in the face of powerful economic and political forces. But efforts must be made to correct at least the obvious deficiencies.

CONCLUSION: IF THE SHOE FITS . . .

I believe that today's corporation is no more capable of riding on one position of this horseshoe than is a horse of stepping on any one part of its shoe. In other words, we need to treat the conceptual horseshoe as a portfolio of positions from which we can draw, depending on circumstances. Exclusive reliance on any one position will lead to a narrow

---

* Of course, a number of these proposals might be worthwhile to pursue in parts of the public and parapublic sectors as well, for example to divide up overgrown hospitals, school systems, social service agencies, and all kinds of government departments.

and dogmatic society, with an excess of concentration of power. The use of a variety of positions, can encourage the pluralism I believe most of us feel is necessary to sustain democracy. If the shoe fits, then let the corporation wear it.

I do not mean to imply that some of the positions do not represent fundamentally different ideologies. Clearly they do. But I also believe that anyone who makes an honest assessment of the realities of power in and around today's large corporation, no matter to which side he or she tilts, must conclude that a variety of positions have to be relied upon.

I tilt to the left of center, as has no doubt been obvious in my comments to this point. Let me summarize my own prescriptions as follows, and in the process provide some basis for considering when it is appropriate to use each of the eight positions.

First "trust it," or at least "socialize it." Despite my suspicions about much of the rhetoric that passes for social responsibility and the discouraging evidence about the behavior of many large contemporary organizations (not only corporations), I remain firmly convinced that without honest and responsible people in important places, we are in deep trouble. We need to trust it because, no matter how much we rely on the other positions on the horseshoe, managers will always retain a great deal of discretionary power. And that power necessarily has social no less than economic consequences.

The positions on the right side of our horseshoe ignore these social consequences, while some of those on the left fail to recognize the difficulties of influencing these consequences in large, hierarchical organizations. Sitting between these two sets of positions at "trust it," managers can use their discretion to satisfy or to subvert the wishes of the public. Ultimately, what managers do is determined by their sense of responsibility as individual members of society.

Although we must "trust it," we cannot *but* "trust it." As I have argued, there is an appropriate and limited role for social responsibility— essentially to get the corporation's own house in order and to encourage it to act responsibly in its own sphere of operations. Beyond that, social responsibility needs to be influenced by other positions around our horseshoe.

Then "pressure it," ceaselessly. As we have seen, too many forces interfere with social responsibility. The best antidote to these forces is the ad hoc pressure campaign, designed to pinpoint unethical behaviors and to raise social consciousness about issues. The existence of the "pressure it" position is what most clearly distinguishes the Western from the Eastern "democracies." Give me one Ralph Nader to all those banks of government functionaries.

In fact, "pressure it" underlies the viability of most of the other positions. Pressure campaigns have, for example, brought about necessary new regulations and have highlighted the case for corporate democracy. And, as we have seen, the "ignore it" position collapses without "pressure it."

After that, try to "democratize it." A somewhat distant third in my portfolio is "democratize it," a position I view as radical only in terms of the current U.S. debate, not in terms of fundamental American values. Pluralistic control of institutions is very much in the tradition of American democracy. And democracy matters most where it affects us directly—in the water we drink, the jobs we perform, the products we consume. How can we call our society democratic when many of its most powerful institutions are closed to governance from the outside and are run as oligarchies from within?

As noted earlier, we have yet to find the means to achieve corporate democracy. But we also know how resourceful people can be when they decide to resolve a problem—and this is a problem that badly needs resolving. Somehow, ways must be found to open the corporation up to the formal influence of the constituencies most affected by it—employees, customers, neighbors, even owners of small numbers of shares—without weakening it as an economic institution. At issue is nothing less than the maintenance of basic freedoms in our society.

Then, only where specifically appropriate, "regulate it" and "induce it." Facing each other on the horseshoe are two positions that have useful if limited roles to play. Regulation is neither a panacea nor a menace. It should be used where the corporation can abuse the power it has and can be penalized for that abuse—especially where externalities can be identified with specific corporations. Financial inducements belong not where a corporation has created a problem but where it has the capability to solve a problem created by someone else.

Occasionally, selectively, "nationalize it" and "restore it," but not in Friedman's way. The extreme positions should be reserved for extreme problems. If "pressure it" is a scalpel and "regulate it" a cleaver, then "nationalize it" and "restore it" are guillotines.

Both these positions are implicitly proposed as alternatives to "democratize it." One offers public control, the other "shareholder democracy." The trouble is that control by everyone often turns out to be control by no one, while exclusive control by the owners—even if attainable—would remove the corporation even further from the influence of those most influenced by it.

Yet, as noted earlier, nationalization sometimes makes sense, namely, where private enterprise cannot provide a necessary mission, at least in a sufficient or appropriate way, and sometimes where the activities of a corporation must be intimately tied to government policy.

As for "restore it," I believe Friedman's particular proposals will aggravate the problems of political control and social responsibility, strengthening oligarchical tendencies in society and further tilting what I see as the current imbalance between social and economic goals. In response to Friedman's choice between "subversive" socialism and "free" enterprise, I say "a plague on both your houses." Let us concentrate our efforts on the intermediate positions around the horseshoe.

However, other forms of "restore it" are worth considering: to "divest it" where diversification has interfered with capital markets, competition, and economic efficiency; to "*dis*integrate it" vertically where a trading network is preferable to a managerial hierarchy; to "strengthen its board" so that directors can assess managers objectively; and to "reduce it" where size represents a power game rather than a means to provide better and more efficient service to the public. I stand with Friedman in wishing to see competitive markets strengthened; it is just that I believe his proposals lead in exactly the opposite direction.

Finally, above all, don't "ignore it." I leave one position out of my portfolio altogether, because it contradicts the others. The one thing we must not do is ignore the large, widely held corporation. It is too influential a force in our lives. Our challenge is to find ways to distribute the power in and around our large organizations so that they will remain responsive, vital, *and* effective.

16

A NOTE ON THAT DIRTY WORD "EFFICIENCY"

The title of this piece may seem cute, its tone whimsical. Don't be fooled. It deals with a critical issue in our society of organizations. The problem is not that people sneer at "efficiency experts"; it's that trying to be efficient can sometimes make us ineffective. Recalling our earlier discussion of analysis and intuition in Chapter 4, what we find here is that an obsession with being "objective" can prove subjective, that professional managers who claim to be "amoral" may find themselves drawn into decidedly immoral behaviors.

The suggestion is that management as conventionally practiced may prove to be the problem, not the solution. It may have worked against our best interests, not only as consumers of the products of organizations who seek quality and economy, but also as citizens who expect organizations to treat us as human beings. This theme underlies our discussion here; it becomes the focus of attention in the next chapter, our last. Thus, "A Note on That Dirty Word Efficiency" helps to set up our closing essay.

Why should "efficiency" be considered a dirty word in so many quarters? It is one thing when assembly line workers or student radicals rail against it, but quite another when a Harvard Business School publication refers to the label "efficiency expert" applied to a manager in one of its cases as "most uncomplimentary in connotation."[1]

Efficiency, Herbert Simon argued in *Administrative Behavior,* is a value-free concept, in his words, "completely neutral." He defined the "criterion of efficiency" as dictating "that choice of alternative which produces the largest result for the given application of resources."[2] In other words, to be efficient means to get the most of whatever goal an organization wishes to pursue—for example the most growth, the happiest employees, or the highest-quality products. Efficiency means the greatest *benefit* for the *cost,* in the words of McNamara's whiz kids at the Pentagon back in the 1960s, "the biggest bang for the buck." And since resources are always constrained in a competitive world, efficiency is a logical goal of every organization, indeed every human endeavor. It too is like "motherhood." How could anyone possibly be against efficiency?

I believe the root of the problem lies not in the definition of the term but in how that definition is inevitably put into operation. In practice, efficiency does not mean the greatest benefit for the cost; it means the greatest *measurable* benefit for the *measurable* cost. In other words, efficiency means *demonstrated* efficiency, *proven* efficiency, above all, *calculated* efficiency. A management obsessed with efficiency is a management obsessed with measurement. The cult of efficiency is the cult of calculation. And therein lies the problem.

A simple experiment demonstrates the point. I asked fifty-nine MBA students, cold, at the start of a class on another subject, to write down the first thing that came into their heads when I said that a restaurant was efficient. (Readers are invited to stop here and record their own answers.) According to Simon's definition, the answers should have varied widely. According to my contention, however, easily quantified goals should have predominated.

In fact, forty-three of the students named that most operational of goals, speed of service, in one form or another (for instance, "fast service," "no delays"). The quality of the food—surely at least as important a goal for restaurants, although less easily measured—did evoke thirteen positive comments (such as "serves good meals," "tasty food"), but also five specifically negative ones (for example, "terrible food," "serves what should be thrown out," "bland, boring, and dehumanizing"; my father, to whom I put the same question, remarked, "I don't see what efficiency has to do with food," but then, on further reflection, added, "If I heard that a restaurant was efficient, I would wonder about the food.")* I polled twenty-two more students a year later, and this time all but two mentioned speed of service (fourteen exclusively).

I also polled both groups of students on the statement that my house was efficient. Forty of the fifty-nine as well as ten of the twenty-two referred to something related to getting around in it or cleaning it up quickly. Seven of the first group and ten of the second commented on its fuel consumption. Issues of comfort, beauty, and warmth (in the psychological sense) were hardly mentioned.

---

* It should be added that a few students made comments on price, cleanliness, and profitability; note also that some made more than one comment.

Thus, in practice, efficiency is associated with criteria that are measurable. An efficient restaurant is one that gets its food on the table in thirteen minutes, independent of, or perhaps in spite of, the quality of that food. An efficient home is one that warms the bodies of its occupants with only 3,000 liters of oil during a frigid Canadian winter, not one that warms their hearts with its charm.

This orientation has three major consequences.

1. Because costs are typically more easily measured than benefits, efficiency all too often reduces to economy. Compared with benefits, costs more easily lend themselves to expression in quantitative terms—in dollars, person-hours, materials, or whatever. For example, university administrators know with some precision how much it costs to train an MBA student. But no one really has a clue how much is learned in such programs, or what effect that learning has on the practice of management.

The all-too-frequent result of an obsession with efficiency, therefore, is the cutting of tangible costs at the expense of intangible benefits. What university administrator cannot cut 10 percent from the cost of training an MBA with no *measurable* effect on the benefits? Even in a business firm, it is a simple matter for a chief executive to cut certain costs without impacting on benefits—that almightly bottom line—not in the short run, at least. One simply reduces spending on research or advertising. The effect on profits may not show up for years, long after the executive has left. All too often, therefore, efficiency just means economy, with benefits suffering at the expense of costs, so to speak. And efficiency gets a bad name.

2. Because economic costs can usually be more easily measured than social costs, efficiency often produces an escalation in social costs, which are treated as "externalities." Business firms in particular like to measure things. Peter Drucker makes this clear: The "task can be identified. It can be defined. Goals can be set. And performance can be measured. And then business can perform."[3] The problem is that some things are more easily measured than others. The dollars spent, the hours worked, the materials consumed are easily quantified. The air polluted, the minds dulled, the scenery destroyed are costs, too, but they are not so easily measured.

In all kinds of organizations, the economic costs—the tangible resources deployed—are generally easier to measure than the social costs—the consequences on people's lives. An emphasis on efficiency thus encourages the attribution of only the tangible costs to the organization; the intangible costs, usually social, get dismissed as "externalities," for which society is considered responsible. The implicit assumption is that if a cost cannot be measured, it has not been incurred. And so it is not the concern of a management responsible for "efficiency." As a result, the economic costs tend to be closely controlled by "efficient" managers, while the social costs escalate. And efficiency gets a bad name.

3. Because economic benefits are typically more easily measured than social benefits, efficiency often drives the organization toward an economic morality which can amount to a social immorality. Human activities create many benefits, ranging from the tangible to the highly ambiguous. A manager concerned with efficiency naturally favors the former; he or she can measure them and attribute them to his or her efforts. The dean who must base his promotion decisions on "hard facts" will be encouraged to count the publications of professors rather than make subjective assessments of their quality.

An obsession with efficiency therefore means that tangible, demonstrable, measurable benefits (such as speed of service) are allowed to obscure intangible, less easily specified and quantified benefits (such as the quality of food). Indeed, the more serious problem is that the former are often allowed to drive out the latter, even when the latter are generally recognized as more important. If one marches to the tune of efficiency, if one is "measured" on one's performance, then there may be no choice. Again, it is those things economic—associated with tangible resources—that best lend themselves to measurement. The social values get left behind.

Pirsig, in his popular book, *Zen and the Art of Motorcycle Maintenance,* helps us to take this point one step further, by suggesting that such social values may be beyond our skills of logic and analysis (and, therefore, measurement): "I think there is such a thing as Quality, but as soon as you try to define it, something goes haywire. You can't do it. . . . Because definitions are a product of rigid, formal thinking, Quality cannot be defined." And yet, "even though Quality cannot be defined, you know what Quality is."[4] But do the efficiency experts? Or at least, do they allow themselves to "know" that which is beyond the power of their tools?

Thus efficiency emerges in practice not as a neutral concept but as one associated with a particular system of values—economic values. In fact, an obsession with efficiency can force the trading off of social benefits for economic ones that can drive an organization beyond an economic morality to a social immorality. In Chapter 9, I cited Ackerman on how the systems of objectives used in large corporations "may actually inhibit social responsiveness" by driving out the less operational social goals.[5] And it is worth repeating here Bower's illustration of this, the turning of the financial screws in one such system, at General Electric, that contributed to the famous price-fixing scandal of 1961. As he noted, in the giant corporation, people

> . . . are rewarded for performance, but performance is almost always defined as short-run economic or technical results. The more objective the system, the more an attempt is made to quantify results, the harder it is to broaden the rules of the game to take into account the social role of the executive.[6]

Thus proeconomic behavior becomes antisocial behavior. And efficiency gets a bad name.

Thus, in practice if not in theory, efficiency is associated with a particular system of values. The call to "be efficient" is the call to calculate, where calculation means economizing, means treating social costs as externalities, and means allowing economic benefits to push out social ones. At the limit, efficiency emerges as one pillar of an ideology that worships economic goals, sometimes with immoral consequences. Thus efficiency, that "completely neutral" concept, as well as the managers and management schools obsessed with it, get a bad name.

17

SOCIETY HAS BECOME UNMANAGEABLE AS A RESULT OF MANAGEMENT

The title is a sentence from a talk I gave in 1982 at a symposium held in St. Gallen, Switzerland. The talk was my diatribe against all the things that bothered me about management and organizations. The audience of businessmen and students received it rather well, I thought. But I never published it, waiting, I guess, for the right moment. This seems to be it. The issue, the integration, the tone all seem appropriate right here, to close and cap this book.

It is interesting that a talk on the problems of management and organizations should bring together so much of my work. But that it does: Virtually every major theme I developed over these last twenty years somehow gets integrated here. I did not set out to do this; it just occurred naturally as I wove together a series of ideas. One consequence is that you will find some repetition here. In my revision and editing of the speech, I chose to leave some of that repetition in, even the occasional quotation that I felt merited being reread, because this last chapter is meant not only to highlight what I believe are critical issues in society but also to summarize the themes of this book.

I have purposely left in the speechlike tone of the discussion as well. It may seem casual in places, but I feel it helps to retain the pace of the presentation and the forcefulness with which the points are made. You might wish to consider this the literary license of an author in the concluding chapter of his book.

What I have to say here may also strike you as pessimistic. I think it is necessarily so. In my opinion, management as contemporarily practiced and organizations as contemporarily run, the two together in a society of large institutions, pose grave dangers for us all. I prefer to overstate my case to bring more attention to it. Clearly the issues are not as one-sided as presented here. But what I have written elsewhere in this book, on planning and the role of analysis in general and on the functional aspects of bureaucracy, among other things, outline my views with more balance. This final presentation is meant to be a polemic.

A business school dean once commented that while the consultants get paid for the answers, the academics get paid for the questions. This sounds like a sensible division of labor to me! It is true, though, that this paper is longer on the problems than it is on the solutions. But I do make a number of suggestions at the end (one colleague managed to identify thirteen proposals buried there). I present them, however, to stimulate thinking about these issues. This is not a finished paper but an intermediate step on the way to understanding and dealing with what I consider to be some serious problems. I suspect I shall never finish writing this article, no matter how often I try.

In the final analysis, I would like to think that the tone of this paper is really optimistic. If we can only understand how our organizations work, how and why they go out of control, and why our conventional managerial interventions have often aggravated this, then we might be able to work toward resolution of these problems. Our organizations must serve us, as workers, consumers, and citizens, by using and reflecting the best of our human qualities—our capabilities, intuitive and emotional as well as analytical, and our fundamental spirit. We need to manage organizations in ways that will make our society manageable.

In time gone by, Inuit* hunters could find their way across dozens of miles of flat white tundra to visit the camp of a friend, guided only by their intuition. A few years ago, the snowmobile of three young Inuit broke down only a few miles from their home and they froze to death because they could not make their way back.

This story disturbed me, and has since come to symbolize for me the problems of our society. I believe we are in danger of freezing to death for the same reason: Our machinery, in the broadest sense, not just our technologies, but our social systems and especially our organizations, has likewise dulled our senses, driving out our intuition and making it increasingly difficult to find our way out of our problems. My theme,

---

* "Eskimo" is actually an Indian word, a pejorative term for their neighbors to the north, meaning "eaters of raw flesh." "Inuit" is the term "the people" use for themselves.

specifically, is that society has become unmanageable as a result of management.

I am an organization theorist, interested in how organizations and the management processes that underlie them really work. I began my research career by studying the work of the managers who run organizations. I found that there were tremendous pressures on them to be superficial and concluded that managers had to learn to be effective in their superficiality. I have since begun to question that conclusion, to wonder how effectively anyone can manage a large, complex organization.

After that, I began research on the processes by which organizations make their strategies—how they establish basic directions for themselves. In my work and that of others, this turned out to be far more complicated than had been generally thought. In fact, the long favored approach, called "strategic planning," proved to be a myth: There turned out to be no systematic way to create strategy. And so I came to describe two less systematic approaches, a centralized one based on entrepreneurial vision and a decentralized one based on "grassroots" learning. But recently I have begun to wonder if either process can really work all that well in a large organization with its pressures of superficiality. Can any leader know enough to conceive a vision in an entrepreneurial way or even to deal with all those initiatives coming up from below?

In parallel work, seeking to make sense of the research on structure and power, I found it necessary to describe organizations as configurations, concluding that they succeed because they put things together in some integrated way—around central leadership or machinelike procedures or professional skills, among other things. In other words, the effectiveness of an organization lay more in integration itself than in the form that a particular integration happened to take. Later I came to realize that each integrated configuration naturally sows the seeds of its own destruction. And so I began to consider life cycle models of organizations, to show how various forms rise and fall over time. In particular, there appeared to be an entrepreneurial form for initial development, a machine or professional form for maturity, and a political form for decline, the latter eventually killing the moribund organization to allow its replacement by new entrepreneurial ones. But increasingly, I see interference with that cycle in our society, as old, spent organizations, incapable of finding new direction or inspiring their people, are sustained through political means, at the expense of the creation of fresh new ones.

Thus I now suspect that superficiality may be the problem, that as a result management may not be capable of providing new direction to our large organizations, and instead of replacing them in natural cycles, we sustain them at the expense of renewal in society.

What I wish to do here is pull together my various concerns, to assail in one place all the things I see as wrong in our highly organized societies. Please bear with me as I do this, because in some sense every sentence that follows is an overstatement (including this one!). My reason is to draw attention to a set of trends in society that I find both consequential and disturbing. I shall proceed through a series of highlighted points.

My first point is that ours is a society of organizations. What happens in our society happens in the context of organizations, from our birth in hospitals to our burial by funeral homes, including most of our work and our recreation in between.

I once looked at something called the *Encyclopedia of Associations*. In fact, it is an encyclopedia of American associations, because Americans are undoubtedly the greatest organizers of them all. (Witness the popularity of that most structured of sports, American football, with its formal field leadership, sharp division of labor, carefully planned procedures, etc.) In that encyclopedia I found, for example, The Flying Funeral Directors of America, an organization that brings together funeral directors "to create and further a common interest in flying and funeral service; to join together in case of mass disaster, and to improve flying safety"! Skipping past the National Horseshoe Pitchers' Association (15,000 member!) and the Pen Fanciers' Club (only 1000), I came to Pickle Packers International, an organization that every two years gives a "Hall of Fame" award to the person who has done the most for the pickle industry. It publishes *Picklepak* bimonthly. Nearby was the Popcorn Institute, which exists to promote the consumption of popcorn. Significant about the Popcorn Institute, according to the Encyclopedia, is that in 1960 it absorbed the Popcorn Processors Association, a harbinger, no doubt, of the wave of mergers that was to sweep across America in that decade.

If you wish to do something in this kind of society, no matter how private or recreational, do it in an organization. Otherwise you will have to explain yourself. If it's work, even the private work of, say, pulling teeth, join an organization of dentists; if it's bicycling, don't just hop on your bike and go, find a touring club that will plan it all out for you. And even if you insist on actually doing it yourself, you probably need to rely on an organization to get you there or at least to provide you with the means of doing it, if not to have informed you about being able to do it in the first place.

My second point is that our society of organizations is in good part a society of large organizations. We swim in a sea of big business, big government, big labor, big education. This has an important consequence for my own field, because it is organization theory that focuses its attention on the organization itself. Indeed, in this kind of society, organization theory may be better disposed to explain social behavior than the more established social sciences to which we have traditionally turned, notably economics and political science.

Every field of research has its central concept: In economics, it is the market, in political science, it is politics. But conventional markets and politics do not tell us a great deal about systems that operate as collections of large organizations. Large business organizations can interact in part free of purely competitive economic markets, taking on more of a political orientation, while, ironically, governments have come to look more and more like conglomerate clusters of organizations somewhat free of the formalities of legislative politics. Thus, considering "rational" entrepreneurs who maximize profit under conditions of competition, as economists traditionally do, reveals little about the behavior of big business, just as studying legislative bargaining among politicians, as in traditional political science, reveals little about the network of interlocking organizations of big government.

Of interest in this society of organizations is what most influences our thinking about how to construct organizations. Picking up on the idea of configuration, a number of different forms of organization seem to be possible, including an entrepreneurial configuration based on personal intuition, a missionary configuration based on ideology, a machine-like configuration (sometimes diversified) based on formal standardization, a professional configuration based on trained expertise, and an innovative configuration based on flexible teamwork.

My third point is that a form of structure called machine bureaucracy dominates our thinking about how organizations should be constructed. This form is familiar to us all, although not necessarily by that name (since we tend to associate bureaucracy with red tape and other dysfunctions, without stopping to realize that "getting organized," "being rational," and "achieving efficiency" are part and parcel of the same package). Machine bureaucracy is characterized by specialized and standardized work, formalized procedure, close control through rules and regulations, clear hierarchy of authority, formalized planning to formulate strategies before implementation, and so on.

I believe that to most people in our society of large organizations, what I am calling machine bureaucracy is not just *a* way to organize, it is *the* way to organize; it's not *one* form of structure, it *is* structure. This thinking dominates not only big government and big business, not just big management consulting, but also big labor, big social service, big fundraising, as well as big pickles and big popcorn.

The question thus arises, why machine bureaucracy? And the explanations are several.

The most obvious explanation—and the most "functional"—is that when operating tasks are simple and repetitive, as in the mass production of automobiles or the delivery of mail, then machine bureaucracy becomes the most natural way to organize. In other words, these conditions make it necessary to formalize, standardize, and rationalize behavior. But if these were the only reasons, then our automobile companies and post offices would be organized as machine bureaucracies but many of our other businesses and government departments might not, our schools would not, our welfare agencies would not. There must, therefore, be other forces that drive organizations to this structure.

One is the notion of countervailing power that John Kenneth Galbraith wrote about some years ago.[1] Since some organizations are big, other organizations must become big in response. And big generally means impersonal, and therefore machine bureaucratic. Big business generates big labor, big business and big labor generate big government, big government generates bigger business and bigger labor and also encourages big school systems, big social welfare organizations, perhaps big popcorn institutes as well. It all becomes one big power game.

The Cree Indians of northern Quebec have not had a tradition of centralized structure; each community, given its historical physical isolation, organized independently. But when the government bureaucrats of the "south" went in to build their dams to suck out the electricity, and, incidentally, flood the Cree lands, the Indians, in order to protest, had to "get organized." The government, being "Liberal," was, of course, willing to negotiate. But in *its* courts, by *its* system of justice. "Take us to your leader," said the government. And so the Cree had to centralize, to strengthen the leadership over its loose network of villages. And to that leadership, the system said, "Make your case. Show us the 'facts.' Collect the data, rationalize them, and present them to impress the judges, our judges." So the Cree had to formalize too—develop procedures and harden their data (count the dead animals, for example).* And centralization coupled with formalization is exactly what machine bureaucracy is. Thus, to save their traditional way of life, the Cree had to forfeit it: They had to organize like us. We didn't set out to bureaucratize the Cree culture. But moving it in that direction was an inevitable consequence of our actions.

Countervailing power is probably behind another factor that drives organizations toward machine bureaucracy: obsession with control. Control is the central driving force in these structures—control of workers, control of markets, control of the future, control of whatever might control them, including, if necessary, owners and elected governments. Bringing things under control is exactly what their planning systems are designed to do. They specify what is wanted and then program whatever is necessary to get it. (In fact, it is the obsession with planning, as a form of control, that explains all the fuss made in our society about "turbulent" conditions, about this so-called "age of discontinuity," and the like. It is not that our world has become any more unstable— quite the contrary, in fact, when anyone considers the 1930s and the 1940s. It is just that any perturbation at all, anything unexpected, such as a new competitor or a changed technology, upsets the carefully honed procedures of the planning systems and so sets the machine bureaucracies into a quivering panic. When the planners run around like Chicken Little crying, "The environment is turbulent! The environment is turbulent!," what they really mean is that something happened which was not anticipated by their inflexible systems.)

Now, in theory, an organization can control its future by being independent of outside forces. But in a society of machine bureaucracies, all obsessed with control, there is hardly anywhere to hide. So to be in control generally means doing the controlling yourself. The organization must grow bigger and try to dominate other organizations to avoid being dominated by them instead.

Consider the waves of mergers that have swept across the United States during the past century, first to consolidate firms of single industries

---

* A friend and former doctoral student, Fritz Rieger, who worked with the Cree, wrote to me in response to my request to review these comments: "The need for harder data reached extremes. I understood that in order to establish that natural foods were an essential part of the Cree diet, not only dietary inputs (quantity of natural foods consumed) but also human waste products (in significant quantities) were collected by native research assistants under direction of some McGill anthropologists and geographers for analysis!"

into giant trusts, then to extend the operating chains of these firms forward and backward in so-called vertical integration, and in more recent times to agglomerate all kinds of diversified businesses into single corporations. Some of the forces that drove these were no doubt economic. But many have also been political, when not representing a sheer lust for power then at least reflecting the reality that to avoid being taken over by another organization, you had better take it over first. How many small, healthy organizations have been destroyed over the years by having been gobbled up by the big bureaucracies (which immediately bureaucratized them—"What, no organization chart?" say the technocrats)? Unless, of course, they voluntarily forfeited that small size to become those voracious bureaucracies themselves.

But there is still another set of forces that gives rise to machine bureaucracy, in my opinion the most fundamental.

My fourth point is that an irrational form of "rationality" underlies our attraction to machine bureaucracy. Certain fields try to control words. The statisticians, for example, have tried to take over the word "significant," and in so doing may have reversed its meaning (since so much that proved "statistically significant" turned out to be trivial). So too, the economists have tried to take over the word "rational," with much the same effect. As human beings, we must above all be "rational," meaning to emphasize a strictly logical, explicit, and analytical—basically linear—form of reasoning. Everything must be worked out in advance, ideally based on numerical calculation.

This notion of rationality really amounts to mental control—mind over matter—and to the "rational" mind, mental control is the most important kind of control. And so organizations obsessed with control become organizations obsessed with this form of rationality.

To be in control in the machine bureaucracy means, above all, to have it down on paper. A market is controlled if a high number appears next to the label "market share"; quality is controlled if a low number appears next to "defects"; work is controlled if its accomplishment has been duly ticked off on a sheet of paper; people are controlled if each is connected to a boss on an organigram; the whole system is controlled if everything that must happen is recorded in a document called a "plan." It matters not that the real world goes its own merry way, so long as the mind controls the records of that world on paper. We deal with the discrepancies that arise through a process known as "creative accounting"!

How rational is this form of "rationality"? If no other form of thinking existed short of the haphazard, or if any other form that did exist was demonstrably inferior, then it would appear to be rational.

In fact, however, there is another form of thinking. We have long sensed it, have even had labels for it, although it has only been in recent years, through the hard science of physiology, that we discovered it. It appears to have been hiding all along in the mute right hemisphere of the human brain. We still do not know much about it—our words for it, "intuition" and "judgment," just label our ignorance—except that it seems to be inaccessible to our conscious ("rational") minds and appears to be neither linear nor analytical in its workings. Processing seems to take place in parallel, in a more holistic manner, oriented to synthesis.

If to be rational really means to use the process that most effectively achieves your goals, then intuition, no matter how mysterious, has never been demonstrated to be any less rational than conventional, formal "rationality"—no one has ever proved it to be an inferior process. Of course, how could they? The concept of proof itself resides in conventional rationality. How can we allow "rational" argument to prove or disprove the inferiority of a thought process that itself is beyond such rationality? That would be like using black-and-white photography to study the colors of the rainbow.

If this is true, then machine bureaucracies, because they accept only the narrow form of rationality, must be considered irrational organizations. Such rationality has been their obsession since Frederick Taylor began his time and motion studies of factory workers a century ago. Taylor's purpose was to root out instinct, intuition, and judgment in favor of this narrow form of rationality. From the factory, this same orientation moved into the office, as "rational" operations research techniques and formal information systems become popular after World War II. It then moved up the hierarchy, to culminate in the use of "strategic planning" in the executive suite. Such "rational" thinking has likewise dominated our business schools, which ostensibly train managers as if their brains had only one hemisphere. That old joke about MBA meaning "management by analysis" is no joke at all.

Bear in mind what "rationality" means in management, whether business, government, or the parapublic sector—it makes no difference. To rationalize almost inevitably means to cut, to reduce, to eliminate, not to integrate or grow or create. In effect, rationalizing is to the contemporary manager what bloodletting was to the medieval physician. No matter

what form it takes—firing workers, cutting budgets, restructuring, etc.—
rationalizing becomes the machine bureaucracy's solution to all of its
problems. Integrating, growing, and creating depend in good part on
the other mode of thinking—on viewing things holistically, from the
perspective of synthesis, processes that seem to be beyond the machine
bureaucracy.

Such rationalizing tends to be promoted by numerically literate people—the technocrats—for whom control means rules not skills, behavior
means standards not norms, decision-making means analysis not intuition.
When the other form of thinking is called for, the machine bureaucracy
usually cannot respond. Thus small firms taken over by large ones are
not allowed to be loose and informal; inspired organizations captured
by conglomerates are not allowed to believe in anything beyond measurable ("bottom line") efficiency; creative and professional organizations
that come under the control of big governments are not allowed to be
innovative or to be proficient. All behavior must come under the technocratic control of the rules, the standards, the analyses.

We see this most clearly—most irrationally—in our school systems,
which in my opinion have become areas of unmitigated disaster. In the
name of rationality, education has been inundated with curricula carefully
planned in offices distant from the classroom and has been forced into
facilities cleverly rationalized to be efficient. Both look wonderful on
paper. Yet both, by imposing forms of control incompatible with the
activities in question (for reasons to be discussed later), have produced
unprecedented alienation. We end up, here and in many other spheres
of human activity, with "rationally" designed organizational machines
that affront us—machines for which people hate to work and from which
people hate to take service.

If formal proof is rooted in the conventional view of rationality, then
"prove it" is the motto of a society of organizations. This means that
you win points by proving it explicitly, quantitatively—by "rational"
argument, analytical and logical, based on "hard," replicable data.
"Sense" doesn't count, not intuitive sense. As an Inuit, you would be
expected to make your way across the tundra with a map and a compass
tucked under the seat of your snowmobile. Even if no one had charted
the territory before and there existed no magnetic field for guidance.
That way at least you could show how you did it, prove it to people
who have never seen snow. If you got out alive. As a Cree, you have
to dress up as a lawyer (or better, hire one of ours) and present logical
arguments, eloquently, supported by facts and figures. And you must

do this in a perfectly orderly courtroom, a thousand miles from the chaos of your swamped land and its dead animals.

"Prove it" manifests itself most pointedly in the question period of parliamentary democracy, where each day opposition members bombard government ministers with embarrassing questions. Under the glare of the television lights (in Canada at least), ministers have to justify to the nation what they have done (or, more often, what some civil servant they never met did in Moose Jaw, Saskatchewan). Imagine the Prime Minister arising in response to a question about why he funded some project or other with the comment, "because it felt good, because deep in my gut I knew it was right." No, he must have facts, formal justifications, logical arguments. The same, of course, holds true for presidential press conferences in the United States.

But how else can you run a modern state, you might wonder? We can't have politicians running around doing whatever they please. True enough. But neither can we have them denying their innate feel for things. Or more to the point, neither can we afford to have people in positions of influence who lack such feelings. Maybe they never had a chance to develop them in the first place; most were, after all, lawyers who spent their careers in those orderly courtrooms, far from the snow and the dead animals. But people with richer experiences do sometimes make it to government too. But how can innate sense work in that environment? What happens to feel and intuition when all these people see around them are facts and figures, files and filibusters, slick technocrats professing analytical arguments and superficial politicians mouthing easy opinions?

Certainly, when there are reliable facts our leaders had better get them right. But how often are the facts reliable? How often do different "facts" contradict each other? And how often do superficial facts suppress deeper wisdom? Where does intuition come in? The parliamentary question period and the U.S. presidential press conference have certainly proved a boon to problem recognition. But they turn out to be a menace to problem solution. They expose problems in a marvelously public way, and then impose superficial solutions on them, solutions that violate our real needs.

If you are in business, you may be inclined to dismiss some of this, attributing it to the pressures of the political process. But that would miss a major point: The problem is fundamentally organizational. It is rooted in a major premise of machine bureaucracy, private no less than public, that it is those people who sit on the top of an organizational hierarchy—whether called manager or minister—who must decide. It is they who are responsible. And the reason is that they know better. All the information comes together right there, at their level. Anyone can see this on the organigram, right there on paper, where all the lines join.

Of course, you might wonder how this can be. How can people who sit in offices wearing shirts and ties all day long know so much about the services rendered in Moose Jaw, the lands flooded in James Bay, the products produced in Saskatoon and sold in Trois Pistoles? Simple, they have a system to inform them. It is called an MIS—management information system. Everything they need to know gets recorded—black figures on white paper. All they have to do to get informed is to read. And if there is too much to read, the system takes care of that too: It aggregates. It combines data, packages them neatly and dispenses them to the leaders in neat periodic reports. In government, it's the opinion poll. So much more convenient than having to talk to real citizens. In business, it's the accounting statement and the marketing research report. A lot quicker and more "rational" than having to visit factories and meet customers. Or it's capital budgeting, a procedure whereby senior managers are expected to approve major proposals on the basis of reviewing aggregated figures of costs and benefits, neatly combined into projections of return on investment. Another form of "prove it."

The problem with all this aggregated rationality is that it drives out judgment and intuition. How can you feel if you cannot see for yourself? How can you sense if you cannot experience firsthand?

Nowhere is this better reflected than in the world of the contemporary MBA. How do we train managers, the leaders of our organizations, where products are hammered out in messy factories and then sold in busy market places? We lock bright and inexperienced people up in austere buildings and inundate them with paper. They never set foot in a factory, never meet a customer. Cases do it for them instead, much like those MIS reports in practice. The cases describe the real world, right there on paper—the products, the personalities, the politics, they're all there, in black on white. The MBAs "know" because they've read it all in a pithy twenty-page report the night before. On a given day it might be General Motors: what that hundred billion dollar corporation should do to secure its future. They all decide together, all those eager young MBAs, all challenging each other to "prove it."

Recently I got into a discussion with a group of MBA students about the excessive reliance on numerical scores to assess applicants to the program. I wondered what that had to do with native managerial ability, including intuition. One student asked: How can you select for intuition if you can't even measure it?! But another raised a more reasonable point: Would not the use of judgment introduce bias into the selection process? Absolutely, I replied, because bias is the other side of judgment. The best way to get rid of bias is to get rid of judgment. But at what price?

Is it not the elimination of judgment that so characterizes the bureaucratic institutions of our age? Is that not in good part why government is so bureaucratic—to ensure that citizens are not discriminated against or that the minister does not sneak his mistress onto the payroll? It's all very efficient at rooting out bias. Too bad it destroys organizational effectiveness.

Let us return to that court of law, where "proving it" is the means to eliminate bias. In the case of a challenge by an employee who has been fired, the courts say to the employer: "Don't tell us that person was incompetent, disagreeable, an impediment to the work of everyone else. No opinions please, just the facts and figures. Prove it. How many days off? How do you know she wasn't sick? Maybe the lighting at work made her sick. He insulted the customers? Well, customers can be disagreeable too. Prove they weren't.'' Better to keep the employee than face all that. (And bear in mind which organizations can afford to keep that employee.) Thus, in seeking to protect the individual from false (biased) dismissal, certainly a proper thing to do, we build bureaucratic systems free of the exercise of judgment that tie everyone else in knots.* Surely we must face the dilemma of having to balance the exercise of judgment with the avoidance of bias. As Solzhenitsyn has commented:

> I have spent all my life under a communist regime and I will tell you that a society without any objective legal scale is a terrible one indeed.

---

* I must add a note on academic tenure here. It, too, was introduced to eliminate bias, in this case the arbitrary dismissal of faculty members with unpopular views by governments or university trustees. Tenure was designed to protect freedom of expression. But today it's effect is exactly the opposite: It suppresses freedom of expression. That is because the threat to the maverick academic now comes not from the outside but from his or her own colleagues. Whereas once *having* tenure may have protected those who spoke out, today *getting* tenure menaces them. Their offended colleagues will seek to deny it to them. Thus tenure works to weed out those who do not toe the accepted line, whether that be conservative economics at one university or radical sociology at another.

But a society with no other scale but the legal one is not quite worthy of man either. A society which is based on the letter of the law and never reaches any higher is taking very scarce advantage of the high level of human possibilities. The letter of the law is too cold and formal to have a beneficial influence on society. Whenever the tissue of life is woven of legalistic relations, there is an atmosphere of moral mediocrity, paralyzing man's noblest impulses.[2]

Thus no matter who wins, it is inevitably *judgment* that the courts strike down, *gut feel* that the government procedures preclude, *intuition* that the corporate systems eliminate. Judgment, gut feel, and intuition can't be justified, not the way "rational" argument can. No matter where you function in a bureaucratic society, then, you have to "prove" your case, even if there are no maps, no compasses, no magnetic fields. And if you have to prove it, you can't feel it, you can't sense it. You forget how to use your intuition. So when the machinery breaks down, you're stranded.

My fifth point is that a society of large, "rational," machine bureaucratic organizations dictates an age of capital letter MANAGEMENT, so-called professional, that often proves thin, superficial, and sometimes immoral. What characterizes this dominant configuration of machine bureaucracy above all is the power of its administrators. The rules, the standards, the data, the rationales, these come from the administrators—line managers as well as staff analysts, the planners, systems people, accountants, and many others of the technostructure. When Robert Michels set out his "iron law of oligarchy" early in this century ("who says organization, says oligarchy") he was talking about the inevitable power of the administrators in machine bureaucracy.[3]

It is not just management that matters in our society of large organizations, but "rational" management, analytical management, management defined as "professional." But what does the word "professional" mean in the context of managing? It surely does not mean the same as in medicine or engineering, for these fields have certified methods for diagnosing and for solving practical problems in particular contexts. We certainly have techniques in management, no shortage of those, but none certified in that way. Indeed, we know a lot more about the failure of our techniques—whether PPBS, "total" information systems, giant models of the firm, or strategic planning—than we do about their successful applications. In other words, we have almost no systematic evidence on the successful practice of management, at least as compared with the complexity of the everyday job of managing. Against the occasional study of what managers actually do, and the no less rare study of how a particular technique actually functioned in practice, are the reams of publications imploring managers to use the latest techniques because they are so elegantly rational. And our universities do no better. A good part of MBA training is devoted to drill in techniques, free of context, most of whose abilities have never been demonstrated in practice. The occasional student who asks the nasty question is likely to be told that the reason the technique is not used is because it is so far ahead of those neanderthal managers practicing out there.

Thus, formal education can hardly be considered a prerequisite to practicing this so-called profession. No one identifies successful managers on the basis of holding an MBA (apart from the fact that it starts them off on that fast track). Indeed, if the success of the Japanese in practicing management compared with their reluctance to teach it is any indication, then conventional MBA training should be considered part of the problem, not part of the solution.

What "professional" means, then, is really "generic," that is, people armed with this arbitrary set of techniques can manage anything. They are specialists in nothing more than the management process itself. The context in which it is to be applied is not relevant. In medicine, this would be equivalent to physicians who, because they know how to cut, assume they can replace hearts as well as remove gallbladders; in engineering, to engineers who, because they know how to design (or more to the point, have a computer-aided program to do so on their desks), assume they can construct nuclear reactors as well as build bridges.

"Professional management" is the great invention of this century, an invention that produced gains in organizational *efficiency* so great that it eventually destroyed organizational *effectiveness*. The idea grew out of Taylor's early time and motion study work. Taylor's idea was that you programmed a task by studying it meticulously so that you could decompose it into clear steps, and then set up a specific procedure for carrying out each one. His work rendered enormous improvements in the efficiency of the highly routine physical work of the factory and equivalent clerical work of the office. This hardly endeared Taylor and the many time study analysts who followed him to the workers in question, but it worked. In other words, it proved *efficient* to treat workers as machines, with arms and legs but no brains. Personal involvement with the task may have been sacrificed, even quality and capacity for innovation, but the effects on the costs of production were dramatic.

Through professional management, Taylor's approach was brought to all areas of organizational activity, from scheduling production and selecting employees to formulating strategy. But not his basic message, because that was in fact misunderstood.

Taylor did not try to program work that he did not fully comprehend. His studies and experiments were meticulous. He described before he prescribed. Many of his imitators never learned that lesson. Strategic planners, for example, leapt into prescription in the face of almost total ignorance about how strategies really do form. We had barely any empirical evidence on strategy-making throughout the 1960s and 1970s, when strategic planning was promoted so aggressively. It was simply assumed that the "rational" approach was better. Now we do have some evidence, and it shows how naïve the assumptions that underlie strategic planning really were. For one thing, strategy-making depends importantly on synthesis, while formal planning offers only analysis. Disaggregating a process into steps and checklists does not reintegrate it. For another, strategy-making is a highly dynamic process, one of slow learning over time in response to unpredictable events. For this, formal planning offered a static sequence of steps, converting a future considered predictable into a set of prescheduled strategies.

In 1979, in order to explain the success of Texas Instruments, Marianne Jelinek published *Institutionalizing Innovation*. Her argument, in essence, was that Taylor's successes in the factory could be replicated in the executive offices by processes that were fundamentally the same, though on a different level of abstraction. "It is through administrative systems that planning and policy are made possible because the *systems* capture knowledge about the task."[4] But those systems captured nothing; they failed soon after the book was published: Texas Instruments' own fancy planning system was subsequently believed to *dis*courage innovation.[5] In fact, there never was any evidence that the company's success stemmed from anything more than a capable leader who knew how to learn and whose own energy and enthusiasm enabled him to attract good people and to invigorate them. Good people, of course, make for good organizations. They also design good systems, at least systems that are good for them. But remove the good people and the systems collapse. Innovation, it turned out, could not be institutionalized.

But strategic planning and other techniques failed not only because of ignorance of the processes they tried to replace. They also failed because Taylor's approach was not suited to other contexts, to situations where the mind and the motivation of the worker mattered more than his or her ability to do simple, routine tasks.

Taylor said, many years ago, "In the past the man has been first; in the future the system must be first."[6] Prophetic words indeed. It is the procedure that counted, not the person who happened to execute it. Now, if you are dealing with the carrying of pig iron—to cite one of Taylor's famous studies—then such an attitude may not matter all that much, at least not to those concerned strictly with an organization's efficiency. The work gets done, quickly, so long as people remain willing to do it, even if it makes them miserable. But when the work requires the thinking of the worker, then it also requires that person's motivation—his or her involvement and commitment. Formal systems do not put the brain into gear; rather they disengage it. Removing control over the work from the worker—as, for example, strategic planning did to the managers expected to carry out the plans—had the eventual effect of destroying that motivation.

Thus professional management, by putting the systems ahead of the people, has had the effect of bleeding out of organizations, slowly and gradually, their capacity to do mental work as it must be done—with energy, vigor, and imagination. Taylor's "scientific management" has exacted its toll not only on the workers who don't care about the products of their labor, but also on the managers and analysts who have been equally dehumanized by the whole effort.

Thus has the cult of rationality, as manifested in so-called professional management, served to destroy the deep-rooted effectiveness of many of our large organizations, by squeezing out their very humanness. In its own form of *reductio ad absurdum,* professional management made organizations so rational, so efficient, that they ceased to function effectively. Alfred Chandler and Oliver Williamson have published highly acclaimed books about the advantages of administrative systems over market relationships.[7] Managers were described as being able to manage certain transactions within their administrative hierarchies (for example, through vertical integration) more efficiently than could trading relationships deal with them in the marketplace. But at what cost in human terms? And in organizational effectiveness? Chandler titled his Pulitzer Prize-winning book *The Visible Hand,* to contrast the power of administration with Adam Smith's "invisible hand" of market forces. "The Visible Claw" might have been a more appropriate title.

Why do we persist in imputing such powers to management systems?

How can we so condemn the centralized management of governments in Eastern Europe while remaining so enamored of the same form of management in our Western corporations? Why do we insist on attributing every human success in organizations to systems, pretending that we can sustain idiosyncratic human initiative by perpetuating the formal procedures that merely aid it? What is wrong with recognizing success as residing in the energy, the intelligence, and the commitment of individual flesh-and-blood human beings?

Two personal stories illustrate well, I believe, the widespread feelings about the effects of impersonalized management. Shortly after I published my article ''The Manager's Job: Folklore and Fact,'' the *New York Times* ran a story on it in which they characterized my description as ''calculated chaos'' and ''controlled disorder.''[8] A few days later I received calls from a radio station in Winnipeg and a television network in Toronto, in both cases from production assistants working on morning programs who requested interviews on the air. Both added a curious comment in those calls, to the effect that ''Are we glad someone finally let managers have it!''

Now one thing my article certainly did *not* do was let managers have it; both women who called had read only the *Times* account, but that did not give such an impression either. Indeed, managers themselves have been the most enthusiastic recipients of my article. Why then the comments? I believe they were a reaction to what those people experienced management to be—the impersonal directives coming down from above. It was not flesh-and-blood managers they saw up there, not people struggling like them to deal with complex problems, but cold, impersonal systems. I was certainly letting *that* have it, if not them. But to the people who called, the two seemed synonymous. And so words like ''chaos'' and ''disorder'' appeared to them to debunk managers rather than to humanize them.

The second story reinforces the first. Some time ago, I was asked to join a group that was screening a series of National Film Board of Canada films called ''Corporation,'' about the Steinberg supermarket chain and especially about its colorful leader, Sam Steinberg. I am hardly a right-wing reactionary, but this was a particularly radical group. (It was shortly after 1968, and this was a retreat on Vancouver Island.) One member of the group referred to the films as ''subversive'' because they made Sam Steinberg seem so affectionately human: Everyone *knew* that managers were really sons of bitches!

Some years ago, a professor named Albert Shapero expressed the point well with an article entitled "What MANAGEMENT Says and What Managers Do." Like him, I believe it is capital-letter MANAGE-MENT that is the son of a bitch, not small-letter managers. "Twenty-five years of MANAGEMENT have resulted in an Analysis in Wonderland outlook where abstractions are reality and where people and things are ciphers or difficulties to be dealt with."[9] It is the impersonal systems that people rail against, the dehumanizing nature of a professional management that believes it can function free of context, free of human initiative. The systems will do it. Of course, there is no shortage of capital-letter MANAGERS who believe they can capital-letter MANAGE by staying in their offices and using their authority to dictate bottom-line performance by playing with numbers on financial statements and boxes on portfolio grids. But we should not forget that there does still exist another form of management, in which very human people work hard to understand their world and those who populate it, people who feel the need to be more rational than the rationality that surrounds them and so find the need to work in calculated chaos. Of course, the reason we sometimes forget this, as did those two production assistants, is that we are so inundated with the systems of MANAGEMENT.

Earlier, I mentioned that I had changed my views on the issue of superficiality in managerial work. In my own study, I found that the pressures of their job drove managers to be superficial; I concluded that the effective managers were the ones who had learned to be proficient at their superficiality. For example, they knew they had to make decisions with inadequate information, that deciding, even superficially, was prefer-able to not deciding at all because that at least enabled their organization to do *something*. Or else, lacking knowledge of the details of specific proposals, they could choose the sponsors of those proposals instead, allowing their intuition to function where they did have knowledge, namely about the character of their people.

Increasingly, however, I have begun to believe that superficiality *is* the problem. To continue with overstatement, but as always in the hope of conveying an important grain of truth, inherent in the job of being a manager is the need to make decisions on things one knows nothing about. Now, of course, the job of the manager is to know things, to get informed. And in small organizations, as well as in larger ones concentrated on a particular business, managers can do that, at least if they have some deep-rooted knowledge of the issues in question (which means that there had to have been life before management, in the factories and with the customers, which probably also means there was no MBA early in the career to project the inexperienced directly into the abstractions of administration). But I would maintain that to be so informed in other organizations has become enormously difficult due to distance and detachment. In other words, to manage at the senior levels of today's large, complex, and especially diversified organization is to have only the most superficial knowledge of the things that must be decided about.

The purpose of the management information system is, of course, to inform the manager. As noted earlier, the professional manager is supposed to sit back in his or her office and read MIS reports. Because there is too much to absorb, the data are aggregated, periodicized, and packaged neatly (thereby magically making the unknowable knowable). That is how professional managers in machine bureaucracies are supposed to "know."

But how much does anyone who reads words and numbers on pieces of paper really know? Not much, I suspect, because there is another kind of "knowing," one more relevant for the management of organizations. Borrowing a word from the anthropologist Clifford Geertz, I shall call it "thick knowing," resulting in "thick management."[10] "Thin management" remains distant from the subject of its efforts, acting as if it moved pieces on a chessboard (the "portfolio" of businesses is one popular conception), making little effort to influence what those pieces really do, even how they relate to each other in any but the most superficial ways. Faced with an organization's lack of innovation, thin management throws cash at a research and development facility; faced with declining profits in a division, thin management sells it or fires its manager; faced with the need to bring the wonders of electronics to its products, thin management acquires an electronics firm and slaps it together with its own activities; faced with public accusations of the organization's social irresponsibility, thin management appoints a vice president in charge of social responsibility to be responsible for everyone else.

A management informed by the MIS, a management whose knowledge consists of black symbols on white paper, is afraid to intervene in any but these most superficial of ways. Epitomizing the "thin" form of information—aggregated, analytical, detached—were the body counts of Vietnam. That is how Secretary of Defense McNamara "knew" what was going on in that unfortunate war. Robert McNamara was, of course, the archetypal professional manager, the hero of a generation of MBAs, just as the U.S. Army was the archetypal machine bureaucracy.

"Thick" information, in contrast, is information rich in detail and color, far beyond what can be quantified and aggregated. It must be dug out, on site, by people intimately involved with the phenomenon they wish to influence. In Vietnam, it was the look on a peasant's face; in business, the will of a customer, the mood of the factory, the intricacies of a technological change; in government, it is the service that actually gets delivered and the citizen's response to that service at the moment of delivery. This is the kind of information, it seems to me, that informs intuition and that allows for "thick management," a management that intervenes deeply to influence and to integrate activities. Those who practice this kind of management bypass the MIS to ensure that they get informed. They drop in on their facilities unexpectedly or, better, work in them periodically; they meet their customers or, better, *are* their customers, consuming their own products and services whenever they can.

Unfortunately, when organizations become large, complex, and diversified, managers can't do these things very easily; they are precluded from managing in thick ways. There is simply too much to do, too much to know. That is why our political leaders live on aggregated opinion polls instead of speaking with ordinary citizens (a recent Canadian news story accused the Conservative government of averaging four polls a *week* for its several years in office!), and why business leaders do the same with market research reports instead of meeting ordinary customers. What they get are abstractions often as deadly as those body counts. The statistic replaces the flesh-and-blood human being, and the managers think they are informed, while the citizens and the customers burn.

Of course, the machine bureaucracy, at least the one with diversified markets, has an answer for this problem too, one rooted in its belief in the division of labor. The managers at headquarters, who cannot be well informed about many diverse businesses, manage the strategic portfolio—they buy and sell businesses. It is the managers of the divisions who manage the individual businesses, where the necessary knowledge can be obtained. Unfortunately, it does not work out quite as planned. The division managers, who are supposed to be looking down to manage their own businesses, feel the gaze from above; they thus get distracted by having to glance up from time to time. There is just something about being controlled superficially, by having to satisfy someone who cannot see beyond that bottom line. To manage is to control, in one way or another. Too many levels of management has to mean too much control. Thus, the administrative arrangements promoted by Chandler and Williamson are not better at all, not after they have squeezed the human energy and involvement out of the people through their continual pressures and rationalizations, through their obsession with controlling performance directly.

This brings us back to the subject of strategy formation, setting the direction for an organization. Now strategy can be viewed as simply *position,* or else as more complex *perspective.* One focuses on the products and markets selected, the other on the business idea conceived, the organization's way of doing things. Portfolio management treats strategy as position, or at least a set of positions loosely coupled. That is compatible with thin management. But it is insufficient, because positions must have substance too; there must be some rich perspective behind each one. And such perspective cannot be developed without thick knowing, without deep-rooted involvement. Put another way, rich, creative strategy formation requires rich knowledge and mental synthesis. But synthesis, as noted, is quite different from rational analysis; it seems to be the province of the brain's mysterious right hemisphere and appears to be fed primarily by soft data. Thus, because our machine bureaucracies, whether or not diversified, are oriented to hard data and analytical thinking, they tend to treat strategy as no more than position. And so they tend to end up with thin strategies, bland and lifeless, at best imitations of the strategies already invented by other organizations—the "Whoppers" of this world in response to the "Big Macs."

For some time, in fact, machine bureaucracies have recognized the problem—that their managers are often incapable of generating rich new strategies. So they have relied on a system to do it for them instead, namely strategic planning. But as suggested earlier, that system has no real substance: It is just another set of black words on sheets of white paper. Each is placed in its appropriate box, labeled, for example, "assess your competitive advantage" or "generate strategies to match strengths with opportunities." But inside, the boxes are empty—no one ever explained how these things are to be done.

Behind the boxes are, of course, the planners. So it is really they who take charge of the process, using the cover of technique to promote their own influence. The "whiz kids"—the "best and the brightest," to use Halberstam's label for those responsible for the Vietnam debacle[11]—claim to do what thin management cannot do. They will pull the strategic rabbit out of an overgrown left hemisphere, so to speak. Of course, they never could. They could read all the documents, all the hard data; they could analyze furiously; they could write eloquently.

But it all lacked substance. Their strategies, like their knowledge, were thin; ultimately there was no wisdom.

Wisdom is a word that seems to have been lost in the English language. It suggests deep knowledge, based on substantial experience—intimate experience. The whiz kids lack wisdom, indeed, in their bias toward systematic analysis, they tend to denigrate it.

I collect definitions of the expert. Best known, perhaps, is: "An expert is a guy from out of town." The whiz kids tend to be from out of the industry. They are professionals; they don't let an ignorance of specifics interfere with their application of analysis. Another favorite definition is: "An expert is someone with no elementary knowledge." This captures the idea that the whiz kids have the facts and figures, all the sophistication that comes out of the computer, but they lack "street sense," wisdom. My own favorite definition is: "An expert is a person who avoids all the many pitfalls on his or her way to the grand fallacy." Pitfalls are sins to be avoided in order to serve the almighty, in this case rational analysis. But the pitfalls claimed by the experts in the "science" of management are superficial, only skin deep, and in any event are blamed on others, never on analysis. For example, planning fails because managers are not committed to it; analytical studies are ignored because organizations are too political. What trips up the whiz kids, however, are not these pitfalls at all (managers have given far more commitment to planning than it ever deserved; and analysis has done its share to politicize organizations), but some more fundamental fallacies, for example that discontinuities can be forecast in systematic ways, that hard data can substitute for soft, that decomposition and rationalization are what matter. The grand fallacy is that analysis magically provides synthesis.

In all these ways, the age of management has become the age of the "quick fix." Call in your technocrats, throw a lot of technique at a problem, drown it in hard data, the data you can get without ever having to leave your comfortable office, and all will be well. Resolve it quickly so that you can get on with the next problem. Better still, call in the consultants to resolve it; they know even less about your industry; you get a slick report from the experts; the board will be impressed (what do they know anyway?). If it's a strategy you need, they have a nice list of generic ones to choose from. If your culture is no longer any good, they have four easy steps to a new one. Quality, you say? Well, they can measure that.

Then, once you have the final answer, let others lower down in the hierarchy work it all out. It is called "implementation." Implementation means dropping a solution into the laps of people informed enough to know it won't work but restricted from telling anyone with power what can. So while administrators in the executive suites are smiling about how "Quality is Job 1" or whatever, the implementers are running around the factories trying to plug the holes. (I was on a panel recently with a top Ford executive who talked about their quality program; I mentioned a report I had seen just before about an awful work situation in a Ford assembly plant. The executive dismissed it as an isolated problem in one factory. After the session, two people came up to tell me of similar situations they had encountered in two other Ford plants. Sometimes I wonder how much such programs—whether or not conceived in good faith—amount to substance and how much to administrative wheel-spinning, and whether a distant management can even tell the difference.)

Occasionally someone does write about the reality of management, and the effect can be stunning. Let me recount two examples. Some years ago, the British Government hired the Boston Consulting Group (BCG) to help explain how it was that the Japanese firms, especially Honda, took over the U.K. firms' markets for motorcycles in the United States. (In 1959, they had a 49 percent market share; by 1966 Honda alone had 63%!) They issued their report in 1975 and it was vintage BCG, and classic rational MANAGEMENT (so much so that the report became the basis for well-known cases used at American business schools to teach the students exemplary strategic behavior). The report was all about experience curves and high market shares and carefully thought-out deliberate strategies and the like, especially how a firm dedicated to low cost, using the scale of its domestic production base, attacked the American market by forcing entry through a new segment—the sale of small motorcycles to middle-class consumers. Very clever, those Japanese. To quote from the BCG report:

> The Japanese motorcycle industry, and in particular Honda, the market leader, present a [consistent] picture. The basic philosophy of the Japanese manufacturers is that high volumes per model provide the potential for high productivity as a result of using capital intensive and highly automated techniques. Their marketing strategies are, therefore, directed towards developing these high model volumes, hence the careful attention that we have observed them giving to growth and market share.[12]

Wondering about all this, Richard Pascale, co-author of *The Art of*

Japanese Management,[13] flew to Japan and interviewed the Japanese managers who had done all this in America. They told a different story.

"In truth, we had *no* strategy other than the idea of seeing if we could sell *something* in the United States." Honda had to obtain a currency allocation from the Japanese Ministry of Finance, part of a government so famous for supporting the competitiveness of its industry abroad. "They were extraordinarily skeptical," said the managers, finally granting Honda the right to invest $250,000 in the U.S., but only $110,000 in cash!

"Mr. Honda was especially confident of the 250cc and 305cc machines," the managers continued about their leader. "The shape of the handlebars on these larger machines looked like the eyebrow of Buddha, which he felt was a strong selling point."

The managers rented a cheap apartment in Los Angeles; two of them slept on the floor. In their warehouse in a rundown section of town, they swept the floors themselves and stacked the motorcycles by hand, to save money. Their arrival in America coincided with the *closing* of the 1959 motorcycle season.

The next year, a few of the larger bikes began to sell. Then, as they put it, "disaster struck." Because motorcycles are driven longer and faster in the U.S., the Hondas begun to break down. "But in the meantime," to use their words, *"events had taken a surprising turn"*:

> Throughout our first eight months, following Mr. Honda's and our own instincts, we had not attempted to move the 50cc Supercubs. While they were a smash success in Japan (and manufacturing couldn't keep up with demand there), they seemed wholly unsuitable for the U.S. market where everything was bigger and more luxurious. As a clincher, we had our sights on the import market—and the Europeans, like the American manufacturers, emphasized the larger machines.
>
> We used the Honda 50cc ourselves to ride around Los Angeles on errands. They attracted a lot of attention. One day we had a call from a Sears buyer. While persisting in our refusal to sell through an intermediary, we took note of Sears' interest. But we still hesitated to push the 50cc bikes out of fear they might harm our image in a heavily macho market. But when the larger bikes started breaking, *we had no choice.* We let the 50cc bikes move.[14]

The rest is history. Sales rose dramatically. Middle-class Americans began to ride on Hondas, first the Supercubs, later the larger bikes. Even the famous ad campaign—"You meet the nicest people on a Honda"—was serendipitous: It was conceived by a UCLA undergraduate for a class project. Shown the idea, the Honda managers—still trying to straddle the market and not antagonize the black leather jacket types—were split. Eventually the sales director talked his more senior colleagues into accepting it!

Well, then, what in the world makes the Japanese so smart? This is a story of success, not failure, yet they seemed to do everything wrong. Indeed, the story violates everything we believe about effective management (and much that BCG imputed to those clever Japanese). Just consider the passive tone of the Japanese managers' comments ("events took a surprising turn," "we had no choice," etc.) compared with the willful vocabulary of the BCG report.

If this story is any indication, then the Japanese advantage lies not in their cleverness at all, but in our own stupidity. While we run around being "rational," they use their common sense. Their secret seems to be as much in what they *avoid* as in what they *have*. Honda avoided being too rational. Rather than believing they could work it all out in Tokyo, they came to America prepared to *learn*. As Pascale put it, "success was achieved by senior managers humble enough not to take their initial strategic positions too seriously." We build organizations so they cannot learn. The formulators lack the information, the implementers lack the power. The Honda managers let the market hit them over the head with its needs until they got the message.

And what the Japanese *have* is a different form of organization. The managers of the Honda story had commitment—they were in America to work it out, without having to report to some silly controller in Tokyo every week or two. (Jay Galbraith, a consultant and researcher in management, tells the story of the headquarters managers who pull up the young shoots that the divisions have planted to have a look with the comment "no roots yet"!) And they had involvement, on site—they met the dealers and customers, drove the motorcycles on the streets of America.

Now imagine two British motorcycle manufacturers wanting to get back into the American market. You give one the BCG report, the other the Honda managers' account. What would each do? In the obvious answers—one going back upstairs to do even more clever strategy analysis, the other buying a pair of jeans and moving to Driggs, Idaho, to ride motorcycles—you get the perfect juxtaposition of thin and thick management.

In fact, the most revealing aspect of this story for me came in a book I recently discovered called *Whatever Happened to the British Motorcycle Industry?* Here, Bert Hopwood recalls as an executive of BSA, one of the principal British motorcycle producers, that "not a soul on the Parent Board [meaning full-time senior executives] knew the first thing about single track vehicles." More significantly, "in the early 1960s," at precisely the moment when the Japanese managers were in America learning,

> . . . the Chief Executive of a world famous group of management consultants tried hard to convince me that it is ideal that top level management executives should have as little knowledge as possible relative to the product. This great man really believed that this qualification enabled them to deal efficiently with all business matters in a detached and uninhibited way.[15]

That is where we were not so many years ago!!

The second story reflects exactly the same philosophy, except that its consequences were far more serious than losing a market for motorcycles. This philosophy was implicated in the most devastating chapter in British military history, the World War I battle of Passchendaele. The chiefs had their plan at headquarters. It was a clever plan. Unfortunately it did not account for the possibility of rain while the battle was fought; 250,000 British troops fell as a result:

> The critics argued that the planning of Passchendaele was carried out in almost total ignorance of the conditions under which the battle had to be fought. No senior officer from the Operations Branch of the General Headquarters, it was claimed, ever set foot (or eyes) on the Passchendaele battlefield during the four months that battle was in progress. Daily reports on the condition of the battlefield were first ignored, then ordered discontinued. Only after that battle did the Army chief of staff learn that he had been directing men to advance through a sea of mud.[16]

To quote Stokesbury's account in his history of World War I, the "great plan" was implemented despite the effect the steady, drenching rain had on the battlefield—despite the fact that guns clogged, that soldiers carrying heavy ammunition slipped off their paths into muddy shell holes and drowned, that the guns could not be moved forward and the wounded could not be brought backward. "Still the attack went on; they slept between sheets at corps headquarters and lamented that the infantry did not show more offensive spirit."

> [A] staff officer . . . came up to see the battlefield after it was all quiet again. He gazed out over the sea of mud, then said half to himself, "My God, did we send men to advance in that?" after which he broke down weeping and his escort led him away. Staff officers . . . complained that infantrymen failed to salute them.[17]

The formulators finished formulating and then the implementers had to implement. One decided, the other saluted. Thus does the age of management become an age of superficiality; thus does efficiency produce ineffectiveness.

Perhaps these officers were well-intentioned, even if misguided. But professional management can sometimes produce not just superficial behavior but immoral behavior as well. The systems simply deflect good intentions, or else encourage bad ones. To quote Singer and Wooton with reference to Albert Speer's seemingly enlightened management of the Nazi wartime production machine, "It's not that managers are authoritarian themselves; rather . . . it may be that the process of management is authoritarian."[18]

The professional manager claims to be a "hired gun," so to speak, there with the technique to apply to any set of needs. "Tell us what you want," such managers claim, "and we can get you the most of it." Professional managers are ostensibly "amoral," their techniques supposedly neutral. But it doesn't always work out that way. The "hired gun" analogy holds up in more ways than one.

Technique is not amoral when its very nature drives organizations to a certain type of morality. Calculation is not neutral when some things are more easily calculated than others—costs more than benefits, tangible costs more than intangible costs, economic benefits more than social benefits. All of this can lead strictly professional managers into all kinds of questionable behaviors. Economizing cuts the needs of the workers and the customers alongside the costs of production (for example, by speeding up assembly lines beyond human capacity, or by eliminating experimentation on new products, which can also reduce the long-term economic viability of an organization by eliminating investments such as research treated as costs). "Rational" accounting slips social costs off the ledgers by treating them as "externalities," which means that society has to foot the organization's bills (for example, by calculating that unsafe gas tanks are cheaper than safe ones, or by letting the health care system pay for the mental breakdowns of the workers on those speeded-up assembly lines). Amorality thus becomes economic morality, and when pushed to the limit becomes social immorality. We end up with a one-dimensional society in which innocent people get run over by professional managers racing down the fast track, trampling whoever gets in the way of serving that almighty bottom line.

In his study at the Harvard Business School, Robert Ackerman[19] noted that the control systems intrinsic to the very functioning of the diversified corporation—bottom-line systems based on quantifiable, specifically financial goals—discouraged consideration of the social goals simply because the latter could not easily be measured. He found this to be the case even when the chief executive sincerely believed in the social goals and wished to promote them. The very control system the leader had to use to run the organization precluded attention to those goals. "Listen, boss, do you want me to treat people nice or meet the targets?"

My sixth point is that machine bureaucratic organizations run by professional management, by emphasizing calculation, drive out commitment, and so reduce human systems to impersonal shells. Earlier, in our discussion of Taylor's procedures, I mentioned the effect that rationalization has on motivation—how it discourages involvement and commitment. Here I wish to pursue at greater length what I believe may be the worst consequence of this syndrome of machine bureaucracy run by professional management: its stifling effect on commitment. James Worthy, once an executive at Sears, Roebuck, attributes this directly to the machine notion of the organization and its emphasis on planning for control:

> The obsession for control springs from the failure to recognize or appreciate the value of spontaneity, either in everyday work or in economic processes. Hence the need for planning. Hence the machine as the idea for human organization. For the machine has no will of its own. Its parts have no urge to independent action. Thinking, direction—even purpose—must be provided from outside or above.[20]

The problem of commitment can be partly attributed to professionalism in management too. A professional is someone who "knows better," who takes care of your needs for you. When I am lying on an operating table with my appendix about to burst, I am hardly inclined to second-guess the surgeon. That person really does know better. But when I am sitting in a classroom or doing difficult work in an organization, having someone above who thinks he or she knows better only impedes my efforts, because I need a good deal of personal control over such work.

That is why I am opposed to the strict notion of professionalism in education. True, it may have helped reduce the influence of educational administrators, whose excessive controls have, in my opinion, had a devastating effect on the process. But professionalism fares no better if it is used to concentrate power over the learning process in the hands of the teacher instead of the student. That is why children who go crazy being forced to learn a language in school turn around and pick it up on the street with no effort at all. (If we could measure it, what would we find to be the efficiency of the average classroom, in terms of the capacity of the students' potential used? Would it get as high as 10 percent? Why do we continue to tolerate this?) To draw on an old expression, a teacher cannot teach children anything, only help them to find it within themselves. And the same holds true for the relationship between managers and people doing difficult work. Managers who claim that as professionals they must take control of that work through planning and other technocratic procedures, like professional teachers who claim they must control the learning process through detailed specification of the curriculum, destroy the need for commitment and spontaneous learning in these activities.

Is that not what we have seen so much of in our organizations—administrative systems that have squeezed the commitment out of those subjected to them? Formal structure, together with these systems, constitutes the bones of an organization. Every system needs its skeleton. But an organization in which these dominate remains no more than an empty shell. Only when it is infused with human spirit—with energy, ideology, culture, call it what you like—does the organization come alive. And that energy cannot reside exclusively at the top of a formal hierarchy, any more than our human energy can flow exclusively from our brains.

Someone once claimed that to be objective is to treat people as objects. "Nothing but the facts, ma'am," Sergeant Friday used to say on television. But that just doesn't work in management, because facts themselves are infused with value, in their content and in their origin as well as in their selection. In an important way, calculation and commitment are mutually exclusive. You can sit back and calculate or you can dive in and commit. The Honda story contrasted these. In the early 1960s, IBM committed to remaking its entire line of computers as an act of faith. It decided to eliminate its traditional lines without being sure what the new ones would look like. "We'll work it out" was the attitude. (Imagine the looks on the faces of MBA students specializing in finance when asked what bottom-line calculations could have informed that decision.) In contrast, an airline we studied introduced a shuttle service without reserved seating. When passengers kept trying to book seats, the airline scuttled the shuttle a few days later. Far from working it out, their attitude was, "We tried, didn't we?"

It is amazing how such attitudes get communicated throughout an organization, how what is inside the heads—really the hearts—of the senior management, the intentions that really drive them, somehow gets conveyed to everyone else. It's almost psychic. Maybe that is why the managers of one organization, who get personally involved, can so fire everyone up, while those of another, sitting back and pontificating through systems, can have such a deadening effect. Consider the toll that has been exacted from so many people in organizations by the obsession with the bottom line. How in the world did the idea spread in management that you make money by managing money, instead of dealing with people and products? It is as if everybody pretends to be managing a bank (although it probably doesn't work even there!). With these kinds of ideas so current in the executive suites—now it is the absurd notion of managing "shareholder value," the assumption of direct links between all the fuzzy decision-making that goes on and the price of the stock in some distant capital market—is it any wonder that so few workers care what is being produced, let alone how or for whose benefit?

Thus, with understanding, intuition, belief, and commitment driven out, along with social concerns, it should come as no surprise that the population at large has become so alienated from its large organizations, private as well as public. As workers, customers, citizens, often even as managers themselves, people have come increasingly to question whether organizations are there to serve them or to enslave them. And that is a formula for failure, economic no less than social.

My seventh point is that every form of organization sows the seeds of its own destruction; in machine bureaucracy devoid of human commitment, that manifests itself as enveloping politicization. Success breeds failure; in strength lie the roots of weakness. Organizations succeed by balancing the competing forces of conflict with the committing forces of ideology. But when the latter get squeezed out, the former take over.

The strength of machine bureaucracy lies in its ability to "buffer" itself from environmental forces, to seal itself off from external perturbations in order to rationalize its operations and so attain a high level of efficiency. But no one need be reminded that "power tends to corrupt, and absolute power corrupts absolutely." In sealing itself off, the machine bureaucracy concentrates its power in its administrators, those people who run its systems of authority and control. Commitment, in the form of culture or ideology, can temper that power. Everyone works for the common good. But when that force is removed, power becomes corrupting. The large bureaucratic organization becomes a closed system in the service of its administrators (despite their self-serving claims of "social responsibility").

When this happens, the whole system begins to deteriorate. Administrators become increasingly greedy, seeking satisfaction through the building of larger personal empires rather than the serving of customers or even owners. That puts pressure on the organization to grow, no matter what the consequences, so that all the demands can be met without excessive conflict. Other insiders get the message too, for example the workers who insist on their share of the spoils. And since the one thing a closed system management cannot tolerate is public challenge, which might expose the fundamental illegitimacy of its power base, it is inclined to give in. More growth can always pay for the excessive wage settlements, or, failing that, greater exploitation of the organization's market power.

But as excess piles upon excess—stories of executive jets and golden parachutes and bonuses growing faster than performance (consider the rise in Fortune 500 executive salaries over the last decade or so compared with industrial profits or workers' salaries)—outsiders take notice too. Some may try to get a piece of the action, while others, further removed, may instead challenge the legitimacy of the whole system of power. "Why is what's good for General Motors good for the country?" they ask, especially when they see the management, not the board, controlling the corporation. And so pressure campaigns arise, and government intervention follows.

All of this ends up, however, less correcting the excesses than further politicizing the organization. Whereas before the large corporation may have looked like an economic entity with political power, now it appears to be a political entity that happens to operate in the economic sphere. It takes on the form of a political arena for some, who use it to fight out their ideological battles, and a fountain of benefits for others, who compete with each other for personal gain. And once the large organization has been so captured by conflict, it is unlikely ever to free itself of it. Which of our giant, highly politicized organizations—in business, government, or any other sphere—is ever likely to be left alone by any of the demanding influencers who surround it?

All this would be fine if politicization served the role that equivalent processes serve in nature. When an animal can no longer function effectively, it becomes prey to attackers and is eventually cut down. The system is brutal but functional—resources get redistributed, and nature wins. Were the dysfunctional animals to survive, then nature would lose, because its resources would be misallocated. That, I maintain, is exactly what is happening in our society of organizations.

My eighth and final point is that large politicized organizations are increasingly allowed to sustain themselves by political means, threatening the destruction, not of the single spent organization, but of the whole society of organizations instead. How can an organization that has lost sight of its central mission possibly survive? The answer is suggested in its own politicization. It acts as a political entity, seeking to sustain itself through the sheer exploitation of its political power.

In a world of large organizations, the competition of Adam Smith's brewer, baker, and butcher becomes the oligarchy of giant corporations, massive governments, and huge trade unions making deals with one another for their mutual convenience. Organizations, especially business organizations, may have grown large because they were sharper, smarter, more competitive—that was "getting there." It was essentially economic. But "staying there" is another matter. Large organizations are often able to sustain themselves in other ways. One is through past successes— not what they do now so much as today's consequences of what they did earlier. For example, a corporation may have locked up the best retailing sites or the cheapest sources of supply, or established the reputation to which purchasing agents must defer. Another way is through sheer exploitation of the power they have, in ways more political than economic. Large organizations can, for example, make reciprocal trading arrangements with each other to preempt competitive markets; they can mount huge advertising campaigns of image to manipulate public opinion; in the airline business, they can use a modern form of "payola" that offers points to private individuals whose companies paid for their tickets, thereby discouraging travel on the smaller carriers with less extensive networks; they can bring the influences of the many people and organizations that depend on them to lobby for favorable government legislation. Even government regulation can be favorable to the large organization, by keeping out smaller would-be competitors discouraged by the paperwork alone.

In Canada, large corporations secure government grants by threatening to close down existing plants. Like their response to the occasional dramatic plane crash as compared with the steady stream of carnage on the highways, governments have become obsessed with job losses and gains large enough to be reported by the press. In America, essentially bankrupt corporations lobby for trade barriers or government loan guarantees, pointing to the consequence on the economy if they fail (short-term, anyway). Lee Iacocca may have turned Chrysler around, but the hidden cost of that may prove to be enormous. That is because every argument that Iacocca used, and every political stop he pulled out—drawing on Chrysler's suppliers and workers to pressure their politicians about the consequences of the jobs and business that would be lost—can be used by any failing large corporation. If it becomes considered proper to have saved Chrysler—and its very survival seems to make that case—then never again can the American government let any large corporation go bankrupt.

The Chrysler episode signifies the growing trend toward mutual relationships among large organizations, public and private, outside the forces of open competition. It is not new, however; President Eisenhower warned when he left office in 1959 of the dangers of the "military–industrial complex." But today such arrangements cut increasingly across, not just large corporations, not just those corporations and their governments, but private and public organizations of all kinds around the world. Many people applaud the cooperation of the huge consortiums of businesses and governments—joint ventures of all kinds—without stopping to think what effect these can have on bureaucratization, on politicization, and on competition. (Consider all the vigorous young organizations that are simply too small to join.)

Of course, all these problems are not those of business alone. They can be found in large organizations in every sector of human activity. The politicization of government departments is widely acknowledged; and here there is often not even a semblance of competition to provide some countervailing force. And so we get festering public bureaucracies that continue to squander public resources. Likewise in other sectors: Powerful unions entrench themselves in political ways, sometime even through the use of physical violence, and large politicized welfare agencies and universities work themselves into positions of invulnerability and then sit back and waste society's resources.

Thus we end up with a vicious circle in our society. An irrational obsession with "rationality" produces a society of large, bureaucratic organizations run by a "professional" management that proves thin, superficial, and sometimes immoral. That drives out human commitment, which in turn leads to the politicization of organizations. This should destroy them, but it does not, for they turn around and use their political power to sustain themselves artificially. Organizations thereby get larger, more bureaucratic, and more politicized, and their managements as a consequence get thinner, more superficial, and less moral. It is an irony of contemporary society that the large organizations designed to serve themselves as closed systems are so stable and those dominated by politics so protected, while younger organizations that respond to creative leadership or that exhibit a strong sense of mission are inherently so vulnerable. Today it almost seems wrong to believe in what is produced, as opposed to how, or, more to the point, for whose personal benefit. Should we not be encouraging the demise of our large, spent organizations, so that they can be replaced in a natural cycle of renewal by younger, smaller, less constrained and more vigorous ones? Does the society that discourages the demise of its spent organizations not risk its own demise instead?

To conclude, we are a world of large organizations in an age of capital-letter MANAGEMENT, and as a result society has become unmanageable. Like those Inuit boys, our machinery has broken down and we cannot find our way home.

Well, this is an awfully bleak picture. We might be consoled by the fact that I have overstated my points. But not for long, I fear. The situation today may not be as bad as I have described, but I believe the trends are evident. Overall, the prognosis is not encouraging.

We do need machine bureaucracies to bring us mass-produced goods and services efficiently. But we do not need them to dehumanize us and to dominate our lives, public and private. Likewise we do need analysis and we do need planning. I am not arguing for a return to the cults of personality of times gone by. Unchecked intuition is as dangerous as unchecked analysis. It is just that I see the latter as the problem today. I am arguing for a return to balance, to allow intuition to function alongside analysis, recognized as a valid and necessary process in organizations. Shapero puts it perfectly in his article cited earlier: "We need to return to a rationality tuned to the natural messiness of life, and not one dedicated to abstractions."[21]

Of course, there are great organizations out there, even great large ones. Rich culture and dedicated management hold many a large organization together and render it effective and humane. But this is accomplished against the natural pressures created by bigness and rationalization. In my opinion, Peters and Waterman's book *In Search of Excellence* attained its enormous success precisely because it was about the exceptions, about organizations that didn't give in to those pressures. It was exciting to read of organizations that managed to maintain their vigor and effectiveness, their very human qualities, despite their growth to large size—typically, it appeared, because of the strong ideologies infused in them by founding leaders still present or recently departed. These organizations seemed so different from the ones we all knew. But that vigor and that humanness are not easy to maintain, not even in the Peters and Waterman organizations, as the subsequent *Business Week* story on the faltering "excellent" companies, with a cover labeled "Oops," pointed out.[22] I see pockets of excellence out there too, but bobbing up and down in a stormy sea of increasing bureaucratization, increasing politicization, increasing alienation. Unless we break that vicious circle, I am not terribly optimistic about our future.

Where to intervene, how to break the vicious circle? Ideally, of course, it would break itself. Small organizations would nip at the heels of the ineffective large ones until the latter collapsed. While we can, of course, see this on many fronts, we also see too much of the opposite—of governments and other organizations coming to the rescue of spent big ones by kicking away the small ones or by building protective shelters around the big ones. Thus, I believe there will have to be concerted intervention, based on a change of attitude. And sooner rather than later. The longer this goes on, the more established our politicized organizations become, and the more we adapt ourselves to them (the final stage of slavery being when you no longer realize that you are a slave).

Milton Friedman's solution, to wind down the role of government and, in his words, allow "free" enterprise to displace "subversive" socialism, is no solution at all, but simply a formula for a particular kind of oligarchy. Today the problem is not private versus public but bureaucracy in all its forms. Who cares if the system that regulates us is owned by thousands of shareholders as opposed to millions of citizens, since neither exercises control over the management. At the limit, the difference between America and the Soviet Union from an organization theory perspective is that one is controlled by a single giant closed system machine bureaucracy while the other is dominated by several hundred. "A plague on both your houses" is my answer to Friedman. Don't compound the problem by compounding the bureaucracies. Give me a system in which all organizations have to be responsive to me, as a worker, a client, a citizen, an owner.

Thus, neither nationalization nor privatization is a fundamental solution, nor is regulation or deregulation, for that matter. We can keep bouncing back and forth between these, perhaps correcting some deficiencies at the margin, but never solving any fundamental problem. Nor is the "democratization" of our large organizations a basic solution, because that won't make them much more responsive, not even the proposals for "self-management," a wonderful idea as soon as someone figures out what it means in places that need a great deal of systematic coordination. (There are not many ways to bolt a bumper onto a Volvo.) Certainly we must work to democratize our large organizations, to open them up to broader forms of social control. That will temper their power and provide them with a certain legitimacy. But let's not pretend that will resolve any basic issue.

As for social responsibility, that is a fine and noble concept. We critically need responsible people in important places. But how can even decent, well-meaning people be responsible in places that are impersonal and that breed alienation by their very nature? If power really does corrupt, then we will have to make some fundamental changes in the nature of our organizations before we can expect them to exhibit greater social responsibility.

Our best hope may lie in subtle and clever interventions where things can be changed in basic ways. We can certainly afford to promote small organizations, ones of a human scale, wherever feasible. We may not be able to afford small petrochemical refineries or small automobile firms, but we can certainly afford human-sized businesses in many other spheres, manufacturing and especially service. And it is not at all clear why we need all those huge hospitals, schools, libraries, social services, and so on. The tradeoff between the commitment and personalized services offered by "human scale" and the cost savings offered by "economies of scale" has never been firmly established. Yet how often do we opt for the latter, in response to the hard data accumulated by the large organization, or else simply as a result of the power game played by its administrators? Who, after all, is in the best position to "prove it"?

To illustrate with an exception, some years ago, a vice principal at McGill University proposed to close our small management library and incorporate its collection into the large general library. Concerned by the thought of having to deal with that big impersonal system, we marshaled our resources to study the issue. On every quantifiable criterion, our little library was two to three times more efficient than the big one. (And imagine what might have been suggested by the nonquantifiable ones!) And why not? It did naturally all those things that big organizations tie themselves in knots trying to accomplish through formal programs: "job enrichment" (everyone naturally pitched in to help do everything), "managerial involvement" (if someone had to step out, the boss became

a worker), "motivation" (the librarians knew the people they were serving), and so on. We saved our library and learned a lesson in the bargain
(and, incidentally, found that we had been "had" by a clever administrator—all he wanted was a free study of library efficiency, and so he got
a group of worried academics to "prove it"!)

If we are to promote small organizations, then we shall have to demote
many large ones. We must not attack them arbitrarily, but we should
challenge their effectiveness. Put the onus on them: "Give us good
reasons why you should be sustained." And when those reasons are
lacking—when they cannot "prove it" beyond questionable numbers
in slick reports, cannot show significant benefits in operating efficiency
and strategic responsiveness to the people they were designed to serve—
then we should pull out every plug that favors them. Especially when
they show signs of pervasive politicization—a form of rot no less evident
than the black spots that appear on a piece of fruit. Size alone gives
large organizations a huge advantage; offering them other advantages,
or even allowing more subtle intrinsic advantages to dominate, simply
throws the whole society of organizations out of balance.

Likewise we should question conglomeration wherever it appears.
The popular arguments about the benefits of hierarchies over markets
notwithstanding, there is no evidence that anyone knows how to manage
effectively a diversity of businesses under one corporate umbrella, except
by the sheer power of personality. (But think how much more productive
such personality could be if dedicated to the development of new focused
businesses. Indeed, think of the consequences of marshaling all that
creative energy now devoted to restructuring and other financial games
toward the production of better products and services!) A great deal of
diversification and conglomeration has been nothing more than a giant
power game played for the benefit of administrators and financial types
who keep score by the number of digits on the bottom line. ("Diversific-
tion," the [Freudian?] slip of a former secretary of mine, better describes
this phenomenon.) Above all, let us get rid of the multiple layers of
management—authority piled upon authority, increasingly detached and
superficial—that serves only to sap the energy of involved, committed
people.

Likewise, let us question vertical integration where a network of trading
relationships involving negotiations among smaller, autonomous units
is superior to a monolithic hierarchy of captive divisions. By the same
token, let us question the trend toward the contractual associations of
organizations, public and private, on an international basis. Some of

this will no doubt serve us well, but much will not: We must scrutinize these relationships carefully. And let us question agglomeration in other sectors too, of "multiversities," huge school systems, large chains of newspapers, huge unions, and on and on. Many of these giant organizations have exacted a cost in human commitment and economic effectiveness far in excess of the benefits to any but the few who rule them.

We should be encouraging young organizations to establish themselves and attain adulthood; we should be encouraging small organizations that involve their people and provide eclecticism in the marketplace; we should be encouraging autonomous, focused organizations that understand their missions, "know" the people they serve, and excite the ones they employ; we should be encouraging "thick" management, deep knowledge, healthy competition, and authentic social responsibility. We need to get back to our basic senses, to feel genuine commitment, to use informal intuition, by promoting forms of organization that encourage these things. Only in these ways, it seems to me, shall we find our way back from the frozen wastes of our strange world of organizations.

Notes

Part I Introduction

1. J.-J. Serven-Schreiber, *The American Challenge* (New York: Atheneum, 1968).

Chapter 1 The Manager's Job

1. F. Andrews, "Management: How a Boss Works in Calculated Chaos," *New York Times,* October 29, 1976.

2. The data from my study can be found in Henry Mintzberg, *The Nature of Managerial Work* (New York: Harper & Row, 1973).

3. Robert H. Guest, "Of Time and the Foreman," *Personnel,* May 1956, p. 478.

4. Rosemary Stewart, *Managers and Their Jobs* (New York: Macmillan, 1967); see also Sune Carlson, *Executive Behaviour* (Stockholm: Strömbergs, 1951), the first of the diary studies.

5. Irving Choran, unpublished McGill MBA thesis, reported in Mintzberg, *Nature of Managerial Work.*

6. Robert T. Davis, *Performance and Development of Field Sales Managers* (Cambridge: Division of Research, Harvard Business School, 1957), and George H. Copeman, *The Role of the Managing Director* (London: Business Publications, 1963).

7. Stewart, *Managers and Their Jobs,* and Tom Burns, "The Directions of Activity and Communication in a Departmental Executive Group," *Human Relations,* February, 1954, p. 73.

8. Richard E. Neustadt, *Presidential Power* (New York: Wiley, 1960), pp. 153–54; italics added.

9. George C. Homans, *The Human Group* (New York: Harcourt Brace & World, 1950), based on the study by W. F. Whyte, *Street Corner Society,* revised edition (Chicago: University of Chicago Press, 1955).

10. Neustadt, *Presidential Power,* p. 157.

11. Peter F. Drucker, *The Practice of Management* (New York: Harper & Row, 1954), pp. 341–42.

12. Leonard R. Sayles, *Managerial Behavior* (New York: McGraw-Hill, 1964), p. 162.

13. James S. Hekimian and Henry Mintzberg, "The Planning Dilemma," *Management Review,* May 1968, p. 4.

Chapter 2 Crafting Strategy

1. Richard T. Pascale, "Perspective on Strategy: The Real Story Behind Honda's Success" *California Management Review,* Spring 1984, pp. 47–72.

2. James B. Quinn, "IBM(A): The System/360 Decision," in J. B. Quinn, H. Mintzberg, and R. M. James, *The Strategy Process: Concepts, Context, and Cases* (Englewood Cliffs, N.J.: Prentice-Hall, 1988), pp. 189–203.

3. See Danny Miller and Peter H. Friesen, *Organizations: A Quantum View* (Englewood Cliffs, N.J.: Prentice-Hall, 1984).

4. See Chapter 11. The term *adhocracy* was coined by Warren G. Bennis and Philip L. Slater in *The Temporary Society* (New York: Harper & Row, 1964).

5. See Danny Miller and Peter H. Friesen, "Archetypes of Strategy Formulation," *Management Science,* May 1978, pp. 921–23.

Chapter 3 Planning on the Left Side, Managing on the Right

1. Richard Restak, "The Hemispheres of the Brain Have Minds of Their Own," *New York Times,* January 25, 1976.

2. Robert Ornstein, *The Psychology of Consciousness* (San Francisco: Freeman, 1975), p. 60.

3. Henry Mintzberg, Duru Raisinghani, and André Théorêt, "The Structure of 'Unstructured' Decision Processes," *Administrative Science Quarterly,* 1976, pp. 246–75.

4. Clyde T. Hardwick and Bernard F. Landuyt, *Administrative Strategy and Decision Making,* 2d edition (Cincinnati: South Western, 1966).

5. This point is elaborated upon in Henry Mintzberg, a forthcoming book on *Strategic Planning.*

6. Ornstein, *Psychology of Consciousness,* p. 10.

Chapter 4 Coupling Analysis and Intuition in Management

1. P. M. S. Blackett, *Studies of War: Nuclear and Conventional* (Edinburgh: Olivier and Boyd, 1962), p. 199.

2. David B. Hertz, "Has Management Science Reached a Dead End?," *McKinsey Quarterly,* Winter 1972, p. 44.

3. Herbert A. Simon, *Administrative Behavior* (New York: Macmillan, first published in 1947); *Organizations* (with James G. March) (New York: Wiley, 1957); *The Sciences of the Artificial* (Cambridge: MIT Press, 1964);

and *The New Science of Management Decision* (New York: Harper & Row, first published in 1960); among others.

4. Herbert A. Simon, *The New Science of Management Decision,* revised edition (Englewood Cliffs, N.J.: Prentice-Hall, 1977), p. 69.

5. Henry Mintzberg, *The Nature of Managerial Work* (New York: Harper & Row, 1973), pp. 132–33.

6. Simon, *New Science*, p. 69.

7. David Halberstam, *The Best and the Brightest* (New York: Random House, 1972).

8. Charles J. Hitch and Roland N. McKean, *The Economics of Defense in the Nuclear Age* (Cambridge: Harvard University Press, 1960).

9. Halberstam, *Best and Brightest,* p. 256.

10. See Robert W. Ackerman, *The Social Challenge to Business* (Cambridge: Harvard University Press, 1975).

11. In Halberstam, *Best and Brightest,* p. 81.

12. Simon, *New Science,* p. 68; italics added.

13. Simon, *New Science*, p. 81; and Roger Sperry, "Messages from the Laboratory," *Engineering and Science,* January 1974, p. 30; italics added.

14. Simon, *New Science*, p. 71; italics added.

15. Herbert A. Simon, "Making Management Decisions: The Role of Intuition and Emotion," *Academy of Management Executive,* February 1987, pp. 58–59, citing with regard to the evidence of the last paragraph, R. H. Doktor, "Problem Solving Styles of Executives and Management Scientists," in A. Charnes, W. W. Cooper, and R. J. Niehaus, eds., *Management Science Approaches to Manpower Planning and Organization Design* (New York: Elsevier North-Holland, 1978), and R. H. Docktor and W. F. Hamilton, "Cognitive Styles and the Acceptance of Management Science Recommendations," *Management Science,* 1973, pp. 884–94.

16. Simon, "Making Management Decisions," pp. 60, 61.

17. *Ibid.,* pp. 61, 63.

18. George A. Miller, "The Magic Number Seven, Plus or Minus Two: Some Limits on Our Capacity for Processing Information," *Psychology Review*, March 1956, pp. 81–97.

19. F. Bello, "The Magic That Made Polaroid," *Fortune*, April 1959, p. 158; italics added.

20. J. T. Peters, K. R. Hammond, and D. A. Summers, "A Note on Intuitive vs. Analytical Thinking," *Organizational Behavior and Human Performance,* August 1974, p. 126, quoting Brunswik.

21. *Ibid.,* p. 129; see also K. R. Hammond, R. M. Hamm, J. Arassca, and

T. Pearson, "Direct Comparison of Efficiency of Intuitive and Analytical Cognition in Expert Judgement," in *IEEE Transactions on Systems, Man, and Cybernetics,* September–October, 1987, pp. 753–768.

22. Polanyi, paraphrased in D. Braybrooke and C. E. Lindblom, *A Strategy of Decision* (New York: Free Press, 1963), pp. 44–45.

23. C. P. Curtis and F. Greenslet, *The Practical Cogitator* (Boston: Houghton Mifflin, 1945), p. 18.

24. F. E. Kast and J. E. Rosenzweig, *Organization and Management: A Systems Approach* (New York: McGraw-Hill, 1970).

25. Jay W. Forrester, "The Counter-Intuitive Behavior of Social Systems," in *Collected Papers of J. W. Forrester* (Cambridge: Wright-Allen Press, 1975).

26. J. McKenney and P. G. W. Keen, "How Managers' Minds Work," *Harvard Business Review,* May–June 1974, p. 84.

27. P. M. Morse, "The History of the Development of Operations Research," in G. J. Kelleher, ed. *The Challenge to Systems Analysis: Public Policy and Social Change* (New York: Wiley, 1970), p. 28.

28. In J. de Montigny, review of speech by Harold Lardner, *Bulletin of the Canadian Operational Research Society,* 1972, p. 5.

29. Aaron Wildavsky, "The Political Essay of Efficiency: Cost-Benefit Analysis, Systems Analysis, and Program Budgeting," *Public Administration Review,* 1968, p. 298.

30. Halberstam, *Best and Brightest,* p. 610.

31. Herbert A. Simon, "The Future of Information Processing Technology," *Management Science,* 1968, p. 622.

32. Aaron Wildavsky, "If Planning Is Everything, Maybe It's Nothing," *Policy Sciences,* June 1973, pp. 127–53.

Chapter 5 Training Managers, Not MBAs

1. R. H. Hayes and W. J. Abernathy, "Managing Our Way to Economic Decline," *Harvard Business Review,* July–August 1980, pp. 67–77.

2. Herbert A. Simon, *The Sciences of the Artificial* (Cambridge: MIT Press, 1969).

3. S. Zalaznick, "The MBA—the Man, the Myth, and the Method," *Fortune,* May 1, 1969, p. 168 ff.

4. J. A. Barks, "Here They Come: Master's Admissions at Sloan," *Sloan Magazine,* Winter 1987.

5. J. Stirling Livingston, "The Myth of the Well-Educated Manager," *Harvard Business Review,* January–February 1971, pp. 79–89.

6. Herbert A. Simon, *The New Science of Management Decision,* revised edition (Englewood Cliffs, N.J.: Prentice-Hall, 1977), p. 44.

7. Abraham Kaplan, *The Conduct of Inquiry: Methodology for Behavioral Science* (San Francisco: Chandler, 1964).

8. C. R. Christensen, K. R. Andrews, J. L. Bower, R. G. Hammermesh, and M. E. Porter, *Business Policy: Text and Cases,* 5th edition (Homewood, Ill.: Irwin, 1982).

Part II Introduction

1. George A. Miller, "The Magic Number Seven, Plus or Minus Two: Some Limits on Our Capacity for Processing Information," *Psychological Review,* March 1956, pp. 81–97.

Chapter 6 Deriving Configurations

1. Pradip Khandwalla, *The Effects of Environment on the Organizational Structure of Firms,* doctoral dissertation, Graduate School of Industrial Administration, Carnegie–Mellon University, 1970.

Chapter 7 The Entrepreneurial Organization

1. Peter Brook, *The Empty Space* (Harmondsworth, Middlesex: Penguin Books, 1968).

2. *Ibid.,* p. 154.

3. Lee Iacocca with William Novak, *Iacocca: An Autobiography* (New York: Bantam Books, 1984), p. 141.

4. Edwin Land, "People Should Want More From Life . . . ," *Forbes,* June 1, 1975, p. 50.

5. "The Most Basic Form of Creativity," *Time,* June 26, 1972, p. 84.

6. D. Wise, "Apple's New Crusade," *Business Week,* November 26, 1984, p. 146.

7. Albert Speer, *Inside the Third Reich* (New York: Macmillan, 1970), p. 16.

8. Brook, *Empty Space,* p. 157.

9. A. H. Cole, *Business Enterprise in Its Social Setting* (Cambridge: Harvard University Press, 1959).

10. Kurt Lewin, *Field Theory in Social Science* (New York: Harper & Row, 1951).

11. Thomas J. Peters, "A Style for All Seasons," *Executive,* Summer 1980, Graduate School of Business and Public Administration, Cornell University, pp. 12–16.

Chapter 8 The Machine Organization

1. Thomas A. Murphy, interviewed in *Executive* magazine, Summer 1980, Graduate School of Business and Public Administration, Cornell University, p. 4.

1a. A. L. Stinchcombe, "Social Structure and Organizations," in J. G. March, ed., *Handbook of Organizations* (Chicago: Rand McNally, 1965), Ch. 4.

2. Studs Terkel, *Working* (New York: Pantheon Books, 1972), pp. 186, 406.

3. Charles Perrow, *Complex Organizations: A Critical Essay* (New York: Scott, Foresman, 1972), p. 199.

4. John Kenneth Galbraith, *The New Industrial State* (Boston: Houghton Mifflin, 1967).

5. James C. Worthy, *Big Business and Free Men* (New York: Harper & Row, 1959), p. 77.

6. H. Constas, "The USSR—From Charismatic Sect to Bureaucratic Society," *Administrative Science Quarterly,* 1961–62, p. 294.

7. Michel Crozier, *The Bureaucratic Phenomenon* (Chicago: University of Chicago Press, 1964), p. 176.

8. H. H. Gerth and C. Wright Mills, eds., *From Max Weber: Essays in Sociology* (New York: Oxford University Press, 1958).

9. Worthy, *Big Business and Free Men,* pp. 67, 79, 70.

10. Quoted in *ibid.,* p. 73.

11. Victor A. Thompson, *Modern Organizations* (New York: Knopf, 1961).

12. James C. Worthy, "Organizational Structure and Employee Morale," *American Sociological Review,* April 1950, p. 176.

13. R. G. Hunt, "Technology and Organization," *Academy of Management Journal,* 1970, pp. 235–52.

14. Danny Miller and Peter H. Friesen, *Organizations: A Quantum View* (Englewood Cliffs, N.J.: Prentice-Hall, 1984).

15. Mihaela Firsirotu, "Strategic Turnaround as Cultural Revolution: The Case of Canadian National Express," doctoral dissertation, Faculty of Management, McGill University, 1985.

Chapter 9 The Diversified Organization

1. D. F. Channon, "The Strategy, Structure and Financial Performance of the Services Industries," working paper, Manchester Business School, 1975.

2. From Richard P. Rumelt, *Strategy, Structure, and Economic Performance.* Boston: Division of Research, Harvard Business School, 1974. Republished as a Harvard Business School Classic (Boston: Harvard Business School Press, 1986). Copyright © 1974, 1986 by the President and Fellows of Harvard College. Used with permission of the publisher and author. (Figure 1.4, p. 21, in source.)

3. L. C. Martin, "How Beatrice Foods Sneaked Up on $5 Billion," *Fortune,* April 1976.

4. Oliver E. Williamson, *Markets and Hierarchies* (New York: Free Press, 1975), and *The Economic Institutions of Captitalism* (New York: Free Press, 1985).

5. R. C. Moyer, "Berle and Means Revisted: The Conglomerate Merger," *Business and Society,* Spring 1970, pp. 20–29.

6. J. L. Bower, "Planning Within the Firm," *The American Economic Review: Papers and Proceedings of the 82nd Annual Meeting,* May 1970, p. 194.

7. L. Smith, "The Boardroom's Becoming a Different Scene," *Fortune,* May 8, 1978.

8. J. Bacon, *Corporate Dictatorship Practices: Memberships and Committees of the Board* (Conference Board and American Society of Corporate Secretaries, Inc., 1973), p. 40.

9. L. Wrigley, "Diversification and Divisional Autonomy," DBA dissertation, Graduate School of Business Administration, Harvard University, 1970, p. V78.

10. Rumelt, *Strategy, Structure, and Economic Performance.*

11. Wrigley, "Diversification and Divisional Autonomy," p. V86.

12. Bower, "Planning Within Firm," p. 193.

13. Robert W. Ackerman, *The Social Challenge to Business* (Cambridge: Harvard University Press, 1975), pp. 55, 56.

14. Bower, "Planning Within Firm," p. 193.

15. John Kenneth Galbraith, *American Capitalism: The Concept of Countervailing Power* (Boston: Houghton Mifflin, 1952).

Chapter 10 The Professional Organization

1. R. Gosselin, "A Study of the Interdependence of Medical Specialists in Quebec Teaching Hospitals," doctoral dissertation, Faculty of Management, McGill University, 1978.

2. F. C. Spencer, "Deductive Reasoning in the Lifelong Continuing Education of a Cardiovascular Surgeon," *Archives of Surgery,* 1976, pp. 1179, 1182.

3. K. E. Weick, "Educational Organizations as Loosely Coupled Systems," *Administrative Science Quarterly,* 1976, p. 8.

4. J. G. March and J. P. Olsen, *Ambiguity and Choice in Organizations* (Bergen, Norway: Universitetforlaget, 1976).

5. W. H. Taylor, "The Nature of Policy Making in Universities," *The Canadian Journal of Higher Education,* 1, 1983, p. 18.

6. M. D. Cohen, J. G. March, and J. P. Olsen, "A Garbage Can Model of Organizational Choice," *Administrative Science Quarterly,* 1972, p. 1; also March and Olsen, *Ambiguity and Choice.*

7. Spencer, "Deductive Reasoning," p. 1181.

8. J. W. Garbarino, "Faculty Unionization: The Pre-Yeshiva Years, 1966–1979," *Industrial Relations*, 1980, p. 229.

9. *Ibid.*, p. 228.

Chapter 11 The Innovative Organization

1. Warren G. Bennis and Philip L. Slater, *The Temporary Society* (New York: Harper & Row, 1964), and Alvin Toffler, *Future Shock* (New York: Bantam Books, 1970).

2. C. Reeser, "Some Potential Human Problems of the Project Form of Organization," *Academy of Management Journal*, 1969, p. 463.

3. Alvin Toffler, *Future Shock*, p. 133.

4. Charles E. Lindblom, *The Policy-Making Process* (Englewood Cliffs, N.J.: Prentice-Hall, 1968), p. 25.

5. Tom Burns and G. M. Stalker, *The Management of Innovation*, 2d edition, (London: Tavistock, 1966), pp. 122–23.

6. C. Reeser, "Some Potential Human Problems," pp. 459–67.

Chapter 12 Ideology and the Missionary Organization

1. Max Weber, "The Three Types of Legitimate Rule," trans. by H. Gerth, in Amitai Etzioni, ed., *A Sociological Reader on Complex Organizations*, 2d edition (New York: Holt, Rinehart and Winston, 1969), p. 12.

2. Philip Selznick, *Leadership in Administration: A Sociological Interpretation* (New York: Harper & Row, 1957).

3. B. R. Clark, "The Organizational Saga in Higher Education," *Administrative Science Quarterly*, 1972, p. 178.

4. B. R. Clark, *The Distinctive College* (Chicago: Aldine, 1970), p. 235.

5. R. A. Scott, "The Selection of Clients by Social Welfare Agencies: The Case of the Blind," *Social Problems*, Winter 1967, pp. 248–57.

6. A. Jay, *Management and Machiavelli* (Harmondsworth, Middlesex: Penguin, 1970), p. 70.

7. D. L. Sills, *The Volunteers* (Glencoe, Ill.: Free Press, 1957).

8. From M. Rosner, "Principal Types and Problems of Direct Democracy in the Kibbutz," working paper, Social Research Center on the Kibbutz, Givat Havina, Israel, 1969.

9. E. Goffman, "The Characteristics of Total Institutions," in Amitai Etzioni, ed., *Complex Organizations: A Sociological Reader* (New York: Holt, Rinehart and Winston, 1961).

10. W. G. Ouchi and A. M. Jaeger, "Type Z Organizations: Stability in the Midst of Mobility," *Academy of Management Review*, 1978, p. 308.

11. *Ibid.*, p. 309.

12. W. G. Ouchi, *Theory Z: How American Business Can Meet the Japanese Challenge* (Reading, Mass.: Addison-Wesley, 1981).

13. W. G. Ouchi and B. Johnson, "Types of Organizational Control and Their Relationship to Emotional Well Being," *Administrative Science Quarterly,* 1978, p. 302.

Chapter 13 Politics and the Political Organization

1. Graham T. Allison, *Essence of Decision: Explaining the Cuban Missile Crisis* (Boston: Little, Brown, 1971), p. 170.

2. M. N. Zald and M. A. Berger, "Social Movements in Organizations: Coup d'Etat, Insurgency, and Mass Movements," *American Journal of Sociology,* 1978, p. 841.

3. David Mechanic, "Sources of Power of Lower Participants in Complex Organizations," *Administrative Science Quarterly,* 1962, pp. 349–64.

4. Aaron B. Wildavsky, "Budgeting as a Political Process," in D. L. Sills, ed., *International Encyclopedia of the Social Sciences* (New York: Crowell, Collier, Macmillan, 1968), vol. 2, and *The Politics of the Budgeting Process,* 2d ed. (Boston: Little, Brown, 1974).

5. D. J. Hickson, C. A. Lee, R. E. Schneck, and J. M. Pennings, "A Strategic Contingencies' Theory of Intraorganizational Power," *Administrative Science Quarterly,* 1971, pp. 216–29.

6. Zald and Berger, "Social Movements," p. 833.

7. David C. McClelland, "The Two Faces of Power," *Journal of International Affairs,* 1970, pp. 29–47.

8. Allison, *Essence of Decision,* p. 145.

9. T. Burns, "Micropolitics: Mechanisms of Institutional Change," *Administrative Science Quarterly,* 1961–62, p. 260.

Chapter 14 Beyond Configuration

1. S. Gordon Redding, *The Spirit of Chinese Capitalism* (Cambridge: Cambridge University Press, forthcoming in 1989).

2. Manfred F. R. Kets de Vries and Danny Miller, *The Neurotic Organization* (San Francisco: Jossey-Bass, 1984).

3. See "Sequential attention to goals" in Richard M. Cyert and James G. March, *A Behavioral Theory of the Firm* (Englewood Cliffs, N.J.: Prentice-Hall, 1963), p. 118.

4. B. R. Clark, *The Distinctive College* (Chicago: Aldine, 1970).

5. Michael E. Porter, *Competitive Strategy: Techniques for Analyzing Industries and Competition* (New York: Free Press, 1980).

6. Quoted in Walter Kiechel III, "Sniping at Strategic Planning (Interview with himself)," *Planning Review,* May 1984, p. 11.

7. Thomas J. Peters and Robert H. Waterman, Jr., *In Search of Excellence* (New York: Harper & Row, 1982).

8. R. Raphael, *Edges* (New York: Knopf, 1976), pp. 5–6.

9. William Starbuck, "Organizational Growth and Development," in J. G. March, ed., *Handbook of Organizations* (Chicago: Rand McNally, 1965), p. 486.

10. Robert Michels, *Political Parties: A Sociological Study of the Oligarchical Tendencies of Modern Democracy* (New York: Free Press, 1958).

11. See, for example, Adolph A. Berle and G. C. Means, *The Modern Corporation and Private Property,* revised edition (New York: Harcourt, Brace & World, 1968).

12. See, for example, T. Hafsi, "The Dynamics of Government in Business," *Interfaces,* July–August 1985, pp. 62–69.

13. "Who's Excellent Now?" *Business Week,* November 5, 1984, pp. 76–78.

14. M. N. Zald and M. A. Berger, "Social Movements in Organizations: Coup d'Etat, Insurgency, and Mass Movements," *American Journal of Sociology,* 1978, pp. 823–61.

Chapter 15 Who Should Control the Corporation?

1. G. D. Garson, "The Codetermination Model of Workers' Participation: Where Is It Leading?" *Sloan Management Review,* Spring 1977, p. 63.

2. J. Bacon and J. K. Brown, *Corporate Directorship Practices: Role, Selection and Legal Status of the Board* (Conference Board and American Society of Corporate Secretaries, Inc., 1975), p. 48.

3. J. Kralj, "Is There a Role for Managers?" *Journal of General Management,* Winter 1977, p. 13.

4. Theodore Levitt, "Why Business Always Loses," *Harvard Business Review,* March–April 1968, p. 83.

5. E. F. Cheit, "The New Place of Business: Why Managers Cultivate Social Responsibility," in E. F. Cheit, ed., *The Business Establishment* (New York: Wiley, 1964), p. 172.

6. Levitt, "Why Business Always Loses," p. 83.

7. D. Braybrooke, "Skepticism of Wants, and Certain Subversive Effects of Corporations on American Values," in Sydney Hook, ed., *Human Values and Economic Policy* (New York: NYU Press, 1967), p. 224.

8. Milton Friedman, "A Friedman Doctrine: The Social Responsibility of Business Is to Increase Its Profits," *New York Times Magazine,* September 13, 1970, pp. 32 ff.

9. S. N. Brenner and E. A. Molander, "Is the Ethics of Business Changing?" *Harvard Business Review,* January–February 1977, pp. 59, 62.

10. Robert W. Ackerman, *The Social Challenge to Business* (Cambridge: Harvard University Press, 1975).

11. I. Ross, "How Lawless Are the Big Companies?" *Fortune,* December 1, 1980, p. 57.

12. Aleksandr Solzhenitsyn, "Why the West Has Succumbed to Cowardice," *Montreal Star, News and Review,* June 10, 1978, p. B1.

13. Friedman, "A Friedman Doctrine," p. 33.

14. Milton Friedman, *Capitalism and Freedom* (Chicago: University of Chicago Press, 1962), p. 20.

15. Albert O. Hirschman, *Exit, Voice and Loyalty: Responses to Decline in Firms, Organizations, and States* (Cambridge: Harvard University Press, 1970).

Chapter 16 A Note on That Dirty Word "Efficiency"

1. Teaching note for "The Rose Company," Case 9–453–002, Intercollegiate Case Clearing House, Graduate School of Business Administration, Harvard University.

2. Herbert A. Simon, *Administrative Behavior,* 2d edition (New York: Macmillan, 1957), pp. 14, 179.

3. Peter F. Drucker, *Management: Tasks, Responsibilities, and Practices* (New York: Harper & Row, 1973), p. 347.

4. Robert M. Pirsig, *Zen and the Art of Motorcycle Maintenance: An Inquiry into Values* (New York: Bantam, 1974), pp. 200, 201.

5. Robert W. Ackerman, *The Social Challenge to Business* (Cambridge: Harvard University Press, 1975), p. 56.

6. J. L. Bower, "Planning and Control: Bottom Up or Top Down?" *Journal of General Management,* 3, 1974, pp. 22–23.

Chapter 17 Society Has Become Unmanageable as a Result of Management

1. John Kenneth Galbraith, *American Capitalism: The Concept of Countervailing Power* (Boston: Houghton Mifflin, 1952).

2. Aleksandr Solzhenitsyn, "Why the West Has Succumbed to Cowardice," *Montreal Star, News and Review,* June 10, 1978, p. B1.

3. Robert Michels, *Political Parties: A Sociological Study of the Oligarchical Tendencies of Modern Democracy* (New York: Free Press, 1958). Originally published in 1915.

4. Marianne Jelinek, *Institutionalizing Innovation* (New York: Praeger, 1979), p. 139. italics added.

5. *Business Week,* September 19, 1983, pp. 56–64, and November 5, 1984, pp. 82–87.

6. Quoted in James C. Worthy, *Big Business and Free Men* (New York: Harper & Row, 1959), p. 73.

7. Alfred D. Chandler, *Strategy and Structure* (Cambridge: MIT Press, 1962) and *The Visible Hand: The Managerial Revolution in American Business* (Cambridge: Harvard University Press, 1977), and Oliver E. Williamson, *Markets and Hierarchies* (New York: Free Press, 1975) and *The Economic Institutions of Capitalism* (New York: Free Press, 1985).

8. F. Andrews, "Management: How a Boss Works in Calculated Chaos," *New York Times,* October 29, 1978.

9. Albert Shapero, "What MANAGEMENT Says and What Managers Do," *Interfaces,* February 1977, p. 107.

10. Clifford Gccrtz, *The Interpretation of Cultures* (New York: Basic Books, 1973).

11. David Halberstam, *The Best and the Brightest* (New York: Random House, 1972).

12. Boston Consulting Group, *Strategy Alternatives for the British Motorcycle Industry* (London: Her Majesty's Stationery Office, 1975), p. 59.

13. Richard T. Pascale and A. G. Athos, *The Art of Japanese Management* (New York: Simon & Schuster, 1981).

14. All quotations above are from Richard T. Pascale, "Perspectives on Strategy: The Real Story Behind Honda's Success," *California Management Review,* Spring 1984, pp. 47–72; italics added.

15. Bert Hopwood, *What Ever Happened to the British Motorcycle Industry?* (San Leandro, Calif.: Haynes Publishing, 1981), p. 173.

16. M. D. Feld, "Information and Authority: The Structure of Military Organization," *American Sociological Review,* February 1959, p. 21.

17. J. L. Stokesbury, *A Short History of World War I* (New York: Morrow, 1981), pp. 241, 242.

18. E. A. Singer and L. M. Wooton, "The Triumph and Failure of Albert Speer's Administrative Genius: Implications for Current Management Theory and Practice," *Journal of Applied Behavioral Science,* 1976, p. 100.

19. Robert W. Ackerman, *The Social Challenge to Business* (Cambridge: Harvard University Press, 1975).

20. James C. Worthy, *Big Business and Free Men* (New York: Harper & Row, 1959), p. 29.

21. Shapero, "What MANAGEMENT Says," p. 108.

22. "Who's Excellent Now?" *Business Week,* November 5, 1984, pp. 76–78.

FOR FURTHER DETAIL

Chapter 1 The Manager's Job

My book *The Nature of Managerial Work* (Harper & Row, 1973; Prentice-Hall, 1980), contains detailed discussion of all the characteristics and roles described in this chapter, as well as the implications of that discussion for managers and management scientists. One chapter also considers variations in managerial work by level, function, and other factors. An appendix to the Harper & Row edition also presents detail on the research method used.

Chapter 2 Crafting Strategy

This material was drawn from various published articles; perhaps most relevant are "Patterns in Strategy Formation," *Management Science,* May 1979, on Volkswagenwerk (as well as on our study of U.S. strategy in Vietnam), "Tracking Strategy in an Entrepreneurial Firm" (with Jim Waters), *Academy of Management Journal,* September 1982, on Steinberg, Inc., and "Strategy Formation in an Adhocracy" (with Alexandra McHugh), *Administrative Science Quarterly,* June 1985, on the National Film Board of Canada. Some of this and related other material will be considered in Part II of this book. In addition, I have discussed different definitions of strategy in "Five P's for Strategy," *California Management Review,* Fall 1987, and different types of strategies (umbrella, process, etc.) in "Of Strategies, Deliberate and Emergent" (with Jim Waters), *Strategic Management Journal,* July–September 1985. An application of these ideas to the public sector is contained in "Emergent Strategy for Public Policy" (with Jan Jorgensen), *Canadian Public Administration,* Summer 1987. My earlier reference to my first article on the subject is "The Science of Strategy Making," published in what is now called the *Sloan Management Review,* Spring 1967. In addition, I am currently completing a rather long paper on "ten schools of thought" on strategy formation, to be published in J. W. Fredrickson (ed.), *Perspectives on Strategic Management* (New York: Ballinger, 1989).

Chapter 3 Planning on the Left Side, Managing on the Right

Aside from references to my other work (cited, or contained elsewhere in this book), further detail can be found in the next chapter.

Chapter 4 Coupling Analysis and Intuition in Management

My review of Simon's book can be found in the *Administrative Science Quarterly,* June 1977; his revised book *The New Science of Management Decision* was published by Prentice-Hall in 1977, while the article from which his passages are quoted, "Making Management Decisions: The Role of Intuition and Emotion," appeared in the *Academy of Management Executive* in February 1987. My ideas on the strengths and weaknesses of analysis and intuition, as well as the role of analysis in strategic decision-making, appeared in "Beyond Implementation: An Analysis of Resistance to Policy Analysis," published in K. B. Haley, ed., *Operations Research '78* (Elsevier North-Holland, 1979), pp. 106–62. *Impediments to the Use of Management Information,* which takes up the role of MIS in management and also provides more detail on the limitations of brains, organizations, and systems in information processing, appeared as a monograph published in 1975 jointly by the National Association of Accountants of the U.S. and the Society of Management Accountants of Canada. My forthcoming book on planning, tentatively entitled *Strategic Planning: An Irreverent Review* and to be published in 1990, goes into considerable detail on the meaning and models of strategic planning, the evidence on its performance over the years, its pitfalls and fallacies, and what seem to me to be the appropriate roles for planning, plans, and planners in various organizational contexts. I am also working with a number of colleagues and doctoral students on a paper entitled "Opening Up Decision Processes: The View from the Black Stool," which, among other issues, probes into the roles of insight and inspiration in decision-making and why these have tended to be slighted in the formal research and literature.

Chapter 5 Training Managers, Not MBAs

The implications of these ideas for management practice will be discussed in the final chapter of this book. A similar paper on research methods in management can be found in my "An Emerging Strategy of Direct Research" (*Administrative Science Quarterly*, December 1979) or, more of a diatribe; "If You're Not Serving Bill and Barbara, then You're

Not Serving Leadership'' (in Hunt et al., eds., *Leadership: Beyond Establishment Views* (Southern Illinois University Press, 1982).

Chapter 6 Deriving Configurations

Every concept, every attribute, every hypothesis presented here has been elaborated in one or the other of two books (which together comprise 1,200 pages), sometimes in a paragraph, sometimes in a section, not infrequently in an entire chapter (as is true for each of the design parameters and sets of conditions as well as the configurations themselves). The material on structure can be found in *The Structuring of Organizations* (Prentice-Hall, 1979), or the shorter version by that publisher, *Structure in Fives: Designing Effective Organizations* (1983), while the material on power can be found in *Power In and Around Organizations* by the same publisher (1983). The full ''Case for Configuration'' of the introduction to Part II, by Danny Miller and myself, can be found in Miller and Friesen's *Organizations: A Quantum View* (Prentice-Hall, 1984), Chapter 1.

Chapter 7 The Entrepreneurial Organization

Most of this chapter has been drawn from *The Structuring of Organizations* (Prentice-Hall, 1979), which devotes one chapter to ''simple structure.'' Some also comes from a chapter in *Power In and Around Organizations* on the ''autocracy.'' The material on strategy formation comes from three papers which present these conclusions in greater depth: ''Visionary Leadership and Strategic Management,'' *Strategic Management Journal*, forthcoming in 1989, co-authored with Frances Westley; ''Tracking Strategy in an Entrepreneurial Firm,'' about Steinberg's, published in the *Academy of Management Journal* in 1982, pp. 465–99; and ''Researching the Formation of Strategies: The History of Canadian Lady, 1939–1976,'' in R. B. Lamb, ed., *Competitive Strategic Management* (Prentice-Hall, 1984) about Canadelle, the last two articles co-authored with Jim Waters.

Chapter 8 The Machine Organization

The structure and conditions as well as the social issues associated with the machine organization are discussed at length in the chapter ''Machine Bureaucracy'' in my book *The Structuring of Organizations* (Prentice-Hall, 1979). A full chapter on both the ''Instrument'' and the ''Closed System'' can be found in my book *Power In and Around Organizations* (Prentice-Hall, 1983). And the material on strategy formation in this type of organization is discussed at greater length in three articles: ''Patterns in Strategy Formation,'' on Volkswagenwerk and U.S. Strategy in Vietnam, *Management Science,* 1978; "Does Planning Impede Strategic Thinking? The Strategy of Air Canada, 1937–1976" (with Pierre Brunet and Jim Waters), in R. B. Lamb and P. Shrivastava, eds., *Advances in Strategic Management, Volume IV* (JAI Press, 1987); and "The Mind of the Strategist(s)" (with Jim Waters), in S. Srivastva, ed., *The Executive Mind* (Jossey-Bass, 1983). Of further interest may be my book *Strategic Planning: An Irreverent Review,* forthcoming in 1990, on the nature and difficulties of formal planning.

Chapter 9 The Diversified Organization

All the points discussed here, especially those of the diversified configuration's social consequences, are developed at greater length in Chapter 20 of *The Structuring of Organizations* (Prentice-Hall, 1979). An article entitled "Diversi*fiction* (what a difference an "a" makes)," on "thick" and "thin" management, is in progress (also further developed in Chapter 17 of this book).

Chapter 10 The Professional Organization

The structure, context, and social issues of the "professional bureaucracy," including considerable detail on the pigeonholing process and other aspects, is discussed at length in Chapter 19 of *The Structuring of Organizations* (Prentice-Hall, 1979). Strategy-making in these organizations—specifically in academia—is discussed at greater length in the paper by Cynthia Hardy, Ann Langley, Janet Rose, and myself entitled "Strategy Formation in the University Setting," published in J. L. Bess, ed., *College and University Organization* (New York University Press, 1984). Finally, the full text of "A Note on the Unionization of Professionals from the Perspective of Organization Theory," including discussion of the U.S. Supreme Court decision concerning the unionization of faculty at Yeshiva University (and why I believe it was the right one for the wrong reason), can be found in the *Industrial Relations Law Journal* of 1983, pp. 623–34.

Chapter 11 The Innovative Organization

The adhocracy structure, including its operating and administrative forms and its contexts and issues, are discussed at length in Chapter 21 of *The Structuring of Organizations* (Prentice-Hall, 1979). Strategy-making in this configuration, especially aspects of the "grassroots" model, can be found in "Strategy Formation in an Adhocracy," co-authored with Alexandra McHugh and published in the *Administrative Science Quarterly* (1985), pp. 160–97, and "Strategy of Design: A Study of 'Architects in Co-Partnership,' " co-authored with Suzane Otis, Jamal Shamsie, and Jim Waters and published in J. Grant, ed., *Strategic Management Frontiers* (J.A.I. Press, 1988).

Chapter 12 Ideology and the Missionary Organization

Chapter 11 of *Power In and Around Organizations* (Prentice-Hall, 1983) discusses "the system of ideology," including its three stages of development, at greater length, while Chapter 21 goes into considerable detail on the goals and power relationships of the missionary configuration as well as the various forms it can take—pure (reformer, converter, cloister), quasi (overlays), and pseudo (only seemingly ideological).

Chapter 13 Politics and the Political Organization

Two chapters in *Power In and Around Organizations* (Prentice-Hall, 1983) elaborate at some length on all the points raised here. Chapter 13, "The System of Politics," discusses each of the political games at length as well as why politics is played in organizations and with what equipment (will, skill, privileged information, privileged access, and so on). Chapter 23, "The Political Arena," then discusses each of the four forms of political organization at length, with a number of illustrations, and also describes in detail the life cycle model of the political organization.

Chapter 14 Beyond Configuration

Much of this discussion is new to this book, although some of the basic ideas (pulls, hybrids, transitions, a simple pentagon) were introduced briefly in the concluding chapter of *The Structuring of Organizations* (Prentice-Hall, 1979). The life cycle model was developed in more detail and in a more academic way in Chapter 24 of *Power In and Around Organizations* (Prentice-Hall, 1983). Examples of all the possible transitions between the configurations and the reasons I consider some intrinsically more natural than others can also be found in that chapter.

Chapter 15 Who Should Control the Corporation?

As noted, this article was drawn from my book *Power In and Around Organizations* (Prentice-Hall, 1983), which devotes one section to this issue, including a full chapter on each of the eight positions. Readers interested in more detail, as well as the support (and published references) behind the arguments presented here, are referred to these chapters. Two of these positions have also been presented in articles in their own right, one called "Why America Needs, but Cannot Have Corporate

Democracy" (*Organizational Dynamics,* Spring 1983), the other "The Case for Corporate Social Responsibility" (*The Journal of Business Strategy,* Fall 1983, although I preferred the paper's original title, "That Naïve and Necessary Concept Called Social Responsibility"). I feel the critique of Milton Friedman's views, discussed under "restore it," really requires the longer, original version for a full understanding; this can be found on pages 632–44 of my "Power" book. Finally, the brief comments on the board of directors, inserted here into the discussion of "democratize it," are drawn from Chapter 6 of my "Power" book, which reviews the directors' roles and powers at some length. A late decision eliminated a full discussion of that subject in its own chapter in this book, but interested readers can turn to the original source. Otherwise, the summary of all this material presented here is similar to an article that appeared by the same title in the *California Management Review* (Fall 1984) or the *McKinsey Quarterly* in 1986.

Chapter 16 A Note on That Dirty Word "Efficiency"

This paper was published in *Interfaces,* October (1982), more or less as presented here. A slightly longer version, under the title "Efficiency as a Systems Goal," can be found in *Power In and Around Organizations* (Prentice-Hall, 1983), on pages 268–73. The same chapter, "Specific Goals in Organizations," also discusses survival, control, and growth as systems goals of organizations, and how these can displace mission as a goal. "The Determination of Organizational Goals," including the argument that organizations do have intrinsic goals, which must be inferred from their actions, and discussion of how conflicting goals are reconciled in organizations, is taken up in the preceding chapter of that book.

Chapter 17 Society Has Become Unmanageable as a Result of Management

No further detail. Go back to Chapter 1!

Credits and Acknowledgments

Chapter 1: Based on, and reprinted by permission of *Harvard Business Review*, "The Manager's Job: Folklore and Fact," by Henry Mintzberg (July/August 1975). Copyright © 1975 by the President and Fellows of Harvard College; all rights reserved.

Chapter 2: Based on, and reprinted by permission of *Harvard Business Review*, "Crafting Strategy," by Henry Mintzberg (July/August 1987). Copyright © 1987 by the President and Fellows of Harvard College; all rights reserved.

Chapter 3: Based on, and reprinted by permission of *Harvard Business Review*, "Planning on the Left Side and Managing on the Right," by Henry Mintzberg (July/August 1976). Copyright © 1976 by the President and Fellows of Harvard College; all rights reserved.

Chapter 4: Excerpts reprinted from Review of "The New Science of Management Decision," by Henry Mintzberg, published in *Administrative Science Quarterly* (June 1977), by permission of *Administrative Science Quarterly*, copyright © 1977 Cornell University; and excerpts from "Making Management Decisions: The Role of Intuition and Emotions," by Herbert A. Simon, in *Academy of Management Executive* (February 1987), used by permission of the publisher and author; correspondence with Herbert Simon used with his permission.

Chapter 6–15: Sections from Henry Mintzberg, *The Structuring of Organizations*, © 1979, and/or Henry Mintzberg, *Power In and Around Organizations,* © 1983; adapted by permission of Prentice-Hall, Inc., Englewood Cliffs, N.J.

Chapter 14: Permission granted by LEGO Overseas A/S, Billund, Denmark, to use the copyrighted word LEGO.

Chapter 16: Reprinted by permission from, with minor editing, "A Note on That Dirty Word 'Efficiency' " by Henry Mintzberg, in *Interfaces,* vol. 12, no. 5 (October 1982), pp. 101–105. Copyright 1982, The Institute of Management Sciences and the Operations Research Society of America.

Figure 4–1: From "A Note on Intuitive vs. Analytic Thinking," by J. T. Peters, K. R. Hammond, and D. A. Summers, in *Organizational Behavior and Human Performance* (August 1974), p. 128. Used by permission of Academic Press, Orlando, Fla., and author.

Figure 7–1: Used by permission of Steinberg, Inc., Montreal.

Figure 9–3: From Richard P. Rumelt, *Strategy, Structure and Economic Performance.* Boston: Division of Research, Harvard Business School, 1974. Republished as a Harvard Business School Classic. Boston: Harvard Business School Press, 1986. Copyright © 1974, 1986 by the President and Fellows of Harvard College. Used with permission of the publisher and author. (Figure 1.4, p. 21, in source.)

Figure 11–1: Used by permission of the National Film Board of Canada, Montreal.

INDEX